Bovine Medicine

Bovine Medicine

Third Edition

Edited by

Peter D. Cockcroft
Professor of Ruminant Health,
School of Animal and Veterinary Sciences,
University of Adelaide, South Australia

WILEY Blackwell

Registered office: John Wiley & Sons, Ltd, The Atrium, Southern Gate, Chichester, West Sussex, PO19 8SQ, UK
Editorial offices: 9600 Garsington Road, Oxford, OX4 2DQ, UK
The Atrium, Southern Gate, Chichester, West Sussex, PO19 8SQ, UK
1606 Golden Aspen Drive, Suites 103 and 104, Ames, Iowa 50010, USA

For details of our global editorial offices, for customer services and for information about how to apply for permission to reuse the copyright material in this book please see our website at www.wiley.com/wiley-blackwell.

Library of Congress Cataloging-in-Publication Data

Bovine medicine / edited by Peter Cockcroft. – Third edition.
p. ; cm.
Includes bibliographical references and index.
ISBN 978-1-4443-3643-6 (cloth)
I. Cockcroft, Peter D., editor.
[DNLM: 1. Cattle Diseases. 2. Animal Husbandry–methods. 3. Cattle. SF 961]
SF961
636.20896–dc23

2015000038

A catalogue record for this book is available from the British Library.

Wiley also publishes its books in a variety of electronic formats. Some content that appears in print may not be available in electronic books.

Cover image: Photo of beef feedlot (3rd image down of inset images) courtesy of Mandi Carr, University of Adelaide. All other photos courtesy of Peter Cockcroft.

Set in 9.5/12pt, MinionPro-Regular by Laserwords Private Limited, Chennai, India

1 2015

This book is dedicated to David

Contents

Section IV: Herd Health

Section V: Dairy Cattle Herd Health

Section VI: Beef Cattle Herd Health

Contributors

Katrine Bazeley
Synergy Farm Health
West Hill Barn, West Hill, Dorchester

Nick Bell
Lecturer in Livestock Veterinary Extension Services, Farm Animal Health and Production Group, The Royal Veterinary College, UK

Andrew Biggs
The Vale Veterinary Centre, Tiverton, UK

Wayne Boardman
Senior Lecturer in Veterinary Biosecurity, School of Animal and Veterinary Sciences, University of Adelaide, South Australia, Australia

George Caldow
Veterinary Services, SAC Consulting, Greycrook, St Boswells, Scottish Borders

John R. Campbell
Professor, Department of Large Animal Clinical Sciences, Western College of Veterinary Medicine, University of Saskatchewan, Canada

Jude L. Capper
Livestock Sustainability Consultant, Adjunct Professor, Department of Animal Sciences, Washington State University, USA

Charles Caraguel
Senior Lecturer, School of Animal and Veterinary Sciences, University of Adelaide, South Australia, Australia

Mandi Carr
Lecturer, School of Animal and Veterinary Sciences, University of Adelaide, South Australia, Australia

Tom Chamberlain
Chalcombe, Wickham, Hants, UK

Peter Chenoweth
Professor, School of Animal and Veterinary Sciences, Charles Sturt University Wagga Wagga, New South Wales, Australia

Peter D. Cockcroft
Professor Ruminant Health, School of Animal and Veterinary Sciences, University of Adelaide, South Australia, Australia

Nigel B. Cook
Professor in Food Animal Production Medicine, University of Wisconsin-Madison, School of Veterinary Medicine, USA

Peter J. DeGaris
SBScibus, Camden, New South Wales, Australia

Kathryn Ellis
Senior University Clinician, University of Glasgow, School of Veterinary Medicine, Glasgow, UK

Richard J. Esslemont
Independent Consultant, Poole, UK

Adele Feakes
Lecturer, School of Animal and Veterinary Sciences, University of Adelaide, South Australia, Australia

Mark A. Holmes
Reader in Microbial Genomics & Veterinary Science, Department of Veterinary Medicine, University of Cambridge, UK

Nick Jonsson
Professor of Production Animal Health, College of Medical, Veterinary and Life Sciences, University of Glasgow, UK

Allan Kessell
Gribbles Veterinary Pathology, Adelaide, South Australia, Australia
Adjunct Senior Lecturer School of Animal and Veterinary Sciences, University of Adelaide, South Australia, Australia

Robert L. Larson, DVM
Professor, Food Animal Production Medicine, Kansas State University Kansas, USA

Ian J. Lean
SBScibus, Camden, New South Wales, Australia

Chris Livesey
Veterinary Laboratories Agency, UK

Alastair Macrae
Senior Lecturer in Farm Animal Health and Production, Dairy Herd Health and Productivity Service, Royal (Dick) School of Veterinary Studies and the Roslin Institute, The University of Edinburgh, UK

Bryan Markey
Senior Lecturer, Department of Veterinary Microbiology and Parasitology, School of Veterinary Medicine, University College Dublin, Ireland

Michelle McArthur
Lecturer, School of Animal and Veterinary Sciences, University of Adelaide, South Australia, Australia

Elizabeth F. McInnes
Toxicological Pathology Consultant, Adelaide, South Australia, Australia

Colin Morgan
Scottish Agricultural College, Scotland

N. Moss
SBScibus, Camden, New South Wales, Australia

Karin Mueller
Senior Lecturer in Reproduction and Animal Husbandry, School of Veterinary Science, Liverpool University, UK

Alan Murphy
Department of Environment Food and Rural Affairs, UK

Jos. P. Noordhuizen
Adjunct Professor, Charles Sturt University, School of Animal and Veterinary Science, Wagga Wagga, New South Wales 2678, Australia, VACQA-International Consultancies, Santarém, Portugal

Peter Orpin
Park Vet Group, Leicester
Special Lecturer Cattle Medicine, Nottingham University, UK

Tim Parkinson
Professor, Institute of Veterinary, Animal and Biomedical Sciences, Massey University, New Zealand

Jo Payne
Animal and Plant Health Agency, UK

Kiro Petrovski
Senior Lecturer, School of Animal and Veterinary Sciences
University of Adelaide, South Australia, Australia

Clive Phillips
Professor, Centre for Animal Welfare and Ethics, School of Veterinary Science, University of Queensland, Queensland, Australia

Emily K Piper
School of Veterinary Science, University of Queensland, Queensland, Australia

A.R. Rabiee
SBScibus, Camden, New South Wales, Australia

Michael P. Reichel
Professor, School of Animal and Veterinary Sciences, University of Adelaide, South Australia, Australia

Richard D. Murray
Institute of Translational Medicine and School of Veterinary Science University of Liverpool, Liverpool, UK

Iain Ridell
Scottish Agricultural College, Scotland

Jamie Robertson
Honorary Research Fellow, School of Biological Science University of Aberdeen, Scotland

Paul Roger
Veterinary Consultancy Services Ltd, Reeth, North Yorkshire, UK

Phil Scott
Reader, Farm Animal Practice,
Royal (Dick) School of Veterinary Studies, University Edinburgh, UK

Rob Smith
Senior Lecturer, School of Veterinary Science, Liverpool University, UK

Jonathan M.E. Statham
Bishopton Veterinary Group/RAFT Solutions Ltd, UK

Mike Taylor
Professor, Veterinary Director, VparST Ltd, Market Weighton, East Yorkshire, UK

Cheryl L. Waldner
Professor, Department of Large Animal Clinical Sciences
Western College of Veterinary Medicine, University of Saskatchewan, Canada

Chris Watson
Wood Veterinary Group, Quedgeley, Gloucester, UK

Brad J. White
Associate Professor, Department of Clinical Sciences, Kansas State University, College of Veterinary Medicine, Kansas, USA

Dai Grove-White
Head of Division, Livestock Health & Welfare, School of Veterinary Science, University of Liverpool, UK

Preface

Many new books on specific bovine medicine topics have been published since the last edition of this book, with the majority of them taking a traditional approach to their structure and content. This book takes a radical departure from this format in order to provide the additional skills and insights required for modern service delivery and practice organisation. To this end, the publishers and I have decided to completely restructure and rewrite the book so that it reflects the shift in the skills sets required for modern cattle practice. This edition does not retain any chapters from the previous editions, and has a new multi-national team of contributors.

The aim of the book is to provide a selection of useful, relevant and practical information for the cattle practitioner, which is not readily available elsewhere, and which supports modern practice and industry needs. The book could equally have been retitled 'Cattle Practice' to reflect the change in scope and emphasis in this new edition. The non-technical skills, such as leadership, marketing, communication and business organisation, are now represented. In addition, the book acknowledges the growing importance of population medicine and herd health management planning. The skills required to support this important shift form the backbone of the book. Key technical skills are also represented, such as: the ability to perform an on-farm post-mortem and to take appropriate samples; the ability to select appropriate antimicrobials; and to optimise pain management.

The book comprises 57 chapters. Each chapter provides a set of learning objectives so the reader is given an insight into the author's intent. It is partitioned into six sections: Modern cattle Practice and Education, Professional Skills, Clinical Skills, Herd Health, Dairy Cattle Herd Health and Beef Cattle Herd Health. The clinical or farm audit has been used as an applied structural framework to integrate husbandry, welfare and health at a group or herd level within the herd health sections. The audit scopes across the management practices, and processes and identifies relevant key performance indicators and target values to measure the strengths and weaknesses of performance. The intent is not to provide all the traditional information about a topic, as this can be found easily elsewhere, but to indicate how knowledge and information can be used in risk assessment and in the formulation of recommendations that have a high impact at population level. Further reference information on cattle diseases is provided in a *Vade Mecum* at the end of the book. The chapters collectively form a toolkit of skills that will support the delivery of cattle practice.

SECTION I

Modern Cattle Practice

CHAPTER 1

Sustainability and One Health

Judith L. Capper

Learning objectives

- Understand future demands for food production and the need for sustainability.
- Appreciate the global impact of bovine production.
- Be aware of the opportunities for mitigation.
- Understand the environmental impacts and public perception.
- Appreciate the role of the veterinarian/animal scientist and future developments.

Introduction

The sustainability of global bovine production systems is currently one of the most highly debated issues relating to food production. Ruminant livestock provide high-quality animal-source foods in conjunction with a myriad of associated economic and social benefits to communities worldwide. Nonetheless, the question is often raised as to whether the consumption of milk and meat is inherently unsustainable.

Sustainability was defined within the Brundtland Report (United Nations World Commission on Environment & Development, 1987) as: *'meeting the needs of the present without compromising the ability of future generations to meet their own needs'*, and this remains the most commonly used definition, implying the need to use resources at rates that do not exceed the earth's capacity to replenish them, while ensuring human food security. 870 million people are currently considered to be food-insecure on a global basis (Food & Agriculture Organisation of the United Nations, 2012), so global food production could be argued to be unsustainable as per the first half of the definition.

Nonetheless, a sustainable food system is not simply dependent upon producing sufficient food but upon delivering and marketing food through an efficient infrastructure with minimal waste. The political and logistical challenges associated with food provision to currently food-insecure populations are beyond the scale of this chapter, so discussion will be confined to the three pillars of sustainability (i.e. economic viability, social responsibility and particularly environmental stewardship), as these relate to bovine production systems.

Within any production system, a balance must exist between environmental stewardship, economic viability and social responsibility; if one of these factors is out of alignment, the system cannot achieve long-term sustainability. For example, the use of hormone implants to improve productivity within US beef production has positive economic and environmental effects (Capper & Hayes, 2012), yet such technologies are not registered for use within the European Union and, as such, are socially unacceptable (Lusk *et al.*, 2003). No 'magic bullet' or suite of production practices exists to achieve global sustainability; individual production systems must be tailored to the resources, climate and culture indigenous to that region and to potential export markets. However, there is no doubt that prevailing global consumer and policy-maker concerns regarding the environmental sustainability of bovine production will have considerable effects on future production systems.

The global population is predicted to plateau at over 9.5 billion people in the year 2050 (Food & Agriculture Organisation of the United Nations, 2009) with disproportionate increases in population growth in the developing world. Concurrent increases in the *per capita* income within China, India and Africa over this time period will result in considerable increases in animal-source food consumption within currently impoverished nations and a projected 70% increase in global food requirements (Food & Agriculture Organisation of the United Nations, 2009; Masuda & Goldsmith, 2010).

The challenge facing global bovine production is to supply the growing population with sufficient economically affordable

Bovine Medicine, Third Edition. Edited by Peter D. Cockcroft.

milk and meat products to maintain dietary choice and human health while minimising environmental impact through reductions in both resource use and waste output. This challenge has myriad implications at the regional level, many of which are dependent on the current state of agricultural research and technology adoption. Despite the highly developed nature of the UK agricultural production system, Leaver (2009) notes that significant investment in research and development, and a greater collaboration between agricultural practice and science, are required in order to meet the rising demand for food in the UK (predicted to increase by 25% over the next 50 years) and to remain competitive on the global market.

What is the global impact of bovine production?

Discussion of animal agriculture's environmental impact is often restricted to greenhouse gas (GHG) emissions. Under the Climate Change Act of 2008, the UK government made a legally binding commitment to reduce GHG emissions by 80% by the year 2050, including a 11% reduction in GHG emissions (based on 2008 emissions) from agriculture by 2020 (HM Government, 2008), underlining the significant political concerns relating to this issue. However, resource scarcity (specifically water, land, inorganic fertilisers and fossil fuels) may be argued to have a greater immediate effect upon food production than climate change. Dairy and beef production also have a variety of direct environmental impacts (including positive and negative effects upon water and air quality, nutrient leaching, soil erosion and biodiversity) that should be included in environmental assessments. Nonetheless, the majority of studies to date have concentrated on GHG as the sole arbiter of environmental impact, so therefore GHG will be assumed to be a valid proxy for environmental effects in the following discussion, unless otherwise stated.

Global GHG emissions from agriculture were estimated by Bellarby *et al.* (2008) to account for between 17% and 32% of all human-induced emissions, with a recent report by the FAO (Food & Agriculture Organisation of the United Nations, 2006), concluding that animal agriculture contributes 18% of GHG emissions. In conjunction with estimates citing animal agriculture's contribution at up to 51% (Goodland & Anhang, 2009), these data have been eagerly adopted by activist groups as evidence for the benefits of a vegetarian or vegan lifestyle (Environmental Working Group, 2011). Due to methodological flaws, the 18% figure cited by the FAO is considered to be an overestimate (Pitesky *et al.*, 2009). Nonetheless, ruminant production systems make a significant contribution to total GHG emissions and resource use, due to having relatively less efficient feed conversion than their monogastric cohorts.

Dairy production accounts for approximately 2.7% of worldwide GHG emissions, with average emissions of 2.4 kg CO_2-eq/kg FPCM (fat and protein-corrected milk) at the farm gate (Food & Agriculture Organisation of the United Nations, 2010). Nonetheless, significant regional variation exists, with emissions ranging from 1.3 CO_2-eq/kg FPCM in North America to 7.5 kg CO_2-eq/kg FPCM in sub-Saharan Africa. Plotting average FPC milk yield against carbon footprint reveals a negative correlation - as production intensity and milk yield decrease with a regional shift from the developed to the developing world, GHG emissions increase (Figure 1.1).

Similar effects of productivity upon GHG emissions would be predicted for global beef production, yet are not borne out by comparisons among studies (Figure 1.2). These exhibit considerable methodological variation, and show that intensive systems have GHG emissions per kg beef ranging from 9.9–36.4 kg CO_2-eq, compared with extensive systems at 12.0–44.0 kg CO_2-eq/kg beef (Capper, 2011b; Cederberg *et al.*, 2011; Ogino *et al.*, 2004; Peters *et al.*, 2010).

Within both dairy and beef production, the environmental mitigation effect of improved productivity is conferred by the 'dilution of maintenance' concept, as shown in Figure 1.3 (Capper, 2011a; Capper *et al.*, 2008).

Every animal in the dairy or beef herd has a daily maintenance nutrient requirement that can be considered as a proxy for resource use and GHG emissions. As productivity (milk yield, meat yield or growth rate) increases, the proportion of daily energy allocated to maintenance decreases and the maintenance requirement of the total animal population decreases. This is exemplified by comparing the US dairy industries in 1944 and 2007: a four-fold increase in milk yield per cow over this time period reduced the national dairy herd from 25.6 million to 9.2 million cattle, with a concurrent 59% increase in milk production (53 billion kg in 1944 vs. 84 billion kg in 2007). This reduced feed use by 77%, land use by 90%, water use by 65% and conferred a 63% decrease in GHG emissions per kg of milk (Capper *et al.*, 2009). Similarly, if growth rate is increased in beef cattle, the population maintenance requirement is reduced because cattle take fewer days to reach slaughter weight. Considerable reductions in feed (19%), land (33%), water (12%) and GHG emissions (16%) were demonstrated by productivity improvements within the US cattle industry between 1977 and 2007 (Capper, 2011a). In this instance, environmental impact was reduced by an interaction between greater slaughter weights (607 kg *vs.* 468 kg) and faster average growth rates (1.18 kg/d vs. 0.72 kg/d) in 2007 compared with 1977 (Figure 1.3).

It is clear that improving system productivity and efficiency has a significant effect upon environmental sustainability. The aforementioned regional comparisons could lead to the conclusion that, for example, all regions should adopt confined

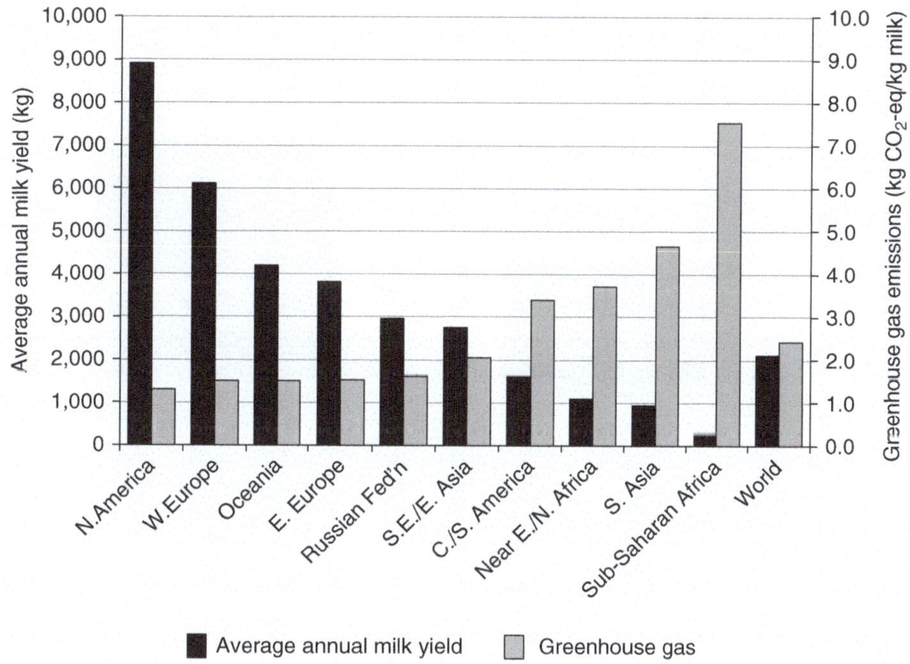

Figure 1.1 Relationship between average annual milk yield and greenhouse gas emissions per unit of milk on a regional and global basis.

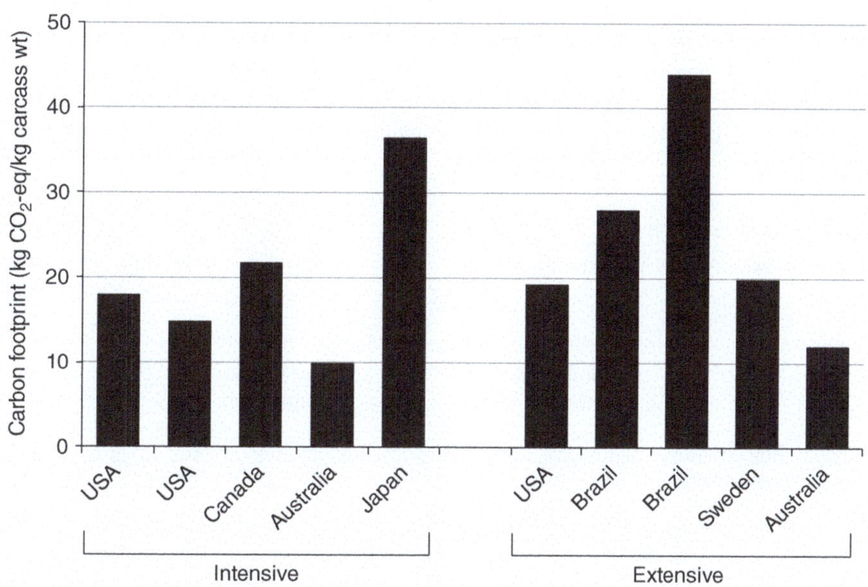

Figure 1.2 Regional and production system (intensive vs. extensive) variation in greenhouse gas emissions per unit of beef.

feeding operations such as those commonly practised in North America, in order to mitigate environmental impact. However, the three-faceted nature of sustainability must be considered; GHG emissions from dairy cattle in sub-Saharan Africa may be considerably higher than those in Europe. However, the nutritional and economic value gained from animal production, in addition to the social status of livestock ownership in developing countries, means that environmental impact cannot and should not be the sole consideration.

However, making the most efficient use of available resources has a two-fold advantage to the producer – efficient use of resources reduces environmental impact and reduces the economic costs of production (Capper & Hayes, 2012), thus contributing to economic viability.

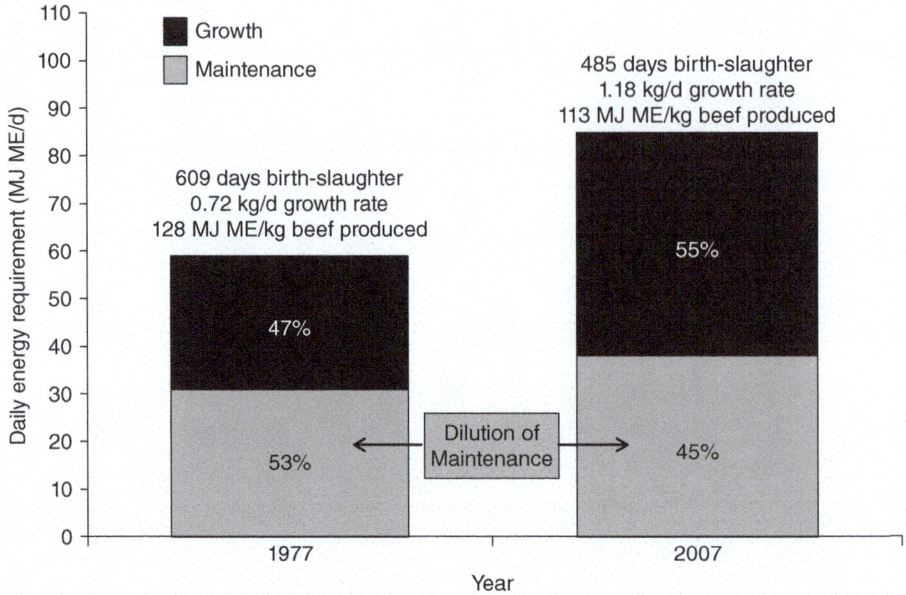

Figure 1.3 An example of the dilution of maintenance effect – comparing US beef production in 1977 and 2007.

What are the opportunities for mitigation?

Improved efficiency is inherently tied to a reduction in waste and losses throughout the system. This may be achieved through management practices that reduce specific environmental impacts, e.g. soil testing to assess fertiliser requirements, slurry injection to reduce nutrient leaching or recycling water for parlour sanitation (Figure 1.4).

However, whole-system approaches may have a greater overall mitigation effect. If a dairy or beef system working at optimal efficiency within every sub-system could potentially produce a set quantity of milk or meat based on animal genetic merit, every productivity loss within the system will reduce the potential yield and increase the environmental impact per unit of food produced. The potential losses from dairy and beef systems that will impact environmental sustainability are presented in Figure 1.5.

Productivity measures such as milk yield (dairy) and growth rate (beef) arguably have the most significant effect upon environmental sustainability, yet other metrics must also be

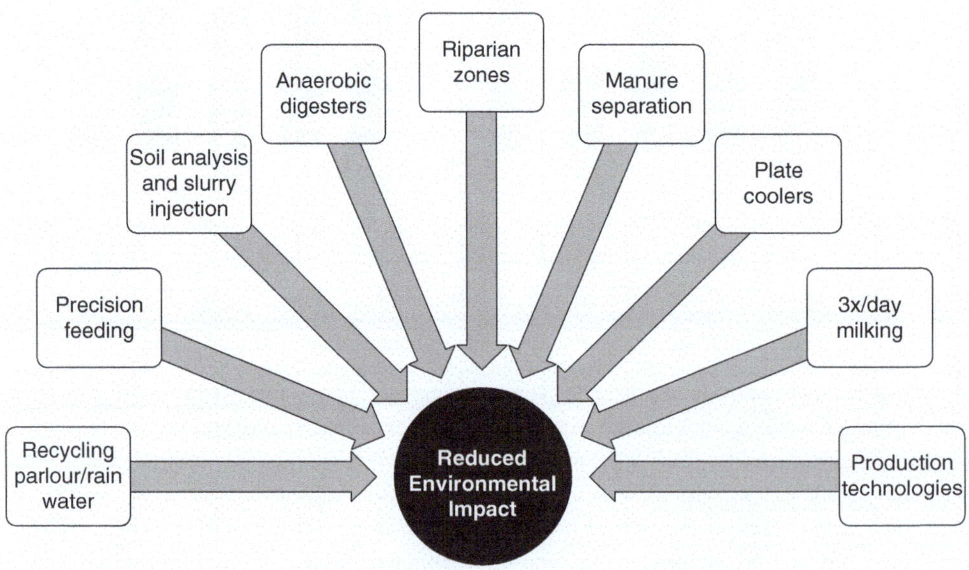

Figure 1.4 Specific management practices targeted to reduce the environmental impact of ruminant production.

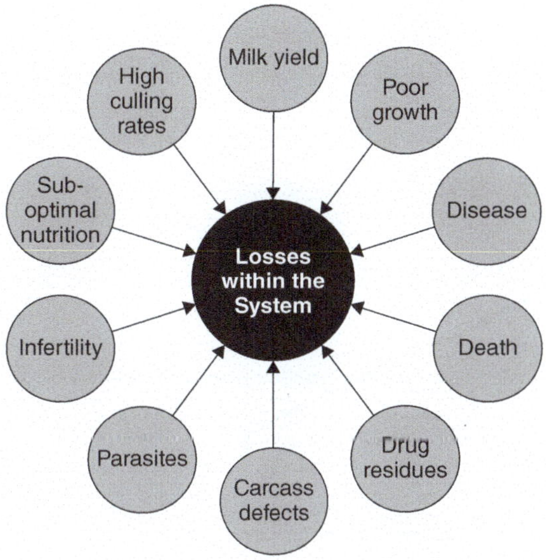

Figure 1.5 Losses within ruminant production systems that potentially increase environmental impact.

considered. To date, the environmental effects of less tangible productivity losses within dairy and beef systems (e.g. fertility, morbidity and growth of heifer replacements) have yet to be quantified.

Across dairy and beef industries, mature cow body weight has often increased concurrently with productivity gains, so daily resource use and GHG emissions per animal have increased (Capper, 2011a; Capper *et al.*, 2008). This may lead to future legislative complications if environmental assessments are based upon the number of livestock units per operation, without consideration of productivity.

In an evaluation of the environmental impact of cheese production from Jersey and Holstein milk, Capper & Cady (2012) demonstrated that land use, water use and GHG emissions were reduced by 32%, 11% and 20% respectively by the use of Jersey cattle. In this instance, environmental savings were conferred by the interaction between an increase in milk fat and protein content, combined with decreases in body weight and milk yield for Jersey cattle. Nonetheless, when breed-specific traits were examined in isolation, the difference in body weight between Jersey (454 kg) and Holstein (680 kg) cattle led to a 74% reduction in population body mass (and thus a reduced population maintenance requirement), despite a 9% increase in the total number of cattle required to produce an equivalent amount of cheese. Within this study, body weight was the most influential factor affecting environmental impact, with milk composition and milk yield following closely behind, yet with little effect of age at first calving, culling rate or calving interval.

These results were echoed by Bell *et al.* (2011), who reported that changing energy-corrected milk (ECM) yield (highly correlated with cheese yield) by one standard deviation conferred a 14.1% decrease in the carbon footprint per unit of ECM compared with feed efficiency, calving interval or culling rate (6.0%, 0.40% and 0.14% decreases, respectively).

Significant interest exists among beef producers in selecting cattle for improved feed efficiency, either as an improvement in residual feed intake (RFI; i.e. reduced feed consumption requirement to support maintenance and production compared with the predicted or average quantity), or through cows that have a lesser body weight, yet still produce calves that reach target weights for weaning and finishing. The development of estimated breeding values (EBVs) for RFI is relatively new, yet appears to show promise as a strategy by which producers may improve environmental impact.

Steers selected for high efficiency (low RFI) consumed less feed over the finishing period compared with low-efficiency cohorts in a large-scale feedlot study by Herd *et al.* (2009), exhibiting a greater dressing percentage and equal finishing weight at slaughter. Furthermore, Hegarty *et al.* (2007) reported that Angus steers showed considerable variation in methane emissions relative to intake, yet those selected for a lower RFI had reduced emissions consistent with reduced dry matter intake (DMI).

If productivity may be maintained on a reduced DMI, as per the aforementioned Holstein vs. Jersey example, resource use and GHG emissions would also be predicted to decrease per unit of output. For example, if mature cow body weight were reduced from 703 kg to 486 kg, while maintaining the final carcass weight of the offspring, GHG emissions per unit of beef would decline by 13% (Figure 1.6).

A negative trade-off exists, whereby selection for increased productivity within dairy cattle is generally considered to have contributed to declining fertility rates. Garnsworthy (2004) demonstrated that restoring fertility levels to those seen in UK dairy cattle c. 1995 reduced methane emissions per unit of milk compared with current fertility levels, and achieving ideal fertility reduced GHG emissions still further through a reduction in the number of heifer replacements required within the herd.

Fertility is arguably the major factor by which global beef producers (specifically seed stock and cow-calf producers) could also mitigate the environmental impact of beef production. Within beef production, conflict may also exist between selection for paternal traits (e.g. growth, carcass weight or frame size) and maternal traits (e.g. fertility, milk yield) under the nutritional limitations of pasture-based systems (Renquist *et al.*, 2006). Within the USA, 89% of cows bear a live calf each year (USDA, 2009), and this number declines to between 50–60% in the extensive systems characteristic of Brazil, Argentina and Chile. Given that the cow-calf operation contributes up to 80% of GHG emissions per unit of beef (Beauchemin *et al.*, 2010), and that productivity improvements post-calving cannot

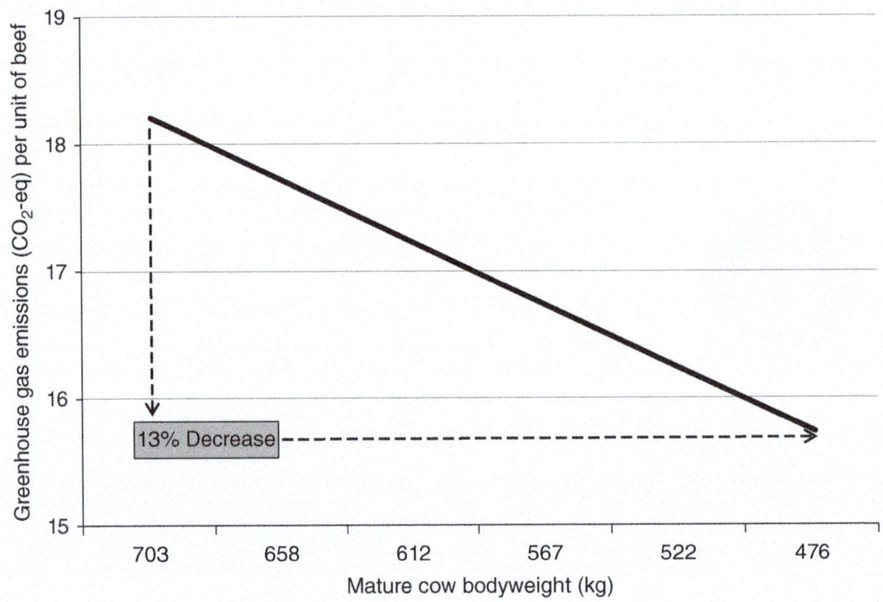

Figure 1.6 The effect of reducing mature beef cow body weight upon greenhouse gas emissions per unit of beef.

compensate for the resource use and GHG emissions associated with maintaining a non-productive cow, management practices and technologies that improve pregnancy rate offer significant opportunities.

Environmental impact and public perception

It is tempting to try to identify so-called 'silver bullets' that will instantly mitigate the environmental impact of dairy or beef production. Such interventions are often targeted by marketing campaigns or media as providing a simple solution, yet they may result in significant negative trade-offs. One example would be the installation of methane digesters which, although effective at reducing total GHG emissions from dairy production, are often economically prohibitive and require significant skilled labour to operate correctly (Chianese *et al.*, 2009). The supposition that transport of feed or fertilisers confers a far greater GHG burden upon grain-fed beef, compared with grass-finished systems, is often propounded in the media. However, recent studies show that GHG from transportation accounts for less than 1% of the carbon emissions associated with a unit of beef (Capper, 2011a; Capper, 2012), and that beef from cattle produced in wholly forage-fed systems is associated with considerable increases in land (80.8%), water (303%) and GHG emissions (70.4%), due to efficiency differences between systems.

In the USA and other developed regions, campaigns such as 'Meatless Mondays' or 'Meat Free Mondays' have emerged in recent years, as consumers increasingly perceive that animal protein consumption is environmentally or physically unhealthy. Scientific credence is lent to the campaign by papers evaluating the environmental impact of reducing meat consumption, with one such paper by researchers from Carnegie-Mellon University concluding that: '*Switching less than one day per week's worth of calories from red meat and dairy products to chicken, fish, eggs or a vegetable-based diet achieves more greenhouse gas reductions than buying all locally sourced food*' (Weber & Matthews, 2008).

Regardless of the underlying motivation for the Meatless Monday campaigns, the claims for a significant improvement in environmental impact appear to be over-exaggerated. To use the USA as an example, the US Environmental Protection Agency cites red meat and dairy production as contributing 2.1% of annual GHG emissions (US EPA, 2013). If we take the simplistic view that a one-day per week reduction in meat consumption would cut animal production by one-seventh, if every one of the USA's 316 million inhabitants adopted such a dietary change, the projected reduction in national GHG emissions would be equal to 0.30%. It is somewhat difficult to view a change that reduces national GHG emissions by less than one-third of one percent as having a meaningful environmental impact.

The claim that the world's nutrient requirements could be met simply using the grains currently fed to livestock is one of the most commonly heard arguments for vegetarianism or veganism and is often accompanied by a claim that it takes 10, 20 or even 30 kg of grain (Palmquist, 2011) to produce a kilogram of meat. Aside from the biological implausibility of the aforementioned numbers (corn only accounts for 7% of the total feed used to produce a kilo of beef in the USA), the implicit assumption is that the human population would be content to survive on a corn-based diet. Yet, when the additional land and resources required to grow other, lower-yielding crops (e.g.

salad leaves, asparagus and Brussels sprouts) to maintain dietary variety is included in the calculation, whole-scale conversion to vegetarianism appears to be a considerable challenge.

In an elegant comparison of resource use for various different diets, Fairlie (2010) notes that converting from the conventional omnivorous diet to a vegan system would reduce overall land use, yet the reduction is almost entirely confined to pasture land. The amount of land used for annual crops is increased in Fairlie's vegan scenario, due both to the lack of animal manures for fertiliser and to the need to provide fats and oils for energy within the human diet. Considerable quantities of pastureland are currently used to raise livestock, leading to the suggestion that the land could be far better employed to raise human food crops. However, only a small proportion of grazed pasturelands is suitable for food crop production, due to terrain, water or nutrient restrictions – indeed, 60% of farmed land in the UK is only suitable for pasture production (Pullar *et al.*, 2011).

The relatively low feed conversion efficiency of plant-based feedstuffs into animal proteins is likely to remain one of the biggest arguments against the omnivorous diet, yet is also one of livestock production's biggest selling points. Considerable quantities of by-products from the human feed and fibre industries are currently used within livestock diets – quantities which are often overlooked by governmental or organisational reports that cite grain-fed production as being unsustainable (Environmental Working Group, 2011; Foresight, 2011). When feed efficiency is quantified as a ratio of human-edible protein input to human-edible protein output, both dairy and grass-fed beef cattle produce a greater amount of human-edible food than they consume (due to the quantities of forage used within the diet), and lamb, swine and poultry have feed efficiency ratios between 1.1 and 2.6 kg human-edible protein input per kg of human-edible protein output (Wilkinson, 2011). Given the amino acid balance and protein quality of animal proteins compared with plant-based foods, this strengthens the rationale for maintaining omnivorous diets.

Role of the veterinarian/animal scientist and future developments

The veterinary and animal science communities have a significant role to play in helping to mitigate the environmental impact of ruminant production (Green *et al.*, 2011). Aforementioned productivity improvements that help to reduce resource use and GHG emissions can only be achieved through collaboration between producers, veterinarians, other allied industry and academia, in order to ensure that animals are bred, fed and cared for using management practices and technologies that will enable cattle to perform to their genetic potential.

Technologies such as ionophores, steroid implants, hormones and beta-agonists have a significant role to play in improving the environmental impact of ruminant production. Capper *et al.* (2008) demonstrated that use of recombinant bovine somatotropin reduced the GHG emissions from dairy production by 8.8%, while removing production-enhancing technology from US beef production was predicted by Capper & Hayes (2012) to increase resource use, to be equivalent to imposing an 8.2% economic tax on beef producers, and to increase global GHG emissions by 3.14 billion metric tonnes over time as a consequence of shifts in exports from countries with less-intensive production systems.

Despite considerable evaluation by national and global health agencies, and the prevailing opinion that no human health threats are presented by the use of such technologies, political and social agendas often oppose the approval or registration of these product within specific regions. Approval has recently been gained for the use of beta-agonists within Brazilian beef production systems and, as Brazil is a major beef producer, it will be interesting to see whether this sets a precedent for use of other technologies. The input of researchers, veterinarians and animal science professionals will be crucial within future debates, in order to ensure that science is not lost amongst public perception or political considerations.

When attempting to improve the sustainability of any system, it is crucial to note that, although productivity indices exist that are consistent across the spectrum, changes in management practice must be implemented with due consideration for the system resources in terms of labour, labour, economics, market and animal characteristics. No 'one-size-fits-all' solution exists yet, if all systems improve efficiency and productivity on a global scale, the challenge of meeting human food requirements for milk and meat products by the year 2050 becomes far more achievable.

References

Beauchemin, K.A., Janzen, H., Little, S.M., McAllister, T.A. and McGinn, S.M. (2010). Life cycle assessment of greenhouse gas emissions from beef production in western Canada: A case study. *Agricultural Systems* **103**, 371–379.

Bell, M.J., Wall, E., Russell, G., Simm, G. and Stott, A.W. (2011). The effect of improving cow productivity, fertility and longevity on the global warming potential of dairy systems. *Journal of Dairy Science* **94**, 3662–3678.

Bellarby, J., Foereid, B., Hastings, A. and Smith, P. (2008). *Cool Farming: Climate Impacts of Agriculture and Mitigation Potential*, Greenpeace International, Amsterdam, The Netherlands.

Capper, J.L. (2011a). The environmental impact of beef production in the United States: 1977 compared with 2007. *Journal of Animal Science* **89**, 4249–4261.

Capper, J.L. (2011b). Replacing rose-tinted spectacles with a high-powered microscope: The historical vs. modern carbon footprint of animal agriculture. *Animal Frontiers* **1**, 26–32.

Capper, J.L. (2012). Is the grass always greener? Comparing resource use and carbon footprints of conventional, natural and grass-fed beef production systems. *Animals* **2**, 127–143.

Capper, J.L. and Cady, R.A. (2012). A comparison of the environmental impact of Jersey vs. Holstein milk for cheese production. *Journal of Dairy Science* **95**, 165–176.

Capper, J.L. and Hayes, D.J. (2012). The environmental and economic impact of removing growth-enhancing technologies from United States beef production. *Journal of Animal Science* **90**, 3527–3537.

Capper, J.L., Castañeda-Gutiérrez, E., Cady, R.A. and Bauman, D.E. (2008). The environmental impact of recombinant bovine somatotropin (rbST) use in dairy production. *Proceedings of the National Academy of Sciences of the United States of America* **105**, 9668–9673.

Capper, J.L., Cady, R.A. and Bauman, D.E. (2009). The environmental impact of dairy production: 1944 compared with 2007. *Journal of Animal Science* **87**, 2160–2167.

Cederberg, C., Persson, M., Neovius, K., Molander, S. and Clift, R. (2011). Including carbon emissions from deforestation in the carbon footprint of Brazilian beef. *Environmental Science and Technology* **45**, 1773–1779.

Chianese, D.S., Harrison, J.O. and Lester, J.C. (2009). Anaerobic digesters: Benefits, barriers and policy implications. In: *Proceedings of 2009 ASABE Annual International Meeting*, ASABE, Reno, NV.

Environmental Working Group. (2011). *Meat Eater's Guide to Climate Change and Health*, Environmental Working Group, Washington, DC.

Fairlie, S. (2010). *Meat – A Benign Extravagance*. Chelsea Green Publishing, White River Junction, VT.

Food and Agriculture Organization of the United Nations. (2006). *Livestock's Long Shadow – Environmental Issues and Options*. FAO, Rome, Italy.

Food and Agriculture Organization of the United Nations. (2009). *How to Feed the World in 2050*. FAO, Rome, Italy.

Food and Agriculture Organization of the United Nations. (2010). *Greenhouse Gas Emissions from the Dairy Sector: A Life Cycle Assessment*. FAO, Rome, Italy.

Food and Agriculture Organization of the United Nations. (2012). *The State of Food Insecurity in the World 2012*. FAO, Rome, Italty.

Foresight. (2011). *The Future of Food and Farming. Final Project Report.*, The Government Office for Science, London.

Garnsworthy, P.C. (2004). The environmental impact of fertility in dairy cows: a modelling approach to predict methane and ammonia emissions. *Animal Feed Science and Technology* **112**, 211–223.

Goodland, R. and Anhang, J. (2009). *Livestock and Climate Change. What if the Key Actors in Climate Change were Pigs, Chickens and Cows?* Worldwatch Institute, Washington, DC.

Green, M., Husband, J., Huxley, J. and Statham, J. (2011). Role of the veterinary surgeon in managing the impact of dairy farming on the environment. *In Practice* **33**, 366–373.

Hegarty, R.S., Goopy, J.P., Herd, R.M. and McCorkell, B. (2007). Cattle selected for lower residual feed intake have reduced daily methane production. *Journal of Animal Science* **85**, 1479–1486.

Her Majesty's Government (2008). *Climate Change Act 2008*. The Stationery Office, London, UK.

Herd, R.M., Piper, S., Thompson, J.M., Arthur, P.F., McCorkell, B. and Dibley, K.C.P. (2009). Benefits of genetic superiority in residual feed intake in a large commercial feedlot. *Proceedings of the Association for the Advancement of Animal Breeding and Genetics* **18**, 476–479.

Leaver, D. (2009). Practice with Science and Agriculture: The Need to Re-Invigorate This Partnership. In: The Royal Society (ed.) *Reaping the Benefits. Science and the Sustainable Intensification of Global Agriculture*. The Royal Society, London, UK.

Lusk, J.L., Roosen, J. and Fox, J.A. (2003). Demand for beef from cattle administered growth hormones or fed genetically modified corn: A comparison of consumers in France, Germany, the United Kingdom and the United States. *American Journal of Agricultural Economics* **85**, 16–29.

Masuda, T. and Goldsmith, P.D. (2010). China's meat consumption: An income elasticity analysis and long-term projections In: *Proceedings of Agricultural & Applied Economics Association 2010 AAEA, CAES, & WAEA Joint Annual Meeting*, Agricultural & Applied Economics Association, Denver, CO.

Ogino, A., Kaku, K., Osada, T. and Shimada, K. (2004). Environmental impacts of the Japanese beef-fattening system with different feeding lengths as evaluated by a life-cycle assessment method. *Journal of Animal Science* **82**, 2115–2122.

Palmquist, D. (2011). Can the World Feed Itself Without Ruining the Planet? Available at: http://blog.nature.org/2011/10/can-the-world-feed-itself-without-ruining-the-planet/ (accessed: October 23, 2014).

Peters, G.M., Rowley, H.V., Wiedemann, S., Tucker, R., Short, M.D. and Schultz, M.S. (2010). Red meat production in Australia: Life cycle assessment and comparison with overseas studies. *Environmental Science and Technology* **44**, 1327–1332.

Pitesky, M.E., Stackhouse, K.R. and Mitloehner, F.M. (2009). Clearing the air: Livestock's contribution to climate change. *Advances in Agronomy* **103**, 3–40.

Pullar, D., Allen, N. and Sloyan, M. (2011). Challenges and opportunities for sustainable livestock production in the UK. *Nutrition Bulletin* **36**, 432–437.

Renquist, B.L., Oltjen, J.W., Sainz, R.D. and Calvert, C.C. (2006). Relationship between body condition score and production of multiparous beef cows. *Livestock Science* **104**, 147–155.

United Nations World Commission on Environment and Development (1987). *Our Common Future: Report of the World Commission on Environment and Development*. Oxford University Press, Oxford, UK.

US EPA (2013). *Inventory of U.S. Greenhouse Gas Emissions and Sinks: 1990–2011*. US EPA, Washington, DC.

USDA (2009). *Beef 2007–08 Part II: Reference of Beef Cow-calf Management Practices in the United States, 2007–08*. USDA:APHIS:VS, CEAH, National Animal Health Monitoring System, Fort Collins, CO.

Weber, C.L. and Matthews, H.S. (2008). Food-miles and the relative climate impacts of food choices in the United States. *Environmental Science and Technology* **42**, 3508–3515.

Wilkinson, J.M. (2011). Re-defining efficiency of feed use by livestock. *Animal* **5**, 1014–1022.

CHAPTER 2

Modern Cattle Practice: a Blueprint for the Future

Jos P. Noordhuizen

Learning objectives

- Present the key recommendations from the Lowe, Frawley and Foresight reports on the need for change in the role of the veterinarian in production animal farming.
- Provide a profile of the characteristics of the entrepreneurial dairy cattle farmer, the client.
- Indicate the need to understand current and future needs of clients, and how the veterinarian can add value by promoting and providing support in cattle health care, welfare, productivity, profitability and sustainability.
- Explain the role of the veterinarian in providing Veterinary Advisory Services (VAS), and how this relates to the implementation of population medicine concepts.
- Indicate the perceived weaknesses in the current veterinary services.
- Explain the importance of targeting our services to farmers within a practice business plan.
- Indicate the range of VAS which veterinarians can provide, including Diagnostic Herd Farm Visits, Herd Fertility Schemes, Herd Health and Productivity Management Advisory Services and Quality Risk Management Advisory Services, and how these can be implemented.
- Indicate how the VAS can contribute to the sustainability of the enterprise.
- Indicate the skills and knowledge required to implement a successful VAS, as well as the need to adopt a 'we' attitude when advising or solving a farm problem together with the dairy farmer.

Introduction

Cattle production has changed over the past decades, not least because the margin between production costs and farm income has become smaller. There is an increasing need for better control of production costs and *production losses* on cattle farms. Such production losses may originate from infectious and non-infectious animal diseases, impaired cattle welfare and lost cow comfort, suboptimal husbandry methods, production-related disorders and failing farm management ('management disorders').

While in dairy cattle, the milk yield has increased dramatically, with productions up to 10.000 or 12.000 litres per cow per year, it seems that farm management quality has fallen behind and is not always (sufficiently) competent to accommodate such high-yielding cows. The latter is indicated by the relatively high incidence and prevalence of production diseases, resulting in poor performance in production, reproduction and health status.

Veterinary assistance to cattle farmers has long been reactive, in response to requests from farmers such as: '*there is an acute sick cow, please come and treat her*'; '*can you vaccinate my herd tomorrow*'; '*please deliver dry cow injectors this week*'; '*please come do a Caesarean*'. This type of assistance costs money, and is commonly considered by farmers as an *economic loss*. Veterinarians in rural practice, in response to these demands, still predominantly focus on individual illness cases, rather than on whole-herd medicine.

Veterinarians rarely market their wide range of knowledge and skills, or are incapable of doing so. At the same time, farmers are not aware of the support that veterinarians could provide them with; moreover, veterinary costs are too often considered as losses (direct costs) and, hence, expensive (Frawley, 2003). However, veterinarians are able to increase farm profitability by addressing farming domains like reproduction, nutrition, udder health, anti-parasite strategies, claw health and genetic improvement. They appear not to invest much time and effort in promoting programs to sell their advisory services; neither do they spread inventory lists like the one presented in Annex 2.1: an inventory of satisfaction of the farmer about his herd performance, which can be found at the end of this chapter.

Bovine Medicine, Third Edition. Edited by Peter D. Cockcroft.

Lowe (2009) again points to the need of changing veterinary practice policies from solely emergencies to more planned herd health programs. Farmers in the UK, too, feel that veterinarians are not focusing sufficiently on solving whole-herd problems. Veterinarians should put more efforts into practice marketing and investigating client needs and expectations. Rural practices should develop and evolve into multidisciplinary teams, implementing whole-farm advisory services (Foresight, 2009).

Changing the type of practice is not always easy for veterinarians or farmers. It takes time to adapt and appreciate the benefits of the new approaches and methods. These would include analysing weak points and strong points in the practice (concerning products and services offered), identifying opportunities and threats to modernise the veterinary practice, and turning the perception among farmers regarding veterinary costs as direct costs into indirect costs (i.e. investments). One of the identified opportunities is that farmers require more than emergency assistance to bring down their production costs and losses. This requires an extension of the services provided from individual animals to *herd level approaches*, so that the main herd problems of economic importance are identified and corrected. Prevention and problem analysis to reduce or prevent losses have become much more important than before to provide assurance and risk management.

Dairy farms these days can be considered as enterprises, and farmers as entrepreneurs. The economic value of such farms is calculated in millions of US dollars. Their number is increasing, while the more traditional farming systems still remain. *Entrepreneur-like dairy farmers* can be characterised by specific features (Bergevoet, 2005). Some of the most important features are presented in Table 2.1.

The success of an entrepreneurial dairy farmer is reflected in the achievement of multiple goals. This type of dairy farmer has professional skills, a commercial and market focus, a farm-economic drive, shows a high level of organisation, is well-skilled in communication and negotiation, is aware of their own abilities and skills, and knows what other service-providers should bring. In fact, this farmer combines the professional skills with managerial qualities and entrepreneurial abilities (Noordhuizen *et al.*, 2006; Noordhuizen *et al.*, 2008[1]). This farmer will not blindly accept a professional's advice; he needs to analyse such advice to fully understand it and to determine whether he will implement it. Discussions between the veterinarian and the farmer should be held in an atmosphere of equality between two professionals. This is quite different from the attitude of, say, more traditional dairy farmers, who sometimes have full confidence and trust in their veterinarian and just simply follow the advice given.

Table 2.1 Some of the most important features of entrepreneurial dairy farmers.

1	This dairy farmer is rather risk-taking in nature.
2	The farmer is capital providing.
3	The farmer is innovative and always prone to new challenges.
4	The farmer finds opportunities to make profit.
5	The farmer feels responsible for the process to create new values.
6	The farmer will enhance changes because he does not stick to 'old' practices.
7	The farmer's decision-making is based on multiple judgments; critical farmer.
8	The farmer is a planner and has ideas, and is professionally well-skilled.
9	The farmer inspires people, is a team-worker and networker, and loves action.
10	Economic profit is not the only drive; pleasure in the work is paramount.

The *Veterinary Advisory Service (VAS)* may assist the farmer to better control production costs and losses, because veterinarians have, in principle, the appropriate knowledge and skills in many farming domains. Farmers are not always aware that veterinarians could provide such services, while veterinarians, in turn, are not always aware of what their clients want, nor are sufficiently proactive to market their services; they act, as in emergency cases, on a 'wait and see, and go' basis. These VAS may cover a wide range of activities, including simple operational farm monitoring activities and subsequent action planning; advisory plans on biosecurity or a health domain (like udder health); holistic herd health and productivity management advice; and the more tactical integrated quality risk management advice. The inventory list of farmers' satisfaction about herd performance (Annex 2.1) is an easy and simple marketing tool, used to discuss poor performance areas with the farmer and compose a tailor-made VAS.

The veterinarian who wants to provide such 'population-oriented' programs needs to acquire knowledge and skills in particular domains, which will be addressed later in this chapter. A large survey of dairy farmers in the Netherlands (Lievaart *et al.*, 2008) identified a range of weaknesses the farmers perceived in their veterinarians (Table 2.2). Being aware of such remarks, the veterinarian may work to improve these points (Eelkman-Rooda, 2006; Noordhuizen *et al.*, 2006).

Of course, the issues listed in Table 2.2 are averaged. Not all veterinarians are deficient in all of the highlighted areas. On the other hand, it is worthwhile to consider the ten points in Table 2.2 to find out whether something strategic has to be changed in the veterinary practice, and whether additional skills or knowledge have to be acquired. A strengths-and-weaknesses analysis of the products and services provided by the practice is a useful exercise (Noordhuizen *et al.*, 2008). One could, for example, use the scheme presented in Figure 2.1, and put the different products and services in each quadrant to find out the best possible choices for the next five or ten years.

Services in the area of 'sleepers' could be developed further, while those in 'winners' should be further emphasised. Products

Table 2.2 Some major points for improvement in veterinarians, as defined by dairy farmers in a 2006 study in the Netherlands.

1	A too dominant attitude, as if the veterinarian seems to know everything.
2	The vet talks too much and listens too little (poor professional communication).
3	The vet does not work by structured protocols; the advice is not structured.
4	The vet has limited knowledge about cattle nutrition and associated issues.
5	The vet has limited knowledge about economics and management on a farm.
6	The vet has little knowledge about entrepreneurs (features; ways to approach).
7	The image of the vet is that the vet is too expensive.
8	The vet does not show the expertise in other fields (housing, climate, etc).
9	The vet does not show what he/she might contribute to the farm performance.
10	The vet shows little empathy, is too much abiding time, little proactive.

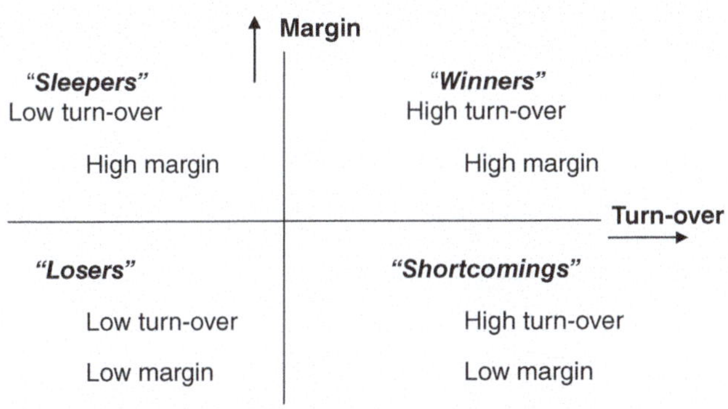

Figure 2.1 Scheme for analysing, positioning and weighing veterinary products and services provided to clients (Noordhuizen *et al*., 2006). Reproduced with permission of Context Products Ltd.

and services in the area of 'losers' should most probably be stopped (unless relevant for certain reasons such as a notifiable disease). The services in 'shortcomings' should be revisited, evaluated, and then adjusted or stopped. Through this method, the veterinary practice may develop a *practice business plan* for the next five or ten years, following trends in the cattle production sector and society.

In this chapter, the development phases of *Veterinary Advisory Services* will be highlighted and, where appropriate, examples of implementation will be provided.

Veterinary advisory services

Diagnostic herd evaluation farm visits

Diagnostic Herd Evaluation (DHE) is the method of routinely monitoring current performance of the herd by observing cows and cow groups while standing at the feed rack, their environment, the management, and farm-related data, during monthly or two-weekly planned farm visits. Table 2.3 presents a range of important parameters that could be monitored.

The process of monitoring requires organisation and time-management. Not all items need to be monitored every month (checking growth in young stock once every six months as a routine; BCS every one or two months; concentrates dispenser once every six months). Hence, a selection has to be made together with the farmer to determine the highest priorities and to define the monitoring scheme for the next 4–6 visits to come.

On the basis of the findings, the veterinarian performs an analysis and draws conclusions which s/he discusses with the farmer. Upon acceptance, measures to control the weaker points are discussed and, if feasible within farm operational management, a plan of implementation is devised for the short term and the mid/long term. These issues are written down in a short *farm visit report*. Figure 2.2 presents an example of such a farm visit report, with the previously described paragraphs.

Through the DHE, the veterinarian identifies risk factors and risk areas, where the threat of potential future economic losses exists on the farm (see Box 1 for an example).

The DHE can function as a stand-alone advisory service, and it takes no longer than 30–45 min for herds up to 100–150 cows. It could be considered as the 'routine technical health check of the farm', just like the compulsory checks on cars many countries. The DHE provides an *instant picture* of the farm situation, visible to the farmer and a *platform for discussion* between farmer and veterinarian. Over the months, trends in farm performance become explicit, especially when the most important performance parameters are listed on a separate *monthly performance list*. The latter is often available in computer software for farmers or veterinary practices. The DHE can also be conducted in combination with other advisory services, such as herd fertility schemes, herd health and production management advisory services, and quality risk management advice.

Herd fertility schemes (HFSs)

HFSs were introduced in the late 1960s and 70s in many countries worldwide (De Kruif, 1975; Williamson, 1980; Esslemont *et al*., 1985). This service has two components (Brand *et al*., 1996):

1 examination of selected cows;
2 evaluation of herd performance and analysis of prevailing problems.

Since the start of these services, many farmers have dropped out, while others have joined the service. Drop-outs were predominantly caused by the fact that veterinarians focused on operational (clinical) matters alone and neglected, or simply omitted, the second component. Hence, they were not able to propose strategic advice on reproductive performance and management. Moreover, reporting in writing appeared not to

Table 2.3 Examples of parameters for routine monitoring during DHE farm visits (Alvès de Oliveira *et al*., 2008; Noordhuizen, 2012).

Cows, calves, maiden heifers	Animal environment & management	Farm-related data
Body condition score, BCS	General hygiene on the farm	Milk recording (L; milk fat; milk protein)
Rumen Fill score, RF	Milking hygiene	Somatic cell counts
Faecal Consistency score, FC	Milking practice	Milk quality issues (Lab parameters)
Undigested Fibre in Faeces score, UFF	Barn climate (humidity; ventilation; draughts; heat stress; cold stress)	Quality of grass and corn silages
Teat-End Callosity score, TEC	Housing (passageways; cubicles; feed bunk; feed table)	Quality of grass
Teat lesions (and mastitis)	Cow comfort (feed; barn climate; housing; behaviour; claw health)	Quality of pastures
Skin lesions	Manure scraping (system; frequency)	Quality of soil
Cows with poor leg posture	Claw trimming and foot bath	Quality of water (source)
Lame cows (and Locomotion Score, LS)	Ration composition (calculations; frequency)	Herd performance parameters
Hock lesions (depilation; abscess)	Concentrate dispenser (check dose)	Laboratory reports
Cow hygiene score, HYG (thighs/udder)	Exercise areas	Sanitary herd book
Typical behaviour (agonistic/antagonistic)	Roads to pasture (quality and risks)	Herd Disease-free Certificates
Growth pattern in calves	Management, hygiene & quality of colostrum	Milk urea (values and trends)
Diarrhoea in calves	Housing and climate for calves	Culling rate (% and reasons)
Respiratory disease in calves	Housing, stress for maiden heifers (parity 1)	Good Dairy Farming code of practice
Results of rectal palpation	Quality of feed bunk and hygiene	Soil quality data
Clinical disease cases as indicator cows (e.g. ketosis : acidosis)	Floor design and maintenance in houses	Surface water quality

Box 2.1 Example: Diagnostic herd evaluation – lameness.

On a dairy farm, the vet has made an inventory of cows with poor hind leg posture (the legs are rotated to the outside, which is a sign of claw lesions potentially being present). The prevalence is about 60% of the cows in the herd. At the same visit to this farm, the vet observes a slippery floor in the barn, a lack of manure scraping, a damp barn climate, and poor forage quality in the feed bunk.

The vet discusses these findings with the farmer, pointing out some of the affected cows and the areas of concern, and proposes management measures to change the situation in order to prevent large losses occurring in the future.

Action plan:

Short term

1 Improve forage quality for high yielding cows and feed the current forage to heifers.
2 Increase the frequency of manure scraping on the day (4-6 times).
3 Functional claw trimming determines the diagnosis of the claw lesions.

Mid/long term:

4 Improve barn ventilation facilities.
5 New strategies to define when claw trimming results are known

The forenamed elements are written in a dated farm visit report.

During the subsequent visits, the vet checks what has been done and what the impact and outcomes are by conducting again a DHE.

be a strong point of the veterinarians. The first component is apparently too close to the classic clinical work of the veterinarian: just do the job, treat whenever you can, and that is it. A standard listing of cows due for examination is given in Table 2.4 (Brand *et al.*, 1996).

Over the past decades, however, it has been stated that herd fertility cannot be considered as completely stand-alone and should be approached in a much more holistic manner (Brand *et al.*, 1996). For example, injecting cows postpartum with prostaglandins F2-α while these cows are in a severe negative energy balance and anoestrus will be futile. See Box 2.2 for some further details.

These limitations have been the starting point for the development of herd health programs and of herd health & production

FARM VISIT REPORT FOR FARM XYZ ON 9 SEP 2014

LOGO
of veterinary clinic

***Strong points**

On entering, the farm premises are clean and well-organised; bulk tank room and milking parlour are very clean.

Cows: Generally, a good BCS, given the milk yield level (BCS around 3); BCS at start of lactation is okay (±3, without too much variation). Rumen Fill score is okay in all lactation stages (2–3); good scores for Faeces Consistency and Faeces fibres (2–3). Score of hygiene and cleanness is good (scores 1–2). Teat end scores are good (1–2). Locomotion score (static and dynamic) is ±acceptable; not for #678 and #955. There are some hock lesions (4 on 20 cows); so **be careful**: recheck next visit.

Environment: Barn has a good volume (see reference standards) and good light (>200 lux). Barn climate and cow comfort is good; temperature is somewhat high (ventilation). Cubicles with straw are spacious for head movements. Distribution of feed to cows is okay; concentrates dispenser dose is well gauged. Farmer is to the point and ambitious.

Farm data: Level of production (L) and milk fat and protein are okay (milk recording). Bulk milk somatic cell counts were historically okay (but alarm in March). Calving peak is between May and December, so today (8 Sep) most of the cows are at the end of lactation. There are about 42% of first lactation cows (= **many!**): check culling policy of farmer. Rather few mastitis cases (5 on 70 cows in July). Milk quality parameters do not show any deviation in the past year.

***Points for improvement**

Cows: BCS after 50 days : too many thin cows; end lactation okay; BCS in dry cows is too high. Rumen Fill score in dry cows is far from the ideal. Level of rumination in the herd (2 tests) was not more than 50% of the cows (norm is >70%). Causes are stress? high temperatures? disease? Too many cows (±50%) show poor leg posture; possibly claw lesions (locomotion score may be slowly shifting to the bad side). Some cows have long claws on front feet; this hampers an appropriate feed intake. Cow #810 shows a metritis at 18 days after calving: **needs follow-up**.

Environment/management: Too few drinking places (3 times 2 × 30 cm)= 180 cm (norm is 45 cm width per 10 cows, so 315 cm in total for 70 cows; in heat periods twice as much).

Farm data: Some cows are suspected of rumen acidosis given the milk recording results of April—May and June—July. These cows must be checked at next recording date. In April, several cows showed a substantial drop in milk yield. In November 2008, there has already been a drop in milk yield. **Precaution**: put to the barn earlier in the season? Smoothen the transition pasture-barn period. There is a group of cows with high SCC; they are a risk for their herd mates with respect to mastitis. How to handle them best within the herd? We need to know their bacteriological profile for better treatment options (so milk samples needed). The yearly culling rate is rather high (38% versus norm of < 30%); main reasons are fertility and lameness. Calving interval is 420 days (distribution to be checked); 30% of cows had more than 3 services (and 20% parity 1 cows, only 7% in maiden heifers).

***Synthesis and conclusions**

(a) Problem of <u>fertility in the herd</u>; needs to be explored in more detail. We may consider an analysis of heat detection after calving and at 3–6–9 weeks after AI. Check the prevalence of metritis and cysts too.

(b) <u>Subclinical claw lesions</u> are present, but diagnosis is not sufficiently reliable. So we need a sample of 20% of the herd to be trimmed for diagnosis, either during routine claw trimming (inventory of primary diagnoses), or during a specific farm visit.

(c) Problem of <u>high SCC cows</u>, which form a risk for other cows.

(d) <u>BCS scores</u> need to be better controlled at the <u>end of lactation</u> and in the <u>dry period</u>, to better avoid problems in reproduction and production in next lactation.

(e) Adapt the number of drinking places; add new ones if necessary ; note that high-yielding cows consume more than 120 L water per day.

***Advice in the short term**

1. Continue <u>routine claw trimming</u> once or twice per year (do not neglect front claws!); cows which show poor locomotion score or have a poor leg posture must be checked. A photo-diagnosis instruction card for the farmer may be of great help for properly diagnosing primary lesions.
2. It would be highly desirable that the farmer <u>writes down all diagnoses</u> of claw lesions that he encounters. This is the only way of having a quick insight into the development of claw lesions. Proper diagnoses are needed to tailor-make the plan of actions (risk factors are different for each diagnosis). At the same time, manure scraping must be more frequent (4–6 times per day), because the floor must be kept dry and clean.
3. Adapt the <u>rations at the end of lactation and in the dry period</u> for better controlling BCS (at 3.5 instead of 4) and subsequent problems (poor feed intake; poor transition; poor ovulation rate).
4. Add <u>drinking places</u> up to a total width of at least 350 cm (in summer the double width).

***Advice in the mid/long term**

1. Analyse first in detail the <u>fertility problems</u> (intervals which deviate, cows with poor performance, cysts, metritis, etc); action plans will then follow.
2. Analyse the cows in the group of '<u>High SCC cows</u>' to better know the details of this problem. A bacteriological profile is indispensable; <u>milk samples</u> must be taken. The samples can be stored in the <u>freezer</u> with labelled cow ID, date, quarter sampled. The samples can be sent to the lab in one batch. On the basis of this profile, the <u>Herd Treatment Advisory Plan</u> can be designed. Other measures are: milk high SCC cows last; separate high SCC cows from other cows; consider culling of chronically high SCC cows.

Figure 2.2 An example of a DHE farm visit report: observations, synthesis and conclusions, proposed interventions and other advice for the short and mid-long term (Noordhuizen, 2012). Reproduced with permission of Context Products Ltd.

Box 2.2 Details on herd fertility.

Cows show a negative energy balance after calving, due to the intake of energy being less than that required for the increased milk yield. This phenomenon causes a ketosis in the cow. Follicles do not reach their state of dominance and do not ovulate. Such cows do not show oestrus, sometimes from calving onward, sometimes after having shown just one oestrus around Day 20 after calving. The phenomenon diminishes when the energy imbalance recedes, resulting in oestrus at Day 80 or more after calving. Management of the transition period, feeding management in general and feed intake after calving are paramount issues in this respect.

If cows after calving are affected by infectious or non-infectious claw lesions, then they may not be able to express oestrus, due to pain. These cows also have a reduced dry matter intake. This, combined with a pre-existing negative energy balance, will reduce the prospect of getting in calf further. Hence, a good claw health in the herd contributes to better reproductive performance.

Table 2.4 A standard listing of cows due for examination during HFS farm visits.

1	Cows for pregnancy diagnosis (by ultrasound at 30 days post AI) or by rectal palpation (around 40–60 days post-AI).
2	Cows freshly calved to be checked around 30 days post calving (check on endo-metritis; ovarian function and cyclicity; cysts).
3	Cows not observed in heat at 50 days post calving (prediction of cycle stage).
4	Cows with abnormal cycles and abnormal oestrus intervals.
5	Repeat breeder cows (with three inseminations or more).
6	Cows with reproductive disorders (e.g. vaginal discharge) or other disorders (e.g. ketosis).

management advisory programs (Noordhuizen *et al.*, 2008; Boersma *et al.*, 2010).

Herd Health and Production Management advisory Service (HHPMS)

Herd health programs which are limited to vaccination schemes or de-worming strategies are outside the scope of this chapter and not further addressed.

HHPMS encompass all farm domains relevant to an individual farmer. Among these are: milk production and nutrition; udder health; claw health; general health status; young stock rearing; welfare and cow comfort; and public health issues.

They are a combination of three components:

1 the monthly diagnostic herd evaluation, DHE;
2 the analysis of prevailing or pending problems and suggestion of solutions;
3 the development of preventative plans (biosecurity; general measures of prevention).

The DHE is the basis for the HHPMS; it provides access to the farm, and facilitates the discussion between farmer and veterinarian and other consultants such as the nutritionist. In its application, a HHPMS is very dynamic and flexible, always adapting to the individual needs and priorities of a farmer, and to the current farm situation. The most important features of HHPMS are that they are following *protocols*, or preset working procedures, and that they are focused on operational management. An example of a general protocol is presented in Figure 2.3, the structured analysis of general claw health problems.

The advantage of such protocols is that the veterinarian will not forget to check certain elements, especially when the protocol details become more complex or when two disorders occur at the same time. They also indicate to the farmer where the farm stands in the analysis process. The farmer will more easily understand what is being done and for what reason; the veterinarian can explain the details.

Such a protocol can be followed by repeated farm audits (such as with the DHE). An example of a farm audit, associated with the protocol in Figure 2.3, is presented in Table 2.5.

Prevention comprises two components:

1 general preventive measures;
2 specific measures.

The former are related to attitude and mentality of people working on the farm; they represent the 'dos' and the 'don'ts' and form part of the *Good Cattle Farming code of Practice* (OIE, 2006; Noordhuizen *et al.*, 2008; Boersema *et al.*, 2010). Examples can be found in the criteria to define a 'closed farm', where high hygiene standards prevail, and no cattle are purchased or visitors allowed unless under strict conditions (see for details Noordhuizen, 2012). Specific measures are commonly concerned with specific diseases, which are considered relevant for the farm, and their associated risk factors. Another example concerns the definition and implementation of biosecurity plans for defined infectious diseases (for details see BAMN, 2000; Boersema *et al.*, 2010). Biosecurity plans are management tools to avoid infectious diseases entering the farm or to reduce their impact once they have entered the farm. Key elements are risk identification and risk management. Details on the development and application of biosecurity plans are presented in Noordhuizen *et al.* (2008).

Herd health and production management advisory programs have now been implemented worldwide, both on smaller (<250 cattle herd) and larger (>1000 cattle herd) farms. Results are varied, possibly due to the variability of veterinary expertise in associated domains. When implemented properly, the benefits are greater than the costs (Sol *et al*, 1984). Veterinarians should learn more about domains such as business management, marketing, professional communication, behavioural economics, quality concepts and assurance, and performing a strengths-and-weaknesses analysis, to render this service truly

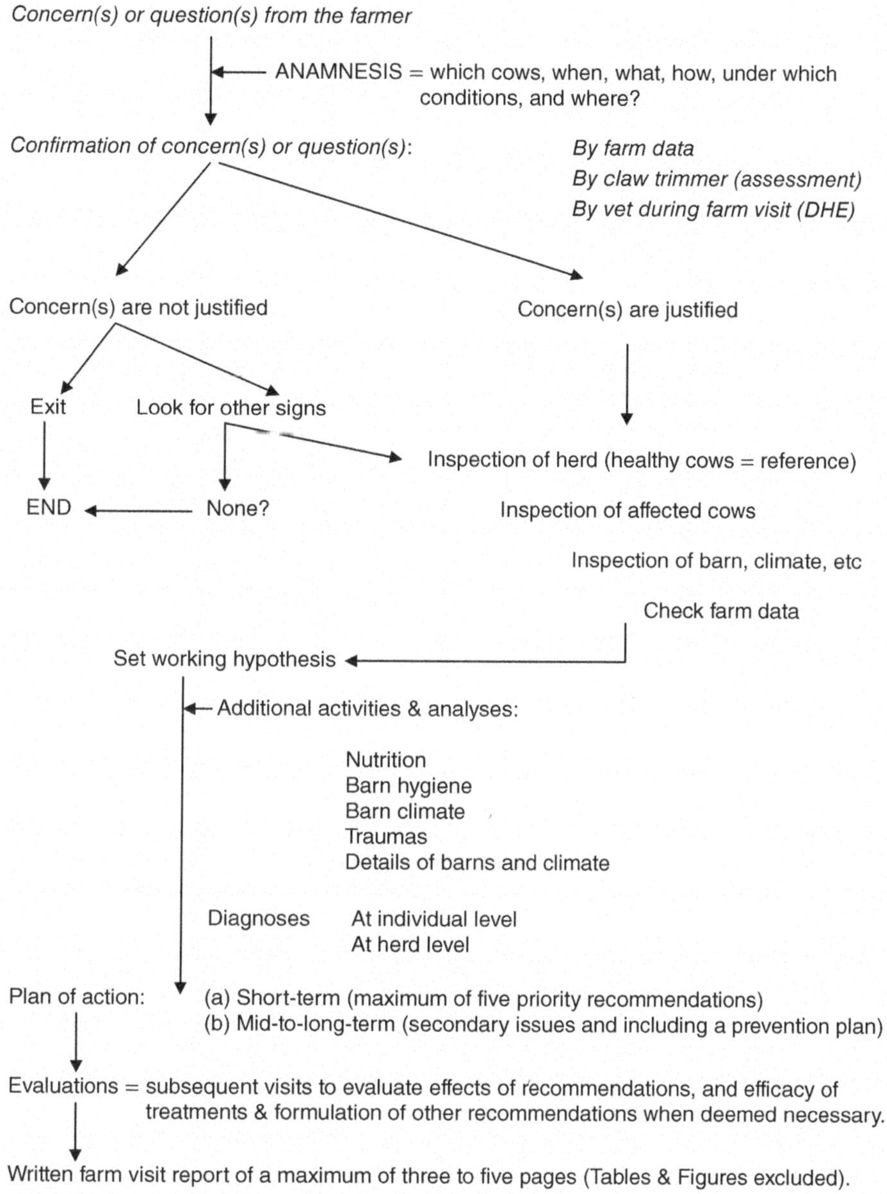

Figure 2.3 A basic protocol for the structured analysis of problems in the area of claw health.

professional. These skills are equally applicable to the veterinary practice, which also should be run like a business (Cannas da Silva *et al.*, 2006).

Quality risk management programs, QRM

The quality of cattle products (e.g. milk) has always been of greatest importance, due to public health concerns associated with milk-borne infections such as brucellosis, but also for the processing of milk into cheese and other products. Current quality parameters of milk include somatic cell count, bacteria count, antibiotic residues and butyric acid bacteria. The general public (consumers) have become more sensitised to the way the milk or meat is produced on the farm, with regards to animal welfare issues. Quality is therefore extended to the *production process* itself.

It has been postulated that quality on a dairy farm can be read from parameters associated with animal health, animal welfare, public health and food safety status of the herd (Noordhuizen *et al.*, 2008). These four domains appear in various governmental directives or regulations (e.g. EC regulation 178-2002; EC directives 852/853/854-2004 in Noordhuizen *et al.*, 2008), and also in quality assurance programs linked to the dairy production chain, where industry takes incentives to optimise quality in its largest sense. Consumer protection has become a

Table 2.5 An example of a farm audit scheme of the current prevalence of interdigital dermatitis, using the protocol in Figure 2.3.

Question	What is the actual prevalence of interdigital dermatitis?
Best practice or gold standard	Monthly prevalence of interdigital dermatitis less than 15% of the adult cow herd
Findings[a]	The prevalence of interdigital dermatitis is 11%
Comments	This seems okay, but it is increasing over time
Associated KPI (target values)[b]	**Prevalence of claw lesions**: digital dermatitis: <10%/year; blood imbibitions in the sole: <15%/year; sole ulcers: <15%/year; panaritium: <10%/year; white line disorders: <15%/year. **Reproduction**: Cows not observed in heat: <10%/month **Milk production**: drop in milk yield between two consecutive monthly recordings <10%/cow
Potential impact on farm profitability (high–medium–low)	Medium to high
Actual impact	Low

[a]Findings as collected during observations in a DHE
[b]Target values are to be defined for each individual farm

crucial issue, not least due to different outbreaks of diseases (e.g. *E. coli* $O_{157}H_7$; leptospirosis; tuberculosis; salmonellosis).

Different *quality concepts* have been described (Evans & Lindsay, 1996). In the dairy food chain, good manufacturing codes of practice (*GMP*) and hazard analysis and critical control points (*HACCP*) are being implemented, but on dairy farms quality assurance programs addressing the production process are very rarely applied. Transportation of dairy products can be assured through implementing ISO-9000 (International Office of Standardisation). Food safety standards can hardly be met in industry by GMP codes, and are replaced by the HACCP approach.

Noordhuizen and Welpelo (1996) have presented the features of and differences between quality control programs such as GMP, HACCP and ISO-9000, if they are to be applied on the dairy farm (Table 2.6). Their conclusion was that a quality risk management program (QRM) based on the principles of HACCP would be the best possible option to serve both the tactical goal of safeguarding the consumer and the quality of the product, as well as the operational management goals of the individual dairy farmer.

The farmer can recognise his/her farm and management style best with HACCP-like applications. The GMP is too general and too vague in nature and not truly certifiable, while the ISO-9000 is too laborious, too costly and not specific enough.

In Table 2.7 are named the subsequent steps in developing a HACCP-like QRM for dairy farms.

An example of a *production process flow diagram* (steps 4 and 5 in Table 2.6) is shown in Figure 2.4. Such flow diagrams facilitate the discussion within the Quality Team, as well as with farm workers.

In step 6 in Table 2.7, the hazards concern diseases and disorders of various nature, already prevalent on the farm or considered important to avoid on the farm. Such diseases usually have associated risk factors. For an individual farm, the risk factors have to be ranked according to their importance to that farm. *Risk weighting* can be done based on published quantitative epidemiological studies yielding odds ratios or relative risks (Noordhuizen *et al.*, 2001), or through qualitative assessment using the formula Probability × Impact, and for each factor, three classes (high; intermediate; low, or 3; 2; 1 points respectively). When a threshold for the outcome of the formula is chosen (e.g. six or more points), the specific risks can be prioritised.

The critical control points (CCPs) in step 7 are commonly related to physical processes (e.g. milking). On a farm, biological processes, with their biological variation, predominantly prevail, rendering it very hard to define true CCPs. Therefore, one could replace certain CCPs by a target value. Note that these target values come close to those defined in HHPMS. Examples are: a target value for yearly clinical mastitis rate of <25%; or a target value for calf diarrhoea of <5% per year. The monitoring system in step 9 is highly comparable to the routine monitoring DHE. The corrective measures of step 10 are, for example, assembled in a mastitis control program, a claw health program or a fertility scheme.

Various field trials have been conducted to evaluate the implementation of these HACCP-like QRM programs. Bell *et al.* (2003) investigated the application of such QRM in the area of lameness, and concluded that it is a practical tool for both farmers and veterinarians. From other field surveys, it was concluded that farmers like the way that the program is structured, that there was a joint effort by veterinarian and farmer to try solve the problem, and that they feel pinpointed to items which are truly relevant on their farms (Boersema *et al.*, 2010; Beekhuis-Gibbon *et al.*, 2011). Noordhuizen and Cannas da Silva (2009) addressed the application of such programs in the area of udder health.

It is beyond the scope of this chapter to detail fully the development and implementation of the HACCP-like QRM. For that purpose, we refer to practical handbooks where these issues have been elaborated for dairy farms and for dairy young stock respectively, together with many examples (Noordhuizen *et al.*, 2008; Boersema *et al.*, 2010).

Table 2.6 Major features of different quality control concepts.

Feature	GMP code of practice	HACCP	ISO-9000
Area of interest	Process	Process + products	The system
Type of approach	Top-down	Bottom up	Bottom up
Health state is demonstrable	No	Yes	Yes
Corrective actions are specified	No	Yes	No
Suitable for certification	No	Yes	Yes
Documentation needed	Yes (as guidelines)	Yes (specific)	Yes (much)
Simplicity in application	Yes	Yes	No
Is farm-specific	No	Yes	?
High labour input needed	No	No	Yes
Self-management possible	No	Yes	N.A.
Expected benefits : costs	Low	High	Intermediate
Can be integrated into quality assurance program	Yes, but limited	Yes in full	n.a.
Functional link with industry	Yes, but limited	Yes	Yes

Table 2.7 The different steps in the development of a HACCP-like QRM (Noordhuizen *et al.*, 2008). Reproduced with permission of Wageningen Academic Publishers.

Step	Short description
1	Assemble a multidisciplinary, farm-based, *quality team, QT,* including the farmer, veterinarian, nutritionist, and another specialist when needed.
2	Describe the products delivered (milk; meat; livestock) and the way they are delivered.
3	Identify the way that the products delivered would be used by the targeted purchaser.
4	Develop flow diagrams of the production process on the farm (facilitate discussions).
5	Verify these flow diagrams on the farm with QT, manager and farm workers.
6	Identify the hazards which are most relevant to the farm, as well as their associated risk factors/conditions. Conduct a risk weighing and prioritise the risks.
7	Identify critical control points (CCP) in the production process, required to reduce or eliminate the hazards/risks. A true CCP should meet several preset criteria. Identify points of particular attention (POPA) when true CCPs cannot be identified.
8	Define tolerance limits for CCPs and target values for POPAs. Deviations should trigger the application of corrective measures.
9	Establish an on-farm monitoring system and its requirements regarding CCPs and POPAs. Monitoring results are used to adjust the QRM and retain process control.
10	Corrective measures should be defined on beforehand and be available in writing.
11	Establish a sound record-keeping system on the farm so the functioning and the effectiveness of the QRM can be proven.
12	Establish internal validation procedures and external auditing for verification.

The great advantages of the HACCP-like QRM programs are that all actions are protocolled, that there is structure, planning and organisation in the advisory program, and that the record system serves the management of the farmer and the evaluation of effectiveness and implementation of the program. This QRM is the formalisation of advisory activities, as named under DHE and HHPMS. If cattle farms should be certified, this QRM is the best possible option.

Veterinary advisory service and sustainability

Sustainability of a (dairy) farm is becoming increasingly relevant. Public opinion and government directives more or less force the farmers to take that route (Smyth & Dumanski, 1994). The sustainability concept comprises four pillars – ethics, economics, society, and ecology – which should all be in mutual balance (Cornelissen *et al.*, 2001; Emanuelson, 2007; Boogaard *et al.*, 2008; Hemme, 2010; Steinfeld *et al.*, 2010).

Sustainability in the dairy sector can be addressed at three levels: the structural level, the technological level and the managerial level (SAI, 2009; Oenema, 2010). The *structural level* is associated with the organisation of the food chain, including all stakeholders, and the related type and size of farming system. This is at a high level and may reflect political decisions. The *technological level* includes buildings, machines, transport, land and equipment, as well as their investments. This level provides the direct environment for the cattle. Instead of focusing on major domains, such as environmental pollution (air, soil, water) or the appropriate investment strategies, the question must be raised of where the farmer and the veterinarian would interact. This would be at the *managerial level.* The latter is, in fact, the proper and timely allocation of resources to achieve the farming goals. This encompasses a broad spectrum: from financial management to health care, to nutrient and land management. Different suppliers play their role with regard to products and services. In Table 2.8, the different domains, where sustainability challenges exist, are listed (Noordhuizen, 2012).

Given the domains named in Table 2.7, it is clear that the veterinarian can indeed assist and advise the farmer in

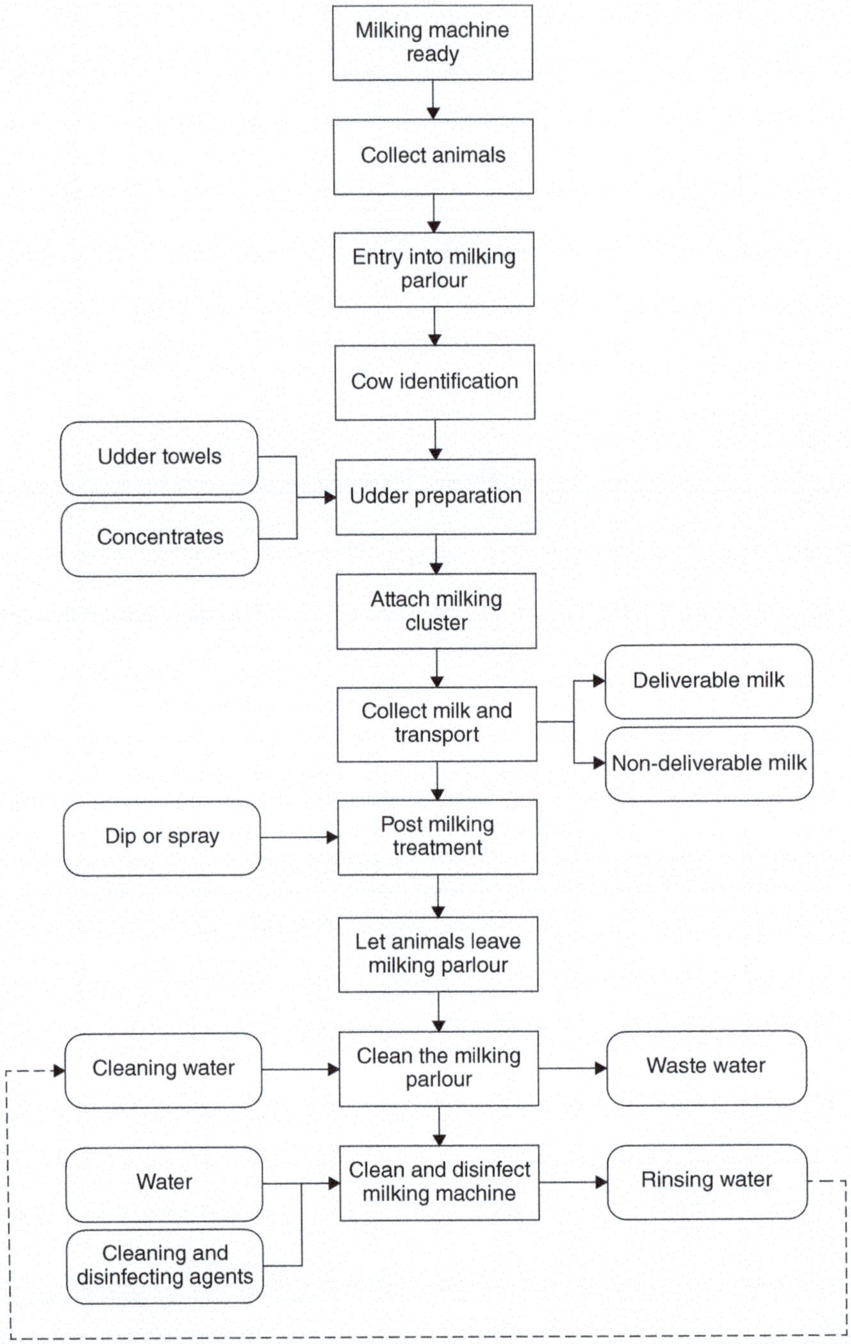

Figure 2.4 An example of a production process flow diagram on a dairy farm. Hazards (e.g. diseases or milk contamination) and their associated risk factors and critical control points can be assigned to their respective location in the flow diagram.

achieving sustainability goals. Note that the domains 1, 3, 4, 5, 6, and 7 already play a substantial role in advisory programs like HHPMS and QRM, as addressed previously. Domains 2, 8 and 9 need additional attention, either from the veterinary advisor, or from a domain-specialist, or both. A further elaboration of these domains can be found in Noordhuizen (2012). A few items from Table 2.8 are further addressed in Box 3.

The economic basis for sustainability within the dairy farm is formed by the combination of:

1 the genetic potential of the herd;
2 a fine-tuned nutrition;

Box 2.3 Some details regarding the domains in Table 7.

Animal selection: instead of focusing on milk yield alone, mixed breeding goals could better safeguard animal welfare and longevity, high health status, or heat stress resistance.

Animal health: sick cows have reduced feed conversion and less milk yield, hence resulting in economic losses. Moreover, nutrient and possibly antibiotic residues will dissipate into the environment.

Pasture exploitation: has a direct effect on milk yield and hence economics of the farm. Moreover, it represents an issue of public image of the farm, because the general public desires to 'see cows in the pasture'. Soil quality and nutrient management refer to precision farming, where the waste and risk of environmental pollution are reduced.

Table 2.8 Major farming domains where sustainability challenges exist (after SAI, 2009; Feenstra *et al*., 2010).

1	Farm economics	4	Animal selection	7	Herd health and production management
2	Relationship with society	5	Animal nutrition	8	Pasture exploitation, nutrient management, soil quality
3	Management planning	6	Animal reproduction	9	Waste management

3 optimal health and welfare conditions;
4 good housing facilities; and
5 high management quality (Oenema, 2010).

If one of these five economic factors is sub-optimal, overall sustainability on the farm will be at risk. The five factors can be put into a multiplicative formula to show that the same great efforts should be done on all five to achieve an acceptable result (Noordhuizen, 2012). Herd health and production management advisory services have been considered as a prerequisite and a key for achieving sustainability (Smith, 2010). Sustainability indexes for agricultural systems resemble those applied in quality assurance programs (SMK, 2009; Spoelstra & Elzen, 2010).

The question is not whether environmental or sustainability disorders could also be part of a veterinary HHPM or a QRM program as outlined above, where hazards and risks are dealt with, but rather how to define sustainability disorders and how to identify the risk factors associated with these disorders. Once these have been identified, one can move to the next phase: monitoring and correction (or rather, prevention of such disorders). Several sustainability disorders are related to diseases at cow and herd level, centred on nutrition and health/welfare of the cattle, and conditioned by issues like poor housing and management. These disorders must already be taken care of through HHPM or QRM in the context of sustainability. However, other sustainability disorders may remain.

Developmental steps should be made slowly; the farmers should not get lost on the way. The best way to do so is by addressing an important area – say, herd health – and improving the health status. At the same time, the farmer will notice that the milk yield will increase, losses will be reduced and income increases. This is a process of coaching by the veterinarian.

Skills and knowledge of veterinarians to comply with the VAS requirements

Different levels of skills and knowledge are required, depending on the advisory service being offered. For example, most veterinarians should be capable of carrying out a routine Diagnostic Herd Evaluation (DHE). The process requires observational skills and a sound knowledge to interpret the observation findings, followed by a synthesis and conclusions. The next step, to formulate an action plan with priorities for the short term and secondary items for the mid-long term, is relatively straightforward.

To carry out a professional HHPMS, the veterinarian needs to be well-organised and structured in approach, and have a well-developed analytical ability. The DHE is still the basis of such service, but the evaluation of herd performance and risk factors are further developed. Appropriate professional communication skills are paramount (Kleen *et al.*, 2011). Short written reports are a must in order to keep the farmer informed and motivated. Discussions between the veterinarian and the farmer are crucial in HHPMS. Extended veterinary-zootechnical disciplines, such as: applied farm economics (e.g. disease loss assessment, and benefits/costs ratio estimation); quantitative epidemiology (odds ratios; diagnostic test characteristics); applied cattle nutrition; farm management; behavioural economics; marketing principles; business administration (for practice and farms); risk identification; and risk management, are a few new areas to address in order to achieve the best performance in HHPMS. Further details can be found in Brand *et al.* (1996) and in Noordhuizen (2012).

Veterinarians need to acquire further skills and knowledge once they have decided to support QRM programs. Among the disciplines are: quality concepts and management; quality assurance principles; applied quantitative veterinary epidemiology (quantitative and qualitative); risk identification and risk management; HACCP concept and principles; the writing of protocols; and GMP guidelines for the farm, as well as: operational work instructions (e.g. how to manage: foot baths, colostrum); professional communication; marketing and business management; farm economics; and behavioural economics. Many examples have been presented by Noordhuizen *et al.* (2008) and Boersema *et al.* (2010).

Although *Professional Communication* (ProCom) ProCom now forms part of some veterinary curricula around the world, it is far from being integrated in all veterinary curricula for large animals (cattle). This is a drawback, because it has been established that, with a proper ProCom, the veterinarian can improve his/her performance with clients, while at the same time the client feels better understood and respected (Kleen *et al.*, 2011)

ProCom comprises three kinds of communication:

1 basal interpersonal communication;
2 the problem-solving type of communication; and
3 solutions-oriented communication.

The first of these deals with day-to-day (private) communication, while the second can be found in curative practice. The third one is the rather continuous kind of communication applied in HHPMS and QRM. Ideally, one needs a balanced mixture of all three.

Pro Com comprises (non-rational) elements like perceptions, emotions, attitude, tone of speech, and avoidance of dominance. Because verbal and written communication is fundamental for HHPMS and QRM, the veterinarian needs to pay close attention to these aspects. The veterinarian should be aware that roughly 70% of an advisory message impact is achieved by this ProCom, and only 30% by its technical contents. Written reports are not only meant to show the farmer what to do, they also serve to evaluate at a later stage the effects of advice given and interventions carried out. Reports and discussions are important references for farmers and their activities.

Behavioural economics is the discipline which studies the elements of non-rationality in decision making. In general, farmers want to pay for (for example) intra-mammary antibiotic tubes to treat a cow with mastitis. However, they are less willing to pay for a proposed udder health control program. This is caused by the perception that losses are to be dealt with, while it is not clear that the money spent for a future udder health control program will guarantee a mastitis-free period in the future and save the farmer money. In general, people do not like change; they have become used to a certain situation (methods of feeding) and live with that. The effort to change a routine appears too great. Next to technical advice and professional communication, the veterinarian needs to become a process-coach for the farmer, providing motivation and support constantly through the process of (management) change.

Concluding remarks

Society is changing and so is the dairy production sector. Instead of considering those changes as threats, they should be seen as opportunities. Farmers are in need of veterinary advisory programs (VAS) (Lievaart *et al.*, 2008); the veterinarian should be able and sufficiently skilled to deliver such a service effectively. The advisory programs should be introduced gradually, in a targeted manner, to reflect the needs and priorities of the farmer. They should be gradually increased and developed, depending on the farmer's wishes and capacities. The progression should be from routine farm monitoring DHE, to herd health and production management service, to HACCP-like QRM (Figure 2.5), then up to advisory programs for sustainable dairy production. Curative practice may run in parallel, and is likely to diminish in task volume as disease risks are reduced and eliminated.

Sustainable Land Management, which is considered to be the summation of new technologies, policies, socio-economic principles and environmental issues, addresses five conditions (Smyth & Dumanski, 1994; Rowarth, 2011):

- it must maintain and enhance farm productivity;
- it should decrease production risks;
- it should protect natural resources and prevent environmental degradation;
- it must economically be viable; and
- it must be socially acceptable.

It should be noted that veterinarians can play a role in each of these five areas.

The VAS addressing dairy farm sustainability is a high-level challenge. It demonstrates the best possible way how the veterinarian can assist farmers in achieving their goals. Moving gradually forward, together with the farmer, represents a mutual learning process for both and is symbiotic; farm workers should never be excluded from that process, and sometimes need short,

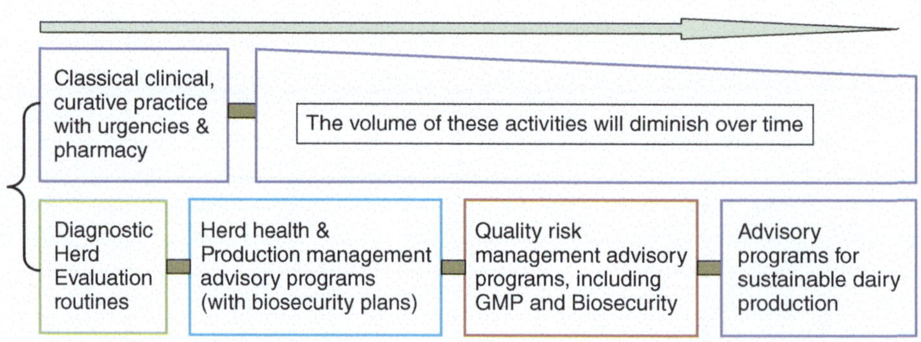

Figure 2.5 Developing veterinary advisory programs, VAS, over time.

on-site training courses. Once VAS is established and viable, the veterinary cattle practice may benefit from being split into two departments:

1 curative services;
2 consultative services.

For the farmer, this would clarify the purpose, contents and costs of farm visits when these two departments act in parallel. Dehorning calves when making a HHPMS or QRM farm visit would trouble the farmer, and would take the veterinarian too far away from the advisory tasks. It is likely that curative services will diminish over time as prevention increases. What remains are specialties and rather rare or difficult cases.

Veterinary practices could further develop (see also Figure 2.1). Already, nowadays, multi species or mono species practices exist, sometimes with up to 20 or 40 veterinarians. This has the advantage that veterinarians can acquire sub-specialisations such as milk harvest and mastitis, cattle nutrition and metabolic diseases and reproduction. In this way, they are complementarily in achieving higher practice performance quality and, moreover, they will have an individual professional identity. Various veterinary practices (e.g. in the Netherlands) have engaged animal science professionals, such as a nutritionist, to deal with zootechnical issues on the dairy farms. Perhaps, in the future, the professional relationship between practitioners and animals science professionals will become closer, to the benefit of the farmer.

Overall, veterinary advisory services, when adequately carried out, will increasingly bring added value to the farmers and to the veterinary practice itself. They should be based on marketing principles (knowing clients' needs and expectations) and positively building on the practice image or brand (car number plates; brochures; calendars; memory sticks; overalls with names and logo; radio interviews; weekly columns in a local journal). Properly executed, such VAS brings professional pleasure and identity to veterinarians while, at the same time, they serve society. In particular, veterinarians are crucial to validating pre- and post-harvest production standards and quality (Rowarth, 2011).

References

Alvès de Oliveira, L., Arcangioli, M.A., Mounier, L., Otz, P., LeSobre, G. and Noordhuizen, J.P.T.M. (2008). Apporter de la valeur au suivi de reproduction. *Le Point Vétérinaire* **289**, 47–52.

BAMN. (2000). An introduction to infectious disease control & biosecurity on dairy farms. *Bulletin of the Bovine Alliance on Management and Nutrition, published by AFIA*, Arlington VI, USA.

Beekhuis-Gibbon, L., Whyte, P., O'Grady, L., More, S.J. and Doherty, M.L. (2011). A HACCP-based approach to mastitis control in dairy herds. Part 1: development; part 2: implementation and evaluation. *Irish Veterinary Journal* **64**(2) & **64**(7).

Bell, N.J., Main, D.C.J., Buncic, S., Whay, H.R., Bell, M.J., Knowles, T.G. and Webster, A.J.F. (2003). Applying principles of the hazard analysis critical control points (HACCP) system to reduce lameness in UK dairy heifers. *Cattle Practice* **11**(4), 385.

Bergevoet, R.H.M. (2005). *Entrepreneurship of Dutch dairy farmers.* PhD thesis, Wageningen University, Dept. of Farm Management, Wageningen, the Netherlands.

Boersema, J.S.C., Cannas da Silva, J., Mee, J. and Noordhuizen, J.P.T.M. (2010). *Farm health and productivity management of dairy young stock.* Wageningen Academic Publishers, Wageningen, the Netherlands, 208 pp.

Boogaard, B.K., Oosting, S.J. and Bock, B.B. (2008). Defining sustainability as a socio-cultural concept. *Livestock Science* **117**, 24–33.

Brand A., Noordhuizen, J.P.T.M. and Schukken, Y.H. (1996). *Herd health and production management in dairy practice*, 1st edition. Wageningen Academic Publishers, Wageningen, the Netherlands, 543 pp.

Cannas da Silva, J., Noordhuizen, J.P.T.M., Vagneur, M., Bexiga, R., Gelfert, C.C. and Baumgartner, W. (2006). Veterinary dairy herd health management in Europe: constraints and perspectives. *Veterinary Quarterly* **28**(1), 23–32.

Cornelissen, A.M.G., vanden, Bergh, J., Koops, W., Grossman, M. and Udo, H.M.J. (2001). Assessment of the contribution of sustainability indicators to sustainable development: a novel approach using fuzzy set theory. *Agricultural Ecosystems & Environment* **86**, 173–185.

De Kruif, A. (1975). *Fertility and subfertility in cattle.* PhD thesis University of Utrecht, Faculty of Veterinary Medicine, Utrecht, the Netherlands.

Eelkman-Rooda, D.C. (2006). *Communication: management problems within the veterinary practice is about communication.* Dier-en-Arts 6/7 (in Dutch with English summary).

Emanuelson, U. (2007). *How can veterinary epidemiology contribute to sustainable animal production?* In: van de, Honing, Y. (ed). Book of Abstracts of the 58th EAAP annual meeting, 26–26 August 2007, Dublin Ireland.

Esslemont, R.J., Bailie, J.H. and Cooper, M.J. (1985). *Fertility management in dairy cattle.* Collins Publishers, London, UK.

Evans, J.R. and Lindsay, W.M. (1996).*The management and control of quality.* West Publishing Company, St Paul, MN, USA.

Feenstra, G., Ingels, Ch., Campbell, D. (2010) at www.sarep.ucdavis.edu /concept.htm accessed January 8th, 2011.

Foresight. (2009). *The future of food and farming.* Final project report. The Government Office for Science, London 211. www.bis.gov.uk /assets/bispartners/foresight/docs/food-and-farming/11-546-future -of-food-and-farming-report.pdf accessed December 8th, 2011.

Frawley, P.T. (2003). *Review of rural veterinary service.* Commonwealth Department of Education, Science and Training. www.daff.gov.au /data/assets/pdf-file/0008/156923/vetreport.pdf p 133. Accessed December 10th 2011.

Hemme, T. (2010). Competitiveness of bovine milk in a world of subsidies and more liberal commodity trade. Updates on Ruminant Production and Medicine. In: Wittwer, F. *et al.* (eds). *Updates of Ruminant Production and Medicine*, ISPAH symposium proceedings, pp 303–309. XXVI World Buiatrics Congress, November 15th 2010, Santiago, Chile.

Kleen, J.W., Atkinson, O. and Noordhuizen, J.P.T.M. (2011). Communication in production animal medicine: modeling a complex interaction with the example of dairy herd health management. *The Irish Veterinary Journal* **64**(8).

Lievaart, J.J., Noordhuizen, J.T.M., Buckley, D. and van Winden, S. (2008). The marketing of herd health & production management services on Dutch dairy farms: perceptions of dairy farmers and their veterinary surgeons. *The Irish Veterinary Journal* **61**(10), 668–676.

Lowe, P. (2009). *Unlocking potential: a report on veterinary expertise in food animal production.* Department of Environment, Food & Rural Affairs. www.defra.gov.uk/animalh/ahws/vservices/pdf/lowe-vets090806.pdf accessed December 11th 2011.

Noordhuizen, J.P.T.M. (2012). *Dairy Herd Health and Management.* Context Products Ltd, Packington, UK. 465 pp.

Noordhuizen, J.P.T.M. and Cannas da Silva, J. (2009). A HACCP-based Quality Risk Management approach to udder health problems in dairy farms. *The Irish Veterinary Journal* **62**, Supplement, 'Focus on Bovine Mastitis' (reflection of the Alltech Dairy Solutions Symposium, Dublin, EI, September 2007).

Noordhuizen, J.P.T.M. and Welpelo, H.J. (1996). Sustainable improvement of animal health care by systematic quality risk management according to the HACCP concept. *The Veterinary Quarterly* **18**, 121–126.

Noordhuizen, J.P.T.M., Frankena, K., Thrusfield, M.V. and Graat, E.A.M. (2001). *Application of quantitative methods in veterinary epidemiology.* Wageningen Academic Publishers, Wageningen, the Netherlands, 2nd edition, 429 pp.

Noordhuizen, J.P.T.M., van Egmond, M.J., van Dellen, D.K.H., Jorritsma, R., Hogeveen, H., van Wervan, T., Vos, P.L.A.M. and Lievaart, J.J. (2006). *Veterinary advice for entrepreneurial dairy farmers – from curative practice to coach-consultant, what needs to be changed?* CD-ROM issued by Pfizer Animal Health, also at www.vacqa-international.com and *Dutch Veterinary Journal (Tijdschrift voor Diergeneeskunde)* (2008), **133**(1): 4–8.

Noordhuizen, J.P.T.M., Cannas da Silva, J., Boersema, J.S.C. and Vieira, A. (2008). *Applying HACCP-based quality risk management on dairy farms.* Wageningen Academic Publishers, Wageningen, the Netherlands, 311 pp.

Oenema, O., Menzi, H. and Lesschen, J.P. (2010). Intensive livestock production and environmental effects: a review. In: Wittwer, F. *et al.* (eds). *Updates on Ruminant Production and Medicine*, ISPAH symposium proceedings XXVI World Buiatrics Congress, November 15th 2010, Santiago, Chile, pp 13–32.

OIE. (2006). Guide to good farming practices for animal production food safety. Office Internationale des Epizooties. *Revue Scientifique et Technique* **25**(2), 823–836.

Rowarth, J. (2011). The future for sheep and beef cattle farming: the role of veterinarians. In: Proceedings of the Society for sheep and beef cattle veterinarians of the NZVA, pp 2.4.1.–2.4.7.

SAI (2009). *Principles and practices for sustainable dairy farming.* The Sustainable Agriculture Initiative (SAI) platform. www.saiplatform.org, accessed July 21st 2011.

Smith, B. (2010). Veterinary Ireland's submission to the 2020 Strategy Committee. *Irish Veterinary Journal* **63**, 396–298.

SMK (2009). In: Spoelstra and Elzen : *Towards a sustainable livestock production.* Proceedings of the ISDA conference, Montpellier, France, 28–30 June 2010.

Smyth, A.J., Dumanski, J. (1994). *Progress towards an international framework for evaluating sustainale land management.* In: Proceedings of the 15th World Congress on Soil Science, Mexico, pp 373–378.

Sol, J., Renkema, J.A., Stelwagen, J., Dijkhuizen, A.A. and Brand, A. (1984). A three year herd health and management program on thirty Dutch dairy herds. *The Veterinary Quarterly* **6**, 141–169.

Spoelstra, S. and Elzen, B. (2010). *Outline of a learning and experimentation system.* In: Proceedings of the ISDA conference 'Towards a sustainable livestock production', 28–30 June 2010, Montpellier, France.

Steinfeld, H., Mooney, H.A., Schneider, F. and Neville, L.A. (eds, 2010). *Livestock in a Changing Landscape: Drivers, Consequences and Responses* (Volume 1). Island Press, Washington, 396 pp.

Williamson, NB. (1980). The economic efficiency of a veterinary preventive medicine and management program in Victorian dairy herds. *Australian Veterinary Journal* **56**, 1–9.

Suggested further reading

Brand, A., Noordhuizen, J.P.T.M. and Schukken, Y.H. (2001). *Herd health and production management in dairy practice*, 2nd edition. Wageningen Academic Publishers, Wageningen, The Netherlands, 345 pp.

Thrusfield, M.V. (1995). *Veterinary Epidemiogy*, 2nd edition, Blackwell Science Publishing, Oxford, UK.

Suggested website consulting (non-exhaustive)

- www.DQACenter.org/university
- www.agri-ed.com/catalog.html
- www.agri-ed.com/heifer.html
- www.agry.purdue.edu/Ext/forages/publications/ID-172.htm
- www.codewalimentarius.net/download/stndards/357/CXG_030e.pdf
- www.dairyherd.com
- www.efsa.europe.eu
- www.europa.eu.int/comm/food/fs/fsp
- www.aphis.usda.gov/animal_health
- www.cdc.gov/ncidod/dbmd/
- www.fao.org
- www.knowmycotoxins.com
- www.foodsafetynetwork.ca/food/zoonoses.html
- www.nahms.usda.gov/
- www.oie.org
- www.vacqa-international.com
- www.vetvice.com
- www.winepi.unizar.es or http://solismail.uu.nl or www.zod.wau.nl/QVE (public domain quantitative epidemiology software for veterinarians).

Examples of software for HACCP applications in industry:

do HACCP by Norback , Ley & Associates LLC, 3022 Woodland Trail, Middleton, WI, USA www.norbackley.com.

QSA software Ltd, POBox 306, St.Albans, Herts AL1 I3W, UK www.qsa.co.uk (demo version available).

Annex 2.1

Inventory sheet to evaluate the degree of satisfaction of farmers about the performance of their own dairy farm (Noordhuizen, 2012).

➔ FARMER NAME =
➔ ADDRESS =
➔ VET =
➔ DATE =

(score 1 = not satisfactory; score 3 = intermediate; score 5 = very satisfactory)

Milk production	1	2	3	4	5	Important remarks
Litres of milk per cow per year (mean)						
Milk fat %						
Milk protein %						
Milk production in first lactation						
Milk production at start of lactation (0–50 days)						
Udder health						
% cows with clinical mastitis per year						
% cows with high cell counts per year						
% cows with subclinical mastitis per year						
Mastitis cases during the dry period						
Outcome of mastitis treatments						
Claw health						
% lame cows per year						
Outcome of routine herd claw trimming						
% cows with foot rot per year						
% cows with laminitis per year						
% cows with Mortellaro disease per year						
% cows with hock lesions per year						
Overall animal health						
% cows with rumen acidosis						
% cows with ketosis						
% cows with infectious diseases						
% cows with skin lesions						
Health of calves and maiden heifers						
% diarrhoea in neonate calves						
% diarrhoea in older calves						
% respiratory disease in calves/heifers						
Reproduction and fertility						
Calving interval						
Age of heifers at first calving						
Interval between calving – first insemination						
Interval between calving – conception						
Detection of heat among cows						
Detection of heat among maiden heifers						
% cows with cystic ovarian disease per year						
% cows with retained afterbirth per year						
% cows with endometritis per year						
Number of inseminations per pregnant cow						
Quality of milk (bulk tank)						
Mean cell count (× 1000/ml)						
Mean bacteria count (× 1000/ml)						
Milk fat %						
Milk protein %						
Butyric acid spores						
Antibiotic residues						

[c] **Other observations worth mentioning** (e.g. nutrition; hygiene; other)

Questions to the dairy farmer:

1. Do you think it is worthwhile to address certain non-satisfactory areas together with your vet?
2. If yes, what would be your priorities to address?
3. If no, is there another specialist you want to consult? Why this person?

CHAPTER 3

Education and Cattle Practice: 'What Do We Do? What Should We Do?'

Peter D. Cockcroft

Learning objectives

- Appreciate the clinical competencies and day one skills expected of entry level veterinarians.
- Appreciate the range of proficiencies that are highly valued by bovine practitioners.
- Appreciate the relative frequency with which a range of procedures are performed in clinical practice.
- Be aware of the expanded skills sets required for the 21st century cattle practitioner.
- Be aware of a practitioner derived curriculum for dairy, cow and calf and feedlot practice.

Introduction

There has been a long-standing interest within the veterinary profession in farm animal veterinarians moving away from providing 'fire brigade' services to sick and injured animals and towards a role as a trusted advisor to the farmer, providing preventative animal health consultancy services (Adam, 2013).

Nordlund (1998) summarised the challenges in delivering cattle practice services in the 21st century. 'Veterinarians sometimes argue as to whether a herd reproductive program is 'production medicine' or 'traditional medicine'. I would contend that it could be either. If a group of cows are examined, pregnancies recorded, abnormalities treated, heats predicted, and left at that point, the reproductive program is traditional medicine directed at correcting problems of many individual cows. On the other hand, if herd performance is summarised and charted, allowing management to make herd-based decisions, the reproductive program is 'production medicine'.

Because of the subtle nuances of these terms, it is more precise to characterise dairy veterinary services as having three components: drugs/supplies; medical/surgical procedures; and management assistance services. The categories are essentially self-explanatory. Drugs/supplies would include any product dispensing or sales. Medical/surgical procedures would include almost all technical services performed on animals. Management assistance would include any informational services that assist the herd manager in analysis, controls, and decision-making'.

Veterinarians have an important role in the provision of services in the dairy and beef industries. They are a trusted source of advice and information for farmers. The role of the veterinarian has expanded from the treatment of individual animals to a more cost-effective holistic role in whole-farm consultancy and herd health management. The need to retain the skills to support our traditional role, while at the same time introducing new skills to service the future needs of the cattle industries, makes veterinary education challenging.

The needs of the industry, individual farmers, veterinary practices as employers and government all need to be met. In addition, an important, but often overlooked, role of cattle veterinarians is their leadership role in promoting change to optimise health, sustainability, welfare, productivity and profitability. However, the profession is often accused of being reactive rather than proactive. Recent reports on the role of rural and livestock veterinarians have highlighted the need to make farmers more aware of the wide range of cost-effective services we can offer (Frawley, 2003; Lowe, 2009). It is often the case that we actively promote only a fraction of the potential range of services that we could deliver and contribute.

This chapter presents some practitioner-defined entry level graduate competencies that are considered to be important. The frequency with which practitioners use a range of cattle practice-related skills and procedures is presented.

Bovine Medicine, Third Edition. Edited by Peter D. Cockcroft.

Table 3.1 AVMA statement on clinical competencies outcomes.

Veterinary graduates must have the basic scientific knowledge, skills and values to practise veterinary medicine, independently, at the time of graduation. At a minimum, graduates must be competent in providing entry-level health care for a variety of animal species.
The school/college must provide evidence that students/graduates have had adequate access to primary care cases and hands-on experiences with live animals, and it must address clinical competencies in the following areas:
1 Comprehensive patient diagnosis and demonstration of problem solving skills (e.g. appropriate use of clinical laboratory testing, and record management).
2 Comprehensive treatment planning, including patient referral when indicated.
3 Anaesthesia and pain management, patient welfare.
4 Basic surgery skills, experience and case management.
5 Basic medicine skills, experience and case management.
6 Emergency and intensive care case management.
7 Health promotion, disease prevention, zoonosis and food safety.
8 Client communications and ethical conduct.
9 Strong appreciation for the role of research in furthering the practice of veterinary medicine.

The Royal College of Veterinary Surgeons (RCVS) and the American Veterinary Medical Association (AVMA) have defined clinical competencies for day one graduates. The RCVS Day One Competencies are under review and can be accessed at the RCVS website. The AVMA clinical competencies are presented in Table 3.1.

The British Cattle Veterinary Association (BCVA) has developed a list of essential and desirable day one skills. This is designed to enable students who wish to develop a career in cattle practice to have guidance when seeing practice during their extra mural studies (EMS). The aim in devising this list was to help undergraduates identify and then attain the skills expected by employers while on EMS. This list is reproduced in Table 3.2.

In a study by Miller (2004), practitioners identified the entry-level knowledge requirements and skills (competencies) needed by new veterinary graduates as they enter food animal practice. The study used focus groups and a validated method of curriculum development. This study included competency lists for dairy, cow and calf and feedlot cattle. The number of practitioners contributing to each of these sections was eight, nine and 13 respectively. The outcomes of this study are reproduced at the end of this chapter. Further details regarding the methodology used to create the lists can be found at the website: CVM.Missouri.edu/FADACUM.

Information about the skills most frequently used by bovine practitioners and the proficiency that practitioners expect of entry-level veterinarians is useful in shaping core curriculum design. Morin *et al.* (2002a; 2002b) reported the outcomes of a survey of veterinarians involved in cattle practice working in the United States in two papers. There were 1030 respondents. A summary of the results reported for 95 individual animal medicine and animal production procedures performed most frequently in bovine practice and the skills expected of entry-level veterinarians are presented in Tables 3.3 and 3.4 respectively (Morin *et al.*, 2002a). The authors concluded that a balance between individual animal medicine and animal production training must be sought because, without good diagnostic and technical skills at the individual animal level, new graduates will be unable to make accurate herd-level diagnoses and institute appropriate cost-effective control measures.

A summary of the results of 53 surgery, anaesthesia, and restraint procedures performed most frequently in bovine practice and the entry-level skills expected of new veterinary graduates are presented in Tables 3.5 and 3.6 (Morin *et al.*, 2002b).

The results of this survey indicated that private veterinary practitioners who work with cattle perform a variety of surgery, anaesthesia, and restraint procedures on a frequent basis (11 procedures, performed at least once a month), and expect entry-level veterinarians to be skilled and to require little supervision in those procedures. The highest rated procedures involved the processing of cattle (castration, dehorning, tattooing, and ear implant placement), anaesthesia (epidural anaesthesia, local anaesthesia of the horn, eye, and orbit, local or regional anaesthesia of the flank, and IV or IM sedation), wound management, hoof examination and treatment, repair of uterine or vaginal prolapse, caesarean section, and removal of supernumerary teats. General (non-specified) surgical skills and general (non-specified) restraint skills, as well as several more specific skills (castration, dehorning, gastrointestinal surgical skills, caesarean section, and uterine prolapse repair), were listed among the five most important skills for entry-level veterinarians in bovine practice by ≥50 respondents. Unfortunately, these same skills were also listed among the most deficient.

Luby *et al.* (2013) performed a survey of practising veterinarians involved in dairy practice to identify the skills they used most frequently and their opinions of the skills required of entry level veterinarians for this sector of the profession. The survey was in western Canada. The ten skills performed at least once a month by the 24 respondents who spent 75% or more of their time in dairy practice are presented in Table 3.7.

The survey asked these practitioners to identify what they thought were the three most important skills new graduates need to have and what three skills new graduates were lacking the most. The five most important skills in ranked order were pregnancy diagnosis, physical examination, general surgery, herd health management and communication. The skills in which

Table 3.2 British Cattle Veterinary Association – day one skills.

Essential Requirements of a Farm Animal Practitioner:

1 Be able to handle and restrain or to direct adequate restraint of the animal to be examined safely and effectively and understand the responsibility for other persons in attendance. This includes:
- the ability to cast and roll a cow
- restrain a foot for examination and treatment
- restrain a cow for stomach tubing

2 Be able to perform a thorough clinical examination with appropriate history taking. This includes:
- thoracic and abdominal auscultation
- rectal and reproductive tract examination

3 Assess the nutritional status of an animal and be able to body condition score and advise appropriately on feeding and husbandry procedures.

4 Be able to assess an obstetrical problem for example a calving or prolapse and perform a thorough examination. Be able to know personal limitations and when to request assistance.

5 Appreciate and advise on animal welfare improvements in conjunction with management, economics and the welfare ethics. Also appreciate the law and codes of recommendations with regards to welfare and welfare ethics.

6 Understand and demonstrate adequate bio-security and be able to advise on bio-security procedures.

7 Be able to advise and administer appropriate treatment for disease in both individuals and groups of animals, with an appreciation of economic and practical challenges.

8 Be able to advise on preventative medicine.

9 Following assessment, be able to safely perform:
- sedation
- general anaesthesia
- analgesia of the bovine animal

10 Be competent in the performance of local anaesthesia including ring blocks and epidurals. Be able to administer for the procedures of:
- castration
- disbudding/dehorning
- uterine replacement
- caesarean section
- abdominal surgery
- teat surgery

11 Be able to sterilise equipment and apply the principles of aseptic surgical techniques in order to carry out basic surgical procedures.

12 Be able to humanely euthanize an animal while ensuring personal safety and safety of assistants. Also advise on carcass disposal.

13 Be able to perform a basic post mortem with sample collection and transportation and be able to interpret and advise on results.

14 Be able to demonstrate an understanding of public health and food production and advise on procedures following the discovery of a notifiable disease and zoonotic diseases.

15 Be able to administer treatment to an animal via all routes of administration. This includes:
- intravenous injection
- uterine irrigation
- stomach intubation
- intramammary infusion

16 Be able to rectally examine an animal and pregnancy diagnose manually from 60 days. Be able to find the cervix and manually palpate ovaries and ovarian structures. Appreciate the importance of practice and to have the confidence to know personal limitations and to recheck at a later date if required.

17 Be able to routinely trim a foot and identify obvious lesions. Also be familiar with types of foot blocks available and be able to apply a preferred type of foot block adequately.

18 Be familiar with animal health statutory requirements and procedures for investigations, i.e. abortion.

19 Be familiar with certification for emergency slaughter on farm and legislation regarding transport of casualty animals.

Desirable Day One Skills for a Farm Practitioner:

1 Be able to perform local anaesthesia in the form of paravertebral nerve blocks and Intravenous Regional Anaesthesia for the performance of abdominal surgery and digital amputation respectively.

2 Have a knowledge and understanding of animal production data and performance indicators and be able to advise on improving welfare and economic performance.

3 Be able to rectally examine an animal and consistently pregnancy diagnose manually from 60 days and with ultrasound from 40 days.

Table 3.3 Frequency with which bovine veterinarians performed procedures and skills pertaining to individual animal medicine or animal production (adapted from Morin *et al*., 2002a).

At least twice each week
- Administration of injections
- Oral administration of medication
- Pregnancy detection by palpation per rectum
- Venipuncture
- Treatment of pneumonia

At least once a week
- Manual extraction of a calf
- Treatment of diarrhoea
- Auscultation of lungs
- IV fluid therapy
- Cardiac auscultation
- Auscultation of the GI tract
- Development of vaccination programs
- Control of a respiratory problem in a herd
- Development of an anthelmintic program
- Breeding soundness examination (cow)
- Faecal flotation

At least once a month
- Necropsy
- Treatment of metritis
- Treatment of bloat
- Control of an off feed problem in a herd
- Development of parasiticide programs
- Oestrus synchronisation
- Control of a diarrhoea problem in a herd
- Treatment of clinical mastitis
- Subconjunctival injection
- IV catheterisation
- Percussion of the thorax
- Residue avoidance program
- Preconditioning/metaphylaxis program
- Body condition scoring
- Sanitation/hygiene program
- Control of an infertility problem in a herd
- Client education
- Colostrum management program
- Control of an abortion problem in a herd
- Breeding soundness examination (bull)

Less than once a month
- Control of a lameness problem in a herd
- Neurologic examination
- Tuberculosis testing
- Control of a nutrition problem
- Milk culturing
- Aseptic milk sampling
- Fetotomy
- Skin scraping or biopsy
- Control of a mastitis problem in a herd
- Uterine detorsion
- Advising about feed additives
- Bacteriologic culturing (not milk)
- Advising about milk replacers
- Urinalysis
- Use of California Mastitis Test
- Quantitative faecal examination
- Somatic cell count analysis
- Tissue aspirate or biopsy
- Assessment of heifer growth
- Assessment of intervention efficacy
- Gram staining
- Cytological examination
- Assessment of housing or ventilation
- Advising about genetics or breeding
- CBC
- Radiography
- Use of computer records
- Forage sampling
- Advising about grazing program
- Ration analysis
- Use of spreadsheets
- Assessment of DHIA records
- Abdominocentesis
- Rumenocentesis
- Retinal examination
- Bulk tank milk analysis
- Blood transfusion
- Assessment of feed particle size
- Assessment of milking procedures
- Feed dry matter determination
- Ration formulation
- Assessment of ration cation-anion balance
- Economic analysis
- Artificial insemination
- Advising about waste management
- Financial advising
- Nasal swabbing
- Transtracheal aspiration

Never performed the procedure or technique
- Pelvimetry
- Transfaunation
- Milking machine performance evaluation
- Ultrasonography
- Ultrasonographic pregnancy diagnosis
- Cerebrospinal fluid collection
- Endoscopy
- Electrocardiography
- Embryo transfer
- Pulmonary artery pressure determination
- Echocardiography

GI = Gastrointestinal. DHIA = Dairy Herd Improvement Association.

Table 3.4 Proficiency expected of entry-level bovine veterinarians for procedures and skills pertaining to individual animal medicine or animal production (adapted from Morin *et al*., 2002a).

Complete knowledge and excellent skills
- Administration of injections
- Oral administration of medication
- Venipuncture
- IV fluid therapy
- Faecal flotation

Working knowledge and good skills
- Treatment of pneumonia
- Auscultation of lungs
- Cardiac auscultation
- Necropsy
- Treatment of bloat
- Treatment of diarrhoea
- Auscultation of the GI tract
- Manual extraction of a calf
- Subconjunctival injection
- IV catheterisation
- Treatment of clinical mastitis
- Pregnancy detection by palpation per rectum
- Control of a diarrhoea problem in a herd
- Control of a respiratory problem in a herd
- Development of vaccination programs
- Development of an anthelmintic program
- Treatment of metritis
- Aseptic milk sampling
- Control of an off feed problem in a herd
- Percussion of the thorax
- Skin scraping or biopsy
- Development of an insecticide program
- Tuberculosis testing
- Oestrus synchronisation
- Residue avoidance program
- Use of California Mastitis Test
- Urinalysis
- Colostrum management program
- Breeding soundness examination (cow)
- Preconditioning/metaphylaxis program
- Body condition scoring
- Tissue aspirate or biopsy
- Gram staining
- Bacteriologic culturing (not milk)
- Milk culturing
- Quantitative faecal examination Control of an abortion problem in a herd
- Control of an infertility problem in a herd
- Sanitation/hygiene program
- Client education
- Neurologic examination
- Cytological examination
- Radiography
- Control of a lameness problem in a herd
- Advising about milk replacers
- Control of a mastitis problem in a herd
- CBC
- Somatic cell count analysis
- Breeding soundness examination (bull)

Some knowledge and basic skills
- Fetotomy
- Uterine detorsion
- Assessment of heifer growth
- Blood transfusion
- Bulk tank milk analysis
- Control of a nutrition problem
- Abdominocentesis
- Forage sampling
- Use of computer records
- Retinal examination
- Advising about feed additives
- Use of spreadsheets
- Rumenocentesis
- Assessment of milking procedures
- Assessment of intervention efficacy
- Ration analysis
- Nasal swabbing
- Feed dry matter determination
- Assessment of housing or ventilation
- Transtracheal aspiration
- Assessment of DHIA records
- Assessment of feed particle size
- Advising about grazing program
- Ration formulation
- Assessment of ration cation-anion balance
- Economic analysis
- Artificial insemination
- Advising about genetics or breeding
- Transfaunation
- Ultrasonography
- Pelvimetry
- Advising about waste management
- Endoscopy
- Financial advising
- Cerebrospinal fluid collection
- Ultrasonographic pregnancy diagnosis

Ability to research and refer
- Milking machine performance evaluation
- Electrocardiography
- Echocardiography
- Pulmonary artery pressure determination
- Embryo transfer

Table 3.5 Frequency with which bovine veterinarians performed surgery, anaesthesia, and restraint procedures (adapted from Morin *et al.*, 2002b).

At least once a week
- Castration
- Epidural anaesthesia
- Dehorning
- IV or IM sedation
- Tattooing

At least once a month
- Wound management
- Hoof examination and treatment
- Ear implant administration
- Local or regional anaesthesia of the flank
- Uterine prolapse repair
- Vaginal prolapse repair
- Casting (for restraint)
- Supernumerary teat removal
- Roping (for animal capture)
- Corrective or cosmetic hoof trimming
- Caesarean section

Less than once a month
- Omentopexy or surgical abomasopexy
- Episiotomy
- Repair of teat obstruction
- Local anaesthesia of the horn
- Nictitating membrane flap
- Umbilical herniorrhaphy
- Local anaesthesia of the eye and orbit
- Excision of interdigital fibroma
- Enucleation or exenteration
- Orthopaedic splinting
- Exploratory laparotomy
- Fracture repair by casting
- Excision of nictitating membrane
- Tail docking
- Digit amputation
- Urethrostomy
- Branding
- Abomasopexy by blind suture or toggle
- Temporary rumenostomy
- IV regional anaesthesia
- Rumenotomy
- Joint lavage or arthrocentesis
- Repair of recto-vaginal laceration or fistula
- Umbilical resection
- Procedures to create teaser bulls

Never
- Hyperthermia treatment for neoplasia
- Cryosurgery
- Ovariectomy
- Corrective penile or preputial surgery
- Tracheostomy
- Intestinal resection and anastomosis
- Urethroplasty
- Liver biopsy
- Fracture repair by means other than casting
- Tracheal intubation
- Inhalation anaesthesia
- Pelvic symphysiotomy

Table 3.6 Proficiency expected of entry-level bovine veterinarians for surgery, anaesthesia, and restraint procedures by practitioners (adapted from Morin *et al.*, 2002b).

Working knowledge and good skills
- Castration
- Epidural anaesthesia
- Dehorning
- Wound management
- IV or IM sedation
- Hoof examination and treatment
- Local or regional anaesthesia of the flank
- Ear implant administration
- Tattooing
- Uterine prolapse repair
- Vaginal prolapse repair
- Supernumerary teat removal
- Caesarean section
- Casting (for restraint)
- Local anaesthesia of the horn
- Local anaesthesia of the eye and orbit
- Nictitating membrane flap
- Repair of teat obstruction
- Episiotomy
- Corrective or cosmetic hoof trimming
- Fracture repair by casting
- Umbilical herniorrhaphy
- Orthopaedic splinting
- Omentopexy or surgical abomasopexy
- Tail docking
- Excision of interdigital fibroma
- Excision of nictitating membrane
- Enucleation

Some knowledge and basic skills
- Exploratory laparotomy
- Digit amputation
- Roping (for animal capture)
- IV regional anaesthesia
- Urethrostomy
- Branding
- Temporary rumenostomy
- Rumenotomy
- Hyperthermia treatment for neoplasia
- Tracheostomy
- Repair of recto-vaginal laceration or fistula
- Abomasopexy by blind suture or toggle
- Umbilical resection
- Joint lavage or arthrocentesis
- Cryosurgery
- Tracheal intubation
- Inhalation anaesthesia
- Intestinal resection and anastomosis
- Liver biopsy
- Urethroplasty
- Procedures to create teaser bulls
- Fracture repair by means other than casting

Ability to research and refer
- Corrective penile or preputial surgery
- Ovariectomy
- Pelvic symphysiotomy

Table 3.7 Skills performed at least once a month by respondents spending 75% or more of their time in dairy practice (n = 24) (adapted from Luby *et al.*, 2013).

Skill
Abdomen examination
Injection
Body condition scoring
Thorax examination
Sedation
Dystocia management
Oral medication
Displaced abomasum surgery

level entry veterinarians seem least prepared, in ranked order, were pregnancy diagnosis, herd health management, general surgery, communication and nutrition. The authors concluded that the design of veterinary curricula should continue to focus on ensuring sufficient training in individual animal skills, but also should ensure that veterinarians possess the skills to adapt to a changing industry. The changing industry includes some task based skills being performed by non-veterinarians and the increasing recognition by larger dairies of the importance of herd health programs.

Adam (2013) reported on the outcomes of a survey of UK veterinarians involved with farm animal work. There were 375 respondents. One of the aims of the study was to identify the main services provided by UK farm animal veterinarians. Respondents were invited to describe the three main services that they provide to their farming clients, The categories of veterinary services described by the respondents were: herd health/advisory; statutory testing (mainly TB testing); fertility; obstetrics; disease investigation; emergency treatment; visiting sick animals; dispensing medication; and technical services (e.g. castration, dehorning and foot trimming).

Fertility services were the most commonly mentioned, with 57% of respondents stating that they provide fertility services, including pregnancy diagnosis, ultrasound scanning, reproductive therapeutics and bull fertility examinations. The second most common class of services was the examination, diagnosis and treatment of sick animals, which was mentioned by 51% of respondents. 32% of respondents mentioned herd health planning and other advisory services. The author concluded that while traditional reactive services are clearly still an important part of farm animal practice, the findings indicate that preventative or advisory services such as routine fertility visits, herd health planning and advisory services are provided by many farm animal vets.

Table 3.8 Attributes that were identified as important or very important by the majority of the non-small animal veterinarians (adapted from Mellenby *et al.*, 2011).

Attribute

- Knowledge about veterinary medicine and surgery
- Good with animals
- Compassion for patients
- Cleanliness
- Good practical skills
- Honesty
- Confidence
- Friendliness
- Compassion for owners
- Good communication skills
- Recognises own limitations and knows when to seek advice
- Good listening skills
- Good at explaining technical terms
- Decisiveness
- Patience
- Clear about cost of treatment
- Politeness
- Ability to work in a team
- A likeable personality
- Professional appearance

The perception of veterinarians and non-small animal (SA) clients which included farm animal veterinarians on what attributes constitute 'a good veterinarian' were examined by a questionnaire survey (Mellenby *et al.*, 2011). The majority of these veterinarians rated the attributes in Table 3.8 as important or very important.

The cattle practitioner-defined competencies (Boxes 3.1 to 3.3) need to be tempered with the broader educational needs of the veterinary graduate and the requirements of the statutory accreditation boards. However, the implications of the studies presented on curriculum design and time allocation are obvious. New graduates need to be proficient in common and important skills and procedures to support individual, as well as herd level, practice. Non-technical skills such as communication, report writing and business management are now being recognised as crucial to the promotion and leadership in bringing about translational change, so that veterinarians can maximise their contribution to herd welfare, health, production, sustainability and profitability in the cattle industries.

Box 3.1 Dairy Competency List (Source: Reproduced with permission from AAVMC).

A. Demonstrate knowledge of general animal husbandry/production

1 Demonstrate an understanding of dairy farm operation from the dairyman's perspective
2 Demonstrate an understanding of dairy farm operations
  a. waste management
  b. feeding management
  c. employee management
  d. herd management
3 Demonstrate a knowledge of dairy cow anatomy and physiology
4 Describe physiology and endocrinology of:
  a. lactation
  b. reproduction
  c. ruminant digestion
5 Identify good husbandry practices to maximise performance
6 Perform animal handling and restraint techniques
7 Describe animal behaviour
  a. normal behaviour
  b. abnormal behaviour
8 Identify production parameters for:
  a. milk production
  b. reproduction
  c. udder health
  d. replacement heifers
9 Explain the importance of public perception of animal welfare (i.e. humane treatment of animals).
10 Describe the life cycle of a dairy animal:
  a. adult
  b. heifer
  c. calf
11 Identify methods to reduce the risk of injury:
  a. personal
  b. to farm workers
12 Demonstrate problem-solving ability

B. Demonstrate knowledge of population medicine/epidemiology

1 Describe the interrelationships between disease, production, and economics (use individual cow problems to identify herd problems)
2 Identify the principles of cow comfort
3 Describe the components of milking systems
4 Demonstrate an understanding of milking machine function
5 Describe a colostrum management program
6 Differentiate between a perceived and actual problem
7 Demonstrate an understanding of oestrus synchronisation
8 Design and build treatment protocols for common diseases
9 Interpret the accuracy of scientific information
  a. demonstrate an ability to apply statistics to dairy-related problems
  b. demonstrate an understanding of epidemiology
10 Demonstrate an ability to evaluate herd production records
11 Develop a diagnostic plan for problems associated with the following:
  a. nutrition
  b. mastitis:
    (1) environmental
    (2) contagious
  c. calf and heifer development
  d. lameness
  e. metabolic diseases:
    (1) milk fever
    (2) ketosis
    (3) indigestion
  f. abortion and infertility

C. Demonstrate an understanding of individual animal medicine

1 Perform a complete physical examination
2 Demonstrate ability to take history and examine the environment
3 Demonstrate ability to determine appropriate lab tests for different situations
4 Interpret laboratory result:
  a. faecal
  b. bacteriology
  c. serology
  d. virology
  e. serum chemistries
  f. cytology
  g. antibiotic sensitivity tests
5 Discuss hormonal therapy
6 Describe the importance of follow-up communications for treatment success
7 Explain how and why to teach clients diagnostic procedures (e.g. auscultation, taking temperature, California Mastitis Test, etc)
8 Perform faecal examination
9 Perform a post-mortem examination and collect appropriate samples
10 Perform bacteriology as related to milk quality
11 Perform bull breeding soundness exam

D. Demonstrate an understanding of anaesthesia/euthanasia

1 Discuss the acceptable methods and proper use of euthanasia
2 Demonstrate an ability to understand and use sedative agents and tranquilisers appropriately
3 Perform local and regional nerve blocks:
  a. epidural
  b. line
  c. inverted L
  d. cornual
  e. retrobulbular
  f. paravertebral

E. Demonstrate an understanding of surgical treatments

1 Perform and demonstrate an understanding for:
  a. caesarean section
  b. teat surgery
  c. claw amputation
  d. eye enucleation
  e. torsions
  f. laparotomy
  g. different approaches for displaced abomasal surgery
  h. umbilical hernia repair
  i. castration
  j. uterine torsion
  k. tail docking
  l. removal of supernumary teats
  m. rumenotomy
  n. draining abscesses tumour removal
  o. third eyelid flap
  p. cryotherapy
  q. Caslick's procedure
  r. uterine amputation
  s. uterine prolapse
  t. vaginal prolapse
  u. wound management
2 Demonstrate an understanding of sterile techniques
3 Identify common surgical instruments
4 Demonstrate the proper use of surgical instruments

5 Describe sterilisation techniques
6 Differentiate between abscesses, seromas and hematomas

F. Demonstrate an understanding of medical treatment techniques

1 Perform medical techniques:
- **a.** bandaging techniques
- **b.** casting procedures
- **c.** artificial insemination
- **d.** transtracheal wash
- **e.** rumenocentesis
- **f.** liver biopsy
- **g.** placement of stomach tube
- **h.** hoof trimming
- **i.** hoof care
- **j.** tattooing
- **k.** rectal palpation

2 Demonstrate competencies in obstetrical procedures, including fetotomy
3 Demonstrate proper use of obstetrical instruments
4 Demonstrate drug administration techniques:
- **a.** intramuscular injection
- **b.** subcutaneous injection
- **c.** intravenous injection
- **d.** oral
- **e.** topical

5 Collect a sterile milk sample
6 Collect blood samples:
- **a.** jugular
- **b.** tail

7 Demonstrate collection of urine samples
8 Perform faecal sample collection
9 Perform IV catheter placement for cows and calves
10 Administer fluid therapy
11 Administer intramammary products
12 Demonstrate an understanding of how and why to teach basic treatment techniques to clients

G. Demonstrate knowledge of clinical pharmacology and regulatory responsibility

1 Discuss the rational use of antibiotics
2 Demonstrate knowledge of cost/benefit analysis of treatment
3 Demonstrate proper storage and handling of pharmaceuticals and biologicals
4 Demonstrate an understanding of potential human abuse of veterinary pharmaceuticals
5 Demonstrate an understanding of the clinical pharmacology of common antibiotics
6 Demonstrate an understanding of the criteria for a veterinary-client-patient relationship
7 Demonstrate an understanding of managing adverse drug reactions

H. Recognise, treat, and/or control common diseases of dairy cows

I. Demonstrate knowledge of business skills and practice management

1 Demonstrate an understanding of:
- **a.** accounts receivable
- **b.** tax liabilities
- **c.** overhead
- **d.** cash flow
- **e.** lifestyle management
- **f.** client complaints
- **g.** employee management
- **h.** benefit packages
- **i.** insurance
- **j.** inventory control

2 Discuss different types of practice structure
3 Demonstrate an understanding for and apply time management techniques
4 Discuss professional record keeping responsibilities:
- **a.** legal
- **b.** professional

5 Explain the importance of prioritising tasks in a practice environment
6 Develop strategies to work with other professionals and/or allied industries
7 Discuss the importance of follow-up for public relations
8 Discuss the legal responsibilities for client/staff safety

J. Demonstrate people skills ability

1 Demonstrate writing and oral communication skills:
- **a.** with clients
- **b.** with staff
- **c.** with colleagues

2 Identify positive stress management techniques
3 Demonstrate ability to use active listening skills
4 Identify techniques to effectively resolve conflicts
5 Demonstrate skills in delegation of tasks
6 Discuss the benefits and responsibilities associated with delegation of tasks
7 Discuss the management structure of dairy farm operation and how to work within the structure to implement changes
8 Discuss the importance of speaking in layman's terminology with clients
9 Describe the importance of recognising teachable moments
10 Discuss the importance of team members' individual roles and their contribution to the team
11 Discuss the importance of recognising cultural and personality traits
12 Identify learning styles
13 Discuss the necessity of a family/work balance

K. Demonstrate an understanding of informatics

1 Describe how to identify and access valid sources of information
2 Identify resources:
- **a.** people
- **b.** periodicals
- **c.** cyberspace

L. Demonstrate an understanding of quality assurance

1 Discuss veterinary responsibilities in maintaining a safe food supply
2 Interpret bulk tank samples and other surveillance methods
3 Demonstrate microbiological skills as they relate to milk quality
4 Demonstrate ability to develop an on-farm HACCP, including ten-point plan for dairy beef quality assurance and dairy quality assurance
5 Discuss the interactions associated with milk quality (i.e. public health, farm finances, and regulations)

M. Demonstrate an understanding of ethics and professionalism

1 Describe the importance of maintaining a professional image
2 Discuss veterinarian/client confidentiality
3 Demonstrate an understanding of work ethics and expectations of veterinary practice
4 Demonstrate self-discipline:
- **a.** dependability
- **b.** positive attitude
- **c.** appropriate attire

5 Demonstrate an understanding of the Animal Medicinal Drug Use Clarification Act

6 Discuss the expectation of the community, the regulatory agencies and the general public for the veterinarian
7 Discuss the importance of continuing education
8 Discuss how to build credibility and rapport with clients
9 Discuss how to separate personal and client business objectives

N. Demonstrate an understanding of public health
1 Discuss principles of meat hygiene
2 Demonstrate an understanding of zoonotic diseases:
- **a.** Salmonellosis
- **b.** *E. coli* H0157
- **c.** Johne's disease: Crohn's disease
- **d.** Bovine spongiform encephalopathy (BSE)
- **e.** Cryptosporidosis
- **f.** Tuberculosis (TB)
- **g.** Brucellosis
- **h.** Listeria
- **i.** Leptospirosis
- **j.** Rabies

3 Discuss disaster relief awareness

O. Explain the benefits and structure of organised veterinary medicine
1 American Veterinary Medical Association
2 State veterinary association
3 Breed specific organisations
4 State and national organisations
5 Identify strategies to develop a peer network

P. Demonstrate an understanding of nutrition
1 Discuss principles of nutrition
2 Evaluate:
- **a.** rations
- **b.** feedbunk management
- **c.** storage of feedstuffs
- **d.** ration preparation and delivery
- **e.** dry cow rations
- **f.** manure

3 Identify health-related problems due to improper nutritional management
4 Describe importance of water

Box 3.2 Cow-Calf Competency List (Source: Reproduced with permission from AAVMC).

A. Demonstrate knowledge of general animal husbandry/production
1 Discuss the function and economics of each segment of the cow-calf industry
- **a.** hobby herds
- **b.** gleaner (crop residue) herds
- **c.** commercial herds
- **d.** seedstock herds

2 Describe the beef cow-calf production cycle and its interactions with the farm community
3 Demonstrate an understanding of veterinary medicine's role in the total cow-calf industry system
4 Demonstrate an understanding of beef cattle terminology (basic vocabulary), e.g. breeds, body types, equipment, nutrition, feeding, etc.
5 Discuss animal breeding systems, line breeding, crossbreeding and terminal crosses
6 Summarise expected progeny differences
7 Demonstrate an understanding of bovine behaviour during handling and transport
8 Demonstrate an understanding of cattle marketing structures
9 Describe components that affect animal welfare, e.g. environment, facilities, etc.

B. Demonstrate a knowledge of population medicine/epidemiology
1 Discuss disease dynamics
2 List risk factors for various types of diseases
3 Apply statistical principles to different practice situations
4 Explain the principles of biosecurity
5 Discuss the pros and cons of metaphylaxis
6 Describe and discuss prophylaxis, prevention, and immunisation strategies
7 Discuss biometrics, statistics, and scientific method
8 Explain the steps and process of record analysis
9 Demonstrate ability to perform a pregnancy examination
10 Conduct a clinical examination
11 Given several situations establish a herd diagnosis for each situation

C. Demonstrate knowledge of individual animal medicine
1 Demonstrate an understanding of cattle restraint
- **a.** physical restraints
- **b.** chemical restraints

2 Perform a physical examination utilising the five senses: subjective/objective/assessment/plan
3 Recognise and discuss the cost effectiveness of laboratory tests
4 Evaluate the cost effectiveness of treatments
5 Recognise the attributes of a normal bovine

D. Administer anaesthesia/euthanasia
1 Explain indications for the use of available local, regional and general anaesthesia agents and demonstrate proper technique of administration
2 Describe the indications for combinations of physical and/or chemical restraint

E. Perform surgical treatments
1 Perform routine emergency surgeries without assistance by professionals
- **a.** Caesarean section
- **b.** Obstetrical procedures
- **c.** Prolapse of vagina, uterus and rectum
- **d.** Urinary calculi and complications
- **e.** Laceration repair
- **f.** Bloat management

2 Demonstrate an understanding of principals of surgery – aseptic technique, suture material, suture patterns, etc.
3 Discuss contamination factors
4 Explain and illustrate the anatomical relationship of various surgical approaches
5 Demonstrate field surgical techniques
6 Diagnose and treat feet problems

F. Demonstrate knowledge of medical treatment and diagnostic techniques
1 Demonstrate ability to perform intravenous (IV), intramuscular (IM), subcutaneous (SQ), intraperitoneal (IP), intradermal (ID), oral (PO), intrauterine (IU) and ear implantation procedures
2 Demonstrate physical restraint techniques
3 Demonstrate breeding soundness examination (BSE), pregnancy determination, palpation, auscultation and ballottement
4 Demonstrate ability to use radiology and ultrasound equipment and interpret produced images
5 Demonstrate ability to use laboratory equipment and interpret findings

G. Demonstrate a knowledge of clinical pharmacology and regulatory responsibility
1 Demonstrate knowledge of resources available today (e.g. *Compendium of Veterinary Products*, textbooks, Food Animal Residue Avoidance Databank, etc.)
2 Describe the mechanisms of action for different antibiotics

3 Discuss factors influencing proper drug choice and treatment protocols
4 Explain cost effectiveness of treatments
5 Describe flexible labelling
6 Explain the factors affecting drug withdrawal times
7 Summarise AMDUCA, i.e. records, labelling, valid veterinarian-client-patient relationship (VCPR)
8 Demonstrate the proper use of prescription writing

H. Recognise, treat, and/or control (RTC) common and exotic diseases of cattle

I. Demonstrate knowledge of business skills and practice management
1 Demonstrate knowledge of basic record-keeping and accounting procedures
   a. Medical
   b. Financial
2 Explain the importance of clean environment as related to clinic, equipment and vehicles
3 Calculate and discuss your financial worth to both practice and client
4 Define a good work ethic and list its components
5 Demonstrate how to teach leadership and team member skills to clinic staff
6 Explain partial budget cost/benefit
7 Discuss and list the costs associated with operating a business
8 Explain the necessity of billing for all services rendered
9 Discuss the principle of total quality management

J. Demonstrate people skills ability
1 Discuss all aspects of communicating with clients
2 Demonstrate how to teach leadership and team member skills to clinic staff
3 Practise listening skills
4 List the basic personality types and explain their significance
5 Demonstrate willingness and ability to work with clients empathetically.
6 Demonstrate an ability to deal with people at their level
7 Explain the process for resolving conflicts

K. Demonstrate an understanding of informatics
1 Demonstrate an understanding of critical review of scientific literature
2 Demonstrate ability to access the internet
3 Demonstrate ability to access and use online databases
4 Explain the importance of continuing education and lifetime learning
5 Demonstrate ability to use appropriate software programs
6 Explain the importance of knowing resources available at colleges of veterinary medicine

L. Demonstrate an understanding of quality assurance
1 Describe beef quality assurance
2 Discuss the veterinarian's role in the delivery of beef quality assurance programs

M. Demonstrate an understanding of ethics and professionalism
1 Explain how the delivery of professional services can convey the correct professional images
2 Explain the importance of state practice acts and discuss the practitioner's role in enforcement
3 Discuss the importance of personal appearance and professionalism
4 Explain the importance of having a sense of community service
5 Explain the benefits of organised veterinary medicine
6 Recognise the importance of personal hygiene
7 Discuss proper disposal of trash and medical waste
8 Explain the benefits of camaraderie rather than competition among practitioners
9 Discuss reasons to maintain written records for each case (examination, treatment, recommendation, etc.)
10 Discuss the importance of appreciating the public's perception of animal welfare

N. Demonstrate an understanding of public health
1 List and discuss the zoonotic diseases of cattle
2 Discuss manure management problems associated with cow-calf operations
3 Explain the structure of the public health system
4 Discuss the role of veterinarians in the public health system

O. Demonstrate an understanding of state and federal regulations
1 Demonstrate an understanding of OSHA regulations that pertain to practice
2 Describe biosecurity environmental concerns
3 Discuss environmental regulations associated with cow/calf industry
4 Explain the responsibility associated with federal accreditation
5 List reportable cattle diseases
6 Demonstrate an understanding of proper procedures for controlled substances
7 Recognise sources of information for State and Federal regulations
8 Discuss carcass disposal regulations

P. Demonstrate an understanding of nutrition
1 Discuss body condition management within the production cycle
2 Discuss the role of minerals in cow-calf nutrition and macro-micro mineral interactions
3 Describe general knowledge of feed sources – commercial product availability
4 Explain role of supplements (energy, protein, mineral)
5 Demonstrate an understanding of:
   a. forages
   b. implants
   c. feed stuffs
   d. feed additives

Q. Demonstrate ability in problem solving
List the five steps of problem-solving

R. Crystal ball
1 Relate an understanding of the changing role of practitioners and clinicians, from medical to commodity economics, based on sound medical principle
2 Discuss the role for consortiums among universities
3 Discuss the local veterinarian as a contractor within a larger structure
4 Describe diagnostics, not treatment, as the income generator – treatment to lowest bidder
5 Recognise the huge pressure in industry to license technicians to practise alone
6 Discuss the trends towards fewer food animal veterinarians doing more of what they are trained for
7 Discuss the expanded use of licensed veterinary assistants to perform pregnancy checks, ultrasound, castrations, etc.
8 Discuss pros and cons of internships – one year pre/post-graduate experience
9 Recognise the trend towards less protectionism for the veterinarian's role
10 Recognise the trend towards enforcement of practice acts only by complaints

Box 3.3 Feedlot Competency List (Source: Reproduced with permission from AAVMC).

A. Demonstrate an understanding of general animal husbandry/production
- **1** Demonstrate an understanding of feedlot terminology
- **2** Demonstrate an understanding of a feedlot production cycle
- **3** Discuss the influencers of performance: (e.g. genetics, nutrition, environment, animal health, cattle handling, facility design, etc.)
- **4** Demonstrate an understanding of the management of a feedlot operation (e.g. health, maintenance, marketing services and cattle, feed mill, and environmental issues)
- **5** Demonstrate an understanding of feedlot economics (e.g. individual animal, pen, profit centres, marketing, etc.)
- **6** Demonstrate an understanding of the desired end product for each of the customers that a calf needs to satisfy during its lifetime (e.g. producer, feedlot, packer, processor, retailer, restaurant, and consumer)
- **7** Demonstrate an understanding of cattle grading and inspection.
- **8** Discuss dark cutters; carcass cuts; grading (quality grade and /yield grade); maturity; cutability; and meat tenderness, juiciness and flavour.
- **9** Demonstrate an understanding of the basics of equipment operation (e.g. feed truck, front-end loader, etc.)
- **10** Design a risk avoidance management program for a feedlot
- **11** Demonstrate an understanding of animal behaviour
- **12** Demonstrate an understanding of cattle and beef marketing
- **13** Recognise the different kinds of forages
- **14** Discuss the nutrient value of the different forages
- **15** Recognise the different kinds of feedstuffs
- **16** Discuss the nutrient value of the different feedstuffs
- **17** Evaluate a feedlot ration

B. Demonstrate an understanding of population medicine/epidemiology
- **1** Discuss disease prevention (e.g. good management practices (GMP), cattle source, immunisation, mass medication by feed or parentally, and biosecurity)
- **2** Demonstrate ability to perform problem solving (e.g. identify problem, gather information, organise results, apply decision tree analysis, rank outcome on decision tree analysis)
- **3** Apply methods and techniques of production problem investigation
- **4** Demonstrate knowledge of data collection, keeping records, and acquisition systems
- **5** Demonstrate ability to transfer individual animal information to herd or population database
- **6** Discuss the methods used to analyse different types of data
- **7** Demonstrate proficiency in the application of epidemiology
- **8** Demonstrate understanding of economic modelling, analysis, and relevant outcomes as it relates to good management practices and source of cattle

C. Demonstrate an understanding of individual animal medicine
- **1** Perform clinical examination pertinent to a given situation and record results to apply to population data
  - **a.** Take history from client
    - **(1)** Develop listening skills
    - **(2)** Develop interviewing skills
  - **b.** Examine environment
    - **(1)** Examine herd, pasture, housing, water, feed, etc.
    - **(2)** Examine client's and premise's environmental history
  - **c.** Perform physical exam for diagnostic purposes
    - **(1)** Determine temperature, pulse rate, and respiratory rate
    - **(2)** Check eyes, ears, nose, and throat
    - **(3)** Perform oral exam
    - **(4)** Determine age of cattle
    - **(5)** Perform rectal exam
    - **(6)** Percuss and auscultate thorax
    - **(7)** Percuss and auscultate abdomen
      - **(a)** Diagnose normality, right displaced abomasum (RDA), ulcers, cecal torsion, rumenatony, hardware, left displaced abomasum (LDA)
      - **(b)** Evaluate rumen function
    - **(8)** Examine musculo-skeletal system
    - **(9)** Interpret thermometer readings (normal and abnormal, values)
    - **(10)** Collect appropriate samples
    - **(11)** Examine skin
    - **(12)** Examine urinary/genital systems
    - **(13)** Examine nervous system
  - **d.** Perform lab tests/special exams
    - **(1)** Perform vena puncture
    - **(2)** Collect and maintain samples
    - **(3)** Determine appropriate tests(s)
    - **(4)** Determine sample(s) needed to support diagnosis
    - **(5)** Determine appropriate laboratory for testing sample(s)
    - **(6)** Interpret lab results and data
    - **(7)** Discuss cost effectiveness of lab tests
    - **(8)** Discuss lab variability vs. individual animal variability
    - **(9)** Describe the sensitivity and specificity of different tests
  - **e.** Demonstrate knowledge of clinical pathology
    - **(1)** Perform faecal exam
    - **(2)** Perform complete blood cell count
    - **(3)** Determine total plasma and packed cell volume
    - **(4)** Use various kinds of lab equipment
    - **(5)** Demonstrate knowledge of gross and microscopic parasitology
    - **(6)** Demonstrate knowledge of clinical bacteriology
    - **(7)** Demonstrate knowledge of cytology
    - **(8)** Demonstrate knowledge of antibiotic residue tests
- **2** Demonstrate knowledge of post mortem examination
  - **a.** Perform a necropsy
  - **b.** Recognise normal tissue
  - **c.** Perform sample collection and submission
  - **d.** Recognise lesions
  - **e.** Discuss the importance of obtaining a complete history
- **3** Demonstrate knowledge of nursing care and hospital pen management
- **4** Recognise good hospital management
- **5** Demonstrate knowledge of necropsy examination appropriate to feedlot standards

D. Demonstrate an understanding of anaesthesia and euthanasia procedures
- **1** Demonstrate an understanding of animal welfare and well-being (e.g. castration, dehorn, eyes, claws, prolapses, abscesses, etc)
- **2** Discuss the importance of understanding the public's perception of how animals are handled (including when dead)
- **3** Discuss the importance of establishing a long-term anaesthesia and euthanasia policy for a feedlot

E. Demonstrate an understanding of surgical treatments

F. Demonstrate an understanding of medical treatment techniques
- **1** Demonstrate an understanding of the methods of administration, equipment maintenance, and sanitation
- **2** Demonstrate an understanding of mass treatment techniques (e.g. injectables, feed or water, topical, and implants)

3 Demonstrate an understanding of individual treatment techniques (e.g. subcutaneous, intravenous, oral (balling gun, stomach tubes) and topical)
4 Demonstrate an understanding of injection site selection, tissue damage and beef quality assurance
5 Demonstrate knowledge in the selection of appropriate treatment methods (e.g. beef quality assurance, regulatory, withdrawal time)

G. Demonstrate knowledge of clinical pharmacology, drug selection, and regulatory responsibility

1 Demonstrate knowledge of AMDUCA and how it impacts feedlots
2 Demonstrate knowledge of The Animal Drug Availability Act of 1996 (ADAA)
3 Demonstrate an understanding of the proper storage and handling of pharmaceuticals and biologicals
4 Discuss the importance of a correct diagnosis on drug selection
5 Demonstrate knowledge of treatment protocols, dosing schedules, prescriptions, other order, withdrawal times, etc.
6 Demonstrate an understanding of efficacious drug selection (e.g. pharmacokinetics, pharmacodynamics, and efficacy data)
7 Demonstrate knowledge of proper selection of medication as to efficacy, route of delivery, withdrawal time, and cost
8 Demonstrate an understanding of proper treatment interval and dosing (amount, route, and site selection)
9 Explain the proper use of withdrawal times
10 Demonstrate knowledge of cost and benefit analysis (performance, management, and safety)
11 Demonstrate an understanding of proper adverse product complaint investigation and reporting
12 Demonstrate knowledge of production enhancement products
13 Demonstrate an understanding of recording and maintaining treatment records
14 Demonstrate knowledge of prescription writing, other orders, and veterinary feed directives

H. Recognise, treat and/or control diseases of feedlot cattle

1 Demonstrate knowledge of microorganisms commonly associated with Bovine Respiratory Disease Syndrome (BRD)
- **a.** Bovine herpes virus 1 (BHV-1) and 3/Malignant Catarrhal Fever (MCF)
- **b.** Bovine Para influenza 3 virus (PI3)
- **c.** Bovine viral diarrhoea virus (BVDV)
- **d.** Bovine respiratory syncytial virus (BRSV)
- **e.** Bovine adenovirus
- **f.** Bovine rhinovirus
- **g.** Bovine corona virus
- **h.** *Mannheimia haemolytica*
- **i.** *Pasteurella multocida*
- **j.** *Hemophilus somnus*
- **k.** *Mycoplasma* spp.
- **l.** *Chlamydia* spp.

2 Demonstrate knowledge of miscellaneous respiratory conditions
- **a.** Atypical interstitial pneumonia
- **b.** Laryngeal abscesses
- **c.** Tracheal oedema
- **d.** Late feeding period BRD

3 Demonstrate knowledge of digestive conditions
- **a.** Rumen tympany (primary and secondary bloat)
- **b.** Acidosis (clinical and sub-clinical)
- **c.** Sudden death syndrome
- **d.** Clostridial diseases
- **e.** Peritonitis
- **f.** Salmonellosis
- **g.** Trichobezoars

4 Demonstrate knowledge of musculo-skeletal ailments
- **a.** Toe abscesses
- **b.** Foot rot
- **c.** Arthritis
- **d.** The 'Buller' syndrome
- **e.** Laminitis

5 Demonstrate knowledge of central nervous conditions
- **a.** Rabies
- **b.** Polioencephalomalacia
- **c.** Thromboembolic meningoencephalitis
- **d.** Nervous coccidiosis
- **e.** Acute severe acidosis associated with grain overload
- **f.** Listeriosis

6 Demonstrate knowledge of urogenital conditions
- **a.** Urolithiasis
- **b.** Pylonephritis
- **c.** Leptospirosis
- **d.** Dystocia
- **e.** Infections of the reproductive tract
- **f.** Castration complication

7 Demonstrate knowledge of ocular conditions
- **a.** Infectious bovine keratoconjunctivitis
- **b.** Infectious bovine rhinotracheitis
- **c.** Foreign bodies and injury
- **d.** Ocular squamous-cell carcinoma

8 Demonstrate knowledge of parasitic diseases
- **a.** Anaplasmosis
- **b.** Coccidiosis
- **c.** Intestinal nematodes and cestodes
- **d.** Flukes
- **e.** External parasites

9 Demonstrate knowledge of miscellaneous feedlot conditions
- **a.** Heat stress
- **b.** Cold stress
- **c.** Ionophore toxicity
- **d.** Organophosphate toxicity
- **e.** Urea toxicity
- **f.** Anaphylaxes
- **g.** Pericarditis and endocarditis
- **h.** Traumatic pericarditis

10 Demonstrate knowledge of disease monitoring in feedlots via slaughter checks
11 Define and discuss the pathogenesis of the conditions represented by the terms used by USDA-FSIS as reasons for condemnation at slaughter
- **a.** Emaciation and miscellaneous degeneration
- **b.** Eosinophilic myositis
- **c.** Nephritis and pyelitis
- **d.** Pyemia
- **e.** Pyrexia
- **f.** Residue
- **g.** Septicemia
- **h.** Toxaemia
- **i.** Uraemia

I. Demonstrate knowledge of business skills and practice management

1 Demonstrate knowledge of the different kinds of insurance (e.g. malpractice, property, etc.),
2 Demonstrate ability to sell professional skills
3 Demonstrate an understanding of how to handle client complaints
4 Demonstrate an understanding of overhead (e.g. solo vs. groups vs. partnerships)

5 Demonstrate an understanding of the principles of inventory control
6 Discuss different methods of collecting overdue accounts and how to prevent overdue accounts
7 Demonstrate an understanding of cash flow in a practice
8 Discuss the different taxes that affect the practice, the individual, and clients
9 Demonstrate an understanding of practice record keeping, required licences, client accounts, sales tax, social security tax, interest, and depreciation
10 Develop a plan for repaying student debt
11 Demonstrate an understanding of basis for setting fees
12 Demonstrate an understanding of the principles of time management
13 Demonstrate an understanding of the value of life style management
14 Demonstrate an understanding of the different types of business structure, (e.g. partnership, corporation)
15 Demonstrate an understanding of records required for controlled substances
16 Demonstrate an understanding of feedlot accounting
17 Demonstrate knowledge of client confidentiality, competitive advantage, and proprietary issues
18 Demonstrate an understanding of separating your personal and client's business objectives
19 Demonstrate an understanding of the importance of how an organisational tree power structure of a feedlot will influence your role as a consultant
20 Demonstrate an understanding of the delicacy of dealing with customers and suppliers of feedlots
21 Demonstrate an understanding of recognising conflict of interests

J. Demonstrate people skills ability
1 Discuss types of client education
2 Identify and understand personality types
3 Speak with confidence to individuals and groups
4 Communicate with people at their level by telephone, in person, and by writing
5 Demonstrate an understanding of how to inspire teamwork in colleagues, employees, and clients' employees
6 Write brief, complete accurate reports
7 Demonstrate an understanding of the principles of conflict management
8 Demonstrate an understanding proper hiring and firing practices.
9 Report case progress to client promptly
10 Demonstrate proper telephone skills and client communications
11 Recognise proper communication practices
12 Demonstrate an understanding of the potential conflicts between family and practice
13 Demonstrate an understanding of the principals of managing people

K. Demonstrate an understanding of informatics
1 Demonstrate ability to perform critical evaluation of scientific literature
2 Explain the need for continuing education
3 Demonstrate computer literacy (e.g. spread sheets, word processing, data bases, literature retrieval)
4 Demonstrate knowledge of computer hardware and operating system
5 Demonstrate knowledge of internet skills (e.g. veterinary medicine, USDA, FDA, commodity market sites, etc)
6 Demonstrate an awareness of appropriate software for feedlot practice
7 Explain the importance of life long learning

L. Demonstrate an understanding of beef quality assurance
1 Apply current concepts of animal welfare to feedlot practice
2 Demonstrate an understanding of methods of residue avoidance and withdrawal times.
3 Demonstrate an understanding of the concept of total quality management including Hazard analysis and critical control points, genetics, nutrition, processing, handling, etc.
4 Explain how to prevent carcass blemishes

M. Demonstrate an understanding of ethics and professionalism
1 Define ethics and professionalism
2 Apply ethics to various situations involving conflicts between veterinary practitioners
3 Apply ethics to various situations involving conflicts between veterinary practitioners and clients)
4 Demonstrate an understanding basic public relations and how to present the profession well in all situations
5 Describe benefits derived from using ethical practices
6 Define professionalism
7 Describe the benefits to be derived from professionalism
8 Demonstrate an understanding of the meaning of client/patient relationship
9 Demonstrate an understanding of the importance of maintaining a professional image
10 Discuss doctor/client confidentiality
11 Demonstrate appropriate situational attire
12 Explain the importance of personal responsibility and reliability

N. Demonstrate an understanding of the feedlot veterinarian's role in public health
1 Discuss drug withdrawal and residue avoidance
2 List the zoonotic pathogens associated with the feedlot environment
3 Discuss the veterinarian's role in improving feedlot worker safety
4 Explain the veterinarian's role in preventing environmental contamination by feedlots

O. Explain the benefits of organised veterinary medicine
1 Describe the benefits derived from belonging to and participating organised veterinary groups
2 Develop a plan to become involved in veterinary organisations (local, state, national, specialty, and support groups)

P. Demonstrate an understanding of nutrition

Q. Demonstrate an understanding of State and Federal regulations pertaining to feedlots
1 Explain the veterinarian's role and obligation to the feedlot, public, government, and self in regards to laws, regulations, and ethics. (FDA, USDA, EPA, DNR-DEQ, OSHA, and zoning)
2 Demonstrate an understanding of the regulatory aspects of interstate, intrastate, and international cattle movements
3 List quarantinable and reportable cattle diseases

R. Demonstrate an understanding of the livestock marketing structure
1 Evaluate different generic sources of feedlot cattle
2 Understand flow of cattle in through the livestock structure
3 Understand intrastate/interstate/international transport regulations
4 Understand responsibility and consequence of marketing low-performing and out-cattle

References

Adam, K., (2013). Farm animal veterinary services in the 21st century: What do vets really do? *Cattle Practice* **12**(2), 127.

Frawley, P. (2003). Review of rural veterinary services, Commonwealth of Australia.

Lowe, (2009). Unlocking Potential; A report on veterinary expertise in food animal production. Department for Environment, Food and Rural Affairs.

Luby, C.D., McIntyre, K., Jelinski, M.D. (2013). Skills required of dairy veterinarians in western Canada: A survey of practicing veterinarians. *Canadian Veterinary Journal* **54**(2), 67–270.

Mellanby, R.J., Rhind, S.M., Bell, C., Shaw, D.J., Gifford, J., Fennell, D., Manser, C., Spratt, D.P., Wright, M.H., Zago, S., Hudson, N.P.H. (2011). Paper: Perceptions of clients and veterinarians on what attributes constitute 'a good vet'. *Veterinary Record* **168**(23), 616–622.

Miller, R.B., Hardin, L.E., Cowart, R.P., Ellersieck, M.R. (2004) Practitioner-defined competencies required of new veterinary graduates in food animal practice. *Journal of Veterinary Medical Education* **31**(4), 347–65.

Morin, D.E., Constable, P.D., Troutt, H.F., Johnson, A.L. (2002a) Individual animal medicine and animal production skills expected of entry-level veterinarians in bovine practice. *Journal of the American Veterinary Medical Association* **221**, 959–968.

Morin, D.E., Constable, P.D., Troutt, H.F., Johnson, A.L. (2002b) Surgery, anesthesia, and restraint skills expected of entry-level veterinarians in bovine practice. *Journal of the American Veterinary Medical Association* **221**, 969–974.

Nordlund, K. (1998) Grumpy Old Vets: The 1960's practice hits the 21st Century. *The Bovine Practitioner* **32**, 58–62.

CHAPTER 4

Evidence-Based Veterinary Medicine and Clinical Audits in Cattle Practice

Peter D. Cockcroft

Learning objectives

- Understand what evidence-based veterinary medicine (EBVM) is.
- Understand the process of EBVM: ask, access, appraise, apply, audit.
- Appreciate the skills and resources required to successfully practise EBVM.
- Understand what a clinical audit is.
- Appreciate why they are important.
- Understand the processes involved in performing a clinical audit.

Introduction

Bovine clinicians are constantly faced with a range of clinical tasks associated with disease in a particular animal, such as: interpreting diagnostic tests; optimising the diagnostic process; judging the efficacy of preventative or therapeutic interventions; trying to predict the harm associated with specific therapies; predicting the course and prognosis of a disease; and estimating the costs of intervention. Veterinary clinicians need to know whether their procedures and judgments are valid.

Society expects that safe and effective treatments and advice are provided by veterinary surgeons. A veterinary surgeon has a moral and ethical obligation to provide treatment and advice for which there is good evidence (Ramey and Rollin, 2001). Primary research papers are the source of science-based evidence. The link or bridge between clinical research and clinical practice is evidence-based veterinary medicine. This bridge is vital if we are to use the output of research to best advantage in the care of our patients.

The application of EBVM can:

- improve and optimise: diagnosis, prognosis, control, treatment of animals;
- provide informed choices for farmers;
- enable veterinarians to: defend their decisions scientifically; provide the user with a methodology for appropriate, patient-orientated life-long, self-directed learning; identify information deficits in the literature; and direct clinical research.

How do you make your decisions in a science-based profession that is rapidly advancing?

• Dogmatism	This is the best way to do it.
• Policy	This is the way we do it around here.
• Experience	This way worked the last few times.
• Whim	This way might work.
• Nihilism	It doesn't really matter what we do.
• Rule of least worst	Do what you will regret the least.
• Defer to experts	How would you do it?
• Defer to patient	How would you like to proceed?

A simple way of assessing your own performance as an EBVM practitioner is to answer the following questions:

- Do I identify and prioritise the problems to be solved (information needs)?
- Do I search for the missing information?
- Do I understand what is meant by the terms Type I error, Type II error, power, sensitivity specificity and number needed to treat?
- Do I appraise new information in terms of scientific validity?
- Do I have the resources to access the internet?
- Am I aware of the veterinary information databases?

Bovine Medicine, Third Edition. Edited by Peter D. Cockcroft.

- Is my application of new information scientifically justified and intuitively sensible for this situation?
- Do I explain the pros and cons of different opinions, taking into account the different utilities to the owner?
- Have I got the all the tools to perform EBVM in my professional toolkit, and do I know what they are?

In human medicine, the application of evidence-based medicine (EBM) has been responsible for a major step up in patient care and appropriate life-long learning.

Developments that have allowed this situation to change are:

- The development of search strategies for efficiently tracking down appraising evidence (for its validity and relevance).
- The creation of systematic reviews and concise summaries.
- The creation of evidence-based journals of secondary publication.
- The creation of information systems to allow fast access.
- The identification and application of effective strategies for life-long learning for improving clinical performance.

What is evidence-based veterinary medicine (EBVM)?

Evidence-based medicine (EBM) has been defined as 'The integration of best research evidence with clinical expertise and patient values' (Sackett *et al.*, 2000). In veterinary medicine, a suitable definition of EBVM might be, 'The use of current best evidence in making clinical decisions' (Cockcroft and Holmes, 2003). Other descriptive terms that have been used include: 'Research into practice', 'Just in time learning', 'A process of life-long self-directed, problem-based learning'.

Rapid advances in knowledge constantly challenge our ability to provide the best and most current clinical information for cattle health care. When faced by uncertainty as to the best and most current approach to a clinical problem, we can choose from several options. These include:

- Relying on our knowledge of pathophysiology, remembering unsystematic clinical observations of a previous case, tossing a coin to decide between two competing options, intelligent guess work, doing nothing to avoid harm, asking colleagues, referring to text books, browsing journals and doing a database search with an unstructured appraisal.
- Proceeding on the basis of our personal experiences or clinical intuition.
- Seeking the advice of an expert in the field.
- Relying on scientific evidence-based veterinary medicine.

The traditional approach suggests that:

- Clinical experience is a valid way of gaining an understanding about diagnosis, prognosis and treatment.
- Pathophysiological rationale is a valid way of guiding treatments.
- Common sense and classical medical training are the only qualities needed to evaluate medical literature.

The EBVM approach suggests:

- personal experience may be misleading;
- randomised studies are required to validate results, because predictions based upon physiology may be wrong;
- reading literature requires more than common sense to evaluate the evidence.

What is evidence?

Evidence is something that serves as proof to support (or refute) a fact, and it may range from weak to strong. Research studies that do not conform to accepted scientific methodologies will produce evidence that is invalid. The best evidence is derived from well-designed clinically relevant research, especially from patient-centred clinical research.

The value of evidence derived from clinical trials is directly related to the statistical power of the study. The power of the study represents the probability that a specified difference will be detected. This allows the construction of a hierarchy of evidence based upon the strengths of the different study designs to answer specific questions.

A typical representation of this hierarchy is the so-called pyramid of evidence illustrated in Figure 4.1. The second pyramid, which is harder to define, is reliant upon evidence from other sources. The use of the second pyramid is not unusual in veterinary medicine.

The process of EBVM is as follows:

- Information needs are identified.
- Information needs are transformed into a series of questions.
- A search is performed for the best available evidence with which to answer the question with maximum efficiency.
- The evidence obtained is critically appraised for its validity (closeness to the truth) and usefulness (clinical applicability).
- The results of this appraisal are used in clinical judgments and actions.
- The outcome of the resulting decisions and actions are evaluated.

This process can be remembered by using the 5 'A's:

1. *Ask* an answerable *clinical question*
2. *Access* (*systematically search*) AND rank the evidence to help answer clinical question,
3. *Appraise* evidence
4. *Apply* the best evidence:
   a. *Amalgamate* the valid evidence with other relevant information to make a good decision; and
   b. *Act on your (or owner's) decision*
5. *Audit* your practice (i.e. check your actual practice – 'actions' – against 'best' evidence-based practice)

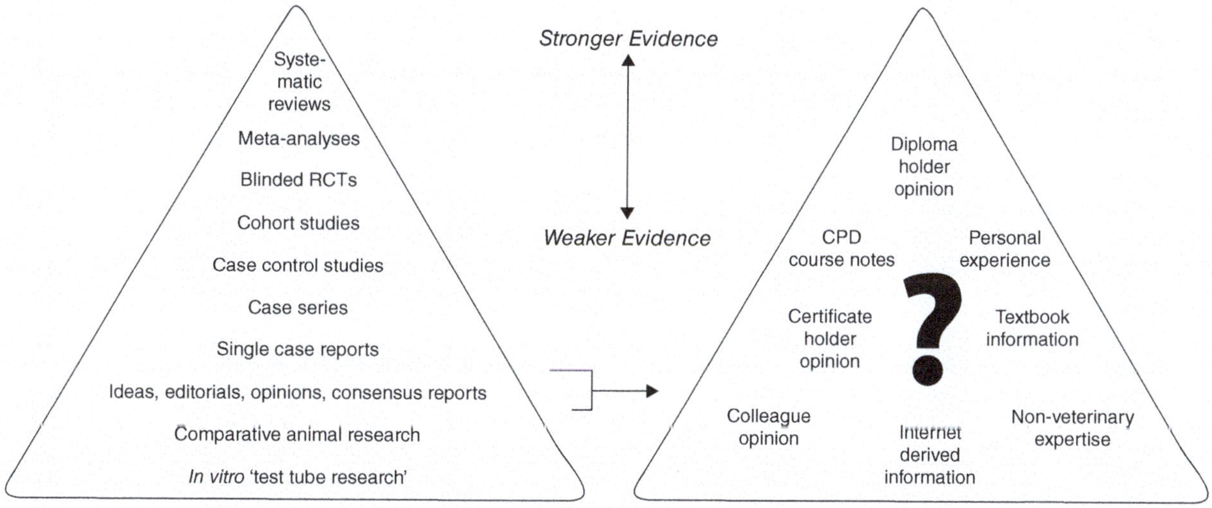

Figure 4.1 An illustration of the hierarchy of evidence. The pyramid on the right shows the difficulty in ranking much of the evidence used in clinical veterinary work.

What skills do I need to practise EBVM?

The starting point is to identify that further information is required. Information needed to solve a problem fall into three categories:

- information that is needed and is known;
- information that is needed but not known;
- information needs that are not recognised.

Turning information needs into scientific questions

The definition and structure of an appropriate question is crucial if the search for appropriate evidence is to be successful. The question should define the clinical problem using scientific terminology that will identify the evidence required and lead us to the most efficient search strategy to locate that evidence.

A clinical question may have the form:

Is this a good treatment for a disease?

An answerable question would be: What is the probability of a cure with the treatment, compared with an alternative standard therapy in a patient that has the disease in a population like mine?

Four main elements of a well-formed clinical question (PICO or PECOT)

The four main elements of a good clinical question can be remembered from the mnemonic *PICO*: **P**atient, **I**ntervention, **C**omparison, and **O**utcome.

Another acronym gaining popularity is *PECOT*: **P**opulation, **E**xposure, **C**omparison, **O**utcome and **T**ime. Exposure includes treatments as well as risk factors for disease.

Example using PICO

Is there an advantage to using ketoprofen when surgically castrating calves?:

- **Patient or problem**
  How would a group of patients similar to mine be described?
  A group of 3 month old Simmental x Holstein-Friesian bull calves which are to be surgically castrated
- **Intervention (a cause, prognostic factor, treatment)**
  Which main intervention am I considering?
  Ketoprofen (Ketofen) 10% 3mg/kg i/m at the time of castration
- **Comparison intervention (if appropriate)**
  What is the main alternative I am considering?
  No analgesia
- **Outcome**
  What are the main benefits or downsides?
  With ketoprofen, compared to untreated animals, is there: a greater growth rate in the month after castration? Is there better food conversion efficiency? Is there a cost benefit? Is there reduced stress and discomfort?

To assist in identifying information needs and translating them into scientific questions, it is useful to categorise the type of question you are asking into one or more of the following categories:

- Epidemiological
- Diagnostic tests
- Treatment
- Harm/aetiology
- Prognosis
- Control and prevention

Prioritising the questions

When you have more questions than time, consider:

- Which question is the most important to the animal's welfare?
- Which question is the most feasible to answer in the time available?
- Which question is most interesting to you?
- Which question are you most likely to encounter repeatedly during the course of your work?
- Which question has the lowest time cost but the greatest cost/clinical benefit?

Sources of evidence

The most reliable evidence is that derived from scientific research using valid methodologies which is published in primary research papers.

Appraising the evidence

The greatest statistical certainty comes from well conducted meta-analyses that incorporate a number of randomised controlled experimental studies. Similarly, systematic reviews also provide strong evidence (see Figure 4.1).

The randomised control trial (RCT) will always have the greatest power when compared to other data collection designs, but it may not be appropriate to answer questions about causation where cohorts or case control studies are more appropriate. Randomised control trials are the design of choice for evidence regarding treatments. Trial designs further down the pyramid produce results that are less transferable to other populations, but may be more applicable to certain types of patient. The object of the evidence hierarchy is to concentrate the effort on those sources most likely to yield the greatest rewards.

When few higher-quality sources of evidence are available representing the apex of the pyramid, we can work down the hierarchy until sufficient information is obtained. In the absence of any other information, individual case reports may be extremely helpful. Alternatively, when searches yield an excessive numbers of articles, we can concentrate on the better evidence by filtering out the results of studies lower in the hierarchy.

Appraising the studies you have selected

Appraisal establishes the validity of the evidence and enables the results to be critically assessed and transformed into useful information. An understanding of randomisation, double-blinding and statistics such as probabilities and odds is required. Specific parameters such as the number needed to treat in therapy studies requires a knowledge that will need to be acquired if the results are to be meaningful. The number needed to treat is the number of animals needed to be treated before an additional animal benefits from the treatment. The ability to analyse studies about tests, therapy, diagnosis, aetiology and prognosis will require you to learn new skills if the evidence is to be identified as clinically relevant.

Future needs

Resources for the practice of EVBM

Outlined below are some of the developments that have enabled EBM to become a reality in everyday medical practice.

Critically appraised topics (CATs)

There are now numerous internet sites that contain a database of CATs. A CAT is a short summary of the evidence to a focused clinical question. The preparation of CATs enables this information to be shared or used at a later date.

Standard protocols have been produced regarding the format of CATS. Any qualified practitioners may submit CATS to these dedicated websites. Some EBM centres use the acronym POEM (**P**atient **O**rientated **E**vidence that **M**atters) as an alternative to CAT. The Centre for Evidence-based Veterinary Medicine at the Nottingham University School of Veterinary Medicine has a BETS (Best Evidence Topic) database, which is a CAT by another name.

High-quality systematic reviews

Systematic reviews of the literature designed to answer a specific clinical question represent a form of secondary scientific literature with a very high evidence value. They enable evidence to be located quickly, in a summarised form, with an objective science-based opinion that addresses the quality of the evidence presented. In human medicine, dedicated resources exist to fulfil this need. The Cochrane Library is a good example of a database of systemic reviews.

Secondary journals

Secondary journals to support the practice of EBM have developed in human medicine. Secondary journals publish structured abstracts summarising the best quality evidence and the most clinically useful recent research from the literature.

What resources do we need for the practice of EBVM?

It is clear that, if EBVM is to succeed, we need (Valori, 2001):

- Systematic reviews.
- Secondary journals.
- A central database of CATs.
- More clinical trials.
- Education at all levels in EBVM skills.
- An audit of commonly asked questions for which there is poor evidence, to identify priority area for clinical research and systematic review.

- Fewer or more uniform databases.
- Better indexing and tagging of controlled trials.
- Tagging of discredited evidence.
- Links to full text papers and reviews.
- Uniformity in the format and criteria used to present summary and primary evidence
- Locally adapted guidelines (practice) from centrally tested evidence (universities, institutes and referral practices).

Conclusion

There will not be time to find answers to every question generated by our information needs, and there is a need to prioritise our information needs to those that have a major impact on our patient care. However, every effort should be made to use the current best evidence in our decision-making if we are to maintain our professional standing. The practice of EBVM should form part of life-long, problem-orientated, self-directed learning, to ensure our knowledge and skills are optimised to match the needs of our clients and patients. National and international co-operation will be required to provide the necessary resources.

The Centre for Evidence-based Veterinary Medicine at the Nottingham School of Veterinary Medicine now has a website which provides useful tutorials to support the practice of evidence-based veterinary medicine. A recent issue of the Veterinary Clinics of North America was entitled 'Evidence-Based Veterinary Medicine for the Bovine Veterinarian' (Buczinski and Vandeweerd, 2012). These developments, in addition to other interest groups, reflect the growing interest and recognition of the importance of the paradigm.

Clinical audits

What is a clinical audit?

A clinical audit has been defined as follows:

> '*Clinical audit is a quality improvement process that seeks to improve patient care and outcomes through systematic review of care against explicit criteria and the implementation of change. Aspects of the structure, processes, and outcomes are selected and systematically evaluate against explicit criteria. Where indicated, changes are implemented at the individual, team or service level and further monitoring is used to confirm improvement in health care delivery.*' (NICE, 2002).

The audit is a performance review, and it measures practice performance. From this, the need for change can be identified. Although often overlooked, it provides a mechanism for identifying learning needs and implementing best (evidence-based) practice. Clinical audits have been shown to be an effective method to change practice behaviour.

The process involves:

- Preparation (what to audit and the team to do it).
- Criteria selection (processes or outcomes).
- Setting standards (evidence-based).
- Measurement of performance.
- Analysis and review of the results.
- Repeat of the cycle to measure impact.

Starting with a perceived important and common problem within the practice is useful to stimulate interest and motivate participants. Examples in cattle practice are mastitis therapeutics, obstetrical interventions, on-farm surgery and therapeutic protocols for improving fertility, protocols for castration, disbudding and de-horning. The treatments and the outcomes derived from practice records should be compared with those available from the best evidence, according to the published literature. Analysis may present trends or just provide information for comparison. Statistical analysis may be appropriate but is not essential. The process should be constructive, blame-free and support self-directed learning. Drawbacks include: lack of time; cost; lack of expertise in audit design and analysis; disagreements between practice members; and the high level of participation required.

Why is it important?

It is important to be able to assure clients and peers that the expertise and service offered is safe, effective and efficient. A clinical audit is a process to assess, evaluate and improve patient care and client services. The process identifies deficiencies and monitors the outcome of any changes made to address those deficiencies. It enables the identification and implementation of current best practice. It can improve practice efficiency, administration, communication and effectiveness and reduce clinical errors (lower the risk of liability) and foster practice change.

Clinical audits and EBVM

Clinical audit must always be evidence-based to ensure that clinical practice and decisions to change it are based upon the best possible evidence of effectiveness. Clinical audits can be used to compare current practice with the best available evidence. They provide a methodology to assess whether the best evidence is being applied within the practice.

Process and outcome clinical audits

There are two types of audit: a process audit and an outcome audit. Both may be addressed in the same investigation. Processes are what you do – for example, a treatment you use for a condition (e.g. antibiotic selection for mastitis), or a surgical procedure that you use (e.g. caesarean section). Outcomes are what happens to the patient following the process – for example, mortality or recovery. With outcome audits, there can be many confounding factors in addition to the process. For example, a poor outcome may result, even after exemplary patient care, because of the patient's underlying health conditions or poor owner compliance with medication. When evaluating outcomes, it is important to remember that the illness itself, the diagnostics tests, the potential treatments, and patient or farmer compliance all play a role in the clinical outcome. A meaningful outcome audit requires a large number of cases and consideration of all the possible confounding factors. However, it can provide an early warning system that the treatment may be sub-optimal. Mortality rates and poor manual pregnancy accuracy are good examples.

Statistics and clinical audits

The big debate is whether statistical analysis should be applied to clinical audits or whether we are just 'eyeballing' trends? When we are measuring a process audit, formal statistical analysis is unnecessary as we are measuring the number of times something is performed. When we are measuring outcomes, statistical analysis give us an indication as to whether our results could be a random event, or whether the results do differ significantly from an accepted or target standard.

One of the problems is if we accept the rigorous standard of scientific research of 95% confidence intervals (a one in 20 chance that the result may be incorrect), we will have to collect a lot of information to make our study powerful enough to demonstrate a statistical difference if one exists. A compromise is to accept a lower standard such as 75% or 60% to indicate if our result might be different than an accepted standard. Most of our results for outcomes will be in the form of a fraction (often termed a proportion). Table 4.1 below illustrates the impact of changing the confidence interval when we have a proportion as a result. Bold text indicates a significant difference (i.e. the confidence intervals do not overlap) when the standard is compared to the result.

A Simple guide to performing clinical audits

Questions to consider (SPVS workshop 2005)

- Who are the stakeholders?
- How can we get the stakeholders on board?
- What resources will be needed?
- How will they be met?

Table 4.1 Confidence intervals and population size.

Standard	Proportion	Confidence intervals		
	%	95%	75%	60%
100/1000	10	8–13	9–12	9–11
Result				
2/10	20	3–55	6–43	8–38
10/50	20	13–28	**13–28**	**15–26**
20/100	20	13–29	**15–26**	**16–24**
20/1000	20	**18–23**	**19–22**	**19–21**

- What will we audit?
- Who should we involve?
- How should we involve them?
- Where and how do we establish the evidence for best practice?
- What criteria will we use?
- How will we establish the appropriate standards?
- Can those standards be compared externally?
- What to measure?
- How will we measure the variable (criteria)?
- Who will measure the variable (criteria)?
- How and where do we get out data from?
- How will we report our results?
- How should the data be analysed?
- How do we decide if the results are significant?
- How do we judge the success of the audit?
- How can we modify behaviour/clinical practices?
- How often should the audit cycle be repeated?
- Should the results be made public?

Step 1: Deciding what to audit (Modified from Cain & Paula, 2005)

Identifying problems and choosing a topic

Choose a subject that you consider to be important or significant.

Ways of spotting audit topics	Examples
Important clinical events	Dystocia
'Significant events'	Deaths following caesarean section
Farmers complaints	The vet is always late
Observation	No system to avoid stocking of out of date drugs
Observations of staff	Client phone calls not recorded
Use of resources	Would another ultrasound machine be useful

Step 2: Setting criteria and standards

Criteria

An audit criterion is the variable that is being measured – for example, expiry date of drugs in our veterinarian's vehicles.

Setting standards

An audit standard is a minimum level of acceptable performance for that criterion – for example, 100% of drugs the drugs in our veterinarians vehicles should be in date.

Step 3: Collecting data and making measurements

The collection of accurate data and qualitative information is crucial to ensure that any conclusions are valid. Information may be available from computer databases, medical records, questionnaires of farmers, staff and veterinarians. Data collection sheets may have to be devised.

Step 4: Compare results with evidence-based standards

For example:

Criteria	Evidence-based standards	Results
All practice phone calls should be answered within 30 seconds	Minimum 70%	45%
Veterinarians should be less than one hour late	Minimum 95%	90%
All dairy farms to receive a monthly fertility report	Minimum 100%	80%

Before you start planning changes, you need to work out possible reasons why the practice has not met the standard you have set.

Step 5: Implementing change

Introducing change is necessary when the audit results indicate that the processes or outcomes do not meet the standard and actions to remedy identified deficiencies. It is important to emphasise what has been achieved and what is being done well, in addition to what needs to change to correct the deficits.

Changes must be practical

How are you actually going to make the changes? Simply saying 'We've got to do better' will not result in change. You need to think through in detail: what needs to be done? Who is going to do it? When will the change begin? How is the impact going to be monitored?

Keep a written audit record

Keep brief written records of the audit, which should include: the reason for doing the audit; the criteria and standards used; the results; the plans for change; the action taken; and when and whether to repeat the audit.

Step 6: Repeating the cycle

Re-evaluate carefully to ensure that any remedial action has been effective.

General comments

Audits may be seen as a threat, as an unpleasant, time-consuming distraction from day-to-day practice. They can antagonise staff if introduced in an insensitive way, and may give the impression of implied criticism. Audits must assist staff and must be effective at improving animal care and services to farmers. They should not be perceived as a menace or a means of discipline. They must have a clear purpose and must be completed. They should respect the individual skills of staff and create an atmosphere in which mistakes can be admitted without blame.

References and further reading (Evidence-based veterinary medicine)

Badenoch, D. and Heneghan, C. (2002). *Evidence-based Medicine Toolkit*. BMJ Books, London.

Buczinski, S. and Vandeweerd, J. (2012). Evidence Based Veterinary Medicine for the Bovine Veterinarian. *Veterinary Clinics: Food Animal Practice* **28** (1), 1–148.

Cockcroft, P.D. and Holmes, M.A. (2003). *Handbook of Evidence-Based Veterinary Medicine*. Blackwell Publishing.

Department of Health (1998). *A First Class Service*. HMSO, London.

Greenhalagh, T. (2010). *How to Read a Paper: The Basics of Evidence-Based Medicine*, 4th Edition, BMJ Books.

Keene, W.B. (2000) Editorial: towards evidence-based veterinary medicine. *Journal of Veterinary Internal Medicine* **14**, 118–19.

McGovern, D.P.B., Valori, R.M., Summerskill, W.S.M. and Levi, M. (2001). *Key Topic in Evidence-based Medicine*. BIOS Scientific Publications.

Ramey, D.W., Rollin, B.E. (2001). Ethical aspects of proof and 'alternative' therapies. *Journal of American Veterinary Medical Association* **218**, 343–346.

Sackett, D.L. , Straus, S.E., Richardson, S.W. and Rosenberg, W. (2000). *Evidence-Based Medicine: How to Practice and Teach EBM*. Churchill Livingston, Edinburgh.

Schmidt, P.L. (2007). Evidence-based Veterinary Medicine. *Veterinary Clinics of North America: Small Animal Practice* **37**, 3.

Valori, R.M. (2001). The Future of EBM. In: McGovern, D.P.B., Valori, R.M., Summerskill, W.S.M. and Levi, M. (eds). *Key Topics in Evidence-based Medicine*. Bios. Scientific Publications Ltd, Oxford.

References and further reading (Audits)

British Orthoptic Society (2002). *Clinical Audit*, Tavistock House North, Tavistock Square, London.

Cain, P. (2005). Department of General Practice, Royal United Hospital, Bath BA1 3NG http://www.gppro.co.uk/contents.htm.

Department of Health (1998). *A First Class Service*. HMSO, London.

NHS (2002). *Principles for Best Practice in Clinical Audits*. Radcliffe Medical Press Limited, Abingdon, Oxford.

NICE (2002). *Principles for Best Practice in Clinical Audit.* National Institute of Clinical Excellence, London.

Moore, D.A. and Klingborg D.J.(2003). Using clinical audits to identify practitioner learning needs. *Journal of Veterinary Medical Education* **30**(1), 57–61.

Mosedale, P. (1998). Introducing clinical audit to veterinary practice. *In Practice* **20**(1), 40–42.

Rayment, Kim 2002 Clinical audit-a means of evaluating quality. *In Practice* **24**(8), 481–484.

SPVS website: Clinical Audit Resources.

Viner, B. (2005). Clinical audit in veterinary practice – the story so far. *In Practice* **27**, 215–218.

CHAPTER 5

Practice-Based Clinical Research

Mark A. Holmes

Learning objectives

- Be able to identify the qualities of a good research question.
- Understand how the number of subjects needed for a study can be calculated.
- Understand the importance of good case definition in clinical research.
- Understand the characteristics of a good outcome measure in clinical research.
- Understand the study design features that reduce the potential for bias and confounders.
- Appreciate the reason for statistical analysis.
- Understand the structure of a scientific publication and the publishing process.
- Be aware of the REFLECT statement and other publishing guidelines.
- Be aware of the GCP guidelines

Introduction

The development of evidence-based veterinary medicine and its widespread adoption has highlighted the value and importance of good clinical research. Much of the published research is based on cattle populations that are readily accessible to researchers working in universities or research institutes. These animals may not represent the animals that we see in general cattle practice, and husbandry practices may vary considerably from country to country. Clearly, we need the results from clinical research to improve veterinary practice; all veterinary graduates have most of the skills and knowledge needed to undertake clinical research; and the best populations to study are those seen in general practice.

The conclusion is obvious: practice-based clinical research is potentially a colossal resource for the veterinary profession. Practitioners have produced some of the best veterinary clinical research, and these individuals have found clinical research to be a rewarding and fulfilling extension of their clinical work. Although practice-based clinical research can involve a tremendous amount of additional work, and may be frustrating when events outside one's control make it difficult to complete a study, it generates the best evidence for subsequent application to cattle practice.

The key to successful clinical research is meticulous preparation and detailed planning. The biggest mistake we can make is to rush into recruiting subjects and collecting data without having addressed fully the design of the study.

The phases of clinical research are summarised in Figure 5.1. We start with an initial idea, design the study, implement the study and then communicate the results.

The research question and study hypothesis

While the success of a study is largely dependent on hard work and attention to detail in the design phase, starting with a good research question is the essential first step. The translation of an idea, or an interest about a clinical phenomenon, into a research question or a testable hypothesis may present a challenge. Good research asks simple, focused questions. It is better to obtain the answer to a single question concerning a clinical problem, rather than to try to investigate every aspect of a disease in a single study. The research question should also be clinically relevant. The relevance can be assessed by asking, 'would knowing the answer to the question affect our clinical decision making in similar cases?' A checklist covering the characteristics of a good research question can be considered using the mnemonic FINER (see Table 5.1).

After deciding on a research question, we need to turn this into the study hypothesis. This is the first critical design step. If

Bovine Medicine, Third Edition. Edited by Peter D. Cockcroft.

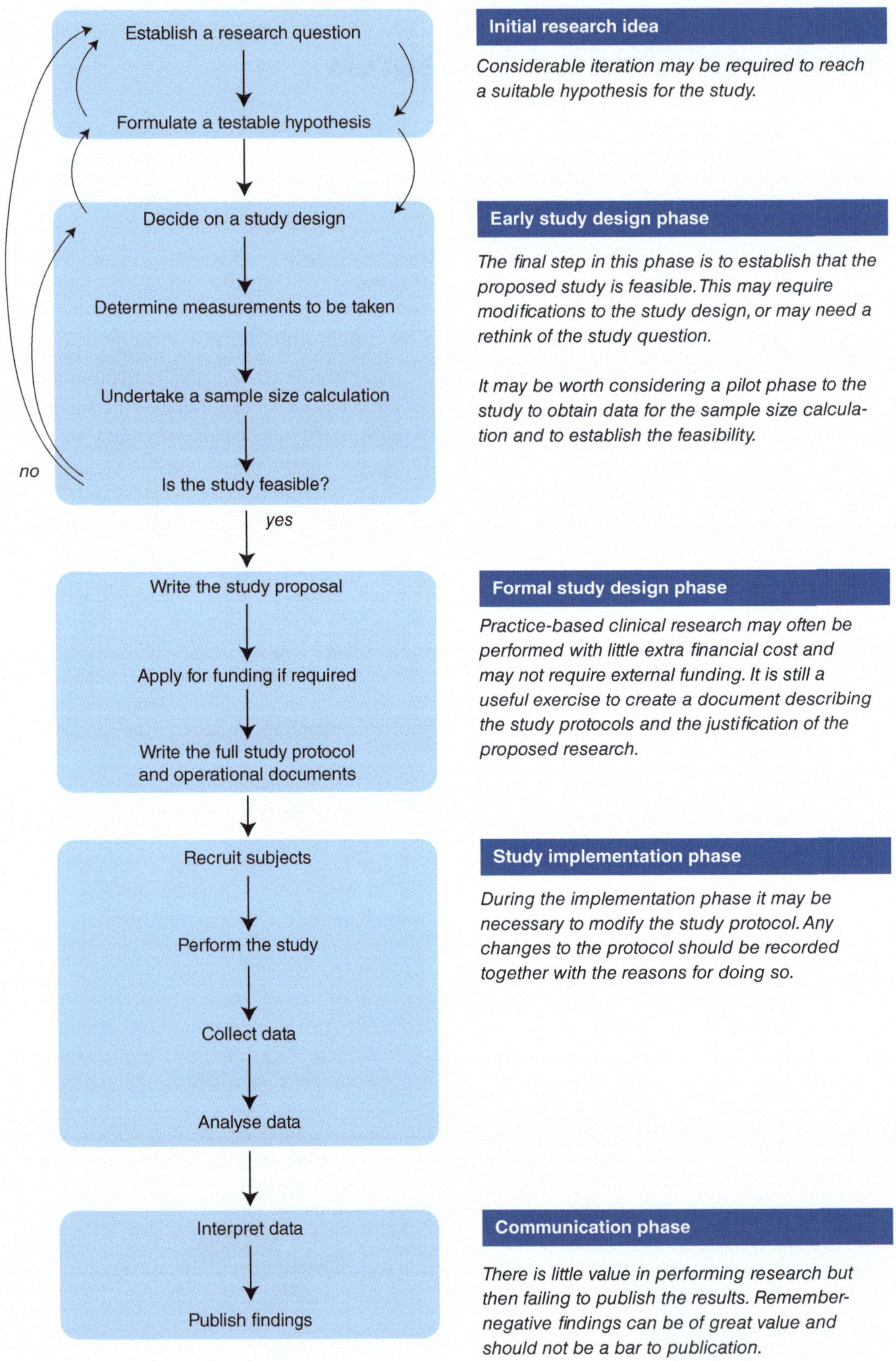

Figure 5.1 A schematic representation of the tasks involved in clinical research studies.

Table 5.1 The FINER checklist for evaluating a potential research question.

Feasibility	Can enough cases be recruited within the planned duration of the study? Is it technically feasible? What are the costs (time or money)?
Interest	There may be a balance between a more feasible narrowly focused question, which may be of less interest to the wider community, and a broader more substantial question that may be more difficult to answer.
Novelty	It is important to remember that any clinical study will have at least one novel feature: it will be studying a different population. One of the weaknesses of veterinary clinical research is the lack of replication of clinical studies, particularly using populations of cattle relevant to general practice. No single study can be expected to find a generally applicable result. Never be afraid to repeat a previously published study. It is both interesting and valuable to attempt to confirm the results of prior published work, and it is an excellent way for inexperienced researchers to start, as much of the design can be obtained from published studies.
Ethics	It is essential to consider ethical and legal issues. Practice-based researchers may have limited access to institutional ethical committees, but it is worth approaching a local university for help. It is also important to give serious consideration about how to ensure that clients are giving informed consent. Simply signing a consent form is not good enough. Investigators need to ensure that owners/stockmen understand the issues and have sufficient opportunity to discuss matters of concern.
Relevance	One way to consider the relevance of a clinical study is to consider how the results of the study can be used. Will knowing the answer make a difference? You may be trying to provide evidence that one particular treatment or diagnostic option is better than another – the results will clearly be relevant. However, even when the study is more narrowly focused, or esoteric, the results may well inform future research by providing data that improves a case definition, determines variation in clinical signs, or provides data from which sample-size calculations can be performed for future studies.

the question was 'Is the use of a teat sealant better than dry cow therapy?' then, in order to formulate the hypothesis, we need to start thinking about the outcome measure that we might use. Should we look at somatic cell counts or incidence of mastitis? Should we look for effects over the whole lactation, or just in the immediate post-partum period? We need a single outcome measure to form the main study hypothesis. This should be feasible to measure and relevant to the clinical scenario that we see in practice.

If our study was focusing on a particular type of mastitis diagnosed by the detection of a pathogen, we might look for that pathogen before and after treatment. In this case, our hypothesis might be: 'That the rate of detection of the pathogen is different in cows receiving teat sealant than those receiving dry cow therapy'. As we progress with the design, we will tightly specify each element in the hypothesis (i.e. the patients, the treatments, the timings and the outcome measures). Once we have a main study hypothesis, we can move on to the design phase.

Study design

The following paragraphs describe some key design issues.

How many patients will be needed?

An important question that needs to be answered is, 'How many subjects do we need?' The easiest way to answer this question is to consult someone with the appropriate statistical knowledge. In order to be able to estimate the number of subjects needed (whether we do it ourselves or ask the statistician), we need three pieces of information:

1 The hypothesis.
2 An estimate of the variability of the outcome measure (e.g. the expected standard deviation or variance of temperatures in healthy cows if temperature was being used as the outcome measure).
3 The smallest difference that if it existed we would want to be able to detect (sometimes called the effect size).

The last of these pieces of information depends on your judgment of clinical usefulness. If we were looking at the efficacy of two treatments using pathogen isolation, we would be expecting a difference in the proportion between the two groups. I might have personal experience of recurrence of infection in about 10% of cases that I treat, and may arbitrarily decide that a treatment that reduced this rate to 8% or less would be worth using. The smaller the difference between the two groups that I want to be able to detect, then the greater the number of subjects I am going to need. Similarly, if the amount of natural variation in the outcome measure is large, then this will increase the number of subjects needed.

What is the case definition?

This is an early design consideration, and is a major consideration on the feasibility of the study. Are we sure that animals we diagnose as having the disease really do have the disease and, similarly, are we sure that any animals in the study described as free of the disease are not falsely negative? What we are trying to achieve is objectivity and reproducibility (i.e. if someone else tried to repeat our study, would their 'cases' be a good representation of our 'cases'?)

Try to think about the 'grey' areas. Most studies rely on a number of inclusion and exclusion criteria to ensure accurate diagnosis and to avoid potential confounders (e.g. concurrent diseases). In veterinary practice-based research, the case definition will often be a compromise between the confidence one has is in the diagnosis and the 'real world situation'. Few practitioners have the luxury of always being able to diagnose definitively the cause of respiratory disease in calves, so a case definition based on clinical signs may be relevant to clinical practice, even if it introduces a level of subjectivity.

Avoiding bias?

It is impossible to avoid letting our own thoughts or beliefs influence our decisions when we are interested in the outcome; either consciously or unconsciously, we introduce bias. We can only avoid this by making it as difficult as possible for us (or others) to affect the outcome being measured. This can be achieved through randomisation and blinding. When patients are randomly assigned to treatment groups, we will avoid the temptation of assigning mild disease or early disease to a particular treatment. If we do not know which treatment was given to a patient, then it will not influence our assessments during the post-treatment examination. Ideally, the blinding should continue throughout the study, with the identification of the groups only being revealed after the statistical analysis has been performed.

What analysis is going to be performed?

One area where practitioners are unlikely to be confident in their knowledge is the statistical analysis of research results. Obtaining statistical advice at an early stage, in order to make some initial decisions about what statistical model or tests are going to be used, is highly advisable. This is closely related to the 'number of subjects needed' calculation. It may save considerable effort, and avoid potential problems, to consider these things at the design stage rather than discover that the study cannot be published when reviewers point out some obvious statistical failure.

If the study hypothesis is that there is a difference between two groups, and the nature of that difference is that of proportion (e.g. proportion of patients with a clinical sign) or of magnitude (e.g. average weight gain of the groups), then there is unlikely to be much difficulty. Complications arise when collecting many different measurements and performing multiple tests. While it is often appropriate to collect additional data to answer secondary questions, good research concentrates on a simple, focused primary question. To make best use of a statistician, it helps to have a well-formed study hypothesis and to be able to provide some sample data. Sample data may be available from existing clinical records, or it may be worthwhile undertaking a pilot study to generate some.

Implementing the study

This should be the most straightforward part of the study, and is often the happiest phase. At first we are carried along by our initial enthusiasm, but this momentum will be rapidly lost if we encounter too many problems that were not anticipated in the design phase. For inexperienced clinical researchers, it may well be worth using the first few cases in a pilot study. This enables procedures to be practised and processes to be tested and refined, and this data may also be of value for a final sample size calculation (as mentioned above).

A frequent observation by clinical researchers is that, once recruitment starts, the number of cases of the disease is less than expected. When considering the feasibility of a study, case recruitment is an important issue. From the outset, it may be worth considering the possibility of recruiting cases from colleagues. You should also base your study duration on a low estimate of the case frequency – there will always be withdrawals or exclusions that affect the number of subjects that can be used in the study. Once again, thorough preparation will reduce the likelihood of major problems in the implementation phase.

Good record-keeping and systematic storage of data greatly simplifies the analysis of results and the writing up of the study. Make sure that backup copies of computer files are made and that original paper documents are filed, so that they can be retrieved if needed. It is also worth remembering that it is far easier to collect data from farmers or stockmen while we are on the farm than to try and obtain it weeks or months later. Have any forms or questionnaires ready and, if necessary, provide any guidance or help that may be needed to fill them in.

Publishing the results of the study

Clinical research is of little value if its results fail to reach those individuals who can best apply those results in their own work. A research project is not complete until the study is written up and published as a paper in a peer-reviewed scientific journal.

Although publication of a journal paper is our aim, there may be value in presenting results at a conference (as a short talk or in poster form) in order to share the knowledge that has been gained. Feedback from conference participants can provide useful guidance about potential flaws in the study that can be addressed in the full publication. Writing up the paper that describes the study can be a daunting task for the inexperienced clinical researcher, but following the style and formats of existing papers describing the results from similar studies is strongly recommended. The conventional paper format is summarised in Table 5.2.

Writing should start with the materials and methods section. Sufficient detail should be included to enable a suitably qualified

Table 5.2 Components of a paper.

Title and authors	Should include the affiliations of the authors (normally their place of work)
Abstract	Summary of the paper (may be structured)
Introduction	Relevant knowledge that preceded the current study. Should normally explain why the question is worth answering.
Materials and methods	A complete description of what was done and how it was done. This must contain sufficient detail to enable the study to be reproduced.
Results	The raw results of the study without any interpretation.
Discussion	Interpreting the results of the study and placing them in the context of our current understanding.
References	Citations are required for any material fact or statement used in the paper for which evidence is not provided by the results of the study.
Declaration of interests	This is required by most clinical journals to indicate sources of financial interest, or other motivation that might not otherwise be evident.

colleague to repeat the study almost identically to your study, using this section for guidance. If you have used diagnostic tests or drugs, you will need to indicate their source (product name and manufacturer). If you have used a method described in another paper, you must provide a citation to that paper.

The next section to write is the results section. As far as possible, a simple description of all the data generated by the study should be included. When numbers of subjects are small, this may include all the data from each subject. When numbers are larger, we may need to summarise the results as averages, with ranges and indications of the variance. It may help to illustrate typical manifestations of individual results, using pictures (e.g. examples of the three types of foot lesion that are included in the data). It is important that the results section should include only the results, and not any interpretation of their meaning or significance.

The discussion section provides the opportunity to put the results into context. What do these results mean, and how should they be applied? It is also important to reflect on the study's strengths and weaknesses. It is important help readers work out how applicable the results are to their own practice. It is generally a good idea to anticipate how a sceptical reviewer may comment, and try to address any potential criticisms from the outset.

Before submitting the paper to a journal, check the submission instructions carefully and adhere to them. Following submission, the journal editor will assign the paper to two (or more) suitably qualified or experienced experts for their comments. The peer-review process can be a disheartening experience both for the newcomer and the experienced author alike. While most of us will happily acknowledge the need for expert scrutiny of scientific papers, it is nonetheless frustrating when one reviewer seems quite happy with your paper while the other seems to find offence in every sentence. The editor should function as a moderator and act upon important flaws in methodology, analysis and interpretation. Such flaws may well lead to rejection. Less important problems, such as failing to include consideration of other important work in the area, or even just differences in opinion, can often be dealt with by some re-writing.

The REFLECT Statement and other reporting guidelines

REFLECT stands for **R**eporting guid**E**lines **F**or randomised contro**L**led trials for liv**E**sto**C**k and food safe**T**y and is an extension of the CONSORT guidelines used in human clinical trial reporting (O'Connor *et al.*, 2010). It is a checklist of items that should be included in the reporting of clinical trials involving animal production, health, and food safety outcomes. The aim of the REFLECT statement is to help authors improve the reporting of livestock trials. Copies of the statement were published in a number of veterinary journals in 2010, and it can be found at www.reflect-statement.org. Although these guidelines are primarily intended to improve the quality of the reporting of clinical trials, they also provide excellent guidance on the best way to design studies and the data that should be collected.

There are a number of other reporting guidelines of relevance to different types of clinical studies. An updated list of these can be found at www.equator-network.org.

VICH Good clinical practice (GCP)

Good clinical practice is the framework upon which standards in clinical research used in drug registration of human pharmaceuticals is based. An equivalent veterinary framework has been incorporated into European and North American veterinary pharmaceutical regulations, called the 'International Cooperation on Harmonisation of Technical Requirements for Registration of Veterinary Medicinal Products' (VICH). VICH is an international program of co-operation between regulatory authorities and the animal health industries of the European Union, Japan and the United States of America that aims to harmonise technical requirements for veterinary medicinal products registration. Australia and New Zealand participate as active observers. An awareness of these guidelines may be of importance if the clinical research being undertaken forms part of the registration of veterinary pharmaceutical products. Relevant documents may be obtained from the VICH website (www.vichsec.org).

Conclusion

Increasing the quantity and quality of practice-based clinical research has enormous potential to improve veterinary practice. It expands the horizons of those who undertake such research, and it provides evidence for what may be the best intervention for the users of the research.

Reference

O'Connor, A.M., Sargeant, J.M., Gardner, I.A. *et al.* (2010). The REFLECT statement: Methods and processes of creating reporting guidelines for randomised controlled trials for livestock and food safety. *Journal of Swine Health and Production* **18**(1), 18–26. (this paper is open access and can be found at http://www.aasv.org/shap/issues/v18n1/v18n1p18.html)

Further reading

Holmes, M.A. and Cockroft, P.D. (2008). *Handbook of Veterinary Clinical Research*. Blackwells Scientific, Oxford.

Petrie, A. and Watson, P. (2006). *Statistics for Veterinary and Animal Science (2nd Edition) Blackwell Publishing*, Oxford.

- www.vichsec.org
- www.equator-network.org
- www.reflect-statemen.org

CHAPTER 6

Expert Witness

Paul Roger

Learning objectives

- To appreciate the role of the expert witness
- To understand the different types of evidence
- To understand what is expected of the expert witness
- To understand how to structure a report
- To appreciate the importance of the statements of truth
- To understand what Independence means
- To understand the importance of establishing and referencing evidence
- To appreciate the importance of changes in the law

Introduction

The invitation to act as an expert witness is not one to be taken lightly. No training course creates this status because, although one may be singularly well qualified and recognised as a specialist backed by years of clinical experience, the only arbiter able to grant expert status is the court before which one appears. The further qualifications held may help to establish expertise, but may not be viewed in the same manner to which peer review would lead us to expect.

This role may be filled by people from a variety of backgrounds, depending on the exact task with which the lawyers perceive they need help. The expert witness is needed to help to explain technical difficulties to the court. The role is to explain, impartially, the facts as they are presented to the court, and to aid the court in understanding technicalities which necessitate expert knowledge. The provision of this witness is complicated further by the complex rules governing evidence, and by the type of case (civil or criminal) in which the involvement is needed.

In the UK, criminal cases are adversarial, so it is of critical importance that the expert is not seen to be partisan. Often, after experts have reviewed the evidence and produced reports, face-to-face meetings may help to resolve issues prior to trial, which can simplify and expedite the trial process by focusing only on those areas of continuing disagreement. In civil procedures, a single joint expert may be used, although each side may retain expert advisors separately. The role of the single joint expert is to produce a report and to answer all questions posed by the court. Experts in both of these situations may find themselves open to examination in court. Where the role is that of adversarial conflict, then examination and cross-examination may be a testing experience.

Types of evidence offered

There are three types of witness which one can be asked to give in court in criminal cases:

1. As a member of the public such as a witness to a car crash.
2. As a professional witness who has attended the scene where the alleged offence has been made or occurred and where the primary role is to gather evidence and report factually on the findings of that evidence.
3. As an expert where a review of the evidence is allowed to explain technical evidence in understandable terms and to offer opinion.

These areas may sometimes overlap, and veterinary surgeons are frequently called as professional witnesses and then asked to convert their evidence into that of an expert by offering opinion. This is dangerous territory, as it is unlikely that the opinion of the professional will seek to undermine his/her own interpretation of his/her findings, and it introduces an unnecessary bias into the evidence before the court. This creates potential problems for the court, as the evidence may be given undue weight by this corroborative construct.

Bovine Medicine, Third Edition. Edited by Peter D. Cockcroft.

What is expected of the expert witness?

First of all, a familiarity and knowledge of the area(s) of technical difficulty involved. This can be evidenced by employment, CPD, further qualifications and recognition, and through publication and delivery of education or information to peer groups (such as specialist species societies or special interest groups). It is an absolute prerequisite and, if this level of expertise does not fall in your remit, then the invitation should be politely declined. Secondly, the expert should have an ability to analyse complex data and also have time to concentrate on the preparation and delivery of a report for those instructing in the case to consider. The lay-out and format of the report needs to be closely structured, and additional information may be added as addenda, rather than kept in the body of the report.

Thirdly, time and patience to deal with other experts instructed, where meetings of experts are deemed advantageous to reducing the time and concentration of the case towards those areas where agreement is not possible. The provision of an evidence base is critical to the production of a balanced report but, frustratingly, this can sometimes be ignored by the judiciary (particularly in welfare offences, where the offences are apparently seen as minor and the strict application of the law may not seem to be the driving force in the continuation of a case).

Where statistical analysis is used, if the expert is not completely at home with the application and understanding of the limitations of particular systems, then this should be stated, so that no misleading or slanted evidence is put before the court. The simple basis for any technical terms or methods used needs to be explained clearly and without obfuscation in order to demonstrate how the court can use the information to come to a clear decision by applying the law to the evidence.

Structuring a report

The report should be clearly titled and should be set out under particular headings germane to the case; an example is given in Figure 6.1.

The pertinent points to consider are:

1 Who is the report for?
2 Who has issued instruction for the creation and delivery of the report?
3 Can the case be summarised?
4 Can the opinion be simply and concisely stated?

The provision of a *Curriculum Vitae* is useful, as well as a summary statement indicating why one is a suitable person to be considered by the court and to be granted expert status.

Immunity from prosecution for misleading clients, or for poor performance, is not part of the present protection offered by the courts to those offering expert witness, so further insurance may be necessary specifically for professional indemnity in this area.

Both the Royal College of Veterinary Surgeons and the British Veterinary Association publish guidelines for those acting as witnesses in legal cases, and these can be accessed through their respective websites. These sites provide convenient and well-summarised advice for those unfamiliar with court procedures and requirements. These guidelines are useful, as instructions may be received from a variety of sources, and the veterinary surgeon supplying an expert witness report must understand the duty of impartiality to the court, despite being retained by one of the two (or more) sides in the case. This can be particularly difficult where witnesses stray beyond the boundaries of their instruction, and where witnesses of fact are asked to provide opinion. It is difficult to see how a witness of fact can offer unbiased opinion in any case, as they would not wish to undermine their evidence which may have been the driving force behind lodging the allegations faced in court.

Statements of truth

Depending on the system, a statement of truth is an integral part of a report and affirms that, although the content may have been discussed with those instructing the expert, the report

Report format

- Title page explaining which case, by who instructed and the author's details
- Index page giving all sections titles and page numbers
- A statement of qualification explaining why the court may consider you as an expert in the area concerned
- Detailed breakdown of the case and evidence and analysis of this under suitable headings
- It is always useful to create a full chronology for the evidence and the particular facts of each case
- It is useful to provide an executive summary at the front of the report
- Following the conclusion, a statement of truth should be included
- Other considerations should include double spacing of lines to allow notes to be made
- Consignment of a full print of the final report signed on each page by the author
- Ensure all documents and evidence on which you have relied to produce the report have been disclosed and are available at court if necessary
- Fully reference any assertions you make where possible and have those references available for the court should there be any wish by the court to view them

Figure 6.1 Format of the report.

Statements of truth

All reports prepared for the courts should conclude with a statement of truth. There is a wealth of guidance on the wording of these and the individual may craft their own or use a standard approach.

Carefully read the statement you are signing.

Examples of the type of wording used are shown below:

1 I understand that my primary duty in producing this report is to the Court and to explain technical evidence in a comprehensible manner, to enable the court to decide this case on the evidence and apply the law.

This statement is true to the very best of my knowledge information and belief. I make it knowing that, if it is tendered in evidence, I shall be liable to prosecution if I have wilfully stated in it anything which, I know to be false or do not believe to be true.

Or

2 1) I understand that my overriding duty is to the Court, both in preparation of reports and the giving of oral evidence.

2) I have provided in my report what I understand from the instructions to be the questions in respect of which my opinion is required.

3) I have done my best to ensure that my report is as complete as I can make it from the information with which I have been presented.

4) I have drawn the attention of the Court to all matters of which I am aware that might adversely affect my opinion of where the information is inadequate.

5) I have neither included nor excluded from the report anything which has been suggested to me by anyone, including those who have instructed me, without forming my own opinion of the matter.

6) Where there is a range of opinion, I have indicated the extent of the range within my report.

7) At the time of writing this report, I consider it to be as complete and accurate as I can make it on the information made available to me. I will notify the Court if, for any reason, I subsequently consider that the report needs correction or qualification.

8) I understand that this report will be evidence that I will give under oath, subject to any correction or quantification, which I may make before swearing to its veracity.

9) I believe that the facts which I state in this report are true, and that the opinions I have expressed are correct.

The final arbiter of the type of statement of truth may be found under guidance from those instructing you or from links through one of the specialist societies. Membership of these would be advised. Rules for civil court procedure include practice directions for expert witnesses and should be consulted before completing any report in this jurisdiction.

Figure 6.2 Statements of truth.

bears the expert's analysis and opinion as the expert's own and has been written by the expert in the expert's own words. It would be an abuse of process if the expert were simply to agree with a statement prepared for them by others and to sign as representing their own opinion. Examples of statements of truth are given in Figure 6.2.

Clarity of instruction

It is useful to ensure that clear, simple, written instructions are supplied and included in the referenced material upon which the report is based. It can help to clarify issues if instructions include specific questions that define key arguments in the case and which may help to simplify the issues before the court.

Meetings of experts can save court time and cost, as well as lessening the undoubtedly stressful experience that a court appearance can bring, by effectively reducing the issues for the court to consider.

Meetings of experts should include a clear note of the agenda for the meeting so that both sides are clear concerning the items that will be discussed. Any summary or joint statement should be issued and signed before the meeting adjourns. These meetings are not privileged, so may be referred to in court or during the trial.

Independence

The expert witness needs to be able to establish his/her independence and to establish his/her credentials to the court. In occasional cases, there may be a challenge to the claimed qualifications presented to the court and documentary evidence of qualifications may be necessary. It is usual that there is notice given if this type of challenge is to be mounted but, occasionally, it is necessary where claims of expertise cannot be matched to particular claims for qualifications or recognition of those qualifications.

Independence may be demonstrated by the expert through the engagement by both prosecution and defence teams over a portfolio of different cases and, equally, by the demonstration of professional expertise in a particular species or area or discipline where this reflects a majority interest in the life of the expert. The expert's continuing and current involvement in the clinical concerns before the court is also a part of the process for establishing the level of credibility afforded to the witness.

Establishing and referencing evidence

When preparing a report, it is a useful discipline to reference factual statements, where possible, and to support opinion, where possible, by reference to the literature. The full reference should be supplied in an appendix to the report so that the court can, if it chooses, inspect and read the relevant sections. This will help to avoid accusations of misinterpretation or bias. It can be frustrating where the tribunal instructs the witness to state his/her own opinion if the referenced material is ignored, and the expert has a duty to explain to the court that, without this level of corroboration, the value of any opinion must be questioned. There are times when the evidential base may be limited and, where this occurs, the expert should acknowledge the limitations put on his/her opinion. Therefore, keep the text as simple as possible, but make sure that it is properly referenced and that the appendices are thoroughly indexed.

Responding to a disclosed report

When responding to a report, it is sensible to avoid entering a slanging match with professional colleagues who may be appearing for other parties involved in the case. It is expected that clinicians offering their services in this area will have a good knowledge of the areas that the case covers. This can be explored by the court when the witness is called. Questioning the expertise or integrity of the other experts appearing before the court is unlikely to gain any favour or weight with the court.

The evidential statements can be compared and differences highlighted. The court may, on occasion, appoint a single joint expert, or ask that a combined expert report is submitted. Where this happens, all parties need to have a clear vision of their evidence and must be prepared to defend their position to demonstrate the areas of disagreement to the court. Joint statements are usually formulated at meetings of experts, so a full agenda and timescale for the production of the statement is needed (and preferably will have been agreed and set by the court).

Appearance in court

The role of the expert in the trial process usually culminates in an appearance at court for the duration of the trial. It may be that the expert is required only to attend to give their evidence, but often the expert is needed by the legal representatives to help them work through the technicalities of the case. Trial work can be irksome, as it is subject to the vagaries of the system, which has a high pressure to deal rapidly and effectively with cases. In the magistrates' court, delays often occur, but they seem to be the norm in the higher courts, as cases are listed for part hearings or reports or sentencing, and are prioritised in front of other cases. This can lead to large amounts of 'dead time' for expert witnesses.

When called to give evidence, the witness will be asked to affirm or give an oath regarding the truthfulness of the evidence to be given, and the usher will ask for an indication of which the expert would rather take. The witness should realise that the court sits in order for the bench to adjudicate on the substance of the case, and he/she should not make any comment on the application of the law, although it may be permissible to explain how the veterinary science base affects the wording involved on the case description (in a criminal case, this would refer to the article(s) under which allegations have been made or charges lodged; in civil cases, it depends on the case alleged).

The questions are put by the advocates to the witness on behalf of the court, and the side instructing you will introduce your evidence and establish your report, which may not be dealt with fully if it has been lodged in the bundle for the court to consider. The other parties have a chance to cross-examine, and the bench can then ask for clarification of any further points after your instructing team has had a chance to redirect your evidence on any points raised in the cross-examination.

The tribunal may then thank you for your evidence and grant you release from the court. This means you may leave, but often the legal team will ask you to remain.

The trial finishes when all the evidence has been heard and the members of the tribunal retire to consider the evidence and formulate a verdict. This may be given at a later date if the trial has been difficult, or it may take place within a reasonable period (bear in mind that this verdict needs to be given with consideration of the evidence and to be written, so that it remains on record). Sentencing then follows the verdict, with whatever mitigation is pleaded being taken into consideration (in criminal cases where probation reports are requested, this may also delay sentencing).

Review

Cases in which veterinary surgeons are likely to be asked to give expert evidence range widely and may stretch your appreciation of areas within which veterinary competence can be demonstrated.

One important aspect of appearing as an expert is to reflect on cases in which the expert has been actively involved. Ethical perception of the behaviour of the expert requires that reflection and justification of the case presented is viewed in terms of the accepted values and mores of society (Mason & McCall Smith, 2006).

In legal cases, it could be argued that critical review forms an integral part of the ethical discourse necessary to justify the expert's action and to guide the expert in the ethical resolution of particular challenges they may face.

It is useful to consider these actions by using the asset of an ethical framework, such as that widely adopted in medical ethics – that is, the four principles (Beauchamp & Childres, 2001).

These are:

1 The principle of respect for individual autonomy (individuals are independent moral agents with a right to choose how to live their own lives).
2 The principle of beneficence (strive to do good where possible).
3 The principle of non-maleficence (avoid doing harm).
4 The principle of justice (treat all fairly – not necessarily equally).

This type of framework can be used to put the actions of the expert into an ethical context and can help to resolve potential dilemmas that will be met in this field of work.

Changes in the law

Our laws change slowly in response to statute, but can be quickly influenced by changes in case law (Brooman and Legge (1996), Radford (2001)). For this reason, it is important to belong to agencies or associations that can help to keep you informed of changes as they occur. Although the expert is not expected to be applying or analysing the law, the expert's own testimony or method of delivery may be challenged by case law (which can change rapidly), even in areas such as the immunity or liability of the witness when giving evidence. Ignorance of the law is not a defence that can be mounted.

A number of societies and associations publish regular newsletters which highlight those areas of change that may be of interest to their members.

Summary

Wilson (1993) expounds that an expert is one who, by reason of education or specialised experience, possesses superior knowledge respecting a subject about which persons having no particular training are incapable of forming an accurate opinion or deducing correct opinion. This implies certain attributes:

- The expert must know the subject.
- The expert should be calm, confident, cooperative and courteous.
- The expert should supply a correct answer structure.
- The expert must act honestly.
- The expert may use notes where permitted and should always examine texts put to them in court.
- The expert must address the jury or tribunal in everyday terminology.
- The expert should not serve on cases in which they do not believe.
- The expert should be able to summarise succinctly.
- The expert should act, speak and dress like an expert.

Rollin (1993) suggests that most people are too busy to consider the moral issues facing their field, and that most scientists fail to recognise that they take moral positions in their day-to-day decisions. In the UK, the RCVS Guide to Professional Conduct shows both morally and explicitly that the highest ethical obligations are laid upon all those working as veterinary surgeons.

Veterinarians, like members of any profession, need to think deeply about the specific role of their profession and what is required of it. In this task, they will need not only to consult amongst themselves, but to be aware of what others are expecting of them and what others are thinking (Legood, 2000, Benson and Rollin, 2004).

Thus, the commitment to prepare and give expert witness requires thought and reflection on ethical as well as scientific and clinical issues, and is a step which should only be taken with this level of due consideration.

The expert witness may find that the ethical and emotional pressures placed on him/her by the circumstances of a case require an approach unlike any experienced in the clinical setting, and that these pressures can be isolating and disturbing and challenge professional skills and knowledge to limits outside their own comfort zones.

It is, however, important that, if there are arguments to be heard, the scientific and clinical basis of these arguments is fully understood by the courts. For that end to be attained, the veterinary expert must continue to be a necessary part of our judicial process.

References

Beauchamp, T. and Childres, (2001). *Principles of biomedical ethics*, 5th Edition). Oxford University Press, Oxford.

Benson, G.J. and Rollin, B.E. (2004). *The Well-Being of Farm Animals (Challenges and Solutions)*. Blackwell Publishing.

Brooman, S. and Legge, D. (1996). *Law relating to Animals*. Cavendish Publishing Ltd.

Legood, G. (2000). Introduction (p.xiv) in Legood, G. (ed.) *Veterinary Ethics – an introduction*. Continuum.

Mason, J.K. and Lawrie, G.T. (2006) *Mason and McCall Smith's Law and Medical Ethics*, 7th Edition. Oxford University Press, Oxford.

Radford, M. (2001). *Animal Welfare Law in Britain*. Oxford University Press, Oxford.

Rollin, B.E. (1993). Animal welfare, science, and value. *Journal of Agricultural and Environmental Ethics* **6**(Supplement 2), 44–50.

Wilson, J.F. (1993). *Law and Ethics of the Veterinary Profession*. Priority Press Ltd.

Further reading

Webster, John (Ed) (2011) *Management and welfare of Farm Animals - The UFAW Farm Handbook*. Wiley-Blackwell.

Further information and useful contacts:

Animal Welfare Science, Ethics and Law Veterinary Association, www.awselva.org.uk

British Cattle Veterinary Association, www.bcva.eu

British Veterinary Association, www.bva.co.uk

British Veterinary Forensic and Law Association, www.veterinaryexpertwitnesses.co.uk

European Board of Veterinary Specialties, www.ebvs.org

Royal College of Veterinary Surgeons, www.rcvs.org.uk

Society of Expert Witnesses, www.sew.org.uk

SECTION II

Practice Management and Professional Skills

CHAPTER 7

Practice Management – Developing a Progressive Veterinary Practice

Peter Orpin

Learning objectives

- Understand the essential requirements to develop a successful practice.
- Appreciate the rate limiting factors.
- Be able to develop a plan for your practice.
- Be able to develop a the business plan.
- Understand the importance of developing the veterinary team.
- Appreciate ways of improving efficiency by organising the veterinary team and pharmacy.
- Be aware of the advantages and disadvantages of different pricing models and health contracts.

Introduction

The purpose of this chapter is to provide guidance to those wishing to develop a progressive veterinary practice, focusing on improving health outcomes while still retaining a profitable business.

Farm practice management has particular challenges. The individual nature of farm veterinarians, combined with lone working, make it particularly difficult to employ the common business principles applied within typical office type environment.

The need, however, to improve the quality of management processes within an increasingly complex and competitive market place, is increasing year on year.

In the last ten years, there have been substantive changes in agriculture and the veterinary profession (deregulation, consolidation, competition, specialisation, increased consumer awareness, etc.) which have created threats and opportunities to farm practitioners worldwide.

Practices that can seek to identify opportunities amongst these changes will thrive.

Essential requirements to develop a successful practice

There are three key steps to developing a progressive farm practice:

- **Define the direction** of the business. What is possible? What is practical? Does the direction meet the needs of the prospective client base?
- **Create a business plan** with SMART targets (Specific, Measurable, Achievable, Realistic and Time-related). Where does the practice see itself in five years' time?
- **Implement practical changes** to make it happen. This requires an effective team approach.

Rate-limiting factors – practice size and structure and livestock density

The ability for the practice to develop may be defined by a number of rate-limiting factors. These will vary according to your own circumstances, but would typically include practice size, stock density, client demands and local competition. The attitude of the partners can also limit progress. The ethos of the business must match the current needs of the farmers and the progressive veterinarian they seek to employ. There has to be a willingness to change the business to meet the demands of a changing environment.

In order for a practice to be successful in delivering an effective preventive medicine-focused practice, the critical mass of committed veterinarians must exceed three veterinarians. In order to provide more specialist services demanded by clients, there must be a sufficient number of veterinarians to provide

Bovine Medicine, Third Edition. Edited by Peter D. Cockcroft.

both emergency and pre-planned work. Once the first opinion practice size falls below this level, it is problematic to provide a decent out-of-hours rota, attend CPD and provide an effective service during periods of holiday and absence (Orpin, 2000, 2003). This factor alone may determine the next steps for the practice. Unless the critical mass of veterinarians is sufficient, the ability to attract and retain veterinary staff will be limited, and the long-term viability of the practice may depend on merger or collaboration for survival.

Livestock density is a key driver for profitability of a practice. As livestock density decreases, the risk of non-chargeable time increases due to driving distances. The ability to provide emergency treatment over larger geographic areas is problematic. The delivery model for practices in these regions depends on longer pre-planned visits and contract arrangements with the practice based on production gains, rather than relying on income from visits to the farm.

Developing a plan for your practice

'*Failing to plan is planning to fail … the only benefit of not planning is avoiding the period of worry before you fail.*' Winston Churchill.

With any change process, establishing where you are now and where the future opportunities may lie is crucial for a business to identify.

The first steps to developing your farm practice are to undertake a SWOT analysis of the farm practice. This teases out the **S**trengths and **W**eaknesses of, **O**pportunities for, and **T**hreats to, the business. This can be performed on a flipchart within the practice. An example SWOT analysis for a typical mixed practice in the UK is illustrated in Figure 7.1.

This effective business technique can help formulate the priorities for the practice and initiate a business planning process, and can at least provide a framework for strategic decision-making.

Developing the business plan

The SWOT analysis is likely to identify a number of opportunities and challenges that will need to be resolved for progress to be achieved (see Figure 7.2).

The opportunities must be 'sanity' checked, to ensure that exploiting the opportunity will be valued by the clients, and be cost-effective for the practice to provide.

Market testing any new idea and seeking opinions from key farmers on future developments is always advisable. The key areas to develop further will be explored further within this chapter.

Creating the expertise pyramid

The services offered by the practice will depend on the level of expertise within the practice and the demands of the client base (see Figure 7.3).

The simplest model is to provide basic clinical services and local pharmacy supply, which typically cross-subsidises the services. However, given the sustained downward pressures on medicine margins, and consumer pressure to reduce the overall usage of medicines, this particular model is not sustainable. There is a compelling need to widen the role of the practice to facilitate a more comprehensive service to the farmer client base.

If there is a repeated requirement for a given procedure (e.g. embryo transfer), then developing in-house expertise and providing this service directly may be the most efficient and effective route. However, if the demands are episodic, outsourcing this work may be more cost-effective

Collaborative working with specialist practices and universities can usefully expand the services offered to the client base. Alternatively, expanding paraprofessional and support services to farmers is an effective way to increase the delivery of healthcare to the farmer and also to improve efficiency of operation of the practice. In many instances, the service provided to the farmer is based on the limitations of the in-house skills and the knowledge/aspirations of the owners. This approach exposes the business to risk, as the farmers will seek to satisfy their needs with other providers, and retaining clinicians becomes challenging within such a limited structure. The focus on developing new services to expand the business is an essential part of practice development.

Strengths	Weaknesses
• Experienced farm veterinarians • Good reputation • Well established • Committed clients	• No new farm partners • Integrating new veterinarians • Lack of expertise with new computer programs • Knowledge gaps • Retention of farm veterinarians
Opportunities	Threats
• Improve marketing • Expand health planning/ preventive programs • Join a buying or marketing group • Consultancy advice • Develop links with consultant practices/universities • Better training and CPD to help retain staff • Gain new clients due to good reputation and service • More services to larger clients • Merge with neighbouring practice	• Declining client numbers • Reduced livestock farmers • Fewer larger clients • Maintaining at least 3 farm veterinarians • Increased competition • Deregulation e.g. TB testing • Changes to medicine regulation • Internet pharmacy • Farm economics • Global competition • Specialist consultancy farm practices

Figure 7.1 A SWOT analysis for a typical mixed practice in the UK.

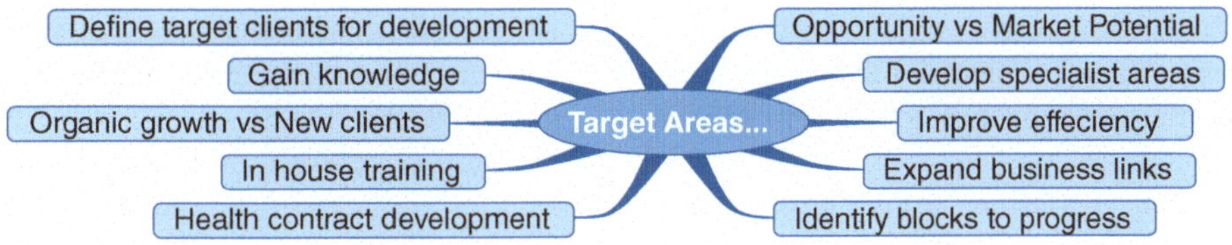

Figure 7.2 Mind map of the target opportunities for an example farm practice.

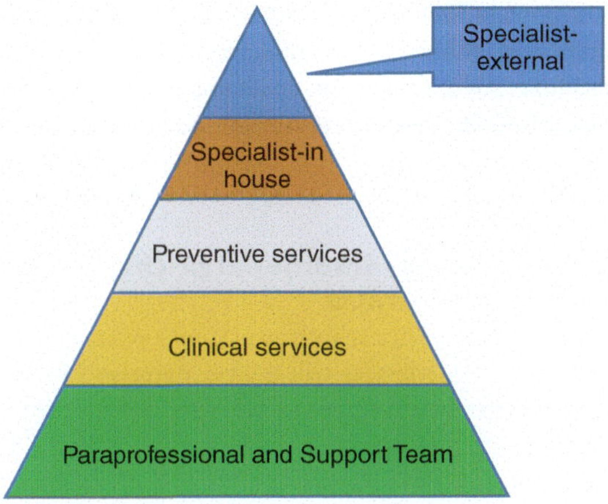

Figure 7.3 The expertise pyramid, illustrating what can be provided by the practice.

Support team - office based	Paraprofessional - farm based
Staff rotas	Body condition scoring
Medicine ordering and supply	Mobility scoring
Stock control (manual or automatic)	Foot trimming
Booking visits, managing the day	Blood testing
Marketing support - newsletters, organising meetings	Veterinary support - surgical
Data management - recording services, report generation	Data gathering
Lab work and lab report management	Paraprofessional tasks delegated from the veterinary team
Invoicing	Project and practice research work
Project and practice research work	Farmer training

Figure 7.4 Potential roles that office-based support team and farm-based paraprofessionals could provide for a veterinary practice.

Developing the veterinary team – veterinarians, support staff and paraprofessionals

The successful farm practice will have a well-organised team to ensure an effective delivery of farm services and medicine supplies to the farmer clients.

Veterinarians are encouraged to focus on providing expertise to the clients. Any simple task or procedure should be delegated to the support or paraprofessional team. The potential roles which can be provided by the support team are shown in Figure 7.4.

In areas of high stock density within larger practices, the development of a paraprofessional team is possible. Farmers committing to higher levels of health monitoring and care will value a more comprehensive practice service, which would include the services delivered by a paraprofessional employed by the practice. In smaller practices, part-time support staff may be used or, as an alternative, closer relations could be developed between the practice and independently employed paraprofessionals.

Lack of time is often cited as the reason why busy clinicians fail to explore opportunities. Closer analysis reveals that reluctance to delegate and train support staff is the root cause of the problem. Developing a cohesive practice team, with clearly defined roles and responsibilities, is the key to success.

Integrating younger veterinarians within the practice team is a crucial step which many practices find problematic. A 'buddy' system, where the senior 'lead' vet providing the pre-planned work to the farm has a junior 'follower' vet, who is responsible for the farm during times of absence or holiday, is a useful method of integrating the younger veterinarians into the higher level work.

Practices that embrace the development of a strong support team are best placed to expand their businesses, as they are more likely to implement any opportunities identified.

Improving efficiency – organising the veterinary team

The primary objective is to ensure that the fee generators are kept fully occupied, with minimal wasted time during the day. The veterinary team comprise the largest fixed cost within the farm practice, and optimising their utilisation will drive the business forward.

The objective should be to achieve over four hours of chargeable work per vet per day for a dedicated farm vet. This will only be achieved with planning and organisation. Increasingly, the cow contact time will reduce with the advent of technological and knowledge improvements. The overall fee charged for veterinary services must, therefore, include time spent by the veterinarian providing analysis, training and consultancy for the farmer.

Achieving this goal requires:

- Trained dedicated support staff which have the responsibility of organising the veterinary diaries.

- An effective practice management system which clearly illustrates and organises the work allocation. Many computer-based systems will effectively manage repeat appointments automatically.
- A fee system which encourages farmers to pre-book veterinary work (discounted visits/contract arrangements) and charges realistically for emergency work.
- Mobile communication systems which link the team together – smartphones allowing work to be allocated by voice, text and email.
- Gaining acceptance from the veterinary team that they will be managed by the support staff and accept centralised management!

Improving efficiency – the pharmacy

Medicine supply is a key function within a farm animal practice in most regions of the world, and is often the largest variable cost for a farm veterinary practice. In some regions, the legal process has diverted medicine supply from the practice, and medicines are supplied from independent pharmacies.

In the last ten years, the medicine to fee ratio for typical dairy farm practices in the United Kingdom has changed from over 2 : 1 to nearer 1 : 1. This has been driven by the advent of internet pharmacies, larger practices with greater purchasing power, and an increase in fees to compensate for reduced medicine margins.

The key requirements for delivering an efficient practice pharmacy are:

- A computerised system for accurate pricing, providing full traceability and recording of medicines from practice to farm.
- A system for accurately defining the net purchase and sale price for each medicine. This can be challenging when there may be a multiplicity of discounts offered by the wholesaler and supplier. A pricing system based on net margins (rather than mark-up) for all products is essential.
- A charging system which ensures prompt payment, using direct debit charging, cash payments, discounts for early payment and penalties for late payment, is crucial to ensure that cash flow targets are met.
- A storage area which meets the regulatory requirements and also facilitates usage of medicines in date order (i.e. the oldest product is used first to avoid out-of-date stock).
- An efficient stock tracking system to ensure the correct stock levels at all times and stock nearing out of date is identified in the pharmacy and vehicles.
- Appropriate refrigeration and temperature management of all areas within the pharmacy.
- Appropriately trained and qualified staff to ensure all legal requirements are met with dispensing and supply.
- An effective system to ensure that stock supplied on farm is correctly billed at the time, using dockets or point of sale computers/tablets.
- Monitoring of stock levels and invoices from veterinarians vehicles to ensure stock is not habitually supplied without an invoice.
- Correct labelling and instructions (verbal and written) for all medicines supplied.

The responsibilities are real, rather than nominal, with a significant cost attributable to the management of medicines.

Alternative mechanisms of medicine supply involve pre-ordering of medicines via prescription and centralised dispensing and delivery from an internet or local pharmacy. This removes the burden of responsibility from the practice.

Veterinary pricing - traditional pricing models versus health contracts

The pricing of any service is both an art and a science. If the pricing is correct, your services will deliver perceived value to the client and will not be a barrier for engagement with the practice. Pricing, however, must generate advantages for both the practice and the client, for it to be a success. The use of creative pricing models to encourage the type of work which is more profitable and efficient for both farmer and practice, such as pre-planned visits, routine fertility work or visits booked in by 9.30 am, can substantively help the practice. Equally, ensuring that the fee and medicine margins are appropriate for the target client base is essential. If the mission is to attract or retain larger dairy clients, then the pricing system must be competitive and attractive to these clients.

Strategic discounts may be offered based on prompt or direct debit payment, or on greater commitment to purchasing services or products from the practice. Similarly, providing clear systems for penalising late payment is good business practice.

The pricing of veterinary work has undergone significant changes in the last ten years. There has been a significant increase in fees, in return for lower margins on medicines, in response to increased competition for medicine supply.

The shift towards a fee-based model, following a more transparent system, has been welcomed by the sectors which used the largest amounts of medicines (dairy, intensive beef). The challenge with increased fees, however, is that they make some procedures traditionally performed by veterinarians, less cost-effective and, also, make slower, less experienced veterinarians less attractive to the farmer.

The pricing of veterinary work is largely based on the 'activity based ambulatory model', whereupon an action is priced (e.g. visit, examination, time or supply of medicine). The more

	Traditional model based on 40% margin on medicines	Traditional model plus monthly fee for advice/ data management	Health Contract 20% margin on medicines and pence per litre charging
Fees (Visits and Time)	£3,000	£3,000	0.4ppl
Medicines	£7,000	£6,000*	£5,600**
Advice	Inclusive	£500	0.05ppl
Meetings	Inclusive	£250	inclusive
Training	Inclusive	£250	inclusive
Data management/ monitoring	Not provided	£500	0.05ppl
Paraprofessional services			0.05ppl
Total income	£10,000	£10,500	£11,100
Estimated profit contribution			

[a] *medicine supply may fall due to advice or improved disease control
[b] **overall use of preventive medicines may increase due to lower overall cost to farmer

Figure 7.5 Potential pricing model for a 130 cow herd supplying 1 million litres of milk per annum, based on traditional, traditional plus advice contract, and full pence per litre health contract.

activities the farmer purchases, the busier the veterinary practice becomes. The traditional model favours disease treatments or activity, but not necessarily health prevention and control.

Alternative models for pricing, based on contractual arrangements between veterinarian and farmer, have developed. These are inclusive arrangements, based on an agreed level of inputs for an agreed price or services and medicine margin. The model can be developed further to include a payment which is linked to productivity, such as the pence per litre charging system (Dobbs, 2001). If the total litres of milk sold increases, due to improvements in the health and productivity of the herd, the veterinary bill increases in line with this increase. The opposite equally applies. The different models are illustrated in Figure 7.5.

The traditional pricing model does not accurately reflect the services provided. Increasingly, more practices are becoming involved in more comprehensive advice and data management, and these cannot simply be included as 'part of the service'. Greater transparency is required, with an ability to charge for the 'health' or advisory component of veterinary practice.

This can be further developed with the pence per litre pricing model. Linking fees to the litres of milk sold allows the veterinary practice to share in the success of the farm, as well as to reduce the overall margin on medicines. The advantages and disadvantages of traditional, traditional plus advice contract, and full pence per litre contract, are shown in Figure 7.6.

Summary

The practice organisation and structure is central to providing a progressive veterinary service within an increasingly

	Traditional – high margin medicines/ lower fees	Traditional plus advice	Health contract Pence per litre model
Advantages	• familiar • popular with smaller or average farmers dependent on emergency services • penalises the larger medicine using farmers • lower fees facilitating more work	• Similar advantages to traditional fee structure with additional ability to add on a monthly payment for advice • useful model for beef breeding herds and smaller farmers not wishing to adopt a full contract	• fixed monthly payment from farmer • practice shares in reward for improved health • lower medicine margins possible • simplifies budgeting for farmer
Disadvantages	• relies on cross subsidies between and within farmers • higher margins on medicines • risk of losing larger key clients • improving health through advice reduces income for the practice	• no ability to reduce medicine margins unless fees and monthly fees are increased to compensate for reduction	• vet practice carries the risk that farmer may not follow advice and become exposed to increased workload for same pay • traditional farmers may fear change and refuse to contract to the practice

Figure 7.6 The advantages and disadvantages of traditional, traditional plus advice contract and full pence per litre contract.

competitive environment. Developing a clear plan for the practice, combined with effective leadership and vision, will allow the practice to develop and expand. An effective 'team approach' is required, with everyone playing to their strengths. This will only be achieved with a culture of development and delegation.

Acknowledgements

To my colleagues within the Park Vet Group, Matt Dobbs, Westpoint Veterinary Services, Dick Sibley, Westridge Veterinary Group and Peter Gripper, Anval.

References

Dobbs. M. (2001). *Role of the specialist vet in production advice, monitoring performance and welfare.* Nuffield Scholarship.

Orpin, P.G. (2000). The future of cattle practice: Possible solutions. *Cattle Practice* **8**, 2.

Orpin, P.G. (2003). Farm practice in areas of low stock density: a blueprint for survival. *In Practice* **25**, 161–165.

CHAPTER 8

Veterinary Leadership and Communication Skills

Michelle McArthur and Adele Feakes

Learning objectives

- Appreciate the leadership roles of the bovine practitioner.
- Appreciate why effective communication is important.
- Understand the process of effective communication.
- Appreciate the three components of gathering information: obtain background information; determine the presenting problem; and discern the client perspective.
- Appreciate the value of written and supplementary communication tools.

Leadership and individualised communication strategies

This chapter will highlight the leadership skills required of the bovine veterinarian. It will also outline an approach to enhance communication with farmers using the Calgary-Cambridge Guides (Kurtz *et al.*, 2003) as a tool. The central tenet of this chapter is the importance of discerning the farming client's perspective and to achieve an individualised approach whether the consultation is curative, advisory or at industry level. It focuses on one technique that will help elicit farmers' perspectives and provide readers with a skill which can be implemented immediately. Such a focus does not imply that it is the only, or the most important, clinical communication technique, but that this particular skill should form part of the practitioner's necessary communication skill set.

All bovine veterinarians are leaders

As professionals, veterinarians are seen by the public as experts in their area – skilled, trained, qualified and leaders. The core expertise of bovine veterinarians is technical proficiency and diagnostic/clinical reasoning ability. However, leadership and management skills are required as adjuncts to diagnostic/clinical reasoning ability (Kristensen & Enevoldsen 2008; Lloyd *et al.* 2005; Lloyd & Walsh 2002).

Veterinarians in bovine medicine undertake leadership roles in a variety of settings, such as:

1 Curative and/or advisory practitioners.
2 Facilitators of regional farm focus groups.
3 Teachers (of farmers or students).
4 Industry or aid organisations.
5 Government or regulatory positions.

In summary, bovine veterinarians assume positions of leadership in all forums of their professional lives.

Bovine veterinarian leadership skills

Bovine veterinarians routinely exemplify leadership skills: they manage, effect, take control, guide, support, strategise and motivate others. Taken together, such leadership skills can be combined as the 'ability to influence process' (Wustenberg, 2006) and, more broadly, the ability to motivate and influence strategy. The ability to influence process depends on the veterinarian's skill in gaining the decision-maker's trust and then communicating the technical and scientific content to the client (Wustenberg, 2006). Therefore, in order to influence process, the ability to build relationships with decision-makers (farming clients), and develop an effective communication skill set, are vital to success. The ability to influence process in more formal communication environments, such as corporate or regulatory activities, is also fundamental to the profession's ability to remain relevant.

Lloyd *et al.* (2005) outlined key leadership skills for veterinarians, including the ability to:

- Develop a clear vision of the future;
- Communicate that vision in a meaningful way;
- Establish trust; and
- Commit oneself to lifelong personal and professional learning.

Accordingly, developing leadership skills, based on good communication and interpersonal skills, is vital to the success of the

Bovine Medicine, Third Edition. Edited by Peter D. Cockcroft.

bovine practitioner. Being effective at the farm level or industry level is essentially the ability to combine clinical reasoning/diagnostic skills with a suite of leadership skills underpinned by skilled communication ability.

Effective communication and bovine veterinarians

The ability to demonstrate effective communication skills is recognised as a core skill for veterinary practitioners. This recognition ranges from the pivotal studies espousing the need for a greater focus on the development of veterinarian's communication skills (Pritchard 1989; Cron *et al.*, 2000), both in practitioners (Mellanby *et al.*, 2011) and veterinary students (Shaw & Ihle, 2006), clearly reporting the importance of such skills in clinical practice. Effective communication is important across all realms of veterinary medicine and while the setting, content and emphasis may change, the required skills and the potential positive sequelae do not.

The studies examining clinical communication and its effects in veterinary medicine are few, but revealing. Similar to the expansive literature in wider healthcare communication research, effective communication skills are related to adherence (Kanji *et al.*, 2012), veterinarian satisfaction (Shaw *et al.*, 2012) and client satisfaction (Coe *et al.*, 2008). These are preliminary studies and involve companion animal patients and their owners but, nevertheless, they do shed light on important clinical and service indicators associated with effective communication in veterinary medicine.

There is scant literature specifically examining the veterinarian's communication skills in large animal medicine. However, studies have examined farmer's attitudes and have found that they value good communication skills in their veterinarian (Chapman *et al.*, 1991). Other studies have appraised farmers' mindsets, categorised farmers accordingly, then tailored specific communication strategies for each identified group (Jansen *et al.*, 2010).

The communication strategies outlined by (Jansen *et al.*, 2010) provide a useful starting point when considering how to adopt a more individualised approach. However, it is important to note that these suggested communication strategies are not intended for individuals, but for members of that specific group. Each member of the group has a unique mindset or perspective that needs to be appreciated and then addressed by the veterinarian, in order to establish a true partnership approach. Therefore, the ideal approach implements fully individualised communication strategies and skills targeted at the particular needs, issues or goal of the farming client.

Effective individualised communication process

Individualising communication approaches requires an understanding of the components of efficient and accurate communication. Effective communication means more than just talking; it involves content, process and perceptual skills (Silverman *et al.*, 2005; see Figure 8.1.)

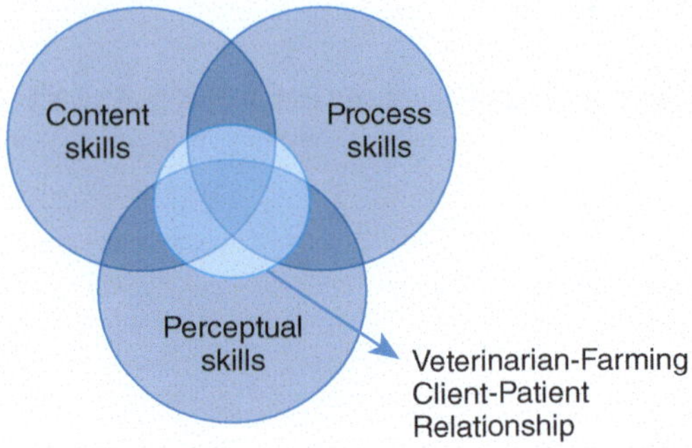

Figure 8.1 Interdependence of the skills of effective communication.

- The first – content skills – relates to the actual content of the information gathered and provided, or the 'what is said' of communication. This entails the medical, preventative or technical information as well as any relevant, the lifestyle-social information.
- The second – process skills – are the 'how' of communication, in terms of how the veterinarian communicates with the farmer, specifically the manner of data gathering and provision of information, relationship building and structuring an efficient consultation. Process skills are constant across settings, while the content and focus changes.
- Third, perceptual skills are associated with thoughts and feelings related to self- and other-awareness. This also includes the individual's thought processes around clinical reasoning.

The three skills outlined above are interdependent, lie at the heart of the veterinarian-client-patient relationship and are key attributes of effective leadership.

Process skills are often packaged in consultation models in order to provide a framework for effective interactions. There are many such published and widely used models, but of particular focus in this chapter are the Calgary-Cambridge Guides (Kurtz *et al.*, 2003). These guides are used extensively in healthcare communication training, and each of its process skills are evidence-based in increasing the effectiveness, accuracy and supportiveness during the consultation (see Figure 8.2).

Importantly, in any consultation, in any setting, many of these skills will be evident, but an effective consultation does not mean all listed Calgary-Cambridge Guides skills are used, nor does it mean that each step of the process is followed. It has been suggested that the Calgary-Cambridge Guides model is only useful for curative consultations, not an advisory role (Kleen *et al.*, 2011). Such a stance predominantly focuses on the content skills of the consultation, but not the generic process skills inherent to all interactions, nor the perceptual skills.

The Calgary-Cambridge Guides are used widely in training veterinary medicine students (Adams & Kurtz, 2006), and the authors believe they demonstrate applicability across various

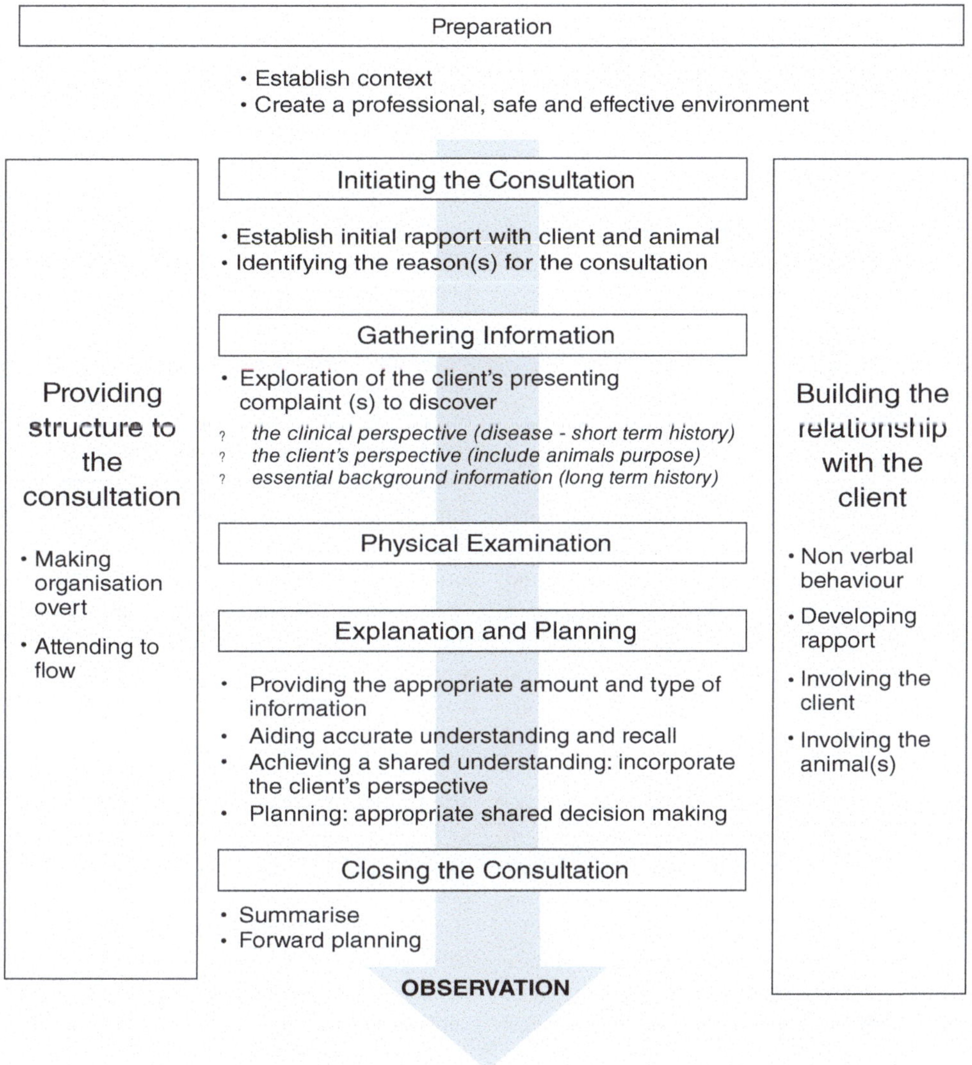

Figure 8.2 The expanded Calgary-Cambridge Guides. Reproduced with permission of Lippincott Williams & Wilkins.

settings and consultation types – a view shared by Adams & Coe (2011). The guides are a tool which has been approved and adapted for use in veterinary medicine (Radford *et al.*, 2006), with the addition of continued observation of the patient/s. However, other consultation models emphasising process skills would be equally applicable.

The Calgary-Cambridge Guides consist of simple steps that can act as a guide for any consultation type. While it is not within the scope of this chapter to discuss each of these skills, nor each step, it is suggested that readers consult Radford *et al.* (2006) for a review of the adapted Calgary-Cambridge Guides for veterinary medicine. Additionally, for a comprehensive review of the literature underpinning the skills listed in these guides, see Silverman *et al.*, (2005). Also, see Shaw (2006) for an in-depth discussion and review of the micro-skills underpinning effective communication in veterinary medicine. For the purposes of this chapter, an important concept emphasised in the Calgary-Cambridge Guides will be reviewed with a focus on obtaining the farmer's perspective when gathering information to achieve an individualised approach to explanation and planning with the farmer.

Gathering information: three components

The two traditional components: obtaining background information and the presenting problem

Traditionally, gathering information in a consultation has focused on two predominant areas: the animal's/herd's presenting

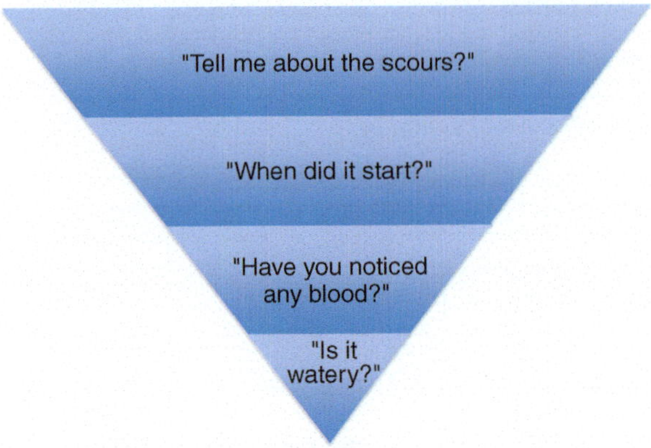

Figure 8.3 A funnel approach to gathering information.

problem and past history/husbandry (See Figure 8.2). Veterinarians are well trained to take such a history. Skills used to elicit such information have also traditionally centred around employing closed-ended questions (Shaw *et al.*, 2004b; McCann & Fitzgerald, 2013). While these types of questions are effective for the clinician gathering information that fits with clinical decision-making models, they can also result in failure of pertinent information coming to light. Overuse of closed-ended questions may also limit client participation in the consultation and can impact rapport (Boyle *et al.*, 2005). Instead, the asking of open-ended questions at the outset and at each line of enquiry is often more efficient while, at the same time, builds the relationship with the farmer as they begin to discuss the issues/needs from their perspective.

A 'funnel approach' is recommended (Kurtz *et al*, 2003; see Figure 8.3). Simple broad open-ended questions begin the gathering information phase, followed up with targeted open-ended questions. At this point, specific closed-ended questions should be used to ensure the veterinarian has all the information they require. Utilising such an approach helps to meet the needs of both veterinarian and farmer.

Interestingly, Shaw *et al.* (2004b) found that open-ended questions are an under-utilised skill, suggested by their absence in 25% of consultations in a companion animal sample. To demonstrate one benefit of the use of open-ended solicitations of client concerns at the outset in companion animal consultations, clients were noted to express significantly more concerns (Dysart *et al.*, 2011). Expressing concerns at the outset limits the likelihood of late-arising issues which can derail the consultation and reduce efficiency. It also permits detailed information gathering and inclusion of the client. Parallel positive outcomes are likely when such purposeful questioning is applied in bovine consultations.

The remainder of this chapter will focus on the skill of using open-ended questions to achieve an individualised approach in any consultation format.

The third component: the client perspective – an individualised approach

There is a third component of the information gathering process; understanding the client's perspective (Silverman *et al.*, 2005; see Figure 8.2). Gaining an understanding of the client's perspective is a central feature of relationship-centred care (Beach & Inui, 2006). Relationship-centred care in veterinary medicine could be viewed as a collaborative partnership between veterinarian and farmer to meet the healthcare needs of the animal(s) (Shaw *et al.*, 2004a). It is a style of communication that has been associated with increased adherence in veterinary medicine (Kanji *et al.*, 2012). The farmer has expectations, opinions, thoughts and an appreciation of their own capacities and limitations related to the management and prospects of their animal(s). Furthermore, farmers have their own personal and professional expertise of farming practice and relationship with the animals on the farm. Additionally, there is a culture within which farmers work and, on an individual level, each farmer has a self-identity or an appraisal of how they see themselves and their values.

These are all elements of the farmer's (client's) perspective. The farmer's perspective is the third piece of the information-gathering process which may be overlooked or gathered incidentally rather than intentionally. Anecdotally, veterinarians discover the value of eliciting this information through experience. A more effective consultation style could be attained through intentional use of this third and integral component of the information-gathering phase and, ultimately, a relationship-centred approach.

Interestingly, there seems to be a misalignment between veterinarians' and farmers' beliefs. A Danish study found that veterinarians perceived that farmers place primary importance on productivity and financial performance, in contrast to farmers' reported desires to enhance teamwork and animal welfare (Kristensen & Enevoldsen, 2008). Farmers preferred a team-based approach, working towards common goals and ambitions – these are both elements of the farmer's perspective. Accordingly, a focus on productivity and profitability alone may not meet the expectations of the farmer, and thus may potentially limit the farmer-veterinarian relationship and uptake of best-practice recommendations. It is therefore essential that, in all consultations, the farmer's perspective is elicited to ensure alignment (Jansen & Lam, 2012), and this should occur during the early phase of the consultation.

The individualised approach: the farmer is an expert, too

Farmers/clients have a great deal of knowledge which can help the veterinarian ensure accuracy of diagnosis and/or effectiveness of herd management problem-solving or advice, and also help in the later stages of the consultation. Studies have shown that farmers value and seek proactive veterinarians who draw on their expertise in medicine and heath management, to identify opportunities for enhancement on the farm (Hall & Wapenaar, 2012). While the bovine farming client has much expertise in their particular area of cattle production and husbandry (e.g. dairy, beef, feedlot) at industry level, as well as being expert in the day-to-day functioning of the particular farm.

Regardless of the extent and type of proficiency, recognising that the farmer has knowledge which the veterinarian cannot fully know is an important and, in many respects, equalising premise; the consultation becomes a meeting of experts (Tuckett *et al.*, 1985). Such a view leads to a natural partnership, in so much as the veterinarian needs the farmer's expertise as much as the farmer requires the veterinarian in order to achieve the best possible outcomes for the animals in their care. This premise is another element of a relationship-centred style of communication. It is also an example of a perceptual skill that can be communicated explicitly to the farmer, which Kristensen & Jakobsen (2011) believe helps validate the positive self-identity of the farmer.

The individualised approach: the role of the animal/s on the farm

The human-animal relationship, in many respects, drives the need for effective communication in veterinary medicine. Furthermore, an appreciation of the role of the animal in the life of the farmer is vital for working in partnership and for tailoring treatment and management strategies. Veterinarians working with farmers will be aware of the relationships that farmers can, and do, develop with their livestock. Farmers develop relationships with their herds that can be influenced by the size, purpose and husbandry practices of the farm. Specifically, they can be influenced by the frequency and intensity of contact, and they vary between and within species (Bock *et al.*, 2007).

In a study of farmers' reported attachment to their animals, Bock *et al.* (2007) found that bovine farmers generally felt closer to their cows and likened them to family members and friends, more so than do pig and poultry farmers. The study found that the attachment ranged from very close to loose and, even among those who described a detached relationship, they still positively regarded the herd over and above their economic potential. Given the diversity of reported relationships between farmers and their cattle, the research suggests that it is important to understand this relationship, in order to best work in partnership with farmers and to appreciate their perspective particularly in terms of their goals, expectations and needs.

Over and above those already mentioned, there are multiple underlying reasons why farmers develop relationships with their herd. Farmers like being close to their animals, and it is a source of satisfaction (Seabrook & Wilkinson, 2000). Being a well-regarded farmer is characterised by taking good care of animals (Dockes & Kling Eveillard, 2006), and this caretaking is important even when economic reasons are the primary motivator (Bock *et al.*, 2007). Being a good farmer forms part of their self-identity. Furthermore, heritage or the personal history of the farmer is an important aspect of the human-animal relationship on the farm. When breeding from old bloodlines, farm, animal and family become connected (Bock *et al.*, 2007).

An evaluation of farmers' attitudes suggested that one group of farmers expected a correlation between animal welfare and herd health with their own subjective wellbeing, and this would be achieved by surrounding themselves with healthy cows (Kristensen & Enevoldsen, 2008). This finding further suggests that farmers can, and do, develop relationships with their herds that may be related to their self-identity and wellbeing. Without having an understanding of the role/s of the animals in the farmer's life, it is difficult to tailor treatment and management approaches that fit with the farmer's perspective and, thereby, meet their goals.

In order to understand the role of the animals in the farmer's life, again the use of open-ended questions is indicated: 'Tell me about the main purpose of the farm?' 'What outcomes are most important for you on your farm?' 'What are your goals for the farm?'

Explanation and planning: connecting it to the farmer's perspective

The client perspective: an integrated, individualised approach

By the explanation and planning phase of the consultation (see Figure 8.2), the bovine veterinarian should have some understanding of the farmer's motivations, expectations, opinions, values, capacity and/or limitations. Therefore, the medical condition or health strategy can be viewed in light of the entire farm dynamic and, as such, treatment and management approaches can be individually tailored and based on mutual understanding. In an analysis of companion animal consultations, Kanji *et al.* (2012) found that eliciting the client's perspective would likely increase adherence. Furthermore, they reported that aligning clinical recommendations with the previously elicited client's expectations and needs is thought to enhance client adherence. Incorporation of the farmer's perspective during this phase of the consultation will likely harness factors which facilitate adherence.

The Health Belief Model is a well-regarded social cognition model that attempts to explain and predict acceptance of healthcare recommendations (Rosenstock, 1974). It is useful to consider these predictors in the context of understanding the farmer's perspective and how this may relate to adherence. The Health Belief Model involves the following dimensions, with associated open-ended soliciting questions, as they might apply to farmers.

- *Perceived Susceptibility*. Perception of vulnerability or risk of being impacted by a health condition: 'How concerned are you about … '.
- *Perceived Severity*. Perception of the seriousness of contracting, or not treating, a condition as it relates to clinical and social issues: 'What's your sense of the impact on your farm if we don't treat this condition/implement this preventative measure?'
- *Perceived Benefits*. Perception of feasibility and effectiveness of recommended strategies: 'You have a busy farm. How feasible is it to implement these recommendations?' 'How can we work together to achieve this?'
- *Perceived Barriers*. Perception of the cost-benefit of the health related action; this requires a review of the negative consequences of action such as expense, side effects and time: 'What might make it difficult for you to implement this?'

Finally, there is a hypothesised factor which may call farmers to action and stimulate the decision-making process. The factor is either an internal (e.g. symptoms) or external (e.g. mass media, discussions with other farmers) cue, and the external cue is of particular relevance to veterinarians, given the mass media promotion of many health-related/promoting strategies in the farming community. Thus, after exposure to external cues, farmers may be ready to discuss such health strategies and require a discussion of:

1 the perceived risks and severity;
2 the perceived benefits and barriers.

It is unlikely that farmers will take action unless both conditions are met (Jansen *et al*, 2010). Moreover, Kristensen & Enevoldsen (2008) recommended that veterinarians understand and integrate individual differences as promoting factors for change. Therefore, inviting farmers to ask questions, to seek clarification or to express doubts or concerns, encourages active participation.

An integrated, individualised approach: the farmer is an expert, too

Farmers have expertise in knowing their livestock and their farming practices, and they may be quite knowledgeable about medical conditions. On the other hand, they may be misinformed, have an incomplete understanding, or may have never heard of certain conditions or practices. Their expertise may have breadth but not depth. To assume the expertise of the farmer and either give them too little information or too detailed information are equally problematic. It is thus vital that information is tailored to the knowledge base of the individual farmer (see Figure 8.2), which is best explicitly elicited. Useful questions can include: 'I don't know how much you know about … Tell me your understanding of this condition?' 'There is a lot of information out there about mastitis. How much information would you like?' 'What additional information do you need?' 'How familiar are you with this condition?'

Having an understanding of the farmer's knowledge base, another element of the farmer's perspective, gives the bovine veterinarian a starting point for the treatment plan and management discussions. Once into the explanation and planning phase of service delivery, confirming or re-checking the expertise of the farmer and underlying knowledge base is equally important. Often, closed-ended questions such as 'Do you understand?' or 'Does that make sense?' are asked, and these do serve as a check-in with the client. This also enables the information to be provided in more manageable amounts (a skill listed in the Calgary-Cambridge Guides as 'chunk 'n' check'). However, a more useful check-in statement is open-ended (e.g. 'How do you feel about this?'), providing the farmer with an opportunity to elaborate and potentially give further perspectives.

Given the complexity and range of information that veterinarians can provide to farmers, multiple methods of communicating may be indicated. Hall & Wapenaar (2012) found, in their study investigating discussions between farmers and veterinarians, that veterinarians overestimated the effectiveness of conversations in many areas of herd health management. The authors note that veterinarians may well be addressing each area, but the amount and, indeed, technical nature of information, may benefit from or require supplemental communication strategies.

Written and supplementary communication tools

The use of models, pamphlets, DVDs, links to online materials, reports and summarising letters, are also aids to the farming client for the integration of information.

For corporate owners or government bodies, the bovine veterinarian will be involved in more formal communication methods, such as submission of 'items for meetings' and 'executive summaries and reports'. Clear, succinct, professionally laid out documents, which are written with the perspective of the particular client or stakeholders in mind, are likely to enhance the role of the veterinarian in advisory or higher-level strategic and/or motivational input.

Conclusion

As bovine production management systems become more complex, engaging effectively with the relevant stakeholders will likely require, and result in, veterinarians utilising more formal communication strategies (Wustenberg, 2006). While this chapter has focused on veterinarian-farmer interaction, the individualised approach based on the client's perspective can be extrapolated to settings where the veterinarian is in a leadership position. For example, it is essential that veterinarians understand the stakeholders' perspectives and expertise, such as the goals and needs of the regional group or the expectations and opinions of the industry board. Acknowledging and incorporating these perspectives into management approaches is integral to effective practice.

Hence, the authors' premise that skilled communication underpins effective leadership, as it is not until the leader understands the perspectives of the farming client that they can then proceed and determine strategy and implementation. Consequently, a focus on leadership skills, with particular emphasis on intentional implementation of evidence-based communication skills, such as those listed in this chapter, is indicated in the education and continuing professional development of all bovine veterinarians. Moreover, these are skills that can, and are, being successfully taught in veterinary medicine.

References

Adams, C.L. and Coe, J.B. (2011). Enhancing udder health with clinical communication skills: evidence based communication frameworks for the 22nd century. In: Hogeveen, H. and Lam, T.J.G.M. (eds). *Udder Health and Communication*. Wageningen Academic Publishers, Netherlands.

Adams, C.L. and Kurtz, S.M. (2006). Building on existing models from human medical education to develop a communication curriculum in veterinary medicine. *Journal of Veterinary Medical Education* **33**(1), 28–37.

Beach, M.C and Inui, T. (2006). Relationship-centred care. A constructive reframing, *Journal of General Internal Medicine* **21**(Suppl 1), S3–S8.

Bock, B.B., Van Huik, M.M., Prutzer, M., Kling Eveillard, F. and Dockes, A. (2007). Farmers' relationship with different animals: the importance of getting close to the animals. Case studies of French, Swedish and Dutch cattle, pig and poultry farmers. *International Journal of Sociology of Food and Agriculture* **15**(3), 109–125.

Boyle, D., Dwinnell, B. and Platt, F. (2005). Invite, listen, and summarize: a patient-centred communication technique. *Academic Medicine* **1**, 29–32.

Chapman, H.M., Copland, R.S., Swan, R.A. and Robertson, I.D. (1991). A survey of farmers' attitudes to services provided by consulting veterinarians to the Western Australian sheep industry. *Australian Veterinary Journal* **68**(6), 196–198.

Coe, J.B., Adams, C.L. and Bonnett, B.N. (2008). A focus group study of veterinarians and pet owners' perceptions of veterinarian-client communication in companion animal practice. *Journal of the American Veterinary Medical Association* **233**(7), 1072–1080.

Cron, W.L., Slocum, J.V.J. and Goodnight, D.B. (2000). Executive summary of the Brakke management and behaviour study. *Journal of American Veterninary Medical Assocation* **217**, 332–338.

Dockes, A. and Kling Eveillard, F. (2006). Farmers' and advisers' representations of animals and animal welfare. *Livestock Science* **103**(3), 243–249.

Dysart, L.M., Coe, J.B. and Adams, C.L. (2011). Analysis of solicitation of client concerns in companion animal practice. *Journal of the American Veterinary Medical Association* **238**(12), 1609–1615.

Hall, J. and Wapenaar, W. (2012). Opinions and practices of veterinarians and dairy farmers towards herd health management in the UK. *Veterinary Record* **170**(17), 441.

Jansen, J. and Lam, T.J. (2012). The role of communication in improving udder health. *Veterinary Clinics of North America. Food Animal Practice* **28**(2), 363–379.

Jansen, J., Steuten, C.D., Renes, R.J., Aarts, N. and Lam, T.J. (2010). Debunking the myth of the hard-to-reach farmer: effective communication on udder health. *Journal of Dairy Science* **93**(3), 1296–1306.

Kanji, N., Coe, J.B., Adams, C.L. and Shaw, J.R. (2012). Effect of veterinarian-client-patient interactions on client adherence to dentistry and surgery recommendations in companion-animal practice. *Journal of the American Veterinary Medical Association* **240**(4), 427–436.

Kleen, J.L., Atkinson, O. and Noordhuizen, J.P. (2011). Communication in production animal medicine: modelling a complex interaction with the example of dairy herd health medicine. *Irish Veterinary Journal* **64**(1), 8.

Kristensen, E. and Enevoldsen, C. (2008). A mixed methods inquiry: How dairy farmers perceive the value(s) of their involvement in an intensive dairy herd health management program. *Acta Veterinaria Scandinavica* **50**, 50.

Kristensen, E. and Jakobsen, E.B. (2011). Challenging the myth of the irrational dairy farmer; understanding decision-making related to herd health. *New Zealand Veterinary Journal* **59**, 1–7.

Kurtz, S., Silverman, J., Benson, J. and Draper, J. (2003). Marrying content and process in clinical method teaching: enhancing the Calgary-Cambridge guides. *Academic Medicine* **78**(8), 802–809.

Lloyd, J.W. and Walsh, D.A. (2002). Template for a recommended curriculum in 'Veterinary Professional Development and Career Success'. *Journal of Veterinary Medical Education* **29**(2), 84–93.

Lloyd, J.W., King, L.J., Mase, C.A. and Harris, D. (2005). Future needs and recommendations for leadership in veterinary medicine. *Journal of the American Veterinary Medical Association* **226**(7), 1060–1067.

Mellanby, R.J., Rhind, S.M., Bell, C., Shaw, D.J., Gifford, J., Fennell, D., Manser, C., Spratt, D.P., Wright, M.J., Zago, S. and Hudson, N.P. (2011). Perceptions of clients and veterinarians on what attributes constitute 'a good vet'. *Veterinary Record* **168**(23), 616.

Pritchard, W.R. (ed.). (1989). *Future Directions for Veterinary Medicine*. Pew National Veterinary Education Program, Duke University, Durham, NC.

Radford, A., Stockley, P., Silverman, J., Taylor, I., Turner, R. and Gray, C. (2006). Development, teaching, and evaluation of a consultation structure model for use in veterinary education. *Journal of Veterinary Medical Education* **33**(1), 38–44.

Rosenstock, I. (1974). Historical origins of the health belief model. *Health Education Monographs* **2**(4), 328–335.
Seabrook, M.F. and Wilkinson, J.M. (2000). Stockpersons' attitudes to the husbandry of dairy cows. *Veterinary Record* **147**(6), 157–160.
Shaw, D.H. and Ihle, S.L. (2006). Communication skills training at the Atlantic Veterinary College, University of Prince Edward Island. *Journal of Veterinary Medical Education* **33**(1), 100–104.
Shaw, J. (2006). Four core communication skills of highly effective practitioners. *Veterinary Clinics of North America – Small Animal Practice* **36**(2), 385–396.
Shaw, J.R., Adams, C.L. and Bonnett, B.N. (2004a). What can veterinarians learn from studies of physician-patient communication about veterinarian-client-patient communication? *Journal of the American Veterinary Medical Association* **224**(5), 676–684.
Shaw, J.R., Adams, C.L., Bonnett, B.N., Larson, S. and Roter, D.L. (2004b). Use of the Roter interaction analysis system to analyze veterinarian-client-patient communication in companion animal practice. *Journal of the American Veterinary Medical Association* **225**(2), 222–229.
Shaw, J.R., Adams, C.L., Bonnett, B.N., Larson, S and Roter, D.L. (2012). Veterinarian satisfaction with companion animal visits. *Journal of the American Veterinary Medical Association* **240**(7), 832–841.
Silverman, J.D., Kurtz, S. and Draper, J. (2005). *Skills for communicating with patients*, 2nd edition. Radcliffe Publishing, Oxford.
Tuckett, D., Boulton, M., Olson, C. and Williams, A. (1985). *Meetings Between Experts: an approach to sharing ideas in medical consultations*. Tavistock, London.
Wustenberg, M. (2006). Veterinarians in the Production Setting: Where Do Veterinarians Fit in? What Can They Provide? What Skills Do They Need? *Journal of Veterinary Medical Education* **33**(4), 489–491.

CHAPTER 9

Marketing, Promotion and Farmer Education

Peter Orpin

Learning objectives

- Understanding the challenges to effective marketing.
- Be able to developing a marketing strategy for the practice.
- Understand the processes that are required to implement the strategy.
- Appreciate the importance of farmer education.

Understanding the challenges to effective marketing

Marketing, promotion and farmer education are key elements of building a successful farm practice. The veterinary practice plays a central lead in helping farmers to adopt the opportunities that exist to improve the technical performance of their herds. We, as veterinarians, have the knowledge to help advance herd health and production of the herd. However, unless we can communicate what we can offer to our farmers in an effective way which can help shape the behaviours and priorities of the farmer, then progress will be slow. Typically, we often view our neighbouring practices as our greatest competitors. The real competitors are more likely to be other, non-veterinary, businesses which are often more efficient at competing for both the attention and resources of the farmer. If our marketing is effective, then animal health should be within the top three priorities for the farmer.

There are several definitions of 'marketing'. The most appropriate definition within a veterinary context appears to be: 'the management process responsible for identifying, anticipating, shaping and satisfying customer requirements profitably'. Marketing embraces the whole process of market research, communication, promotion and, ultimately, altering farmers' purchasing decisions and behaviour. Confusion often exists between selling, advertising and marketing. 'Selling' is part of the process, but does not define the whole process of marketing. There is a real risk that the veterinarian who dislikes the process of 'selling' then avoids marketing as a consequence. The practice can then become totally reactive, and simply responds to the current demands of the farmer, rather than shaping future opportunities for both farmer and the vet.

Farmer education is also an essential part of the marketing mix. Education helps with providing a context for any solutions that may exist to improve health. With understanding, we have compliance. Without understanding, we have confusion. The explanation of the benefits of health improvements and how these can be achieved is a 'central plank' of creating a successful health-orientated veterinary practice.

The pressures of clinical work and "time poverty" can often constrain the ability of the practice to market the services and solutions that it provides effectively. A common limitation of practice marketing is that the marketing activity is designed to suit the plans of the supplier or sponsor, rather than the needs of the client or the practice. Suppliers are keen to work with veterinarians to help promote income opportunities and endorsements for their own products. Adopting a marketing approach driven by your suppliers is likely to be more fragmented and without a coordinated narrative. A clearly thought-out marketing process, with defined clear aims and objectives matching the needs of your own practice and clients, will be much more effective. The present chapter seeks to illustrate how a more cohesive approach could be adopted, following some basic steps.

Developing a marketing strategy for the practice

To optimise the impact of any marketing approach there needs to be a marketing plan which should dovetail in with the overall business plan for the practice.

Bovine Medicine, Third Edition. Edited by Peter D. Cockcroft.

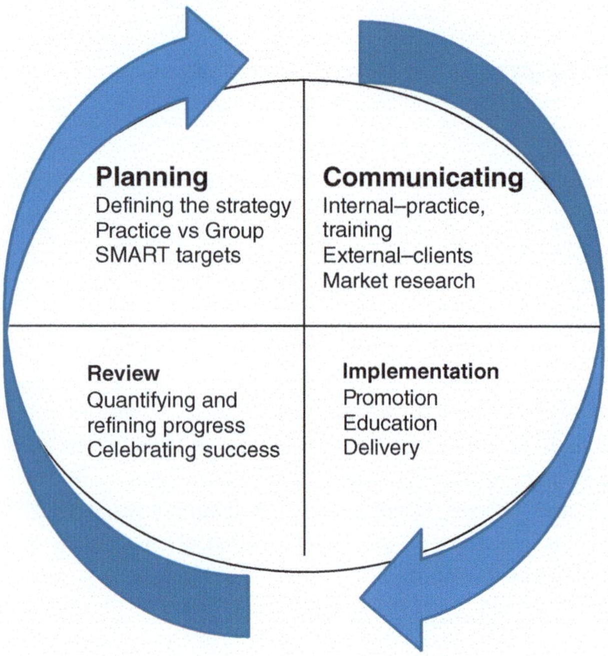

Figure 9.1 The process of creating a marketing plan.

The successful marketing plan will achieve two main aims: satisfying client needs; and delivering a profitable and sustainable result for the practice. The process of creating a marketing plan can be broken down into four distinct phases – planning, communicating, implementation and review – which are highlighted in Figures 9.1 and 9.2.

A mind map (Figure 9.2) of the methodology of the process illustrates the level of detail required to create a successful marketing plan for a veterinary practice. The process can be broken down into a series of logical steps. In this particular example, we will focus on a marketing campaign primarily directed at existing clients, with the intention of developing a health-orientated practice.

The planning phase

Define your strategy

The marketing strategy should be linked to the overall business plan for the farm practice and the most recent SWOT analysis. What are the key objectives of the marketing process? To deliver more profit or secure a closer bond with the client? What are the most important areas to develop? Services? Products? Consultancy? Absolute clarity is required. A series of individual marketing tactics can be delivered, but ideally these should all meet the main marketing plan objectives. The strategic delivery of a marketing plan is classically defined as the 'eight Ps' of marketing (Lovelock & Wirtz, Lovelock and Wirtz, 2007), as illustrated in Figure 9.3.

Objectives and targets

Once you have established a plan, it is useful to clarify the specific objectives and targets. Are there SMART targets (Specific, Measurable, Achievable, Realistic and Targeted) for the marketing program, which will allow us to evaluate the marketing program and celebrate success if the targets are achieved? For example: 'To

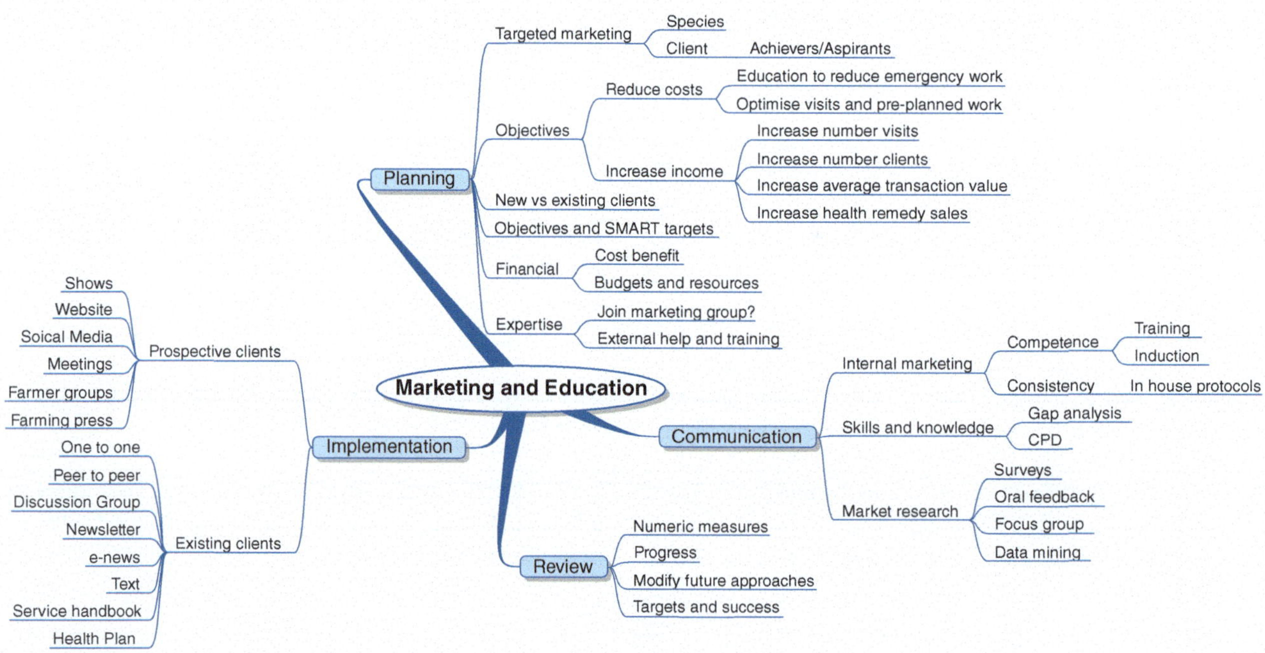

Figure 9.2 Mind map of the key steps to an effective marketing and farmer education process.

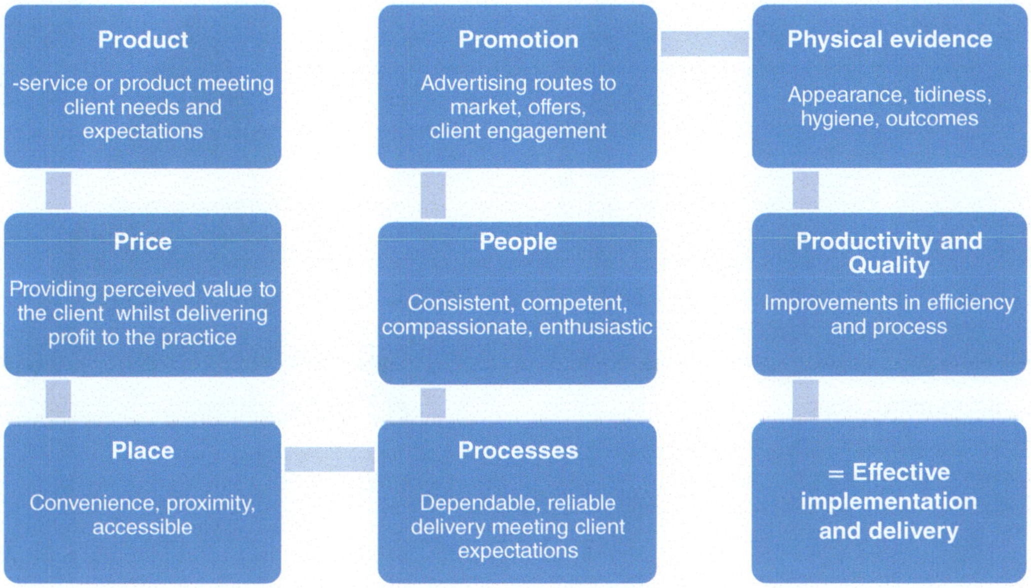

Figure 9.3 The 'eight Ps' of marketing.

increase the uptake of farmers using your fertility program by 20% by July 2013' is much SMARTer than 'having a promotion on fertility with our farmers this year'.

Establish your marketing partners

Who will help you with your marketing? Are you going to join a marketing group? Do you require external consultancy to help build your skills, or are you going to depend on the marketing skills of your suppliers? In the UK, practices are gathering together in buying and marketing groups in order to share expertise and develop common marketing opportunities which all practices can utilise. For example, a marketing group called XLVets has been established which allows for the sharing of expertise and costs (Black & Schmitt, Black and Schmitt, 2012). This allows common themes to be developed within the group and a sharing of resources (printing, shows, exhibitions; see Figure 9.4). Ansoff's matrix suggests four alternative marketing strategies, which hinge on whether products are new or existing. They also focus on whether a market is new or existing. This is illustrated in Figure 9.5.

What are you going to market?

The relative ease of the strategy will depend on the client group, and whether the system is tried and tested. For instance, it is considerably easier to sell an existing service (e.g. an established fertility program) to an existing client, rather than a completely novel hi-tech solution to a prospective or new client. The most successful marketing campaigns identify areas which are tried and tested, with potential for long-term gains and repeat business for both farmer and vet (e.g. fertility programs). In most veterinary practices, the greatest gains are in the areas of market penetration and product and service expansion within their existing clients. These are lowest risk and cost to deliver.

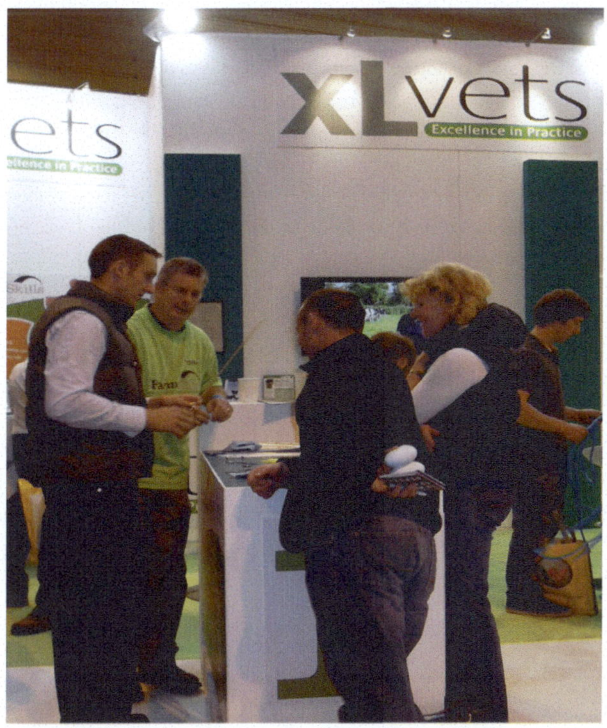

Figure 9.4 XLVets' stand at the European Dairy Event (2010).

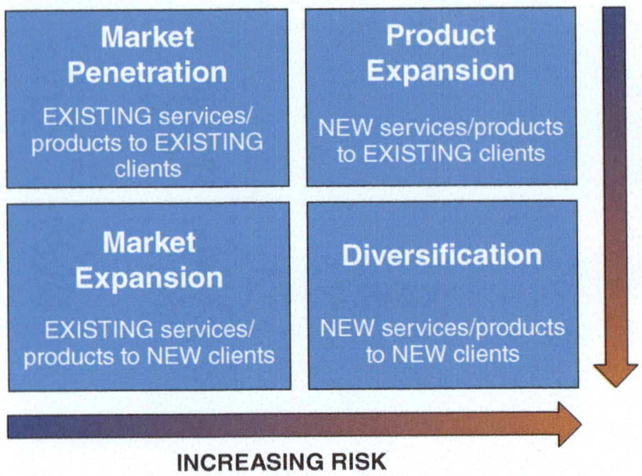

Figure 9.5 Ansoff's marketing matrix, illustrating the relative ease of promotion according to service and client type.

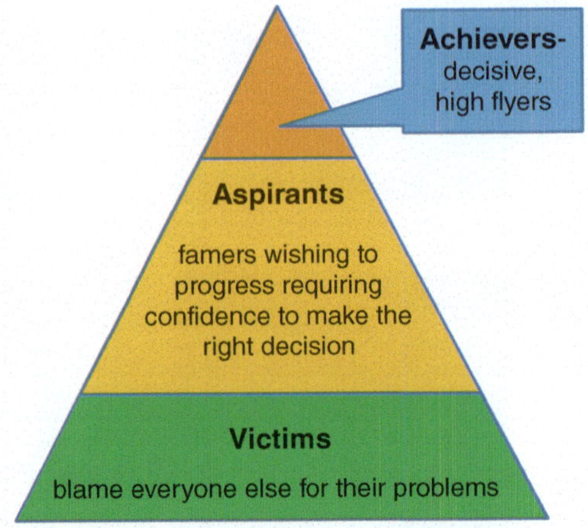

Figure 9.6 The 'achiever, aspirant and victims' methodology of dividing a customer group.

Define the target group

Analyse your existing database to establish where the greatest growth potential exists. Are you targeting all clients equally, or particular key clients or species groups? The more targeted the approach, the more effective the campaign will be. Focusing on clients who have previously shown an interest, or have committed to previous practice developments, is a productive approach. Ranking clients according to overall purchases will allow you to identify the typical 20% of the clients which deliver 80% of the income for your practice (the Pareto principle). A simple list of clients, followed by a series of columns indicating what services and key products they purchase from you, will help you identify and perform a 'gap' analysis of your client base.

Client segmentation: focusing on the receptive groups

Another useful concept to use is the 'victim, aspirant and achiever' profiling approach (see Figure 9.6). Clients can be divided up according to their attitude to investing in health. The aim should be always to appeal to the 'achievers' and 'aspirants', and to ensure limited time is spent on the 'victims'. With the correct environment, the achievers will encourage aspirants to progress. This forms the basis of organising successful discussion groups or meetings where the focus is to establish a mix of aspirants and achievers.

Communicating

The success of the marketing program is totally dependent on achieving compliance with all those involved. Work by the American Animal Hospital Association (AAHA) developed the knowledge, attitude and behaviour models used in human healthcare compliance to produce the CRAFT formula for effective client communications: Compliance = Recommendation + Acceptance + Follow Through. Nothing happens unless a clear recommendation is made, acceptance is achieved in the mind of the receiver of this recommendation, and steps are put in place to ensure that follow-up is taken to ensure something happens. This model equally applies to the challenges of internal marketing.

Internal marketing – involving the team

Internal marketing is a key step which is often omitted during the planning stage. If an influential member of the farm team is not engaged with the process, there is a risk that most of the good work may be undone later. Spending time early in the process managing objections and gaining acceptance is time well spent. Communication within farm practice teams is not easy. Geographic 'lone' working can often limit or delay progress, preventing agreement and engagement with the marketing plan. Building effective communication systems within the practice are vital, using smartphones, intranets, social media or email, which will greatly help information flow.

Meetings and decision-making

For effective decision-making, meetings will be required, with defined agendas and outcomes. Preparation for meetings is essential, with typically twice as much time preparing for meetings than in the meeting itself. Meetings are often poorly managed within practices, resulting in a discussion focused on anecdotes and destructive criticisms, rather than proactive planning opportunities. A section of every practice meeting should be devoted to marketing and improving client service.

Skills and knowledge

Do we know enough to deliver the service or promote the health remedy? Identifying gaps in knowledge will help prevent a premature or poorly developed promotion. Who will champion the program? Does everyone else know enough about the features and benefits of the project to answer any queries a farmer might raise and help to promote the program?

The Veterinary Group Beef Services Questionnaire

As a practice, we are aiming to improve the service we offer to our beef clients. We are therefore interested to know what it is that you would like us to be able to provide for you in the future.

We would greatly appreciate it if you could spare a few moments of your time to complete the questionnaire below:

Name and Farm: ______________________________

1. What would you perceive as the main limitation to improving profitability to a beefherd?

2. Please rank the following in order of importance to you (1 = most important, 4 = least);
   - Improving fertility
   - Reducing calf mortality
   - Improving live weight gain
   - Achieving a tighter calving pattern
   - Other ....

Figure 9.7 An excerpt from a beef client survey conducted in the author's practice in 2012.

Market research: test the market and identify farmer needs

Market research conducted at an early stage will prevent you from wasting time delivering a plan which does not meet the need of the farmer. Farmer needs can be achieved by 'one to one' discussion with the target group of clients, structured farmer surveys, or focus or discussion groups. If you can correctly identify the most important health topics which concern the client and rank these by importance, you can help to prioritise the marketing plan. Use open questions such as: 'What is your greatest health concern?' or 'Which health problems are costing you the most money, and how can we help you reduce these losses?' to help get a closer understanding of the clients' needs. The concept of 'active listening' ensures that you tease out from your farmers what is most important to them, and the results can help sharpen up your marketing campaign, as the features and benefits will be more closely aligned to the farmers' concerns.

Farmer surveys

Getting professional help with the construction of any farmer survey is always advised. The success is largely dependent on the asking the right questions (see Figure 9.7). A useful technique is to combine the open questions with some that provide potential answers for ranking in order or importance.

Implementation: farmer education and marketing delivery

Practical delivery of the plan

One of the most effective ways to manage a marketing plan is by using a Gantt chart methodology (Figure 9.8). This can be simply done in a spreadsheet, where the months are the columns and the rows are the key activities required to deliver the plan (defining the target market, in-house training, newsletters, farmer meetings, follow-up). This ensures that the key steps of the campaign are not forgotten, and the whole process can be tracked through in a coordinated way. Free web-based versions are also available, with options to share between users via the web (e.g. Smartsheet). For simple marketing campaigns, a wall chart or calendar may suffice. The approach, however, is the same where the marketing 'timeline' is split into time specific components, with clear lines of individual responsibility as to who does what when.

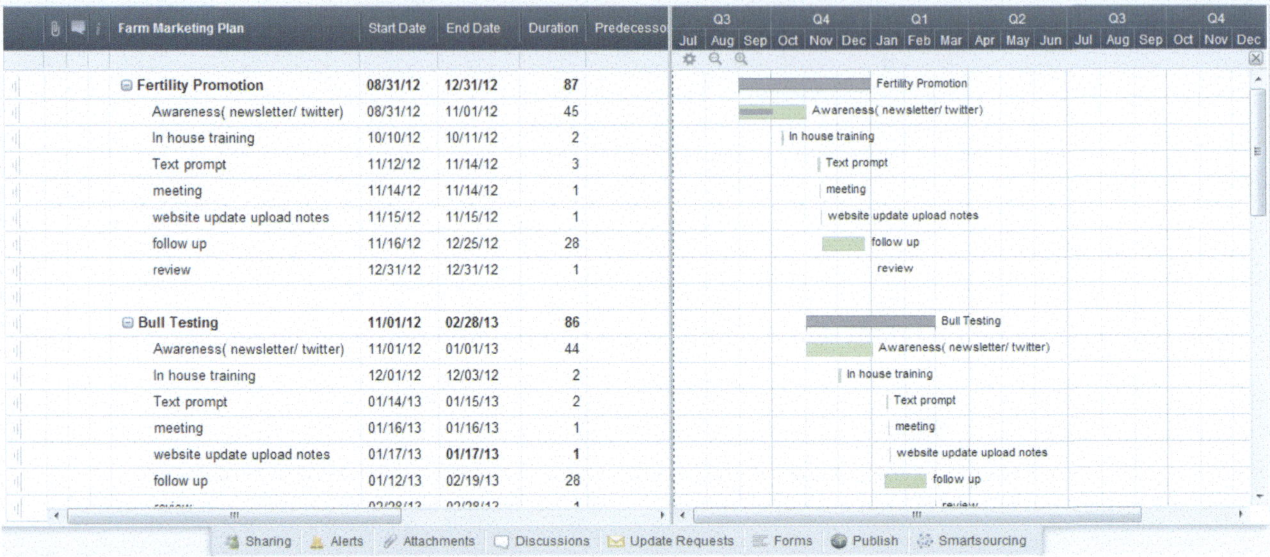

Farm Marketing Plan	Start Date	End Date	Duration	Predecesso
Fertility Promotion	**08/31/12**	**12/31/12**	**87**	
Awareness(newsletter/ twitter)	08/31/12	11/01/12	45	
In house training	10/10/12	10/11/12	2	
Text prompt	11/12/12	11/14/12	3	
meeting	11/14/12	11/14/12	1	
website update upload notes	11/15/12	11/15/12	1	
follow up	11/16/12	12/25/12	28	
review	12/31/12	12/31/12	1	
Bull Testing	**11/01/12**	**02/28/13**	**86**	
Awareness(newsletter/ twitter)	11/01/12	01/01/13	44	
In house training	12/01/12	12/03/12	2	
Text prompt	01/14/13	01/15/13	2	
meeting	01/16/13	01/16/13	1	
website update upload notes	01/17/13	01/17/13	1	
follow up	01/12/13	02/19/13	28	

Figure 9.8 A Gantt chart illustrating the key components and timelines for delivering a successful farmer training program.

'Shaping' farmer needs prior to promotion

Before a solution is embraced, clients have to believe that the solution will be of benefit to them, and there is a need for this solution to be adopted. In some situations, the need for your solution has not been explained well enough. A good example of this may be a farmer who totally underestimates the cost of hypocalcaemia. Unless this is explained, then it is highly unlikely they will sign up to a hi-tech solution to prevent milk fever. Avoid delivering solutions until the need is firmly established in the farmer's mind.

Tactics and delivery

What is the mechanism you will use to communicate your marketing campaign to your farmer clients? What medium will you use? Who are you targeting? Farmer owners or the herdspersons? What will be the most effective mechanism for delivery? Large group meetings? On-farm discussion groups? One-to-one discussions?

The small farm discussion group is by far the most effective medium for changing behaviours, especially if this can be combined with on-farm real demonstration of the benefits for participation in the program. Peer-to-peer communication is a more effective method of behaviour change than vet-to-farmer in most instances. Typically, the use of multiple routes is the most effective way of ensuring efficient knowledge transfer and the triggering of action on the farm.

Communication methods

The farmer education program is often combined with the overall marketing program for the practice. The choice of delivery and route of knowledge transfer is heavily dependent on the topic and message you are wishing to impart and the client type you are targeting. The relative advantages and disadvantages of the various routes are highlighted in Figure 9.9 and described in more detail in Orpin (Orpin, 1993).

Selling health – features and benefits

The final stages of the marketing program generally involve a coordinated communication process with the farmer. This typically requires a combination of creating awareness, defining the features and benefits of any solution, objection handling and, finally, securing commitment ('closing the deal') (Figure 9.10). Unless all steps are followed in a logical order, the outcome will not be secured.

For the marketing process to be successful, all elements must be managed. Unless the members of the practice team are fully aware of the features and benefits of the product or concept you are aiming to sell, it is highly unlikely that the marketing program will be as successful as it could have been. Too often, the expectation is that a farmer's change of behaviour or buying decisions will occur, based on a single newsletter or meeting. Further one-to-one discussion and follow-up is required. A useful methodology to follow is the 'feature and benefit' sales process.

The process is achieved by highlighting a topical issue in a newsletter or via social media. This generates an opportunity for discussion. Through dialogue, the needs of the farmer are established and an opportunity is taken to explain the 'features and benefits' to the farmer if he were to commit to the program

Method	Advantages	Disadvantages
'One to one' vet-farmer	Moderate cost, occurs on the farm visit, able to listen to concerns and manage objections and secure commitment.	Often perceived as direct 'selling' by client, limited visual aids, dependent on the vet's ability to communicate features and benefits clearly to farmer.
Discussion Group/ Small Group	Achievers can be mixed with aspirants. Effective route to delivering behaviour change, especially with practical demonstration of results.	Higher cost than large group meetings, results dependent on quality of facilitation and participants discussions.
Large Group Meeting	Useful for simple messages which can be illustrated using PowerPoint or flip-chart. Can be run 'off' farm in the evening.	Can become boring and less likely to influence behaviour. Raises awareness but often requires follow up for action to occur.
Newsletter or E-News	Low cost if delivered at time of invoice. Creates awareness and reinforces key health messages. Highly valued by clients.	Unlikely to generate behaviour changes alone. Requires follow-up. No opportunity for interaction. May not be read.
Social Media	Appealing to the more technology- or computer-savvy farmer who is familiar with the medium; low cost.	Not all clients may be familiar with social networking.
Text	Useful for reminders and disease alerts, easy access via mobile.	Limited information transfer.
Health Plan	A bespoke platform for defining health treatments, advice and services.	Higher cost, requires individual inputs for each farm.
Practice Protocols	Standard protocols and advice which can be 'plasticised' and placed on farm office walls/ booklets. Simple and effective.	Generic and non-specific to the farm.
Practice Handbook	Defines what the practice offer can complete, with features and benefits. Simple and low cost. Can be integrated with practice protocols.	Generic and non-specific to the farm.
Practice Web site	Common portal for clients and prospective clients to access information and guidance.	Requires frequent updating, depends on clients being referred to the site via Twitter/ newsletter/work.

Figure 9.9 Table illustrating the advantages and disadvantages of different communication methods.

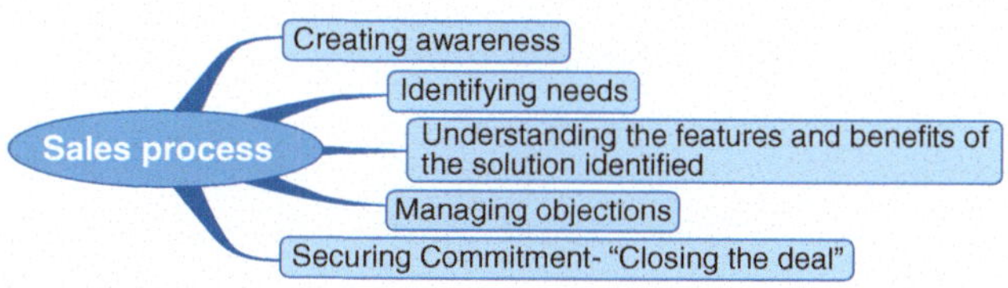

Figure 9.10 Graphic of the feature and benefit sales process.

or product. The benefits must be closely aligned to the needs or drivers of the farmer. If there are any concerns or objections to the solution identified, then these are discussed. Finally and most importantly, the farmer is asked whether s/he would like to commit to the program. This methodical approach will allow the vet to provide effective solutions for the farmer and will avoid the risk of a 'bad' or perceived 'hard sell'.

The traditional approach of *ad hoc* marketing and communication is to be avoided, as it risks priming the market by creating awareness and then failing to follow through and deliver a practical solution for the farmer. The lack of an agreed follow-up procedure by the practice may result in other competitor suppliers ultimately providing the service or product to the farm, when all the hard work in creating the market has been provided by the practice.

Review

If SMART objectives have been set at the outset, the review process allows the practice to re-evaluate progress with marketing campaigns and to record and celebrate success if agreed targets have been achieved. The aim is to look at what worked well, what could have worked better, and what will we do differently or aim to repeat successfully next time. Missing out this step is a common failing with practice marketing processes. Creating simple rewards and opportunities for recognition and acknowledgement are crucial areas to get right for continued success.

Summary

Marketing can be hugely satisfying part of veterinary practice and, if it is done well, it can help to secure a sustainable future for both the farmer and the practice. Effective marketing is a philosophy that determines the way that a practice is set up and run. Utilising effective marketing plans and communications will help focus the team, aid staff retention and, most importantly, provide a sound platform from which high health and welfare can be delivered to the farmer clients by working in close partnership, rather than just being seen as one of many suppliers to the farm.

References

Black, D. and Schmitt. E. (2012). Veterinary Practice as a Business. What, How, When, Why. Round Table Discussion. *Proceedings World Buiatrics*.

Lovelock, C. and Wirtz, J. (2007). *Services Marketing: People, Technology, Strategy*. 6th Edition, pp 22–23. Pearson, New Jersey, USA.

Orpin. P.G. (1993). Farm Animal Practice and Promotion. *In Practice* **15**(2), 100–110.

Useful web links

www.business-fundas.com
www.aahanet.org

CHAPTER 10

Veterinary Equipment in Ambulatory Practice

Karin Mueller

Learning objectives

- Be aware of the range of equipment useful for ambulatory cattle practice.
- Understand what may govern individual choices of equipment used or carried.
- Know the equipment required to provide first aid and deal with urgent cases.
- Recognise other requirements such as equipment care or drug storage.

Introduction

With most cattle veterinary work being carried out on an ambulatory basis, the practitioner needs to ensure that the equipment and supplies required for the common range of tasks is carried in the vehicle or present on farm. It is personal preference whether the entire range of equipment is carried at all times, or whether certain 'task boxes' and larger pieces of equipment (such as an ultrasound machine) are taken on an as-and-when-needed basis for pre-scheduled tasks. The geographical area covered by the practice will, in part, influence this decision. Equipment suggestions in this chapter are listed in Boxes 10.1 to 10.11 below, grouped by type of activity (e.g. fertility work) to aid setting up 'task boxes'. Surgical kits and instruments for different procedures are indicated in Table 10.1. The selection of suture materials and needles are presented in Table 10.2. How to care for various pieces of equipment is shown in Table 10.3. Figures 10.1, 10.2 and 10.3 presents, respectively, the basic equipment required for catheterisation, bandaging and obstetrics.

Equipment for emergency first aid should always be carried. The range of emergencies one should be able to address includes soft tissue damage (wound lavage, bandaging, suturing, antibiosis, analgesia), fractures (materials for limb immobilisation), haemorrhage (suture material, artery forceps, pressure bandages) and acute metabolic disease (calcium borogluconate, magnesium sulphate). Prompt attention to obstetrical cases should also be enabled. To facilitate dealing with emergencies, a method of sedation should be available, as should a method of euthanasia. Lastly, consideration should be given to carrying a base line of drugs, in order to be able to attend to individual medical cases (for example, pneumonia) without having to go back to the practice base.

The suggestions in this chapter are based on the years the author has spent in practice. Various types of equipment suitable for the same task exist, and each veterinary surgeon will have his/her own preferred option. The type of cattle practice (i.e. whether predominantly dairy or beef) and clients' preferences will also influence one's choice.

The range, type and amount of drugs carried will depend on:

(a) The type of work carried out (e.g. a practice with predominantly beef youngstock will probably carry a different selection than a practice with predominantly dairy farms).
(b) Country-specific licensing regulations.
(c) Practice policy (e.g. on the use of fluorquinolons or third/fourth generation cephalosporins).
(d) Whether a mobile dispensary is provided.

The practice vehicle must enable storage of drugs at the correct temperature. Protection from freezing can easily be achieved by drug drawers or compartments insulated, for example, with Thinsulate™ or polystyrene. To stay below the maximum storage temperature (25–28°C for most drugs), refrigeration will be necessary (either as an in-built compartment or a stand-alone chiller box plugged into the vehicle battery). Even in temperate climates, like the United Kingdom, the inside temperature of a vehicle commonly exceeds 45°C on warm days. Vaccines that are carried in the vehicle will always require refrigeration.

Various options exist for the organisation and storage of drugs and equipment inside the vehicle, from built-in compartment units to free-standing plastic boxes. Equipment must be stored securely to avoid forward propulsion during an emergency stop.

Bovine Medicine, Third Edition. Edited by Peter D. Cockcroft.

Table 10.1 Surgery kits and instruments for different procedures.

	C-Section Kit	Laparotomy	LDA-surgical methods, Rumenotomy	LDA-Grymer-Sterner Method	Small procedure kit[§]
Tail tie	√	√	√		
Clippers or razor and blades	√	√	√	√	√
Cotton wool or gauze swabs (non-sterile)	√	√	√	√	√
Disinfectant[1]	√	√	√	√	√
Methylated spirit (spray bottle)	√	√	√	√	√
Scrubbing brush	√	√	√		
Gloves, surgical, sterile	√	√	√	√	√
Gown, ideally sterile[2]	√	√	√		
Long sleeves, sterile	√	√	√		
Face mask	√	√	√		
Surgeon's cap	√	√	√		
Scalpel blade, no. 22	2	2	2		
Scalpel blade, no. 10					2
Scalpel handle, no. 4	2	2	2		
Scalpel handle, no. 3					1
Mayo scissors, straight	1	1	1		1
Mayo scissors, curved	1	1	1		
Suture scissors	1	1	1	1	
Metzenbaum scissors	1	1	1		
Tissue forceps, toothed	1	1	1		1
Tissue forceps, plain	1	1	1		
Artery forceps/haemostats, assorted sizes, straight & curved	10	5–10	5–10	2	4
Allis tissue forceps	4–5	4–5	4–5		2
Needle holder	2	2	2		1
Gauze swabs, sterile, pack of 5	min. 4	min. 4	min. 4		1
Drape, sterile (e.g. Buster, ≈120 × 250 cm)	1–2	1	1		
Towel clips	8–10	8–10	8–10		
Uterus holding forceps	1–2				
Roberts embryotomy knife	1				
Bowel clamps		2–4			

[§]Instruments in plastic or metal kidney dish;
[1]e.g. chlorhexidine, povidone iodine;
[2]e.g. Krutex disposable sterile coat

Table 10.2 Suture material and uses.

Type	Material	Strength		Length	Needle			Uses
		Metric	USP		Point	Shape	Size	
Absorbable	Pg910 or Pgc25	4–5	1–2	90–100 cm	Round	½ circle	50–80 mm	AW, SW, U
		3	2–0	90 cm	Tapercut	½ circle	35 mm	SW, L, T, A
		2	3–0	45 cm	Cutting	½ circle	22 mm	T
		4	1	90 cm	Cutting	½ circle	50 mm	Sa
	Catgut	6–7	2–3	Reel				AW, U
	PDS	4	1	90 cm	Tapercut	½ circle	50 mm	UH
Non-absorbable	Nylon 6 and 6.6, mono-filament[a]	5	2	100 cm	Cutting	⅜ circle	90 mm	S
		6–7	3–5	Reel				S

Pg910 = Polyglactin 910 (multifilament); Pgc25 = polyglecaprone 25 (monofilament)
[a]e.g. Ethilon®
AW = abdominal wall: muscle layers; SW = soft tissue wound closure; U = Uterus; L = ligature of vessels/haemostasis; T = Teat surgery; A = Anastomosis of intestine; S/Sa = skin/absorbable suture; UH = umbilical hernia

Table 10.3 Equipment care.

Item	Routine care	Additional care
Surgical instruments	Clean and disinfect as soon as possible after use. Then thoroughly rinse and dry, before packing up for autoclaving. N.B. (a) Do not allow body fluids or tissues to dry on instruments. If they cannot be processed immediately, soak in plain water (without disinfectant). (b) Do not exceed 45°C water temperature to avoid protein coagulation.	Lubricate all joints, ideally after every cleaning cycle. Send scissors for sharpening.
Disbudding iron	Allow to cool before returning to vehicle. If this requires dipping into water, take care to only immerse the very tip, otherwise the jet may block.	Check for leaks in gas tubing. Tighten loose parts. Unblock jet with thin wire if required.
Fetotome	Thoroughly rinse and disinfect, making sure that no hair or tissue remains in the barrels. Allow to dry.	Sharpen guarded knife. Lubricate joint on Krey's hook.
Calving ropes	Wash in 60°C machine cycle. Dry and autoclave.	
Protective clothing	Wash in 60°C machine cycle.	
Footcare equipment	Clean and disinfect before leaving premises.	Sharpen hoof knives
McLintock syringe	Clean barrel and plunger with cotton wool soaked in spirit. Sterilise by boiling. In hard water areas, remove lime with cotton wool soaked in spirit.	Calibrate regularly.

Box 10.1 Restraint & examination (including sample collection).

Restraint

Rope halter
Rope (leg restraint), thick, eye splice, 1.8 m (6.5')
Rope (casting), thick, 12 m (39')

Optional
Nose grip/bulldog
Anti-kick bar
Dart gun or stick
Mobile crush

Sample collection
Universal container, sterile, 30 ml (milk culture)
Universal container, 100 or 150 ml (faeces)
Transport swab (charcoal & plain)
Vacutainer (or sample pot):
7 or 10 ml, EDTA, heparin, plain (for blood)
1 or 2.5 ml, EDTA, plain (for centesis fluids)
Vacutainer needles, 18–20 g
2.5 cm (1''; coccygeal vein)
3.75 cm (2''; jugular vein)
Vacutainer needle holder:
Scalpel blades, no. 10 and 22

Optional
Interdental brush (ocular swab)
Jugular vein tourniquet
Butcher's/Post-mortem knife
Pots, large, with 10% buffered formalin

Examination

Stethoscope
Thermometer, rectal (digital or mercury)
Watch
Gloves, long-sleeve
Gloves, disposable, non-sterile (e.g. nitrile)
Lubricant, 500 ml bottle
Artery forceps (neurological examination)
Mouth gag (e.g. Drinkwater)
Pen torch
Fluorets (ophthalmology)
Urine dipsticks
Cow-side Ketosis diagnostics[1]
California Mastitis Test: tray & reagent
Tote tray (to carry equipment & drugs)

Optional
Pleximeter & percussion hammer/plexor
Ophthalmoscope
Mare urinary catheter
Dog urinary catheter
Torch, large
Cow-side diagnostics (viral, bacterial, serological)
pH meter (rumen fluid analysis)
Blood gas analyser (e.g. i-STAT®)
Mobile x-ray machine

[1]For example: Ketostix test strips (Bayer), KetoCheck powder (Great States Animal Health), Rothera's powder, KetoTest (Elanco), PortaBHB test (PortaCheck Inc.), Precision Xtra™ meter and blood ketone test strips (Abbott Laboratories)

Box 10.2 Drugs[1] and drug administration (including fluid therapy: see Figure 10.1).

Drug administration

Syringes, sterile: 1, 2, 5, 10, 20–30, 50 ml
Hypodermic needles:
1.6 cm (5/8″) in 23–25 g
≥ 5 cm (2″) in 18–20 g
3.75 cm (1.5″) in 14–16 g, 18–19 g, 20–22 g
2.5 cm (1″) in 14–16 g, 18–19 g, 20–22 g
Drenching bottle, 700–1000 ml capacity
Intravenous flutter valve

Optional
Syringe, catheter-tip, 50 ml
Tourniquet (jugular, limb vein)
Needle-free dispensing pins (for drug bottles)
Dart gun

Antimicrobials
Penicillin, procaine
Penicillin, potentiated (e.g. clavulanic acid)
Macrolide (short and long-acting)
Trimethoprim-Sulfonamide
Tetracycline (short and long-acting)
Cephalosporin
Fluorquinolon
Aminoglycoside
Intra-mammary preparation
(narrow and broad spectrum)
Eye ointment
(Cloxacillin- and tetracycline-based)

Anti-inflammatory
NSAID, short and long-acting (e.g. flunixin, ketoprofen, meloxicam, carprofen)
Dexamethasone, short and long-acting

Sedation, analgesia, anaesthesia
Alpha-2 agonist (e.g. xylazine, detomidine HCl)
Local anaesthetic[3] (procaine HCl, lidocaine HCl)
Ocular anaesthetic (e.g. amethocaine HCl)

Optional
Atipamezole hydrochloride
Butorphanol tartrate
Ketamine HCl
Cotton buds for topical anaesthetic application

Other[2]

Euthanasia preparation (e.g. Pentobarbitone sodium)
Vitamin solutions (B1, B-complex, D_3, E)
Calcium borogluconate, 20% and 40%
Magnesium sulphate
Glucose 40% or Dextrose 50%
Phosphorus preparation
(e.g. toldimphos, calcium hypophosphite)

Optional
Selenium injection
Anthelmintics (endo- and ectoparasites)
Etamiphylline camsylate
Hyoscine butylbromide
Bromhexine HCl
Calcium chloride and sulphate oral bolus
Rumen probiotic preparation
Fly repellent ointment
Captive bolt or Humane killer/pistol
Bolus applicators (anthelmintic, mineral etc.)

Fluid therapy
Stomach tube, 2.5–3 m length, 15–20 mm Ø
Funnel to fit stomach tube
Mouth gag
Oesophageal feeder tube (calf)
I/v administration set (straight or spiral)
I/v catheters, short-stay (e.g. Intraflon)
Adults: 12–16 g, min. 80 mm (3 1/4″)
Calves: 16–20 g, min. 50 mm (2″)
Scalpel blade (no. 11 or 22)
Superglue
Suture material with cutting needle
Sodium chloride, 0.9% (1 litre, 3–5 litres)
Sodium chloride, 7.2% (3 litres)
Hartman's solution (1 litre, 3–5 litres)
Sodium bicarbonate solution, 8.4% (200 ml)
Oral rehydration preparations (calf and adult)

Optional
Stomach pump
T-Connector
Stoppers, male luer-lock (e.g. Vygon)
Medium to long-stay catheter
Blood administration set (for plasma)
Heparin sodium and water for injection (flush)
Anti-coagulant for blood transfusion

[1] Choice and range will vary depending on national regulations on drugs use in food-production animals.
[2] See also Boxes 10.3 and 10.6 (drugs used specifically in fertility work and obstetrics)
[3] A product containing adrenaline may be used for local infiltration and paravertebral blocks. However, for epidural and IVRA the solution should not contain adrenaline.

Cargo nets are useful to achieve this. Depending on practice type, the practitioner may wish to carry hot and cold water.

Cattle stocks or crushes are typically provided by clients, and the standard device present on farm is usually adequate. Mobile restraining devices exist and the veterinary surgeon may wish to bring task-specific devices, such as a Wopa foot-trimming crush or tilting table (see Box 10.1). For breeding soundness evaluation of bulls, a race is usually sufficient. However, for this task, the client needs additionally to provide a sheltered secure area with an electrical power point for microscopy. A standard crush may have to be adapted for young or small cattle for certain tasks (e.g. CSF collection) to prevent sideways movement. This can be achieved by hanging tyres or 5–10 litre plastic containers on the inside of the crush.

The practitioner should also consider the means to lift recumbent cattle. This is useful both for examination as well as treatment purposes. Several types of cow lifting harnesses are available, as are purpose-made mobile flotation tanks.

Typical bovine work requires some additional equipment to be available at the practice base. Examples are a microscope, various stains (for example polychrome methylene blue, Gram-stain, Diff-Quik), supplies to carry out faecal egg counts and milk bacteriological cultures, and a blood biochemistry and haematology analyser.

Explanatory notes on drug administration (Box 10.2)

A range of hypodermic needles is suggested to accommodate different types of cattle, viscosity of drugs and speed of administration. The following may serve as an aid in choosing an appropriate needle:

- For intra-muscular injections, a length of 2.5 cm (1") is suitable for calves and yearlings, and adults up to a body condition score of 3 (on a scale of 1 to 5).
- For adults in higher body condition, a 3.75 cm (1.5") needle ensures correct deposition into muscle.
- For intravenous injections using the jugular vein, a 2.5 cm (1") long needle is suitable for pre-weaned calves, with a 3.75 cm (1.5") needle used in older cattle.
- Subcutaneous injections are administered using a 2.5 cm (1") needle.
- Drugs of lower viscosity (e.g. NSAIDs, trimethoprim sulphonamide, reproductive hormones) and volumes up to 5 ml can easily be administered using a 21 gauge needle, with volumes up to about 10 ml given through a 18 or 19 gauge needle.
- For larger volumes, or drugs with higher viscosity (e.g. penicillins), a 16 gauge needle is preferable.
- A 14 gauge needle is suitable for the administration of very large volumes (e.g. calcium borogluconate).
- For infiltration of local anaesthetic, 20 or 21 gauge is preferred. The length of needle depends on the local block, with 2.5 cm (1") suitable for a cornual block, IVRA or scrotal infiltration, while a length of at least 5 cm (2") being more suitable for line infiltration of the flank.
- For sub-conjunctival injections, a short 23–25 g needle is most useful.

Explanatory notes on intravenous fluid therapy (Box 10.2)

The suggested lengths for intravenous catheters should be read as the minimum. In particular in calves, the relative looseness and mobility of the bovine skin over the jugular groove requires an i/v catheter of good length, to prevent its dislodgement during normal movements of the animal.

Unfortunately, it is becoming increasingly difficult to find short-stay catheters longer than 50 mm, particularly in the smaller gauges. An alternative is to use mid- to long-stay catheters, but these are somewhat more difficult to place, and are more expensive. With regard to different catheter types, for most applications in cattle work, a short-stay catheter with a dwell-time of up to 72 hours will suffice. Securing the catheter to the skin with superglue is a convenient method for dwell-times of a few hours, causing relatively little trauma to the bovine skin on removal. For longer dwell-times, suturing is recommended. In addition to conventional suturing material and needles, this can also be achieved with a 20 to 21 gauge hypodermic needle with fine suture material threaded through. Good anchoring is greatly aided by wings on the catheter. If these are not present, they can be manufactured from zinc oxide tape placed in a butterfly fashion around the hub of the catheter.

Ready-prepared intravenous fluids suitable for cattle work are now almost universally available at reasonable costs. Nevertheless, some practices may prefer to carry weighed-out sachets of salts and electrolytes to prepare fluids on farm. For this, two things should be noted: only sterilised or tap water should be

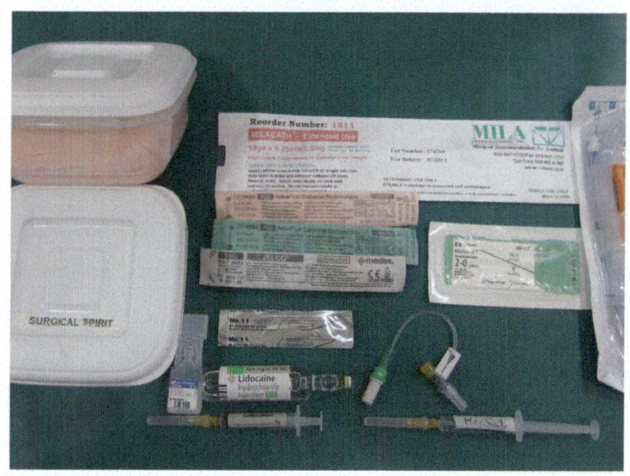

Figure 10.1 An i/v catheter kit containing, in a clockwise direction from lower left: local anaesthetic and syringe; scalpel blade; swabs for surgical scrub (chlorhexidine and surgical spirit); i/v catheters of different lengths and gauges; suture material; fluid administration set; heparin saline flush; T-port. Not shown are means of clipping the area.

Box 10.3 Fertility work.

Female fertility visit

Gloves, disposable, non-sterile (e.g. nitrile)
Gloves, long-sleeve
Lubricant (2–5 litres)
Paper towels (vulva area cleaning)
Prostaglandin $F_{2\alpha}$ (e.g. cloprostenol)
GnRH (e.g. buserelin acetate)
Progesterone, intravaginal:
devices and applicator
Disinfectant
(chlorhexidine, povidone iodine solution)
Syringes, sterile: 2, 5 ml
Hypodermic needles: 2.5 cm (1'') in 19–21 g
Recording sheets
Clipboard

Optional
Ultrasound machine, linear probe, 7.5 MHz
Vaginal speculum and light source
Chorionic gonadotrophin
Intra-uterine antimicrobial (endometritis)
Progesterone ELISA kit (bench-top)

Male fertility examination
Rope halter (XL)
Microscope with heat-stage and phase-contrast

Power lead and extension power cable
Immersion oil
Lens cleaning tissues
Gloves, disposable, non-sterile (e.g. nitrile)
Gloves, long-sleeve
Lubricant (0.5–2 litres)
KY Jelly
Scrotal circumference tape
Test tubes[1], clear, graduated, 15 ml, with top
Insulation sleeves for test tubes
(e.g. pipe lagging)
Test tube rack

Syringes[2], sterile, 1 ml

Needles, 1.6 cm (5/8'') in 25 g
Sample pots, plain, plastic, 5 ml
Pipettes, plastic, disposable
Microscope slides
Cover slips
Marker pen/small labels (ID of slides)
Slide holders
Morphology stain (e.g. Nigrosin-Eosin)
Formol saline (100–200 ml)
Saline (ideally phosphate-buffered)
Transport swabs, sterile (charcoal, plain)
Sharps container

Optional
Desk tally
Water bath
Haemocytometer with cover slip
Micro-pipettes, 5 ml and 40 µl, plus tips
Watch glass (for semen staining)
pH paper/meter
Ultrasound machine, linear probe, 7.5 MHz

For EEJ collection:
EEJ machine
Probe, 75 mm[3]
Power cable for probe (and spare)
Power cable/spare battery for machine
Collection handle (and two elastic bands)
Collection cones, disposable
(closed or open-ended)

For AV collection:
Artificial vagina
AV Liners (min. 2×)
AV Collection cones (min. 2×)
Elastic bands
Test tubes with rim
Thermometer, laboratory standard
Funnel

[1]For AV collection, and if open-ended collection cone is used for EEJ collection.
[2]Syringes must either be without a rubber seal, or the rubber must be non-spermaticidal.
[3]For yearling bulls use 60 mm, for Bos indicus-types use 90 mm diameter.

Box 10.4 Foot, limb and wound care (see Figure 10.2).

Foot care

Hoof knife, left-handed, 2× pairs
Toe-clippers (pincers), 1× pair
Hoof knife, right-handed, 2× pairs
Claw blocks & adhesive & mixing utensils
  (e.g. Demotec®, Cowslips™)
Gloves, disposable, non-sterile (e.g. nitrile)
Cotton wool, roll
Methylated spirit
Antibiotic spray (e.g. oxytetracycline)
Probe, sterile, 2 mm Ø × 12–15 cm

Local block / IVRA:
Tourniquet
Local anaesthetic (without adrenaline)
Syringe, sterile, 20–30 ml
Hypodermic needles:
  2.5 cm (1″) 19–21g

Optional
Gloves, anti-cut / protective
Hoof tester
Rasp
Angle-grinder

Bandaging and wound care

Bandages, 7.5–10 cm width, 4 rolls of each
Bandage, poultice (e.g. Animalintex®)
  Elastic adhesive (e.g. Tensoplast®)
  Cohesive (e.g. Vetrap™)
  Conforming (e.g. Knit-Firm)
  Padding (e.g. Soffban®)
Dressing, non-adhesive, 10 × 20 cm
  (e.g. Melolin™, Allevyn™, Primapore™)
Tape, adhesive (e.g. zinc oxide, 2 cm width)
Scalpel blade, no. 22
Bandage scissors, pair
Casting material, min. 6 rolls
  Fibreglass and resin[1] or plaster of Paris
  Widths of 7.5, 10, 12.5 cm

Optional
Stockinette
Casting tape (e.g. Vet-Lite)
Gamgee™
Intrasite™ gel, 15 g
Skin conditioning ointment
(e.g. udder cream, Vaseline, Dermisol®)

[1] For example, Vetcast™ or Dynacast®. If an oscillating saw is not available, also required are lengths of tubing (e.g. from administration set) and of fetotomy wire to aid cast removal with (wire fed through tubing and buried under cast).

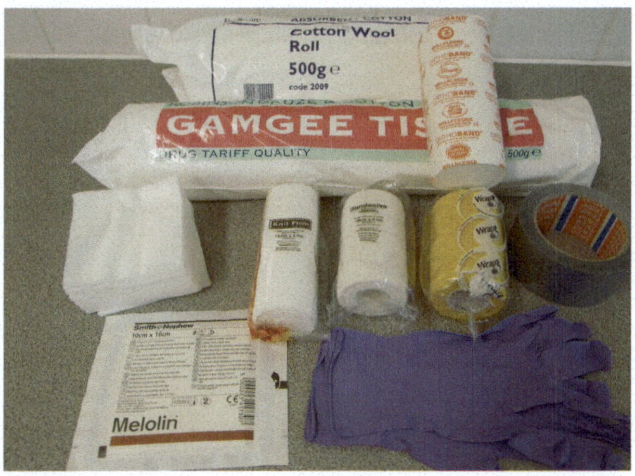

Figure 10.2 Useful material for bandaging, showing from top to bottom (and left to right): padding material (cotton wool, Gamgee™, OrthoBand®, gauze swabs); conforming, elastic adhesive and cohesive bandages (in widths of 10 and 7.5 cm); commercial duct tape; non-adhesive dressing; disposable gloves.

used for dilution, and the ingredients should have chemical grade standard (e.g. sourced through a pharmacy or scientific laboratory supplier). The latter is to avoid unwanted, and sometimes unknown, ingredients like the anti-caking agents or potassium chloride in some table salts. For the fluids commonly used in cattle practice, the following types and quantities are useful. Amounts need to be weighed out accurately, using a set of letter or laboratory scales:

(a) 9 grams sachets of sodium chloride, each to make one litre of isotonic 0.9% saline.
(b) 216 grams sachets of sodium chloride, each to make three litres of hypertonic 7.2% saline.
(c) 16.8 grams sachets of sodium bicarbonate, each to make 200 ml of molar 8.4% solution.
(d) Sachets containing 3.1 grams sodium lactate, 6 grams sodium chloride, 0.3 grams potassium chloride and 0.2 grams calcium chloride, each to make one litre of Hartman's.

Any vessels or bags used to prepare and administer the fluids with must be thoroughly cleaned (e.g. using diluted

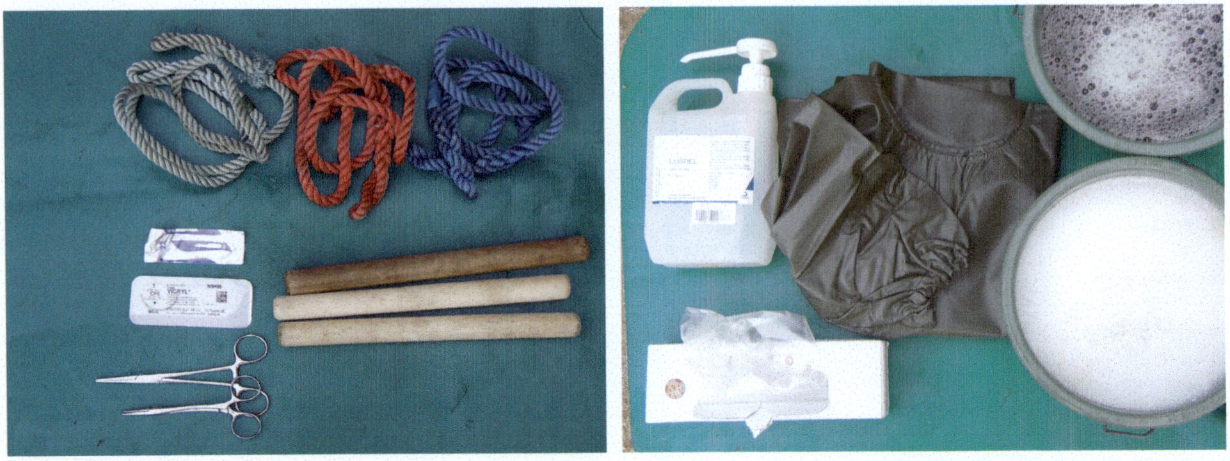

(a) (b)

Figure 10.3 Basic obstetrics kit, showing in a clockwise direction from top left in: (a): three calving ropes, ideally of different colours to aid placement identification; rope handles; and episiotomy equipment (artery forceps/needle holders, suture material, scalpel blade). (b): obstetrical lube; parturition gown; clean water with mild disinfectant for both obstetrician and patient; disposable long-sleeve gloves.

Box 10.5 Castration, disbudding and dehorning.

Rope halter
Animal marker spray
Scalpel blades, no. 22
Blade holder, no. 4
Artery forceps, pair
Gloves, disposable, non-sterile (e.g. nitrile)
Disinfectant (e.g. chlorhexidine)
Gauze swabs or cotton wool
Disbudding iron
Matches
Embryotomy wire & handles & wire cutter
and/or Scoop-Dehorner (e.g. Barnes-type)
Bucket, clean, ≈10 litres capacity

Depending on age/technique:
Emasculator
Burdizzo
Suture material for ligation

Sedative, alpha-2 agonist
(e.g. xylazine, detomidine hydrochloride)
Local anaesthetic (procaine HCl, lidocaine HCl)
Antimicrobial, injectable (penicillin-group)
Antimicrobial, spray
NSAID, short-acting (e.g. ketoprofen)
Syringes, sterile: 5, 10, 20 ml
Hypodermic needles:
3.75 cm (1.5″) in 21 g
2.5 cm (1″) in 16 g, 18–19 g, 21 g

Optional
Gloves, sterile surgical
Clipboard & recording sheets
Spare gas bottle

Box 10.6 Obstetrics (See Figures 10.3 a/b).

Either 'Calving' or 'Normal assistance'

Rope halter
Calving ropes or chains, sets of 3
Handles for ropes/chains
Gloves, long sleeve
Lubricant, obstetrical, min. 10 litres
Calf resuscitator (e.g. Cox's)

For epidural:
Scissors, curved (for clipping)
Methylated spirit
Gauze swabs or cotton wool
Syringe, sterile: 5 ml
Needle, hypodermic, 3.75 cm (1.5''), 19g
Local anaesthetic without adrenaline

For episiotomy:
Scalpel blade, no. 10 or 22
Suture material, cutting needle
Needle holder or artery forceps

Optional
Rope and tackle pulley
Calving jack/calf puller

Doxapram hydrochloride Fetotomy:
Fetotome, 2-barrel, stainless steel
with introducer probe (and cleaning brush)
Embryotomy wire (min. 3 reels)
Wire cutter
Wire introducer (e.g. Sand's)
Wire handles

Calving chains (2×)
Krey's hook
Eye hook, sharp & blunt pairs, plus rope
Guarded knife
Scalpel blade, no. 22
Caesarean section (Figure 10.4):
C-Section surgery kit (see Table 10.1)
Suture material and needles (see Table 10.2)

Drugs:
Sedative (e.g. alpha-2 agonist)
Local anaesthetic (procaine HCl, lidocaine HCl)
Clenbuturol
Oxytocin
Antimicrobial, injectable, broad-spectrum
NSAID (e.g. ketoprofen, meloxicam)
Syringes, sterile: 5, 10, 20–30 ml
Hypodermic needles:
5 cm (2'') in 20–21 g
2.5 cm (1'') in 16 g, 18–19 g, 21 g

Other:
Saline for irrigation, min. 1 litre

Optional
Spinal needles 75–90 mm (3–3.5'') in 18 g
(for paravertebral)
Rope (leg restraint), thick with eye splice,
1.8 m (6.5')
Antimicrobial, spray
Antimicrobial, intra-abdominal
(e.g. crystalline penicillin, dihydro-streptomycin)

Box 10.7 Selected surgical procedures.

General supplies
Syringes, sterile: 2, 5, 20–30 ml

Surgery kits (see Table 10.1)
Suture material and needles (see Table 10.2)
Fly repellent
Anti-inflammatory (NSAIDs)
Antimicrobial (systemic)

Teat lesions and injuries
Various models of:
Slitter, papillotome, lancet, dilator, extractor
Teat cannula, metal
Teat cannula, plastic, with plug
Local anaesthetic (without adrenaline)
Hypodermic needles: 1.6–2.5 cm (5/8–1″) in 23 g
Elastic band, household (as tourniquet)
Antimicrobial, intra-mammary
Wound spray (e.g. Leukopor®)
Teat bandaging tape (e.g. Leukopor®)

Soft tissue wounds
Wound protection during clipping (e.g. KY Jelly)
Wound irrigation:
Saline (min. 1 litre)
±0.1% Povidone antiseptic solution
Syringe, sterile, 30 ml
Hypodermic needle, 2.5 cm (1″) in 19 g
Local block/IVRA:
Tourniquet
Local anaesthetic[1]
Syringe, sterile, 20–30 ml
Hypodermic needles: 2.5, 5 cm (1″, 2″) 19–21g
Bandage material and wound dressings (see Box 10.4)
Optional

Medicated ointments

Rumen tympany
Local anaesthetic
Hypodermic needles: 2.5 cm (1″) in 21–23 g
Scalpel blade, no. 22

[1]Without adrenaline for IVRA

Rumen trocar:
Screw-in (e.g. 'Red Devil')
or Cannula (12–15 cm length)
Suture for cannula, on cutting needle
Surfactant (e.g. poloxalene)

Optional
Probang and gag

Bull ring application
Rope halter (XL)
Nose tissue punch
Nose ring & locking screw
Antimicrobial, topical
For infra-orbital or infiltration block:
Local anaesthetic
Hypodermic needle: 2.5 cm (1″) in 21–23 g

Laparotomy/displaced abomasum/
Rumenotomy/umbilical hernia repair
Local anaesthetic
Hypodermic needles: 5 cm (2″) in 19–21 g
or Spinal needles 75–90 mm (3–3.5″), 18 g
Tubing, sterile, Luer-connector
Hypodermic needles for deflation:
2.5 or 3.75 cm (1″ or 1.5″) in 16 g, 20 g

Optional:
Sterile sleeve for ultrasound probe

<u>Depending on LDA correction method:</u>
Grymer-Sterner Toggle kit
Suture needle, cutting, straight, 12–15 cm
Suture, absorbable, 5 metric/2 USP
(min. 300 cm length)
For rumenotomy:
Temporary anchor of rumen wall to skin:
Weingart frame, Steinman pins, stay sutures

For umbilical hernia repair
Prolene® mesh

Box 10.8 Special diagnostic procedures.

General supplies
Clippers/razor & blades/curved scissors
Surgical scrub
Gauze swabs/cotton wool
Gloves, surgical, sterile
Local anaesthetic
Hypodermic needle:
2.5 cm (1'') in 21–23 g (local block)
Syringe, sterile, 5 ml

Cerebro-spinal fluid collection (lumbo-sacral)
Hypodermic needles, 5 cm (2''), 20–21 g (calves)
Spinal needles, 9 cm (3.5''), 18 g (adults)
Syringes, sterile, 10 ml
Sample pots, EDTA and plain, 2.5–5 ml

Liver biopsy
Biopsy needle, 14 g (e.g. TruCut)
or s/s trochar, 4 mm OD (e.g. Shoof)
10 cm for calves, 25 cm for adults
Scalpel blade, no. 22
Syringe, sterile, 20 ml (if using trochar)
Suture material, cutting needle
(or skin staples and applicator)
Needle holder
Suture scissors
De-ionised water and syringe (to rinse blood off tissue sample)
Sample pots:
10% buffered formalin (histopathology)
Plain (mineral/heavy metal analysis)
Antimicrobial (e.g. penicillin-based)
Re-sterilisation of instruments between patients:
Quick-action disinfectant (e.g. chlorhexidine gluconate) and sterile saline

Broncho-alveolar lavage/Tracheal wash
Syringe, sterile, 50 ml, catheter tip
Saline, sterile, 50–100 ml
(ideally phosphate-buffered)
Sample pots, sterile, plain & VTM[1]

Intra-nasal approach
Local anaesthetic gel (e.g. xylocaine)
Flexible tube, 40–50 cm, 8–10 mm OD
Flexible, tube, 90 cm, 5–6 mm OD

Intra-tracheal approach
Hypodermic needle, 2.5 cm (1'') in 12–14 g
Tomcat catheter, 3–5 Fr

Tuberculosis testing (intra-dermal)
McLintock syringe, 1–2[2]
Record or Schimmel Needles:
0.4–1 cm (5/32''–3/8''), 22 g
Needle adaptors & washers
Spanner
Skin callipers
Scissors (curved) or clippers
Test chart or book
Tuberculin (bovine +/- avian)
Holster belt
Cotton wool
Spirit-based disinfectant
Optional
DNA tags and applicator

[1]VTM: Virus transport medium.
[2]Depending on whether comparative (avian and bovine) or single test is applied. Calibrated to deliver 0.1 ml tuberculin. For comparative test, also clear identification of syringes (e.g. blue and red thumb knob).

Box 10.9 Biosecurity and personal care.

Sharps bin
Clinical waste bags
Cable ties
Protective clothing (plus 1× change)
Gloves, disposable, non-sterile (e.g. nitrile)
Disinfectant for hands (e.g. chlorhexidine, povidone iodine)
Towels (paper or cloth)
Disinfectant for boots and equipment, approved to required standard (e.g. iodophor)
Bucket and brush
First Aid kit

Optional:
Knapsack sprayer
Goggles

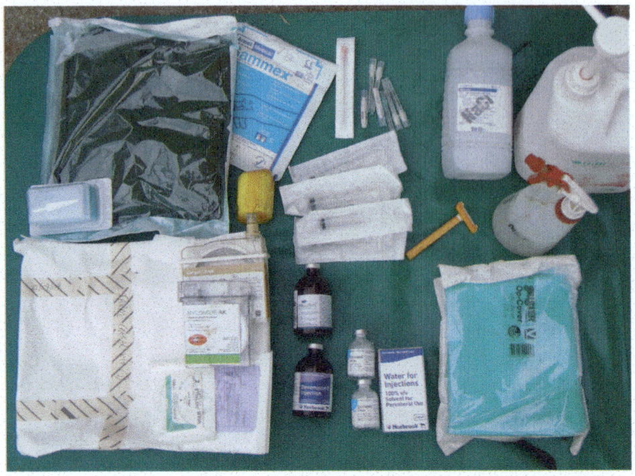

Figure 10.4 Caesarean-section kit, showing in a clockwise direction from top left: nail brush; surgical gown; surgical gloves; tail bandage; needles and syringes for local/regional anaesthesia; saline for irrigation; razor for clipping; disinfectants for surgical site and surgeon (chlorhexidine, surgical spirit); drape; intra-peritoneal antimicrobrials; local anaesthetic; instrument kit; suture material.

bleach), rinsed and dried after every use. They must be regularly inspected for signs of mould or other contaminants, the presence of which should trigger immediate disposal and replacement.

In areas where blood parasites are common, anti-coagulants to allow quick-response blood collection and transfusion are also useful. Options include carrying sachets of sodium citrate in crystalline form, to mix with sterile isotonic saline at the point of use (for example 3.8 grams dissolved in 100 ml saline for each litre of blood, or 15 grams of sodium citrate in 400 ml sterile saline for 4–5 litres of blood). Alternatively, 5000 IU of heparin sodium in 25 ml sterile isotonic saline per litre of blood can be used.

Box 10.10 Record keeping and reference material.

Maps of practice area/satellite navigation system
Mobile phone (and charger)/RT-system
List of contact numbers (incl. police, government authorities, slaughterman, veterinary poisoning service)
Drug compendium
Drug labels (+/- label printer, barcode reader)
Electronic recording device (e.g. laptop)
Paper visit recording forms
Pens
Reference books

Box 10.11 Vehicle equipment and care.

Vehicle documents
Driving licence
Fuel card
Contact for breakdown service
Spare wheel, jack, wheel brace
Tow bar/rope
Fire extinguisher
Hazard triangle/light/hi-visibility vest
Chilled compartment for temperature-sensitive drugs

Explanatory notes on obstetric equipment (Box 10.6)

For dystocia cases, both calving ropes and chains may be used. Ropes tend to be less traumatic on both the calf's limbs and veterinarian's hands. Having ropes of different colours in each set is useful to clearly identify which rope has been applied to which body part of the calf (e.g. red on right limb, green on left limb, blue on head). A disadvantage of ropes is that they cannot be effectively cleaned and disinfected on farm. Therefore, chains are more useful in practice areas with seasonal calving patterns and potential consecutive dystocia visits. Several models of chain handles can be purchased. For ropes, handles can be manufactured by cutting a household broomstick into three parts of equal length, rounding off the ends with sandpaper. As knots in calving ropes make placement difficult, the ropes are secured to handles or calving aids using a clove hitch.

CHAPTER 11

The Practice Laboratory

Allan Kessell

Learning objectives

- To appreciate the range of tests and techniques that may be usefully performed in-house, and the equipment required.
- To be able to perform some basic laboratory procedures.
- To be able to decide which tests/procedures will suit the practice.
- To be able to design and equip an in house laboratory for the practice needs.

Introduction

There has been, in recent times, a demand for the establishment or expansion of the capabilities of the practice laboratory, and for relying less on commercial laboratories. This may be due to a number of reasons:

1 The development of in-house blood and biochemistry machines with increasing capability.
2 The development of tests in kit form, based on ELISA or other technologies, that are fast and reported to be accurate.
3 Possibly the increasing expectations of the veterinary public, in concert with the increasing level of post-graduate education available to the practitioner.
4 The aggressive marketing of companies that offer these test modalities.

This is especially so in small animal practice, such that a large percentage of practices may now have in-house haematological and biochemical analyses delivering a comprehensive range of test results, as well as some limited ability to examine urine and faeces. However, when researching this chapter, I could find few guidelines on setting up a practice laboratory for veterinarians predominantly in cattle practice.

If your practice wants to set up a laboratory, there must be careful consideration given to ensuring the quality of the results. Precise and accurate results are useful; inaccurate results are not. The most important component in a successful practice laboratory that generates quality results is the staff. At least one of the veterinarians should oversee the laboratory, and preferably have an interest in diagnostic testing and quality assurance (QA).

The practice laboratory should not replace the external accredited laboratory. A close relationship between the practice veterinarians and the pathologists at an accredited laboratory is very useful for both advice and guidance. The actual day-to-day running of the laboratory should be the responsibility of a trained nominated person – usually a veterinary nurse. Ensuring quality testing should include a reliable QA program for all in-house diagnostic testing and equipment.

Some in-house instruments come with internal quality controls; those that do not require internal and external monitoring QA systems. Maintenance of the laboratory equipment should at least be in accordance with the manufacturers' recommendations. Protocols for all laboratory procedures should be documented for reference, so that there is a standard operating procedure (SOP). Recommendations for laboratory SOPs have been provided by:

- Royal College of Veterinary Surgeons Practice Standards Scheme Manual,
- College of Veterinarians of Ontario Guideline: Ordering, Performing and Interpreting Laboratory Tests in Veterinary Clinical Practice
- American Animal Hospital Association, Accreditation.

In addition to the desktop analytical machines, portable hand-held veterinary machines are available which can measure blood gas, electrolyte, chemistry and haematology from 2-3 drops of whole blood in the practice laboratory or at cowside. Depending upon the cartridge used they can provide values for haematocrit, haemoglobin, BUN, creatinine, ionised calcium, glucose, Na, K, pH, pCO_2, HCO_3, TCO_2, anion gap, base excess and lactate. The results are available within a minute or two.

Bovine Medicine, Third Edition. Edited by Peter D. Cockcroft.

My aim is to provide an overview for the practitioner, with some practical information about the practice laboratory that is hard to find in standard texts. I will cover: tests and techniques that may be useful in clinical pathology; microbiology and parasitology; the type of equipment required; and, finally, some suggestions about planning the practice laboratory.

Clinical pathology

Haematology

Measuring the packed cell volume (PCV), total protein concentration (TP) and fibrinogen concentration

Fill two haematocrit tubes with EDTA blood until each is three-quarters full; wipe excess blood from the outside of the tubes; stopper one end with plasticine.

Both tubes are placed in the centrifuge, with the stoppered end against the outer rim, and are then centrifuged (see section 11.6 for information on speeds and times with various fluids). The percentage of packed red cells (PCV) is measured, using the PCV reader. One tube is then scored just above the buffy coat (bc) with the edge of a glass slide. The tube is carefully broken here, several drops of plasma are placed on the refractometer, and the total plasma protein concentration measured (plasma latescence will falsely elevate this reading; high plasma urea/glucose/cholesterol will also do so, but to a lesser degree).

The other haematocrit tube is placed in a 55–57° C water bath for three minutes (you can use a simple tap water bath), which causes the fluid column to become opaque, due to precipitation of fibrinogen. The tube is then re-centrifuged. This process compacts the fibrinogen above the buffy (bc) layer (see Figure 11.1). The fibrinogen concentration is then calculated by measuring the height (to the nearest 0.1 mm) of the compacted fibrinogen layer over the total height of the fibrinogen/plasma layer, expressed as grams/litre (Millar *et al.*, 1971). This is illustrated in Figure 11.1.

This may be difficult, and prone to parallax error, so in our laboratory we measure the protein content in the plasma, both before and after water bath incubation, with the refractometer. The difference between total protein before and after incubation is also a good estimate of fibrinogen, and possibly easier to perform.

Calculation: method 1

$$\text{Fibrinogen (g/L)} = \frac{\text{length fibrinogen (mm)}}{\text{length fibrinogen + plasma (mm)}}$$

$$= \frac{AB}{AC} \times 100$$

Calculation: method 2

Fibrinogen (g/L) = plasma total protein before heating − plasma total protein after heating

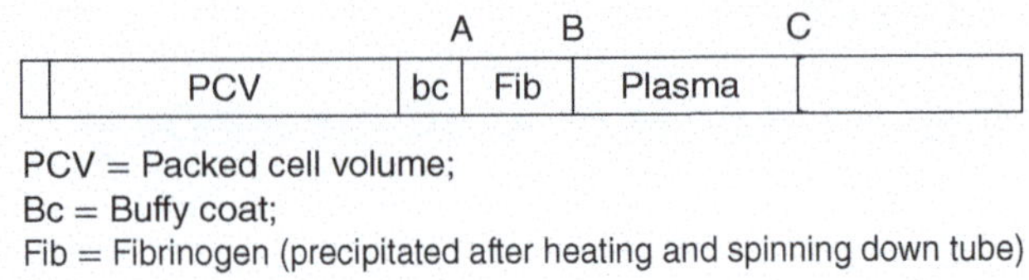

Figure 11.1 Calculation of fibrinogen.

Haematology machine

Total white cell count (WBC)

Most modern machines use impedance and/or laser technology to count cells. These machines can provide an accurate total white blood cell (WBC) count.

Differential white cell count

There is little information on the accuracy of in-house machine generated WBC differentials using bovine blood, (Deprez *et al.*, 2009; Goldmann *et al.*, 2011) but there is sufficient on machine derived differentials in other species to indicate that a manual differential is required (Wenger-Riggenbach *et al.*, 2006; Becker *et al.*, 2008; Deprez *et al.*, 2009; Welles *et al.*, 2009; Goldmann *et al.*, 2011; Riond *et al.*, 2011). Most private laboratories perform manual differentials in all common veterinary species, even though much more expensive haematology machines are available. The platelet count should also be done manually, or at least the smear checked to validate the machine count (platelet clumps at the end of the smear will invalidate a machine or manual count, and likely indicate adequate platelets). The actual PCV should be used in place of the calculated PCV (the haematocrit), as it is more accurate. An examination of the blood film, as well as providing a more accurate differential, will also allow some comment on WBC toxic changes and RBC morphology (including possible RBC parasites), and the presence of abnormal cells.

Blood film preparation

A properly made blood smear is essential for an accurate assessment of haematological changes. If there is a delay in processing (more than four hours), or the blood is kept at high temperature (e.g. in the practice vehicle on a hot day), quite significant degenerative changes can occur in the WBCs, resulting in misclassification of band and mature neutrophils. Under these circumstances, it is best to keep the blood sample cool, or preferably make a blood smear at the time of collection.

A small drop of blood is placed at one end of the glass slide, just above the labelled frosted end, and a 'spreader' (you may use a clean glass slide) is placed just in front of the drop at 45° to the slide. The spreader is then drawn back into the drop, and the blood distributed evenly along the leading edge of the spreader by using an up-and-down see-saw motion. The spreader is then pushed in a smooth, controlled motion towards the opposite end of the glass slide. If the correct amount of blood, correct angle of the spreader, and even distribution of the drop along the edge has occurred, the blood film should finish approximately half to three-quarters of the way down the slide, and have a well-formed 'feathered' edge at the end of the smear (which is absolutely essential).

The blood film is dried quickly by waving it in the air. A hair drier should not be used for this purpose, as the cells can be damaged before fixing. The dried blood film is then fixed for at least 30 seconds (can stay in fixative for a prolonged time if busy), and Diff Quick stained. The stain is then washed off immediately and the slide dried using a hair dryer, which should take 10–15 seconds (this makes the slide available for immediate viewing, and cuts down on RBC artefact).

This staining technique is used for all cytology, keeping in mind that a monolayer of cells has to be formed to allow the viewing of individual cells. With a blood film made this way, the monolayer is just back from the feathered edge.

Using a Microscope: the basics to optimise performance

The distance between the two eyepieces is adjusted to the distance (mm) between your pupils. Each eyepiece may be individually focused (usually the right, with the microscope fine focus, and the left directly on the eyepiece itself).

The sub-stage diaphragm is left up for stained slides, and variably down for unstained preparations (urine sediment, etc.), and the iris diaphragm is usually opened.

The 40× lens is designed to view cells through a cover-slip. Since all lenses can view through a cover slip (including the 100× lens), a cover slip is placed over a drop of oil on the slide prior to any stained examination. It is best to place a drop of immersion oil over the area to be viewed first, and then apply and gently compress a cover slip to spread the oil evenly.

The slide is examined by using the lowest power lens first (4×, 10×, 20×, 40×), with a final examination at 100× (if required – RBC/WBC morphology, bacteria in cytology preparations). The 100× lens is an oil immersion lens. After focusing at 40×, a single drop of oil is placed on top of the cover slip and the 100× lens rotated into the oil for viewing. The reason the 100× lens is used last is that the 40× lens is the same length as the 100× lens and, if it is rotated through the drop of oil while changing lenses, the 40× lens becomes coated with oil, and cannot then give a clear view of the slide. If oil is not immediately cleaned from the 40×, it can form a semi-permanent coat and be very difficult to clean off; if left long enough, the lens may be damaged. This is the usual reason why 40× lenses are not useable in practice. Thus, the following simple protocol is suggested:

- Always place a cover slip over a drop of oil prior to any stained cytological examination.
- Always use the 100× lens as the last step in examination, by looking through a single drop of oil on top of the cover slip.
- Always wipe the oil off the 100× lens immediately after use, being careful *not* to rotate the 40× lens through the oil. If you need to re-examine at 40× after 100×, half-rotate the lens head, wipe the oil off the 100× lens, remove the cover slip with oil on top, and replace with a clean cover slip.

If you need to clean the 40× lens after oil contamination, use fine tissue paper soaked in alcohol. If the oil has been on the lens for some length of time, this cleaning will sometimes take up to a minute of rubbing the lens with alcohol-soaked tissues.

Microscopic examination of a blood smear (Figure 11.2)

1 Feathered edge overview of slide (remember you already have a cover slip on): peruse the feathered edge at 100–400× magnification i.e. using 10–40× lens for platelet clumps (even small numbers of clumps will invalidate any platelet count, either machine generated or manual; if moderate numbers of clumps are present, then platelets are classed as adequate). Also, look for abnormal cells.
2 Monolayer (where RBCs are not quite touching): perform WBC differential at 400–1000× magnification. Using the battlement method, differentiate 100 WBCs (sufficient in ruminant species for an accurate differential, although if the animal is markedly neutropenic, you may wish to count only 25–50 WBCs and correct to 100%).
3 Monolayer: examine the morphology of RBCs and WBCs at 100×.
4 Monolayer: do platelet estimation at 1000× magnification if no (or very few) clumps at end of smear.

Count number of platelets in five 1000× fields and calculate the average/field.
For each 1/field = 20×10^9/l platelets.
e.g. you count 15, 20, 25, 21, 19 platelets in each of five fields; average, 20/100× field;
platelet estimate = $20 \times 20 = 400 \times 10^9$/l

Biochemistry

The biochemistry machine

A large number of machines are available to the clinician for use in-house. Again, most have been validated for small animals and horses (Little *et al.*, 1992; Pinches, 2006; Milne & Scott, 2006; Siska *et al.*, 2011; Rishniw *et al.*, 2012), with fewer for bovines (Rishniw *et al.*, 2012). In a recent comparison survey of a large number of practice and commercial laboratory biochemistry machines, using standard quality control material, practice machines did not perform as well as the more expensive laboratory machines, especially when measuring creatinine and chloride (Welles, 2009). Instruments that were not calibrated daily (some older in house instruments) did not perform as well as those calibrated daily (e.g. IDDEX Catalyst and Abaxis Vetscan). Older papers make reference to the unreliable nature

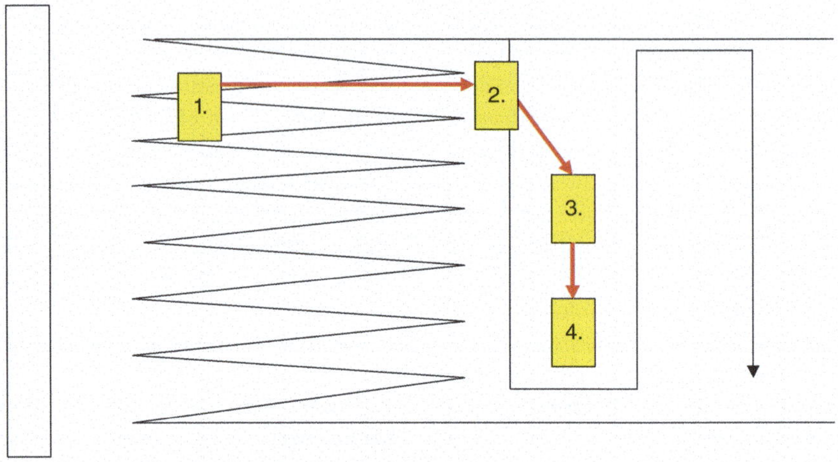

1. Feathered edge (100× magnification)
2. WBC differential - in area where RBCs almost touching (400–1000× magnification)
3. RBC/WBC morphology (1000× magnification)
4. Platelet estimation (1000× magnification)

Figure 11.2 Model blood film (with exaggerated feather edge); see text for explanation.

of calcium results from the older VetTest instrument (Little *et al.*, 1992), but this was not confirmed in more recent assessments (Rishniw *et al.*, 2012).

Panels

There are some well defined profiles that are commonly used in bovine medicine that could be performed in-house on both individual animals and in herd investigations. In valuable individual animals with poorly defined disease presentations, a complete blood count and biochemistry panels can be useful in both ruling out some diseases and identifying others. These are offered by private pathology companies at very competitive prices, and often have the luxury (for which you usually pay) of pathologists' comments and interpretation.

Table 11.1 Tests than can be used to monitor metabolic/nutritional conditions.

Test	Cows tested	Decision level; alarms
NEFA (serum) [a,b] – non-esterified fatty acids	2–14 days before calving	>0.4 mmol/L; > 10% of group
Ketones (*serum) [a–c] – β hydroxybutyrate (BOHB)	type I ketosis: 21–50 days in milk type II ketosis: 5–50 days in milk	>3000/mmol/L >1400 mmol/L; >10%
Urinary pH [d]	Pre-calving after >24 hours on anionic diet	Optimal pH 6–7
Serum Ca [d]	Immediate post parturient, as required	< 2 mmol/L
Ruminal pH [a,b,e]	Lactating cows, about 5 to 150 days in milk (dependent on feeding system) subacute ruminal acidosis	 <5.5 <5.5; >25% of group
Urea nitrogen in blood (BUN) or milk (MUN)[b,f]	Lactating cows at any stage of lactation; measure three hours after protein meal	4.3–5.7 mmol BUN/L 240–330 mg MUN/L

[a]Iwerson *et al.* (2009),
[b]Cook *et al.* (2006a),
[c]Cook *et al.* (2006b),
[d]Le Blanc (2010),
[e]Oetzel (2004),
[f]Rollon (2006).

However, there are some limited profiles that can be generated on in-house machines, reasonably accurately and in a timely fashion. Such disease states include metabolic disease (β hydroxyl butyrate-BOHB, Ca, Mg, phosphate, glucose); myonecrosis (CK, AST – there is prognostic value in downer cows in the degree of elevation); GGT for adequacy of colostral transfer; renal function parameters (creatinine), especially combined with knowledge of hydration status and urine specific gravity. Additional analytes used may be total protein/albumin (useful in inflammatory and protein losing states, to assess degree of dehydration, severe hepatic disease and parasitism).

Most in-house machines do not offer GLDH and SD. If hepatocellular necrosis is suspected, a commercial laboratory can be used. The enzyme AST may be used (if offered on your machine) if there is no evidence of muscle necrosis (normal CK) or haemolysis. Most in-house biochemistry instruments do not offer BOHB. However, hand-held meters that measure BOHB, similar to those used for glucose monitoring in diabetics, have been validated for use on bovine whole blood (Pinches, 2006).

Metabolic disease

Nutritional assessment: there are a variety of disease states in the pre- and post-partum dairy cow that are often linked to imbalances between metabolic demand and energy, protein or mineral intake. These will be covered in detail elsewhere in this text, but a variety of in-house or cowside tests may be used to monitor these conditions (Table 11.1).

1 Metabolites that measure energy balance in transitional cows:

   Non-esterified fatty acids (NEFA): taken in the last two weeks of pregnancy, this reflects the magnitude of mobilisation of fat from storage, and as such will reflect dry matter intake (DMI). Kits have been available in the past (DVM NEFA test, Veterinary Diagnostics) that were reported to give acceptable results and to be cost-effective in large herds (Oetzel, 2004), but they are no longer available. Therefore, serum has be taken and sent to an accredited laboratory for this analyte.

   Ketones: these are the intermediate metabolites of fatty acids such as NEFAs, and will also increase in animals with a negative energy balance. The gold standard test is the level of BOHB in serum or plasma tested within the first two weeks *post partum* (Iwerson *et al.*, 2009). Tests are also available for urine and milk, which are less sensitive and specific (Table 11.2)

2 Measures of peri-parturient hypocalcaemia:

   Blood calcium: clinical and subclinical hypocalcaemia occur most commonly soon after calving, and the gold standard is serum taken in this period for serum-ionised Ca or, more commonly, serum Ca. Serum-ionised Ca can be tested cowside with several hand-held instruments, although these have been designed for use with humans and have not been validated in bovines. Many in-house biochemistry machines will accurately measure serum Ca, but it is also worthwhile testing serum albumin at the same time to check for the likelihood of a true hypocalcaemia (approximately 50% of Ca is associated with albumin, and thus low albumin states can result in low total Ca, but not low ionised Ca).

   Urinary pH: determination of urinary pH can be used on a herd basis to monitor the efficacy of anionic diets fed pre-partum in an attempt to limit the development of clinical and subclinical hypocalcaemia. A urine pH of 6–7 is associated with a low risk compared with higher pH values. Measuring urine pH with narrow-range (scale of 0.3 unity of pH) pH indicator paper is usually sufficient, although a calibrated portable pH meter is more accurate and, therefore, preferable (Rollon, 2006).

Urea nitrogen (UN)

Blood urea nitrogen (BUN) or milk urea nitrogen (MUN) are closely related, and are indirect measures of protein and energy nutritional balance in lactating cows. Cows with high BUN concentrations are a risk factor for infertility and body condition score loss, due to the energy cost of detoxifying excessive ruminal ammonia into urea by the liver. In-house machines can perform BUN or urea tests. The conversion relationship of mmol/L and mg/L is that 1 mmol/L urea = 28 mg/L BUN. Monitoring bulk milk has been suggested, as long as wet chemistry is used (Cook *et al.*, 2006a; Rollon, 2006). Most in-house biochemistry analysers use dry (not wet) chemistry, and I know of no in-house machine validated using milk.

Cytology

Cytology can be useful to diagnose the presence, and sometimes the cause, of inflammatory lesions. It is often used when investigating mastitis and abscesses, but may also be used as part of a fluid analysis when inflammation may be suspected (e.g. peritonitis, pleuritis). The secret of a good cytology preparation is the creation of a monolayer that is properly stained, as with the preparation of a blood smear. Staining preparations with Diff Quik is adequate to demonstrate an inflammatory cells, although additional staining with gram stains allows the morphology and gram reaction of any bacteria to be identified.

Urinalysis

A complete urinalysis requires gross examination, urine specific gravity (USG), dipstick chemistries and unstained sediment examination. The dipstick chemistries are often used cowside (e.g. ketones (BOHB)). The strips that indicate a USG range or inflammation are not accurate for these analyses in animals. The USG is best measured with a refractometer, and WBCs by sediment examination. If there is a delay in processing the sample, it is best kept cool to preserve cytological features.

Table 11.2 Performance of cowside tests for detection of subclinical ketosis (after Le Blanc, 2010). Reproduced with permission of Society for Reproduction and Development.

	Blood	Milk	Urine
Preferred test	Precision XTRA[a] (Medisense Abbott)	Keto-test (BOHB)[a,b] (Sanwa Kagaku Kenkyusho Co.)	Ketostic (AcAc)[b,d] (Bayer)
Sensitivity	87–93%	– at 100umol/l on strip: 83%[b] – at 200umol/l on strip: 30[a] – 54%[b]	– 'small' level, when read after 5 sec 79%; 4–90%[c]
Specificity	93–100%	– at 100 umol/l on strip: 82%[b] – at 200 umol/l on strip: 94%[b] :98%[a]	96%
Approximate cost	$3/test Meter $40	$2/test	$0.25/test
Comments	BOHB strips more accurate in bovines than glucose	– some powders lack sensitivity and are not recommended – colour change assessment may be subjective, and prone to error[a]	– typically only induce 50% of cows to urinate – Acetest lacks specificity –↑[AcAc]→↓ sensitivity[c]

$=USA (2010);
[a]Iwerson *et al.*, 2009;
[b]Oetzel, 2004, 20;
[c]Rollon, 2006;
[d]Carrier.

Often in cattle practice, the sediment examination is not completed, but it can be useful in cases of haematuria, pyuria or crystalluria. It requires spinning down 5 ml of urine, discarding 90% of the supernatant, and re-suspending the sediment button in the remaining fluid. A drop is then placed on a slide under a cover slip, and examined with 10× and 40× lens (unstained, so drop the condenser) for RBCs/WBCs (< 5/40× field), casts (< 2/10× field) and crystals. More details can be found in the text references at the end of the chapter.

Microbiology

Conventional microbiology

Mastitis investigations are achievable in-house, but require an incubator, media to isolate organisms, and a small range of tests to identify the most important bacterial pathogens. Five organisms cause the majority of udder infections, and a flowchart (Figure 11.3) is provided to assist in working through what is required for accurate identification. A good text on veterinary microbiology (see text references), basic instructions on aseptic sample collection, plating, and use of the inoculating loop is required. Unusual or less common causes of mastitis will require the services of an external accredited laboratory, as may antimicrobial sensitivity testing.

Gram stains are essential to subdivide bacterial species into two broad groups (positive and negative), and they may be used, along with cytology, to demonstrate the presence of a bacterial organism associated with inflammation. I have concentrated on the work up required to identify common mastitic organisms here (Figure 11.3). If wider investigations are envisaged, appropriate texts should be consulted and professional advice sought. It is important to note that if in-house microbiology is planned, aseptic technique, proper handling and disposal of materials and cultures is required, and state and country laws should be followed. Antibiotic sensitivity testing is outside the realm of most in-house laboratories, and should be referred to an accredited laboratory.

Tests for mastitis culture (see flowchart, Figure 11.3)

There is a lot of information on the internet for all these tests, including live demonstrations. Suppliers will vary, depending on where you practise, but all these test materials are widely available.

Catalase test: the presence of this enzyme can be demonstrated by placing a drop of 3% hydrogen peroxide (purchased at any chemist) on a slide, and mixing into it a portion of a single bacterial colony you wish to test. If the catalase enzyme is present, it will cause the formation of oxygen from the hydrogen peroxide, resulting in a visible bubbling of the mix (catalase positive).

Oxidase test: used to determine if a bacteria contains cytochrome oxidase. The test uses either a disc or strip of filter paper impregnated with an indicator system (keep in the cool part of refrigerator between tests), which turns blue to dark purple when smeared with the bacterial colony:

- wet paper with about 1–2 loops of water;
- transfer and rub into wet area a single colony of bacteria;
- wait three minutes: positive = area becomes dark purple; negative = area remains uncoloured.

Lancefield grouping: used to demonstrate the type of group specific cell wall polysaccharide antigen (C-substance) in pathogenic *Streptococci* spp. Commercially available latex

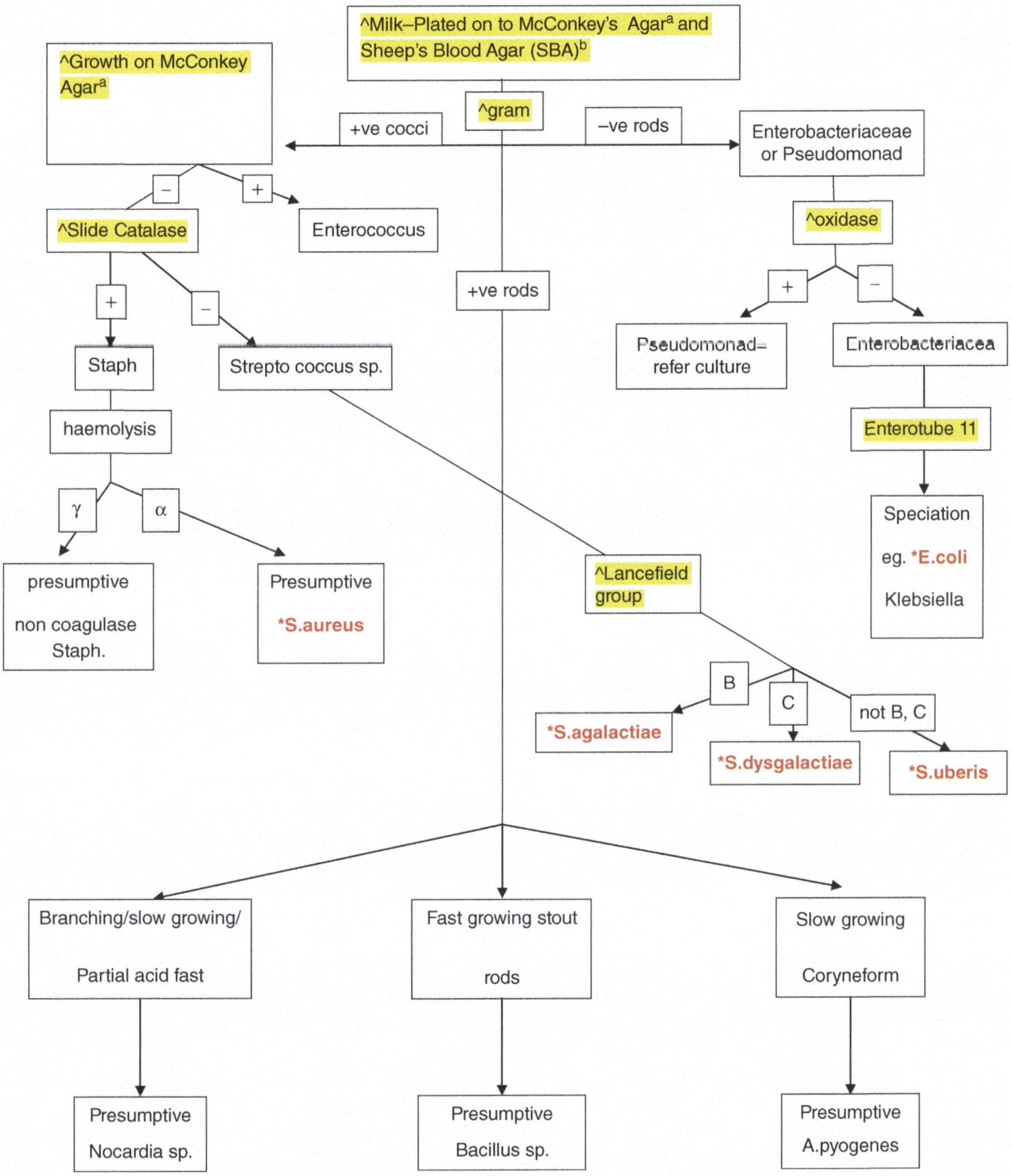

***Most Important Species, ^Tests used,** [a]**McConkey's Agar** is a selective media for Gram-negative, enteric bacteria, [b]**Sheep's Blood Agar** is a non-selective media, good for culturing many bacterial species including Gram negative and Gram-positive species including Staphylococci and Streptococci

Figure 11.3 Flowchart for mastitis culture.

agglutination test kits are available, which will contain group B and C antisera coated onto latex spheres. These tests are not difficult to perform, and come with full directions.

Enterotube II test (Becton-Dickinson and Company): this test is easy to use, but there are a number of test kits available that may be used to speciate the Enterobacteriacea. The test chamber is divided into a series of smaller chambers containing media with different sugars/indicators, which are inoculated from a single bacterial colony using the supplied wire loop. Air is let into some of these chambers and the unit is incubated for approximately 24 hours at 37°C. The resulting colour changes allow speciation of the bacterial colony. The test system comes with full instructions and tables.

Slide coagulase: coagulase is a protein that enables the conversion of fibrinogen to fibrin, and as such requires the use of plasma (usually rabbit). It is used here to identify *S. aureus* more definitively than using just the pattern of haemolysis around the colony alone. It is optional, but advised.

Gram stain method:

- Make smears of tissue/fluid/colony on a dry slide and allow to air dry completely.
- Only heat fix if a smear is from a colony from a culture plate; tissues/fluids contain enough protein to 'stick' the material to the slide and do not require heat fixation.
- Stain with 1% Crystal Violet solution (30 sec), rinse in tap water and drain.
- Stain with Lugols iodine solution, rinse in tap water and drain.
- Rapidly decolourise by dripping acetone/alcohol decolouriser over angled slide until all blue colour is removed from the slide.
- Immediately wash thoroughly in running tap water (you do not want to over-decolourise)
- Counterstain with 0.25% Safranin (1 min), rinse in tap water and drain.
- Dry with hair dryer and examine under microscope.

Test Kits

For the bovine practitioner, kits that test calf faeces for potential pathogens are attractive from a cost and time point of view. The positive and negative predictive value of these tests will depend on their sensitivity, specificity, and prevalence of the disease in the population being tested. The sensitivity and specificity will depend on the detection limit of the 'gold standard' used to calculate them, and can thus vary from study to study. Choice of test will also be dictated by its proposed use, either as a screening test (high sensitivity required) or a diagnostic test (high specificity), as well as frequency of use and cost.

It will be important to research impartial evaluations of the test being considered, and sometimes claims by manufacturers may be based on small sample numbers and/or less sensitive 'gold standards' than some impartial evaluations. Recently, reverse transcriptase PCR (RT-PCR) and real time reverse transcriptase PCR (qRT-PCR) have become the gold standards; the latter is quantitative and more sensitive, and it is important to keep in mind that these techniques are detecting genetic material, not proteins (as with the ELISA tests).

It is also advisable to check with the pathology laboratory you are using – some laboratories will have highly sensitive and specific tests, such as qRT-PCR assays/multiplex PCRs, which offer better accuracy and possibly cost benefit when testing for complex disease states. Space does not allow an exhaustive list or review of all kits available. However, some examples are offered which may be helpful:

- K99 *E. coli*: test kits are available that use ELISA, and LAT. ELISA has been used for some time and has a similar performance to bacterial culture between 1–6 days old (van Zijderveld & Overdigk, 1983). The LAT is usually simpler, easier, and quicker to perform, and in clinical cases is said to give reliable results when compared to the ELISA because of the large number of organisms usually excreted (Nussbaum *et al.*, 1999).
- Coronavirus/Rotavirus: these are often tested together with a number of assays available. ELISA and LAT may be used in-house . In one study (Zijderveld and Overdigk, 1983), LAT and ELISA were compared to RT-PCR for coronavirus and rotavirus. They showed a high specificity (96.4% and 95.3%, respectively), but a relatively low sensitivity (60.0% and 71.9% respectively). In contrast, another recent paper that compared ELISA and LAT with qPT-PCR for coronavirus and rotavirus (Izzo *et al.*, 2012), reported low sensitivity and specificity, as well as low positive and negative predictive values, and questioned its use for diagnostic samples.
- Crytosporidium: Acid-fast staining (AF- Kinyoun method) may be used to demonstrate the presence of Cryptosporidial cysts in calf faeces, but is not as sensitive as immunochromografflic/latex agglutination (LAT). In-house testing may use AF and LAT techniques, which are often compared with the gold standards of floatation sedimentation staining (SF) and PCR. (Nussbaum *et al.*, 1999; Paul *et al.*, 2009; Klein *et al.*, 2009). All tests are reasonably specific (> 92%), but sensitivity varies. One paper reports a sensitivity of 65% and 82% when AF and SF are compared to PCR as a gold standard (Paul *et al.*, 2009); another paper reports a sensitivity of 100% for the LAT when compared to SF as the gold standard (Klein *et al.*, 2009). This would suggest that LAT would be the in-house test of choice.
- Multiple test strips are available that use faecal samples which can test for Cryptosporidium, parvum rotavirus, corona virus, *E. coli* (K99) in outbreaks of calf diarrhoea.
- Bovine viral diarrhoea antigen snap test kits are now available (IDEXX SNAP® BVDV Antigen Test), which help to identify BVDV-infected cattle. This kit can use both serum and ear-notch tissue samples.

Parasitology

Faecal worm egg count (FEC) method

Introduction

Following is a simple method for performing a FEC on bovine (or ovine) faeces. Most methods make use of a set amount of faeces, mixed thoroughly with a saturated salt solution so that the eggs are, theoretically, evenly spread throughout the resultant faeces/saline suspension. This suspension is then quickly sub-sampled (before the eggs start floating to the top) and loaded into a standard counting chamber, which is left for ten minutes so that all the eggs have floated to the same plane of examination in the chamber. The number of eggs in a set area of the chamber are then counted and multiplied by a dilution factor to calculate the number of worm eggs/gram of faeces (FEC).

Equipment needed

1. A jar that holds 60 ml comfortably, with marks on side at 30 and 60 ml (yellow top urine sample jar may be used)
2. An open ended 10 ml syringe (fill with 3 ml – 3 g – of faeces)
3. Some saturated salt solution. This will have a specific gravity (SG) of 1.18–1.20. Preparation: heat water to below boiling, stir in salt until no more will dissolve (some will start settling at the bottom of the container). After the salt has settled and the solution cooled, check specific gravity (100 ml of solution should weigh between 118–120 g).
4. A 1 mm mesh insert, shaped to sit into the jar approximately one-quarter the way down (at about 50 ml).
5. A stirrer/mixer.
6. A 1 ml disposable pipette.
7. A Whitlock universal four-chamber counting slide.
8. A microscope.

Procedure:

1. Place 3 g of faeces in jar.
2. Add 30 ml of salt solution.
3. Mix gently until you have an even suspension (vigorous mixing will result in too many bubbles).
4. Add salt solution to 60 ml mark, and evenly re-suspend faeces/solution mix (i.e. have 3 g of faeces evenly mixed in 57 ml of salt solution).
5. The next step must be done quickly, so that the eggs do not start to all float to the top of the suspension. Place the mesh into the jar so that the top part of the fluid is free of faecal debris. Pipette off approximately 0.5 ml of this fluid, expel air from the pipette, and load the Whitlock chamber by placing the tip of the pipette against the front opening of the chamber and gently squeezing the pipette bulb.
6. Allow ten minutes for the eggs to float to the top of the chamber.
7. At 4× magnification, count all eggs (number = a in calculation below) within the grid lines of the chamber; lowering the condenser will improve contrast.
8. Calculate eggs/gram of faeces =

$$\frac{\text{number of eggs counted} \times \text{total volume}}{\text{volume counted} \times \text{weight of faeces}} = \frac{a \times 60}{0.5 \times 3} = 40a$$

i.e. FEC = $40a$.

Reproduction

There are test kits available to measure milk progesterone concentrations which can be used in the clinical laboratory or cowside. One type of test consists of a dipstick that is dipped into milk and develops a colour change result in five minutes, indicating a high or a low progesterone concentration (Rapid 4, Ridgeway Science).

The IDEXX Bovine Pregnancy Test detects pregnancy with 99.3% sensitivity and up to 95.1% specificity (provided the cow is at least 60 days post-calving and at least 28 days post-conception). This ELISA test detects the pregnancy-associated glycoproteins (PAGs) in serum or plasma EDTA, and a visible colour change provides the result in 2.5 hours. This test can be performed in the practice clinic.

General laboratory equipment

Microscope

This is a major purchase, but a good microscope encourages use and is a pleasure to look through. The microscope should have a binocular head, with iris diaphragm and sub-stage condenser matched to the lens (especially the 100×), a halogen or LED light, a genuine course and fine focus that operates through totally metal gears, and a minimum of four lenses (4×, 10×, 40×, 100×). The minimum acceptable lens quality is achromatic (colour-corrected), and should be DIN standard (which allows the use of lenses from other brands). It is well worth considering upgrading the 40× lens, as this is the lens used most often for cytology/haematology. Basic achromatic lenses have only the central 60% of the field in focus, which can be irritating and frustrating when using the 40× lens. Semi-plan achromatic lenses have 80% of the field in focus, and plan-achromatic 100% of the field in focus. Upgrading the 40× lens can be expensive, with plan achromatic lenses costing between £400–650.

Good microscopes can be purchased for less than £3000 (often with all lenses plan achromatic) and, with proper care, will last a lifetime. Recognised brands are often more expensive, but are likely to last longer, be of better quality and have better service support. New base level ('student') models suitable for in-house labs will generally cost around £2000 (these might have the fully plan achromatic 40× lens). Care should be taken if considering purchasing second hand – there is a risk that gears, lenses, etc. may be damaged.

Centrifuge

If you plan to spin down fluids (urinalysis, fluid analysis etc), as well as performing PCVs, centrifuges with interchangeable heads (one for haematocrit tubes and one for fluid tubes) are available. Acceptable sturdy models are on the market for approximately £1000. If these are operated in a small area, or where excess noise is to be avoided, the more expensive models are usually quieter. You may also consider a separate bench for this machine- they can be associated with considerable vibration.

Haematology consumables

- PCV reader, haematocrit tubes, plasticine.
- Glass slides (double sided frosted one end), pencil.
- Romanowsky stain variant (e.g. Diff Quik stain).
- Hair dryer.
- Cover slips, oil, tissues; alcohol (for cleaning lens).

Cell counter

Capacity for five different cell types and total are adequate. These allow recording of a cell differential when counting cells in blood or fluids. Manual machines are available (approximately £300), while digital are more expensive (approximately £1000), although I have seen phone apps adapted for this use.

Haematology and biochemistry machines

This is often the most expensive piece of equipment if purchased outright, but rental and leasing options are also available; all have advantages and disadvantages (Jaros *et al.*, 2007). A range of technologies is available (e.g. impedance versus optical for haematology, wet versus dry chemistry for biochemistry), but several brands of machine now on the market offer acceptable operational accuracy, and no one recommendation can apply in all situations.

The purchase of these instruments must come with a cost benefit analysis that takes into account: the number of samples processed; provision for individual tests, as opposed to packaged profiles; a comparison of cost/sample and turnaround time using the proposed machine compared to an external laboratory; provision of standard operating procedures (SOPs); operator time and expertise; lost revenue with out-of-date reagents (biochemistry machines are often programmed not to read these); and the provision of some sort of reliable QA.

Incubator

If bacterial culture is considered. Most basic models allow temperature adjustment (you will usually be culturing at 37°C).

Microbiology consumables

These include: sheep blood agar, McConkey's agar, disposable inoculation loops, Bunsen burner, disinfectant pots, H_2O_2, oxidase strips, rabbit serum (for coagulase), gram stain set, Lancefield kit.

Refractometer

These are relatively inexpensive, at approximately £200, and allow an estimation of total protein in serum, plasma and peritoneal fluid, as well as USG using a single drop of fluid on the prism. Those that allow temperature correction and include different USG scales for feline and large animals/canine, are preferred.

pH meter

For the best results, ruminal fluid pH should be determined using a pH meter operated at room temperature. They are inexpensive and highly portable. They are battery operated and include calibration solutions. There are many on the market, they are inexpensive, and they can be used cowside with instant results.

McMaster slide for FEC

Commercial sources of McMaster slides:

1. Chalex Corporation 5004-228th Ave SE, Issaquah, WA. USA 98029, http://www.vetslides.com/
2. Focal Point, Mr. Eddy Krecek, St. Kitts, West Indies http://www.mcmaster.co.za/ email: eddy@mcmaster.co.az
3. Prof. Antanas Vysniauskas, M.Marcinkevičiaus N^0, 17–14, Vilnius LT-08412, Lithuania, Cell phone +370-618-24502, email: n.vysniauskas@gsm.lt.

Centrifuge time/speed needed for different fluids

To calculate the speed (RPM) of the centrifuge for any particular fluid, you need to know the radius of the centrifuge, and the recommended RCF (g) and time spun for that fluid.

To measure centrifugal radius, find the centrifugation centre of the rotor. Measure out to the point where the bottom of the tube will sit at full revolution (take into consideration swing-out rotor versus fixed angle). To calculate RPM from RCF:

$$\text{RPM} = \sqrt{\frac{\text{RCF}}{1.118 \times 10^{-6} \times \text{radius (mm)}}}$$

For example, centrifuge A has a radius = 160 mm.

So long as you know the centrifugal radius (160 mm) and the RCF (see list below), you can calculate the required RPM for any centrifuge rotor.

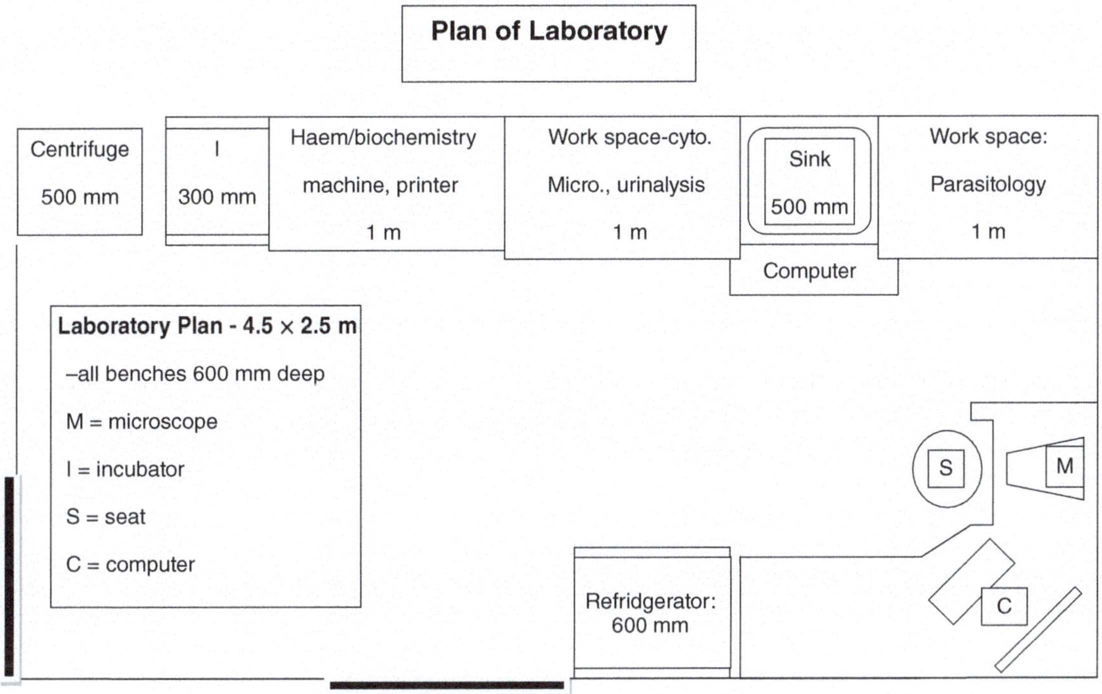

Suggestions for laboratory layout:

1) Microscope/computer workbench – this should have an absolutely dedicated space, with comfortable, adjustable seating, and an open space for legs under the bench to encourage comfortable use (sitting, not standing). It should also be on a bench separate from the work bench, as ideally it is at a lower height than workbench (750 mm vs. 920 mm), and so that vibration from other machines (e.g. centrifuge) does not affect their functioning.

2) Haematology and biochemistry machines – they are often designed to work side by side, and print to a common printer. The footprint of these machines needs to be taken into account, as does power supply, waste disposal, and storage space for supplies.

3) A dedicated laboratory refrigerator/freezer is required, with space for holding samples, storing reagents/consumables.

4) Cytology/urinalysis/microbiology workspace – an area where kits may be used, plating bacteriology, PCV/TP, fibrinogen, gram/Diff Quik staining, etc. is done. This is best placed to one of side of the sink and covered with disposable placticised white paper (used to create a disposable clean worktop).

5) Parasitology – this area can become contaminated and is best placed in the corner, again with plasticised work top.

6) Incubator – this is best placed next to the workspace.

7) Centrifuge – if possible, this should have its own bench, to lessen the effect of vibration on other instruments.

Figure 11.4 Plan of laboratory.

Recommended centrifugation speeds for particular samples are then calculated for centrifuge A, using the recommended RCF (g) and time for fluid type:

- Peritoneal fluid: 5 min @ 200–400 g = 1000–1500 rpm
- CSF: 5 min @ 200 g = 1000 rpm
- Synovial fluid: 5–10 min @ 500–1500 g = 1550–2700 rpm
- Urine: 5 min @ 450 g ~1500 rpm
- Blood: 10 min @ 3000 g = 4000 rpm

Design of the practice laboratory (Figure 11.4)

Decide on which tests your clinic will perform. This will vary from clinic to clinic, and will depend on the mix of clients seen, the expertise/interests of the clinic and the cost/benefit analysis.

1 Compile a list of equipment needed.
2 Plan the physical space to house the equipment. This is a very important consideration, and one that is often overlooked. Surgery, consulting, and radiographic rooms are all carefully planned and, if the practice is to have a laboratory, it must be given a dedicated space where one can work in comfort, free from distractions.

Some basic considerations are:

1 Benches are best covered with stain-resistant material, available from cabinet/ kitchen companies:
   - Standard laboratory work bench: 900–940 mm high, 600 mm deep.
   - Microscope bench: 750 mm high, 600 mm deep.
2 Adjustable height and back seating.
3 Adequate aisle width.
4 Storage areas: cupboards are best placed under the bench, and frequently used consumables in drawers, or on narrow shelves above the bench. Large stocks of chemicals are best placed in a secure area.
5 Water and sink: a large stainless steel sink with a movable goose neck tap and hot and cold running water is required. A staining rack can be placed over the open sink. Most in-house machines will run on mains water, but check specifications of both machine and mains water in your area, especially if water with high mineral content is used.
6 First aid cabinet: most clinics will have some first aid facility. Included should be a suitable eye wash apparatus.
7 Waste disposal: haematology/biochem machines may come with dedicated receptacles for storing used reagents and contaminated water. Disposal of other materials will vary from state to state, county to country, but must be considered. A dedicated sharps container is required. Potentially infectious samples, or culture plates, are best incinerated.
8 Power: does not generally require phase 3, but numerous power points may be necessary. A UPS (uninterruptable power supply) should be considered for some instruments if there are frequent random fluctuations or interruptions to the power supply.
9 Adequate number of data points: remember to think about changing technology.
10 Ventilation/air conditioning: external windows should be insect-screened. Some instrumentation requires a set temperature range for optimal functioning, and freezing of fluid reagents within machines may have operational and wear and tear implications. Generally, temperature ranges between 15–25°C are acceptable for most instruments (and people).
11 Light: the laboratory must be well lit.

References and further reading

Becker, M., Moritz, A. and Giger, U. (2008). Comparative clinical study of canine and feline total blood cell count results with seven in-clinic and two commercial laboratory hematology analysers. *Veterinary Clinical Pathology* **37**, 373–384.

Carrier, J.S., Stewart, S., Godden, S., Fetrow, J. and Rapnicki. P. (2004). Evaluation and use of three cowside tests for detection of subclinical ketosis in early postpartum cows. *Journal of Dairy Science* **87**, 3725–3735.

Cook, N., Oetzel, G. and Nordlund, N. (2006a). Modern techniques for monitoring high-producing dairy cows 1. Principles of herd-level diagnoses. *In Practice* **28**, 510–515.

Cook, N., Oetzel, G. and Nordlund, N. (2006b). Modern techniques for monitoring high-producing dairy cows 2. Practical applications In Practice **28**, 598–603.

Deprez, P., Bauwens, C., Van Schandevijl, K., Lefère, L., Nollet, L.H., Clercq, D. and van Loon, G. (2009). Evaluation of the pocH-100iV DIFF hematology analyzer for use in horses and cattle. *Vlaams Diergeneeskundig Tijdschrift* **78**, 105–109.

Goldmann, F., Bauer, N. and Moritz, A. (2011). Comparison of the Procyte diagnostic analyzer to the Advia 2120 and manual differential for validation of equine and bovine hemograms. *Journal of Clinical Pathology (abstracts)* **40**, 578.

Iwerson, M., Falkenberg, U., Voigtsberger, R. and Heuwieser, W. (2009). Evaluation of an electronic cowside test to detect subclinical ketosis in dairy Cows. *Journal of Dairy Science* **92**, 2618–2624.

Izzo, M.M., Kirkland, P.D., Gu, X., Lele, Y., Gunn, A.A. and House, J.K. (2012). Comparison of three diagnostic techniques for detection of Rotavirus and Coronavirus in calf faeces in Australia. *AVJ* **90**, 122–1129.

Jaros, M.L., Lifshitz, M.S. and De Cresce, R.P. (2007). Financial Management. In: McPherson, R.A. and Pincus, M.R. (eds). *Henry's Clinical Diagnosis and Management by Laboratory Methods*, 21st edition, pp. 122–133.

Klein, D., Kern, A., Lapan, G., Benetka, V., Möstl, K., Hassle, A. and Baumgartner, W. (2009). Evaluation of rapid assays for the detection of bovine coronavirus, rotavirus A and Cryptosporidium parvum in faecal samples of calves. *The Veterinary Journal* **182** , 484–486.

Le Blanc, S. (2010). Monitoring Metabolic Health of Dairy Cattle in the Transition Period. *Journal Reproduction and Development* **56** (suppl), 29–35.

Little, C.J., Gettinby, G., Downs, J. and Marshall, C.B. (1992). Consistency of results from the Vettest 8008 clinical biochemistry analyser. *Veterinary Record* **130**, 419–424.

Millar, H.R., Simpson, J.G. and Stalker, A.L. (1971). An evaluation of the heat precipitation method for plasma fibrinogen estimation. *Journal of Clinical Pathology* **24**, 827–830.

Milne, E. and Scott, P. (2006). Cost-effective biochemistry and haematology in sheep. *In Practice* **28**, 454–461.

Nussbaum, D.J., Salord, J.R. and Rimmele, D.D. (1999). Evaluation of quantitative latex agglutination for detection of Cryptosporidium parvum, E. coli K99, and rotavirus in calf faeces. *Journal of Veterinary Diagnostic Investigation* **11**, 314–318.

Oetzel, G.R. (2002). *Herd-Based Biological Testing For Metabolic Disorders*. American Association of Bovine Practitioners 36th Annual Conference, Preconvention Seminar 7: Dairy Herd Problem Investigation Strategies.

Oetzel, G.R. (2004). Monitoring and Testing Dairy Herds for metabolic disease. *Veterinary Clinics of North America: Food Animal Practice* **20**, 651–674.

Paul, S., Chandra, D., Tewari, A.K., Banerjee, P.S., Ray, D.D., Boral, R. and Rao, J.R. (2009). Comparative evaluation and economic assessment of coprological diagnostic methods and PCR for detection of *Cryptosporidium* spp. in bovines. *Veterinary Parasitology* **164**, 291–295.

Pinches, M. (2006). Getting results in clinical pathology. Pros and cons of in-clinic biochemical testing. *In Practice* **28**, 80–83.

Riond, B., Weissenbacher, S., Hofmann-Lehmann, R. and Lutz, H. (2011). Performance evaluation of the Sysmex pocH-100iV Diff hematology analyzer for analysis of canine, feline, equine, and bovine blood. *Veterinary Clinical Pathology* **40**, 484–495.

Rishniw, M., Pion, P.D. and Maher, T. (2012). The quality of veterinary in-clinic and reference laboratory biochemical testing. *Veterinary Clinical Pathology* **41**, 92–109.

Rollon, F. (2006). *Tools for a Prompt Cowside Diagnosis: what can be implemented by the bovine practitioner?* World Buiatrics Congress (http://www.ivis.org).

Siska, W.D., Rosen, N.K., Christian, J.A., Taddeo, D.A. and DeNicola, D.B. (2011). Validation of the Idexx Catalyst Dry Chemistry analyzer for in-house biochemical analysis. *Journal of Clinical Pathology* (abstracts) **40**, 593.

van Zijderveld, F.G. and Overdigk, E. (1983). Experiences with ELISA for the detection of the E.coli K99 antigen in calf faeces *Annals of Veterinary Research* **14**, 395–399.

Welles, E.F., Hall, A.H and Carpenter, M. (2009). Comparison of canine CBC results from 4 different in-office hematology instruments with results from Advia 120 hematology instrument. *Veterinary Clinical Pathology* **38**(1), 20–29.

Wenger-Riggenbach, B., Hässig, M., Hofmann-Lehmann, R. and Lutz, H. (2006). Evaluation of the LaserCyte: an in-house hematology analyser for dogs and cats. *Comparative Clinical Pathology* **15**, 117–129.

Institutions providing recommendations for standard operating procedures for veterinary laboratories

Royal College of Veterinary Surgeons Practice Standards Scheme Manual. Available at: http://www.rcvs.org.uk/document-library/practice-standards-manual/. Accessed November 21, 2011.

The College of Veterinarians of Ontario Guideline: Ordering, Performing and Interpreting Laboratory Tests in Veterinary Clinical Practice. Available at: http://www.cvo.org/uploadattachments/Laboratorytests guideline.pdf. Accessed November 21, 2011.

American Animal Hospital Association, Accreditation. Available at: http://www.aahanet.org/accreditation/index.aspx. Accessed November 21, 2011.

Recommended list of texts

Clinical pathology

Stockham, S.L. and Scott, M.A. (2008). *Fundamentals of Veterinary Clinical Pathology*, 2nd edition, Blackwell Publishing.

Latimer, K.S. (2011). *Duncan and Prasse's Veterinary Laboratory Medicine – Clinical Pathology*, 5th edition, Wiley Blackwell.

Rosenfeld, A.J. and Dial, S.M. (2010). *Clinical Pathology for the Veterinary Team*. Wiley Blackwell.

Reagan, W.J., Rovira, A.R.I. and DeNicola, D.B. (2008). *Veterinary Hematology: Atlas of Common Domestic and Non-Domestic Species*. John Wiley and Sons.

Carolyn, A., Sink, C.A., Nicole, M. and Weinstein, N.M. (2012). *Practical Veterinary Urinalysis*. Wiley Blackwell.

Microbiology

Quinn, P.J., Markey, B.K., Leonard, F.C. *et al.* (2011). *Veterinary Microbiology and Microbial Disease*, 2nd edition. Wiley Blackwell.

Parasitology

Georgi, J.R. and Bowman, D.D. (2008). *Georgi's Parasitology for Veterinarians*, 9th edition. Elsevier Health Sciences.

CHAPTER 12

Safety: Handling and Restraint of Cattle

Mandi Carr

Learning objectives

- Understand how cattle behaviour can be used to facilitate the movement of cattle.
- Understand how good design of handling yards will facilitate cattle movement.
- Understand the important design features of a crush.
- Understand how head ropes and nose tongs may be used to improve head restraint.
- Appreciate the potential hazards of handling cattle and how risk of injury to handler and animal can be reduced.

Introduction

This chapter will highlight the facilities and restraint equipment required to work with cattle, as well as highlight the important behavioural characteristics of cattle that allow for easier handling.

A summary into the design of cattle handling facilities is best provided by Ohio State University (2002): '*to get cattle to do what you want takes knowledge of animal behaviour, access to good facilities, and proper handling techniques*'.

Understanding cattle behaviour

Understanding the principles of cattle behaviour through experience and training helps to predict the way that an animal will behave in any given situation. The greater the handler's knowledge of cattle behaviour, the better will be their ability to predict the animal's responses. The better their ability to predict the animal's responses, the quicker and easier the process will be, reducing the chance of injury to both animal and handler. Being able to read the body language of an animal and predict its probable response is one of the most important controls to reduce risk and prevent injury.

Cattle are very social animals and if separated from other animals, isolated animals will show clear signs of stress, including increased heart rate, vocalisation, defecation and urination (Rushen *et al.*, 1999). Social order within a mob of cattle is established and maintained by both aggressive and affiliate behaviour. Aggressive behaviour includes lowering the head, head-butting or physical contact with the body of another individual. Bulls tend to vocalise, paw or rub at the ground, or stand to make themselves look larger (turning side-on to their challenger to display their full height and length). Affiliate behaviour includes licking or grooming the neck of another individual. Dominant animals tend to feed and drink first and are often the animals which lead the mob through gateways and into handling yards.

Cattle try to maintain other animals within their field of vision, and have the ability to see threats from almost all directions with their 330° panoramic vision. Cattle have slit-shaped pupils and weak eye muscles which inhibit their ability to focus quickly on objects. They have poor depth perception, resulting in refusing to cross a shadow or a drain grate. They have sensitive hearing and become stressed by loud noises. Cattle can be calmed by scratching under the neck or behind their ears, both areas they cannot reach.

Cattle will generally remain immobile when first threatened, standing still to assess the situation. If frightened, their natural instinct is to escape, fleeing from danger. Controlling the level of 'arousal' and keeping the animal calm allows the handler to remain in control of the animal and the situation.

The flight zone is the comfort zone around the animal; in other words, the animal's personal space. Penetrate the flight zone and the animal moves away. Remain outside the flight zone and the animal remains stationary. Flight zones vary between animals, and may be 1–5 m for dairy or feedlot cattle and up to 20–30 m

Bovine Medicine, Third Edition. Edited by Peter D. Cockcroft.

for wild beef cattle. Understanding the flight zone of an animal is essential for controlling the speed at which an animal moves. In order to predict the direction in which an animal will move, an understanding of the point of balance of an animal is required. From the side, the point of balance is the shoulder. This means that pressure applied from behind the shoulder will move the animal forward. Pressure from in front of the shoulder will move the animal back. From the front, the point of balance is the centre of the head. To move the animal sideways, the handler must be either side of an imaginary longitudinal line which bisects the animal down the midline.

By alternating between entering and retreating from the flight zone, and being in front or behind, to the left or right of the point of balance, the handler can keep the animal moving in the desired direction and at the required pace.

Handling facilities – the yards

Cattle yards should be designed to make maximal use of the natural behaviour of cattle (Table 12.1). Individual yards should be scaled down gradually in size towards the crush, and use a flow-through design which allows cattle to be worked freely without having to be forced. Allowing cattle to see each other helps the flow of movement, and strategically placed cladding can offer directional signals to the animals. The race should lead to the crush in a straight line, so that cattle are invited to the non-threatening view through the head bail. To encourage cattle to enter the crush, cattle should be able to see at least 6 m of unobstructed space beyond the crush. Incorporating a gentle bend can encourage cattle to move toward the cattle they see moving and disappearing. Yards that are poorly designed and do not encourage a good flow of cattle will result in baulking and an increase in the level of anxiety. This may result in an increased risk of injury to animals and handlers.

Long, narrow handling pens, rather than large, wide pens, make it easier to move cattle through the exit gate. Recommended dimensions are 15–20 m long and 3.5–4 m wide, with a holding capacity of 30–35 adult animals. A combination of a curved race and a circular forcing pen, both with sheeted sides, have been shown to reduce the time needed to move cattle by up to 50% in Australia (Vowles & Hollier, 1982). Forcing pens are most efficient when they handle no more that 8–10 cattle. The race should be 660–710 mm wide for adult cattle and 510 mm wide for calves, to avoid the animals turning around. For British breeds, a fence height of 1.52 m has been recommended in the UK, increasing to 1.67–1.83 m for Continental breeds (Grandin, 2009). A curved forcing race funnels animals into a race more effectively than a straight-sided forcing pen.

Drafting gates at the front of the crush should be around 3 m long, to offer a gentle angle to cattle exiting the crush.

Table 12.1 Principles of yard design.

Provide the appearance of clear space
Minimise distractions
Remove the need for the handler to be in direct contact with the animal – incorporate a catwalk
Size of yards to match number of cattle in herd (minimum 1.5 m^2 per adult)
Ensure that gates shut easily and securely, can be fully opened and lie flat against a fence line or yard panel
Use material that is strong enough to withstand the pressure from the cattle that are being handled
Minimise noise and dust
Minimise points where limbs can be trapped
Incorporate a gentle bend to encourage cattle to move towards cattle they see moving and disappearing (minimum radius 5 m)
Ensure adequate drainage but avoid slopes of > 5%
Ensure ease of access for trucks
Ensure adequate lighting – both natural and artificial
Avoid 90° corners
Incorporate a loading ramp angle of 15° and consider a horizontal docking area at the end of the loading ramp

A cattle-free area around the crush should be designated as a safe work area to prevent damage to equipment and injury from loose cattle.

Loading ramps with an angle greater than 22° will create slipping and should be avoided. Creating a ramp with a maximum angle of 15° is preferable. A horizontal docking area of around 1.5 m long at the end of the ramp will prevent cattle from slipping as they are unloaded from the truck. A loading ramp should be no wider than the width of the truck likely to use it. They should be constructed of material that is not going to move when walked on, and should not create excessive noise.

Handling facilities – the crush

For many cattle veterinarians servicing the cattle industry, the crush is their primary worksite. A poorly designed, poorly maintained, poorly built crush is a dangerous place. Add to this poorly handled animals, and the situation can be horrendous. Danger comes from the sudden and unplanned movement of cattle in and around the crush, the environment (tripping hazards, electrical hazards, slippery conditions due to rain or mud, inadequate lighting), and the tiring repetitive nature of the work. Choosing a crush involves consideration of the stock to be restrained, the procedures to be performed, staffing levels and experience, and cost (Beggs, 2009).

A crush consists of the following basic parts:

- the head bail or front gate;
- the side gates;
- the vet gate or 'kick gate';
- the back gate;
- the floor.

The head bail, also known as the front gate, is located at the front of the crush and is designed to restrain the animal by applying pressure to the neck. There are two types of head bails: the walk-through bail, which allows the animal to travel forward through the front of the crush after being restrained, and the guillotine-type bail that requires the animal to be released from the head bail and backed out before the front gate can be opened, to allow the animal to move forward through the front of the crush. Some head bails have the ability to incorporate a head restraint which allows the head to be lifted and restrained. Blocking or baulk gates can be fitted to the front of both types of head bails to prevent stock running through the head bail, should the animal not be caught.

Cattle will struggle excessively in a head bail that chokes, or that does not hold the head and neck in line with the back. If the head is held too low, the animal tends to go down on its knees and kicks with its back feet; the head held too high results in the animal attempting to rear, with the back legs going down under the body (Evans, 1986).

The control lever for the operation of the head bail can be either at the front, at the back, or both. Preference for position of the control lever is based on operator experience and skill but, for single operators, it is often more convenient to have the control lever at the back to avoid walking in front of the animal that is being moved into the crush. It is recommended that control levers that release the head bail when it is under pressure are used.

The side gate(s) allows for access to the side of the animal for procedures such as vaccination, surgery, examination of the lower limbs and semen collection, as well as drafting or release of animals into side yards. The side gate should close to within 20 mm of the floor, to prevent the animal's feet from slipping laterally, and should have sheeted or closed rails up to at least 1 m above the floor in order to prevent the animal from kicking laterally. Side gates should be vertical rather than v-shaped, as narrow bases have been shown to cause cattle discomfort and are more likely to cause cattle to lie down, becoming wedged in the crush. Side gates that are split horizontally are advantageous, as they allow access to the top or bottom of the animal independently while, at the same time, preventing the animal from moving sideways out of the crush. The lower level of the top gate and the upper level of the bottom gate should be approximately level with the animal's stifle (750–800 mm from the floor), to minimise the chance of being kicked while either the top or bottom gate is open.

Side gates can be hinged at the front, the back, or both, but must be able to be opened fully without being obstructed. Removable panels within the side gates can be useful to allow good access when animals are particularly fractious. The ability to squeeze the side gates towards the animal, allowing various sized animals to be restrained, is advantageous.

Locking mechanisms used on side gates are usually bolt mechanisms which can be manually shut or 'slammed' shut (they automatically lock when the gate is shut, but are opened manually). They must be placed as far back from the end of the gate as possible, to reduce the risk of injury from a fast-moving gate opened under pressure, and they must be well maintained to ensure that they lock securely.

The vet gate or 'kick gate' is an additional side gate behind the main side gate that allows access to the back of the animal, providing protection from being kicked or crushed, should the animal escape from the head bail. It is essential for procedures such as rectal examinations. The vet gate should be horizontally split to the level of the stifle of the animal (750–800 mm), with the lower gate sheeted, and a secure locking mechanism must be used. The vet gate should be well maintained to allow for easy opening and closing, to the extent that the lower gate should be able to be 'kicked' closed.

The back gate serves two purposes: to prevent animals from backing out of the crush when not caught in the head bail; and to prevent animals in the race from entering the crush. The back gate must be solid (so an animal cannot break it or a foot/hoof protrude through it), sturdy (so an animal cannot open it), and be of sufficient height so that an animal cannot jump over it. The locking mechanism must ensure that the gate is secure in the closed position.

The floor of the crush should be hard, non-slip and designed for easy cleaning and drainage. Temple Grandin found the use of v-shaped grooves to a depth of 2.5 cm, arranged in a 20 cm diamond or square pattern, was effective to prevent cattle slipping on concrete floors. A similar effect was found with 2.5 cm diameter steel rods raised slightly above the level of a concrete floor.

Handling facilities – equipment

A rope halter is a basic tool of restraint for cattle. The nose loop is made larger than the poll loop. The poll loop then placed behind the ears, allowing the nose loop to drop down over the nose and under the chin. The halter is then tightened under the chin. The rope can then be secured to the side of the crush with a quick release knot.

Table 12.2 Checklist for avoiding injuries when working with cattle.

Avoid handling cattle when tired.	A lack of concentration will increase the risk of injury.
Know the cattle you are working.	A percentage of the mob may be flighty or aggressive, and may react differently under pressure compared with others within the mob.
Keep the cattle calm and give them time to adjust to the new surroundings.	Cattle need at least 30 minutes to adjust when mustered into the yards (Jephcott, 2009).
Assess the type of stock and their behaviour.	Breed, age, sex, horns/polled, number in mob, weather conditions (cattle can be difficult to handle in cold, wet, windy conditions).
Identify an escape route if cornered.	Always keep an eye on what is going on around you.
Know the yards and check for hazards.	Identify stray posts, nails, bolts, gates, shadows, bad smells (e.g. blood).
Know how to operate the crush.	Head bail, side gates, vet/kick gate, back slide gate.
Wear PPE.	Long pants, long-sleeved shirt, boots, hat, sunglasses.
Practise good hygiene.	Wash hands, ensure cattle are vaccinated against leptospirosis, ensure humans are vaccinated against Q fever.

A nose tong (also called a nose grip or a nose plier) clamps the sensitive nasal septum and can severely restrict the movement of the head. The nose tong has two round-edged prongs that are inserted into each nostril. When closed, a space of about 3.5 mm should remain between the prongs, to avoid necrosis of the septum. A rope applies tension to keep the nose tong in place. The nose tong should never be tied, as the nasal septum can be permanently damaged.

Avoiding injuries

Increased awareness of techniques for handling large animals during occupational encounters, such as moving cattle more calmly, being aware of surroundings, and ensuring that the animal is properly restrained, have been suggested as a positive means of reducing the incidence of large animal-associated trauma (Grandin, 1999). Ensuring that equipment is properly maintained, and clearing obstacles around the work area, are actions that can also be taken to decrease the risk of injury associated with cattle work (Table 12.2).

Cattle have been previously shown to account for 23–72% of injuries reported by veterinarians (Thigpen & Dorn, 1973; Landercasper *et al.*, 1988; Poole *et al.*, 1999; Nienhaus *et al.*, 2005; Kabuusu *et al.*, 2010). Injuries sustained in stockyards or handling facilities accounted for the majority of these injuries (82% of cattle-associated injuries to Australian veterinarians were sustained in stockyards or handling facilities (Lucas *et al.*, 2013)). Injuries sustained included fractures, dislocations, sprains, soft tissue damage and wounds, and were the result of being kicked, crushed, struck or stood on by the animal. Muscle and tendon injuries of the upper limb are the most common injuries sustained, and injuries associated with performing obstetrical procedures (mainly pregnancy testing) are the most commonly reported injury. Lucas *et al.* (2013) identified that of those veterinarians reporting serious cattle-associated injuries, 62% reported the use of some safety precaution at the time of injury, ranging from the use of a crush, restraint, sedation or personal protection equipment (PPE).

Conclusion

Knowledge of cattle behaviour is essential when designing cattle handling facilities that save time and reduce stress for cattle and people. There is no such thing as the 'ideal' yard, as it depends on personal preference and the type of cattle being handling. However, there are certain features that can be included in the yard design that will make the yards easier to work than others.

References and further reading

Beggs, D. (2009). *Crush Design and Safety*. Australian Cattle Veterinarians publication.

Evans, P. (1986). *Cattle Yards: Design, Material and Construction*, pp 43–55. QLD DPI Information Series Q186014: Veterinary Crushes and Head Bails.

Grandin, T. (1999). Safe Handling of Large Animals. *Occupational Medicine, State of the Art Reviews* **14**, 195–212.

Grandin, T. (2009). *Beef cattle behaviour*. www.grandin.com.au.

Jephcott, S. (2009). *Crush Design and Safety (A Review of Current Literature)*. Australian Cattle Vets Publication.

Kabuusu, R.M., Kekn, E.O., Kiyini, R. and McCann, T.J. (2010). Prevalence and Patterns of Self-Reported Animal-Related Injury amongst Veterinarians in Metropolitan Kampala. *Journal of Veterinary Science* **11**, 363–365.

Landercasper, J., Cogbill, T.H., Strutt, P.J. and Landercasper, B.O. (1988). Trauma and the Veterinarian. *Journal of Trauma* **28**, 1255–1259.

Lucas, M., Day, L. and Fritschi, L. (2013). Serious Injuries to Australian Veterinarians Working with Cattle. *Australian Veterinary Journal* **91**, 57–60.

Nienhaus, A., Skudlink, C. and Seidler, A. (2005). Work-related Accidents and Occupational Diseases in Veterinarians and their Staff. *International Archives of Occupational and Environmental Health* **78**, 230–238.

Ohio State University Extension (2002). *Beef Quality Assurance Cattle Handling and Working Facilities*. Bulletin 906, Ohio State University Extension.

Poole, A.G., Slone, S.M., Kearney, M.T. and McConnell, D.A. (1999). Survey of Occupational Hazards in Large Animal Practices. *Journal of the American Veterinary Medical Association* **215**, 1433–1435.

Rushen, J., Boissy, A., Terlouw, E.M.D.C. and de Passille, A.M.B. (1999). Opiod peptides and behavioural and physiological responses of dairy cattle to social isolation in unfamiliar surroundings. *Journal of Animal Science* **77**, 2918–2924.

Thigpen, C.K. and Dunn, C.R. (1973). Non-Fatal Accidents Involving Insured Veterinarians in the United States, 1967–1969. *Journal of the American Veterinary Medical Association* **163**, 369–374.

Vowles, W.J. and Hollier, T.J. (1982). The influence of yard design on the movement of animals. *Proceedings from the Australian Society of Animal Production* **14**, 597.

SECTION III

Clinical Skills

CHAPTER 13

Herd Health Investigations in Cattle Practice

Cheryl L. Waldner and John R. Campbell

Learning objectives

- Understand how to define the problem.
- Understand how to investigate the epidemiology and clinical characteristics of the outbreak.
- Be able to evaluate potential risk factors and identify key determinants.
- Be able to develop recommendations for treatment, control and prevention.
- Understand the importance of monitoring the outcomes to assess the effectiveness of the intervention.

Introduction

Managing and dealing with disease outbreaks in cattle herds can be a challenging proposition for the practising veterinarian. The demands of practice often make it difficult for the local practitioner to devote significant time to an outbreak when it occurs. The herd manager may be frustrated and may also be unwilling to invest more finances in a situation that has already had significant losses. The practitioner needs an efficient, systematic approach to outbreaks, in order to maximise the value of their services to the producer and to provide an effective method of dealing with and preventing future losses.

An outbreak is defined as an increase – often sudden – in the observed number of cases of a disease, compared with the expected number for a given place or among a specific group of animals over a particular period of time (MacDonald, 2011). General strategies for managing outbreaks have been presented by several authors (Schwabe *et al.*, 1977; Kahrs, 1978; Blood, 1982; Lessard, 1988; Ribble *et al.*, 1998; Waldner, 2001a; MacDonald, 2011). Others have developed guidelines for investigating specific disease problems and productivity shortfalls (Wikse, 1988; Mickelsen, 1990; Wikse *et al.*, 1992; Ruegg, 1993; Wikse *et al.*, 1994; Sanderson & Christmas, 1997; Waldner, 2001b).

The immediate goal of the practitioner is to take steps to minimise additional herd losses (Ruegg, 1996). After any necessary actions have been taken to address the immediate threat, the next step is to identify the factors that contributed to the development of disease or change in productivity. The practitioner must then determine which of these factors can be controlled by management to reduce further losses and the risk of future outbreaks. These objectives can be achieved by addressing the following questions for each outbreak (W5: what, who, when, where, and why) (Schwabe *et al.*, 1977):

- define the problem – what and how much?
- identify groups for comparison – who, when, and where?
- evaluate potential risk factors and identify key determinants – why ?
- develop recommendations for treatment, control and prevention where appropriate with follow up to assess the effectiveness of the intervention

Define and describe the problem: What? Is it worth investigating? How much?

The first and most critical task early in the investigation is to clearly define the problem (Ribble *et al.*, 1998). The initial complaint could include unexplained mortality; clinical disease (Waldner *et al.*, 1999; Gow *et al.*, 2005); sub-clinical disease; impaired performance and negative trends in productivity (Waldner *et al.*, 2001a, 2001b; Waldner, 2002); or potential public health concerns related to food safety (Ruegg, 1996; Pritchard *et al.*, 2000) and environmental issues (Waldner *et al.*, 1998).

The development of a case definition is an important step in describing the problem. This case definition is critical when comparing cases with non-cases, to determine the importance

Bovine Medicine, Third Edition. Edited by Peter D. Cockcroft.

of potential risk factors for disease. This definition will be re-evaluated and refined as more information become available. The case definition can be very sensitive (identifying all possible cases), such as 'calves with diarrhoea that require treatment', or it can be more specific and detailed (identifying cases only associated with the outbreak), such as 'calves less than one week old with watery diarrhoea and clinical evidence of dehydration'. Case definitions can also include laboratory verification. A simple, easily recognised and applied definition facilitates the consistent reporting of cases by the herd owner, other farm workers, and cooperating veterinarians.

After developing a working description of the clinical disease or impairment in productivity, the practitioner must decide 'how much', or define the extent of the problem. The answer to this question will determine if there is a substantial problem, and the level of effort and resources to allocate to the investigation. Herd productivity and disease frequency are measured and then compared to published benchmarks, historical expectations, goals of the farmer, or to the performance of neighbouring herds (Wikse *et al.*, 1992). The appropriate benchmarks will vary, because of economic constraints, physical restrictions, time and management limitations. Confirming the existence and severity of the problem will minimise any expenditure of time and resources on the investigation of epidemics that do not exist (Lessard, 1988).

The nature and extent of the problem can be defined during the herd visit by collecting a detailed history and examining the herd records, animals, management, and environment. Photographs can be particularly useful for recording subjective observations, including body condition score and farm hygiene. Changes over time can be monitored by comparing representative pictures from two different dates. All records should be in ink, dated and signed. Record where and when the pictures were taken, and include detailed voice narration on video describing what was seen.

History and collection of herd records

Have the herd owner restate the presenting complaint and encourage them to clarify the time sequence of events. Carefully worded 'open-ended' questions allow the possibility of answers not previously considered by the investigator. Unnecessary industry jargon and scientific terminology should be avoided. Each question should ask for one piece of information at a time, and all questions should contain unambiguous time references (Wilson, 1992). 'Loaded' or 'leading' questions can suggest that one answer is better than another, and bias the interview. Referencing a prepared list of questions after the herd owner has told their story can identify potentially important points not covered in the initial disclosure of information.

A management history obtained with simple questions having 'yes' or 'no' answers provides limited and superficial information on herd management practices. For example, asking whether cattle are vaccinated for BVDV and IBR might seem like a relatively straightforward question. However, the producer answering 'yes' provides no information on what type of vaccine was used, when it was administered, and whether label directions were followed.

The next step is to collect herd records that could provide insight onto the current problem. Ask the herd owner for any livestock-associated records which, in addition to breeding, calving, treatment, and performance records, could include veterinary service, supply, or drug bills, auction mart receipts, old calendars, pocket diaries, calving books, feed and supplement bills, financial records of animals bought and sold, and bulk tank receipts showing somatic cell count and bacterial numbers (Hancock & Wikse, 1988).

Raw data are often more reliable than summarised performance measures. For example, the number of cows that were pregnant and the number of cows pregnancy tested is more reliable than a percentage pregnancy rate. Definitions of production and health measurements must be clear and used consistently throughout the investigation. Be consistent when comparing findings from other investigators, as there is very little standardisation of terminology or in methods of calculation. For example, stillbirth has been defined both as 'calves dead within the first hour after birth' (Waldner, 2005) and 'calves dead within 24 hours of birth' (McDermott *et al.*, 1991).

The initial exam: animals, environment and management

Distant observations should be made of the group and individual animals before the animals are confined and restrained for detailed exams (Radostits *et al.*, 2000). A visual check of the herd during feeding or grazing can be a valuable tool that should not be overlooked. When animals cannot be confined, visual body condition scoring can be successful from a reasonable distance, and is comparable to palpation, except when cattle have long hair (Wikse, 1988).

Climate, housing, population density and air quality are potential determinants of disease risk and herd productivity (Radostits *et al.*, 2000). Historical weather data can be obtained from local meteorological stations, if necessary, to confirm herd owner observations. Specific observations for indoor environments include: air quality and ventilation; sanitation and hygiene; the type and condition of the flooring; the barn cleaning and waste disposal system; stall design and dimensions; bedding type and adequacy; the ease of movement for both animals and attendants within the unit; and the adequacy of the lighting.

Management is best assessed through repeated first-hand observations. Very few of the disease problems important in food animal practice require only the infectious agent to cause substantial herd losses. Almost all outbreaks or sub-optimal productivity problems result from a number of factors including management. In some cases, the disease outbreak can provide a unique 'teachable moment' for the veterinarian, to emphasise the importance of management changes that were suggested in the past and ignored.

Generate hypotheses to identify potential causes for the outbreak by identifying groups for comparison – Who, When, and Where?

This is a good point at which to review and refine the case definition and estimate the extent of the herd problem based on initial observations. This step should be repeated as new information becomes available. Given that there is sufficient evidence to proceed with an investigation, the immediate goal is to identify risk factors that can be manipulated to resolve the outbreak or improve herd production and profitability. The risk factors over which management has control, and which can be altered to affect disease rates or production levels, are sometimes referred to as 'key determinants' (Wikse *et al.*, 1992).

The first steps in identifying these risk factors are to tabulate and orient the available case data by time, place and animal (MacDonald, 2011). This allows the investigator to determine which groups of animals are affected (the host characteristics, such as age, sex and breed), when they became affected (time, particularly the date of onset), and where the problem was reported (place or location of affected animals or groups) (Radostits *et al.*, 1994; Smith, 1995).

The investigator should collect all relevant available information on the diseased animals, which could include: identification numbers; age, sex, breed and colour; origin; feed and water source; housing type; stage of reproductive cycle; lactation status; parity; relevant clinical, pathological, or laboratory reports; and processing, vaccination, and treatment histories (Lessard, 1988). Where herds are managed in distinct groups, much of this information might only be available at the group level. Often, the herd owner can describe the count and general characteristics of animals in a pen or pasture group and the number affected, even when there is no record of the specific animals affected. Information should be collected for unaffected, as well as affected, animals and groups within the herd (Lessard, 1988).

The temporal pattern of disease can provide important clues about the origin of the disease (Lessard, 1988). The pattern of disease can be described by plotting the time of onset of each case in appropriate time intervals, against the number of cases recognised in each interval (epidemic curve). The distribution of cases can suggest whether the problem resulted from a single point source exposure, or is caused by an infectious agent. For example, an epidemic curve that has a relatively short time span of new cases, and a dramatic upward slope, is consistent with a point source exposure (Gregg, 1996). A less steep upward slope, followed by a more defined down slope and often one or more additional peaks, can suggest a propagated infection (Gregg, 1996). The location and identification of the first or index case can also provide clues to the source of the problem.

Differences in where affected animals were housed and pastured in relation to unaffected animals, the timing of group movement between different housing facilities or pastures, and the movement of individual animals among different management groups, can also provide important information (Lessard, 1988). A point map of the farm (Thursfield, 1995) should include a sketch of housing facilities, corrals, pastures (including details of cross-fencing), feeding facilities and watering sources. Online mapping programs and aerial photographs can greatly improve the ease and accuracy of location data.

Collect additional data to test your hypotheses: necropsy, clinical examination, sample collection

Necropsy examination

Detailed instructions for post-mortem examination will not be reviewed here, as these are available from most diagnostic labs, as well as other sources (Andrews, 1986). The results from both gross and histological examination can be critical to refining the case definition (Radostits *et al.*, 2000). All available cadavers should be examined when possible, as one or two cases from a major disease outbreak might not be representative (Ribble *et al.*, 1998).The submission of samples to the same laboratory, and a single pathologist, should improve communication, consistency of interpretation, facilitate comparisons between individual cases, and identification of trends during the outbreak (Ribble *et al.*, 1998).

A consistent protocol for sample collection and a log of all samples collected will minimise the risk of missing important information. Tissues from all important systems should be submitted for histopathology, rather than relying on the gross evidence of abnormalities. Call the laboratory for any non-routine samples to verify the amount, appropriate sample container, storage conditions, preservation, and shipping instructions. *Banking tissue samples* for future analysis is appropriate if the factor to be analysed is stable for a known period, and if costs of collection and storage are not prohibitive.

Use a camera to record gross pathological abnormalities. The identity of the subject animal, the date, a size reference scale marker, and the identity of the pathologist, should be included in each photograph where litigation is an issue (Wobeser, 1996). Inform the laboratory before sending the samples for potential legal cases. Many laboratories have special '*chain of custody*' protocol documentation that will assist you in ensuring that any sample results will be admissible in court (Wobeser, 1996).

There are several common errors that must be avoided in 'medico-legal' examinations (Jaffe, 1991; Wobeser, 1996), including: incomplete examination; inadequate documentation; delay in preparation of the report; failing to collect samples for supplementary analysis; improper collection of samples; accidental damage to specimens; confusion of artefacts with important lesions; failure to consult with other experts; and bias from too much emphasis on the case history.

Clinical examination of individual animals

Individual animals can be confined and examined during the initial visit or later, combined with other routine processing activities. An individual animal listing of identification, body condition score and current reproductive status are particularly important if the problem will require monitoring over time, or there is potential for ongoing losses in the herd. The procedure for detailed examination of individual animals has been well documented and will not be reviewed here (Wilson, 1992; Smith, 1995; Radostits *et al.*, 2000). The animals examined might include examples of early cases, severely affected, moderate or mildly affected, and 'normal', or not apparently affected, animals from the herd.

Refine the hypotheses and then collect appropriate clinical and environmental samples

Laboratory examination of strategically submitted samples can help rule out or confirm the diagnosis, monitor exposure to potentially important risk factors, determine the necessity for and appropriate level of intervention and, finally, assess the success of control measures (Hancock *et al.*, 1988). The only laboratory analyses that should be considered in most investigations are those where the results are likely to affect management decisions directly (Hancock *et al.*, 1988). Appropriate samples might include blood, milk, faeces, urine, nasal and ocular swabs, biopsies or tissue from slaughter animals or cadavers, other fluids, feed, water, and soil.

Cost will often prohibit laboratory testing of every animal in the herd. The most common approach to testing is to submit samples comparing cases, and a sample of appropriate control (non-affected) animals. Samples can also be submitted to compare results between animals with acute and chronic disease, or among animals from different age cohorts, management groups, or history of exposure to some other risk factor of interest. The required number of animals is based on:

(a) the acceptable degree of uncertainty in the final estimate;
(b) the expected prevalence, or, for continuous measurements, the expected variation; and
(c) the size of the herd (Thrusfield, 1995; Cameron, 1999).

The number of samples required also depends on the question being asked and the minimal important difference between groups. If the number of cases is limited, there is an advantage to having up to four controls for every case. Serum or sample banking should be considered in order to minimise initial laboratory costs (Moorhouse & Hugh-Jones, 1981).

The investigation of nutritional disorders has been reviewed by Swecker and Thatcher (1988). Nutritionally related or toxicological herd outbreaks are a common occurrence, and investigating the nutritional history of the herd is a crucial part of many investigations. Expensive laboratory analysis alone will not determine whether the nutrition programme is adequate for the type of animal and environment.

Before collecting any feed samples, have the herd owner prepare an inventory of all forages, grains, and purchased supplements. The samples submitted for analysis must be representative of what is being fed. Collect, pool, and thoroughly mix five to ten samples for grain or concentrate, and 20 individual samples for hay or silage from each lot of feed before submission. Silage samples should be placed in airtight plastic bags, stored on ice, and shipped to the laboratory as soon as possible. Ask the laboratory to dry and grind the entire sample before analysis (Swecker & Thatcher, 1988; Holland & Kezar, 1995). Record the visual appearance and physical characteristics of the feed observed during sample collection (Swecker & Thatcher, 1988). Toxic plants can be photographed and then collected and dried for expert identification.

Obtain bottles for water sampling directly from the laboratory where possible. Improperly cleaned containers can contaminate the sample. This is particularly important for trace mineral or organic analysis. Proper sampling technique, special preservatives and rapid transportation are required for samples being tested for potentially volatile components.

Evaluate your hypotheses using clinical findings, herd records and diagnostic test results to identify the 'key determinants' by comparing groups within the herd – Why?

The analysis begins with organising and summarising the data. A simple spreadsheet can list animal identifications and other information such as breed, age, performance data, clinical exam findings, laboratory results, and pen location or management group. The first step is to characterise the problem using descriptive statistics.

Groups should be identified within the herd, based on whether or not the animal is a case, and the presence or absence of risk factors determined by animal characteristics, time and location. Comparisons between these groups can answer the final question – why did the outbreak occur? Sometimes these comparisons will identify one or more key determinants for the disease outbreak, or this process might suggest more questions that can be addressed by obtaining further information from the herd owner or additional laboratory testing.

Attack rate tables can be used to help organise the comparison of different risk factors across groups. The attack rate is the proportion of a group that is affected during a given period.

Table 13.1 Partial attack rate for an abortion problem in a cow-calf herd.

Suspected risk factors	Exposed animals (positive)				Unexposed animals (negative)			
	Number affected (not pregnant)	Number not affected (pregnant)	Total number	Attack rate (%)	Number affected (not pregnant)	Number not affected (pregnant)	Total number	Attack rate (%)
Neospora antibody positive: negative – All cows	122	160	282	43%	7	58	65	11%
– Heifers	38	30	68	56%	2	9	11	18%
– Mature cows	84	135	219	39%	5	49	54	9%

The attack rate can be compared between those that are, and are not, exposed to each individual potential risk factor. To easily visualise this comparison across many different risk factors, an attack rate table is used to help identify the exposures most likely to be associated with disease. Alternatively, a table can be constructed to compare the frequency of exposure to each potentially important risk factor between case and control animals. An example of an attack rate table, comparing the attack rate for abortion between cows that were serum antibody positive and negative for *Neospora caninum*, is shown in Table 13.1.

The importance of different risk factors can be objectively compared by measuring the strength of the association between each exposure and the outcome of interest or disease. Two common indices used to measure the magnitude of effect are the relative risk and odds ratio:

- The relative risk is the ratio of the attack rates (or cumulative incidence or risks) of disease in the animals exposed to the factor of interest to the comparable value in those that were not exposed. It is used in comparing to groups or cohorts, based on their exposure history. If the relative risk < 1, then the exposure is associated with a decreased risk of disease. If the relative risk $= 1$, then there is no association between exposure and disease status. If the relative risk > 1, then the exposure is associated with an increased risk of disease.
- The odds ratio can be used to measure the association between exposure and disease for any study type, but is the method of choice for case-control comparisons. The interpretation of the odds ratio is similar to that of relative risk.

Applying an appropriate statistical test to the comparison between groups will minimise over-interpreting differences between groups that could have been due to chance (Hancock & Wikse, 1988; Gregg, 1996).

Statistical significance alone does not prove that the identified risk factor is a cause of the outbreak (Schwabe *et al.*, 1977; Ruegg, 1996). For a risk factor to be considered a potential cause of disease or sub-optimal productivity, the risk factor must always precede the outcome in time. Other supporting evidence for a causal association would include a relatively strong association between the risk factor and the outcome, a biologically reasonable link between risk factor and outcome, evidence of increasing effect with increasing exposure or that removing or decreasing exposure decreases the risk of disease, and consistency of the reported association across different studies.

Develop recommendations, provide a written report, and follow up to determine the effectiveness of the intervention

The basic process of defining the problem, orienting the problem by animal, time and space, and analysing the data, is common to all outbreak investigations. The steps in this process may occur in a different sequence, will often overlap, and parts of the process may have to be repeated to successfully resolve the problem. Incremental recommendations for control can be provided throughout the investigation as more information becomes available. Control options might include changes to the environment, client education, quarantine of affected and suspect animals, test and slaughter, mass vaccination and treatment and, in extreme circumstances, herd depopulation (Schwabe *et al.*, 1977; Ribble *et al.*, 1998).

A preliminary report should be issued shortly after the first herd visit, with a final report after all laboratory analyses are completed. The report must be designed for the intended audience. Most reports are prepared for the herd owner, but in some cases will need to be accessible to a banker or a lawyer. The report should be as direct and concise as possible (Gay, 1999). The purpose of the investigation should be clearly stated, and the results should be summarised using simple tables and graphs. The action list for the herd owner should be clearly prioritised and should include very specific details for any treatment and management recommendations.

The report should provide a plan for follow up and future monitoring. Many investigations are done retrospectively, with insufficient information to reach definitive conclusions

(Waldner *et al.*, 1999). In these cases, protracted herd health and productivity monitoring and occasionally planned follow-up studies are required to address outstanding questions (Waldner *et al.*, 2001a, 2001b; Waldner, 2002). Where the effectiveness of proposed control measures cannot be predicted with certainty, one infrequently used but potentially invaluable strategy for evaluating the effectiveness of control measures in the herd is the randomised controlled trial (Perry, 1988).

The investigator must consider the potential for future litigation in all statements and recommendations. The report should also present the risks of the recommendations, describe any risks from the current problem to public health and, finally, promote realistic expectations of the results for any interventions. If the disease is contagious, consider what risk the herd poses to other livestock producers in the area, and consult with the herd owner on minimising the potential for transmission beyond the herd. If the exposure could potentially result in food residues, contact the appropriate authorities for direction and advise the herd owner of their legal and ethical responsibilities. If the disease is potentially reportable, the appropriate regulatory officials should be advised of the results of the field investigation as soon as possible.

Summary

Because each outbreak and livestock operation is different, there is no 'recipe for success' that will cover all possible situations in the field. The approach outlined here does not have to be followed in the order presented and, often, individual steps are repeated many times before the information necessary to implement a successful control process becomes apparent. The introduced techniques will be sufficient in many investigations, but some will require consultation with specialists, including epidemiologists and laboratory diagnosticians.

The role of detective or outbreak investigator can be a refreshing break from the routine of daily practice. The investigation of disease outbreaks provides an opportunity for the herd veterinarian to show the client the advantages of a herd health programme and the value of a good record-keeping system. Despite the benefits, the resources required for a thorough herd investigation can seem difficult to justify. The decision to conduct an in-depth investigation should depend on the severity of the problem, the opportunity to control the current outbreak and minimise the potential for future losses, and the risk to other producers.

References

Andrews, J. (1986). Necropsy techniques. *Veterinary Clinics of North America: Food Animal Practice* **2**, (1).

Blood, D. (1982). The clinical examination of cattle. Part II: Examination of the herd. *Bov Proc* **14**, 14–21.

Cameron, A. (1999). *Survey toolbox for livestock diseases: A practical manual and software package for active surveillance in developing countries*. ACIAR Monograph No 54; vii +330 p.

Gay, J. (1999). *Student guidelines for written recommendations* [Online]. Available at: www.vetmed.wsu.edu/courses-jmgay/outbletter.htm [22 Aug 1999].

Gow, S., Waldner, C. and Ross, C. (2005). The effect of duration of treatment on weaning weights in a cow-calf herd with a protracted severe neonatal scours outbreak. *Canadian Veterinary Journal* **16**, 418–425.

Gregg, M. (1996). *Field epidemiology*. Oxford University Press, New York.

Hancock, D. and Wikse, S. (1988). Investigation planning and data gathering. *Veterinary Clinics of North America Food Animal Practice* **4**, 1–16.

Hancock, D., Blodgett, D. and Gay, C. (1988). The collection and submission of samples for laboratory testing. *Veterinary Clinics of North America Food Animal Practice* **4**, 33–60.

Holland, C. and Kezar, W. (1995). *Pioneer forage manual: A nutritional guide*. Pioneer Hi-Bred International, Des Moines, Iowa.

Jaffe, F. (1991). *A guide to pathological evidence for lawyers and police officers*, 3rd edition. Thomson Professional Publishing, Scarborough, Ontario.

Kahrs, R. (1978). Techniques for investigating outbreaks of livestock disease. *Journal of the American Veterinary Medical Association* **173**, 101–103.

Lessard, P. (1988). The characterization of disease outbreaks. *Veterinary Clinics of North America Food Animal Practice* **4**, 17–32.

MacDonald, P. (2011). *Methods in Field Epidemiology*. Jones & Bartlett, Burlington, MA.

McDermott, J., Alves, D., Anderson, N., and Martin, S. (1991). Measures of herd health and productivity in Ontario cow-calf herds. *Canadian Veterinary Journal* **32**, 413–420.

Mickelsen, W. (1990). Investigating the causes of low pregnancy rates in beef cattle herds. *Veterinary Medicine* **85**, 418–420, 422–427.

Moorhouse, P. and Hugh-Jones, M. (1981). Serum banks. *Veterinary Bulletin* **51**, 277–290.

Perry, B. (1988). The design and use of supportive epidemiological studies. *Veterinary Clinics of North America Food Animal Practice* **4**, 79–96.

Pritchard, G., Willshaw, G., Biley, J., Carson, T. and Cheasty, T. (2000). Verocytotoxin-producing Escherichia coli O157 on a farm open to the public: Outbreak investigation and longitudinal bacteriological study. *Veterinary Record* **147**, 259–264.

Radostits, O., Leslie, K. and Fetrow, J. (1994). *Herd Health: Food Animal Production Medicine*, 2nd edition. W.B. Saunders Company, Philadelphia.

Radostits, O., Blood, D. and Gay, C. (2000). *Veterinary Medicine*, 9th edition. Bailliere Tindall, London.

Ribble, C., Janzen, E. and Campbell, J. (1998). Disease outbreak investigation in the beef herd: Defining the problem. *Bov Proc* **31**, 121–127.

Ruegg, P. (1993). Use of basic epidemiologic principles in dairy production medicine. Part II. Investigating herd problems. *Compendium on Continuing Education* **15**, 309–313.

Ruegg, P. (1996). Investigating herd problems and production on dairy farms. *Bov Proc* **29**, 96–101.

Sanderson, M. and Christmas, R. (1997). Investigation of depressed weaning weights in beef cow-calf herds. *Compendium on Continuing Education* **19**, 395–399.

Schwabe, D., Riemann, H., & Franti, C. (1977). *Epidemiology in veterinary practice*. Lea & Febiger, Philadelphia.

Smith, R. (1995). *Veterinary clinical epidemiology. A problem-oriented approach*, 2nd edition. CRC Press, Boca Raton.

Swecker, W. and Thatcher, C. (1988). The investigation of nutritional disorders. *Veterinary Clinics of North America Food Animal Practice* **4**, 127–144.

Thrusfield, M. (1995). *Veterinary epidemiology*, 2nd edition. Blackwell Science Ltd, Oxford.

Waldner, C. (2001a). Investigation of disease outbreaks and suboptimal productivity in herds. In: Radostits, O.M. (ed). *Herd health: Food animal production medicine*, 3rd edition, pp.189–210. WB Saunders Company, Philadelphia.

Waldner, C. (2001b). Investigation of reproductive problems in beef herds. *Large Animal Veterinary Rounds* **1**, 5–6.

Waldner, C. (2002). Precolostral antibodies to Neospora caninum in beef calves following an abortion outbreak and associated fall weaning weights. *Bovine Practitioners* **36**, 81–85.

Waldner, C. (2005). Serological status for N. caninum, Bovine Viral Diarrhea Virus, and Infectious Bovine Rhinotracheitis Virus at pregnancy testing and reproductive performance in beef herd. *Animal Reproductive Science* **90**, 219–242.

Waldner, C., Henderson, J., Wu, J., Coupland, R., & Chow, E. (2001). Continued reproductive losses in a cow-calf herd associated with Neospora caninum following an abortion epidemic. *Canadian Veterinary Journal* **42**, 355–360.

Waldner, C., Janzen, E., Henderson, J., & Haines, D. (1999). An outbreak of abortion associated with Neospora caninum infection in a beef herd. *Journal American Veterinary Medical Association* **215**, 1485–1490.

Waldner, C., Ribble, C., & Janzen, E. (1998). Evaluation of the impact of a natural gas leak from a pipeline on productivity of beef cattle. *Journal American Veterinary Medical Association* **212**, 41–48.

Wikse, S. (1988). Investigation of impaired fertility in beef cattle herds. *Compendium on Continuing Education* **10**, 1225–1231, 1240.

Wikse, S., Kinsel, M., Field, R., & Holand, P. (1994). Investigating perinatal mortality in beef herds. *Veterinary Clinics of North America Food Animal Practice* **10**, 147–166.

Wikse, S., Kinsel, M., Toombs, R., & Holand, P. (1992). An epidemiologic approach to solving beef herd production and disease problems. *Veterinary Medicine* **87**, 495–506.

Wilson, J. (ed) (1992). *Physical Examination. Veterinary Clinics of North America Food Animal Practice* **8**(2). W.B. Saunders, Philadelphia.

Wobeser, G. (1996). Forensic (medico-legal) necropsy of wildlife. *Journal of Wildlife Disease* **32**, 240–249.

CHAPTER 14

Diagnosis and Clinical Reasoning in Cattle Practice

Peter D. Cockcroft

Learning objectives

To be able to:
- describe which method of clinical examination being used.
- describe hypothetico-deductive reasoning.
- describe the three principal methods of pattern recognition.
- understand deductive and inductive reasoning .
- understand abstraction and logic.
- appreciate that clinical signs can be considered tests with sensitivity and sensitivity values.
- identify information needs in the diagnostic process.

Introduction

A five year old high-yielding dairy cow is three weeks post-calving and presents with a history of a 30% daily drop in milk yield over the past four days. The cow has a condition score of 2.5 (range 0–5). The animal is slightly dull, but otherwise appears normal by observation. You collect a urine sample following manual stimulation of the perineum, and confirm that the animal is ketotic by using a urine test stick with a ketone patch. Percussion and auscultation with a stethoscope of the left side of the body from elbow to the tuber coxae reveals a consistent 'ping' over ribs 10–12. You diagnose a left displaced abomasum with a high level of certainty. This is a familiar scenario, but one that involves a complex series of clinical reasoning steps that few of us could articulate easily.

An accurate diagnosis is usually essential to ensure that treatment, control, prevention and the welfare of the patients are all optimised. Diagnosis is a task of classification. It is the determination of the disease, or diseases, producing the clinical abnormalities in the patient. The process of diagnosis involves two components; the identification of clinical abnormalities and disease risk factors, and clinical reasoning that generates a diagnosis or differential diagnoses. This involves sorting out the most likely hypothesis or hypotheses (differential diagnoses) from what is often a wide range of possibilities.

If the process of diagnosis is understood, the collection of appropriate data is likely to be more efficient and clinical reasoning performed more effectively, with more accurate outcomes. The aim of this chapter is to present some of the strategies and concepts which may be used in clinical reasoning, and which can direct the collection of additional information.

The diagnostic process

The steps in the diagnostic process are:

Step 1: Collection of data (clinical examination, laboratory tests).

Step 2: The recall of possible differential diagnoses (hypotheses).

Step 3: Ranking of competing differential diagnoses.

Step 4: Further investigations to enable differentiation of the competing hypotheses.

Go back to step 1 if there are strongly competing differential diagnoses. Go to Step 5 if the diagnosis is confirmed as a result of evidence strongly in favour of a particular diagnosis.

Step 5: Closure

The clinical examination

The purpose of the clinical examination is to identify the clinical abnormalities that are present and the risk factors that lead to manifestation of disease in the individual or a population. Clinical reasoning may be integrated within the clinical examination and thus drive the scope and direction of the clinical examination. Further investigations may follow if there is insufficient evidence for a diagnosis to be made with an accepted level of certainty. The latter may be influenced by cost and the impact of the diagnosis.

Bovine Medicine, Third Edition. Edited by Peter D. Cockcroft.

From this information, the following may be derived:

- the organs or systems involved;
- the location of the lesion;
- the type of lesion present;
- the pathophysiological processes occurring;
- the severity of the disease;
- the most likely cause;
- the epidemiology of the outbreak.

There are several different approaches to the clinical examination: the complete clinical examination, the general clinical examination, and the problem-orientated clinical examination:

- **The complete clinical examination** consists of checking for the presence or absence of all clinical abnormalities and predisposing disease risk factors. From this information a ranked list of differential diagnoses is deduced. This ensures no abnormality or risk factor is missed. The exhaustive approach includes all routine laboratory tests as well. This approach can be expensive in terms of time and cost. The amount of information can be overwhelming if clinical reasoning is delayed until the examination is complete.
- Many clinicians begin their examination by performing a **general clinical examination** consisting of a broad search for abnormalities. The system or region involved is identified, and is then examined in greater detail.
- **The problem-orientated examination** (hypothetico-deductive method) combines clinical examination and clinical reasoning, resulting in the early generation of differential diagnoses. The sequence of the clinical investigation is dictated by the differential diagnoses generated from the previous findings. This results in a limited, but focused examination. The success of the method relies heavily on the background knowledge of the clinician, and it usually assumes that a single condition is responsible for the abnormalities. It is an approach that is highly motivating, as there is a higher probability of identifying an abnormality.

Hypothetico-deductive reasoning

In hypothetico-deductive reasoning, the initial hypotheses are derived from the early clinical findings or presentation. Subsequent data collection is guided by the leading hypothesis and the competing hypotheses (differential diagnoses) being considered. The leading hypothesis may change, depending on the new information acquired, and may prompt further investigation. The competing hypotheses are usually compared, one by one, to the leading hypotheses. This process continues recursively, until a critical level of confidence has been reached. The final step is usually the validation of the diagnosis. Hypothesis generation and recall is critical. A correct diagnosis cannot be made if it has not even been considered.

Aggregation or collation of the individual clinical findings from the initial data into a single pathophysiological process will simplify the diagnostic process. For example signs, consistent with congestive heart failure in cattle, such as an increased heart rate, bilateral jugular distension, sub-mandibular and brisket oedema and diarrhoea, would result in the veterinary surgeon seeking causes of congestive heart failure rather than causes for each of the component signs. The generation of the initial list of possible diagnoses is sometimes selected by using an individual piece of data as a pivotal or key sign. The pivotal sign (or pivot) is usually a sign which can be confidently recognised as an abnormality resulting from disease. The list of differentials will then include all the diseases that contain that pivotal sign.

The diagnostic process includes discriminating between close competitors, pursuing highly likely but unproven possibilities, ruling out less likely competitors and, occasionally, including new hypotheses when additional unexpected findings are obtained. Signs or tests with a high specificity and sensitivity are selected to confirm or rule out a diagnosis. Each piece of information is considered with respect to all hypotheses under consideration before a diagnostic judgment is made. Findings are not sought if they are not related to one of the diagnostic possibilities under consideration.

This method produces a very specific and highly efficient search for discriminatory information, and induces a high level of motivation in the clinician when compared to the use of a complete clinical examination as a first approach. The sign being investigated has a higher probability of being found when compared to a complete clinical examination. Complete clinical examinations yield a higher proportion of negative findings, which may induce a reduction in abnormality recognition due to investigator fatigue.

The number of hypotheses under consideration by the veterinarian at any one time is usually four or five with a maximum of six or seven. The recall of possible diagnoses and the ranking of competing hypotheses use a function called pattern recognition. Pattern recognition is the process used to the generate a list of ranked differential diagnoses from a list of clinical abnormalities.

Recall and ranking

The recall strategies may include the recall of:

- conditions consistent with the age, sex, breed, and class of animal;
- diseases which contain all the signs observed;
- diseases which contain only pivotal signs;
- diseases which contain at least one of the signs observed;
- diseases which contain most of the signs observed;

- diseases which contain an important sign;
- common diseases only.

Pattern recognition

There are three broad categories of pattern recognition: pattern matching, probabilities, and pathophysiological reasoning.

Pattern matching

Pattern matching of facial features to recognise an individual is an example of this method of pattern recognition. In clinical profile pattern matching, the clinical signs observed and disease risk factors are compared to profiles or descriptions of diseases we hold in our memory. Pattern matching ability will increase with experience, because the archive in memory will be more complete and accurate. It is also better developed for common diseases because of exposure and reinforcement.

The differential diagnosis list is constructed according to which of the disease profiles that most closely match the clinical profiles observed in the patient. The pattern matching process is frequently restricted to common diseases in the initial hypothesis generation. The pattern matching may be extended to less common diseases if the matching is poor.

Probabilities

Given the prevalence of cattle diseases in the population under investigation, and the frequency of occurrence of the sets of clinical signs observed within those diseases, the probability of a disease being the diagnosis can be generated. The ranked differential list can then constructed from the disease probabilities. Studies in human medicine have demonstrated a lack of ability to use probabilities even in the simplest applications. The human inability to perform the mathematical computations required and the availability of data are important limiting factors. Clinicians often think they are using probabilities but, in reality, they are considering common diseases and using pattern matching of clinical signs and risk factors to generate a ranked list of differential diagnoses.

Pathophysiological reasoning (functional reasoning)

Using the clinical signs observed the system and the lesion within the system is identified using knowledge of disease mechanisms (pathophysiology and anatomy). A differential list is then constructed, using diseases which could explain the disease processes identified. An important clinical sign, in this context, is one that has an important role in the pathophysiology of the disease under consideration which may be responsible for many of the clinical manifestations of the disease (e.g. rumen pH in ruminal acidosis or severe calf diarrhoea). This method is commonly used by new graduates.

Which method of pattern recognition is used?

A study performed by Cockcroft (1998) included an investigation on the diagnostic methods used by different groups of clinicians. The conclusions of this study were:

- Veterinary students use pathophysiological reasoning most often.
- Experienced veterinary surgeons use pattern matching most often.
- Both groups use all three methods some of the time, and those different methods of pattern matching may be used concurrently in some cases.

Clinical signs as diagnostic tests for the presence or absence of a given disease

Clinical signs, or combinations of signs, can be considered as a test for a given disease, such as the ELISA for Johne's disease. For each given disease, the specificity and sensitivity for each clinical sign or set of signs could be defined:

- **Sensitivity** is the proportion of animals **with the disease with the sign(s)**
- **Specificity** is the proportion of the animals **without the disease that do not have the sign(s)**

For example, the detection of a 'ping' on from the left flank of a cow has both a high sensitivity and specificity for the diagnosis of a left-displaced abomasum (LDA). Ketosis occurs in most cows with an LDA, and also has a high sensitivity for an LDA. However, ketosis is present in several other diseases and is not exclusive to LDA. The specificity is therefore relatively low.

The selection of a sign with a high sensitivity and specificity for a given disease can be used to confirm or rule out a diagnosis, as the sign is likely to be present if the disease is present (high sensitivity) and does not occur in other diseases (high specificity). If the sign is absent, the disease may be ruled out of further consideration.

The absence of a sign with a low sensitivity for a given disease does not rule in or rule out that disease and, therefore, coveys little additional information. For example, it would be unwise to rule in or rule out calf meningitis if excitatory neurological signs were absent.

The presence of a sign with low specificity does not help differentiate the disease from other competing differential diagnoses. For example, reduced appetite is a clinical sign that is common in many diseases.

Predictive values for the presence of a disease, given the absence or presence of a sign, can be computed for a given disease, provided the prevalence of the target disease and competing diseases within the population of interest are known. The positive predictive value is the probability of the patient having the disease when the sign(s) is present. The negative predictive value is the probability of the patient having the disease when the sign(s) is absent.

Logical exclusion of a disease

If an animal presents with a clinical sign that is never observed in a disease (sensitivity 0%), then that disease can be excluded from further consideration. This is a common event and excludes many diseases. We would not expect jaundice in a case of milk fever.

If an animal presents without a clinical sign that is always observed in a disease (sensitivity 100%), then that disease can be excluded from further consideration. Hypomagnesaemia would be expected in a case of grass staggers (hypomagnesaemia).

Logical exclusion is a powerful strategy, but may exclude the true diagnosis if the observation on which the exclusion is based are inaccurate. Logical exclusion should be reserved for observations made with a high degree of certainty. The presence of signs generally has a greater discriminatory power than the absence of signs. Thus, a list of differentials based on the presence of signs will be shorter than one based solely on the absence of signs. However, considering both produces the shortest list overall.

Inductive and deductive reasoning

Deductive reasoning and **inductive** reasoning can be used alternately to investigate a hypothesis:

- **Deductive reasoning:** If a cow is pale then the cow may have haemolytic anaemia.
- **Inductive reasoning:** If the cow has haemolytic anaemia the cow may have haemagloninuria.

This method of reasoning can be used to test the strength of a hypothesis against competing hypotheses. It is a very powerful and common process.

Prevalence

> *'If you hear hoofbeats, think cattle – unless you are in a zoo, then think buffalo.'*

The relative prevalences of competing differential diagnoses are important information in the diagnostic process. By using broad bands of different prevalence values, it is possible to confine the initial search to disease that are known to occur commonly in the population under investigation.

The prevalence of a disease usually represents an average for a defined population, which may be inappropriate for a given individual, where different risk factors may have a large impact on disease occurrence. It is important to determine the risk factors operating on the animal in question at the time of the disease onset. For example, milk fever is a common condition in peri-parturient high-yielding older cows on an inappropriate transition diet, but the prevalence among dairy cows in general is relatively low.

Common errors in clinical reasoning

The most common cause of incorrect diagnoses is a failure to generate, and therefore consider, the correct diagnostic hypothesis. Other errors include.

- The collection of extraneous information which does not lead to the confirmation or testing of a hypothesis.
- Failure to correctly retrieve the correct hypotheses from memory.
- Data collection driven by an inappropriate hypotheses.
- New data being considered in relation to the hypothesis that is being tested and not in relation to alternative hypotheses.
- Information that does not fit the differential diagnoses under consideration may be ignored in preference to generating alternate hypotheses.
- Inexperienced clinicians tend to seek confirmatory information, rather than rule out information reducing their diagnostic efficiency further.

Bias and saliency

Saliency bias occurs in diagnosis when a recent clinical presentation leaves an impression that is disproportionate to the prevalence. A bias is introduced which causes an overestimate of the probability of disease. For example, a recent case of lead poisoning may result in this being the leading hypothesis in the next few investigations, where neurological signs have been observed which may be inappropriate.

Clinical reasoning exercise

Clinical scenario

A five year old Holstein cow, which calved one month ago and was previously yielding 42 litres/day, presents with a poor appetite and milk yield which has fallen steadily over the past three days to 22 L/day. The rectal temperature is 39°C, the respiratory rate is 25/min and the rumen rate is one/min. The cow has a gaunt appearance, with sunken left sub-lumbar fossa consistent with a reduced appetite. There are 200 milking cows in the herd.

Above is a case scenario to consider. Some diagnostic information is provided in Tables 14.1 to 14.4 and Figure 14.1 below. Consider the information, then use the clinical reasoning audit that follows to reflect upon the clinical reasoning pathway you might follow in this case.

Clinical reasoning audit checklist

Clinical examination

Which method of clinical examination would you use?

- Complete clinical examination.
- Problem oriented (hypothetico-deductive) approach.
- General examination followed by a complete examination or problem-orientated approach of the affected system/topographical area.

Clinical reasoning

When using the hypothetico-deductive method, did you follow the following steps?

1. Collection of data (clinical examination, laboratory tests).
2. The recall of possible differential diagnoses (hypotheses).
3. Ranking of competing differential diagnoses.
4. Further investigations to enable differentiation of the competing hypotheses:
   - evidence strongly in favour of particular diagnosis. Go to 5
   - Still unable to decide on a diagnosis Go to 1.
5. Diagnosis confirmed, closure.

When formulating a differential diagnosis list do you:

- Recall of diseases which contain all the signs observed?
- Recall diseases which contain only signs you are confident about?
- Recall diseases for each sign?
- Recall diseases which contain most of the signs observed?
- Recall diseases which contain an important sign?
- Recall only common diseases?

When ranking the differential diagnosis list which method of pattern recognition did you use:

- Pattern matching?
- Probabilities?
- Pathophysiological reasoning?

Which of the following strategies did you use?

- The specificities and sensitivities of clinical signs.
- Logical exclusion of a disease.
- Aggregation.
- Deductive and inductive reasoning.

Conclusion

If the process of diagnosis is understood, the collection of appropriate data is likely to be more efficient and clinical reasoning performed more effectively, with more accurate outcomes. This chapter has presented some of the strategies and concepts which may be used in clinical reasoning and which can direct the collection of additional information with improved efficiency and diagnostic acumen.

References and further reading

Radostits, O.M., Tyler, J.W., and Mayhew, I.G.J. (2000). *Making a diagnosis in Veterinary Clinical Examination and Diagnosis* In: Veterinary Clinical Examination and Diagnosis, Radostitis, O.M., Mayhew, I.G.J. and Houston D.M. (eds), 11–52. W.B. Saunders, London.

Blood, D.C. and Brightling, P. (1988). *Veterinary information management*. Balliere-Tindall, London.

Campbell, E.J.M., Scadding, J.G. and Roberts, R.S. (1979). The concept of disease. *British Medical Journal* **29**(2), 757–762.

Cockcroft, P.D. (1996). *Pattern Matching Models of Veterinary Diagnosis*. DVM&S thesis, University of Edinburgh.

Cockcroft, P.D. (1998). A survey of pattern recognition methods in veterinary diagnosis, *Journal of Veterinary Education* **25**(2), 21–23.

Miller, R.A. and Geissbuhler, A. (1999). Clinical Diagnostic Decision Support Systems: An overview. In: Berner, E.S. (ed). *Clinical Diagnostic Decision Support Systems*, pp. 3–34. Springer, New York.

Smith, R.D. (1995). *Veterinary Clinical Epidemiology*. Butterworth-Heineman, London.

White, M.E. (1988). Diagnosis, information management, and record coding using the Consultant database. *Canadian Veterinary Journal* **29**, 271–273.

Table 14.1 Similarities and differences between the case profile and the differential diagnoses.

Condition	5 year old high-yielding dairy cow	One month post-calving	Sudden drop in milk yield	Normal temperature	Normal respiratory rate	Normal rumen rate	Gaunt appearance	Prevalence
Caecal dilatation/torsion	Yes	Some increased risk	Yes	Yes (elevated in torsion)	Yes (elevated in torsion)	Yes	Sometimes	Rare – but can get outbreaks
Left displaced abomasum	Yes	Increased risk	Yes	Yes	Yes	Yes sometimes can't auscultate	Yes	Common
Liver disease (Fatty Liver Syndrome)	Yes	Usually immediately post-calving	Yes	Yes	Yes	Yes	Sometimes	Rare – but can get outbreaks
Oral lesions	Yes	Slight increased risk	Yes	Yes	Yes	Yes	Yes	Rare
Perforating abomasal ulcer	Yes	Increased risk	Yes	Sometimes elevated (inflammation)	Sometimes elevated (pain)	Often rumen stasis	Yes	Intermediate-rare
Primary ketosis	Yes	Increased risk	Yes	Yes	Yes	Yes	Yes	Common
Pyelonephritis	Yes	Usually spontaneous or post-bull mating	Yes	Elevated (inflammation and pain)	Often elevated (pain)	Yes	Sometimes	Rare
Right displaced abomasum	Yes	Increased risk	Yes	Yes	Yes	Yes	Yes	Intermediate
Ruminal acidosis	Yes	Increased risk	Yes	Normal/ subnormal	Sometimes elevated (metabolic acidosis)	Rumen stasis	Sometimes	Intermediate
Traumatic reticulitis	Yes	Increased risk	Yes	Sometimes elevated (inflammation)	Sometimes elevated (pain)	Often rumen stasis	Yes	Intermediate-rare

Table 14.2 Examples of differential information for the conditions.

Further Investigation	Primary ketosis	LDA	RDA	Abomasal ulcer	TRP	Acute acidosis	Caecal dilatation /torsion	Pyelo-nephritis	Oral lesions	Liver disease (FLS)
History										
Transition cow diet inappropriate	+	+	+							
Condition score dry cows high										+
Access to highly fermentable carbohydrate						+				
Access to sharp objects					+					
Caustic soda used on straw									+/-	
Specific and sensitive clinical signs										
Loss of weight	+									+
Nervous signs	+/-					Depressed				
Abdominal pain				+ (right)	+ (ant/left)			+		
Ping L ribs 10–12	+									
Ping R ribs 10–12		+								
Ping R sub-lumbar fossa							+			
Dehydration			+			+	+			
Diarrhoea			+/-			+				
Rectal examination			+/-				+	Pain		
Left sided Laparotomy/ Rumenotomy		LDA			Adhesions Wire	Fluid filled		Painful kidney		
Right sided Laprotomy/ Rumenotomy			RDA	Adhesions			Dilated caecum	Painful kidney		
Samples and tests										
Urine sample Ketones	+	+	+							
Urine sample Gross morphology								Turbid, contains blood and pus.		
Rumen fluid sample pH						pH < 5.0				
Peritoneal tap				+ inflamm.	+ Inflamm.		+/-	+/-		
Liver biopsy										Very high lipid content
Serum biochemistry	Ketone	Ketone alkalosis (metab.)	Ketone			acidosis (metab.)				Elevated NEFA Hypo-glycemia Elevated AST Elevated SDH, LDH
Haematology: Inflammation				+	+		+/-		+/-	

Table 14.3 Pathophysiological processes.

Condition	Pathophysiology
1. Primary ketosis	Negative energy balance: Hypoglycaemia with beta-oxidation of fats
2. Left displaced abomasum	Negative energy balance: Hypoglycaemia with beta-oxidation of fats. Sequestration of electrolytes and H^+ in abomasum
3. Right displaced abomasum	Negative energy balance: Hypoglycaemia with beta-oxidation of fats. Sequestration of electrolytes and H^+ in abomasum Dehydration
4. Perforating abomasal ulcer	Localised peritonitis
5. Traumatic reticulitis	Localised peritonitis
6. Ruminal acidosis	Metabolic acidosis and ruminal/intestinal osmotic dehydration
7. Caecal dilatation/torsion	Sequestration of electrolyte and fluids in caecum +/− peritonitis
8. Pyelonephritis	Localised peritonitis and nephritis
9. Oral lesions	Stomatitis
10. Liver disease (Fatty Liver Syndrome)	Liver failure

Table 14.4 Differential diagnosis.

Possible differential diagnoses and rank (according to their likelihood of being the diagnosis based upon the case description, identified risk factors and the prevalence)	**Clinical profiles with high specificities and sensitivities**
1. Primary ketosis	Ketosis and no pings
2. Left displaced abomasum	Ketosis, and a left side ping (ribs 10–12)
3. Right displaced abomasum	Ketosis, and a right side ping (ribs 10–12)
4. Perforating abomasal ulcer	Right side anterior abdominal pain with a peritoniteal fluid sample indicating peritonitis
5. Traumatic reticulitis	Anterior abdominal pain with a peritoniteal fluid sample indicating peritonitis
6. Ruminal acidosis	Rumen pH < 5.0 and metabolic acidosis and dehydration and diarrhoea
7. Caecal dilatation/torsion	Ping right sub-lumbar fossa and rectal examination – distended viscus
8. Pyelonephritis	Turbid discoloured urine and pain on palpation of affected kidney
9. Oral lesions	mouth lesions
10. Liver disease (Fatty Liver Syndrome)	Liver biopsy has high lipid content on histopathology and serum biochemistry indicates increase in liver enzymes, NEFA and hypoglycaemia

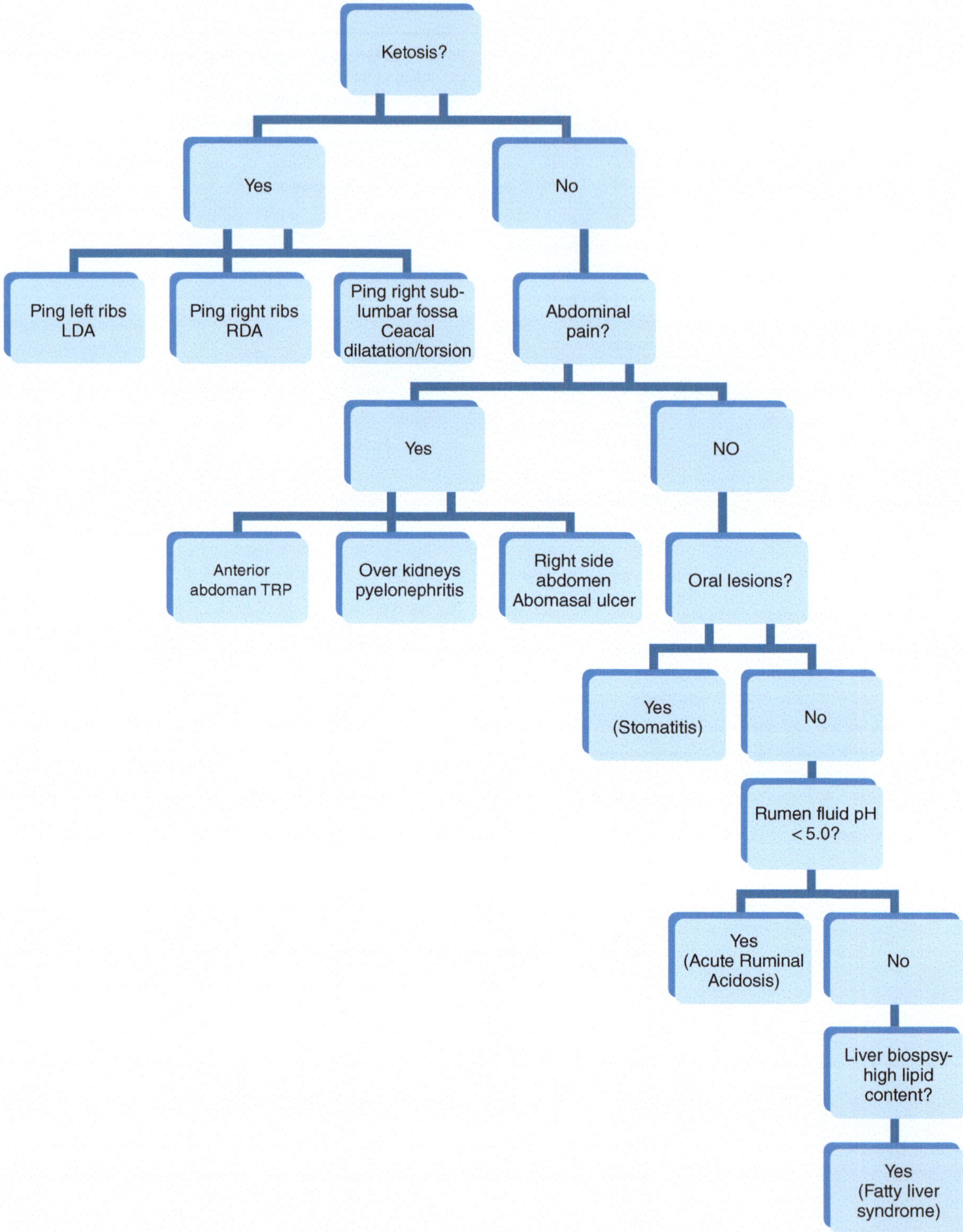

Figure 14.1 Algorithm using highly sensitive and specific signs as nodes in a decision tree.

CHAPTER 15
Special Diagnostic Procedures

Phil Scott and Peter D. Cockcroft

Learning objectives

- Be aware of the range of further investigative techniques available to the cattle practitioner.
- Appreciate the technical skills that are required to perform these techniques.
- Appreciate the additional information that can be derived from the samples obtained.

Skin

Bacterial culture – the normal bovine skin has a large population of bacteria, including staphylococci, streptococci, *Trueperella pyogenes* and coliforms that live symbiotically with their host but can also be opportunist pathogens. Swabs from suspicious lesions should be taken with care to avoid contamination and should be processed quickly. Pustular material from abscesses may be aspirated by sterile needle and syringe for culture. Skin biopsies may also be cultured.

Skin scrapings – these are particularly useful in the diagnosis of mange infestation and should be taken from the periphery of the lesion in the early stages of the disease, because few mites may be present later as the host responds. The scraping is best taken with a scalpel blade to a depth at which signs of capillary bleeding just appear. The scraping may be examined microscopically before or after potassium hydroxide treatment.

Skin biopsy – this is the most useful diagnostic test. Hairs should be clipped short and the skin gently cleaned with 70% alcohol before injection of local anaesthetic solution around and under the proposed biopsy site. The biopsy, by excision or by punch biopsy, should be at least 5 mm in size and should be fixed in 10% buffered formalin at least ten times the volume of the biopsy.

Soft tissue swellings – needle aspirates may reveal an abscess or a hematoma. Ultrasonography can also be useful to differentiate the aetiology. Abscesses have a 'snowstorm' appearance whilst hematomas have a segmental structure (Figure 15.1)

Other diagnostic tests include direct electron microscopy for virus infections such as bovine papular stomatitis.

Cardiovascular

Diagnostic tests

Percussion of the heart – the heart lies beneath the third and sixth ribs on the right, and beneath the third and fifth ribs on the left and extends approximately one-third up the ribs on both sides. Thoracic ultrasonography with portable 5 MHz sector scanners is now readily available and, unlike percussion, it accurately differentiates pleural effusion, cardiac enlargement, pericardial effusion and consolidation of the ventral margins of the lung lobes.

Electrocardiography – electrocardiography is rarely undertaken in farm animal practice, because the important cardiac diseases are more readily diagnosed by ultrasonography.

Ultrasound (US) evaluation – A 3.5 or 5 MHz sector probe with a field depth up to 20 cm is suitable for examining the heart. Good visualisation of the heart is facilitated by placing the animal's ipsilateral foreleg on a block raised 15 cm from the ground and drawing the leg forward. Ultrasonography can readily detect abnormalities of the pericardium (particularly fluid accumulations), epicardium and myocardium, and heart valves. Pericardial effusion appears as an anechoic (black) area surrounding the heart that may extend up to 10–15 cm. Septic pericarditis appears as an anechoic area with multiple hyperechoic dots caused by minute gas bubbles within the exudate. Vegetative endocarditis lesions appear as marked irregularities and thickening of the heart valves.

Doppler flow sector scanners produce more detailed information, including the direction and pressure of blood flow. This information is helpful in cases of congenital cardiac abnor-

Bovine Medicine, Third Edition. Edited by Peter D. Cockcroft.

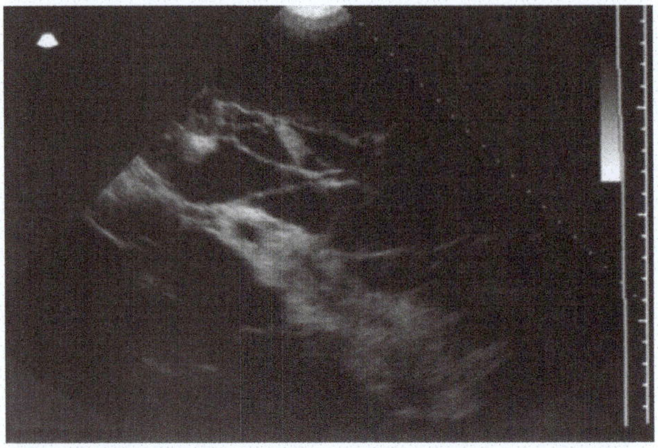

Figure 15.1 Ultrasonography: flank hematoma with a hyper- echogenic segmental appearance.

mality, but it is not essential. It is important to note that large ventricular septal defects may result in no audible murmur.

Radiography – is of very limited value in assessing bovine cardiac morphology, because the size and mass of the bovine heart prevents clear demonstration of the internal divisions of the heart. Radio-opaque foreign bodies (such as wires) may be detected as they pass through the diaphragm from the reticulum to the pericardium, but such information is more readily gained by ultrasonography, without the health and safety concerns of radiography on farm.

Pericardiocentesis – in the absence of ultrasonography, pericardiocentesis can be useful in confirming a septic pericarditis and obtaining a sample of pericardial effusions for further analysis. Ultrasongraphy-guided pericardiocentesis improves the precision of sampling. Large accumulations of transudate within the pericardial sac are rare in cattle. A 9 cm, 19 g spinal needle is inserted under local anaesthesia through the chest wall into the pericardial sac, when fluid can be aspirated for cytology and culture.

Blood culture – blood for culture may be taken aseptically from the jugular vein in cases of endocarditis, but repeated samples may be needed, as bacterial release from valve lesions is intermittent.

Respiratory system

Auscultation and percussion are insufficient to characterise many chronic respiratory diseases. Bronchoalveolar lavage (BAL) is particularly helpful in determining the viral cause(s) of outbreaks of calf pneumonia. Further investigations may include paired serology, nasopharyngeal swabs, faecal sampling for lungworm larvae, and ultrasonography. Fibre-optic endoscopy, radiography, blood gas analysis, thoracocentesis and lung biopsy have few applications in cattle practice.

Bronchoalveolar lavage (BAL)

A BAL sample can be used for the rapid identification of viral antigens by indirect fluorescent antibody tests (IFAT), and for bacteriological culture and cytology. In an acute outbreak of respiratory disease, four to six febrile cattle are selected; severely affected animals should be avoided. The equipment required includes a 50 ml catheter tip syringe, disposable gloves, a sterile 90 cm small diameter flexible tube (6 mm), 20 ml of warm sterile buffered saline, viral transport medium, and topical local anaesthetic gel.The animal is restrained in cattle stocks, a halter applied, and the head pulled forward, extending the animal's neck. Local anaesthetic gel is applied to the inner surface of nostril. The distance to the larynx and the base of the thoracic inlet are marked and the tube is gently passed via the ventral nasal meatus to the larynx, then quickly pushed forward through the glottis into the trachea during inspiration. When successful, breathing will be felt and heard at the end of the tube, accompanied by some mild coughing. If entry to the trachea has not been successful, the tube may have to be withdrawn a few centimetres and advanced again. The tube is then advanced to the bifurcation of the major bronchi (the carina). 20 ml of warm phosphate buffered saline is then injected and immediately withdrawn; about 10 ml of frothy (surfactant-rich) fluid are usually retrieved. The fluid is then decanted into viral transport medium, a sterile tube for bacterial culture, and EDTA for cytological examination. Analyses may include tests for PI3, RSV, IBR, BVD antigens, and bacterial culture for Mannheimia haemolytica, *Pasteurellae* spp. and *Haemophilus somni.*

Diagnosis of lungworm

Examination of faeces (Baermann technique) and bronchoalveolar samples for L1 stage larvae may confirm a diagnosis of a patent lungworm infestation. Prior exposure to lungworm can also be confirmed by an ELISA test on serum.

Acute and convalescent sera

Rising serological titres give a retrospective indication of exposure and the possible causal agent(s) of an outbreak of viral pneumonia. Serological samples are collected from a minimum of five affected animals at the beginning of the outbreak and 4–6 weeks later.

Nasopharyngeal swab

Naso-pharyngeal swabs from early clinical cases may be useful in identifying the etiological agents of pneumonia in cattle; however, *Mannheimia haemolytica* and *Pasteurella* spp. isolates may be commensals.

Radiography

Radiography is of very limited value, especially in older animals, where thoracic ultrasonography is much quicker, cheaper and more informative. Chemical restraint to facilitate positioning of the animal in lateral recumbency may lead to an unacceptable risk. Radiography has limited application in the examination of reticular wires which have penetrated the thorax, and rib fractures.

Ultrasonography

The pleurae and pulmonary surfaces of both lung fields are examined between the 5th and the 7th ribs intercostal spaces. This topographical area usually provides the most useful information. The 5MHz sector transducers are the most useful, but linear transducers are more readily available and can still provide diagnostic images. Systematic ultrasound examination of both sides can be performed quickly.

Ultrasonographic examination of the chest is most helpful in the diagnosis of chronic suppurative pneumonia, where the dorsal margin of the lung pathology is represented by numerous hypoechoic columns extending 2–8 cm into the lung parenchyma, which are bordered distally by bright white (hyperechoic) lines when the transmitted sound waves contact normal aerated lung. Moving the probe head ventrally, there are large hypoechogenic areas, with the echogenic appearance of liver (hepatoid) corresponding to lung consolidation.

Pleural effusions are present in varying quantities in individual cases of dilated cardiomyopathy, thymic, and diffuse fibrosing alveolitis.

Pleural effusion is readily identified as an anechoic area which increases in depth as the probe head is moved ventrally with consequent dorsal displacement of the ventral margins of the lung lobes, which may be consolidated.

Metastases to the lungs appear as discrete 2–3 cm diameter hypoechoic areas without a marked capsule, and are present throughout all lung lobes at necropsy.

Blood gas analysis and PCV

Blood gas analysis needs to be performed rapidly once the sample is taken. Pen-side hand held biochemical/blood gas analysers are becoming increasingly available and cheaper. Blood gas analysis is very helpful in defining the extent of hypoxia and characterising acid/base disorders. Arterial samples are the most useful, and the auricular or coccygeal arteries can be sampled.

The percentage oxygen saturation of arterial haemoglobin can be measured using a pulse oximeter. The sensors are attached to shaved non-pigmented skin of the tail, the non-pigmented areas of the scrotum or the vulva. Pulse oximeters are portable, non-invasive, easy to use, inexpensive, and can be used with success in field conditions.

Thoracocentesis

Samples of pleural fluid can be obtained by ultrasound-guided thoracocentesis at the 5–6th intercostal spaces under local anaesthesia. Equipment required includes hair clippers, a lumbar spinal needle gauge 18, 9 cm, skin disinfectant, alcohol, swabs, EDTA and plain collection tubes.

Lung biopsy

Lung biopsies of areas defined ultrasonographically may be useful to identify pathological changes in lung tissue but should be reserved for cases of respiratory disease in which less invasive techniques have failed to establish a diagnosis. The biopsy can be performed in the standing animal. The hair is shaved or clipped over the lesion(s), and the site aseptically prepared. Local anaesthetic is injected subcutaneously then into the intercostal muscles. A stab incision is made with a scalpel blade into the anaesthetised skin. The skin is then moved caudally, and the Tru-cut needle thrust through the cutaneous stab incision and through the intercostal muscles and pleura into the lung lesion. This approach ensures that the skin incision will not directly overlay the deeper wound and helps reduce the possibility of pneumothorax. The Tru-cut needle is then removed, and the biopsy placed in 10% formal-saline and submitted for histopathology.

Clinical pathology

Metabolic acidosis may occur in carbohydrate engorgement (grain overload). Hand-held biochemical and acid-base analyses are available in small animal hospital practices, and can be used in farm animal practice. Metabolic alkalosis can occur in abomasal conditions due to sequestration of hydrogen ions, and in urea poisoning. Electrolyte measurements may indicate hypokalaemia, which may be present in abomasal distension/volvulus. A low PCV may indicate a haemorrhaging abomasal ulcer, and a raised PCV may indicate dehydration.

A leukocytosis with a relative neutrophilia may indicate an inflammatory process. Alternatively, a leucopaenia and a neutropaenia may be found in severe cases, due to sequestration or endotoxaemia/septicaemia. Hypoalbuminaemia may be a feature of a protein-losing enteropathy, such as paratuberculosis, or a reduction in hepatic production. A high serum globulin and plasma fibrinogen concentrations are useful indicators of chronic and acute inflammation, respectively.

Abdomen

Rectal examination

Rectal palpation is an important investigative procedure. The systematic palpation of the internal anatomical structures (Figure 15.2) and an assessment of the faeces should not be overlooked (Figure 15.3). Table 15.1 describes some of the gastro-intestinal abnormalities that may be detected on rectal palpation, and Table 15.2 indicates the range of gross

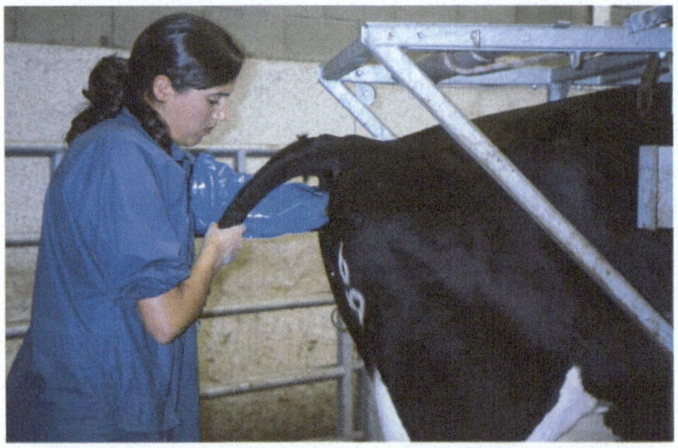

Figure 15.2 Rectal examination is an important investigative procedure.

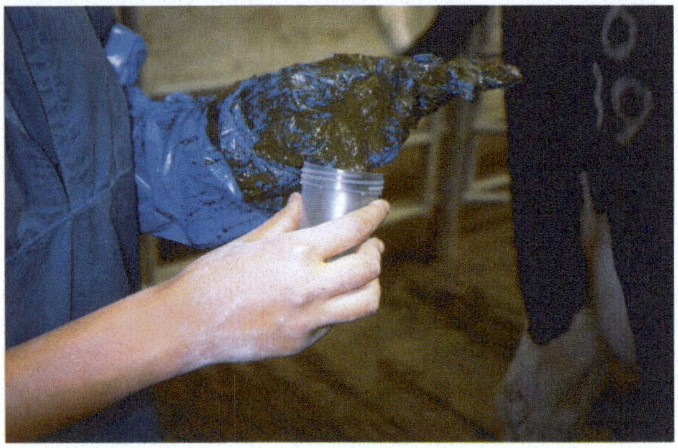

Figure 15.3 Gross examination: faecal sample.

Table 15.1 Rectal palpation findings and possible interpretation.

Rectal examination finding	Condition
Dorsal sac packed with fibre	Vagal indigestion
Dorsal sac distended and tympanic	Bloat
Dorsal sac cannot be palpated	Collapsed dorsal sac
Tense gas filled viscus arms length laterally on the right hand side	Right displaced/dilated abomasum
Large hard sausage-shaped structure on the right	Intussusception
Tense gas filled viscus, shaped like a long balloon with blind end caudally immediately on right laterally	Distended/dilated caecum
Large focal mass(es) which may surround the intestines	Fat necrosis
Thickened small intestines (highly subjective)	Johne's disease

Table 15.2 Gross faecal appearance and possible interpretation.

Faecal samples	Associated condition
Faeces dry, dark brown, ball shaped, shiny (covered in mucous)	Slow gut passage/dehydration
Faeces dark green colour	Increased bile salt content (e.g. haemolytic anaemia)
Faeces pale olive green	Decreased bile salts (e.g. anorexia)
Undigested grains in faeces	Normal cattle fed on unprocessed grain
Dysenteric faeces A mixture of undigested blood mucous and watery faeces usually with an offensive fetid smell sometimes with yellow grey castes (fibrin)	Salmonella, winter dysentery, mucosal disease
Blood and sloughing mucosa	Intussusception (ischemic necrosis)
Melaenic (black) faeces	Digested blood Abomasal ulceration, oesophageal tumour Caudal vena caval syndrome
Frank blood or blood clots	Cocidiosis or mucosa damaged during the rectal examination
Diarrhoea	Enteritis or osmotic (ruminal acidosis)

abnormalities of the faeces and possible interpretations of these findings.

Rumen fluid collection

A sample of rumen fluid may be obtained using a naso-gastric tube or an oral stomach tube to assess rumen health and function. Rumenocentesis avoids possible contamination with saliva. Analysis is best performed within one hour of collection.

Naso-gastric/oral stomach tube – the length of the naso-gastric tube required to reach the larynx and rumen from the nose is marked on the tube. The naso-gastric tube is advanced slowly through the ventral meatus to the pharynx, then into the oesophagus during expiration when the animal swallows (Figure 15.4). Coughing, then breathing, indicates entry into the trachea. When the tube passes into the oesophagus, then rumen, gas with a characteristic odour, escapes. If necessary, blow forcefully down the tube and auscultate the rumen at the left sublumbar fossa for bubbling sounds as the gas penetrates the rumen fluid. Negative pressure is applied with a stirrup pump, or by sucking the end of the tube, to obtain a sample of rumen fluid. If this fails, bend and withdraw the tube and decant the rumen fluid in the distal tube. A sample can be collected into a universal sample pot. The only difference between using a

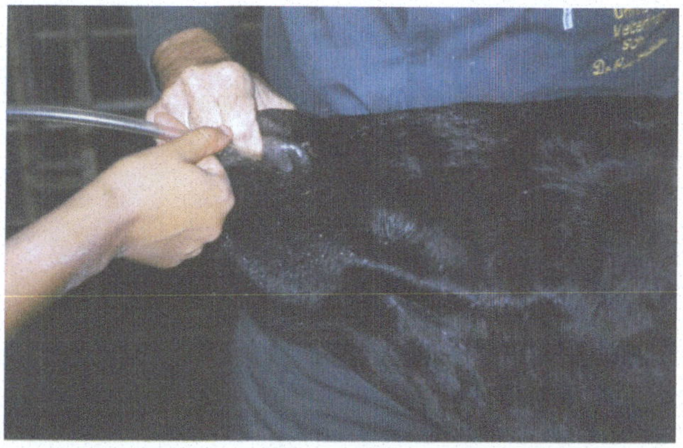

Figure 15.4 Rumen fluid collection: the naso-gastric tube should be directed through the ventral meatus.

stomach tube and a nasogastric tube is that the tube is advanced through the gagged mouth. Contamination of the rumen fluid sample with saliva should be avoided by discarding the first part of column of rumen fluid in the tube.

Ruemocentesis – the equipment required to perform a ruminocentesis includes clippers, surgical antiseptic, alcohol and a 9 cm 18 gauge spinal needle with a stylet. Some practitioners use a 5 cm gauge 14/16, as obstruction by rumen debris is common. The rumen contains a dorsal gas cap, a fibrous raft, and fluid in the ventral sac. A small area of skin in the left ventral quadrant of abdomen is surgically prepared. A tail cinch or an anti-kick bar is then applied and the prepared area infiltrated with local anaesthetic. This greatly facilitates the sampling procedure and is highly recommended. The needle/ lumbar spinal needle is then pushed through the skin at the anaesthetised and prepared site. A syringe is attached to the needle, and a sample is withdrawn. A blocked needle can be cleared by injecting air.

Rumen fluid analysis

Evaluate the rumen fluid sample as soon as possible, as cooling and exposure to air alters protozoan and bacterial activity.

Colour – normal rumen fluid is usually olive green or greenish-brown. In ruminal acidosis, the fluid may appear milky grey.

pH – the rumen fluid pH can be measured immediately by using pH (litmus) paper (range 3.0–9.0) or, ideally, electronic hand-held cow-side pH meters, which are cheap and readily available (normal is 6–7 in cattle on roughage-based diet, and 5.5–6.5 on a concentrate-based diet). In ruminal acidosis (carbohydrate engorgement), the pH will be 5.0 or less. In sub-acute ruminal acidosis, the pH will be in the range 5.1–5.7. In anorexic cattle, the pH will be alkaline (7.5–8.0); higher pH values can occur with urea poisoning.

Sedimentation/flotation – this test for complete sedimentation of solid particles must be performed within a short time following collection, and is an indirect measure of microflora activity. The finer particles sink and the coarser particles float, supported by gas bubbles of fermentation (4–8 minutes in healthy cattle). Inactive microflora results in rapid sedimentation, with little floating material.

Redox potential (methylene blue reduction time) – this test is a measure of the reduction-oxidation activity of the rumen microflora, and reflects anaerobic fermentation by rumen bacteria. One ml of 0.03% methylene blue is mixed with 20 ml of rumen fluid, and the time taken to decolourise the methylene blue is measured (normal around three minutes; around 15 minutes indicates poor microbial activity).

Protozoal activity – a drop of rumen fluid is placed on a warm glass slide under a cover slip and vigorous protozoan activity (10–20 motile protozoa per field) observed using low power (× 10 objective microscope lens). Large protozoa are more sensitive to rumen disturbances. All protozoa are killed when pH drops below pH 5.0. There are reduced numbers in samples with low fermentation activity.

Gram stain – gram-stained smears reveal mainly gram-negative bacteria in normal rumen fluid, but gram-positive streptococci and lactobacilli predominate in ruminal acidosis.

Rumen fluid chloride concentration – in healthy cattle, rumen fluid has a chloride concentration <30 mmol/L; much higher concentrations indicate reflux of abomasal fluid into the rumen. High levels may also occur in ruminal acidosis and prolonged anorexia.

Exploratory laparotomy and rumenotomy

Exploratory laparotomies should only be undertaken after all other ancillary tests, particularly trans-abdominal and trans-rectal ultrasonography, have failed to yield a specific diagnosis (Figure 15.5).

Abdominocentesis (peritoneal tap, paracentesis)

Abdominocentesis is easy and inexpensive to perform, and requires little equipment. In normal healthy cattle, there is usually only 15–20 ml of peritoneal fluid in the abdominal cavity. As a consequence, a sample is not always obtained and the lack of a sample should not be interpreted as abnormal. The only exception to this is during late pregnancy, when the volume markedly increases. Abdominocentesis is best performed after demonstration of peritoneal tranusdate/exudate by trans-abdominal ultrasonography. It is important to recognise that abnormal peritoneal fluid, particularly in cases of local peritonitis, may be confined to a localised area by the enveloping omentum, and is not always collected by abdominocentesis.There are several potential sites to perform an abdominocentesis. A common site is in the ventral anterior abdomen, midway between the xiphisternum and the umbilicus in the midline (Figure 15.6). This

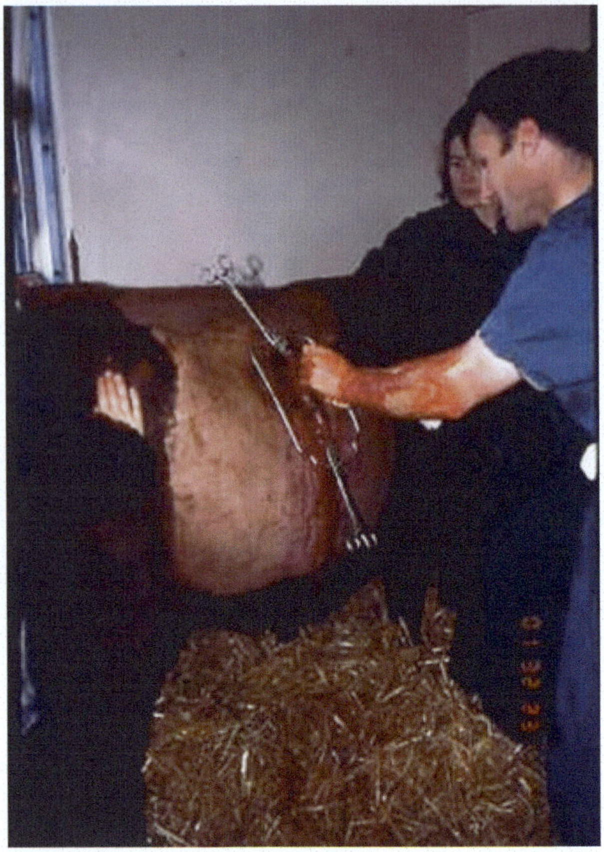

Figure 15.5 Laparotomy and a rumenotomy.

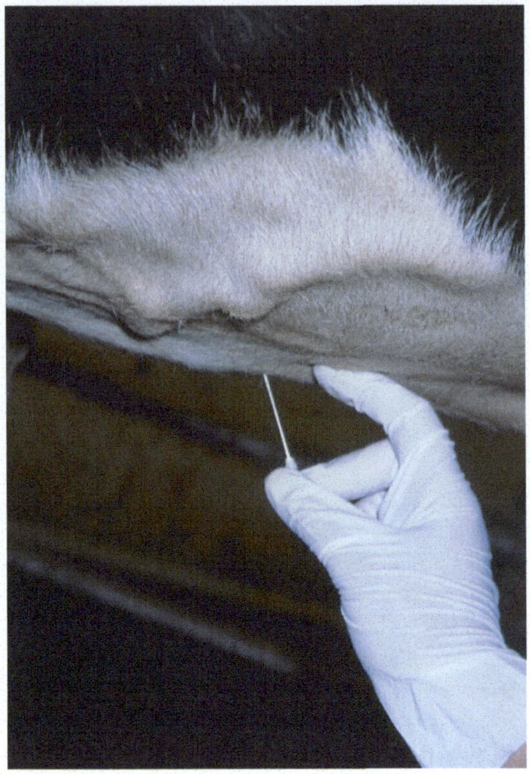

Figure 15.6 Peritoneal tap: midline between the umbilicus and xiphisternum.

site is easy to identify and carries no risk of accidental puncture of the milk vein. An alternative site in the anterior abdomen is 5 cm caudal to xiphisternum and 5 cm to the left or right of midline. Other sites are on the left or right posterior abdomen, just anterior to attachment of the mammary gland to the body wall.

The preparation and procedure is the same for both sites. Ideally, hair is clipped or shaved at the site, and the skin aseptically prepared. Restraint, using a cinch or an anti-kick bar, can improve operator safety. A 5 cm gauge 19 needle is gently pushed into the peritoneal cavity of the abdomen through the skin, musculature and parietal peritoneum. If no peritoneal fluid is obtained, the needle can be rotated and the depth of penetration increased. The rumen is sometimes penetrated in ventral sites, and a dark gritty sample obtained. If no sample is obtained, a new site should be selected. Samples should be collected into a plain tube for bacteriology and an EDTA tube for cytology. Examination of the sample includes colour, viscosity, turbidity, cell number and type, specific gravity, protein concentration, preparation of stained smears for bacteria, and bacterial culture. Table 15.3 indicates some of the interpretations of grossly abnormal peritoneal fluid. The colour of normal peritoneal fluid is clear, straw-coloured or yellow. If the sample is green in colour, this suggests the presence of food material and may indicate a gut rupture, or that a gut sample (a rumen sample being the most common) has inadvertently been obtained. An intense orange/green colour indicates rupture of the biliary system, but this is rare. A pink to red sample indicates presence of haemoglobin and/or red blood cells, which may indicate iatrogenic penetration of a blood vessel, gut infarction or perforation. A red-brown colour indicates necrosis of gut wall. Frank blood indicates haemorrhage into the peritoneum (heamoperitoneum), which may be pathological but may have been caused by the abdominocentesis procedure puncturing a blood vessel. Repeating the procedure at a different site may allow differentiation of the various possibilities.

A turbid sample indicates an increased cellular content. Large quantities of yellowish-coloured turbid fluid (sometimes with fibrin tags) suggest peritonitis. A sample that forms a generous stable froth after vigorous shaking indicates a high protein concentration (exudate) and an inflammatory process. Clotting of the sample indicates an increase in the viscosity of the peritoneal fluid, due to inflammatory processes. More detailed laboratory analysis may include measurements of specific gravity and protein content. A high specific gravity and high protein content suggests vascular damage and leakage of plasma proteins, in cases of peritonitis or ischemic necrosis

Table 15.3 Interpretation of peritoneal fluid gross findings.

Peritoneal fluid	Interpretation
Volume in excess of 10 ml	Pathological process or late pregnancy
Green (+/– particulate matter)	Gut contents (gut rupture or puncture of gut during sampling usually rumen)
Vivid orange	Rupture of bile duct (rare)
Pink/red	Presence of haemoglobin and or red blood cells which may indicate, the iatrogenic penetration of a blood vessel, a gut infarction or perforation
Red/brown	Necrosis of gut wall (e.g. intussusception)
Blood	Haemorrhage into the peritoneum (heamoperitoneum) which may be pathological or puncturing a blood vessel during sampling
Stable head of froth on shaking	Increase in protein content (inflammation)
Increased viscosity	Increase in protein content (inflammation)
Turbid (sometimes with fibrin tags)	Inflammatory products: increased protein and cellular content and fibrin
Clotting	Presence of an inflammatory process

of the bowel. Microscopy may indicate the presence of particulate food material from a ruptured bowel. Cytology may indicate: an increased white cell count (WBC) of the peritoneal fluid, with increased polymorphonuclear cells (PMN), which indicates inflammation (sterile or infectious); the presence of degenerative PMNs, which suggests infection; and increased monocytes, which suggests the presence of a chronic inflammatory process. Table 15.4 provides a classification of normal, transudate, modified transudate and exudate. *A transudate* may be present in Johne's disease as a result of hypoalbuminaemia. *A modified transudate* may be observed in lymphosarcoma of the gastrointestinal tract or congestive heart failure. *An exudate* may be septic or non-septic. Conditions causing a septic exudate include a ruptured uterus and traumatic reticuloperitonitis. Bladder rupture causes a non-septic exudate.

Radiography

Radiography of the anterior abdomen may be useful in the diagnosis of traumatic reticulitis caused by a penetrating wire. However, powerful machines are usually only available in referral veterinary centres.

Metal detectors

Many normal cattle give positive results due to the presence of harmless metal fragments such as anthelmintic boluses, nuts and bolts in the reticulum. A negative result will indicate the absence of a wire in the reticulum/thorax.

Ultrasonography

A 5.0 MHz linear transducer connected to a real-time, B-mode ultrasound machine can be used for all abdominal ultrasonographic examinations except examination of the right kidney where a 5.0 MHz sector transducer is necessary to ensure good contact with the concave flank of the right sublumbar fossa. The field setting of 10 cm on the linear scanner is appropriate for most common abdominal disorders. Occasionally, the 20 cm field depth afforded by certain 5.0 MHz sector scanners more accurately determines the extent of fluid accumulation and bladder diameter but this does not significantly alter the clinical diagnosis. Examination of the entire bovine liver may necessitate using a 3.5 MHz convex transducer but results in loss of definition and image quality.

Sites for ultrasonographic examination

Ultrasound examination is an aid to diagnosis and should be targeted at particular organs, depending upon clinical findings; thereby, the time taken to prepare the site(s) is greatly reduced. A 15 cm by 15 cm area of skin is adequate for most sites, and is the best compromise between the cost of the veterinary surgeon's time and the area examined. The site is preferably shaved, rather than clipped, and ultrasound gel applied.

The abdominal wall is 2–5 cm thick, depending upon the site and body condition score. There is scant peritoneal fluid

Table 15.4 Differentiation of normal, transudative, modified transudative and exudative peritoneal fluid.

Type	Colour/ volume	Total proteing/l	Specific gravity	WBC cells × 106/l	Differential WBC
Normal	Amber clear 1–5 ml	<25 Does not clot	1.005–1.015	<1000	Neutrophils: monocytes 1 : 1
Transudate	Clear pale straw 10–20 ml	>25 Does not clot	>1.018	<1000	Non-degenerate neutrophils
Modified Transudate	Clear straw 10–20	>25 Does not clot	>1.018	<5000	Non-degenerate neutrophils
Exudate Non septic	Amber to pink Turbid	>25 Clots	>1.018	>5000	Non-degenerate neutrophils
Exudate Septic	Pink to red Turbid	28–58Clots	>1.016	>5000	Degenerate neutrophils

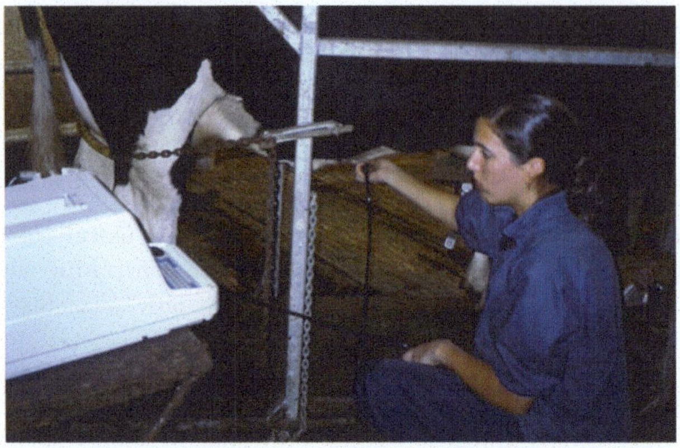

Figure 15.7 Ultrasonography: ventral abdomen.

in normal cattle, which cannot be visualised during ultrasonographic examination.

Cranial ventral abdomen – with cattle adequately restrained in stocks, the reticulum is imaged from the ventral midline immediately caudal to the xiphisternum (Figure 15.7).

Right side: right kidney and liver – examination of the right kidney necessitates shaving an area of the right sublumbar fossa immediately caudal to the last rib. The sector transducer head is firmly held against the skin, to ensure good visualisation of the right kidney juxtaposed the caudal lobe of the liver. Small intestine and caecum are examined from the lower right sublumbar fossa.

In cattle, the liver is readily identified in the ninth to eleventh intercostal spaces on the right side at the level of a line joining the right wing of the ileum with the right elbow. In cases of hepatomegaly, the liver can be imaged immediately caudal to the costal arch at this level, with the 5 MHz sector probe head pointed toward the opposite elbow. A 3.5 MHz convex transducer is necessary for measurements of the liver in cattle, but results in loss of definition and image quality.

Left side: left displaced abomasum – examination for a LDA necessitates shaving an area over the 9th to 12th intercostal spaces, two-thirds the way up the left side.

Transrectal examination – transrectal examination of the bladder is readily achieved in adult cattle.

Ascites – ascites can prove difficult to quantify on clinical examination by ballotment, especially in animals with fluid-distended intestines, but is readily identified during ultrasonographic examination, even when the patient is recumbent. Ascites can be present without significant accumulation of fluid at other sites, such as subcutaneous tissue in the submandibular region (bottle-jaw) and brisket. In standing animals, ascitic fluid appears as an aechoic area with abdominal viscera displaced dorsally. The intestines are clearly outlined as hyperechoic (bright white) lines/circles, containing material of varying echogenicity.

Traumatic reticulitis and associated localised peritonitis – the normal reticulum is in contact with the diaphragm and ventral body wall, and is examined form the ventral midline site immediately caudal to the xiphisternum. Forceful reticular contractions, lasting 3–5 seconds, are observed 1–2 times per minute by holding the probe head stationary.

Traumatic reticulitis is common in cattle, where ultrasonography can readily identify, in chronological order of the disease process: reduced/absent reticular motility; increasing volumes of peritoneal fluid in the anterior abdomen; the development of fibrinous adhesions between the reticulum and abdominal wall; and abscess formation and enlargement.

Significant quantities of peritoneal exudate, often up to 8–10 cm between peritoneum and reticular wall, and thick fibrin deposits on the reticular wall, are commonly observed in traumatic reticulitis where the cow has been sick for more than one week. The hyperechoic latticework appearance of the fibrinous reaction in the anterior abdomen contrasts with the anechoic peritoneal fluid. Involvement of the spleen is common in advanced cases.

Ultrasonographic examination is strongly recommended when considering surgical retrieval of the penetrating foreign body, because the normal vigorous reticular contractions are greatly impaired by adhesions. While the wire may be successfully removed, prognosis for a return to full production is guarded. Indeed, return to normal milk production takes up to four weeks, even in those dairy cattle which have been ill for less than 24 hours.

Localised peritonitis – peritoneal reaction may be limited to focal fibrinous/fibrous adhesions and localised accumulation of peritoneal fluid which has become enveloped by the greater omentum. In this situation, the localised peritonitis will not be imaged unless the lesion is in contact with the abdominal wall.

Occasionally, the peritoneal reaction is limited to a few fibrinous adhesions causing constriction that cannot be visualised. In this situation, the intestines proximal to the lesion are grossly distended with fluid (anechoic appearance, rather than containing normal digesta (anechoic appearance containing multiple bright dots), and there are no propulsive intestinal contractions.

Generalised septic peritonitis – cattle with acute septic peritonitis are dull and depressed, with an increased pulse often in excess of 100 beats per minute, due to circulatory compromise, and are anorexic with a painful expression. They are reluctant to move and are slow to rise. Peritonitis involving small intestine results in abdominal distension, due to fluid sequestration within the intestines. Excessive accumulation of inflammatory exudate and fibrin deposition over several days/weeks causes abdominal distension, despite a poor appetite.

Abomasum – the position and diameter of the abomasum are determined by percussion, and interpreted in context with other clinical findings. Abomasal ulcers cannot be detected by ultrasonography, where volume and consistency of faeces and presence of meleana and other clinical signs are more useful findings.

Left-displaced abomasum (LDA) – the distended abomasum occupies the craniodorsal area of the left side of the abdominal cavity (under the rib cage), and auscultation and succusion reveal high-pitched metallic 'pinging' sounds. Rumen movements can be heard caudally in the sublumbar fossa.

Theoretically, paracentesis of the displaced abomasum contents, aided by ultrasonography to reveal the presence of fluid with no protozoa, and a pH around 2.0 (range 1.5–4.5), confirms the clinical diagnosis, but this approach is rarely undertaken in farm practice because the abomasum and rumen cannot readily be distinguished, and the procedure can be time-consuming.

Small intestine – the wall of the small intestine is 2–3 mm thick, with a diameter of 2–4 cm throughout its length. Normal intestinal content is hyperechoic, containing multiple dots which are regularly propelled by peristaltic waves.

Ileus – ileus most commonly results from peritonitis, with resultant fluid distension of some sections of the intestine up to 6–10 cm diameter, with the contents appearing more anechoic than normal, and no peristalsis. In the case of an obstruction, sections of intestine proximal to the lesion are dilated, while those distal to the lesion are empty.

Intussusception – there is initial mild colic, followed by inappetance and constipation. Palpation *per rectum* in adult cattle of an elongated mass in the lower right abdomen is reported. Ultrasound images of single cases of intussusception are reported in the literature, where fluid distension of the intestine cranial to the lesion, and narrowing caudally, may help localisation, but diagnosis is much more commonly based upon clinical examination in practice.

Caecal dilation – the distended caecum can readily be palpated *per rectum* as a blind-ended sac, except for the rare occasion when it becomes retroflexed. Ultrasound examination reveals only the wall of the gas-filled caecum adjacent to the right flank as far forward as the tenth intercostal space.

Liver – ultrasonographic examination of the liver can reveal abscessation (Figure 15.8), tumours, cholestasis, and fatty change in individual cattle. Liver abscesses can readily be identified when close to the capsule surface, but systematic examination may prove time-consuming in many situations in farm practice. It is difficult to quantify the impact of the lesion(s) on liver function, because the liver can compensate by increased size/weight in most situations. It is also easy to generate artefacts from overlying/adjacent intestine, and miss subtle changes in echogenicity.

Ultrasound-guided aspiration of bile from the gall bladder has been recommended for the detection of liver fluke eggs in cattle, but such examinations are not necessary to establish a diagnosis of a clinically significant patent infestation.

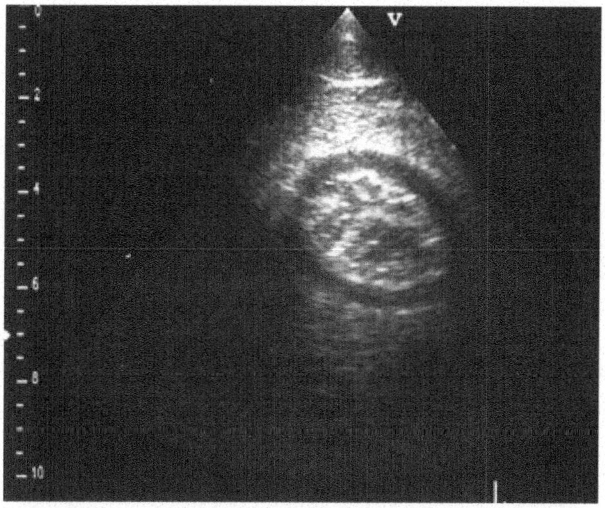

Figure 15.8 Ultrasonography: well encapsulated 4 cm diameter liver abscess.

Liver biopsy

Prophylactic antibiosis and tetanus anti-toxin should be considered. Checking the prothrombin time before proceeding may be a wise precaution. The equipment required is 10 % buffered formalin, a Tru-cut biopsy trocar, local anaesthetic, scalpel blade, syringe, needle, antiseptic and alcohol. The site is best identified ultrasonographically or 15 cm below the transverse processes in the eleventh right intercostal space. The site is also defined by imaginary lines from the wing of the ileum to the point of the elbow and the point of the shoulder. The site is the area of the eleventh intercostal space enclosed by these lines.

The hair is clipped and aseptically prepared. Local anaesthetic is infiltrated subcutaneously and more deeply into the intercostal muscles beneath. A stab incision is made through the skin at this site. The biopsy needle is pushed through the skin incision and aimed towards the opposite elbow. The needle is then pushed into the stroma of the liver. Ultrasonography should be used to guide the placement of the biopsy needle. The passage of the needle through the edge of the diaphragm and the liver gives a slight grating sensation. A biopsy is then taken and the needle withdrawn. The sample can then be placed in 10% formal-saline for histopathology, or the fresh sample used for specific gravity tests and chemical analysis for lipid content. Liver pathology, such as fatty liver syndrome and a fibrotic liver from ragwort poisoning, can be detected.

BSP and propionate liver function tests

BSP function test is now rarely performed, and is contraindicated when there is hypoalbuminaemia or high bilirubin concentration. BSP is injected intravenously as a bolus at a dose rate of 2 mg/kg. A healthy control animal is useful for comparison, although not essential, in view of legislation in many countries worldwide. Blood samples should be taken after 5, 10, 15, 30 and

45 minutes In most normal cattle, the dye has been cleared from the blood after 30 minutes, allowing the half-life of the dye to be calculated. In cattle with liver dysfunction, the dye is still present after 45 minutes (normally less than five minutes).

At 30 minutes, the interpretation of liver dysfunction is based upon the serum concentration as a percentage at the start of the test: 5–10 % mild, 10–25% moderate, and >25% severe. Propionic loading may be used to assess liver function. In a healthy liver, this will cause a rise in blood glucose following increased hepatic gluconeogenesis. Sodium propionate, at a dose rate of 3.0 mmol/kg, is administered intravenously. In healthy animals, there will be a rise in blood glucose of at least 2.0 mmol/l after 30 minutes. Values less than this indicate a reduced liver function.

Atropine test

Bradycardia (40–60 beats/ minute), caused by an increase in the vagal tone (vagotonia) has been recognised in vagal indigestion, cattle deprived of food, and bovine spongiform encephalopathy, and it can be confirmed by an increase in the heart rate following the administration of atropine. Atropine is administered slowly by the intravenous route or subcutaneously. If the intravenous route is to be used, an indwelling catheter should be placed some time before the administration in order to avoid tachycardia induced by stress. The dosage of atropine is administered subcutaneously, 0.06 mg/kg or 30 mg for a 500 kg animal. A dosage of 0.02 mg/kg, or 10 mg for a 500 kg animal, is given by slow intravenous injection. A rise in heart rate of 20 beats/minute is highly suggestive of increased vagal tone. The response following intravenous administration is usually observed within two minutes and persists for up to 30 minutes. Using the subcutaneous route the response is usually seen within ten minutes.

Urinary system

Urolithiasis is more common in yearling bulls, allowing rectal examination, which reveals pulsation in the urethra and marked bladder enlargement, extending well over the pelvic brim, such that ultrasound examination is not necessary to establish the diagnosis. Use of a transrectal linear ultrasound probe reveals a distended bladder with thickened wall in cattle with pyelonephritis, but images of the left kidney are not always so helpful. Similarly, trans-abdominal ultrasound examination via the right sublumar fossa seldom provides convincing evidence of renal pathology. Dilation of renal calyces, echogenic flocculent material within the renal pelvis and renal enlargement, are suggestive of pyelonephritis. Urine samples may be obtained by perineal stimulation with the back of a gloved hand (Figure 15.9), or by catheterisation of the urethra with a 18 g dog catheter. A speculum with a light source is useful, and a finger over the urethral diverticulum to divert the catheter into the urethra is advisable.

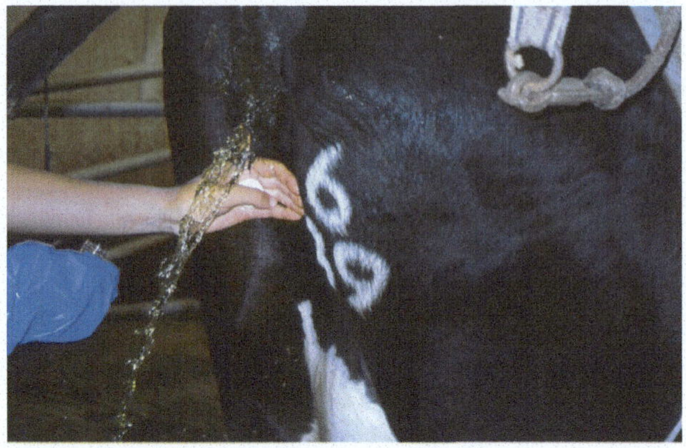

Figure 15.9 Collection of a urine sample: perineal stimulation.

Further tests on milk

Californian Milk Test (CMT)/Rapid Milk Test (RMT)

The CMT measures the quantity of DNA in a milk sample, and gives an indirect measure of the number of somatic cells present. This test is cheap, easy to perform and is often used by herdsmen. A milk sample from each quarter is placed into four wells of a plastic paddle supplied with the test. The volume of the sample is adjusted by pouring off the excess, using a marker in the paddle. An equal volume of detergent is added to each well, and the paddle is gently swirled. The more viscous the mixture becomes, the greater is the somatic cell count. Interpretation is provided in Table 15.5. Cell counts over 200 000 cells/ml indicate the presence of mastitis. There is also a pH indicator present, which turns from purple to yellow with an acidic pH. However, although a decrease in pH is associated with some types of mastitis, lack of colour change does not rule out mastitis and, often, the colour remains purple in the presence of mastitis.

Conductivity

There is an increase in sodium chloride concentration and electrical conductivity 24–36 hours before the rise in somatic cell count. Hand-held conductivity meters are available and can also be fitted in-line in the parlour. Conductivity is usually measured relative to the other quarters in the affected cow, although high absolute values often indicate early mastitis.

Collection of mastitis milk samples for bacteriology

Contamination of the sample is common following poor sampling technique, so consequently the result is often misleading or meaningless. The following protocol is suggested:

- The teat should only be washed if obviously dirty then dried immediately.
- Wash hands and dry thoroughly.
- The end of the teat is cleaned with cotton wool swabs dampened with surgical spirit.

Table 15.5 Interpretation of the Californian Milk Test/Rapid Milk Test.

CMT score	Interpretation	Visible reaction	Total cell count/ml
0	Negative	No reaction	0–200 000 0–25% neutrophils
T	Trace	Slight precipitation	15 000–500 000 30–40% neutrophils
1	Weak positive	Distinct precipitation but no gel formation	400 000–1 500 000 40–60% neutrophils
2	Distinct positive	Mixture thickens with gel formation	800 000–5 000 000 60–70% neutrophils
3	Strong positive	Viscosity greatly increased. Strong gel that is cohesive, with a convex surface	≥ 5 000 000 70–80% neutrophils

- The end of the teat is cleaned until the swab is no longer discoloured.
- A pair of new disposable latex gloves should be worn.
- Two draws of foremilk are discarded.
- Remove the top from a wide-necked universal sample bottle, with the lid held in the crook of the little finger.
- The sample bottle is held away from the udder to avoid contamination from the udder skin.
- The teat is held angled towards the sample bottle and milk withdrawn and directed towards the open mouth of the sample bottle.
- The bottle is filled with milk and the lid replaced.
- The bottle is labelled with the cow number, quarter, and date.

Milk samples for bacteriological culture can be frozen and batched to reduce the cost. Storage for up to three months results in a small reduction in successful cultures. Addition of glycerol increases storage time up to 6–12 months, with little reduction in cultural sensitivity.

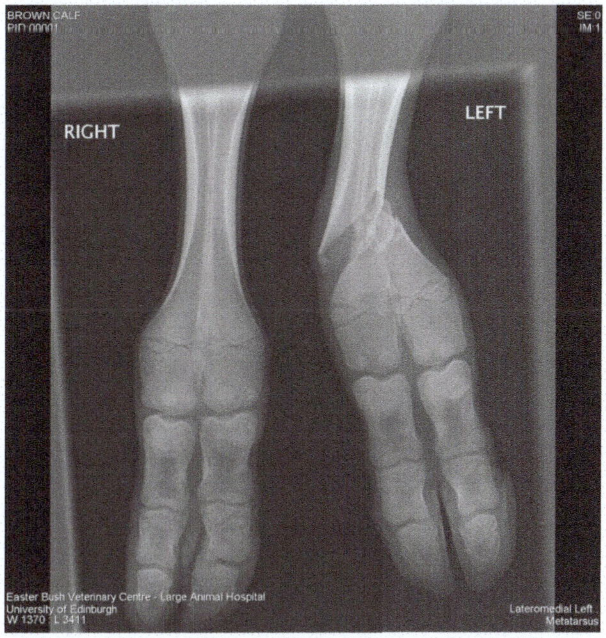

Figure 15.10 Dorso-plantar view of both hindlegs of a calf reveals a mid-shaft fracture of the left third metatarsal bone.

Musculoskeletal system

Most cases of bovine lameness can be diagnosed without recourse to radiography, ultrasonography, scintigraphy, thermography, arthroscopy, muscle biopsies and histopathology and sampling joint fluid, but these ancillary tests are invaluable in particular pathologies.

Radiographs of the lower limbs can be taken using portable sets available in general practice (Figure 15.10) but upper limb investigations may need more powerful machines in veterinary referral centres.

Ultrasonographic scans are useful for evaluation of soft tissue structures, including joints, abscesses/cellulitis, muscle and tendon injuries. Scintigraphy uses radioactive technetium to detect focal areas of inflammation, and it is particularly useful for conditions of the hip joint in large animals, where radiography can be difficult. Availability is restricted to veterinary referral centres. Thermography uses a heat-seeking camera to detect infra-red rays. It can detect small temperature differences, identifying the presence of inflammation, but availability is restricted to referral centres (Figure 15.11a and b).

Muscle biopsies and histopathology are occasionally used to identify white muscle disease and neurogenic disuse, such as femoral nerve paralysis. Arthroscopy can be used to identify cruciate rupture, degenerative joint disease and osteochondritis dissecans; however, general anaesthesia is required, with availability restricted to referral centres. Nerve blocks are seldom used in practice, because most lesions are within the foot. Intra-articular anaesthesia and intravenous regional anaesthesia (IVRA) are sometimes useful to identify the source of lameness.

Arthrocentesis (joint tap)

The technique is as follows:

The hair on the site over the selected joint is clipped and aseptically prepared to avoid introducing infection. A sterile 11/2" 19

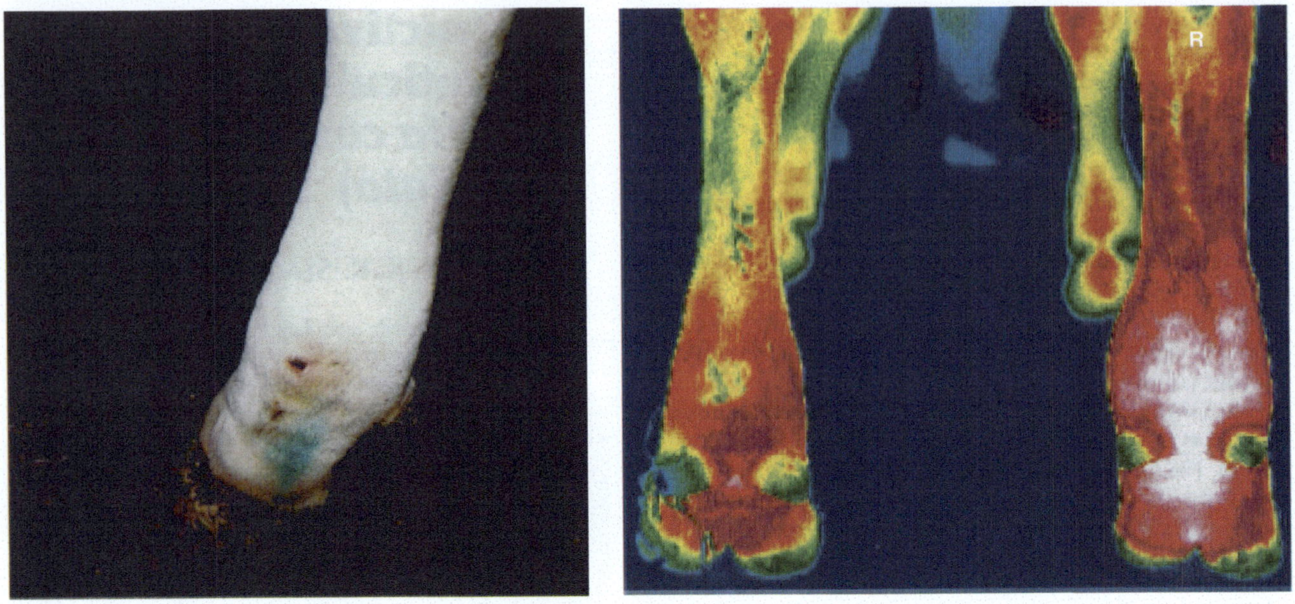

(a) (b)

Figure 15.11 a. Joint penetration wound. b. Thermography: inflammation (white = hot) on the right hind leg.

Table 15.6 Distinguishing characteristics of synovial fluid from a normal joint, a joint with septic arthritis and a joint with degenerative osteoarthritis.

Synovial fluid	Appearance	Clot	WBCX10^9/l	% neutrophils	Protein (g/L)
Normal joint	Clear	–	<0.25	<10	<18
Septic arthritis	Turbid	+	10.00	95	>40
Degenerative	Clear	–	<0.25	<15	<20
Osteoarthritis	+/– turbid				

gauge hypodermic needle is introduced into a distended pouch of the joint capsule, avoiding ligamentous structures, and a sample of synovial fluid is obtained by aspiration using a syringe. The sample is then placed into an EDTA (for cytology and protein content) and a plain tube (for bacteriological culture).

Table 15.6 indicates distinguishing characteristics of synovial fluid from a normal joint, a joint with septic arthritis, and a joint with degenerative osteoarthritis. Ultrasonographic demonstration of joint distension is useful where the joint effusion cannot be palpated.

CNS

Cerebrospinal fluid (CSF) collection and analysis provides rapid, in some situations instant, information to the veterinary clinician investigating a disease problem in the living animal. Cerebrospinal fluid analysis is particularly useful with respect to confirming the presence of an inflammatory lesion involving the leptomeninges, such as bacterial meningo-encephalitis, and investigating potential compressive lesions of the spinal cord. When correctly performed under local anaesthesia, lumbar CSF collection in ruminants is a safe procedure, and there are no harmful sequelae. There are no primary indications for cisternal CSF collection in cattle practice other than at post-mortem, when restraint is no longer a problem.

For CSF collection and examination, it is necessary to puncture the subarachnoid space in the cerebellomedullary cistern (cisternal sample) or at the lumbosacral site (lumbar sample). While theoretically it may be desirable to collect CSF from the site nearer the suspected lesion, this is not possible in

Table 15.7 Guide to needle length and gauge for lumbar CSF sampling.

Calves <100 kg	1 inch19 gauge
Calves 100–250 kg	2 inch 19 gauge
Cattle >250kg	4 inch 18 gauge + internal stylet

Table 15.8 Cerebrospinal fluid from normal cattle and cattle with bacterial encephalitis.

Parameter	Normal CSF	Bacterial encephalitis
Specific gravity	1.004–1.008	Increased
Colour	Colourless (non-clotting)	Turbid (yellow/red)
Protein (g/L)	0.2–0.4	Increased >2
Albumin (g/L)	0.1–0.2	Increased
Globulin (g/L)	0.02–0.08	Increased
Leukocyte count cells × 10^6/L	0–3	>30
Leukocyte differential.	95% lymphocytes	Mainly neutrophils
Magnesium mmol/L	0.86	0.86

field situations. In the absence of a focal compressive spinal cord lesion, there are no substantial differences between the composition of cisternal and lumbar CSF samples.

Collection of lumbar CSF is facilitated if the animal can be positioned in sternal recumbency with the hips flexed and the pelvic limbs extended alongside the abdomen (typically calves and recumbent adults).

The site for lumbar CSF collection is the midpoint of the lumbosacral space, which can be identified as the midline depression between the last palpable dorsal lumbar spine (L6) and the first palpable sacral dorsal spine (S2). The site must be clipped, surgically prepared, and between 1–2 ml of local anaesthetic injected subcutaneously. Sterile surgical gloves should be worn for the collection procedure. In cattle, less than 250 kg hypodermic needles should be used because they are sharp and can be discarded after a single use, and CSF wells up as soon as the needle point enters the dorsal subarachnoid space; internal stylets are unnecessary. In adult cattle, the 4" spinal needle can be guided through a 2" 14 gauge disposable needle for the proximal part of its length.

The needle (Table 15.7) is slowly advanced (over 10 seconds) at a right angle to the plane of the vertebral column, or with the hub directed 5–10° caudally. It is essential to appreciate the changes in tissue resistance as the needle point passes sequentially through the subcutaneous tissue and interarcuate ligament, then the sudden 'pop' due to the loss of resistance as the needle point exits the ligamentum flavum into the extradural space. Once the needle point has penetrated the dorsal subarachnoid space, CSF will well up in the needle hub within 2–3 seconds. Failure to appreciate the change in resistance to needle travel may result in needle puncture of the conus medullaris. This causes unnecessary pain to the animal, which must be avoided at all times.

Between 1–2 ml of CSF is sufficient for laboratory analysis and, while the sample can be collected by free flow over 1–2 minutes, it is more convenient to employ very gentle syringe aspiration over 10–20 seconds. Table 15.8 indicates the differences between cerebrospinal fluid from normal cattle and cattle with bacterial encephalitis.

The normal range for CSF protein concentration quoted for cattle is <0.3 g/L. Normal CSF contains less than 10 cells/μL, which are predominantly lymphocytes with an occasional neutrophil. As a general rule, a predominantly polymorphonuclear intrathecal inflammatory response is found in acute CNS bacterial infections, whereas a mononuclear response is seen in viral CNS infections.

Gross pathology and histopathology are useful in the provisional diagnosis in neurological cases. Vitreous humour or CSF samples can be used to check for magnesium concentration in cases of sudden death; magnesium concentrations of <0.55 mmol/L in vitreous humour within 48 hours of death is diagnostic for hypomagnesaemia.

Radiography, electromyography and electroencephalography are used in some veterinary referral centres.

Further reading

Jackson, P. and Cockcroft, P. (2002). *Clinical Examination of Farm Animals*. Wiley-Blackwell.

Radostits, O. Mayhew, I. and Houston, D. (2000). *Veterinary Clinical Examination and Diagnosis*. Saunders.

CHAPTER 16

Bovine Haematology and Biochemistry

Allan Kessell

Learning objectives

- To appreciate the range of tests routinely available in a bovine complete blood count and biochemistry panel, as well as those suggested in more limited/specific panels.
- To understand how patterns and degree of change in analyte values away from the reference interval can be used to help formulate a differential diagnosis/diagnosis, and suggest other test modalities.
- To understand the responsibilities of the veterinarian when collecting and submitting samples to the laboratory, with relation to quality of result.
- To understand the responsibilities of the laboratory in test analysis and reporting, with respect to quality of result.

Introduction

When combined with history and clinical examination, haematology and biochemistry can offer a relatively non invasive, economical method of assessing the health status of a number of organ systems in the bovine. There are several excellent reviews on bovine biochemistry and haematology available (Suttle, 2004; Jones & Allison, 2007; Russell & Roussel, 2007; Malmo *et al.*, 2010; Otter, 2013). Stockham & Scott (2008) is a useful text on the basics of veterinary clinical pathology.

Sample collection, transport

It is the responsibility of the attending veterinarian to ensure that samples for clinical pathological testing are collected, identified, stored and transported correctly, so that they arrive at the laboratory in a condition that eliminates, or at least limits, changes in analyte values that can occur after sampling. It is important that laboratory results reflect values that are as close as possible to those within the animal at the time of sampling, as post-sampling changes can lead to erroneous analyte values and interpretation.

Blood for haematology and biochemistry can be collected from the coccygeal (in adult) or jugular veins.

A haematological assessment of blood is really a fluid assessment that involves the same broad steps involved in the assessment of all conventional body fluids that have recorded normal values (urine, blood, thoracic/abdominal fluid, joint, cerebrospinal fluid). These are gross appearance; objective assessment of cell numbers (in blood RBCs, WBCs, and platelets); cytology (to assess type of cell and their morphology); and, finally, a measure of protein concentration.

The blood and fluids must arrive at the laboratory suitably preserved, so that the cells can be accurately counted and assessed and an accurate *in vivo* protein concentration obtained. A traumatic collection into an anticoagulant (purple top tube – EDTA), and thorough mixing at the point of collection, are required to inhibit clotting and iatrogenic hemolysis immediately after sampling. A correctly made unstained blood smear at the time of collection is especially important with bovine blood, as it greatly enhances the accuracy of the WBC differential and morphological assessment. This method is described in Chapter 6: The Practice Laboratory. Degenerative changes in cells may be minimised by keeping the sample cooled in transport at 4°C. Acute phase protein (APP) fibrinogen is removed by clotting, and a plasma sample is required (EDTA, Li heparin). Coagulation tests require a citrate tube (blue top).

The analytical methods used to determine most biochemical parameters and serological tests are performed on serum (red top tube), although an accurate glucose requires a grey top (fluoride oxalate) tube. Most trace element analysis is performed on

Bovine Medicine, Third Edition. Edited by Peter D. Cockcroft.

a purple top tube (Li hep), except Zn (glass and plastic stoppers may contaminate the sample with Zn). Special biochemical tests (e.g. lead) may require different samples, and the receiving laboratory should be contacted to ensure that the appropriate samples are collected for the assay available at that laboratory. Serum is best harvested after the blood sample has clotted and contracted. This requires approximately 30 minutes. The serum can either be carefully poured from the tube, leaving the clot behind, or centrifuged and decanted. The harvested serum sample should kept cooled (4°C) until analysis. This will preserve most of the analytes for about 24–48 hours. If there are going to be lengthy delays in processing, freezing at −20°C is suggested.

It is essential that all samples are correctly identified, and that they come to the laboratory with a fully completed sample submission form.

Sample packaging must conform with state and country laws and, for blood and biochemical analysis, this usually requires adequate packaging so as to prevent leakage, often involving 2–3 layers. Regulations and instructions regarding the 'International Carriage of Dangerous Goods by Road', published by the United Nations Economic Commission (UNECE) for Europe, can be found at the following website: http://www.unece.org/trans/danger/publi/adr/adr2005/05contentse.html, but are summarised here as they pertain to likely clinical specimens. Samples can be categorised as:

Category A: an infectious substance which is carried in a form such that, when exposure to it occurs, it is capable of causing permanent disability, life-threatening or fatal disease to humans or animals; or

Category B: an infectious substance which does not meet the criteria for inclusion in Category A. These generally include diagnostic or clinical specimens that concern us here, and are assigned to UN 3373. Packaging required for this class is covered under ADR Packing Instruction P650, and can be summarised as:

1 The primary receptacle holding the sample must be leak-proof for liquids and sift-proof for solids.
2 The primary receptacle is placed within a secondary receptacle which is big enough to allow enough absorbent material to be placed around the primary receptacle/s to absorb a full volume spill or leak. If there are multiple primary receptacles, they must be separated from each other by packing within the secondary receptacle.
3 The paperwork should be placed between the secondary receptacle and the outer packaging, ideally within a waterproof bag.
4 Outer packaging with suitable cushioning material is required to secure the secondary receptacle, and should clearly display the UN3373 marking.
5 Packaging should be clearly labelled with the delivery address and sender's details, in addition to telephone contact details.

Laboratory procedures

Once the sample arrives at the laboratory, it is then the responsibility of the laboratory to process the sample and report accurate results in a speedy and efficient manner. Laboratories use internal quality controls to continually assess the accuracy of results, and most laboratories participate in external proficiency testing schemes. As well larger laboratories are accredited and assessed by various official organisations (e.g. NATA in Australia, UKAS in the UK).

Most analytes will be reported with reference intervals. These have usually been established by the laboratory, using their own machines and analytical methods, on samples from a large number of healthy animals (usually 60–120), and the top and bottom 2.5% of results discarded. This is important, as different methods, different machines and methodology, as well animal characteristics (breeds, age) may result in variation of the reference interval (Knowles *et al.*, 2000). Reference ranges may even change with time (George *et al.*, 2010).

Haematology

Laboratory reference values, with additional comments, are presented in Table 16.1. Haematology is the study of blood and blood forming organs. This section will consider changes within the peripheral blood parameter values that provide useful information on the state of health of the animal. Haematology allows the clinician to assess for the presence of inflammation and anaemia and, in combination with biochemistry, may provide a diagnosis or differential diagnosis and/or suggest other test modalities.

Laboratories have machines that use laser and/or impedance technology to count red blood cells (RBCs), white blood cells (WBCs) and platelets, but WBC differential, RBC/WBC morphology, and the platelet counts are assessed manually by a trained haematologist. This allows the calculation of the absolute number and morphology of different types of cells, which can inform the degree and severity of inflammation, and the classification or cause of the anaemia, as well as check for platelet clumping. The latter will invalidate a machine or a manual platelet count.

Red blood cells

Red blood cells are produced in the bone marrow under the influence of various cytokines and growth factors, the most important of which is erythropoietin (EPO), which is produced by the kidneys. In health, the bovine peripheral RBC has an average life span of 150 days, and accumulated aging changes result in the removal of nearly 1% of aged RBC by splenic macrophages/day (extravascular hemolysis). Thus, extravascular hemolysis and medullary erythropoiesis result

Table 16.1 Bovine haematological and biochemistry reference intervals.

Parameter	Reference Interval	Comments
RBC Count	5–10 × 10^{12}/L	Laser/impedance countered
Haemoglobin	80–150 g/L	Measured
PCV	0.24 – 0.46 L/L	Packed cell volume – measured
Haematocrit	0.24 – 0.46 L/L	= calculated PCV = MCV (fl) × RBC(× 10^{12}/L) /1000; prone to error
MCV	40–60fL	– indices used to classify anaemia as microcytic (↓MCV), hypochromic (↓MCHC): usually Fe deficiency → chronic blood loss (usually)
MCHC	300 – 360 g/L	
MCH	11–17 pg	Mean corpuscular haemoglobin
Reticulocytes	0	Requires polychrome methylene blue stain and manual count to enumerate
WBC count	4–12 ×10^9/L	Laser/impedance countered
Neutrophils	0.6–4.0 ×10^9/L	Absolute number = WBC count × manual % of each WBC – ↑ no. immature (band) neutrophils = inflammatory demand, but fibrinogen a more reliable indicator of inflammation
Band neutrophils	< 0.2 ×10^9/L	
Lymphocytes	2.5–7.5 ×10^9/L	
Monocytes	< 0.9 ×10^9/L	
Eosinophils	< 0.8 ×10^9/L	
Platelets	150–650 × 10^9/L	Significant clumping will invalidate machine and manual counts
Plasma protein	60–80 g/L	Estimated–refractometry
Fibrinogen	3–7 g/L	Acute phase protein – measured, often via the Miller method (see chapter 6)
Serum protein	58–80 g/L	= albumin + globulins (α, β, γ)
Albumin	22–36 g/L	↑= dehydration;↓= loss (GIT, urine, third space) or lack of production (end stage liver disease, severe malnutrition)
Globulin	24–40 g/L	Calculated = TP – albumin; ↑ = antigenic stimulation, dehydration
Sodium	132–152 mmol/L	Anion gap = (Na^{2+} K^+) – (Cl^-+ HCO_3^-) = an approximation of the unmeasured anions – these are usually anions produced in metabolic acidotic states[1] e.g. Ruminal acidosis, lactic acidosis, shock, renal failure
Potassium	3.9–5.8 mmol/L	
Chloride	95–110 mmol/L	
Bicarbonate	20–30 mmol/L	
Anion gap	14–26 mmol/L	
Calcium	2.0–3.0 mmol/L	Clinical hypocalcaemia Ca usually < 1.5; extreme levels Ca < 0.25
Phosphate	1.29–2.26 mmol/l	phosphate levels usually <1 with milk fever; Reflects current dietary intake
Magnesium	0.6–1.1 mmol/L	Hypomag: CUM[2] <12; Tetany –serum Mg < 0.4
BOHB	<1.0 mmol/L	Levels will vary depending of degree of fat mobilization
NEFA	See Table 16.3	Good indicator of level of fat mobilization
Urea	2.1–9.6 mmol/L	50% excreted into GIT/saliva; blood urea N = urea × 2.14
Creatinine	90–120 umol/L	Not resorbed from renal tubules; good estimate of GFR
CK	50–400 U/L	Muscle specific enzyme; level can be used prognostically (see Table 16.4)
AST	60–150 U/L	Muscle and liver; longer half-life than CK
GLDH	< 20 U/L	Hepatocellular specific; increase indicates hepatocellular necrosis
GGT	< 36 U/L	High levels in colostrum – can be used as a measure of passive transfer (Table 16.4)
Bilirubin	2–18 μmol/L	Tissues noticeably yellow(jaundice) when bilirubin > 45 μmol/L

[1] Ewaschuk *et al.* (2003), Malmo *et al.* (2010).
[2] CUM = corrected urinary magnesium = urinary Mg/urinary creatinine (Sutherland *et al.*, 1986).

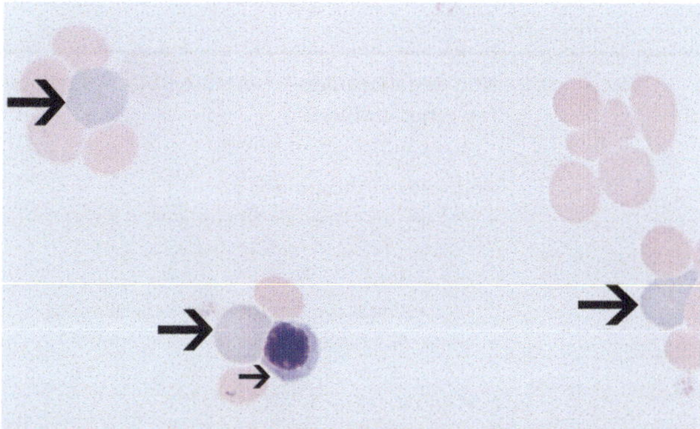

Figure 16.1 High power view of peripheral blood smear from a bovine with a regenerative anaemia. This is suggested here by the presence of polychromatophils (large arrows) and nRBCs (small arrow).

in adequate numbers of healthy RBCs in the blood, capable of meeting the oxygen demands of the animal. In the face of increasing oxygen demand or loss of functioning RBCs (e.g. animals at altitude or undergoing RBC loss), healthy bone marrow will increase the rate of erythropoiesis.

Anaemia

Anaemia is diagnosed when there is a decreased RBC count, packed cell volume (PCV) or haemoglobin concentration in the peripheral blood. If the anaemia is caused by blood loss or haemolysis, the anaemia is said to be 'regenerative', as the bone marrow is able to respond to the anaemia by increased production of RBCs. This takes 2–4 days to be measurable in the peripheral blood and, in most mammals, detection of signs of regeneration relies on the presence of increased numbers immature RBCs within the peripheral blood. Healthy bovines do not normally have detectable immature RBCs (polychromatophils and reticulocytes) within the peripheral blood. In the event of blood loss or haemolysis, they respond by increasing the output of immature RBC. These include larger and nucleated RBCs, reticulocytes with polychromasia and anisocytosis, and basophilic stippling. Some of these changes are illustrated in Figure 16.1 and Figure 16.4. If these responses are not observed within four days of the onset of the event which caused the anaemia, then the anaemia is 'non regenerative', as the bone marrow has not responded adequately.

The assessment of anaemia as regenerative or non-regenerative is important, as it aids in the diagnosis of the cause. Both are common, and the morphologic assessment of RBCs can be helpful in further defining the cause. The commonest cause of a non-regenerative anaemia is 'anaemia of inflammatory disease', largely mediated by the secretion of hepcidin from hepatocytes, which causes both the inhibition of iron absorption from the GIT and export of iron from macrophages and hepatocytes (Fry, 2010). Common causes of bovine regenerative and non regenerative anaemia are presented in Table 16.2.

Polycythaemia

Polycythaemia refers to a true increase in the circulating RBC mass, and is diagnosed by an increased RBC count, PCV and haemoglobin concentration in the absence of dehydration. Spurious (or relative) polycythaemia, better referred to as haemoconcentration, is common in ruminants and is usually caused by dehydration. Dehydration can increase the value of other analytes, including total protein. If dehydration is not present, the animal may have true polycythaemia or secondary polycythemia. Primary polycythaemias are caused by rare, primary, inherited defects, resulting in bone marrow hyperplasia and neoplasia (polycythaemia vera). Secondary polycythaemia is due to conditions that result in increased EPO secretion by the kidneys. This may occur in response to hypoxia, which may be caused by lowered oxygen at altitude, cardiac diseases (e.g. ventricular septal defect and congestive heart failure), severe pulmonary conditions (sever chronic pneumonia) or inappropriate renal EPO secretion (some renal neoplasia, occasionally polycyctic/hydronephrotic kidneys).

White blood cells

Adult healthy bovines have a ratio of one neutrophil to two lymphocytes in their blood count although, in animals less than six months old, neutrophils are predominant, and they may have higher total WBC counts than adults. All WBCs arise from a common precursor in the bone marrow, although maturation and proliferation of lymphocytes takes place in a number of lymphoid organs outside the bone marrow and they can circulate between tissues and blood via the lymphatic system. Assessment of the absolute numbers of different types of WBCs, as opposed to just the WBC count, is useful in bovines to differentiate the responses due to inflammation, stress, excitement and neoplasia. However, the degree of change is often less than that seen in other species.

Neutrophils and inflammation

Whilst neutrophilia with a left shift is the prototypical response to an acute inflammatory insult in most domestic animals, bovine bone marrow contains only a small pool of mature neutrophils available for export to the blood (and tissues) when placed under a sudden inflammatory demand. Thus, acute inflammatory responses in bovines are often characterised by a neutropenia, as demand initially exceeds supply. Neutropenia is also seen in endotoxaemia, due to increased movement of neutrophils from the circulating (sampled) pool to the marginating pool. Within 24–48 hours, immature band-form neutrophils may appear. These can be seen in Figure 16.2.

Band-form neutrophils are an important indicator of an inflammatory response when neutrophils are below or within normal range. It is not uncommon, at this stage of the inflammatory response, to see morphological changes within neutrophils that are referred to as 'toxic changes'. These

Table 16.2 Common causes of regenerative and non-regenerative anaemia in bovines.

Regenerative – immature RBCs may be present	**Non Regenerative – immature RBCs not present**
Blood loss • *Internal* ruptured uterine artery, vessel erosion (abscess) • *External* castration, dehorning, abomasal ulcer, haemorrhagic enteritis, trauma, blood sucking parasites (ticks, lice) • *Acute* – may see ↓total protein • *Chronic* – primarily GIT loss with developing Fe[1] deficiency and microcytic (↓MCV) and hypochromic (↓MCHC) anaemia **Coagulopathy** ↓primary haemostasis =↓platelet number or function • *Marked thrombocytopaenia* = platelets < 20 × 10^9/L, e.g. BVDV type 2, bone marrow failure secondary to pterquiloside poisoning (bracken ferns) • *Reduced platelet function* (can be congenital in cattle) ↓ secondary haemostasis(↑PT/PTT), e.g. dicourmarol in mouldy sweet clover, factor XI deficiency (Holsteins), DIC **Haemolysis** –extravascular/ intravascular[2] • RBC parasites[3] • Heinz body : plants (*Allium* sp., *Brassica* sp, onion[6]) toxins: Cu, chronic lead • ↓phosphate (IV haemolysis, Heinz body) • Bacteria : Bacillary haemoglobinuria (*Cl. novyi* type D – IV hemolysis); *Leptospira pomona* (calves) • Other – has been added to list following ◦ Water intoxication ◦ Bovine congenital erythropoietic porphyria ◦ Copper poisoning (calves) ◦ Postparurient haemoglobinuria ↓phosphate ◦ Selenium deficiency	**Pre-regenerative** • Acute blood loss or hemolysis < three days duration **Reduced erythropoiesis** • *Primary bone marrow disease* (less common) ◦ toxic : bracken fern, mycotoxins, lead ◦ neoplasia ◦ congenital dyserythropioesis (Poll Hereford)[7] • *Secondary bone marrow disease* (common) ◦ chronic inflammatory disease (common) ◦ end stage renal failure (↓ EPO) ◦ malnutrition – ↓Fe[1], Cu[4], Co[5]
Regenerative – immature RBCs may be present	Non-regenerative – immature RBCs not present

[1] Fe deficiency – anaemia will be regenerative at first, but when Fe becomes limiting to haemoglobin production within the bone marrow, the anaemia will become non-regenerative. Microcytosis/hypochromasia develops as the RBC precursors within the bone marrow continue to divide in an attempt to reach the 'correct' haemoglobin concentration.
[2] Intra-vascular hemolysis – will also see haemoglobinaemia/uria (red plasma/red urine) EV hemolysis – usually more pronounced jaundice.
[3] Anaplasma central/marginale, *Babesia bovis* and *bigemmina*, *Theileria* sp. (esp. *T. orientalis* subsp. *ikeda*).
[4] Cu is involved in the incorporation of Fe into heme, and so may present similar to Fe deficiency anaemia.
[5] Co (Vitamin B12): required for DNA synthesis
[6] Lincoln *et al.* (1992).
[7] Steffen *et al.* (1992).
PT (Prothrobin time), PTT (Partial Thromboplastin Time), DIC (Disseminated intra-vascular coagulation), EPO (erythropoietin).

result from an accelerated release of immature neutrophils, characterised by cytoplasmic vacuolation, granularity and variable nuclear fragmentation. These changes can be observed in Figure 16.2. With time, left-shift neutrophilia or mature neutrophilia may develop if the inflammatory stimulus persists, sometimes with a monocytosis.

The degree of elevation in the absolute neutrophil count is smaller than is seen with other common domestic species. For instance, descriptors of mild, moderate or marked neutrophilia may be assigned to neutrophil counts of <8 × 10^9/L, 8–15 × 10^9/L, and >15 × 10^9/L respectively in cattle, as opposed to <15 × 10^9/L, 15–25 × 10^9/L, and >25 × 10^9/L in the horse, or <20 × 10^9/L, <30 × 10^9/L and <50 × 10^9/L in dogs. Inflammation may not always be reflected in elevated WBC numbers, left shift or toxic change, especially if the focus of inflammation is encapsulated, or blood sampling is done later in the disease process. Other measures or indicators of inflammation, such as fibrinogen and other APPs and globulins, may be helpful in these conditions.

Stress

Stress may also cause mature neutrophilia, but a left shift and toxic changes are not seen. There is also a lymphopenia and eosinopenia (although this latter cell is present in low numbers in normal leucograms). The degree of increase in absolute neutrophil numbers is, again, less than in other species with stress, so that the total WBC count may be within normal reference limits.

A physiological response to epinephrine can cause an 'excitement' leucogram pattern, in which there is a mild neutrophilia

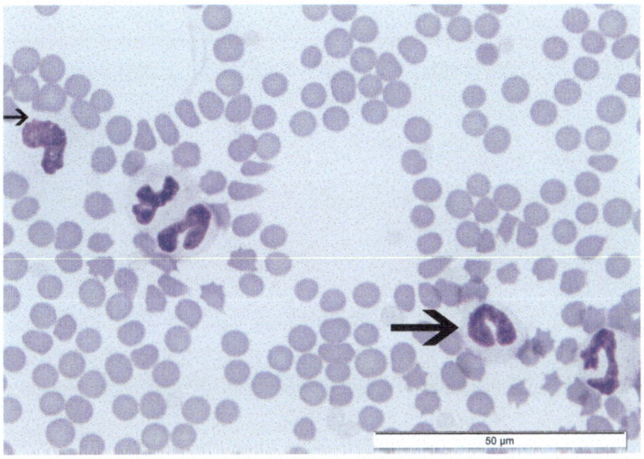

Figure 16.2 High-power view of a peripheral blood smear from a cow, showing a toxic left shift within the neutrophil line. Note the band-form neutrophil (large arrow) with increased staining and granularity of the cytoplasm, and some nuclear fragmentation (small arrow).

and mild to moderate lymphocytosis. This is seen in young animals although, again, the response is less than in other species.

Monocytes

Monocytosis may develop in the face of a chronic inflammation, but may also be seen with necrosis and increased hemolysis. However, its presence is inconsistent.

Lymphocytes

The size of lymphocytes within the peripheral blood is normally variable in the bovine, and small to medium lymphocytes are common. Figure 16.3 is a peripheral blood smear, showing the variability in size and morphology of bovine lymphocytes. In disease states that result in antigenic stimulation, large activated lymphoid cells with intra-nuclear nucleoli can be present, resembling neoplastic lymphoid cells. Persistent lymphocytosis is often seen with bovine leucosis virus infection, although only a small number of these animals go on to develop lymphoma with leukemoid expression (Ferrer *et al.*, 1979). In these cases, neoplastic lymphocytes may be seen in the peripheral blood.

Eosinophils

Accepted wisdom is that eosinophils increase in the peripheral blood and affected tissue in allergic or parasitic conditions. However, although eosinophilia can be seen, it is inconsistent and may be seen with other inflammatory conditions, and it may be absent in allergic and parasitic infections.

Dehydration

The total plasma protein concentration is easily estimated with refractometry and, along with the PCV, is a useful baseline parameter to assess for detection of dehydration and anaemia.

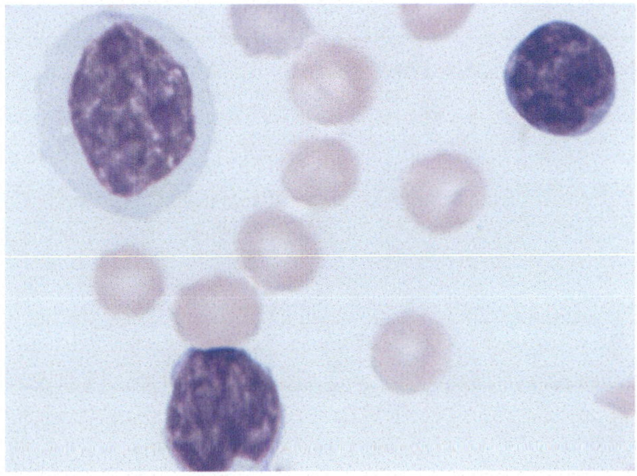

Figure 16.3 High power view of a peripheral blood smear showing the variability in size and morphology of bovine lymphocytes.

Fibrinogen and acute phase proteins

Fibrinogen, along with haptoglobin and serum amyloid A (SAA), is an APP made by the liver under the influence of cytokines released from macrophages during inflammation, and can be used as a non specific indicator of inflammation. Fibrinogen is relatively easy to calculate in the clinic laboratory (refer to Chapter 6), and is often a more reliable indicator of inflammation than total or differential WBC counts; thus, its calculation is mandatory. However, it takes 36–48 hours to increase in the circulation following an inflammatory event, so, in acute inflammatory situations, fibrinogen may be within normal range, and other APPs (haptoglobin and SAA) may be more sensitive indicators of inflammation (Horadagoda *et al.*, 1999; Chan *et al.*, 2004; Petersen *et al.*, 2004). However, they are not generally available at the moment in diagnostic laboratories.

Biochemistry

Normal references ranges for a comprehensive list of biochemical analytes are provided in Table 16.1. Limited biochemical profiles include analytes that offer diagnostic information in common bovine disorders. Examples of bovine biochemical panel profiles are in Table 16.3. These certainly have their place but it is also useful, at times, to more broadly assess health status with a more complete set of results, especially when presented with a disease of unknown aetiology. Analytes measured in isolation do not allow a more holistic appraisal of what is occurring in these situations where, often, patterns of change are important, and where normal results may prove as useful as abnormal results in ruling in and ruling out important pathophysiologies.

It is useful here to briefly discuss each of the analytes listed in a complete profile, and attempt to give some quantitation to what may be considered mild, moderate or marked changes away

Table 16.3 Bovine biochemical profiles.

Panel	Analytes included	Analyte	Mild[1]	Moderate[1]	Marked[1]	Extreme[1]
Downer Cow	Ca, Mg, PO_4, CK, (BOHB, urea)	Ca (mmol/L)	< 2	< 1.5	< 1	<0.5
		CK	< 5 ×	< 10 ×	> 50 ×	> 100 ×
Muscle	CK, AST	AST	< 2 ×	< 3 ×	> 5 ×	> 8 ×
Liver	GLDH (or SDH), GGT; (bilirubin, total protein, albumin, bile acids)	GLDH	< 2 ×	< 4 ×	> 8 ×	> 20 ×
		GGT	< 2 ×	< 4 ×	> 6 ×	> 20 ×
		Bilirubin	< 2 ×	< 3 ×	> 5 ×	> 8 ×
Renal	Creatinine, urea USG	Creatinine	< 2 ×	< 3 ×	> 5 ×	> 8 ×
		USG >1.025 when dehydrated → indicates adequate renal function (azotaemia prerenal)				
Metabolic	Ca, Mg, P, BOHB +/– urea, NEFA, glucose	**BOHB**: mmol/L[2] Dry-off < 0.6 post-calving – subclinical ketosis > 1.4 – ketosis > 3.0			**NEFA** : mmol/L[2] Pre-calving < 1.4 Peak lactation< 0.7	
Electrolytes	Na, Cl, K, HCO^{3-}	↓Cl – often seen with stasis of forestomachs, e.g. – mild : LDA[3] – moderate to marked : RDA[4](< 70 mmol/L): often results in metabolic alkalosis with paradoxical aciduria – ↓K – anorexia, metabolic acidosis (calf diarrhoea)				
Trace element (Suttle, 2004)	Cu, Se, Co (vitamin B12), Zn	Cu : serum screening (liver biopsy preferred) Se : GSH-Px – EDTA/heparin blood Co: serum cobalamine, chilled and light protected Zn: special blood tubes required (ring lab)				

Ca – Calcium; PO_4 – Phosphate; Mg – Magnesium; BOHB – β hydroxybutyrate; AST – Aspartate aminotransferase; GGT – γ glutamyltransferase; GLDH –Glutamate dehydrogenase; SD – Sorbital dehydrogenase; Cu – Copper; Co – Cobalt; Se –Selenium; Zn – Zinc; GSH-Px – Glutathione peroxidise.

[1] degree of elevation: numbers represent multiple of the upper reference limit, except Ca, which is in mmol/L

[2] Oetzel (2004)

[3] RDA – Right displaced abomasum

[4] LDA – Left displaced abomasum

from the reference interval. These often relate to the severity, type and, sometimes, distribution of histopathological change, and thus are diagnostically important.

Total plasma protein

Total plasma protein is composed of albumin and globulins, the value of the latter being derived from the difference between total protein and albumin (both of which are measured). Changes in all of the fractions are useful diagnostically. There are a large number of globulin fractions, most of which are not individually measured in a normal profile (with the exception of fibrinogen). These may be separated by electrophoresis and other methodologies, and are broadly grouped into α globulins (e.g. transport molecules for thyroxine/cortisol/lipids/copper/haemoglobin; antithrombin III; plus $\alpha_2$macroglobulin), β globulins (e.g. transport molecules for Fe – transferrin, ferritin; plus C reactive protein, C3/C4, plasminogen, fibrinogen, clotting factors) and γ globulins (primarily IgG).

Relative increases in all fractions occur with dehydration, and dehydration is the only cause of an elevated albumin. Some proteins increase in inflammation – in particular, the APPs fibrinogen (can reach 10–15 g/l) and the immunoglobulins (some β and the γ globulins). Fibrinogen and the immunoglobulins can increase enough to significantly elevate the total protein measured. To correct an increased fibrinogen for possible dehydration, the total protein-to-fibrinogen ratio can be calculated. A ratio of < 10 : 1 indicates an absolute increase in fibrinogen and suggests inflammation as the cause of the increased fibrinogen. However, globulins also often increase with inflammation, increasing the total protein and, possibly, decreasing the usefulness of this ratio.

Decreases in total protein concentration may be seen in conditions in which either albumin and/or globulins are lost, or fail to be produced. Near end-stage liver disease is required to result in decreased albumin, cholesterol and clotting factors (these are all synthesised by the liver), because of the large functional reserve of the liver. These changes are seen in those conditions that result in diffuse severe hepatic loss, such as pyrrolizadine alkaloid poisoning. Albumin may be lost in protein-losing enteropathies (e.g. Johne's disease, parasitic gastroenteritis), protein-losing nephropathies (e.g. amyloidosis), or into third spaces (e.g. pleuritis, peritonitis). In some of these conditions, it is primarily albumin that is lost (e.g. amyloidosis); in entropathies and effusions, it can be both albumin and globulins which are lost. If inflammation is the cause of the loss, the total protein can actually increase because of the inflammatory stimulus to globulin production. Dehydration may mask these changes.

Serum enzymes

Serum enzymes are proteins that catalyse chemical reactions within the cell, and increased levels within the serum of those routinely measured are largely due to release from damaged cells (CK, AST, GLDH, SD). Some membrane enzymes are inducible (ALP, GGT), and some may increase where there is cellular hyperplasia (GGT – bile ducts). Some of these enzymes are considered tissue-specific when elevated within serum, for example CK (heart and skeletal muscle) and GLDH/SDH (hepatocellular necrosis). The enzyme GGT is associated with the brush border of hepatocytes, biliary epithelial cells, renal tubular cells and mammary epithelial cells (Latimer, 2011; Kaneko *et al.*, 2008). Raised levels in the serum are largely due to cholestasis, as renal tubular damage/induction will result in raised levels of GGT in urine, and raised levels within mammary epithelial cells are reflected by raised levels in colostrums and, therefore, in post-suckled calf serum. In fact, the level of serum GGT can be used to assess the adequacy of passive transfer of immunoglobilins to the calf (see Table 16.4)

Other enzymes are less specific (AST – muscle, liver and RBC), and some are rather non-specific, found in significant amounts in a wide range of tissues (ALP), and may be left out of the normal complete biochemistry panel for that reason by some laboratories. However, the pattern of change may allow deductions to be made with regard to specific tissues. For example, in the absence of haemolysis, a raised AST with normal CK and elevated GLDH indicates that elevated AST is secondary to hepatocellular necrosis and not myonecrosis.

The degree of elevation in particular enzymes may have prognostic value. In Table 16.4, the degree of elevation in muscle specific CK is used as a predictor of outcome in downer cows. The half-life of the enzyme is important as well. The enzyme SDH has a short half-life and, thus, may be of limited value in assessing hepatocellular necrosis unless sampled soon after the insult. The pattern of rise and fall of CK (short half-life) and AST (longer half-life) may allow an assessment of the temporal persistency of ischaemic necrosis in the downer cow.

Urea and creatinine

Urea and creatinine are waste products of protein catabolism. Creatinine arises from the breakdown of the muscle energy storing compound phosphocreatine, and is removed from the body via filtration of plasma at the glomerulus. Creatinine is not significantly resorbed or excreted elsewhere, and thus its plasma level is a good estimate of glomerular filtration rate (GFR), which may be affected by prerenal (hypovolaemia, dehydration, shock), renal (various) or post-renal (usually obstructive) causes. Urea is produced by the liver from ammonia produced by bacteria in the GIT from protein breakdown; however, ruminants re-excrete urea into the saliva and GIT, where rumen microorganisms incorporate it into protein. Thus, plasma urea levels are an unreliable measure of GFR in ruminants. In bovines, it has been used as a measure of protein catabolism.

Bilirubin

Bilirubin is a by product of heme breakdown, and elevations in the blood may be secondary to pre-hepatic causes (e.g. increased hemolysis, especially extravascular), hepatic causes (decreased clearance of unconjugated bilirubin by hepatocytes from the blood, decreased excretion of conjugated bilirubin from hepatocytes into the bile) or post-hepatic causes (cholestatic). If

Table 16.4 Use of serum GGT levels in calves to estimate passive transfer, and CK levels in downer cows to estimate prognosis for recovery.

Day	GGT U/L[1]	CK × URI[2]
1	196	50
2	136	44
3	112	38
4	99	29
5	90	23
6	84	17
7	79	10
8	75	–
9	71	–
10	69	–

[1]Estimate the serum GGT activity that would be equivalent to a serum IgGl (RID) concentration of 10g/L in calves ≤ 3 days old (after Parish *et al.*, 1997), i.e. numbers less than those recorded against each day measured may indicate suboptimal passive transfer.

[2]Elevations of CK (in multiples of the upper reference limit – URI) on days 1–7 above which there is a < 5% chance of recovery (after Clark *et al.*, 1987).

hemolysis is the cause, this will be accompanied by anaemia, which will be regenerative if of more than three days duration. If there is intravascular hemolysis, the plasma and urine may be discoloured red. Hepatic insults resulting in reduced clearance of bilirubin often affect the biliary tract as well. This results in cholestasis, with elevations in hepatocellular (GLDH) and cholestatic (GGT) markers concurrently. In the experience of the author it is extremely difficult to try to separate or quantitate which process is primary based on the degree of change within these markers. In some chronic, near-end stage hepatic diseases, elevations in these enzymes may be minimal, as there may be little residual normal tissue left.

Complicating the assessment of rises in bilirubin in cases of moderate to marked acute anaemia are increases in hepatocellular enzymes secondary to anoxic necrosis of periacinar hepatocytes. Bilirubin rises in these instances may be due both to hemolysis and hepatic causes. In bovines, mild increases in bilirubin may be seen with anorexia. Elevations in indirect (unconjugated) bilirubin occur in haemolytic anaemia, and those in direct (conjugated) bilirubin occur in bile duct obstruction cholangiohepatitis.

Energy metabolism

Energy metabolism in bovines is an extremely important and complex topic, especially in dairy cows during the transition period from late pregnancy to the early part of lactation. There are also some excellent reviews available (Whittaker, 2004; Oetzel, 2004; Maas, 2007 Radostits, 2007; Malmo *et al.*, 2010). Some bovine tissues have the ability to use ketones rather than glucose as a source of energy, but not the brain. Glucose is also required to allow the oxidation of non-esterified fatty acids (NEFA). These are derived from mobilisation and breakdown of triglycerides from adipose tissue, and subsequent production of ATP via the TCA cycle (especially important in times when energy demand exceeds supply).

Bovines derive only approximately 10% of their blood glucose directly from the GIT, as most dietary carbohydrate is converted to volatile fatty acids (acetic, butyric, proprionic) by the ruminal microflora. Hepatic gluconeogenesis, largely using proprionic acid or amino acids as a precursor, supplies the large majority of blood glucose, while acetic acid is more usually incorporated into fat. When fatty acids cannot enter the TCA cycle because glucose is limiting, or the degree of fat mobilisation is excessive (both of which can occur in times of high metabolic demand), the liver accumulates excessive fat (fatty liver), and increased amounts of ketones are formed (resulting in subclinical or clinical ketosis).

Thus, glucose, β hydroxybutyrate (BOHB- a ketone body) and NEFA all have relevance in assessing energy balance, especially in high producing dairy cows within the transition period. Glucose and BOHB are two analytes routinely measured in complete bovine profiles, and NEFA may also be requested during the transition period. These analytes can also be measured as part of a metabolic profile (Table 16.2). For the BOHB and NEFA interpretation, it is important that laboratories have well-established reference intervals for the different stages of late pregnancy and early lactation that are valid for their machine and methods. BOHB is the main ketone found in serum, and the most stable in serum; it is not excreted into urine and, thus, urinary tests for ketone bodies detect acetoacetate and, to a lesser extent, acetone.

Disorders of Ca, Mg and phosphorus

It is important to remember that biochemical profiles measure the total Ca and Mg in the serum, not the ionised free (and biologically active) forms. This may be important with measures of total Ca, where conditions that result in low albumin may affect the total Ca but less so the free, ionised Ca. However, the degree of protein binding is not linear over a physiologic range of albumin, and total calcium may often be used (Bienzle, 1993). Inorganic phosphorus (routinely measured in serum) is excreted from the body via the kidney, and thus may also be elevated when GFR is decreased by whatever cause.

Electrolytes

Sodium is the most abundant extracellular fluid (ECF) ion and is a major contributor to the ECF ionic concentration. Hypernatraemia and hyperchloraemia occur in patients with salt toxicity and water deprivation, but are uncommon in dehydrated animals, due to the loss of electrolytes as well as water.

Potassium is mostly intracellular, and so serum measurements may be falsely elevated in haemolysed samples. Potassium can move between physiological compartments to provide a buffer against changes in pH; thus, serum K^+ levels must be interpreted in conjunction with acid-base status. Acidosis is usually accompanied by hyperkalaemia as K^+ moves from the intracellular fluid (ICF) to the ECF, even though total K^+ may be unchanged or even depleted. In contrast, alkalosis frequently results in hypokalaemia, as K^+ moves into ECF and is excreted by the renal tubule in favour of retaining hydrogen ions.

There is a high turnover of electrolytes within the gastrointestinal tract during normal function. Sodium and HCO_3 are secreted in saliva, H^+ and Cl^- are secreted in the abomasum and HCO_3^- is secreted in the small intestine. The small intestine absorbs dietary K^+ and the large intestine absorbs Na^+, HCO_3^-, Cl^- and H_2O. One common cause of imbalance is diarrhoea, where decreased transit time reduces absorption and leads to dehydration, metabolic acidosis, Na^+ and K^+ loss. Another example is upper gastrointestinal obstruction, where H^+, Cl^- and K^+ become sequestered

Table 16.5 Interpretation of acid-base parameter values.

Acid-base status	Blood pH	pCO_2	HCO_3
Normal	Normal (venous 7.35–7.50)	Normal (venous 34–45 mmHg)	Normal (venous 20–30 mmol/L 20–30 mEq/L)
Metabolic acidosis			
Uncompensated	L	N	L
Compensating	L	L	L
Respiratory acidosis			
Uncompensated	L	H	N
Compensating	L	H	H
Metabolic alkalosis			
Uncompensated	H	N	H
Compensating	H	H	H
Respiratory alkalosis			
Uncompensated	H	L	N
Compensating	H	L	L

L (low), H(High), N (Normal)

Disorders of acid-base

Deviation from normal pH only occurs once physiological buffering mechanisms are exhausted. Bicarbonate is the major pH buffer. The buffering system can be summarised by the Henderson-Hasselbach equation, as follows:

$$H^+ + HCO_3^- \leftrightarrow H_2O + CO_2$$

Acidosis and alkalosis can be metabolic or respiratory. Respiratory acidosis results from increased pCO_2, and the compensating metabolic response is to increase HCO_3^-. A metabolic acidosis may arise from H^+ absorption, H^+ production, H^+ loss or HCO_3 loss. It is characterised by a low HCO_3, with a compensatory low pCO_2. The reverse is true for alkalosis.

There can be different multiple types of acid-base pathophysiologies occurring at the same time, so interpretation can be challenging although, in most cases, there are single disturbances and interpretation is usually straightforward.

Naturally compensatory mechanisms never overcompensate, and the pH will always be in the direction of the primary component. An increase in pH is caused by alkalosis (metabolic or respiratory), and decrease in pH is caused by an acidosis (metabolic or respiratory). Compensatory changes always occur in the opposite direction to the pH. These changes are shown in Table 16.5.

Metabolic acidosis (Low pH, low HCO_3)

The most common causes of metabolic acidosis include ruminal (lactic) acidosis, urea (ammonia) poisoning, ketoacidosis, gastrointestinal loss of HCO_3^-, due to diarrhoea or loss of saliva, hypovolaemia with tissue hypoxia and renal failure. There is exchange of intracellular K^+ for extracellular H^+ to reduce the extracellular pH. This exchange is called the cation shift, and it can result in hyperkalaemia, even though the total body K stores may have been depleted due to renal or gastro-intestinal losses loses.

Respiratory acidosis (Low pH, high pCO^2)

Respiratory acidosis develops due to a decreased in effective alveolar ventilation. This is most commonly seen severe pulmonary disease, bloat and depression of respiratory centre in newborn apnoea.

Metabolic alkalosis (high pH and high HCO_3)

The most common cause of increased H^+ loss, inducing a metabolic alkalosis, is the sequestration of H^+ and Cl^- ions when the abomasum becomes displaced to the left or right, or a right-sided torsion occurs.

Respiratory alkalosis (high pH, low CO_2)

This condition is caused by hyperventilation, which may be stimulated by hypoxaemia or thermoregulation. Hypoxia is associated with pulmonary disease, congestive heart failure and severe anaemia. Hyperventilation may be observed extreme high temperatures.

The anion gap is an estimate of the unmeasured anions in plasma. It is calculated as follows:

$$\text{Anion gap} = (Na^+ + K^+) - (Cl^- + HCO_3^-)$$

Changes in the relative concentrations of the measured ions will alter the magnitude of the gap, and must be taken into consideration when interpreting findings. In the normal state, the

Table 16.6 Interpretations of white blood cell abnormalities.

Abnormality	Interpretation
Neutrophilia	Stress Inflammation – often infectious
Neutropaenia	Endotoxaemia – increased margination Acute inflammation Bone marrow depression or failure
Lymphopaenia	Stress Corticosteroids
Lymphocytosis	Excitement (young animals) Lymphocytic leukaemia
Monocytosis	Chronic bacterial infections
Eosinophilia	Parasites Allergies
Thrombocytopaenia	Increased consumption – bleeding, DIC Deceased bone marrow production (e.g. bracken fern)

Table 16.7 Interpretations of blood protein abnormalities.

Abnormality	Common diagnoses
Hyperproteinaemia	Dehydration Hyperglobinaemia – usually secondary to chronic infection
Hypoproteinaemia	Protein loosing enteropathy: • Johne's disease • Parasitic gastro-enteritis • Salmonellosis Protein loosing nephropathy: • Amyloidosis Hypoalbinaemia: • End-stage liver (chronic pyrrolizadine alkaloid toxicosis) Hyperalbinaemia: • Dehydration Hypoglobinaemia: • Failure passive transfer calves

Table 16.8 Interpretation of serum enzymes abnormalities.

Increase in enzyme	Common diagnoses	Other diagnoses
GLDH (from hepatocytes)	Diseases causing hepatocellular necrosis	Specific for hepatocytes in bovines
AST (from hepatocytes, muscle cells and RBCs))	• Vitamin E/selenium deficiency (white muscle disease) • Ischaemic muscle necrosis (downer cows) • Plant toxicities, e.g. ragwort, green cestrum • Cholangiohepatitis (liver fluke)	Intravascular haemolytic anaemia Fatty liver disease Diseases causing myonecrosis : will also see ↑CK
GGT (hepatic bile ducts)	Acute and chronic liver disease Plant toxicities, e.g. ragwort Cholangiohepatopathies	Neonatal (ingestion of colostrum)
CK (Skeletal and cardiac muscle)	• Vitamin E/selenium deficiency (white muscle disease) • Ischaemic muscle necrosis (downer cows) • Clostridial malignant oedema • Clostridial blackleg	Intra-muscular injections

Table 16.9 Interpretation of urea and creatinine abnormalities.

Abnormality	Common diagnoses	Other diagnoses
Increased creatinine	Pre-renal (e.g. hypovolaemia). Renal (e.g. acute or chronic renal failure). Post-renal (e.g. obstructive urolithiasis, ruptured bladder).	
Decreased creatinine	Over-hydration.	Starvation (reduced muscle mass)
Increased BUN	Pre-renal (e.g. hypovolaemia). Renal (e.g. acute or chronic renal failure). Post-renal (e.g. obstructive urolithiasis, ruptured bladder). Dietary. Incorrect balance of ruminal energy and protein.	
Decreased BUN	Hepatic insufficiency. Incorrect balance of ruminal energy and protein.	Low protein diet

Table 16.10 Interpretation of bilirubin and bile salts abnormalities.

Abnormality	Common diagnoses	Other diagnoses
Increased total bilirubin	Pre-hepatic: haemolytic anaemia	Hepatic disease or post-hepatic bile duct obstruction
Decreased total bilirubin		Over-hydration
Increased bile salts	Hepatic insufficiency Bile duct obstruction	
Decreased bile salts	Malabsorption	Over-hydration

Table 16.11 Interpretation of energy (glucose, NEFA and ketones) abnormalities.

Abnormality	Common diagnoses	Other diagnoses
Hyperglycaemia	Stress Exogenous glucocorticoids Xylazine administration	Diabetes mellitus (rare) i/v administration of glucose
Hypoglycaemia	Neonatal calf malnutrition Neonatal systemic illness Neonatal diarrhoea Primary ketosis Fatty liver syndrome Endotoxic shock	Pregnancy toxaemia
Increase in NEFA	Ketosis Fatty liver syndrome Starvation	
Decrease in NEFA	Extreme emaciation	

Table 16.12 Interpretations of blood mineral (Ca, Mg, P) abnormalities.

Abnormality	Common diagnoses	Other diagnoses
Hypercalcaemia (total)	Hyperalbuminemia (dehydration) Hypervitaminosis D Excessive or rapid administration of calcium	Pseudoparathyroidism (neoplasia) Hyperparathoidism
Hypocalcaemia (total)	Hypoalbinaemia Milk fever (clinical and subclinical) Grass tetany Acute renal failure Anorexia (high yielding dairy cows)	Hypoparathyroidism Oxalate toxicity Tetracycline therapy Excessive bicarbonate therapy Fat necrosis
Hyperphosphataemia	Acute/chronic renal failure Excess dietary phosphorus	Hypervitaminosis D Ruptured bladder
Hypophophataemia	Malnutrition Post-parturient haemaglobinuria Milk fever	Inadequate dietary intake Starvation Chronic wasting diseases Brassica toxicity Pseudoparathyroidism (neoplasia) Hyperparathoidism
Hypermagnesaemia		Excessive administration $MgSO_4$ (Epsom salts) overdose
Hypomagnesaemia	Grass tetany Milk fever Calves on milk only, Mg-deficient diet Excess dietary Ca^{2+}, P, NH_3 or K^+ Ruminal alkalosis	Under-nutrition

Table 16.13 Interpretation of electrolytes abnormalities.

Abnormality	Common diagnoses	Other diagnoses
Hypernatraemia	Dehydration Water deprivation	Thermoregulation (panting) Burns Salt poisoning
Hyponatraemia	Diarrhoea Blood loss Peritonitis Gastro-intestinal sequestration (volvulus, torsion)	Incorrect fluid therapy
Hyperkalaemia	In vitro haemolysis Prolonged sample storage Acute renal failure Metabolic acidosis Tissue necrosis (ischemic muscle necrosis)	Diabetes mellitus
Hypokalaemia	Diarrhoea Vagal indigestion Peritonitis Gastro-intestinal sequestration (volvulus, torsion, LDA/RDA)	Prolonged anorexia Metabolic alkalosis
Hyperchloraemia	Water deprivation Thermoregulation panting Metabolic acidosis Hypertonic fluid therapy	Diarrhoea Burns Diabetes insipidus Respiratory alkalosis compensation
Hypochloraemia	Diarrhoea Blood loss Peritonitis Gastro-intestinal sequestration (volvulus, torsion, LDA/RDA)	Metabolic alkalosis Respiratory acidosis compensation

gap is accounted for by the overall negative charge of plasma proteins. Abnormal production of other anions, such as lactate, ketoacids or phosphate, will increase the gap. The normal value for the anion gap is 14–26 mEq/L or 14–26 mmol/L.

Interpreting results

Abnormality interpretation tables are presented as follow: Table 16.6, white blood cells; Table 16.7, proteins; Table 16.8, serum enzymes; Table 16.9, urea and creatinine; Table 16.10, bilirubin and bile salts; Table 16.11, energy (glucose, NEFA and ketones); Table 16.12, minerals (Ca, Mg, P); Table 16.13, electrolytes; and Table 16.14, acid-base disturbances. The interpretation tables are intended to provide a list of possible aetiologies for abnormal values of a single parameter. They are not exhaustive, and should only be used as a guide; definitive diagnosis demands the full clinical picture to be assessed and the pattern of changes considered.

Factors that should be considered when interpreting results are:

1 Is the reference range provided by the laboratory appropriate?
2 The degree of change: note that 5% of values from normal animals will be outside the normal range, but likely not far out. Thus, small changes should be viewed with caution, and experience is needed to try and gradate the severity of change to assess significance and check for laboratory error.
3 Sensitivity, specificity, prevalence, positive and negative predictive value: these concepts are central to interpretation of results. Sensitivity and specificity are values that are calculated using carefully chosen, artificial populations (animals

Table 16.14 Interpretation of acid-base disturbances.

Abnormality	Common diagnoses	Other diagnoses
Acidosis – Metabolic	Acute ruminal acidosis Ketosis Hypovolaemic shock Diarrhoea Peritonitis	Pregnancy toxaemia Renal failure Urea toxicity Uroperitoneum
Acidosis – Respiratory	Upper airway obstruction Laryngeal oedema Pneumonia General anaesthesia Deep sedation CNS disease	Neonatal apnoea Tetanus Botulism
Alkalosis – Metabolic	Abomasal displacement Abomasal torsion Hypochloraemia Hypokalaemia	Excessive bicarbonate therapy
Alkalosis – Respiratory	Hyperventilation (hypoxia, heat stress, CNS disease)	Excessive positive pressure ventilation
Increased anion gap	Increased lactic acid (ruminal acidosis, diarrhoea, anaerobic exercise) Ketoacidosis Hypochloraemia Hypernatraemia	Uraemia Decrease HCO_3 Hyperkalaemia
Decreased anion gap	Hypoalbinaemia Over-hydration Hyperchloraemia Hyponatraemia	Increased HCO_3 Hypokalaemia

all positive or negative, respectively, when tested against a 'gold standard' test), and do not indicate the predictive value or believability of a test result. This is affected by prevalence, which is often unknown or roughly estimated, in the population being tested. If a test is being used as a screening test (i.e. the prevalence is likely to be low), the positive predictive value of the test is low, but the negative predictive value is high. Experienced clinicians will be able to increase the prevalence of a true positive test by testing only animals from the general population that are more likely to have the disease (or abnormality being tested for), thus increasing the prevalence and positive predictive value of the test.

4 Most importantly, if a test result(s) do not make clinical sense, it is worthwhile phoning the lab to discuss the result. There may include poor sample preservation, laboratory error and poor test selection.

A case example

The animal, an 11-year-old female Aberdeen Angus cow, was part of a group of animals that has been purchased one month ago, and several of the animals appeared depressed. This animal was weak, and jaundiced. Blood samples were taken, and the haematology and biochemistry results are shown in Table 16.15, 16.16 and 16.17. The analytes out of reference range are in bold type. A photomicrograph of the peripheral blood smear is shown in Figure 16.4.

Table 16.15 Case example: red blood cell parameters (abnormalities are in bold).

Red cell parameters	Patient result	Adult reference interval
RBC	**1.15 × 10¹²/L**	5.0–10.0 × 10¹²/L
HGB	**33 g/L**	80–150 g/L
HCT	**0.11 L/L**	0.24–0.46 L/L
MCV	**79 fL**	40–60 fL
MCH	**29 Pg**	11–17 pg
MCHC	**367 g/L**	300–360 g/L
Reticulocyte count (%)	**3.6 %**	0
Reticulocyte count (absolute)	**41 × 10⁹/L**	
nRBC/100 WBCs	**71**	0
PLT	171 × 10⁹/L	100–600 × 10⁹/L
Fibrinogen (g/L)	7	3.0–7.0 g/L

Table 16.16 Case example: white blood cells (abnormalities are in bold).

White cell parameters	patient result	Normal reference interval (adult)
WBC (Corrected for nRBCs)	6.4 × 10⁹/L	4.0–12.0 × 10⁹/L
Neutrophils	4.4 × 10⁹/L (69%)	0.6–4 .0 × 10⁹/L
Lymphocytes	**1.7 × 10⁹/L** (26%)	2.5–7.5 × 10⁹/L
Monocytes	0.3 × 10⁹/L (5%)	0.0–0.9 × 10⁹/L
Eosinophils	0.0 × 10⁹/L (0%)	0.0–0.8 × 10⁹/L

Interpretation

There is a marked anaemia, which is noticeably regenerative (marked polychromasia, basophilic stippling, nRBCs, ↑MCV), indicative of either blood loss or haemolysis. There is hyperproteinemia secondary to both dehydration (hyperabuminemia) and, likely, antigenic stimulation (hyperglobulinemia). There are moderate numbers of an intraerythrocytic organism consistent with *Theileria orientalis* (likely subsp. *ikeda*) and this, along with the presence of an elevated protein and a marked hyperbilirubinaemia, indicates that the anaemia is secondary to haemolysis, not blood loss.

The mild to moderate elevations in GLDH and AST (with a normal CK) is indicative of some hepatocellular necrosis, likely of periacinar hepatocytes secondary to anoxia. The degree of regeneration indicates that the process has been of > 3–4 days duration, but that the animal is likely still eating (normal BOHB

Table 16.17 Case example: biochemistry results (abnormalities are in bold).

Analyte	Patient results	Adult reference intervals
Total protein	**83 g/L**	58–80 g/L
Albumin	**38 g/L**	22–36 g/L
Globulin	**48 g/L**	24–40 g/L
A : G ratio	**0.7**	0.8–1.9
Urea	6.5 mmol/L	2.1–9.6 mmol/L
Creatinine	110 μmol/L	90–120 μmol/L
Bilirubin	**101 μmol/L**	2.0–18.0 μmol/L
AST	**310 U/L**	60–150 U/L
CK	198 U/L	50–400 U/L
GGT	21 U/L	0–36 U/L
GLDH	**57 U/L**	0–20 U/L
Glucose (Fl oxolate)	**8.0 mmol/L**	2.3–4.1 mmol/L
Sodium	136 mmol/L	132–152 mmol/L
Potassium	4.7 mmol/L	3.9–5.8 mmol/L
Anion gap	**25.7 mmol/L**	8–20 mmol/L
Chloride	101 mmol/L	95–110 mmol/L
Bicarbonate	**14 mmol/L**	20–30 mmol/L
Calcium	2.41 mmol/L	2.0–3.0 mmol/L
Phosphorus	1.30 mmol/L	1.29–2.26 mmol/L
Ca : Phosphorus ratio	2	1.8–3.8
Magnesium	0.77 mmol/L	0.70–1.20 mmol/L
B-Hydroxybuterate	0.71 mmol/L	0.0–0.9 mmol/L

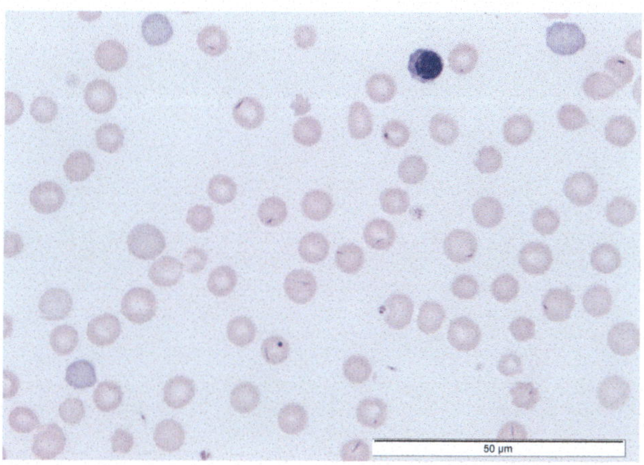

Figure 16.4 High-power view of peripheral blood smear from case example (*Theileria orientalis ikeda*). Interpretation: note the moderate polychromasia, mild to moderate anisokaryosis, and the presence of a nRBC, all indicative of a regenerative response. There is also a single round Howell Jolly body, and numerous slender intra-erythrocytic protozoa within RBCs (consistent with *Theileria* spp.)

indicates there is either minimal fat mobilisation or, possibly, the animal is cachectic and has little fat to mobilise), and that there are not significant periods of recumbency (no elevation in CK). The leucogram pattern, and the hyperglycaemia, are likely stress-related. The low bicarbonate and mildly increased anion gap may reflect a metabolic acidosis secondary to anoxia.

References

Bienzle D., Jacobs R.M. and Lumsden J.H. (1993). Relationship of serum total calcium to serum albumin in dogs, cats, horses and cattle. *Canadian Veterinary Journal* **34**, 360–4.

Chan J.P.W., Chu C.C., Fung H.P. *et al.* (2004). *Serum haptoglobin concentration in cattle.* **66**(1), 43–6.

Clark, R.G., Henderson, H.V., Hoggard, G.K., Ellison, R.S. and Young, B.J. (1987). The ability of biochemical and haematological tests to predict recovery in periparturient recumbenty cows. *New Zealand Veterinary Journal* **35**, 126–133.

Ewaschuk, J.B., Naylor, J.M. and Zello, G.A. (2003). Anion gap correlates with serum D- and DL-lactate concentration in diarrheic neonatal calves. *Journal of Veterinary Internal Medicine* **17**, 940–2.

Ferrer, J.F., Marshak, R.R., Abt, D.A. *et al.* (1979). Relationship between lymphosarcoma and persistent lymphocytosis in cattle: a review. *Journal of the American Veterinary Medical Association* **175**, 705–8.

Fry, M.M. (2010). Anaemia of Inflammatory, Neoplastic, Renal, and Endocrine Diseases. In: *Schalm's Veterinary Hematology*, 6th edition, pp. 246–247.

George, J.W., Snipes, J. and Lane, V.M. (2010). Comparison of bovine hematology reference intervals from 1957 to 2006. *Veterinary Clinical Pathology* **39**(2), 138–148.

Horadagoda, N.U., Knox, K.M.G., Gibbs, H.A., *et al.* (1999). Acute phase proteins in cattle: discrimination between acute and chronic inflammation. *Veterinary Record* **144**, 437–41.

Jones, M.L. and Allison, R.W. (2007). Evaluation of the Ruminant Complete Blood Cell Count. *Veterinary Clinics of North America* **23**, 377–402.

Kaneko, J.J., Harvey, J.W. and Bruss, M.L. (2008). *Clinical Biochemistry of Domestic Animals*, 6th edition, pp. 351–378. Elsevier Academic Press.

Knowles, T.G., Edwards, J.E., Bazeley, K.J., Brown, S.N., Butterworth, A. and Warriss, R.D. (2000). Changes in the blood biochemical and haematological profile of neonatal calves with age. *Veterinary Record* **147**, 593–598.

Latimer K.S. (2011). *Duncan and Prasse's Veterinary Laboratory Medicine*, 5th edition, p. 216. Wiley Blackwell.

Lincoln, S.D., Howell, M.E. and Combs, J.J., *et al.* (1992). Hematologic effects and feeding performance in cattle fed cull domestic onions (*Allium cepa*). *Journal of the American Veterinary Medical Association* **200**(8), 1090–4.

Maas, J. (2007). Diagnostic Considerations for Evaluating Nutritional Problems in Cattle. *Veterinary Clinics of North America* **23**, 527–539.

Malmo, J., Vermunt, J.J. and Parkinson, T.J. (2010). Diseases of Cattle In Australasia, pp. 60–66; 503–548. Vetlearn.

Oetzel, G.R. (2004). Monitoring and testing dairy herds for metabolic disease. *Veterinary Clinics of North America* **20**, 651–674.

Otter, A. (2013). Diagnostic blood biochemistry and haematology in cattle, *In Practice* **35**, 7–16.

Parish, S.M., Tyler, J.W., Besser, T.E., Gay, C.C. and Krytenberg, D. (1997). Prediction of Serum IgG Concentration in Holstein Calves Using Serum Gamma Glutamyltransferase Activity. *Journal of Veterinary Internal Medicine* **11**(6), 344–347.

Petersen, H.H., Nielsen, J.P. and Heegaard, P.M.H. (2004). Application of acute phase protein measurements in veterinary clinical chemistry. *Veterinary Research* **35**,163–187.

Radostits, O.M., Gay, C.C., Hinchcliff, K.W. and Constable, P.D. (2007). *Veterinary Medicine. A textbook of the Diseases of Cattle, Horses, Sheep, Pigs and Goats*, pp. 1618–1626. Saunders Elsevier.

Russell, K. E. and Roussel, A. J. (2007). Evaluation of the ruminant serum chemistry profile. *Veterinary Clinics of North America: Food Animal Practice* **23**, 403–426.

Steffen, D.J., Elliott, G.S., Leipold, H.W. *et al.* (1992). Congenital dyserythropoiesis and progressive alopecia in Polled Hereford calves: hematologic, biochemical, bone marrow cytologic, electrophoretic, and flow cytometric findings. *Journal of Veterinary Diagnostic Investigation* **4**(1), 31–7.

Sutherland, R.J., Bell, K.C., McSporran, K.D. and Carthew, G.W. (1986).: A comparative study of diagnostic tests for the assessment of herd magnesium status in cattle, *New Zealand Veterinary Journal* **34**(8), 133–135.

Suttle, N. (2004). Assessing the needs of cattle for trace elements. *In Practice* **26**, 553–561.

Stockham, S.L. and Scott, M.A. (2008). *Fundamentals of Veterinary Clinical Pathology*, 2nd edition. Blackwell.

Whitaker, D.A. (2004). Metabolic profiles. In Andrews, A.H., Blowey, R.W., Boyd, H. and Eddy, R.G. (eds). *Bovine Medicine. Diseases and husbandry of cattle*, pp. 804–817. Blackwell Science.

CHAPTER 17

Post-Mortem Examination and Sample Taking in Cattle

Elizabeth F. McInnes

Learning objectives

Know and understand:
- the reasons for post-mortem examinations of dead cattle;
- the equipment required for a effective bovine post mortem examination;
- the exact sequence of events in a post-mortem examination;
- the correct procedures for examining various organ systems in cattle;
- the recognition of post-mortem lesions which could be confused with actual lesions during the post-mortem examination;
- the correct methods for collection of fresh and fixed tissue samples from a cattle post-mortem;
- the correct procedures to use during the packaging and posting of post-mortem samples.

Introduction

The usual reason for performing a post-mortem examination on cattle is to establish the cause of illness or death (Howie, 2007). A post-mortem examination may, however, be performed on dead cattle for a number of reasons, including health surveillance, supporting an insurance claim (Whitenack & Johnson, 1986) and the investigation of disease. The process may involve collection of tissues for pathology, as well as the collection of appropriate samples for microbiological and parasitological examinations for disease identification.

Ideally, all cattle post-mortem examinations should be performed in a well-equipped necropsy room but, if this is not possible, they may be carried out in the field (Griffiths, 2005). Griffin (2012) describes a method of post-mortem examination which encourages the veterinarian not to remove organs from the carcass unless necessary, thereby making carcass removal more efficient and minimising the cleaning of the post-mortem area. Veterinarians should not be dissuaded from performing post-mortem examinations in the field, since the information yielded is of considerable value.

Autolysis after death begins immediately after the onset of hypoxia as a result of cessation of blood flow (Slauson & Cooper, 2000). Autolysis of the small intestine will commence within ten minutes of the death of the animal, resulting in the swelling of villus tips and epithelial denudation of the villi in a bovine calf (Pearson & Logan, 1978a, 1978b). Storage of bovine carcasses in a refrigerated storeroom (2–4°C) is, therefore, recommended to avoid the rapid autolysis which may occur in the warm atmosphere outside (Myers & McGavin, 2007).

The veterinarian performing the post-mortem examination should obtain the history of the dead animal before beginning, as it may indicate which organ systems require special attention, what disease is suspected and which tissue samples will require harvesting. Protective clothing, boots and rubber gloves are required for all necropsies. Cut-proof gloves, dust masks and safety goggles may be advisable, particularly in the case of suspected transmissible encephalopathies (Howie, 2007). Two particular risks associated with cattle post-mortem examinations include the risk of zoonoses and the possibility of trauma due to sharp instruments (Howie, 2007). Possible zoonotic infections in cattle include anthrax, salmonellosis and listeriosis (Andrews *et al.*, 1986).

Before commencing the post-mortem, the veterinarian should label all sample containers clearly with the identification number of the animal and the date of the post-mortem. All the samples should be labelled using a waterproof marker, since stick-on labels often come off during transport. The correct identification of the animal is very important. The veterinarian must examine the information on the tattoo or the ear tag of

Bovine Medicine, Third Edition. Edited by Peter D. Cockcroft.

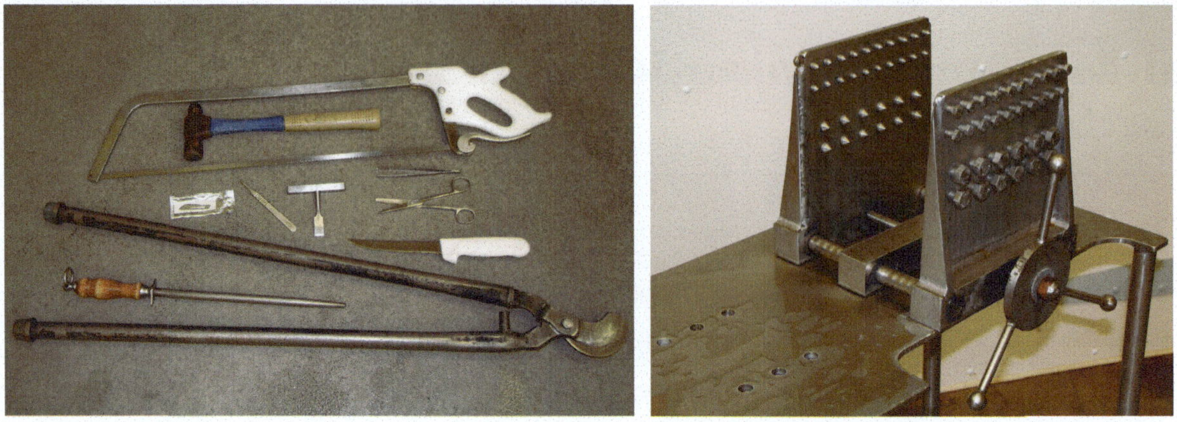

(a) (b)

Figure 17.1 a. Equipment required to complete a post-mortem examination of cattle, including cam lock saw, large bone cutters, a steel, a sharp, pointed knife, sharp scissors, a rat-toothed forceps, orthopaedic chisel and hammer. b. A vice is used for securing the head, in order to open the cranium to remove the brain in cattle.

the animal in order to determine the exact identification of the animal that is to be examined post-mortem. Retaining the identification (ear tag or microchip) with the fixed organs in the pot of formalin is good practice, and acts as a safeguard to ensure that organs can be accurately identified if the external labelling becomes damaged. It is advisable to prepare all instruments, sample collection materials, camera and forms before beginning the necropsy post-mortem. If photos are taken during the post-mortem examination, they should include the animal's identification tag in each photograph (Griffin, 2012).

Useful equipment (Figure 17.1a) includes a cam lock saw, large bone cutters, a steel, vice (Figure 17.1b), a sharp, pointed knife, sharp scissors, a rat-toothed forceps, orthopaedic chisel, hammer and paper towels (Griffiths, 2005). All material from the post-mortem should be retained until the end of the process, to ensure that all samples necessary to make a diagnosis are collected (Howie, 2007).

Post-mortem examinations should be conducted in a well-lit, safe environment which may be easily and effectively cleaned and disinfected. In general, cattle are placed on their left side or on their backs. External examination of the animal includes examining the ears, eyes (Figure 17.2a), oral cavity (Figure 17.2b), rectum (Figure 17.3), skin (Figure 17.4), digits (Figure 17.5) and urogenital openings for the presence of haemorrhage or discharges such as purulent material. Lesions associated with ringworm commonly affect young calves on the skin of the head (Johnson, 1986). Although weighing equipment may not be present, the veterinarian should be able to note down the general body condition (Griffiths, 2005).

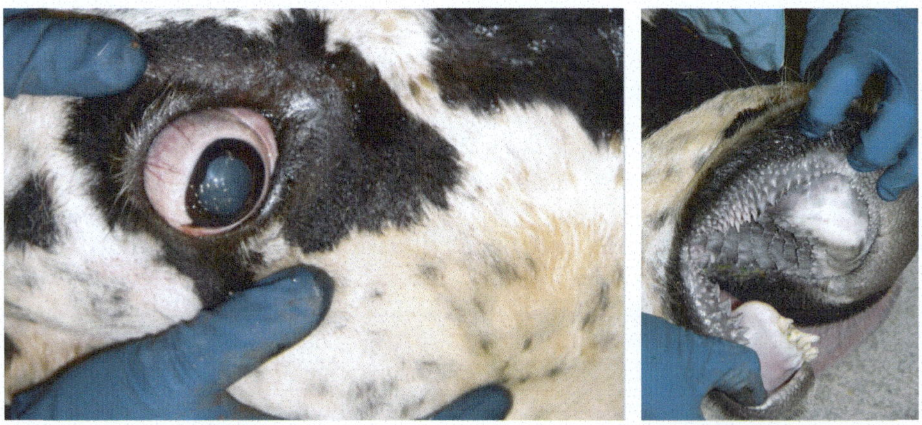

(a) (b)

Figure 17.2 a. Examination of eyes before commencement of the post-mortem examination. b. Examination of the mouth before commencement of the post-mortem examination.

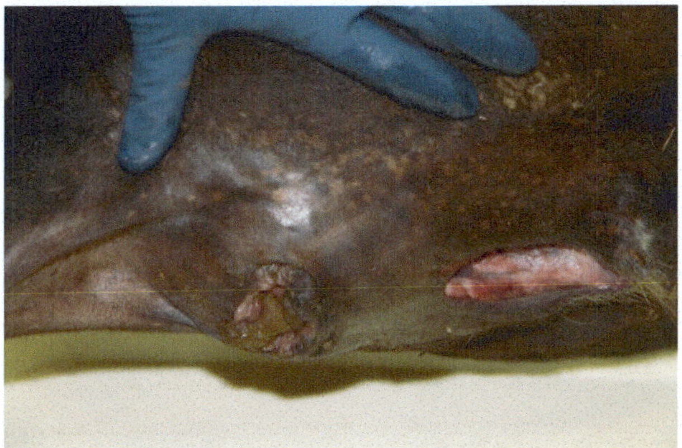

Figure 17.3 Examination of rectum and urogenital openings before commencement of the post-mortem examination.

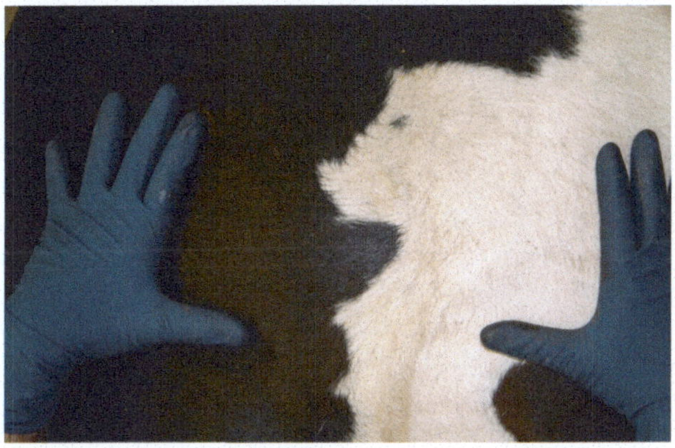

Figure 17.4 Examination of skin before commencement of the post-mortem examination.

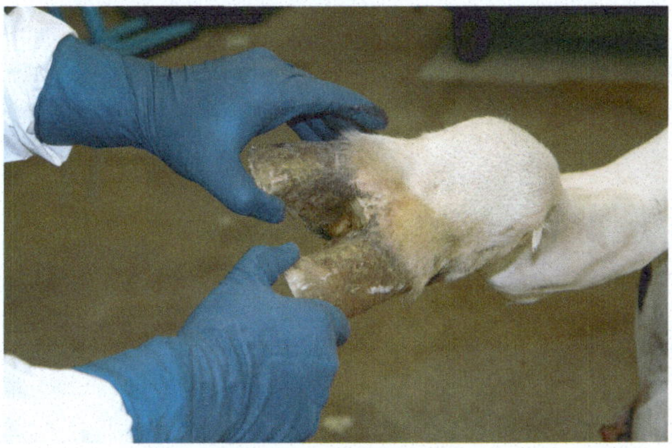

Figure 17.5 Examination of the digits before commencement of the post-mortem examination.

An initial incision is made into the right axilla of the bovine carcass, and the skin incision is extended cranially to the symphysis of the mandible along the midline. The right axillary incision is also extended caudally along the midline to the symphysis pubis. The external genitalia, including the penis or

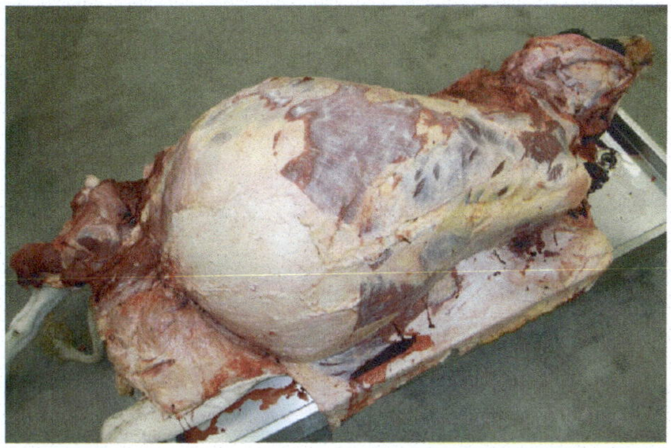

Figure 17.6 The skin is reflected on the right side and both fore and hind limbs are completely abducted.

the udder, may require reflection at this point. It is important to examine the jugular veins *in situ* for the presence of inflammation or thrombosis. The skin is reflected on the right side, and both fore and hind limbs are completely abducted by cutting through the muscular attachments of scapula and cutting into the hip joint in order to expose the femoral head (King *et al.*, 2005). The skin is reflected by using a sharp necropsy knife to cut the subcutaneous tissues. The skin of the thorax and abdomen to the right and left of the midline will require reflection.

When cutting back the skin, it is safer to direct the sharp edge of a knife towards the skin and the back end of a knife towards the body (King *et al.*, 2005; Figure 17.6). Before proceeding further, it is advisable to make multiple incisions into the udder, to expose the teat canals and to examine the udder carefully for the presence of necrosis and possible tumours. If the animal is in lactation, it may be advisable to take milk samples from each teat (Griffiths, 2005).

After examination of the external organs, an incision should be made along the midline, through the abdominal musculature, in order to open the abdominal cavity. The abdominal muscle walls are reflected by cutting down the edge of the caudal ribs and exposing the abdominal organs. The gastrointestinal tract should be examined at this stage, for the presence of abomasal or intestinal torsion (Johnson *et al.*, 1986). Intestinal loops may occasionally be present in the thoracic cavity in the case of a diaphragmatic hernia.

The diaphragm may be visualised near the sternum. A stab incision is made into the diaphragm, and it is important for the veterinarian to note whether an audible intake of air occurs into the thoracic cavity, indicating the presence of negative pressure. If no audible intake of air is heard, it is possible that pneumothorax may exist. The thoracic cavity is now opened with a saw, or bone cutters (Figure 17.7) are used to cut through the costochondral junctions in order to reflect and remove the rib cage. Before removing the thoracic or abdominal organs, it

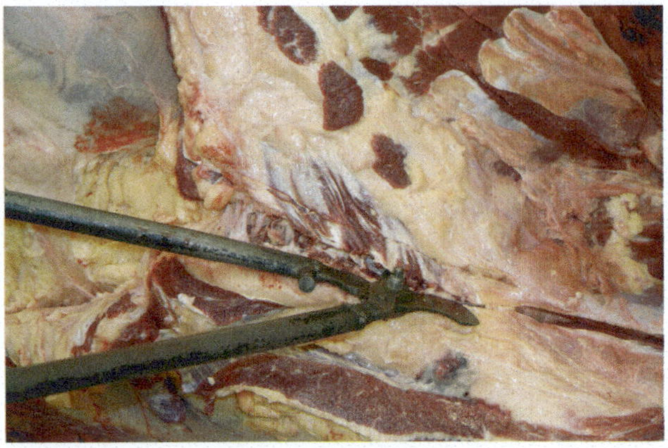

Figure 17.7 The thoracic cavity is now opened with a saw or bone cutters used to cut through the costochondral junctions.

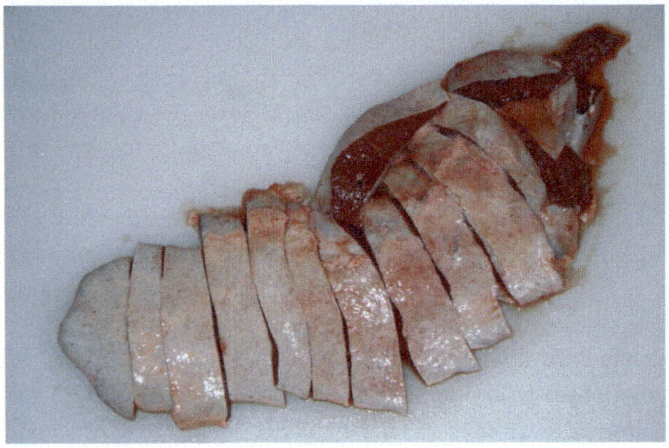

Figure 17.8 Several transverse incisions are made into the spleen to examine the red and white pulp.

is advisable to examine these cavities for the presence of clear fluid, blood or purulent material. The presence of an acute inflammation is often indicated by yellow, non-adherent, fibrin strands. Adhesions may be present in either the thoracic or abdominal cavities, and are characterised by the presence of adherent, white, fibrous strands.

The spleen (Figure 17.8) is located on the underside of the rumen, and should be removed. Several transverse incisions are made into the spleen to examine the red and white pulp and to check for the presence of enlargement, thrombosis and focal infarction (King *et al.*, 2005). Enlargement and congestion of the spleen may be caused by the use of pentobarbitone euthanasia.

Patency of the gall bladder may be checked by applying gentle pressure to the gall bladder (Griffiths, 2005), and it is advisable to incise and inspect the gall bladder *in situ*. Abnormal findings in the gall bladder include excessive dilatation and the presence of viscid, dark bile which may indicate inanition before death (Ruth, 1986). After examining the surface of the liver *in situ* for the presence of masses and adhesions, the pancreas is

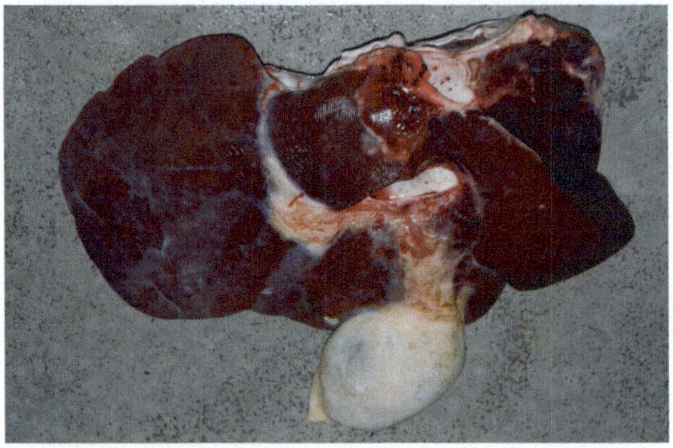

Figure 17.9 Examine the surface of the liver for the presence of masses and adhesions and check the patency of the gall bladder.

located in the mesentery at the level of the cranial duodenum, and blunt dissection should be used to remove both liver and pancreas. Multiple transverse incisions are made into the liver (Figure 17.9) to examine the cut surface for the presence of fatty liver (yellow colour), hepatomegaly (enlargement), tumours and a nutmeg liver (a reticulated pattern with alternating yellow, red and brown areas which may indicate chronic heart failure).

In order to remove the forestomachs and small intestine, the small intestine is pulled towards the veterinarian whilst cutting through the mesentery (King *et al.*, 2005). At this point, the veterinarian may examine the mesenteric lymph nodes for enlargement or the presence of lymphoma. It may be advisable to place ligatures around the oesophagus and the pylorus before removing the forestomachs, in order to prevent rumenal content spillage. Before removing the small and large intestine from the abdominal cavity, it is advisable to locate the duodenum (adjacent to the pancreas) and the ileum by locating the caecum and finding the entry of the ileum into the caecum (Andrews *et al.*, 1986).

The gastrointestinal tract should be laid out in a cranial to caudal order (i.e. from the forestomachs to the abomasum and extending into the duodenum, jejunum, ileum, caecum, colon and rectum). Both the forestomachs and the abomasum should be opened along the greater curvature, and the internal mucosa and contents of each stomach should be examined thoroughly. The feedstuff, colour, liquid and pH are all important features of the rumen contents (Ruth, 1986). Conditions such as rumenal acidosis are characterised by the presence of severe reddening and possibly ulceration of the luminal mucosa. The abomasum should be opened and the surface should be examined for ulceration and the presence of a cobbled surface, which may indicate the presence of *Ostertagia* spp.

Although it is recommended that the entire small and large intestine are opened and examined using blunted-ended scissors

(Howie, 2007), the prosector may wish to open only representative lengths in order to save time. The veterinarian should pay particular attention to the surface of the mucosa of the intestines (looking for conditions such as ulceration and tumours), as well as the contents of the lumen (these may be liquid, malodorous, hemorrhagic or fibrinonecrotic). The thickness and the consistency of the intestinal wall may be increased in conditions such as Johne's disease. The caecum should be examined for the presence of helminths, and a few loops of the spiral colon should be opened to look for necrosis, ulcers and pseudomembranous inflammation. Finally, a faecal sample should be taken from the rectum if required.

After removing and inspecting the gastrointestinal tract, the veterinarian should examine the abdominal organs that have not been removed. The adrenals should be visualised *in situ* and examined for the presence of excessive of enlargement, atrophy and tumours. The adrenal glands are extremely friable, and care should be taken when making a transverse incision in order to examine the cortex and medulla ratio. The right kidney is generally situated more cranially than the left kidney, and the adrenals are situated medial to the cranial poles of each kidney (King *et al.*, 2005).

The veterinarian may wish to examine the ureters at this stage. Abnormal findings in the ureters include excessive urine dilatation. which may indicate an obstruction in the urinary bladder outflow or the urethra, caused by uroliths. Uroliths are often present at the ischial arch or sigmoid flexure of the urethra (Whitenack & Johnson, 1986). The kidneys are now removed separately, and a single longitudinal incision should be made into each kidney to expose the cortex medulla and pelvis. The veterinarian should grasp the kidney capsule with a pair of rat-toothed forceps, and peel away the capsule to expose the cortical surface of the kidney. If the capsule is adherent and difficult to remove from the cortical surface, this is often an indication of underlying chronic inflammation, such as chronic interstitial nephritis. The ovaries, uterine horns, cervix and the cranial portion of vagina may be removed together; however, care must be taken not to damage the underlying aorta and the vena cava.

The pelvic cavity may now be opened by using a saw or bone cutters to cut through the pubis to the obturator foramen and then through the ischium on both sides. The symphysis pubis should then be removed from the pelvic cavity, which may now be visualised. Organs in this area include the caudal aspects of the rectum, reproductive tract, urinary bladder and urethra. The bladder should be opened and the urethra should be checked for the presence of uroliths and inflammation. If the bladder contains urine, it is advisable to collect a urine sample before examining the urinary bladder and possibly testing the urine for the presence of protein and blood using a urine dipstick. In newborn animals, the umbilical arteries will be present on either side of the bladder and the omphalomesenteric veins extending from the umbilicus to the liver will be present. These structures may be inflamed if the young calf has omphalophlebitis.

Once the ovaries, uterine horns, cervix and vagina (cranial portion) have been removed, it is important to incise the ovaries longitudinally to look for the presence of cysts and masses. Both uterine horns, the cervix and vagina should be opened, and the lumen and its contents should be examined. In male animals, the scrotum should be cut open and the testis examined and incised, as well as the accessory sex glands. Major vessels, including the aorta, should be examined for the presence of thrombosis or aneurysm.

While the heart and lungs are still *in situ*, the pericardium should be opened and the pericardial contents examined for the presence of purulent material, foreign bodies, blood or clear fluid. Serous atrophy of the adipose tissue in the coronary groove is generally an indication of starvation or chronic illness (Johnson, 1986). The heart muscle should be examined for white muscle disease lesions, as well as the presence of vegetative endocarditis of the valves (generally characterised by the presence of a friable, yellow, proliferative growths on the valves (Johnson, 1986). The veterinarian should assess the cardiac walls for atrophy or hypertrophy.

There are many different ways in order to examine the heart in detail, but a useful system is to follow the route of the blood flow through the heart (i.e. an inflow-outflow method of dissection (Maxie & Robinson, 2007)). First, the apex of the heart is sectioned and checked for hypertrophy, dilatation, necrosis, mineralisation and fibrosis. Then, the right atrium, from the caudal vena cava to the tip of the atrial appendage, is opened to look for thrombosis and to examine the right atrioventricular valve (tricuspid valve). The lateral side of the right ventricle is cut through adjacent to the ventricular septum and the internal surface of the right ventricle is examined, as well as the endocardial surface and the chordae tendinae. The prosector should check that there are no ventricular septal defects (Griffiths, 2005).

The rostral wall of the right ventricle is sectioned and the pulmonic valves are opened and examined for the presence of stenosis. The pulmonary arteries are examined for thrombosis, particularly in animals with an indwelling jugular catheter (Maxie & Robinson, 2007). The left atrium is opened by cutting into the atrial appendage, in order to examine the foramen ovale/fossa ovalis and the left atrioventricular valve (mitral valve). The left ventricle is opened by cutting along the caudal border of the left ventricle adjacent to the ventricular septum, and the left atrioventricular valve is examined before being incised (Maxie & Robinson, 2007). Finally, the flow of blood is followed by cutting through the aortic valve and along the aorta.

It is advisable to remove the tongue, pharynx, larynx, oesophagus, trachea, lungs and heart together (often called the 'pluck') (Figure 17.10). In order to do this, the veterinarian should cut along the medial sides of both mandibles, close to the bone.

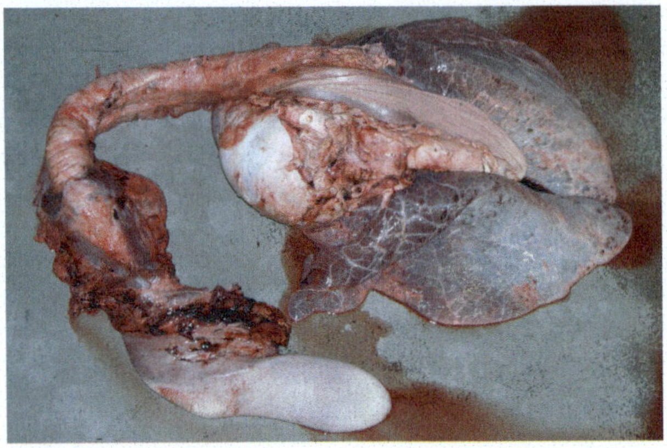

Figure 17.10 It is advisable to remove the tongue, pharynx, larynx, oesophagus, trachea, lungs and heart together (the pluck).

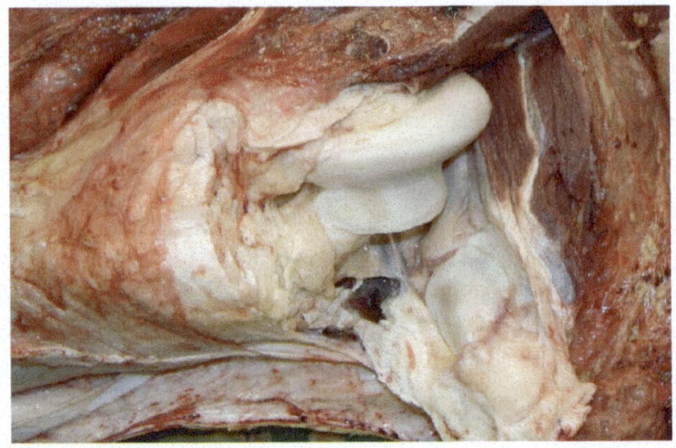

Figure 17.11 The stifle joint has been opened to examine for the presence of haemorrhage and purulent exudate.

The symphysis of the mandible may need to be separated, for easy removal of the tongue and examination of the oral cavity. The tongue is then grasped manually by the prosector and exteriorised between the two mandibles. The prosector continues to pull the tongue down and back, cutting through the hyoid bones (this may require bone cutters) on both the left and right sides. The veterinarian continues to grasp the tongue and to remove the entire trachea, oesophagus, lungs and heart. At this stage, it is possible to palpate the vertebral bodies along the vertebral column, looking for evidence of asymmetry, fracture and osteomyelitis. Several cuts should be made into the large muscles of fore and hind limbs, the external/internal back muscles and the tongue and diaphragm, looking for haemorrhages, protozoan cysts, gas bubbles (possible Clostridial infections) and necrosis. A skeletal muscle sample taken parallel to the muscle fibres as well as a peripheral nerve (such as the sciatic nerve) may be placed on cardboard to prevent contraction during the fixing process (Howie, 2007).

The lips, teeth, tongue and oral cavity should be examined (Andrews *et al.*, 1986), and then transverse sections should be made into the tongue, looking for the presence of granulomas, which may indicate wooden tongue (*Actinobacillus* spp. infection). The size of the thymus at the thoracic inlet should be noted (Andrews *et al.*, 1986), and the parathyroids and thyroids should be isolated on either side of the larynx; these should be examined for the presence of cysts, enlargement and tumours. The full length of the oesophagus should be cut open, and the surface of the oesophageal mucosa should be examined for the presence of ulceration. The lungs should be palpated in order to evaluate the consistency, which should be spongy and elastic. The presence of excessive amounts of air (emphysema), or the presence of pneumonia (hard, firm consistency), are abnormal findings. The veterinarian should cut down the trachea and the major bronchi, and the tracheobronchial lymph nodes should to be examined for the presence of enlargement and lymphoma.

The joints should be routinely examined, particularly in young animals, for the presence of haemorrhage or purulent exudate (Figure 17.11). This includes the right hip joint, the left and right stifle joints, right shoulder joint, the atlanto-occipital joint and the right and left hock joints. In the case of the stifle joint, the ligaments should be cut and patella should the reflected away from the joint surface (Andrews *et al.*, 1986).

Peripheral nerves, such as the sciatic nerve, should be examined and sampled if necessary, and the large lymph nodes, such as the mammary, mesenteric and cervical lymph nodes, should be examined. After the examination of the joints, the skin should be removed from the head and the salivary glands should be examined. The atlanto-occipital joint should be located by moving the head up and down, and cerebro-spinal fluid (CSF) may be collected at this time if it is required. The knife should then be inserted into the atlanto-occipital joint to cut the spinal cord and ligaments, and to remove the head. A small portion of skin should be left around the eyes, which can be used to grasp with forceps in order to loosen the eyeball from the orbit. If required, the eyeballs can be removed and fixed in modified Davison's fixative. This may be done before the necropsy has commenced, in order to prevent autolysis. The major muscle masses should be removed from the cranium, and the foramen magnum should be examined.

Veterinarians should consider the request to remove the brain carefully, since there is risk of the possible presence of transmissible spongiform encephalopathies (TSEs). Extra precautions, such as the use of airflow helmets, should be used if the animal is suspected of being infected with a TSE agent (Griffiths, 2005). The brain is removed by sawing transversely through the frontal bone (Figure 17.12) caudal to the zygomatic process of the frontal bone. The next cut is saggital, medial to the left occipital condyle (Figure 17.13). This is repeated on the other side. The cranium is removed, using a chisel and hammer to loosen the bone (Figure 17.14). The head is tilted so that the

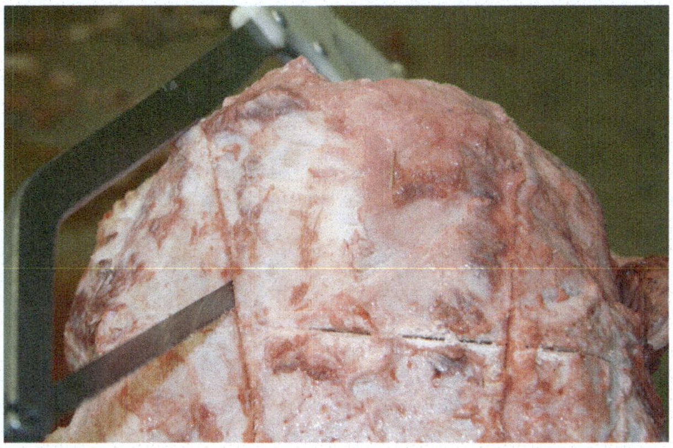

Figure 17.12 Removal of the brain starts with sawing transversely through the frontal bone, caudal to the zygomatic process of the frontal bone.

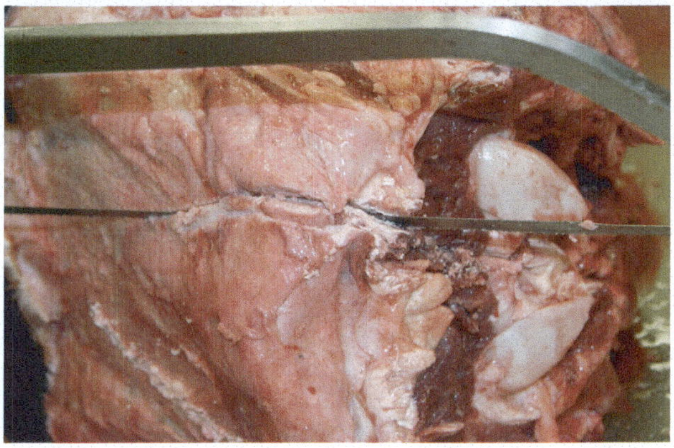

Figure 17.13 The next cut is saggital, medial to the left occipital condyle and this is repeated on the other side.

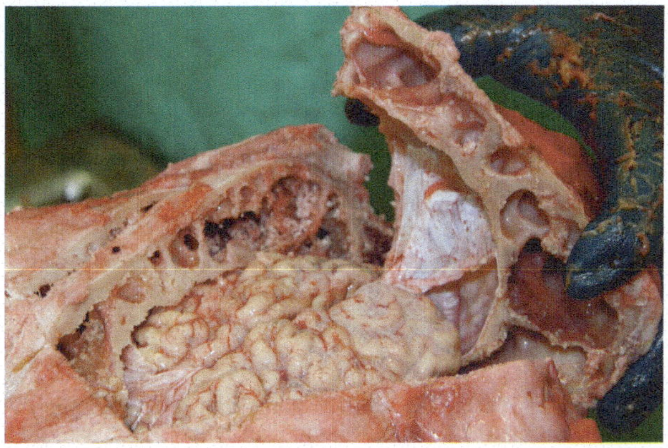

Figure 17.14 The cranium is removed using a chisel and hammer to loosen the bone.

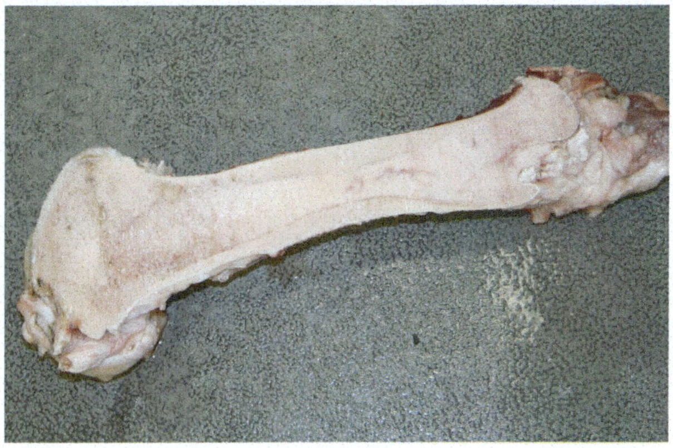

Figure 17.15 A long bone such as the femur should be split in half to examine the growth plate and bone marrow.

brain can be loosened from its attachments and allowed to fall out gently onto the surface of the table or into a container of formalin. The dura mater can be incised and reflected using scissors and forceps (Griffiths, 2005).

The pituitary gland is present within the sella tursica. The external, middle and inner ear canals should be examined if otitis is suspected. If central nervous system disease is suspected, a saw may be used to cut alongside the midline of the vertebral column (Griffiths, 2005) in order to expose the spinal cord. When fixing the spinal cord, the dura mater should be incised along its length, and the cord can be divided up into short sections within the dura (Howie, 2007).

A bone marrow sample, or a bone marrow smear, may be taken from the epiphysis of a long bone such as the femur. A long bone such as the femur should be split in half (Figure 17.15) to examine the bone marrow and the growth plate in younger animals, and a rib may be broken to assess bone strength.

The mandible should be removed from the head, which allows the nasopharynx to be examined. The head should be sawn longitudinally, in order to examine the nasal turbinates. The nasal septum may require removal before examination of the nasal turbinates and sinuses (King *et al.*, 2005). The sinuses should be examined, particularly in calves, where purulent inflammation of the frontal sinus may occur as a consequence of dehorning (Johnson, 1986).

During the necropsy, the veterinarian must record, in some form, all observations made during the necropsy examination. Voice recorders can be helpful in this regard. This will provide a valuable aid at the end of the necropsy and after the histopathological examination of the slides has been conducted, and it will allow conclusions to be drawn about what abnormalities were observed. These observations may be written down on a specific form designed for that purpose, or they may be entered into a computer data collection program. It is a good idea to develop a checklist for the cattle post-mortem procedure, which is referred to each time.

The prosector should make a note of the characteristics of the abnormalities observed. The abnormal organs should be identified and information about the size, site, shape (e.g. wedge-shaped), colour (always use an actual colour rather than the term 'pale'), the consistency (whether the organs are hard or soft to the touch) and borders (sharp demarcation between normal and abnormal tissue or diffuse borders) of the lesion should be recorded. In addition, the appearance of the cut surface of the abnormality should be described as should the normal or abnormal contents of some of the hollow organs, such as the bladder and the small and large intestines. Information on whether the lesion is focal, multifocal, focally disseminate or diffuse should be included. If abscesses or tumours are observed, the size, number and location of each should be recorded. At the end of the post-mortem process, the remains of the carcass should be disposed of responsibly using either incineration, burial or rendering (Howie, 2007).

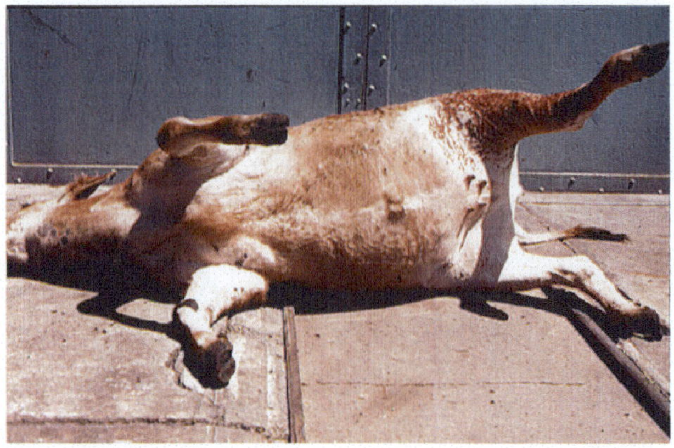

Figure 17.16 *Rigor mortis* is the contraction of muscles after death.

Post-mortem lesions

Post-mortem changes are normal or artefactual lesions which need to be distinguished from the actual lesions of disease in a dead animal. Post-mortem autolysis refers to the degeneration of cells after somatic death caused by hypoxia (Myers & McGavin, 2007). These changes are exacerbated by bacterial decomposition. The bacteria enter tissues shortly before or just after death, migrating from the gastrointestinal tract lumen and into the blood. Post-mortem putrefaction produces changes in colour, texture and gas production, and these changes may interfere with accurate interpretation of both macroscopic and histopathological changes. The longer the period of time between death and the fixing of tissues, the greater the autolysis.

Post-mortem changes (onset, rate, severity) vary greatly depending on the cause of death, the body and environmental temperature, the microbial flora and the particular tissue type. Tissues with high contents of proteolytic enzymes undergo very rapid autolysis (e.g. pancreas). In ruminants, ingesta in the forestomachs will continue to undergo bacterial fermentation after death, and the heat production caused by the formation of gas will result in greater autolysis (Myers & McGavin, 2007). In addition, high body temperatures, high metabolic rate, heat stroke and exercise before death will speed up autolysis (Myers & McGavin, 2007).

Rigor mortis (Figure 17.16) is the contraction of muscles after death and occurs within two to four hours in young, well-conditioned animals that die during intense muscular activity in a warm environment (Ruth, 1986). Rigor mortis will persist for one to two days or slightly longer in a cool environment (Ruth, 1986). Animals with severe malnutrition will have depleted energy stores (ATP and glycogen) and thus no muscle contraction is possible and rigor mortis will be absent (Myers & McGavin, 2007). *Livor mortis* (Figure 17.17) is the gravitational pooling of blood (hypostatic congestion) on the dependent side of the body (the side resting on the hard surface of the table), and may result in distinct, red areas in the skin on the side on which the animal was lying (Myers & McGavin, 2007). If the ribs obstruct the process of gravitational pooling, then pale white areas may be visible on the surface of these organs immediately below the ribs.

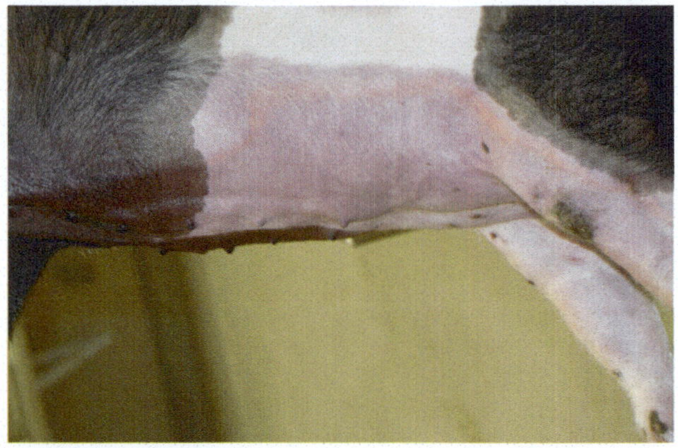

Figure 17.17 *Livor mortis* or hypostatic congestion is the gravitational pooling of blood on the dependent side of the body (shown here in a pig).

Post-mortem clotting occurs in the heart and large vessels because the erythrocytes settle to the base of the heart or large blood vessel. This results in a distinctive clot with two portions (Myers & McGavin, 2007) – that is, an upper portion of yellow, clotted serum and a lower portion of red, clotted erythrocytes. This is referred to as a chicken fat clot. Post-mortem clots are unattached to vessel walls, in contrast to ante-mortem clots, which are attached to vessel walls and tend to be dry and dull in colour (Myers & McGavin, 2007).

Haemoglobin imbibition (Figure 17.18) is the red staining of tissues (particularly of the endocardium of the heart and inner surface of the aorta, as well as the gastrointestinal tract), and it may mimic the appearance of haemorrhage (Myers & McGavin, 2007). This is a common change in carcasses, and it results from haemoglobin from lysed erythrocytes leaking from the blood vessel walls into the surrounding tissues. Bile

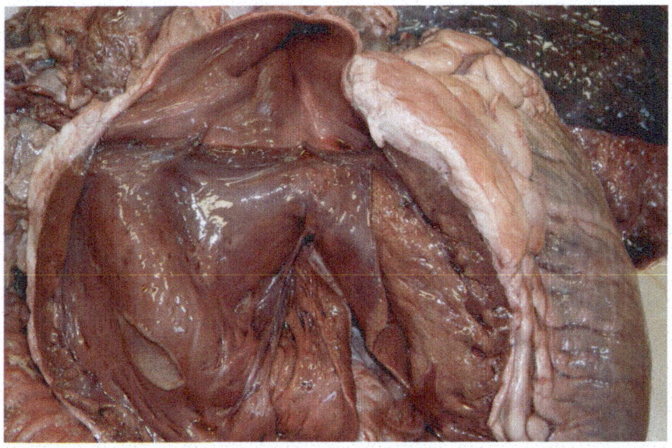

Figure 17.18 Haemoglobin imbibition is the red staining of tissues particularly of the endocardium of the heart.

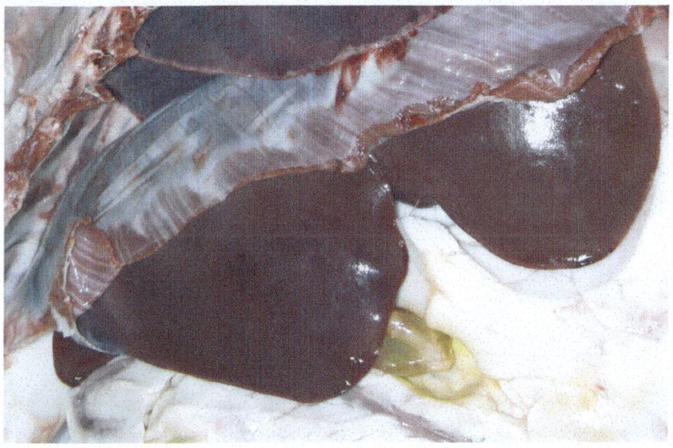

Figure 17.19 Bile imbibition occurs within hours after death when bile leaks from the gallbladder and stains the surrounding tissues yellowish-green.

imbibition (Figure 17.19) occurs within hours after death, when bile leaks from the gall bladder and stains the surrounding tissues yellowish-green and, later, brown (particularly the liver and small intestine) (Myers & McGavin, 2007).

Pseudomelanosis is the green, blue and black discoloration of the carcass tissues due to the presence of iron sulphide. The change results in the post-mortem discoloration of various tissues, including the liver, kidneys, spleen and intestine walls. The iron sulphide is formed by the reaction of hydrogen sulphide from putrefactive bacteria, and iron released from haemoglobin by lysed erythrocytes (Myers & McGavin, 2007).

A bloody nasal or oral discharge (Figure 17.20) is a common post-mortem artefact, due to nasal congestion at death and subsequent increased pressure on the diaphragm due to rumenal bloat (Myers & McGavin, 2007). A further common finding after death is the presence of gastrointestinal or rumenal contents within the respiratory passages (Figure 17.21), due to the relaxation of the cardiac sphincter (King *et al.*, 2005) after death. Tracheal froth is a common artefact of euthanasia (Whitenack & Johnson, 1986). Pulmonary emphysema (Figure 17.22) is also

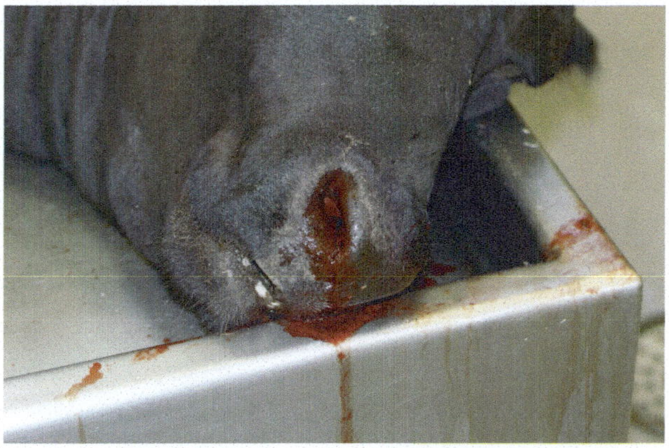

Figure 17.20 A bloody nasal or oral discharge is a common post-mortem artefact.

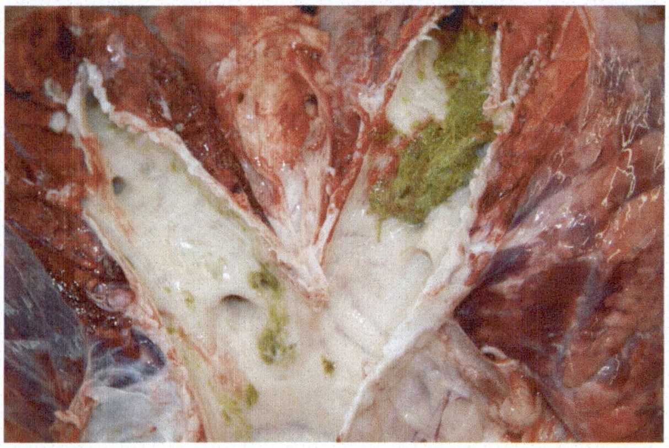

Figure 17.21 The presence of gastrointestinal or rumenal contents within the respiratory passages due to the relaxation of the cardiac sphincter.

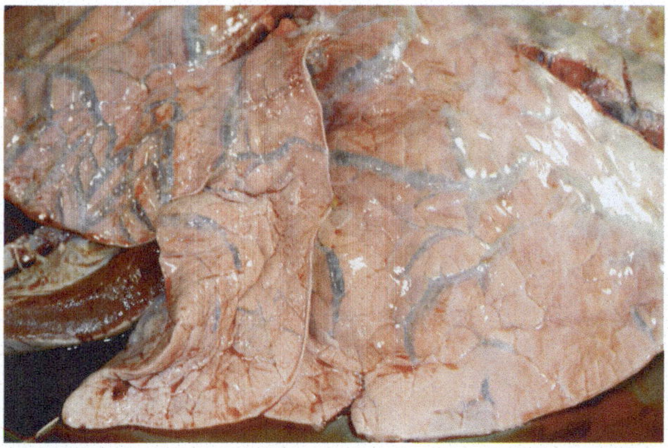

Figure 17.22 Post-mortem pulmonary emphysema may be the result of terminal (agonal) gasping, and one may see large bullae in the lung.

common in cattle that die of various causes. It may be the result of terminal (agonal) gasping, and one may see large bullae in the lung (Whitenack & Johnson, 1986). This lesion is usually of limited significance unless there is an ante-mortem history of

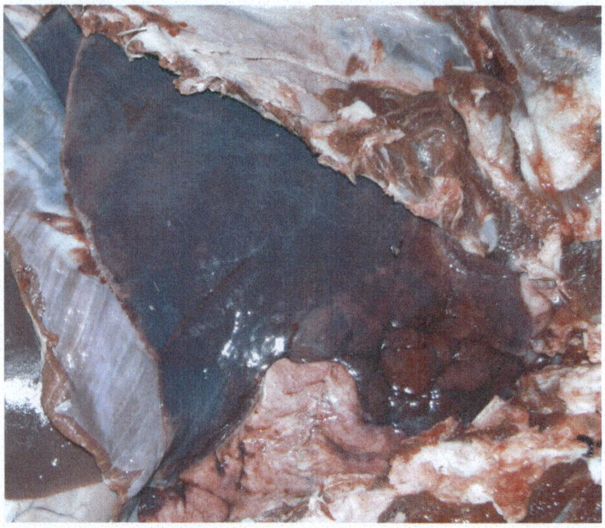

Figure 17.23 Post-mortem changes in the lung also include severe congestion and oedema.

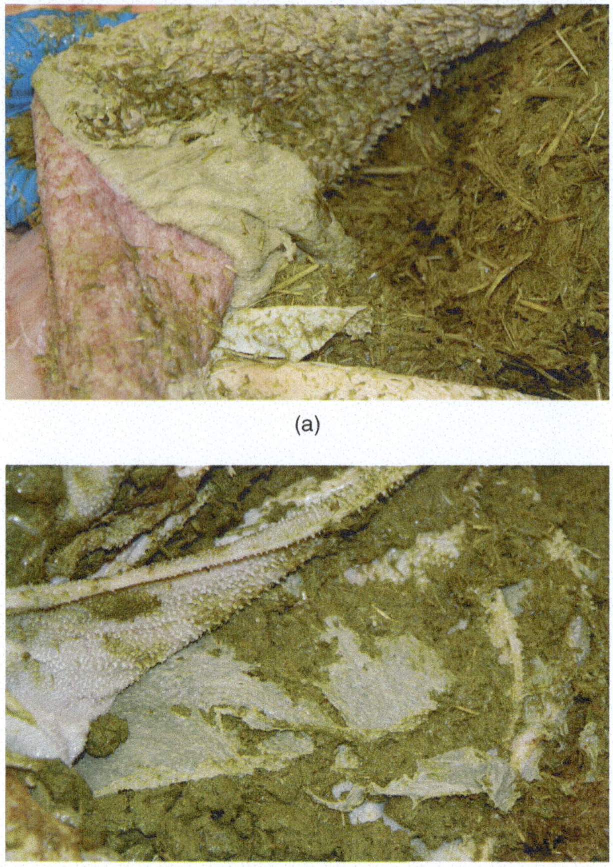

(a)

(b)

Figure 17.24 a. The lining of the rumen may quickly slough (within 20 minutes) and peel off in large strips, leaving a white submucosa underneath. b. The lining of the omasum may quickly slough and peel off in large strips.

dyspnoea. Post-mortem changes in the lung also include severe congestion and oedema (Figure 17.23).

Pneumonia is common in cattle, and useful tests to perform at the post-mortem examination are palpation of the lung tissue. If the lung is not firm and consolidated, the lesion is probably not pneumonia. In addition, the veterinarian may place the lung tissue in formalin or water to see whether the tissue floats. Pneumonic lung tissue will sink, while unaffected lung tissue will float. A normal anatomical feature of the bovine lung pleura, particularly the caudal lobes of the lungs of cattle, is the presence of white, fibrous plaques on the surface. This is a normal feature and should not be confused with pleural adhesions (King *et al.*, 2005). Rectal and vaginal prolapse may be noted as an artefactual lesion caused by gas distension of the rumen, particular if the animal has been fed highly fermentable feeds (King *et al.*, 2005). The prolapsed tissues may be cannibalised by dogs, rodents or birds.

Bloating of the gastrointestinal system occurs as a result of post-mortem bacterial gas formation in lumen (Myers & McGavin, 2007). In ruminants, post-mortem bloating may be severe, and it may result in rupture of the diaphragm or the rumen with no evidence of concomitant inflammation. The most reliable indicator of ante-mortem bloat is the presence of a 'bloat line' in the oesophagus (proximal congestion, distal pallor), which occurs before death due to the increased pressure on the thoracic contents with subsequent blanching of the lower oesophagus (Whitenack & Johnson, 1986). Curved, firm papillae are found at the distal end of the oesophageal groove and omasum in ruminants. These are normal structures, which may be white in young milk-fed animals and are dark brown in older animals (King *et al.*, 2005).

The lining of the rumen and omasum may quickly slough (within 20 minutes of death) (Figure 17.24a and 17.24b), and peel off in large strips, leaving a white submucosa underneath (Ruth, 1986). No oedema or haemorrhage is present in these areas which indicate that this is a post-mortem lesion.

In acute, rumenal acidosis, the mucosa of the papillae is brown and friable, especially in the ventral sac, and if rumenitis has occurred, the mucosa may not detach easily (Ruth, 1986). It is advisable to check the pH of the rumen contents at post-mortem examination. The normal range is between 5.5–7.5 with a pH of below 5.0 considered to be evidence of acidosis (Whitenack & Johnson, 1986). Autolysed intestines may become diffusely reddened, and may contain pink contents (Whitenack & Johnson, 1986). These changes could be confused with hemorrhagic enteritis. Agonal intussusception may occur when intestinal hypermotility has existed before death (e.g. parasites) (Ruth, 1986). However, there will be no concomitant signs of inflammation such as fibrin strands. Gut-associated lymphoid tissue (GALT), including Peyer's patches, in the small intestine

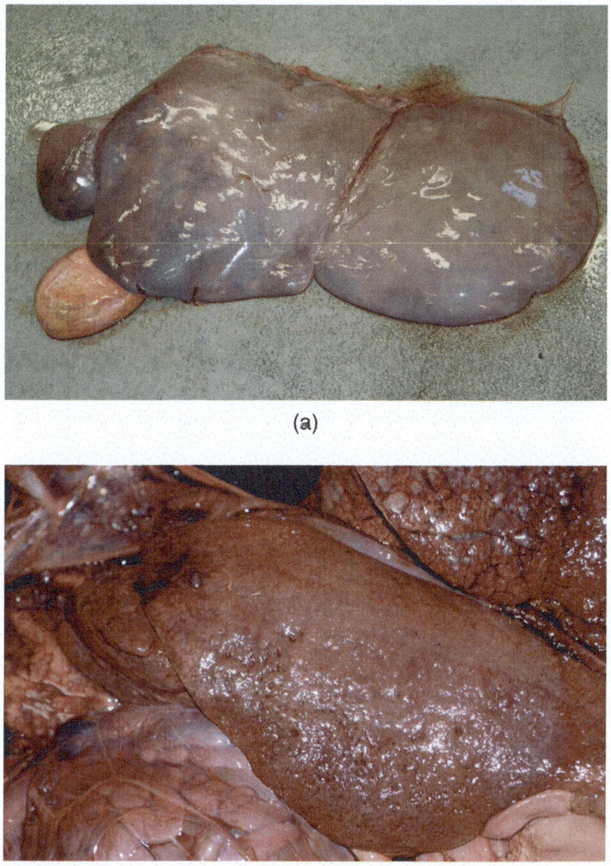

(a)

(b)

Figure 17.25 a. Disseminated irregularly-shaped, pale tan areas in the liver may mimic necrosis or fatty change, but are a normal post-mortem change. b. In advanced autolysis of the liver, gas bubbles produced by autolytic bacteria may be observed.

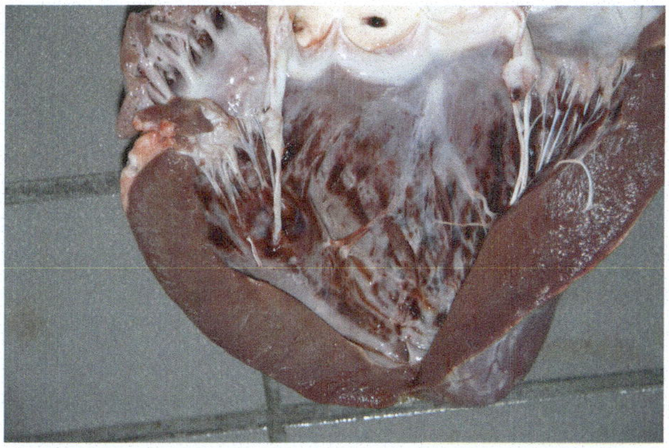

Figure 17.26 Epicardial, endocardial and myocardial petechiae and echymoses are haemorrhages noted as post mortem changes.

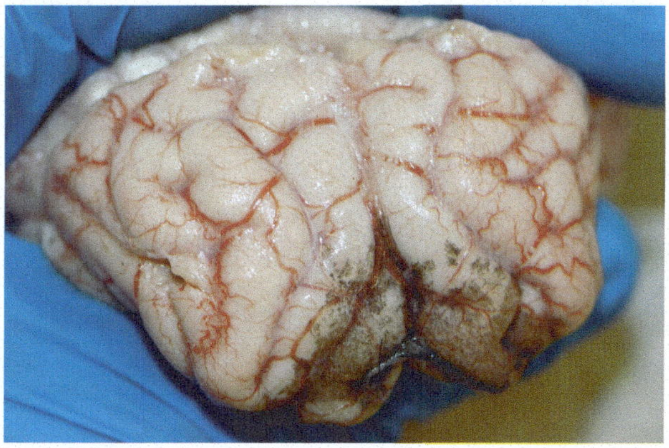

Figure 17.27 Congenital melanosis is the greyish-black coloration of various organs including the meninges and the brain.

and the colonic tonsil (visible distal to the ileum entrance), should not be confused with areas of ulceration.

Disseminated irregularly-shaped, pale tan areas in the liver (Figure 17.25a) may mimic necrosis or fatty change, but are a normal post-mortem change (Whitenack & Johnson, 1986), due to the lysis of hepatocytes by saprophytic bacteria. In advanced autolysis of the liver, gas bubbles produced by autolytic bacteria may be observed (Figure 17.25b). Epicardial, endocardial and myocardial petechiae (Figure 17.26) and echymoses are haemorrhages noted in the heart, thymus and trachea of cattle, particularly after prolonged agonal death (Whitenack & Johnson, 1986). Although they may be observed in septicaemia/toxaemia, these findings should not be considered diagnostic, and other evidence of septicaemia should be sought.

Congenital melanosis (Figure 17.27) is the greyish-black coloration of various organs, including the meninges, brain, lung, pulmonary artery and aorta. This change is often seen incidentally in young animals. Mesenteric lymph nodes may display a gray-green medulla due to the presence of accumulated plant pigment (Ruth, 1986), and lens opacity occurs when the carcass is very cold or frozen (Myers & McGavin, 2007).

Tissue sampling – fresh tissues

The samples collected and submitted from a post-mortem examination depend on the clinical signs, herd history and the findings noted at post-mortem examination. In general:

- nasal or nasopharyngeal swabs should be collected from animals with respiratory diseases;
- faecal samples from animals with enteric diseases;
- cerebrospinal fluid (CSF), nasal secretion and faeces from animals with central nervous system clinical signs;
- vesicular fluid and biopsies from animals with skin lesions (http://vetmed.iastate.edu).

The veterinarian should always take a swab or tissue sample of a lesion such as an abscess or necrotic focus, and should note the number of such lesions present in the animal. Fresh (non-fixed) tissue samples are required for bacterial culture, viral isolation, polymerase chain reaction (PCR) (e.g. *Chlamydia* sp.), serology, toxin testing, trace element assays, worm counts and faecal egg counts. If a single lesion is encountered, fresh samples should be taken for microbiological culture, and samples should be placed in formalin for histopathological examination. If no gross lesions seen, then blanket sampling for microbiology and histopathology is advised. This should include liver, lung, kidney and one segment of small and large intestine.

Microorganisms are killed by heat, desiccation, light and extremes of pH, so microbiological samples should be protected during transport and the correct transport medium should be selected (Howie, 2007). Sterile, dedicated equipment including scalpel blades and forceps should be kept for collection of specimens (Howie, 2007; Figure 17.28). Tissues should be very fresh and collected aseptically, and specimens should be collected prior to antibiotic treatment. The veterinarian should not contaminate the samples with surfaces which have resident anaerobic bacteria, and exposure to air for more than 20 minutes may be detrimental.

The numbers of infectious agents are usually highest at affected sites and during the early stage of disease (Howie, 2007) and generous portions of tissue (a cube of approximately 20 mm or a slice of tissue of approximately 10 mm wide) and several millilitres of pus, exudate or faeces should be submitted. If a lesion is present, it should be included in the sample.

Microbiological samples should be submitted individually in separate bags or jars, with correct and clear identification. They should be maintained at refrigeration temperature (4°C) and sent with ice packs. Freezing and loose ice during transport is generally not recommended; instead, icepacks should be used for cooling during transport.

Milk samples should be collected in sterile screw cap tubes. A 3 ml sample of urine should be collected by cystocentesis, catheter, or mid-stream catch if cystitis is suspected. Pustules and vesicles should be disinfected with alcohol, allowed to dry, and the material should be aspirated using a syringe and needle. Hair, skin scrapings and scab material should be submitted in the case of suspected fungal infections. Samples of the small and large intestine should be 30–40 mm in length and should include content. Faeces will be used for microbiological culture (Figure 17.29), the PCR (Figure 17.30) and faecal egg counts, and should be packed into a screw-capped container, leaving no air, and should be kept cool.

If joints show evidence of arthritis, then joint fluid should be submitted in a sterile container as well as in an EDTA tube for cytology, and a dry swab (Figure 17.31) of the joint fluid should be submitted for the PCR if *Chlamydophila* or *Mycoplasma* spp. is suspected. If body cavity fluids appear exudative (fibrin strands present), these should be submitted in a sterile container. However, clear transudative fluids are not useful and should not be submitted for microbiological testing. Veterinary pathologists suggest taking tissue samples from all major body systems (lungs, liver, heart, kidneys, spleen, rumen, omasum,

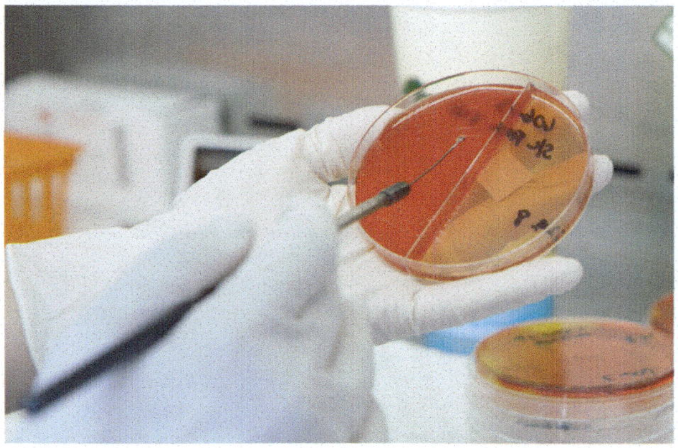

Figure 17.29 Swabbing the microbiological culture plate with faecal content.

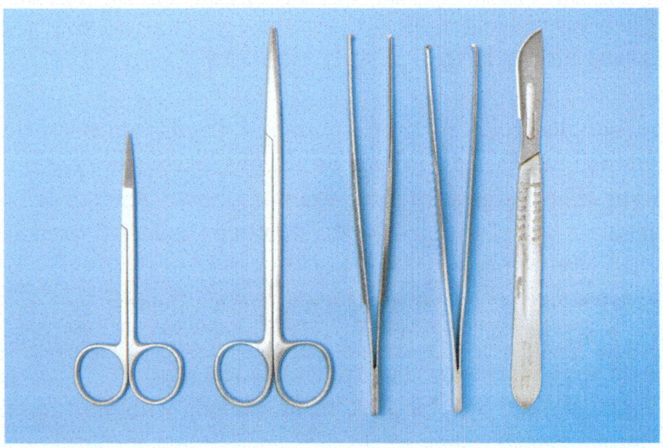

Figure 17.28 Sterile, dedicated equipment, including scalpel blades and forceps, should be kept for collection of specimens.

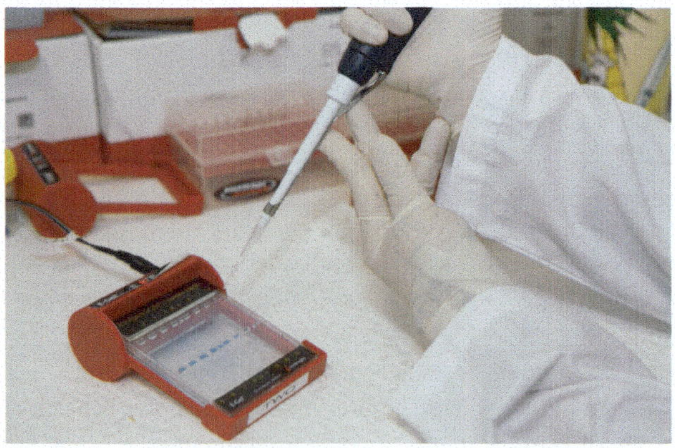

Figure 17.30 Loading a polyacrilamide gel with the product of the polymerase chain reaction.

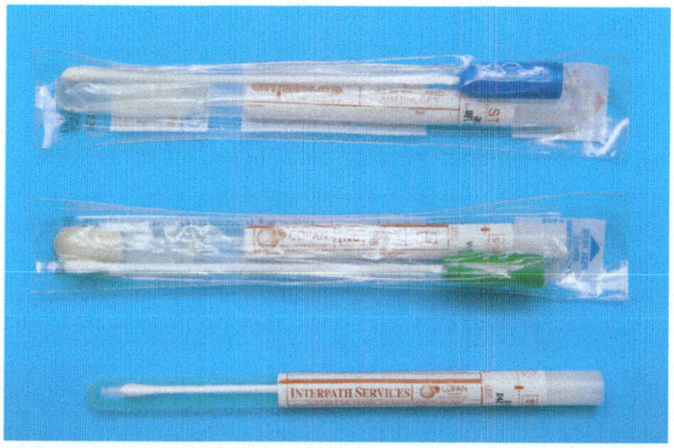

Figure 17.31 A dry swab should be submitted for the PCR and transport medium swabs should be submitted for microbiological examination.

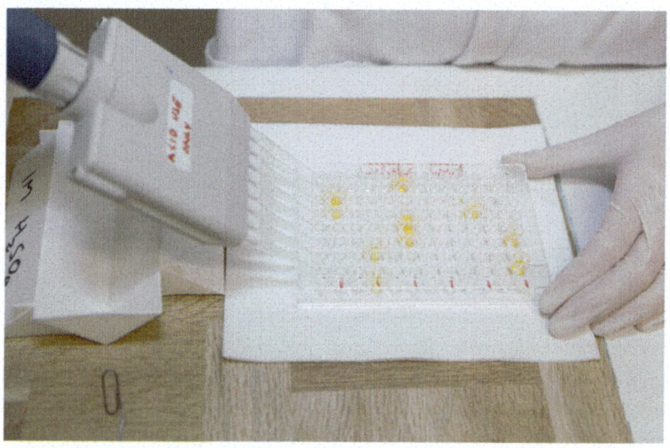

Figure 17.32 Yellow colour reaction in 96 well plates, indicating positive serological ELISA tests.

reticulum, abomasums, duodenum, ileum, caecum, colon) and associated lymph nodes (only if changes are noted in the organs draining particular lymph nodes) (Griffin, 2012).

The polymerase reaction and serology (Figure 17.32) are the most important tests for ruminant viral diagnostic testing, and viral isolation is used less commonly. A dry swab should be used to submit tissue for PCR testing, and clotted and non-clotted blood should be submitted for serology, since these sometimes require plasma. Samples for pesticides and heavy metal (arsenic and lead) testing are required in large amounts, and it is recommended that between 70 and 125 ml of rumen content, 5–10 g of liver and kidney, a 70 ml container of adipose tissue and one side of the cerebral cortex should be submitted. Serum may also be submitted for heavy metal testing.

Environmental samples include feed, drinking water, plants, soils, paint, unidentified substances (Howie, 2007). Feed, grass and water samples are submitted for mycotoxins, ionophores and algal testing, and 1–2 kg of feed, a $20 \times 30\,\text{cm}^2$ bag of grass and a 1 litre water sample are required for adequate testing. Samples for a faecal egg count should include a 70 ml container of faeces (preferably not colonic contents), submitted within 24 hours of collection. A serum pepsinogen is very useful to detect ostertagiosis in cattle younger than two years.

Tissue sampling – fixed tissues

Rapid fixation in 10% neutral buffered formalin is essential to avoid autolysis of tissues taken at post-mortem examination. Tissue samples for histopathological examination should be no more than 0.5–1.0 cm thick (Figure 17.33), and a sharp blade and not scissors should be used to cut the tissue (Howie, 2007).

Ideally, a ratio of 1 : 10 between the sample and the volume of 10% neutral buffered formalin should be maintained, and the correct container and volume of formalin should be selected (Figure 17.34). If clinical signs of the central nervous system have been reported, a two-litre container will be required for fixation of a bovine brain, which may take several days. Nerves may be pinned to a tongue depressor and immersed in formalin (http://vetmed.iastate.edu).

Tissues (apart from the brain) should be fixed in large formalin volumes for 24–48 hours, and replacement of the formalin during fixing process may be necessary (Howie, 2007). Tissues from one animal may be included in the same formalin container, and there should not be any need to label tissue sites individually, unless the lesion occurs in a particular lymph node or a specific site of the intestine. Lesions should be sampled at their margin to include normal tissue and to ensure that, where appropriate, both the cortex and medulla are sampled (e.g. kidney) (Howie, 2007).

The gastrointestinal tract may be fixed on cardboard, with the serosal surfaces down, before immersing the card and sample in

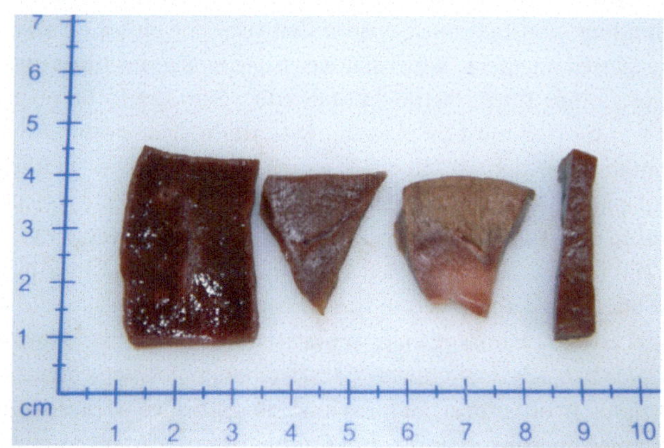

Figure 17.33 The correct size and width of tissues for optimal formalin fixation, including a rectangle of right side liver, a triangle of left side of liver, a piece of the cortex and medulla of the kidney, and a long piece of kidney that includes the entire nephron.

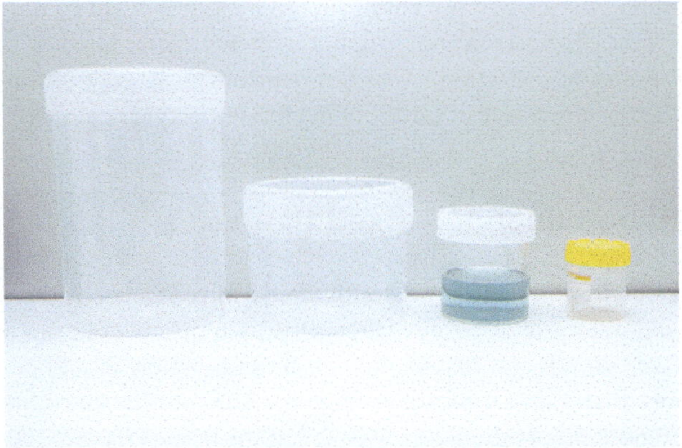

Figure 17.34 The correct container and volume of formalin should be selected for the fixation of tissues.

the formalin (Howie, 2007). This method may also be used for the skin, where the sample is placed epidermis side up onto the cardboard (Howie, 2007). Alternatively, formalin may be flushed through the intestine before placing it in the fixative to ensure that the mucosal surface does not undergo autolysis (Andrews *et al.*, 1986). Samples for electron microscopy will be rare; they should be 1–3 mm^2 in size and should be fixed in glutaraldehyde for 1–3 hours (Howie, 2007).

General guidelines for packaging and posting of tissue specimens

It is extremely important to prevent leakage of specimens during transport, and icepacks are advised for the transporting of fresh tissue specimens (http://vetmed.iastate.edu). Double-bagging of tissues and containers prevents leakage. The containers within a package, as well as the outside of the package, should be identified. It is advisable not to place blood tubes loose in a container, and one must ensure that tubes of blood or serum are placed in racks, with dividers to separate the tubes from one another (http://vetmed.iastate.edu). Samples to be posted or transported must be placed in watertight, leak-proof sample containers which are, in turn, wrapped in absorbent material and placed in a second leak-proof container and then placed within a plastic bag (Howie, 2007; Allen, 1991; Harvey, 1998).

The history and competed form should be placed in a plastic bag, sealed and taped to the specimen. The parcel should be labelled with 'Pathological specimens, handle with care' (Howie, 2007). It is advisable not to pack fresh samples with formalin samples, in order to avoid formalin leakage/fumes, as these compromise microbiological culture results.

References

http://vetmed.iastate.edu/diagnostic-lab/user-guide#bacteriology-submission-guidelines

Allen, M. (1991). Sampling and despatch. *In Practice* **13**, 59–68.

Andrews, J.J., Van Alstine, W.G. and Schwartz, K.J. (1986). A Basic approach to food animal necropsy. *Veterinary Clinics of North America: Food Animal Practice* **2**, 1–29.

Griffin, D. (2012). Field necropsy of cattle and diagnostic sample submission. *Veterinary Clinics of North America: Food Animal Practice* **28**, 391–405.

Griffiths, I. (2005). Post-mortem examination of cattle and sheep. *In Practice* **27**, 458–465.

Harvey, R.G. (1998). Posting pathological samples. *Veterinary Record* **142**, 375–376.

Howie, F. (2007). Necropsy and sampling techniques. In: Aitken, I.D. (ed). *Diseases of Sheep*, 4th Edition, pp 580–597. Blackwell Publishing.

Johnson, D.D. (1986). Necropsy of the suckling calf. *Veterinary Clinics of North America: Food Animal Practice* **2**, 85–96.

King, J.M., Roth-Johnson L. and Dodd, D.C. (2005). *The Necropsy Book*, 4th edition. pp. 1–100. Charles Louis Davis DVM Foundation, Gurnee, IL.

Maxie, M. and Robinson, W.F. (2007). Cardiovascular system. In: Maxie M. (ed.). *Jubb, Kennedy and Palmer's Pathology of Domestic Animals*, vol. 2 , 5th edition, pp. 8–9. Saunders, Philadelphia.

Myers, R.K. and McGavin, M.D. (2007). Cellular and tissue responses to injury. In: McGavin, M.D and Zachary, J.F. (eds). *Pathologic Basis of Veterinary Disease*, 4th Edition, pp. 25–27. Mosby Elsevier.

Pearson, G.R. and Logan, E.F. (1978a). Scanning electron microscopy of early postmortem artefacts in the small intestine of a neonatal calf. *British Journal of Experimental Pathology* **59**, 499–503.

Pearson, G.R. and Logan, E.F. (1978b). The rate of development of postmortem artefact in the small intestine of neonatal calves. *British Journal of Experimental Pathology* **59**, 178–82.

Ruth, G.R. (1986). Necropsy of adult cattle. *Veterinary Clinics of North America: Food Animal Practice* **2**, 119–127.

Slauson, D.O. and Cooper, B.J. (2000). Hypoxic cell injury. In: *Mechanisms of disease. A textbook of comparative general pathology*, pp. 45–53. Mosby, St Louis.

Whitenack, D.L. and Johnson, B. (1986). Necropsy of the feeder and stocker calf. *Veterinary Clinics of North America: Food Animal Practice* **2**, 97–118.

Acknowledgements

The author would like to acknowledge the kindness and generosity of Prof. John Edwards of Texas A and M university who provided most of the photographs used to illustrate this chapter.

CHAPTER 18

Microbiology for Cattle Practitioners

Bryan Markey

Learning objectives

- To appreciate the reasons for testing.
- To be aware of the important aspects of sample collection.
- To appreciate the importance of the postal regulations and storage requirements of diagnostic samples.
- To understand the principles of different types of microbiological tests in common use.
- To understand the criteria used in the interpretation of laboratory test results.

Introduction

Cattle are affected by a range of infectious agents, including bacteria, fungi, viruses and prions. The diseases caused by these microorganisms frequently have an important effect on production and may, in some cases, cause mortality. They may affect the economic viability of a beef or dairy enterprise in a very dramatic way, through the loss of a valuable animal or, more often, through losses incurred as a result of infertility, decreased milk production, poor growth rates and impaired feed conversion. Laboratory testing is both expensive and time-consuming, so it is important to ensure that both the sample collected and the tests requested are appropriate. Equally important is the interpretation of laboratory results and, in general, accurate interpretation can only be achieved through evaluation of both clinical and laboratory information.

Reasons to test

There are many reasons for undertaking the expense and effort of sampling animals and submitting samples for microbiological testing. The principal reasons are:

- Identification of the infectious cause of a clinical disease that has come to the notice of the farmer or veterinary surgeon, particularly where several animals or groups of animal are considered to be at risk.
- To confirm the disease-free status of individual animals. This may be done to facilitate the sale of an animal, or of the herd. It may be done as part of a national or regional accreditation program for particular infectious microorganisms such as *Mycobacterium avium* subsp. *paratuberculosis*.
- Screening of purchased animals before their introduction into a disease-free herd. In addition, it is advisable to quarantine such animals for four weeks and to test again prior to assimilation into the herd.

Diagnostic sample collection

Individual circumstances and the condition suspected will influence the most appropriate sample(s) to collect. However, there are a number of general guidelines that may be helpful in the selection and collection of samples for submission. Most samples will probably be submitted from living animals, and should be collected from the affected site(s) as early as possible after the appearance of clinical disease. This is particularly important for viral infections, because viral titres present in tissues and, being shed, are usually highest early in the course of the infection. It is also an important consideration where secondary opportunist infections may occur and obscure the identity of the primary pathogen involved, such as frequently occurs in respiratory or enteric tract infections. If an animal has died, then samples need to be collected quickly following death, in order to avoid significant degeneration of quality and to limit the possibility of post-mortem invasion by a range of opportunistic bacteria and fungi. In general, samples from animals dead for longer than four hours are not suitable for culture, due to invasion of the tissues

Bovine Medicine, Third Edition. Edited by Peter D. Cockcroft.

by intestinal anaerobes, but the timing is significantly affected by ambient temperature.

Samples should be collected as aseptically as possible, to avoid bacterial and fungal contamination. A guarded swab may be helpful in bypassing a large population of normal flora, such as at the nasal meatus. Samples should be from the edge of lesions, where microbial replication will be maximal. In cases where there is less certainty about the likely infectious agent, as wide a range of samples as possible should be collected in order to permit greater flexibility by laboratory personnel in choosing the most appropriate assays. The administration of antimicrobial treatment may negatively impact on isolation and detection, so samples should be collected before such treatment is begun. The use of highly sensitive assays could be compromised if cross-contamination occurs between samples, or between the sample and the environment, and steps need to be taken to avoid this. In the case of zoonotic infections, it is the attending veterinarian's responsibility to take appropriate steps to ensure that farm, veterinary and laboratory personnel are not put at risk as a result of contact with the animal or samples obtained.

Abortion

Ideally, the placenta and a whole foetus should be submitted. Alternatively, try to send a piece of affected placenta (two or more cotyledons), abomasal contents, liver, lung, spleen, brain and any tissue with gross lesions. A swab of any uterine discharge is useful, as well as paired serum samples from the dam.

Mastitic milk

It is important to collect milk samples as soon as the signs of mastitis are noticed, to collect the samples aseptically and to avoid collecting from animals that have received either intramammary or parenterally administered antibiotics. Do not wash the teats unless they are grossly dirty, and dry with paper towels. Decontaminate the teats with 70% ethanol, paying particular attention to the teat sphincter. Discard the first couple of squirts of milk before collecting some milk from each quarter into your sterile container.

Urine

The preferred methods of collection for bacteriological culture are, in order of preference, by catheter or by mid-stream sample. It is common to find small numbers of bacteria in urine, and it may be necessary to carry out a viable bacterial count. Numbers in excess of 10^5 bacteria/ml are indicative of clinical bacteriuria.

Skin lesions

Intact pustules or vesicles should be surface disinfected with 70% ethanol before aspirating material. The edge of a lesion should be scraped with a scalpel blade until blood begins to appear. Plucked hairs and scab material should also be submitted with the scraping. This will allow examination for dermatophytes and mites, as well as the inoculation of agar plates for bacterial and fungal culture.

Abscesses

Collect about 3 ml of purulent material, along with scrapings from the wall of the abscess. Note that the purulent material in the centre of an abscess may yield no bacterial growth.

Blood cultures

Purpose-designed commercial blood culture bottles are available for the isolation of bacteria from blood where bacteraemia is suspected. Special care must be given to the aseptic collection of the blood, with preparation of the site of venipucture as for a surgical procedure. Otherwise, contamination of the sample with bacterial skin flora is likely. Bacteraemias can be intermittent and repeat sampling over a 24-hour period is advisable. Inoculation of the blood culture bottle should be carried out as soon as possible after sampling.

Single or pooled sample

Samples from individual animals are appropriate for confirmation of a clinical diagnosis or in the case of animals to be introduced into a herd. However, cattle are herd animals and it may be more convenient and cheaper to consider using pooled samples. Pooled samples are frequently used to carry out an initial screening of a herd for the presence of an infectious agent. On dairy farms, there is the option to carry out bulk milk tank testing. This provides a crude, but cost-effective, means of assessing a dairy herd for infection without the need to sample a statistically valid number of individuals. Different age or husbandry management groups can be tested separately if a more comprehensive picture of infection status within the herd and the pattern of spread is required. Test sensitivity is reduced in the case of pooled samples, particularly where herd size is large and the dilution effect is large.

Number of samples

The number of animals sampled will vary according to the information that one is trying to glean. In the case of clinical disease investigation, it is always advisable to collect samples from both clinically affected and in-contact animals. Comrade animals may be at an earlier stage in the disease process and, possibly, shedding the causal agent in substantially greater amounts. As a guide, a minimum of three to six animals should be sampled.

In cases where the determination of disease prevalence or the monitoring of disease status is the goal, then the number of samples required from a herd needs to be determined by a sampling strategy designed to take account of herd size, expected prevalence, the precision of the estimate (margin of error) and the desired confidence level. The required sample size is largest when the expected prevalence is 50%, while it is smallest when the expected prevalence is close to either 0 or 100%.

A sampling strategy may be designed at the whole herd level, or it may take account of epidemiologically distinct groups within the herd, such as young female calves reared in isolation. These animals may go on to develop disease as heifers, following introduction to the main dairy herd. The statistical calculations involved assume random selection of the animals to be tested, and it is important that animals are not chosen on the basis of convenience or some other factor that could introduce an inherent bias. Cannon & Roe (1982) provide a very useful and concise reference for guidance on sample numbers. The review article by Van Winden & Pfeiffer (2008) is also helpful.

Diagnostic sample submission

It is important to provide laboratory staff with a context for the sample(s) being submitted. A complete case or herd history, and tentative diagnosis or rationale for the testing, will greatly assist the laboratory personnel in ensuring that the most appropriate test(s) will be applied, and in ensuring that urgent cases are expedited.

Preservation

Frequently samples cannot be processed within a few hours of collection, and there is a delay due to the time required for the sample to reach the laboratory or because of the need to batch samples for testing. Material on plain swabs, or tiny amounts of sample, are liable to desiccation. Where possible, the sample amount collected should be reasonably generous, such as blocks of tissue approximately 2 cm^3, or several millilitres of exudate, pus or faeces.

Samples intended for histopathology should be placed in 10% formalin, while smears to be tested by immunofluorescence need to be air-dried and fixed in acetone or methanol for about ten minutes to preserve antigenicity. At least 5 ml of blood is recommended for serology, to permit sufficient serum for a number of tests to be carried out as necessary, and for a quantity to be stored for future testing.

In general, samples are best stored for short periods at +4°C rather than frozen in a domestic freezer at −20°C, which tends to have a detrimental effect on enveloped viruses. For longer term storage in the laboratory, a −70°C freezer is suitable. Serum should be separated from whole blood prior to storage, as freezing will lyse the erythrocytes. Bacterial specimens for anaerobic culture should be cultured within a few hours of collection, and are best kept at ambient temperature rather than in the refrigerator, as oxygen absorption is increased at lower temperatures. The use of transport media will enhance the survival of bacteria and viruses. It should be noted that bacterial transport medium is not suitable for viruses, while viral transport medium usually contains antibiotics to suppress contaminating bacteria. Specialist transport media are available for fastidious bacteria, such as chlamydiae and mycoplasmas.

Packaging

The United Nations (UN) Economic and Social Council issues the UN Recommendations on the Transport of Dangerous Goods, also known as the Orange Book. These recommendations are implemented by regulatory bodies in each country, such as Transport Canada or the United States Department of Transportation, and they have been adopted by the regulatory organisations responsible for the different transport modes, for example International Air Transport Association (IATA). In the European Union, the relevant regulations are referred to as the ADR (European Agreement for Transportation of Dangerous Goods).

An infectious substance (Hazard Class 6.2) is one which is known, or could be reasonably expected, to contain pathogens. For the purpose of transportation, such substances are categorised as category A or category B, and must be labelled with the appropriate UN identification number. Category A refers to an infectious substance that is capable of causing permanent disability, life-threatening or fatal disease in healthy humans or animals (biohazard level 4 microorganisms). These materials must be sent using a courier. A category B infectious substance does not meet the criteria for category A (in essence, effective treatment and preventive measures are available; biohazard levels 2 and 3 microorganisms). These samples, collected for diagnostic or investigative purposes, are considered to be "diagnostic specimens" and are labelled "category B biological substances UN3373". They must be packaged according to IATA packing instruction P650, which involves a triple packaging system comprising:

- A primary leak-proof container that is labelled and contains the specimen. This container must be wrapped in sufficient absorbent material e.g. cotton wool, to contain all fluid if breakage occurs. Vials with flip top lids should not be used, screw-topped containers are ideal.
- A secondary leak-proof package such as a plastic container or sealable plastic bag.
- Outer shipping package with suitable cushioning material. A padded envelope is usually sufficient for postage while a rigid cardboard box is more suitable for larger or overseas packages.

The outer package must be labelled with the receiver's (consignee) details, the shipper's (consignor) details, a UN3373 label and the words "biological substance", "pathological specimen", or "diagnostic specimen".

Types of tests

Infectious diseases are often diagnosed on the basis of the case history and clinical signs, or following post-mortem and

Table 18.1 Selection of significant infectious diseases of cattle, their aetiology, suggested samples and confirmatory laboratory tests.

Infectious Disease	Aetiology	Suggested samples	Laboratory tests	Comments
Anthrax	*Bacillus anthracis*	Peripheral blood from tail vein	Microscopy: M'Fadyean reaction Culture PCR	Do not open a suspect carcass in case of release of sporulating organism
Blackleg	*Clostridium chauvoei*	Affected muscle	Microscopy: IFAT Culture: anaerobic	Characteristic pathology
Bluetongue	Bluetongue virus (*Reoviridae*)	Heparin blood, spleen, lymph node Serum	RT-PCR Serology	Several species of *Culicoides* suitable as vectors. Infections usually more severe in sheep
Bovine spongiform encephalopathy (BSE)	BSE agent (Prion)	Brain stem	Immunoblotting ELISA Electron microscopy: scrapie-associated fibrils	Confirmation by IHC staining and histopathological examination
Bovine viral diarrhoea (BVD)	BVD virus 1, 2 (*Flaviviridae*)	Ear notch samples Heparin blood: buffy coat Spleen, lymph node, GIT lesions Serum, milk	RT-PCR Antigen detection: ELISA IFAT on cryostat sections Serology	Persistently infected (PI) animals will be seronegative and virus positive
Brucellosis	*Brucella abortus* (*B. melitensis, B. suis*)	Placenta, abomasal contents, uterine discharge Serum, milk	Microscopy Culture PCR Serology	Zoonosis
Calf diarrhoea	Rotavirus *Eschericihia coli* *Cryptosporidium parvum* *Salmonella* Bovine coronavirus	Faeces	Culture RT-PCR Viral antigen detection Microscopy	Stained smears may reveal *Cryptosporidium* while electron microscopy may reveal virus particles. Many of these agents may also be found in faeces of clinically normal calves
Contagious bovine pleuropneumonia	*Mycoplasma mycoides* subsp. *mycoides* (small colony type)	Bronchoalveolar lavage fluid, lung, pleural fluid Serum	Culture PCR Serology	Characteristic pathology
Enzootic bovine leukosis	Bovine leukaemia virus (*Retroviridae*)	Serum	Serology	Pathological examination necessary. High blood lymphocyte counts may be suggestive
Enzootic pneumonia of calves	Bovine respiratory syncytial virus Bovine parainfluenza virus 3 *Mannheimia haemolytica* *Pasteurella multocida* *Trueperella pyogenes* *Histophilus somni* *Mycoplasma bovis* *Mycoplasma dispar*	Bronchoalveolar fluid Guarded nasal swab Lung Serum	Viruses: IFAT RT-PCR Virus isolation Serology Bacteria: culture	Multiple aetiology, multi-factorial. Frequently an initial viral infection is complicated by secondary bacterial involvement
Foot-and-mouth disease (FMD)	FMD virus (*Picornaviridae*)	Vesicle fluid, epithelium Serum	RT-PCR Antigen detection Virus isolation Serology	Characteristic vesicles, salivation, lameness
Heartwater	*Ehrlichia ruminantium*	Brain	Microscopy: Giemsa stained squash preparation PCR	*Amblyomma* species of tick are the main vectors. Characteristic pathology.
Infectious bovine rhinotracheitis (IBR) – Infectious pustular vulvovaginitis (IPV)	Bovine herpesvirus 1 (*Herpesviridae*)	Swabs of eyes, nares, genitalia Fetal tissues Tracheal lesions Serum, milk	PCR Antigen detection: ELISA IFAT on cryostat sections Virus isolation Serology	Wide range of clinical signs including respiratory disease, abortion, nervous disease, vulvovaginitis. Characteristic lesions, viral inclusions
Infectious bovine keratoconjunctivitis	*Moraxella bovis*	Lacrimal secretions	Culture	Very labile organism

Table 18.1 (*continued*)

Infectious Disease	Aetiology	Suggested samples	Laboratory tests	Comments
Joint-ill	*Escherichia coli,* *Mycoplasma bovis* *Staphylococcus aureus* *Streptococcus* species *Trueperella pyogenes*	Joint aspirate	Culture	May be associated with omphalitis or following septicaemia in young calves
Johne's disease	*Mycobacterium avium* subsp. *paratuberculosis*	Rectal scrapings Mucosa at ileocaecal valve, lymph nodes Faeces Serum, milk	Microscopy: acid-fast bacilli (Ziehl Neelsen stain) PCR Culture Serology	Confirmation by pathological examination
Leptospirosis	*Leptospira interrogans* serovars	Urine, kidney Serum	Microscopy: darkfield, IFAT Culture, PCR Serology	Carrier state is common, shedding in urine
Listeriosis	*Listeria monocytogenes* (*L. ivanovii*: abortion only)	Swabs/smears from lesions Affected tissues: liver, spleen Brain, cerebrospinal fluid Placenta, abomasal contents, uterine discharge	Microscopy Culture	Range of forms including neural, septicaemia, abortion, ocular. Histopathological examination of brain is useful in neural form
Lumpy skin disease (LSD)	LSD virus (*Poxviridae*)	Skin lesion material/biopsy Serum	Electron microscopy Antigen detection: ELISA PCR Serology	Generalised skin nodules
Malignant catarrhal fever	Ovine herpesvirus 2 Alcelaphine herpesvirus 1 (*Herpesviridae*)	Heparin blood: buffy coat Affected tissues	PCR	Clinical signs suggestive. Confirmation by histopathological examination
Mastitis	*Staphylococcus aureus* *Escherichia coli* *Steptococcus uberis* *Steptococcus agalactiae* *Steptococcus dysgalactiae*	Milk	Culture	Many other causes including *Mycoplasma bovis*, *Trueperella pyogenes* and fungi
Mycotic abortion	*Aspergillus fumigatus* *Lichtheimia* sp. *Mortierella wolfii* *Rhizopus* sp. *Mucor* sp. *Rhizomucor* sp.	Placenta, abomasal contents	Culture	Histopathological examination is required to confirm invasion of tissues by the fungus
Pyelonephritis	*Corynebacterium renale* group	Urine	Culture	Enlarged kidneys may be felt upon rectal palpation
Pneumonic pasteurellosis	*Mannheimia haemolytica* *Pasteurella multocida* Bovine parainfluenza virus 3	Bronchoalveolar lavage fluid Lung	Culture	Associated with various stressors including transport ('shipping fever')
Rabies	Rabies virus (*Rhabdoviridae*)	Brain	RT-PCR IFAT	Histopathology: non-suppurative encephalitis and viral inclusions (Negri bodies)
Salmonellosis	*Salmonella enterica* serotypes	Faeces	Culture	Numerous serotypes; Typhimurium and Dublin are of particular importance in cattle
Thromboembolic meningoencephalitis	*Histophilus somni*	Cerebrospinal fluid Lesions	Culture	Characteristic pathological lesions
Tuberculosis	*Mycobacterium bovis*	Heparin blood Lymph node, lung, tissue lesions, milk	Gamma interferon assay Culture Microscopy: acid-fast bacilli (Ziehl Neelsen stain)	Cattle may be screened using an intradermal skin test ('tuberculin test')

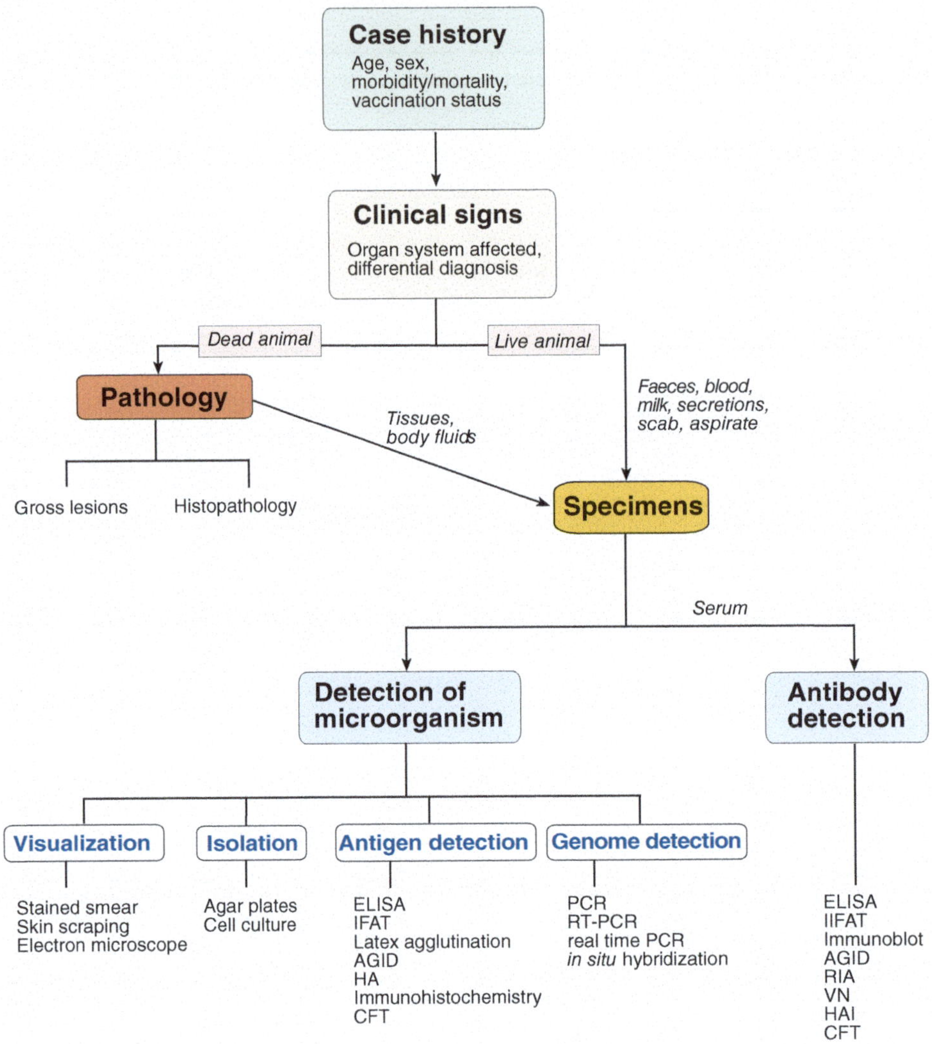

Figure 18.1 Outline of approach to diagnosis of infectious diseases in cattle. AGID agar gel immunodiffusion; CFT complement fixation test; ELISA enzyme-linked immunosorbent assay; HA haemagglutination; HAI haemagglutination inhibition; IFAT immunofluorescent antibody test; IIFAT indirect immunofluorescent antibody test; PCR polymerase chain reaction; RT-PCR reverse transcriptase PCR; RIA radioimmunoassay; VN virus neutralization.

histopathological examination. However, in other cases, the use of confirmatory, laboratory-based diagnostic tests are required (Table 18.1). These laboratory tests fall into two broad categories (Figure 18.1):

- Direct detection of the infectious microorganism.
- Indirect detection of the presence of an infectious organism through evaluation of the immune response of the animals exposed, typically the humoral response (as detected by serological tests).

The choice of the most appropriate test to use in a given situation is important. For example, the testing of bulk milk tank samples for viral-specific antibodies is a good way to identify infected herds. However, animals within an infected herd that are persistently infected (PI) with bovine viral diarrhoea (BVD) virus are immunotolerant to the virus circulating in their bodies and do not produce antibodies. Clearly, a virus detection assay is required to indicate such carrier animals in a herd.

Detection

Visualization of the infectious microorganism in smears, skin scrapings or clarified suspensions/tissue homogenates may be possible, provided large numbers are present in the sample. Staining is used to highlight morphology or particular characteristics such as cell wall type (Gram-stain). Presumptive identification may be possible purely on morphological grounds, or following the use of specific labelled antisera (immunochemistry). An electron microscope is required for visualisation of viruses. Electron microscopy is rapid, but it is a relatively insensitive means of detecting viruses. An increase in sensitivity and specificity can be obtained by using immuno-electron microscopy, which employs antibodies directed against the virus of interest to help concentrate the viral particles onto the copper specimen grid, or to facilitate pelleting by centrifugation.

The detection of key antigens, unique to a particular microbial species, may be accomplished using a variety of formats such as enzyme-linked immunosorbent assay (ELISA), latex agglutination, or immunochromatography. At the heart of these techniques is the use of antibodies directed against antigens specific to the microbial agent in question. In order to visualize the binding of antibody to target antigen, it is necessary to increase the bulk of the antigen : antibody complexes through a latex carrier or, alternatively, to label the antibody with either a fluorochrome dye, such as fluorescein isothiocyanate, or an enzyme such as horseradish peroxidase. The former will fluoresce under particular wavelengths of light, generated and visualised using a special microscope, while the latter will convert a colourless substrate into a coloured product visible to the naked eye. Washing steps are essential in the protocols for all such techniques, in order to ensure removal of unbound antibody and thus avoiding false positive reactions.

Isolation of microbial agents has traditionally been the mainstay of diagnosis and the gold standard against which other diagnostic methods are evaluated. This is still largely the case for bacteria and fungi, but molecular methods have largely supplanted virus isolation as the method of choice. It is relatively inexpensive to culture bacteria and fungi. The inoculation of a standard series of agar plates (typically blood agar, MacConkey agar and Columbia-CNA agar for bacteria; or Sabouraud's dextrose agar for fungi) will permit the isolation of a wide range of bacterial and fungal species. Special selective agars or incubation conditions can be used where particularly fastidious species are suspected.

Once isolated, the particular bacterial or fungal species must be identified, usually on the basis of phenotypic properties or through the sequencing of a conserved gene such as the 16S rRNA gene. A major advantage of isolation is the fact that further analysis, such as antimicrobial susceptibility testing or strain typing, can then be carried out. In contrast, viruses are obligate intracellular pathogens and must be isolated in cell cultures or fertile eggs. This is relatively expensive, particularly in terms of labour. Typically, several cell lines must be continually maintained and diagnostic material passaged a number of times before a result can be given. As a result, there has been a move to employ faster, more specific methods of detection, such as immunohistochemical staining or, increasingly in recent years, genome amplification methods. Proper preservation of samples during transportation, to ensure the microorganism's viability, is essential if isolation is to be successful, whereas organism viability is not necessary for antigen or genome detection.

Nucleic acid amplification techniques are numerous and varied, and the most popular and widely used is polymerase chain reaction (PCR). A PCR assay is essentially a process of DNA copying involving stepwise heating and cooling in a thermal cycler. The three essential steps in each amplification cycle are denaturation of the double stranded DNA, the annealing of short synthetic oligonucleotide primers to specific genome sequences or target sites, and the extension of these primers to form complementary DNA strands. A heat-stable DNA polymerase such as *Taq* polymerase is used to catalyse this primer extension reaction. Typically, each PCR cycle is repeated 30 to 40 times, and the resulting amplified DNA target sequence can then be visualised as a band in an agarose gel following electrophoresis. In order to amplify RNA target sequences, for example to facilitate the detection of RNA viruses, the enzyme reverse transcriptase is first used to produce a complementary strand of DNA (cDNA) before carrying out the PCR assay in the usual way. These assays are referred to as reverse transcriptase PCR (RT-PCR).

Real-time PCR refers to the detection of the progressive accumulation of the amplified DNA target in real time through the detection of fluorescent signal at the end of each cycle. Advantages of real time over conventional PCR include the ability to quantify the initial amount of target sequence present in a sample and the elimination of the electrophoresis step. This saves time and reduces the risk of contamination with amplified product (amplicon), as there is no handling of material post-amplification. The advantages of nucleic acid amplification techniques include exquisite sensitivity, rapid results, small sample size, detection of non-viable or non-culturable microorganisms, and ease of genotyping.

Serological testing

The measurement of humoral responses, the production of antibody, for diagnostic purposes is generally referred to as serology, on account of serum being the most commonly used sample for such purposes. In addition to sample convenience (blood or milk), serological tests are popular because they are less expensive and generally easier to perform than direct detection methods. Antibodies usually appear in the blood (IgM initially, followed by a larger IgG response) from about seven days post-exposure, peaking at 10–14 days. This is termed the primary response. The generation of memory B lymphocytes means that further exposure to the same antigen results in an anamnestic response, whereby antibodies appear within two to three days and titres rise to much higher levels than during the primary response.

Following dilution and testing of the sample, the serological titre is defined as the highest dilution giving a demonstrable effect. Several assay formats can be used to detect the binding of antibody in the sample to the antigen used in the assay. The detection of the resulting immune complex can be through a biological effect (virus neutralisation or haemagglutination inhibition), or through a physical effect (precipitation, complement fixation). However, the most common detection method involves the use of labelled anti-species antibodies. The label used may be an enzyme (enzyme-linked immunosorbent assay, immunoblotting), a radioisotope (radioimmunoassay) or a fluorochrome (immunofluorescent antibody test, IFAT).

Serological tests are an invaluable means of screening animals for exposure to infectious agents as part of a herd investigation, or in order to determine those infectious agents circulating on a farm. The testing of single samples is usually suitable for animal screening, on account of the long periods that antibody titres tend to remain elevated following exposure. However, a single serological result provides little information as to the timing of infection. In theory, the detection of IgM will indicate recent exposure but, in practice, IgM assays have not always proven as reliable as testing paired samples to determine a rising titre of IgG.

The first sample (acute sample) should be obtained as early as possible following the onset of infection. The subsequent sample (convalescent sample) should be obtained 3–4 weeks later. A fourfold or greater rise in antibody titre is indicative of recent, active infection. The main drawback is that the resulting confirmation of a clinical diagnosis is retrospective and, although it may be too late to influence the treatment of the affected animal, the information may be of great usefulness in future control.

Interpretation of laboratory test results

An accurate diagnosis requires the consideration of both clinical and laboratory data. The quality of the dialogue between the veterinary practitioner and laboratory staff will greatly influence the effectiveness of the process. The wrong conclusion, in terms of an animal's true disease status, can be reached if a laboratory test result is relied on solely, without consideration of the clinical signs and the pathological changes.

The isolation of certain infectious agents is not always significant *per se*. There are numerous examples of opportunist pathogens whose presence alone is not sufficient to confirm a diagnosis. In some cases, the quantity of microorganism detected ("pure, heavy growth" of a particular bacterial species) may be of some significance, or the presence of known virulence factors, such as the enterocyte attaching and effacing (*eae*) gene of certain strains of *Escherichia coli*. The presence of some microorganisms can be explained as contamination of samples or post-mortem invasion.

The history of a case may also have a significant bearing on the interpretation of a particular test result. For example, prior use of antibiotics or of vaccines may help to rule out certain infectious causes. On the other hand, their use will certainly affect the results of diagnostic tests, in terms of bacterial isolation and serological titres, respectively. A negative test result does not necessarily confirm that the infectious agent suspected of involvement is not the aetiological agent. Reasons for a negative result could include cessation of shedding, intermittent shedding, loss of viability, degradation of sample, poor test sensitivity and inappropriate sample.

Interpretation of serology

Various factors influence antibody production following exposure to an infectious agent, including agent factors (antigenicity, route of exposure, amount) and animal factors (age, immune status). In addition, there are sample factors (sample type, quality of sample) and test factors (assay format, antigen used, sensitivity, specificity) which will all influence the titres obtained.

In general, serological tests do not distinguish between antibody titres induced following infection from those obtained following vaccination or as a result of the passive transfer of maternal antibody through colostrum. There are a few serological tests that can distinguish between vaccinates and infected animals, known as DIVA (differentiate infected from vaccinated animals) tests. An example of such a test is the ELISA used to detect antibodies to glycoprotein E (gE) of infectious bovine rhinotracheitis (IBR) virus. This test can discriminate between the antibody response produced following vaccination with IBR virus marker vaccine and the antibody response produced following natural infection. This is possible because the virus used in the associated marker vaccine lacks a surface glycoprotein (gE), and therefore induces an antibody response lacking in antibodies specific to this particular glycoprotein.

Sensitivity/specificity

Laboratory diagnostic tests are not perfect; no test is 100% sensitive and specific. Ideally, tests with high sensitivity and specificity characteristics should be employed. However, such tests are not always available, and it is important to understand these and related terms in order to understand the limitations of test results correctly. The sensitivity of a test is a measure of the test's ability to give a positive result when the animal is diseased (i.e. the proportion of animals with the disease that give a positive result). The specificity of a test is a measure of the test's ability to give a negative result when the animal is not diseased (i.e. the proportion of animals free of disease that give a negative result). For a given test, the sensitivity and specificity are usually inversely related. The relationship between a test result and the true disease status of an animal is illustrated in Table 18.2.

For clinicians, the predictive value (validity) of a test is of more relevance than its sensitivity or specificity. The predictive value of a positive test is high where the prevalence of the disease in a population is high. However, in the course of control programs where the disease prevalence is being reduced and the incidence of false positives in the population remains unchanged, the predictive value of a positive result declines. Even very good

Table 18.2 Relationship between test result and health status.

	Health Status	
	Diseased	Not diseased
Test Positive	a	b
Test Negative	c	d

N (total population) = a + b + c + d
a: true positives
b: false positives
c: false negatives
d: true negatives
Sensitivity of test = a/(a + c)
Specificity of test = d/(b + d)
Predictive value of a positive test = a/(a + b)
Predictive value of a negative test = d/(c + d)

tests will falsely designate a few animals as positive in a healthy population.

Conclusion

Microbiological laboratory testing is an extremely powerful and useful tool when interpreted in the light of the case history, the clinical signs, the pathogenesis of the disease and the characteristics of the test being used. An understanding of the principles underpinning sample collection and laboratory tests will greatly assist veterinary practitioners in getting the most from this essential adjunct to the clinical diagnosis of infectious diseases of cattle.

References

Cannon, R.M. and Roe, R.T. (1982). Livestock Disease Surveys. *A Field Manual for Veterinarians.* Bureau of Resource Science, Department of Primary Industry. Australian Government Publishing Service, Canberra.

UN Recommendations on the Transport of Dangerous Goods. Model Regulations (15th edition), New York and Geneva: United Nations, 2007, ISBN 978-92-1-139120-6, ST/SG/AC.10/1/Rev.15

Van Winden, S. and Pfeiffer, D. (2008). Sampling programs to establish and monitor the infectious disease status of cattle herds. *In Practice* **30**, 30–35.

Further reading

Burr, P. and Snodgrass, D. (2004). Demystifying diagnostic testing: serology. *In Practice* **26**(9), 498–502.

Jones, P. (2001). Bovine paratuberculosis: ongoing challenges, renewed concerns. *In Practice* **23**(7), 402–411.

Otter, A. and Cranwell, M. (2007). Differential diagnosis of diarrhoea in adult cattle. *In Practice* **29**, 9–19.

Paxson, J. (2008). Polymerase chain reaction test interpretation. *Compendium: Continuing Education for Veterinarians May:* 186–196.

Pierce-Hendry, S.A. and Dennis J. (2010). Bacterial culture and antibiotic susceptibility testing. *Compendium: Continuing Education for Veterinarians* **32**(7) E1–E6.

Pritchard, G. (2001). Milk antibody testing in cattle. *In Practice* **23**(9) 542–549.

Yeary, T.J. and Kapil, S. (2004a). A primer on diagnostic virology: specimen selection and serology. *Compendium: Continuing Education for Veterinarians August:* 646–658.

Yeary, T.J. and Kapil, S. (2004b). A primer on diagnostic virology: direct and molecular-based detection of viral pathogens. *Compendium: Continuing Education for Veterinarians, September:* 730–740.

CHAPTER 19

Epidemiology: the Important Concepts

Michael P. Reichel

Learning objectives

- Understand basic, yet important terms of veterinary epidemiology.
- Know the difference between analytical, and diagnostic sensitivity and specificity.
- Understand the impact of prevalence on test performance.
- Be able to use Fagan's Nomogram.
- Understand important measures of association.
- Be able to establish appropriate sample sizes for testing.

Introduction

Quite often in veterinary, and also in cattle practice, we rely on support from the diagnostic and laboratory services. The interpretation of these test results is not always straight forward, and an appreciation of some of the basic epidemiological principles can be useful. The following chapter works through some important (yet quite simple) concepts that a bovine practitioner might encounter through their daily work. A glossary of the basic terms, formula for calculation and definition is provided at the end of this chapter.

Diagnostic test evaluation

A lot of the work of the bovine practitioner relies on diagnosing the problem/condition/ disease at hand with accuracy and confidence. Diagnostic sensitivity (DSe) describes the ability of a test (laboratory-based or otherwise) to detect a target condition/disease. When DSe is first established for a diagnostic test we need to know the true status of the animals (by use of a reference or 'gold' standard), and are assessing how good the test is at being a proxy to the true disease/infection status. For example

Table 19.1 Diagnostic sensitivity (DSe) and diagnostic specificity (DSp) of a test.

		Disease		
		Diseased	Not diseased	Total
Test	Positive	10	20	30
	Negative	30	40	70
		40	60	100
		DSe = 0.25	DSp = 0.66	

(refer to Table 19.1), if a test detects ten out of a total of 40 diseased animals, the test identified a quarter of the truly affected animals as infected/diseased, DSe is therefore 0.25 or 25%.

Generally, we also want to know how good a test is at identifying non-diseased animals, a term that is called diagnostic specificity (DSp). In our example in Table 19.1, the test has 40 out of 60 animals correctly identified as non-diseased – therefore, DSp equals 0.66 or 66%. DSe and DSp should not be confused with the analytical sensitivity and specificity. The analytical sensitivity is the ability of a test to detect a condition, or an analyte, down to a certain level (e.g. the ability to detect one persistently infected milking cow with bovine virus diarrhoea virus (BVDv) in a milk sample taken from a bulk tank with contributions from 500 lactating cows). The analytical specificity is the ability of the assay to distinguish the disease or analyte in question from similar ones (e.g. the ability to distinguish between the closely related pestiviruses, BVDv and Border disease (McFadden *et al.*, 2012)).

In a 2 × 2 contingency table (refer to Table 19.1), we are looking at the performance of the test down the columns of the table for the values of DSp and DSe. In real life, however, practitioners are given a test result and do not know the true infection/disease status of the animal. The test result comes as a proxy for the true disease status, but the test results are made up of true positives or negatives (test agrees with the true status of the animal) and false test results (test results and status do not agree for either

Bovine Medicine, Third Edition. Edited by Peter D. Cockcroft.

Table 19.2a Predictive values of a test result with a disease prevalence of 40%.

		Disease			
		Diseased	Not diseased	Total	Predictive values (PV)
Test	Positive	10	20	30	PV+ = 10/30 = 0.33
	Negative	30	40	70	PV − = 40/70 = 0.57
		0.25	0.66	100	

Table 19.2b Predictive values of a test result with a disease prevalence of 4%.

		Disease			
		Diseased	Not diseased	Total	Predictive values (PV)
Test	Positive	10	320	30	PV+ = 10/330 = 0.03
	Negative	30	640	670	PV − = 40/670 = 0.96
		0.25	0.66	1000	

Table 19.2c Predictive values of a test result with a disease prevalence of 80%.

		Disease			
		Diseased	Not diseased	Total	Predictive values (PV)
Test	Positive	20	7	27	PV+ = 20/27 = 0.74
	Negative	60	13	73	PV − = 13/73 = 0.18
		0.25	0.65	100	

positive or negative animals). Here, we start looking at the so called 'predictive values' of the test. The predictive value is the probability of the status of the animal (has the disease, does not have the disease), given a test result. The predictive value allows the clinician to interpret the test diagnostically.

If we again go to a 2 ×2 contingency table (refer to Table 19.2a) and fill that with data, we are now looking along the rows for the value of the predictive value parameters. Thus, using the same example as previously, now in Table 19.2a, only a third (10) of the 30 test-positives are actually truly diseased, and only 57% of the non-diseased animals come up negative in the test.

Predictive values, however, are dependent on the prevalence of the condition in a studied population. In the previous example, our disease had a reasonably high prevalence of 40% (10 + 30 diseased animals out of a total of 100; Table 19.2a), but let us look at an example where the prevalence drops to just 4% in Table 19.2b.

As the prevalence falls from 40% to 4%, the predictive value of a positive test result falls as well; only 3% of test positive animals are now truly diseased. At the same time, however, the predictive value of a negative test result has dramatically improved, from 57% to 96% (i.e. we are now 39% more confident that a negative test result comes from a non-diseased animal). This situation is often encountered in disease eradication programmes where, as the prevalence of disease falls with eradication, the test appear to be less accurate and the reactors identified by testing appear to consist of more and more false-positives (now you know why).

The same is true in reverse. If the prevalence of the condition is much higher, we are then more confident in a positive test result than in a negative test result. This is illustrated in Table 19.2c, with an increase in the prevalence of disease to 80%. Here, the positive predictive value increases (we are more confident that a positive test result comes from a diseased animal), and the negative predictive value has dropped to 18%. All the while, the test characteristics have not changed; DSe and DSp are still as originally described.

In simple terms, the probability of picking a diseased animal out of a pool with lots of diseased animals (high prevalence situation), regardless of the test performance, is higher than in a pool that has few diseased individuals (low prevalence situation). The problem with many publications on diagnostic test performance is that they often state predictive values for the tests without acknowledging that the prevalence of the condition being tested for might vary considerably, depending on the population/situation in which the test is being used (so one should be wary of papers that state predictive values without any reference to the prevalence in the target population).

One way around this is to use *Likelihood ratios* associated with diagnostic tests. This measure of the test performance is independent of prevalence, and it allows pre-test probability (prevalence) to be easily converted into post-test probability. In addition, the strength of ratio also gives an indication of how much the particular test improves the post-test probability, the further away from 1 and the higher the values for the *LRs*, the bigger the contribution of the test.

In the example used here (Figure 19.1), a test with a positive likelihood ratio of 10 improves post-test probability over the pre-test probability (prevalence) by a factor of ten. The equation can also be put into a diagram (see below) and can be visually solved – the whole construct being called 'Fagan's Nomogram' (Caraguel & Vanderstichel, 2013). Choosing test thresholds based on likelihood ratios can be used effectively to improve test performance (Reichel *et al.*, 1999).

Quantitative assessments

It would be just too simple if Koch's principles applied themselves consistently throughout our diagnostic approaches and all animals (and only those) that are infected with a particular pathogen develop the disease – or all animals, and only those, that are exposed to a particular risk, develop a certain condition. In most diagnostic situations, however, we see some overlap (i.e. not all animals exposed to the causative agent develop the condition, and some others that had no exposure also do so).

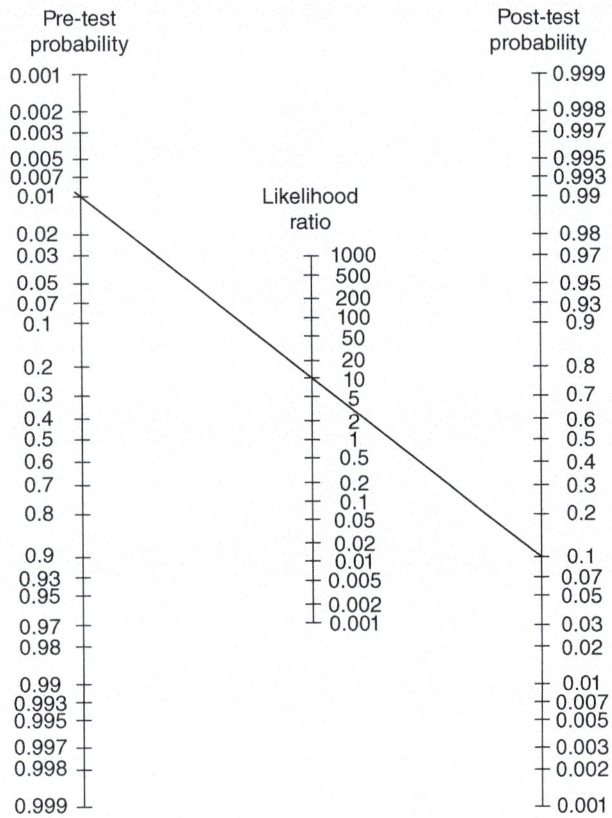

Figure 19.1 Likelihood ratio.

Infection in cattle with *Neospora caninum* might be a good example; it is a cause of mid-gestation abortion, but not all infected cattle abort – in fact, abortion as an outcome is probably the exception, rather than the rule. Many chronically infected dams pass their *N caninum* infection on to the offspring via vertical transmission *in utero*, and a clinically unaffected calf is born (Dubey *et al.*, 2007). In order to be able to tease out whether *N caninum* was causally involved with an abortion outbreak, we may have to employ the use of a 2 × 2 contingency table again and calculate the quantitative contribution that *N caninum* made to the abortion outbreak. We will use an example that has already been published previously from an abortion outbreak in a larger dairy herd in New Zealand (Pfeiffer *et al.*, 2002). This herd experienced an abortion outbreak of epidemic proportions and, over a period of three months, approximately 70 cows and heifers aborted. Serology was performed for a variety of things, but we just want to focus on the ELISA results carried for specific anti-*N caninum* antibodies. The data is presented in Table 19.3a.

Not all animals that had *N. caninum* antibodies aborted; in fact, only 61/481 (12.5%) did. However, some cows that were negative for *N. caninum* antibodies also aborted, although fewer of them, compared to the first group (9/263 (3.4%)). The first

Table 19.3a A 2 × 2 contingency table of abortions and *Neospora caninum* ELISA test results.

		Abortion			
		Diseased	Not diseased	Total	
N caninum ELISA	Positive	61	420	481	$R_{e+} = 0.125$
	Negative	9	257	263	$R_{e-} = 0.034$
		70	677	747	

Relative Risk = Re+/Re− = 0.125/0.034 = 3.7

percentage the epidemiologists call the risk (of abortion in the exposed), Risk $_{\text{Exposed}}$ (R_{e+}), the latter the Risk $_{\text{Unexposed}}$ (R_{e-}). R_{e+} divided by R_{e-} gives us the relative risk, a measure of the strength of the contribution of *N. caninum* status to the risk of abortion (i.e. cows that are *Neospora* positive are more than three times more likely to abort). This value actually agrees extremely well with the published literature, which suggests that *N* caninum-infected cattle are, on average, three times more likely to abort than uninfected ones (Moen *et al.*, 1998).

Another important quantitative measure is the *risk difference*, or *attributable risk* (AR; $R_{e+} - R_{e-}$), which tells us that, out of the 12.5% of aborting cows, 9.1% (12.5% − 3.4%) were attributable to *N. caninum* and the remainder due to other causes (or the 'normal' background of a range of causes that may terminate a pregnancy). Expressed as a fraction $\left(\frac{9.1\%}{12.5\%}\right)$, this gives us the *attributable fraction*, telling us that just on three-quarters of the abortions (72.8%) that we observed in this herd are due to *N. caninum* (Table 19.3b).

Another measure of the strength of an association between a putative causal agent and the outcome is the odds ratio, very similar to the relative risk, which is calculated by multiplying and dividing across the 2 × 2 contingency table (see Table 19.3c). The odds ratio gives the factor by which the pre-test probability is multiplied to get the post-test probability for a given test result. The higher the odds ratio, the higher will be the post-test probability. In this case, the odds ratio is 4.15 for a positive test result. This parameter is independent of the prevalence.

For most of those calculations, there are online calculators or apps available that also automatically offer to calculate the 95% confidence intervals (CI) for the abovementioned quantitative measures – if the 95% CI includes 1 (i.e. the lower limit of the interval drops below 1), this would suggest that the effect is not statistically significant.

Sampling

Frequently, a practitioner is called out and asked to investigate a condition/disease in a herd. Statistical approaches can be used to optimise the use of financial resources when sampling a herd or group within the herd, so you do not take more than the necessary number of samples (and waste the client's money), or

Table 19.3b Risk, relative risk, attributable risk and attributable fraction.

		Abortion						
		Diseased	Not diseased	Total	Risk	Relative risk	AR	AF
N. caninum ELISA	Positive	61	420	481	0.125	3.67	0.091	0.728
	Negative	9	257	263	0.034	(0.125 ÷ 0.034)	(0.125–0.034)	(0.091 ÷ 0.125)
		70	677	747				

Table 19.3c Odds ratios.

		Abortion			
		Diseased	Not diseased	Total	
N caninum ELISA	Positive	61	420	481	OR = (61x257/(9x420) = 4.15
	Negative	9	257	263	
		70	677	747	

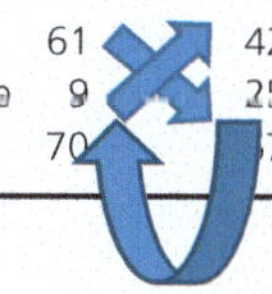

not enough (and risk missing the condition and not making a diagnosis).

Two main considerations drive the number to sample. The first is the need to identify the presence of disease if, it is in fact, occurring, so the sampling must have sufficient *power*. By convention, the value for *power* is often set at 0.8 (i.e. the study design has a 20% chance of missing the condition, even if it is there).

The second consideration is to be sure that any observed presence has not occurred by chance, that the result is statistically significant, and frequently a value of $p = 0.05$ is assumed (i.e. we allow for a 5% chance occurrence of the event).

Table 19.4 Listing of commonly required sample sizes.

Target prevalence (%)	Confidence level	
	95%	99%
1	298	458
5	59	90
10	29	44
20	14	21
30	9	14
40	6	10
50	5	7

Sampling for disease

If we sample a population for the presence (or absence) of a particular condition or disease, we want to test a sufficient number of animals to be sure that we detect it when the condition is truly present (or absent). A target prevalence is often assumed (or taken from previous reports or the literature) – for example, we make an assumption about the level of disease that we want to detect, or we expect to find. As an example, in *N. caninum* infected herds that experience outbreaks of abortion, the within-herd prevalence of infection (i.e. the percentage of individual cattle in the herd infected with the parasite) is often reported to be about 30%.

Thus, if we wanted to be sure that we detected a herd that had *N. caninum* infected individuals, we would want to know how many animals we have to test to determine whether a herd is either *Neospora* infected or free from the disease.

There are various calculators available online, and some are now also available as apps for smartphones. They will calculate that, if we wanted to be 95% confident about our result, we would have to sample nine animals (at random) to detect at least one positive. The size of the population we test from makes very little difference to the calculated result, as the assumed (30%) prevalence (i.e. the probability of being infected) is the driver for the calculation. The level of confidence required is also a driver, higher confidence (99% versus 95%) requiring a larger number of samples to be taken. Table 19.4 gives sample sizes for different levels, prevalence and confidence.

Conclusion

A basic understanding of epidemiological concepts can help direct and shape the diagnostic pathway in cattle practice investigations. For example, appreciating the relationship between the DSe and DSp of a test, and the impact of the disease prevalence on the predictive value of a test result, are important concepts. Equally, quantitative assessments give a measure (of the strength) of the association (but not necessarily yet 'causation') between certain risk factors and the probability of a condition occurring.

Effective sampling in the diagnosis of diseases in cattle practice is cost-effective and ensures that, within defined statistical boundaries, the sample size has the 'power' to be confident that the conditions in question are not missed.

References

Literature cited

Caraguel, C.G. and Vanderstichel, R. (2013). The two-step Fagan's nomogram: *ad hoc* interpretation of a diagnostic test result without calculation. *Evidence-Based Medicine* **18**, 125–128.

Dubey, J.P., Schares, G. and Ortega-Mora, L.M. (2007). Epidemiology and control of neosporosis and *Neospora caninum*. *Clinical Microbiology Reviews* **20**, 323–367.

McFadden, A., Tisdall, D., Hill, F., Otterson, P., Pulford, D., Peake, J., Finnegan, C., La Rocca, S., Kok-Mun, T. and Weir, A. (2012). The first case of a bull persistently infected with Border disease virus in New Zealand. *New Zealand Veterinary Journal* **60**, 290–296.

Moen, A.R., Wouda, W., Mul, M.F., Graat, E.A. and van Werven, T. (1998). Increased risk of abortion following *Neospora caninum* abortion outbreaks: a retrospective and prospective cohort study in four dairy herds. *Theriogenology* **49**, 1301–1309.

Pfeiffer, D.U., Williamson, N.B., Reichel, M.P., Wichtel, J.J. and Teague, W.R. (2002). A longitudinal study of *Neospora caninum* infection on a dairy farm in New Zealand. *Preventive Veterinary Medicine* **54**, 11–24.

Reichel, M.P., Ross, G., Drake, J. and Jowett, J.H. (1999). Performance of an enzyme-linked immunosorbent assay for the diagnosis of *Brucella ovis* infection in rams. *New Zealand Veterinary Journal* **47**, 71–74.

Further reading

A simple, but comprehensive introduction:

Pfeiffer, D. (2009). *Veterinary Epidemiology: An Introduction*. ISBN: 978-1-4051-7694-1, Wiley-Blackwell.

Slightly more advanced:

Smith, R.D. (2005). *Veterinary Clinical Epidemiology*, 3rd Edition. ISBN: 978-0849315664. CRC Press.

Link to online calculators

http://itunes.apple.com/us/app/epical/id557537942?mt=8&ign-mpt=uo%3D4

Glossary

2 × 2 contingency table and terminology, formulae and definition of commonly used epidemiological terms:

		Disease		
		Diseased	Not diseased	Total
Test	Positive	a	b	a + b
	Negative	c	d	c + d
		a + c	b + d	a + b + c + d

Term	Formula	Definition
(Diagnostic) sensitivity	$\left(\frac{a}{a+c}\right)$	Proportion of truly diseased animals that test positive
(Diagnostic) specificity	$\left(\frac{d}{b+d}\right)$	Proportion of non-diseased animals that test negative
Positive predictive value (PPV)	$\left(\frac{a}{a+b}\right)$	Proportion of test-positives that are actually diseased
Negative predictive value (NPV)	$\left(\frac{d}{c+d}\right)$	Proportion of test negatives that are not diseased
Prevalence (pre-test probability)	$\left(\frac{a+c}{a+b+c+d}\right)$	Proportion of diseased animals in the population
Likelihood ratio positive (LR+)	$(Sensitivity/(1-Specificity))$	Likelihood of a positive test result/signifies the strength of a positive test result with disease.
Likelihood ratio negative (LR−)	$((1-Sensitivity)/Specificity)$	Likelihood of a positive test result/signifies the strength of a positive test result with disease.

CHAPTER 20

Biosecurity

Wayne Boardman

Learning objectives

- Define biosecurity, bio-containment and bio-exclusion.
- Describe the components of biosecurity at the international, national, regional and farm level.
- Define the basic components of risk assessment in the biosecurity context.
- Describe the use of risk analysis techniques for making sound biosecurity decisions.
- Define the benefits of a farm biosecurity plan.
- Describe the important components of a farm biosecurity plan.

Introduction

Biosecurity has attracted significant attention in recent years, prompted in part by high-profile global movement of exotic diseases such as foot and mouth disease, bluetongue and besnoitia, the emergence of new diseases such as bovine spongiform encephalopathy and Schmallenberg virus, and the continuing impact of existing infectious diseases (Enticott *et al.*, 2012).

According to Waage & Mumford (2008), there is a broad consensus that biosecurity is growing in importance owing to globalisation and, specifically, due to growing trade, travel, transportation and tourism – the 'four Ts'.

Globally, the World Organisation for Animal Health (OIE) leads the way in standard-setting on the international field when it comes to infectious disease management. Nationally, each country has its own systems of mitigating opportunities for trans-boundary diseases to take hold and also to manage and control endemic and exotic diseases. Regionally, there are specific measures which are important locally. At the farm level, the costs to farmers of a specific infectious disease being introduced to a herd free of the disease can be considerable, in some instances meaning the difference between a good living and bankruptcy.

This chapter will explore the definition of cattle biosecurity and how it is achieved at the global, national and regional levels, and highlights the importance of including biosecurity within a health management plan to minimise the impact of infectious diseases on any cattle property effectively and efficiently. A checklist will be provided as an *aide memoire* for farmers and veterinarians when developing a farm biosecurity plan (FBP).

What is biosecurity?

According to Beale (2008), national biosecurity is the protection of the economy, environment and human health from the negative impacts associated with the entry, establishment or spread of exotic pests and diseases. While robust response arrangements should be in place to combat outbreaks, preventing pest and disease incursions in the first place should remain a priority.

At the farm level, biosecurity can be described as the set of precautions taken to minimise the risk of introducing and spreading an infectious disease within an animal population.

Biosecurity in relation to cattle enterprises can be defined as a set of management practices to prevent the introduction of disease and pathogens to the herd, and control their spread within the herd, with the ultimate aim of minimising damage to the health or productivity of a herd or the safety and quality of food products. Commercial herds can never be totally biosecure, but major biosecurity risks can be managed to minimise the risk of disease entering the herd (Sibley, 2010).

Within this paradigm are two specific biosecurity terms coined today. 'Bio-containment' refers to efforts to control the spread of disease within a herd. The control of any existing disease depends on limiting the spread of the disease and

Bovine Medicine, Third Edition. Edited by Peter D. Cockcroft.

minimising its impact on herd health, welfare and productivity (Sibley, 2010). 'Bio-exclusion' refers to efforts to prevent disease from entering the herd. Both are essential components of an effective biosecurity system.

Infectious disease can threaten all cattle herds even in the most economically sustainable establishments. Farmers and veterinarians need to be aware that a disease incursion can occur at any time and have devastating effects.

Biosecurity at the global level

At the global level, The World Organisation for Animal Health (OIE; http://www.oie.int/) is an intergovernmental organisation with a mandate from its 178 member countries and territories to improve animal health, disease and welfare throughout the world.

The OIE develops standards and guidelines according to the Sanitary and Phytosanitary Agreement of the World Trade Organisation and for use by its member countries, to protect themselves against incursions of diseases or pathogens during trade in animals and animal products, while avoiding unjustified sanitary barriers.

It is responsible for ensuring transparency of the animal disease situation worldwide and for training and producing appropriate material and human resources, especially for developing countries.

OIE Members have a legal obligation to report their animal disease situation, including zoonoses, in a timely and transparent manner. In order to help members fulfil this duty, the OIE has developed the World Animal Health Information System and the World Animal Health Information Database. These tools improve the transparency, efficiency and speed with which global animal health information is disseminated throughout the world.

Biosecurity at the national level – border protection

National biosecurity is important for preventing and then managing the incursion of trans-boundary diseases of economic importance. National, regional and local layers of biosecurity all help protect the health of a cattle herd, with the strength of each layer determining the overall biosecurity of the herd and the country. There are some particularly infectious diseases that cannot be readily or practically prevented at a local level, and these rely on a more communal national strategic approach to biosecurity.

Effective border protection requires a large investment in infrastructure, including high quality diagnostic laboratories and laboratory technicians, well-trained, knowledgeable and experienced personnel, and effective systems. Comprehensive Import Risk Analyses (IRAs) allow for the safe importation of animals and their by-products, and is based on a standardised risk analysis framework.

In order to have an effective nationally directed disease outbreak response capability, it is important to be properly prepared. This requires substantial commitment, experienced personnel, education programs and communication systems. Emergency disease preparedness can include manuals and planning meetings, but one of the most effective ways is to undertake simulation exercises, which are intended to test and improve national capability and readiness to deal with an outbreak of a trans-boundary disease.

Building on this preparedness, effective animal health surveillance is essential for early detection and warning of infectious disease incursions. Surveillance strategies are reviewed regularly, depending on the changes in the disease landscape.

An effective means of reducing the transmission of endemic infectious diseases, which can be centrally or regionally coordinated, is to formulate assurance health programs, accreditation standards or health certification standards to assist primary producers in developing disease-free status farms. This, of course, only holds true if the property complies with the biosecurity measures for the duration of the program.

Once the domain of many governments, the longstanding financial support and strategic direction of animal disease management is increasingly being devolved to farmers and landowners (Enticott *et al.*, 2012).

Biosecurity at the regional level

The risk of transmission of disease on occasions when animals are gathered from different places is high. Impromptu exchange of animals outside markets contributed significantly to the spread of foot and mouth disease outbreak in 2001. In order to curb this, recent legislation in the UK (http://animalhealth.defra.gov.uk/managing-disease/gatherings.html) has sought to reduce the risk of disease transmission at animal gatherings such as markets, shows and exhibitions, and onward consignment where a licence is required. The new regime sets standards of cleansing and disinfection, the time a premise can be open to hold a gathering, and guidance on best practice at livestock markets.

Biosecurity can also be managed at a regional level to maintain the health status of groups of animals or herds within a specific geographic area. The movement controls imposed on animals moving between areas within the UK, for example, to reduce the risks of spreading bovine tuberculosis, is an example of regional risk management.

Regional disease control programmes require regional biosecurity, including movement controls and specific risk management measures that protect the status of the region. There is potential to establish regional disease control programs within the country, which will include biosecurity management between zones of different disease status.

Regionally, local jurisdictions play an important part in education, training and emergency preparedness, and it will often be the regional staff on the ground who will be at the forefront of outbreak response and disease management.

Biosecurity at the farm level – farm biosecurity plans

Benefits of a farm biosecurity plan

Recently, there have been several research papers which have investigated why farmers do not incorporate the principles of biosecurity on their farms (Heffernan *et al.*, 2008; Gunn *et al.*, 2008; Benjamin *et al.*, 2010; Brennan & Christley, 2012). Some of the reasons cited include cost (in time and money), lack of proven efficacies of practices and lack of relevant education of veterinary surgeons, producers and other herd health specialists (Brennan & Christley, 2012).

In the wake of the foot and mouth outbreak in the UK in 2001, bovine tuberculosis was introduced into regions previously unaffected by the disease, such as Cumbria and parts of Scotland (Holliman, 2003). An increase in endemic diseases such as BVD, IBR and Johne's disease was also reported, which may have reflected poor biosecurity practices in place on these farms (Holliman, 2003). Holliman (2003) concluded that many of the problems encountered could have been prevented or minimised with planning and discussion with the local veterinarian.

Veterinarians surveyed in a study by Gunn *et al.* (2008) in the UK did not see themselves as the primary providers of biosecurity information to farmers. The veterinarians viewed the main constraints to be: farmers were not willing to or could not afford to, invest in biosecurity; they shared their clients' scepticism on the efficacy and practicality of biosecurity measures; and they felt they did not have the resources or expertise to provide biosecurity support to their clients (Gunn *et al.*, 2008).

The main obstacles to the implementation of improved farm biosecurity have to be overcome at farm level, and the responsibility for this ultimately must rest with the farmer and their veterinary advisors. It is suggested that improved decision support tools, which make the benefits of improved biosecurity more apparent, are needed. Research into the real efficacy of a range of potential biosecurity measures would also be required to convince veterinarians (Gunn *et al.*, 2008).

However, absolute data to demonstrate the measurable benefits of effective biosecurity management are becoming more available. Work in the Netherlands has shown that there are significant economic benefits of a closed dairy herd a closed dairy herd with good biosecurity, the main benefits being better fertility and reduced culling rates (Van Schaik *et al.*, 1998).

In the USA, Johne's disease-positive herds experienced an economic loss of almost US$ 100 per cow (at 1999 levels), when compared to Johne's disease-negative herds due to reduced milk production and increased cow-replacement costs. Averaged across all herds, Johne's disease cost the US dairy industry, in reduced productivity, US$ 22–27 per cow or US$ 200–250 million annually in 1999 (Ott *et al.*, 1999).

The combined direct and indirect costs of an outbreak of bovine viral diarrhoea in an Australian dairy herd of 320 milking cows were estimated to be $AUD 144,700 (Lanyon *et al.*, 2012). Costs incurred were due to production losses (calves, milk), the need to replace cows, the veterinary costs related to diagnostic testing, and the losses incurred from secondary infections. The indirect costs, primarily related to an increased incidence of mastitis, exceeded the direct costs (Lanyon *et al.*, 2012).

Incursion of an infectious disease onto a farm can have an effect on individual animal health and welfare, and can have long-term impacts on reproduction, longevity, behaviours and population viability. Subclinical and chronic diseases can exert their effects for years and even decades. Ill health, death and reproductive failure in collection animals leads to greater costs (husbandry, veterinary, acquisition), and reduces the financial viability of the farm as a business. The social consequences of managing disease outbreaks should also not be underestimated.

The implementation of biosecurity on cattle farms can only serve to improve cow health, welfare and productivity. Encouraged by the economic benefits of infectious disease control, limited resources can be directed at the most appropriate biosecurity procedures to good effect and can help to achieve the aspirations and objectives of a herd health plan (Sibley, 2010).

It is important that veterinarians develop strong working relationships with farmers, and encourage them to see the improved benefit of a sound biosecurity plan which is part of an over arching herd health plan, including calving management, breeding management, nutrition and productivity targets for the farm.

Assessing and prioritising the level of risk

In order to develop an effective biosecurity plan, veterinarians need to be able to follow a risk analysis process, consisting of risk identification, risk assessment, risk communication and risk management, which has been the standard method underpinning international plant and animal biosecurity for some time (Waage & Mumford, 2008).

A biosecurity plan ideally should be implemented using a risk-analysis approach that assesses the risk of introducing disease, consequences of introduction (e.g. economic, reputation, labour), cost of a mitigation program, and effectiveness of the mitigation program (amount of risk is decreased). Adequate understanding of the epidemiology and ecology of particular disease agents is necessary in order to strategically manage the issues (Sanderson, 2009).

A specific approach used commonly is the hazard analysis and critical control points (HACCP) system (Villaroel *et al.*, 2007). The HACCP system is a risk-assessment approach that focuses on manageable risk factors identified as critical control points – a point at which some control can be applied and, as a result, a hazard can be prevented, eliminated or reduced to an acceptable level. The strength of the system is its flexibility of implementation through progressive improvement (Villaroel *et al.*, 2007). The HACCP system is based on five principles:

1 Identifying hazards – infectious disease pathways.
2 Identifying critical control points.
3 Mitigation procedures – what is required and how can this be done.
4 Designing a monitoring system to evaluate the effectiveness of any control method.
5 Recording information.

Visual representation of the farm and the critical control points within each area, using a map, can be a valuable aid in preventing unintentional introduction of diseases and avoiding the spread of disease agents among areas of a dairy farm. Flowcharts can be used to describe the biosecurity protocol to personnel that work on the farm, and using calendars can help with implementation (Villaroel *et al.*, 2007).

Another excellent system which takes a slightly different approach to biosecurity management is included in the UK website www.myherdhealth.com for cattle farmers and veterinarians. Risks are coded using a 'traffic light' system for ease of understanding.

An effective biosecurity program needs to be decision-focused and flexible enough to adapt to the unique situations of individual enterprises. This requires an understanding by the veterinarian of biosecurity principles and the goals of disease prevention and avoidance, as well as specific information relative to the biology and epidemiology of specific pathogens of interest (Sibley, 2010). It needs to be based on the particular herd's current disease status, the particular disease to be controlled, cost of prevention, likelihood of an outbreak, impact of an outbreak, and risk aversion of the producer.

When developing a Farm Biosecurity Plan, it is good to have a checklist of items (outlined below) under the sub-headings general procedures; bio-exclusion (minimising the risk of introducing infectious diseases onto the property); and bio-containment (minimising the risk of spreading disease on the property).

Farm biosecurity plan

General procedures

Establishing the disease status of the resident herd

Veterinarians should work with the farmer to develop protocols for the routine monitoring, diagnosis and treatment of common diseases. Development of protocols in this manner ensures that planning takes place with input from all of the important players, and also ensures that this plan is communicated to everyone involved.

The first level of monitoring is the recording of clinical cases of disease (Wells *et al.*, 2002).

Routine diagnostic evaluations of clinically abnormal animals are also recommended, using diagnostic protocols developed with the herd veterinarian.

Ideally dead animals, including young stock and adults, should be routinely necropsied by the veterinarian, and appropriate samples should be submitted to the local veterinary diagnostic laboratory. It is important to receive abattoir feedback on any animals that have lesions/diseases found at slaughter.

Farmers should be encouraged where possible to work towards disease-free accreditation for specific diseases. The costs may be offset by higher premiums for animals when sold.

Record-keeping and animal identification

All animals should be identified, without which a record-keeping system cannot work. Record-keeping systems should be in place, with all cases of morbidity and mortality, and all animal movements on or off the farm, routinely recorded. The management team, including the veterinarian, should review records of production and disease on a regular basis. Only by having such monitoring and record-keeping programs in place will producers be able to detect early occurrences of unusual disease incursions in the herd.

Staff training

Staff training on biosecurity measures should be instituted, and the economic and welfare reasons explained to all staff. They should appreciate the urgent response needed when the following clinical signs maybe seen (e.g. clinical signs of targeted diseases, unexplained deaths, sores ulcers on feet, drooling, reduction in milk yield in many animals, discharges with blood). They should know about the importance of good levels of personal hygiene to prevent potential fomite transmission of diseases.

Hotline telephone numbers for emergency animal disease should be readily available, should there be a suspected incursion of an exotic disease. All training should be documented, and any local rules on animal health-related issues should be adhered to.

Emergency biosecurity response plan

In the case of an emergency animal disease, and where applicable, standard operating procedures should be implemented in line with the relevant authorities. Knowing what to do and how to scale up bio-exclusion procedures needs to be considered ahead of time, and may include placing signs to prevent visitation, ensuring that gates are padlocked so vehicles cannot drive onto the property, cleaning and disinfecting of vehicles onto the farm.

Bio-exclusion (minimising the risk of introducing infectious diseases onto the property)

New incoming animals joining the herd can pose a considerable disease risk (see Figure 20.1). A list of diseases for bought in dairy cows would include: BVD, IBR, leptospira, Salmonella, Johne's disease, mastitis pathogens such as *streptocoocus agalactiae* and *staphylococcus aureus*, digital dematitis, ringworm, liver fluke, lungworm, anthelmintic resistant parasites, camplylobacter, *Neospora caninum* and bovine tuberculosis.

In order to formulate an appropriately costed bio-exclusion program, the disease status of the resident herd and the herd of origin needs to be established. A knowledge of the following are all required: the availability of disease vaccines, diagnostic tests, and prophylactic treatments; the clinical signs associated with the diseases; the disease characteristics (epidemiology, prevalence transmission, and incubation period); and the potential cost of an outbreak.

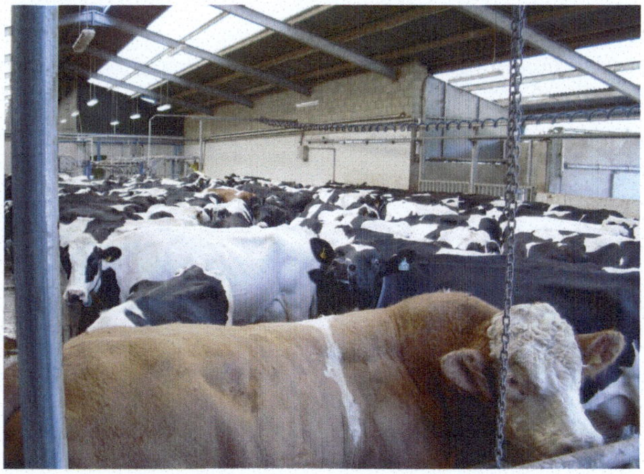

Figure 20.1 Incoming animals may introduce new diseases into the herd with devastating results.

The purchase of a new dairy stock bull may pose a number of biosecurity risks. Diseases of interest may include BVD, leptospirosis, IBR, bovine TB, Johne's disease, trichomoniasis and campylobacter. We may wish to perform some tests before movement onto the farm for BVD, IBR, TB and Johne's disease. We may also want to consider the vaccination history, and which vaccines we need to give during the quarantine period. We may wish to perform preputial sheath washings and send samples off to be tested. We may also prophylactically treat the sheath washing positive bull with effective antibiotics for campylobacter, and inject the animal with streptomycin in case of leptospirosis. Faecal egg counts to determine endoparasite species and load (including fluke and lungworm) is important to avoid bringing resistant parasites onto the farm. Signs of digital dermatitis should sound alarm bells, and lice infestations are common, so prophylactic treatment should be standard.

Stock provenance

Without doubt, the introduction of cattle into a herd is the most significant biosecurity risk for most diseases. The ideal situation is to have a disease-free herd and a closed system, where no animals come onto the property and replacement heifers are reared using semen AI from reputable firms with good disease control programs (Wells *et al.*, 2000). Even if heifers are reared at a separate facility, preventing their exposure to cattle from other herds during this period maintains a closed-herd system (Wells *et al.*, 2000).

If this is not possible, in the case where livestock need to be brought onto the property, animals should be purchased from reputable and biosecurity-conscious suppliers with a history of vaccination where necessary, and preferably from suppliers who maintain a quality assurance program which includes a biosecurity component.

A vendor's declaration should be obtained as to the property of origin and the identification, health status and treatment history of the stock. Preferably, animals should be inspected prior to purchase in order to assess their health status. This may mean asking for specific tests to be done for particular diseases of concern.

Quarantine

A further important aspect of a sound biosecurity plan is to quarantine animals for a period of time. This is rarely done on farms, as the facilities are often not in place, nor is it considered sufficiently important.

Quarantine is a period of isolation for newly arrived animals and, thus, potentially diseased animals are isolated from the rest of the animals on the property for the purpose of detecting and eliminating (where appropriate) disease. It allows an opportunity for acclimatisation, close observation of animals, animal health checks to be carried out, permanent identification, and confirmation of medical history and provenance.

Ideally, this period should be 30 days, but is particularly dependent on the incubation periods of specific diseases under consideration and, in some cases, may be longer. For diseases such as Johne's, brucellosis, leptospirosis, neosporosis, salmonellosis, BVD in persistently infected individuals, and leucosis, quarantine is not an effective biosecurity measure because of the unapparent carrier state (Sanderson, 2009). In these cases, the animals will need to be tested to distinguish individual carriers of disease agents (Sanderson, 2009).

From a practical perspective, and if necessary, ensure that new cows are milked after the resident animals have been milked, and visit and service these isolated animals after the resident animals have been checked. Ideally, wear separate clothes and boots or clean boots before moving back to the resident herd.

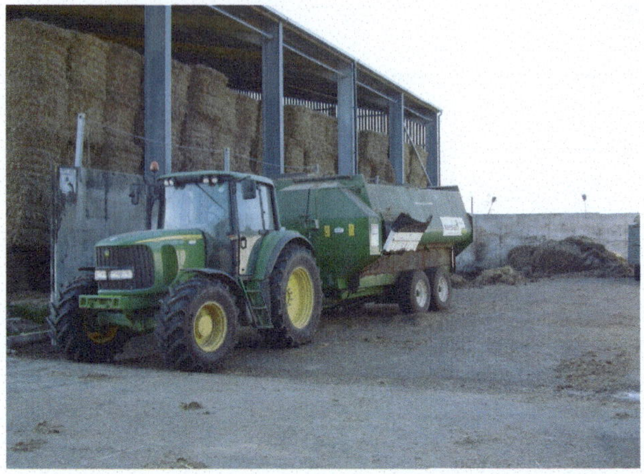

Figure 20.2 Vehicles can act as fomites spreading disease around the farm.

Disease testing

Disease testing of incoming cattle can be useful in decreasing the risk of introducing disease into a herd (Sanderson, 2009), and it is often done in conjunction with a period of quarantine. Ideally, testing should be done on the vendor's farm in case there are any positive cases. The tests used must be carefully evaluated, particularly for their specificity and sensitivity to ensure they achieve the desired goal of decreasing risk of disease entry (Sanderson, 2009).

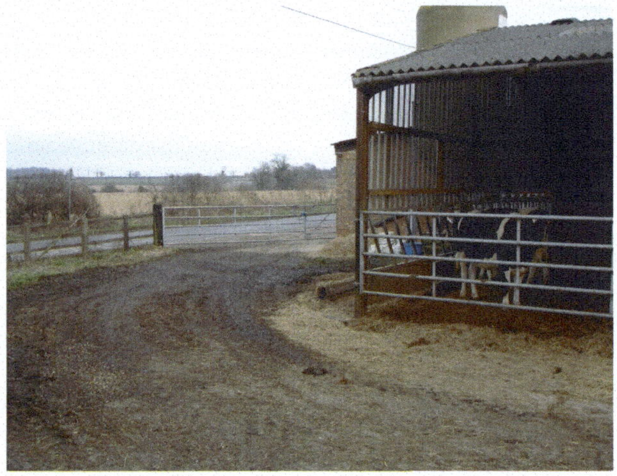

Figure 20.3 The farm boundary should be a well-planned biosecurity interface with notices, boot washing facilities and wheel dips.

Vaccination and immune status

The use of vaccination for maintenance of immunity in the resident herd is another way to manage risk from incoming cattle (Sanderson, 2009). The deployment of vaccines is based on the risk of disease under consideration, and can be an insurance policy if biosecurity is less than optimal. However, it should not be considered as the only, or even the primary, method of decreasing risk (Sanderson, 2009). Even under optimal conditions, not all cattle will respond to vaccination, but overall it can be considered as a useful ally to support improved biosecurity. In addition, sub-optimal nutrition and, in particular, failure of passive immunity in calves, can make them more susceptible to many infectious diseases. Management of potential pathogen loads in housed cattle should be carefully considered.

Fencing and buffer zones

Boundary fences should be appropriate and adequately maintained to ensure that animals of unknown disease status cannot come into physical contact with the resident herd. A buffer zone, whereby animals are not contiguous with animals of unknown disease status, should also be considered. Double fencing is advocated, with at least a 3 m gap, to reduce the risk of aerosol contamination, but this comes at a cost.

Vehicle/people/equipment movements and use

Vehicles moving within the farm can carry diseases between different groups of cattle (Figure 20.2). Where there is regular movement of vehicles, machinery and people onto the property (e.g. tankers, veterinarians, tanker drivers, contractors), the vehicles should be directed to a defined area of the property, preferably on the periphery, ensuring that animals cannot not have access to this area at any time (Figure 20.3). This area should be an impermeable surface (e.g. concrete), so that cleaning and disinfecting procedures can be efficiently and effectively performed.

Dead stock collectors should be considered high risk, as it is likely they will have been to farms where animals have died of infectious causes. Hauling the animal to the periphery of the property, to ensure that the dead stock collector does not come onto the main part of the farm, requesting cleaning and disinfection of the vehicle before arriving, and the use of tyre disinfectant systems, should all be seriously considered.

Where movement of vehicles, machinery and equipment is necessary outside the defined areas (e.g. hay and silage contractors), ensure that the equipment and vehicle is pressure-hosed to minimise disease spread. Designating a specific entrance onto the farm where visitors must arrive affords an opportunity for visitors to routinely clean their boots (and put on overalls and wash hands as necessary). A sign-in, sign-out protocol for visitors will assist traceability.

Stockfeed

There should be monitoring of compliance with any legislation prohibiting the feeding of animal materials to ruminants. In some countries, purchase feed commodities must come from approved suppliers. These approved suppliers must maintain a quality assurance program that includes a biosecurity component which has agreed protocols, to avoid contamination of stock feed by livestock, vermin, feral and domestic animals, and traceability.

Careful consideration should be given to systems for feed storage, feed delivery, feed bunk design, and feeding management. Commodity loads should be inspected on delivery for visible evidence of spoilage or mould, and the presence of animal droppings (e.g. rodents). All feed delivery equipment should be cleaned between deliveries and farms. All feeds should be inspected routinely for moulds or spoiled material and, if spoiled matter is present, the feed should be discarded and not fed to animals.

The risks posed by other animals

Feral animals, wildlife, farm dogs and cats can introduce disease into the farm. For example the farm dog may provide a transient risk of spreading *Neosporum caninum* (Figure 20.4).

Feral animals and wildlife can potentially transmit many diseases to cattle, including leptospirosis, bovine tuberculosis, salmonellosis and campylobacteriosis (Ward *et al.*, 2006).

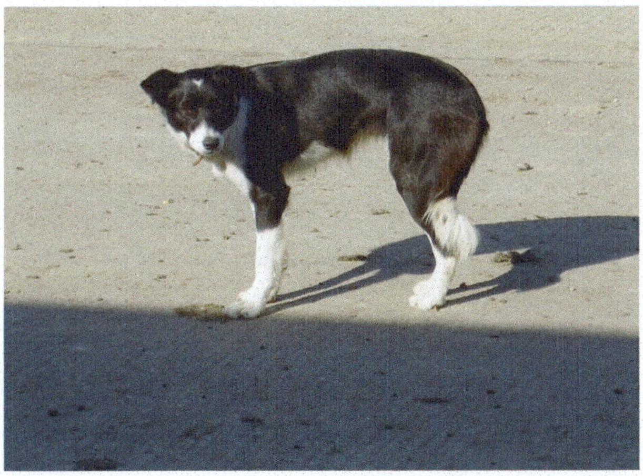

Figure 20.4 Farm dogs may be responsible for an outbreak of *Neosporum caninum* abortion.

With due regard to national legislation, appropriate trapping, baiting and exclusion procedures should be coupled with eradication of nesting sites and spilt food. Simple measures such as these can have a significant effect on reducing the likelihood of contact between feral/wild animals and cattle.

This can be illustrated by the case of bovine tuberculosis in the UK. European badgers (*Meles meles*) have been implicated in the transmission and maintenance of bovine tuberculosis since the 1970s. Recent studies have provided evidence of frequent visits by badgers to farm buildings, during which there is potential for close, direct contact with cattle and contamination of cattle feed (Ward *et al.*, 2006).

Badger exclusion measures include: closing all buildings; sheet metal gates; adjustable metal panels for gates; sheet metal fencing; feed bins; silage clamp fencing; and electric fencing. Elevating food and water troughs to 80 cm above the ground have been 100% effective in preventing badger entry into farm buildings (Ward *et al.*, 2006). This, combined with fencing off badger setts and latrines, can reduce the likelihood of contact with cattle, thus reducing the potential for transmission of bovine tuberculosis.

Bio-containment (minimising the risk of spreading disease on the property)

Sick animal investigation and isolation

All staff involved in the daily monitoring and handling of animals should be aware of the importance of early detection of exotic and endemic diseases and should know what to do if they suspect an animal may be exhibiting signs of such a disease. They should be aware of the need to report cases of unusual illness or death, particularly if there is a sudden outbreak, to their veterinarian or the local government veterinary officer.

Clinically ill animals should be examined and treated as soon as possible. They pose a major reservoir of infection for other animals, so it is important to isolate them by housing them away from other animals. It is especially important not to house these clinically ill animals in or near the maternity facilities, to avoid exposure of newborn calves to these pathogens.

Ideally, unexplained deaths should be investigated and the animals necropsied by a veterinarian as soon as possible. Appropriate hygiene standards should be followed, and the environment cleaned and disinfected where the necropsy has taken place. There should be appropriate handling and disposal of the carcasses in order to avoid interference from wildlife and feral animals and further contamination of the active areas of the farm. If pits are used, they should be covered quickly and effectively. Carcass collection should occur at a designated area on the periphery of the farm.

Disease control and eradication

If important endemic infectious diseases are present on the farm, a risk assessment and a control cost benefit analysis should be performed. This may require testing to establish the prevalence and the identification of the infected animals. Depending on the prevalence and the epidemiology of the disease, biocontainment of the diseased animals may be possible and cost-effective. Vaccination may be helpful, if available. Eradication programmes need to be costed carefully, and the risk of re-introduction carefully considered. The challenges posed by Johne's disease and bovine viral diarrhoea control and eradication programmes provide useful examples.

For example, eradicating Johne's disease is costly and time-consuming, but is feasible when one considers the need to minimise exposure of young calves contaminated milk or manure from the adult herd. Multiple strategies are used to limit this exposure risk. Effective control begins with the birth of calves in a clean, uncontaminated maternity pen or outdoors. Calves should be promptly removed from cows. Pooled colostrum should be avoided, and colostrum to be fed to calves should be from cows that test negative for Johne's disease, and hygienically collected to ensure no faecal contamination.

After colostrum, milk fed to calves should be pasteurised. This can be accomplished by the use of on-farm pasteurisation equipment, or by simply purchasing powdered milk replacer, since these products are pasteurised in the course of being manufactured. Water provided to calves should be free of contamination from the manure of the adult herd. Likewise, solid feeds should be fed to young cattle in the most hygienic manner possible, to avoid manure contamination. Practices such as using the same equipment for removing manure from barns and for moving feed to heifers must be avoided (Collins & Stabel, 2011).

Housing and hygiene practices

By providing good quality bedding, which is regularly changed, and the effective movement of slurry, contamination of the environment can be minimised. Deep litter bedding has been used effectively but, with all areas, regular cleaning and disinfection will minimise disease. Ensuring that buildings are well-ventilated is also an important component in reducing pathogen load (Figure 20.5).

It is also very important to ensure that equipment used to handle manure should not be used to provide feed to animals.

It is essential for all staff to have a clear understanding of, and comply with, good standards of hygiene, in order to minimise cross contamination.

Regular hand washing, boot cleaning and disinfection, and overall washing, are all necessary practices on the farm to minimise disease transmission. Regularly maintained footbaths, situated between areas of differing biosecurity systems on the farm, can be utilised, with the additional aspect that all personnel realise that biosecurity is taken seriously.

All equipment should be cleaned and disinfected where necessary, particularly when moving between areas of differing biosecurity on the farm. The use of one needle per animal should be encouraged at all times. Veterinarians should set an example by exhibiting the highest standards of hygiene and the use of effective disinfectants between animals, between different parts of the farm and between farms.

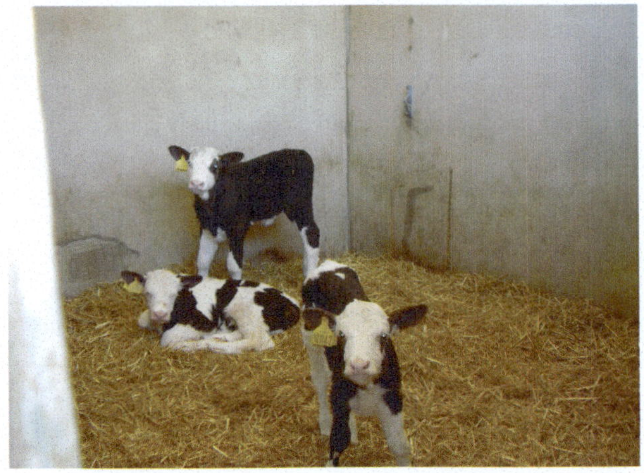

Figure 20.5 Well-designed housing can reduce pathogen loads and facilitate disinfection between batches of calves using the all-in all-out principle.

Traffic control on the farm

In the event of a disease outbreak on a farm, it is very important to minimise the fomite spread of infectious agents around the farm by reducing vehicular movements.

Water quality and management

Many pathogens can be spread through contaminated drinking water. Many cattle farms use surface water (such as lakes, ponds, or rivers) as a water source. Surface water may carry disease agents from other animal facilities as well as bird droppings, urine and faeces from wildlife, and human waste (Villaroel *et al.*, 2007).

Manure management

Because faecal-oral transmission is the most common route of infection for common gastrointestinal diseases, manure systems must be designed to minimise for faecal contamination of feed and water sources. Regardless of the system in place, manure should be removed regularly and in the direction away from the most susceptible animals (i.e. calves, youngstock, maternity pens) (Collins & Stabel, 2011).

A farm biosecurity checklist is provided in Table 20.1.

Acknowledgements

I thank my wife, Katrina and son Jamie for their endless patience and support.

Table 20.1 Farm biosecurity plan checklist.

General procedures:
1. Establishing the disease status of the resident herd
2. Record-keeping and animal identification
3. Staff training
4. Emergency biosecurity response plan
Bio-exclusion:
1. Stock provenance
2. Quarantine
3. Disease testing
4. Vaccination and immune status
5. Fencing and buffer zones
6. Stockfeed management
7. Vehicle/people/equipment movements and use
8. Feral animals, insects and wildlife management
Bio-containment:
1. Sick animal investigation and isolation
2. Disease eradication practices
3. Housing and hygiene practices
4. Traffic control on the farm
5. Water quality and management
6. Manure management

References

Allen, A.R., Skuce, R.A. and McDowell, S.W.J. (2011). *Bovine TB (TB): a review of badger-to-cattle transmission*. http://www.dardni.gov.uk.

Anderson, J.F. (1998). Biosecurity – a new term for an old concept-how to apply it. *Bovine Practitioner* **32**, 61–70.

Barrington, G.M., Gay, J.M., Evermann, J.F. (2002). Biosecurity for neonatal gastrointestinal diseases. *Veterinary Clinics of North America, Food Animal Practice* **18**, 7–34.

Beale, R., Fairbrother, J., Inglis, A. and Trebeck, D. (2008). *One Biosecurity: a working partnership*. The Independent Review of Australia's Quarantine and Biosecurity Arrangements. Report to the Australian Government.

Benjamin, L.A, Fosgate, G.T, Ward, M.P., Roussel, A.J., Feagin, R.A. and Schwartz, A.L. (2010). Attitudes towards biosecurity practices relevant to Johne's disease control on beef cattle farms. *Preventive Veterinary Medicine* **94**, 222–230.

Brennan, M.L. and Christley, R.M. (2012). Biosecurity on Cattle Farms: A Study in North-West England. *PLoS One* **7**(1), e28139. doi:10.1371/journal.pone.0028139.

Collins, M.T, and Stabel, J.R. (2011). Diseases of Dairy Animals Infectious Diseases: Johne's Disease. *Encyclopedia of Dairy Sciences*, 2nd Edition, pp. 174–18. Academic Press.

Enticott, G., Franklin, A. and Van Winden, S. (2012). Biosecurity and food security: spatial strategies for combating bovine tuberculosis in the UK. *The Geographical Journal*, doi: 10.1111/j.1475-4959.2012 .00475.x.

Gunn G.C.C., Heffernan, C., Hall, M., McLeod, A. and Hovi, M. (2008). Measuring and comparing constraints to improved biosecurity amongst GB farmers, veterinarians and the auxiliary industries. *Preventive Veterinary Medicine* **84**, 310–323.

Heffernan, C., Nielsen, L., Thomson, K. and Gunn, G. (2008). An exploration of the drivers to bio-security collective action among a sample of UK cattle and sheep farmers. *Preventive Veterinary Medicine* **87**, 358–372.

Holliman, A. (2003). Restocking problems post-FMD. *Cattle Practice* **11**, 311–312.

Judge, J., McDonald, R.A., Walker, N. and Delahay, R.J. (2011). Effectiveness of Biosecurity Measures in Preventing Badger Visits to Farm Buildings. *PLoS One* **6**(12): e28941. doi:10.1371/journal.pone.0028941.

Lanyon, S., Rogers, J., Kessell, A. and Reichel, M.P. (2012). Economic analysis of an acute outbreak of bovine viral diarrhoea virus (BVDV) in a South Australian dairy herd – a case study. *Australian Cattle Veterinarian* **63**, 13–17.

Maunsell, F. and Donovan, A. (2008). Biosecurity and Risk Management for Dairy Replacements. *Veterinary Clinics of North America: Food Animal Practice* **24**, 155–190.

Ott, S., Wells, S. and Wagner, B. (1999). Herd-level economic losses associated with Johne's disease on US dairy operations. *Preventive Veterinary Medicine* **40**, 179–192.

Sanderson, M. (2009). Biosecurity for Cow-Calf Enterprises. Chapter 113 in *Current Veterinary Therapy Food Animal Practice.*

Sibley, R. (2010). Biosecurity in the dairy herd. *In Practice* **32**, 274–280.

Smith, D.R. (1999). *Biosecurity risk management to improve heifer health and value*. Professional Dairy Heifer Grower's Association, Proceedings from the third annual conference, Bloomington, MN, pp 87–92.

Van Schalk, G., Dijkhuizen, A.A., Benedictus, G., Barkema, H.W. and Koole, J.L. (1998). Exploratory study on the economic value of a closed farming system on Dutch dairy farms. *Veterinary Record* **142**, 240–242.

Villarroel, A., Dargatz, D.A., Lane, V.M., McCluskey, B.J. and Salman, M.D. (2007). Suggested outline of potential critical control points for biosecurity and biocontainment on large dairy farms. *JAVMA* 808–819.

Waage, J.K. and Mumford, J.D. (2008). Agricultural biosecurity. *Philosophical Transactions of the Royal Society B* **363**, 863–876, doi:10.1098/rstb.2007.2188.

Ward, A.I, Tolhurst, B.A. and Delahay, R.J. (2006). Farm husbandry and the risks of disease transmission between wild and domestic mammals: a brief review focusing on bovine tuberculosis in badgers and cattle. *Animal Science* **82**, 767–773.

Wells, S. (2000). Biosecurity on Dairy Operations: Hazards and Risks. *Journal of Dairy Science* **83**, 2380–2386.

Wells, S., Dee, S. and Godden, S. (2002). Biosecurity for gastrointestinal diseases of adult dairy cattle. *Veterinary Clinics of North America, Food Animal Practice* **18**, 35–55.

Further reading

For further information on farm level biosecurity plans, refer to Sibley (2010); Maunsell & Donovan (2008); Sanderson (2009); Wells *et al.* (2002); Villaroel *et al.* (2007).

CHAPTER 21

Applied Clinical Parasitology for Cattle Practitioners

Mike Taylor

Learning objectives

- Be familiar with important endoparasites and ectoparasites in cattle.
- Appreciate the pathogenicity, epidemiology and immunological responses of important parasites.
- Understand the different diagnostic techniques that can be used and how they can be applied to monitoring programmes.
- Have a working knowledge of the different types of antiparasitics available.
- Understand the control strategies that may be used as part of herd health planning programmes and how they impact on the development of resistance.

Introduction

Outbreaks of bovine parasitic diseases are the result of the interplay between cattle and their ability to resist disease (immunity), the parasites' biology and abilities to cause disease (pathogenicity), and the environment in which the cattle and parasites co-exist. The basic principles of parasite disease control are to avoid or reduce parasite exposure by:

1 preventing parasites from coming onto a farm;
2 implementing good management practices aimed at reducing levels of parasite contamination; or
3 strategic interventions to limit or reduce parasite exposure.

Cattle can be affected by a number of different parasites, and other diseases, at any time in their lives. Approaches to parasite control therefore require a complete understanding of the interplay between all the factors that may precipitate disease, and what steps need to be taken to prevent or limit disease from occurring.

Many parasites affect different age groups of cattle, and exposure may lead to disease if levels of challenge are sufficiently high. In this respect, intensive systems of management can lead to increases in parasite numbers by providing larger numbers of susceptible hosts and more heavily contaminated environments. If the animals survive, exposure eventually leads to protective immunity and a consequential reduction in parasite burdens as the animals become older. Incumbent husbandry systems, and how the cattle are managed on a particular farm will, therefore, have a big influence on the balance between parasite challenge, host resistance and disease.

To achieve control, a certain amount of information and knowledge is required before deciding on appropriate intervention strategies. In many situations, a number of control options may have to be considered and integrated into wide-ranging or diverse farm husbandry systems and management practices. Generally, prescriptive parasite control practices will have to be adapted to suit individual farm needs.

Cattle husbandry and management

The management systems under which the world's cattle population (estimated at about 1.3 billion head) are kept vary considerably worldwide. Cattle are primarily raised for meat (beef production) or milk and other dairy products (dairy production), but they may also be used as draft animals in many developing countries. In many parts of the world, nomadic herds of cattle are grazed over large extensive areas, or ranched over large open ranges, such as the grassland plains of the USA and Canada. In many westernised countries, cattle are grazed intensively, requiring the use of grassland management systems, application of fertilisers and higher livestock stocking density levels.

Generally speaking, the cattle industries can be divided into two distinct farming systems of production. In beef herds, cows usually calve in spring or the autumn. Dairy herds can also follow a similar seasonal pattern of calving although, in many

Bovine Medicine, Third Edition. Edited by Peter D. Cockcroft.

dairy herds, calving increasingly occurs all year round, with only minor seasonal peaks. On dairy farms, calves are removed from their dams at, or soon after, birth, while on beef breeding farms the calves typically remain with their dams until weaning, at around 6–9 months of age. On non-breeding beef farms, calves destined for beef production are purchased either from beef breeding herds or dairy herds, for fattening either as calves, at just a few weeks of age, or older store cattle for finishing. Feedlot systems are common in a number of the larger beef-rearing countries, and here beef cattle spend approximately four to six months in a feedlot and fed a grain-based diet prior to slaughter.

Systems of production for both dairy and beef cattle vary from country to country, and also in different regions within the same country. Farm topography and land terrain, and local prevailing, climatic conditions all play a major role in determining the most appropriate management system for a given farm. Thus in hot, dry climates typical of southern Mediterranean countries, little grass grows and cattle are kept and fed indoors all year round. In wetter, western and northern climates, grass growth is lush and cattle can graze outdoors, usually throughout late spring and summer, and even all year round in milder climates. In mountainous and northern latitudes, where cold weather and snow cover may last for months, then cattle are housed for up to six months of the year or even longer. Housed cattle have to be fed either conserved forage (hay and silage), or cereal-based concentrates.

Management systems not only reflect farm location, but also local traditions and consumer preferences for the farm produce. Local culinary tastes can dictate breed type, weaning times, age and weight to slaughter. Farm size, stocking densities, type and availability of cattle feeds, level of stockmanship, and availability of labour, all dictate the type and level of on-farm husbandry and need to be assessed when investigating or implementing parasite control strategies.

Cattle parasites

Cattle are affected by a whole range of parasites and it is not possible to cover all parasites of cattle in detail in this chapter. For a more comprehensive overview of cattle parasites readers are referred to standard parasitological textbooks such as Veterinary Parasitology (Taylor *et al.*, 2007).

Many closely related parasite species will behave similarly, both in terms of their parasitic and non-parasitic phases of their life cycles, but there are some notable exceptions. Even within the same genus, some parasite species will affect different organs in the body, have longer or shorter prepatent and patent periods, and differ in their pathogenicity. Species differences are also found in the development and survivability of free-living and infective stages in the environment. Many parasites have environmental-resistant stages capable of surviving drought or extreme cold; others survive less well outside the host. The balance between free-living stages in the environment (refugia populations), and parasitic stages in the host, can have significant effects on the rate of development of resistance to antiparasitic drugs and the subsequent ability to control parasite populations through chemotherapy.

Endoparasites

Parasitic gastroenteritis

Parasitic gastroenteritis, due to the presence of large numbers of gastrointestinal nematodes, is commonly encountered in cattle in many countries where cattle are grazed outdoors. Over 18 species of nematodes are found in the abomasa and the small and large intestines of cattle. Nematodes in the abomasum are generally considered to be the most pathogenic, with the most predominant and economically important species, *Ostertagia ostertagi*. Nematodes in the small intestine are generally of lesser importance, with *Cooperia oncophora* and *Nematodirus helvetinaus* the commonest species encountered in temperate areas.

Parasitic bronchitis

Parasitic bronchitis (Husk, Dictyocaulosis), is caused by the lungworm *Dictyocaulus viviparus*. Lungworm infection is characterised by bronchitis and pneumonia, and typically affects young cattle during their first grazing season on permanent or semi-permanent pastures. In northern Europe, outbreaks of disease occur from June until November, but are most common from July until September. Parasitic bronchitis may also be seen in adult cattle as a herd phenomenon, or in a particular age group within a herd, if animals have failed to acquire immunity through natural challenge in earlier years. Such animals may develop the disease if exposed to heavy larval challenge, as might occur on pasture recently vacated by calves suffering from clinical husk. The disease is most commonly encountered in the patent phase, although the other forms have been recognised. In addition to coughing and tachypnoea, a reduction in milk yield in cows is a common presenting sign.

Faciolosis

Fasciolosis in many countries is caused by the trematode parasite *Fasciola hepatica*; other species may also be involved. Liver fluke disease arises from the migration of large numbers of immature flukes through the liver or, more usually in cattle, from the presence of adult flukes in the bile ducts, or both. Liver fluke can infect all grazing animals, but mainly affects sheep and cattle, and is generally less pathogenic in cattle. The pathogenesis of fluke infections varies according to the number of metacercariae ingested and the phase of parasitic development in the liver. *Fasciola* infections may cause a loss of production in milking cows during winter. Clinically, these are difficult to detect, since the fluke burdens are usually low and anaemia is not apparent.

Coccidiosis

At least 13 different species of *Eimeria* have been reported to infect cattle. Clinical signs of diarrhoea are associated with the presence of the two main pathogenic species, *E. zuernii* or *E. bovis*, which occur in the lower small intestine, caecum and colon, causing severe enteritis and diarrhoea, or dysentery with tenesmus in heavy infections. *E. alabamensis* has been reported to cause enteritis in yearling calves in some Northern European countries. Bovine coccidiosis is primarily a disease of young animals, normally occurring in calves between three weeks and six months old, but it has been reported in cattle aged one year or more. The disease is usually associated with a previous stressful situation, such as shipping, overcrowding, feed changes, severe weather or concurrent infection with parvovirus.

Cryptosporidiosis

Cryptosporidiosis is common in young calves, and is characterised by anorexia and diarrhoea, often intermittent, which may result in poor growth rates. Several species of *Cryptosporidium* are now reported in cattle, but the main species of importance is *C. parvum*, which is zoonotic. The primary route of infection is mainly by the direct animal-to-animal faecal-oral route. Thus, in calves, overcrowding, stress of early weaning, transport and marketing, together with low levels of hygiene, will increase the risk of clinical infections.

Blood parasites

Blood protozoan parasites, such as *Babesia* and *Theileria* spp., can be locally significant, particularly where tick populations are abundant, but are not discussed in detail here.

External parasites

Flies

A number of species of flies may feed on blood, sweat, skin secretions, tears, saliva, urine or faeces of cattle, to which they are attracted. Flies feed by either puncturing the skin directly, in which case they are known as biting flies (e.g. blackflies (*Simulium* spp.) and midges (*Culicoides* spp.)), or by scavenging at the surface of the skin, wounds or body orifices, in which case they may be classified as non-biting or nuisance flies, such as house flies and face flies (*Musca domestica* and *M. autumnalis*), stable flies (*Stomoxys calcitrans*), head flies (*Hydrotaea irritans*) and horn flies *Haematobia* spp.).

The activity of both biting and non-biting species of fly results in marked defensive behaviour ('fly-worry'). Flies are usually active during the summer months but, if temperatures are high enough, they may also be active in the spring and autumn. Their life cycles, appearance and feeding behaviour vary from species to species. Biting flies are also of importance as vectors of a range of diseases. Biting midges (*Culicoides*) are vectors to over 50 arboviruses, and have become of increasing importance in Europe as vectors of bluetongue (BTV) virus and Schmallenberg virus.

Lice

Louse infestations (pediculosis) are associated with a chronic dermatitis, and in small enough numbers are well tolerated. However, louse populations can increase dramatically, reaching high densities. In heavier infestations, there is pruritus, with rubbing and licking, but if sucking lice are present in large numbers there may be anaemia and weakness.

Blood-sucking lice have been implicated in the transmission of disease. Transfer of lice from animal to animal or from herd to herd is usually by direct physical contact. The most rapid annual increase in louse populations is seen when cattle are winter-housed, and lice can build up in numbers very quickly. In late spring, there is usually an abrupt fall in the numbers of lice, as most of the parasites and eggs are shed with the winter coat.

Mites and ticks

Infestations with mites (ascariosis) can result in severe dermatitis, known as mange, which may cause significant welfare problems and economic losses. A wide range of ticks can affect cattle, causing and spreading disease. Ticks have developed a variety of complex life cycles and feeding strategies, which reflect the nature of their habitats. The various genera of ticks have different thresholds of temperature and humidity within which they are active and feed, and these thresholds govern their distribution. Generally, ticks are most active during the warm season, provided there is sufficient rainfall but, in some species, the larval and nymphal stages are also active in milder weather. Ticks are also capable of transmitting a number of viral, bacterial, protozoal and rickettsial diseases to cattle.

Parasite pathogenicity

The mere presence of a parasite, or group of parasites, does not necessarily indicate the presence of disease. Not all species of parasitic worms or coccidia, for example, are pathogenic, and not all flies are harmful or are potential vectors. Different species of nematodes are more pathogenic than others, and only certain species of coccidia in cattle are pathogenic. Louse infestations need to be differentiated from mite infestations, so a correct and appropriate treatment regime can be instigated. In most situations, proper and correct identification of potential parasites and pathogens is important when devising integrated disease control programmes at the farm level. Diagnosis of parasitic infections should always be based on a combination of farm history, clinical signs and observations, supported where possible by post-mortem or abattoir results and appropriate laboratory-based tests.

Parasite epidemiology

A complete understanding of the epidemiology of individual parasites is essential for their control. Some parasites, such as liver fluke, require an intermediate host that greatly influences both the numbers and appearance of infective stages on pasture which, in turn, is driven by extrinsic climatic factors, particularly heavy rainfall. For those parasites that have a seasonal life cycle, knowing when populations increase or decline determines optimal intervention times for strategic treatments, or application of appropriate control measures

Geographical distribution and bionomics

The geographical spread and distribution of cattle parasites, and their significance in terms of pathogenicity and importance within individual countries, will vary considerably, depending on a number of both intrinsic and extrinsic factors that favour individual parasites' abilities to survive and reproduce. Climate, land terrain and the presence, or absence, of intermediate hosts, all directly influence the survivability and bionomics of free-living parasite stages. Cattle population densities, age, breed, purpose (dairy or beef), and systems of cattle management and production also play a significant part in determining incidence, prevalence and, ultimately, the significance of different parasite species within countries, regions and even individual farms.

Biotic potential refers to the reproductive capacity or fecundity of parasites. Some parasite species are more fecund and have a higher biotic potential than others. Fecund species tend to produce more heavily contaminated farm environments and, therefore, a greater risk of disease through higher levels of parasite exposure and challenge. Assessing the potential risks from levels of contamination and infectivity forms part of the disease control planning process.

Age susceptibility

Age is a factor in the appearance of the different parasitic diseases of cattle (Table 21.1). Many animals become more resistant to primary infections with many parasites as they reach maturity. If infected at an older age, the parasites either fail to develop or are arrested as larval stages in the tissues.

Resistance and immunity

Broadly speaking, resistance to parasitic infections falls into two categories. The first of these, often termed innate resistance, includes species resistance, age resistance and, in some cases, breed resistance – which, by and large, is not immunological in origin.

The second category, acquired immunity, is dependent on antigenic stimulation and subsequent antibody and cellular responses, and plays a highly significant role in protecting animals against infections and in modulating the epidemiology of many parasitic diseases.

Parasites typically have an aggregated distribution within their hosts. A small percentage of animals (≈20%) carry the bulk of the parasite population, while the remainder (≈80%), carry small burdens. This pattern may in part be due to genetically determined differences in host susceptibility. The relationship between parasite burdens and performance can vary, and leads to the concepts of 'resistance' and 'resilience'. Resistance describes individuals that carry lower burdens of parasites, while resilience indicates individuals that may still carry higher parasite burdens, but whose performance is largely unaffected by their presence. As a general rule, resistant animals can alter parasite epidemiology by reducing contamination, transmission and exposure within a system.

Thus, for example, following repeated exposure, calves generate an acquired immunity to gastrointestinal nematodes. Calves in their first grazing season, exposed to *C. oncophora* infections, appear to mount a rapid immune response to this parasite after about 8–12 months of exposure. Immunity to *O. ostertagi* is slower to develop, and cattle are not normally considered to be immune until they have been exposed to infective larvae over two grazing seasons. The response is, to some extent, genetically controlled, and individual animals vary in their ability to mount an immune response. Using FEC as an indicator, it has been shown that about 25% of calves have an innate resistance to worm infections, 50% generate an acquired immunity during their first grazing season, and 25% have an inadequate response, fail to show a reduction in FEC and may still carry relatively high worm burdens at the end of the first grazing season.

Calves exposed to *Dictyocaulus viviparus* rapidly acquire patent infections, readily recognisable by the clinical signs. After a period of a few weeks, immunity develops and the adult worm burdens are expelled. On subsequent exposure in succeeding years, such animals are highly resistant to challenge although, if this is heavy, then clinical signs associated with the re-infection syndrome may be seen. However, this is an acquired immunity that is dependent on sufficient exposure to the parasites, and at this age it is not as strong and effective as in adult animals.

Coccidia are normally present in cattle of all ages, and usually cause no clinical signs, as immunity is quickly acquired and maintained by continuous exposure to re-infection. However, intensification may alter the delicate balance between immunity and disease, with serious consequences for young calves. It has been shown that once young calves have been infected with coccidia, they develop a strong species-specific protective immunity.

Table 21.1 Age-related parasitic diseases of cattle.

Age range	Parasitic diseases	Causative agents	Comments
1–4 weeks	Cryptosporidiosis	*Cryptosporidium spp.*	Usually seen in housed, weaned dairy calves
<6 months	Coccidiosis	*Eimeria spp.*	Indoors or at pasture
	PGE	*Ostertagia ostertagi, Cooperia spp etc.*	Weaned calves turned out to pasture summer to autumn
6–12 months	PGE	*Ostertagia ostertagi, Cooperia spp* *Trichostrongylus spp* *Nematodirus helvetianus*	Calves at pasture summer to autumn
	Coccidiosis	*Eimeria bovis* *Eimeria zuernii*	Can occur in older calves subject to stress
	Parasitic bronchitis	*Dictyocaulus viviparus*	Calves at pasture usually mid-summer
	Liver fluke	*Fasciola hepatica*	Calves at pasture late summer and autumn in endemic fluke areas
	Lice	*Bovicola bovis* *Haematopinus eurysternus* *Linognathus vituli*	Housed or out-wintered yearlings in autumn and winter
>12 months to adult	PGE	*Ostertagia ostertagi, Cooperia spp etc.*	Can occur in second year grazing cattle
	Parasitic bronchitis	*Dictyocaulus viviparus*	Can occur in second year grazing cattle
	Liver fluke	*Fasciola hepatica*	Cattle at pasture late summer and autumn or out-wintered cattle winter and spring in endemic fluke areas
	Warble fly	*Hypoderma bovis* *Hypoderma lineatum*	Fly activity in summer; larvae subcutaneously in late winter and early spring
	Lice	*Bovicola bovis* *Haematopinus eurysternus* *Linognathus vituli*	Housed or out-wintered cattle in autumn and winter
All ages	Flies	Various	Mainly in summer outdoors but extended periods depending on climatic conditions
	Mites	*Psoroptes bovis* *Chorioptes bovis* *Sarcoptes scabei*	Mite populations highest in winter
	Ticks	Various	Spring to autumn while at pasture

Regardless of any maternally derived immunity, most animals will have had enough exposure to pathogenic *Eimeria* in the intestinal tract to rapidly develop natural immunity, usually by six months of age. This immunity still allows for limited cycling of parasites in the intestinal tract and the shedding of oocysts into the environment. The resulting low-level infection pressure will continually boost host immunity, creating a state of endemic stability. The degree of this acquired immunity depends on the number of oocysts ingested during primary infection. Exposure to too few oocysts may not be enough to stimulate adequate immunity to prevent future disease. Other factors can also prevent the development of protective immunity, including concurrent infections such as bovine virus diarrhoea (BVD), or trace element deficiencies. If infection pressure is overwhelmingly high, disease is possible even in animals with acquired immunity.

With all the ectoparasites affecting cattle, there has been little research on resistance to infection and, generally speaking, all ages of cattle are exposed and are equally susceptible to the various arthropod infections. Repeated exposure may, in fact, lead to hypersensitivity to bites and acute allergic reactions. Biting arthropods, particularly biting flies and ticks, are also responsible for transmitting a range of diseases.

Nutrition

Calves' nutritional status, and mineral and vitamin deficiencies, can influence resistance to parasite infections. In single suckle beef systems, suckling calves, in addition to benefiting from colostral intake, may forage less and, hence, pick up fewer parasites from pasture. Additionally, well-nourished animals may simply be able to fight off infection more readily.

Diagnostics

The range, standard, and availability of diagnostic tests used in monitoring parasite infections will vary from country to country, and from even region to region. Specialist laboratories offering a full range of tests described below may not exist in some localities, and monitoring of on-farm parasite levels will often entail a combination of clinical evaluation, responses to therapy, and use of available support tests where appropriate.

Faecal egg counts

Worm FECs have some limitations, and should be viewed as 'additional diagnostic information' to be considered along with history and clinical signs. Careful interpretation is particularly important where the FEC is low, as nematode genera and species vary in their fecundity and pathogenicity. As cattle grow older, they develop an immunity that reduces worm fecundity, so egg count becomes a less reliable indicator of the size of a worm burden because:

1 faecal egg production per worm varies with the time of year, particularly those present in fit, healthy animals in good body condition and with a strong immunity;
2 generally, egg production is highest when larval intake is lowest;
3 during the winter months, high levels of arrested worm burdens may be present, but the FEC is zero.

Despite these limitations, FECs can be used to help decide if anthelmintic treatment is necessary, or can be safely delayed or omitted. On some farms, FEC monitoring may allow anthelmintics to be better timed and, therefore, used more efficiently rather than less frequently. On other farms where anthelmintics are used excessively, FEC monitoring may provide a farmer with the necessary additional information to reduce anthelmintic frequency, while continuing to manage the risk of disease outbreaks or lost productivity.

It is often useful to know whether worms of one particular genus dominate FECs or not. If required, larval culture and differentiation can be performed, usually using the faeces left over from the FEC. This technique takes a further 7–10 days. Larval differentiation involves hatching the eggs in the sample and identifying the larvae. Usually, 50 or 100 larvae are counted, and the percentage of each genus reported. However, the eggs of each genus may not hatch equally, because the temperature at which the culture is performed may favour the hatching rates of one genus over others. It is safer, therefore, to use the larval culture results as a general indication of the worm genera present, rather than a precise determination of the proportion of the FEC contributed by each genus.

Diagnosis of liver fluke infection in cattle is based primarily on clinical signs, seasonal occurrence, prevailing weather patterns, and a previous history of fasciolosis on the farm or the identification of snail habitats. On post-mortem with chronic fluke infections, the liver has an irregular outline and is pale and firm, the ventral lobe being most affected and reduced in size. The liver pathology is characterised by hepatic fibrosis and hyperplastic cholangitis. The pathology in cattle has the added features of calcification of the bile ducts and enlargement of the gall bladder. The calcified bile ducts often protrude from the liver surface, giving rise to the term 'pipe-stem liver'.

When an outbreak of coccidiosis is suspected, it is essential to obtain an adequate history and, for a definitive diagnosis, a post-mortem is usually required. Histological studies may be of value in establishing the type and location of tissue lesions and possible species involved. Diagnosis must, therefore, take into account a number of epidemiological and clinical factors supported by laboratory investigations. It should also be remembered that many other conditions may be confused with coccidiosis, such as colibacillosis, salmonellosis, cryptosporidiosis, rotavirus, coronavirus, as well as trichostrongylosis in young animals at grass. Faecal oocysts counts (FOC) can help support the diagnosis, but it is important to identify the species, as not all are pathogenic. It must be stressed that, particularly in ruminants, very high faecal oocysts counts ($>10^7$/gram faeces) can occur in healthy animals while, conversely, sick or dying animals may have low or even zero oocysts counts.

Box 21.1 Faecal Oocyst Count (FOC)

The following should be born in mind with FOCs:
- Healthy animals can pass large numbers of oocysts
- Symptoms can manifest before oocysts are shed
- Oocyst output may be transient
- Not all species are pathogenic

Estimations of the numbers of oocysts in faeces are made using the modified McMaster method similar to that used for worm faecal egg counting (FEC). This technique gives a rough indication of the severity of infection, but is difficult to interpret. In general, the presence of oocysts in faeces has little clinical significance, as even adult immune animals will shed small numbers of oocysts.

Serological diagnosis

An *Ostertagia* ELISA has been developed that can be used to detect worm infections in adult milking cattle and potential effects on milk production. A number of potential disadvantages exist with such ELISAs that are based on crude worm extracts, as cross-reactions with other helminths may occur. Some cross-reaction with *Cooperia* spp. occurs, but this is not considered a disadvantage if the aim is to estimate the overall burdens. However, cross-reactions with *Dictyocaulus viviparus* and *Fasciola hepatica* can pose difficulties where these co-infections co-exist. The test may require further standardisation and repeatability before it can be used in the field to determine the need for worm treatment of adult milking cows.

Several lungworm ELISAs have been developed to detect lungworm-specific antibodies. Most are based on the use of native lungworm antigen but, more recently, recombinant proteins have been developed for use in commercialised 'dipstick' ELISAs such as the Ceditest™ Lungworm ELISA (Cedi-Diagnostics Lelystad, The Netherlands). The presence of antibody indicates exposure, but not necessarily active infection or immunity to the disease. This means that ELISA results used to diagnose infection in individual animals must be interpreted with care, and it is more appropriate to submit a representative number of blood samples from a suspect herd. A number of positive results provide an indication of herd exposure and the need for further investigations and/or possible treatment.

Diagnosis of liver fluke infections in cattle is normally based on *Fasciola* eggs in faeces. However, this is not possible during the prepatent period, and FEC suffers from poor sensitivity during the patent period due to the relatively low number of eggs shed in cattle faeces. To improve diagnosis during both early and chronic phases of infection, several ELISA techniques have been described. Some of these tests rely on antibody detection using crude somatic extracts or excretory/secretory (E/S) products of *F. hepatica*. The specificity of antibody responses to *F. hepatica* varies during the course of infection and, as a result, several antigens have been identified for use in serological tests. Whilst ELISA antibody tests can identify animals with prepatent infections, a disadvantage with these tests is that a positive result does not necessarily indicate a current infection but, rather, a history of exposure. It has been shown, for example, that antibodies persist in fluke-infected cattle after treatment with triclabendazole for up to seven months. As with the lungworm ELISA, results used to diagnose infection in individual animals must be interpreted with care.

Monitoring worm infections in adult cattle can be used to evaluate the effectiveness of worm control measures and to target anthelmintic treatments where required. In dairy cows, research has focused on the detection of parasite antibody levels in individual or bulk tank milk, because this medium is less costly to sample than blood samples and, therefore, is potentially more suitable for monitoring.

Milk ELISAs

Factors such as milk yield, age of the cow, stage of lactation and the level of mastitis in a herd can all influence milk antibody levels. The ELISA has a reported good repeatability, and results suggest that the ELISA can be used to assess whether GI-nematode infections are potentially affecting milk yield in a herd. However, monitoring worm infections in adult cattle by this means has not yet been routinely adopted. Reasons for this may be incomplete knowledge on the effects of GI nematodes on milk yield, the fact that *O. ostertagi* ELISA has only recently become available, or that subsequent evaluation in the field has only recently been initiated in some countries.

An ELISA for the detection of antibodies against the bovine lungworm, *Dictyocaulus viviparus*, in milk has been reported. The reported test specificity and sensitivity were 100% and 97.5% respectively, and the test offers the potential for routine veterinary diagnosis of lungworm exposure using milk samples instead of sera.

The milk ELISA has been reported as an effective alternative to the serum ELISA for diagnostic and surveillance purposes. The test may be more cost-effective, since veterinarians are not required to collect milk samples, and farmers can submit samples. It has been adapted and validated from the serum ELISA for use with samples of bulk tank milk. The reported sensitivity is 96%, with a specificity of 80%, which is comparable to the serum test in terms of its diagnostic sensitivity and specificity.

Antiparasitics

The choice of the most appropriate treatments for these parasites identified in the farm health plan will vary depending on availability, efficacies (including potential resistance issues), preferences and cost. Only generic names are provided, as trade names, availability and distributing company names will vary from country to country.

Anthelmintics

A wide range of cattle-worming products is available worldwide. As trade names vary from country to country, wormers will be referred to throughout the text by their generic compound name. Most products marketed for the control of gastrointestinal nematodes and are used for both treatment and prevention. The broad-spectrum anthelmintics, currently available for cattle, can be divided into three groups on the basis of chemical structure and mode of action (Table 21.2.).

The main group of anthelmintics now used in cattle are the macrocyclic lactones, which includes the avermectins (abamectin/ivermectin/doramectin/eprinomectin) and the milbemycins (moxidectin). These compounds are highly lipophilic and, following administration, are stored in fat tissue,

Table 21.2 Anthelmintics for cattle.

Compound	Spectrum of activity	*Activity against Ostertagia Cooperia*	*Lungworm*	*Tapeworm*	*Fluke*	Comments
Group 1 - BZ, Benzimidazoles, Probenzimidazoles ¥						
Albendazole	Broad	+	+	+	+ > 10 weeks	50% higher dose rate for fluke.
Netobimin ¥	Broad	+	+	+	+ > 10 weeks	50% higher dose rate for fluke.
Fenbendazole	Broad	+	+	+	–	Some activity against tapeworms segments
Oxfendazole	Broad	+	+	+	–	
Triclabendazole	Narrow	–	–	–	+ > 2 days	
Group 2 – LV, Imidazothiazoles						
Levamisole	Broad	+	+	–	–	Injectable and oral formulations. Incomplete activity against inhibited L_4
Group 3 – ML, Macrocyclic lactones						
Ivermectin	Broad	+	+	–	–	Endectocidal activity. Injectable and Pour-on
Doramectin	Broad	+	+	–	–	Endectocidal activity. Injectable and Pour-on
Eprinomectin	Broad	+	+	–	–	Endectocidal activity. Pour-on only
Moxidectin	Broad	+	+	–	–	Endectocidal activity. Injectable and pour-on

from which they are slowly released. A number of macrocyclic lactone compounds are available for use in cattle and are active against a wide range of nematodes and also some ectoparasites, and are therefore often referred to as endectocides. Doramectin, ivermectin and moxidectin are available in injectable and pour-on formulations, while eprinomectin is only available as a pour-on product. All have variable persistent anthelmintic activity against abomasal nematodes, some intestinal nematode species, lungworms and some ectoparasites. Their persistent activity means that they can be used at extended treatment intervals in strategic dosing strategies. The recommendation for ivermectin products is a 3-8-13 week early season dosing strategy and a 0-8 strategy is recommended for doramectin products. A long-acting injectable preparation of moxidectin has persistent activity of between 90 and 150 days for various parasite species.

Flukicides

Substituted phenol (nitroxynil) and the salicylanilides (oxyclozanide, closantel) are narrow spectrum anthelmintics. They are effective only against fluke and some blood-sucking nematodes (e.g. *Haemonchus, Bunostomum*). Oxyclozanide is also active against rumen fluke (*Paramphistomum* spp). In the host, they bind to plasma protein, which increases the duration of activity against blood-sucking parasites. The benzimidazoles, albendazole and ricobendazole (albendazole sulphoxide) are active against fluke at higher dose rates, as is the pro-benzimidazole, netobimin, which also has activity against the small lancet fluke, *Dicrocoelium dendriticum*. Triclabendazole has high activity against adult and immature flukes > 1 week old. Clorsulon (a benzenesulphonamide) is active against immature liver flukes over eight weeks of age, and adult liver fluke. It inhibits enzymes in the glycolytic pathway by blocking the oxidation of glucose to acetate and proprionate, leading to a gradual suppression of motility and paralysis.

Antiprotozoals

A number of anticoccidials have been used in the control of coccidiosis in ruminants. Anticoccidials may be coccidiostatic (arrest parasite development) or coccidiocidal, and they kill coccidia by acting on different stages of the parasite life cycle, suppressing development of asexual (meronts) stages, sexual stages (gamonts), or both.

Diclazuril (an asymmetrical triazone) has a strong anticoccidiocidal activity when given as a single dose at 1 mg/kg (1 ml/2.5 kg), and it is used in the treatment and prevention of coccidiosis in calves. Toltrazuril (a symmetrical triazone) is given as a single dose at 15 mg/kg (3 ml/10 kg) of 50 mg/ml oral suspension for the treatment and prevention of coccidiosis in calves. Decoquinate is also licensed in several countries for the treatment and prevention of coccidiosis in calves, and is administered incorporated into feed for at least 28 days at the recommended dose rate of 0.5–1.0 mg/kg b.w./day. The polyether ionophores, lasalocid and monensin, which are used to increase feed efficiency and weight gains, are in use in some countries for the prevention of coccidiosis in calves.

Ectoparasiticides

The choice and use of ectoparasiticides depends, to a large extent, on husbandry and management practices, as well as the type of ectoparasite causing the infection. Parasites that live permanently on the host, such as lice and mites, are relatively easily controlled and, once they are eradicated, re-infection only occurs following contact with infected animals. Non-permanent parasites (ticks, flies) are less easily controlled, because only a small proportion of the population can be treated at any one time, and other hosts may maintain them. Many ectoparasite infections are seasonal and predictable, and can be countered by prophylactic use of ectoparasiticides. As an example, in temperate countries, flies occur predominantly from late spring to early autumn, tick populations increase in the spring and autumn, and lice and mites during the autumn and winter months. Treatments can, therefore, be targeted at anticipated times of peak activity, as a means of limiting disease and parasite populations.

Available chemicals used in the treatment of ectoparasites of veterinary importance act either systemically, following uptake of the compound from the hosts' tissues, or by direct contact with the target parasites following external application. Systematically acting chemicals may be given parenterally (by subcutaneous or intramuscular injection), or applied topically to the skin, from where the active ingredient is absorbed through the skin and taken up into the bloodstream. Topically applied chemicals have a direct effect on the target parasite on the surface of the skin. Due to differences in pharmacokinetic behaviour and uptake from application sites, different formulations of a drug preparation may be indicated for different target parasites.

Activity of ML compounds against ectoparasitic infections in cattle varies with individual products, and is dependent on the active molecule, the product formulation and the method of application. MLs are administered to cattle either by injection, or topically as pour-on applications. In general, pour-on products are more effective against sucking lice (*Lignonathus*, *Haematopinus*) and, to some extent, chewing lice (*Bovicola*), as well as headfly (*Haematobia*) infestations on cattle, when compared with equivalent compounds administered by injection. The MLs are also extremely effective against warble fly larvae (*Hypoderma* spp) present in the oesophagus (*H. lineatum*) or epidural fat (*H. bovis*) during their resting phases over the winter months, and third instars present in their subcutaneous site in the spring. MLs are also used in the control of tick infestations in some countries.

Synthetic pyrethroids (SPs) such as cypermethrin, deltamethrin, flumethrin and permethrin are available in many countries as pour-on, spot-on, or spray formulations with activity against biting and nuisance flies and lice on cattle, and with some products for tick control. Some SPs are also available as ear tags for use on cattle, providing protection against biting and nuisance flies for several months during the fly season. Another widely used application is their use in environmental sprays in cattle sheds, barns and dairies, both to kill and repel flies.

Parasticide resistance

Reports of resistance to anthelmintics in cattle nematodes are relatively uncommon in comparison to reports of nematode resistance in sheep and goats worldwide. Anthelmintic resistance has been reported in cattle parasitic nematodes around the world, with some reports of multiple resistant cattle nematodes in USA, New Zealand and South America.

Many reports of ML resistance in cattle nematodes have been with *Cooperia* species, following the identification of a positive faecal egg count (FEC) or faecal egg count reduction test (FECRT), particularly after the use of pour-on treatments. Poor absorption of pour-on ML anthelmintics, and subsequent reduced efficacy against *Cooperia* species, which are the dose-limiting species for the ML group, provides a more likely explanation for positive post-treatment FEC than acquired resistance. However, in the longer term, shedding of *Cooperia* spp. eggs during the prepatent period following treatment with topical ML anthelmintics has been shown experimentally to select for AR, and may lead to increasing AR reports in these species.

Continuous use of anticoccidials has led to ineffective treatment due to drug resistance in the target parasite populations. This is perhaps best exemplified by the situation with anticoccidial compounds used in intensive poultry production, where the emergence of resistance to all chemical groups has been rapid. In contrast, anticoccidial resistance in ruminant coccidia has been only rarely suspected or reported, due to the less intensive selection pressures placed on anticoccidials and their usage in ruminants.

Modern ectoparasiticides are highly effective at removing susceptible individuals, but they can impose strong selection pressure for the development of resistance if used incorrectly. The development of resistance may reduce the effectiveness of the treatment applied and, thereby, increase the frequency of application and the dose required, in turn increasing the costs and adding to the environmental impact. Despite these concerns, there are few reports of pesticide-resistant cattle parasites, with the possible exception of some reports of acaricide-resistant ticks.

Farm health planning

The farm environment and conditions under which cattle are kept will vary greatly and depend on a number of factors. Management and husbandry systems present on a particular farm subsequently influence the presence or absence of parasitic infections and associated levels of disease. Ideally, farms should have a herd health plan detailing preventative healthcare and protocols, as well as a recording system to monitor herd health. The records should chronicle the incidence of specific health conditions and reflect prevalence by assessing progress of each condition over time. The farm should also have biosecurity measures in place to minimise the risk of spread of disease within the farm and between other farms. Within the herd health plan should be a parasite control plan.

Biosecurity refers to those measures taken to keep diseases out of herds where they do not currently exist, or to limit the spread of disease within the herd. The responsibility for farm-level biosecurity belongs to the producer or herd owner. A successful biosecurity plan must address isolation of new animals brought to the farm, isolation of sick animals, regulation of the movement of people, animals and equipment, and procedures for cleaning and disinfecting facilities. Having established a parasite control plan as part of the farm health planning exercise there remains the choice of the most appropriate control strategies, as well as available antiparasitics and diagnostic tests for identified parasite risks.

Box 21.2 Biosecurity Measures

As with other diseases the greatest risk of introducing parasites is by bringing new animals onto the farm. Producers should purchase animals from sources with a sound herd health program and in addition should:

- Isolate new animals ideally to a separate facility but otherwise use a separate pen or pasture that does not permit nose-to-nose contact or shared feed/water supplies.
- Have new animals either tested before mixing them with the existing herd or administered appropriate quarantine treatments for identified diseases.
- Work out a herd health program that includes control for identified parasitic diseases most likely to be a problem. Each farm plan should have a parasite control plan that specifies strategies and worming programmes, including target animals and any medicines to be used.
- Isolate animals showing signs of disease for appropriate tests and treatment.

Parasite control strategies

The control options available for each type of parasite are generalised and will, in many cases, need to be adapted to regions, areas, or even down to individual farm level. As such, parasite control strategies should form an integral part of the farm health planning process and should be based on knowledge of parasite presence and status.

Endoparasites

In many countries where cattle are grazed outdoors, there is a seasonal pattern to the presence of numbers of infective, parasitic nematode larvae on pasture. Parasite contamination of the pasture at the start of the grazing season is derived from surviving, over-wintered infective larvae on pasture, and eggs deposited by older cattle carrying worm burdens acquired the previous year. Build-up of infestations of parasitic gastrointestinal worms on the pasture results from recycling through non-immune calves, and leads to peak pasture contamination from mid-summer onwards.

As a consequence, calves that are turned out in spring follow the classic sequence of events of acquiring infection from over-wintering infection and subsequent pasture contamination. Depending on rainfall and temperature conditions, this results in a build-up of pasture infectivity from mid-July onwards and, if pasture infectivity overwhelms immunity, a high risk of disease and production losses can occur.

Strategies for the control of parasitic nematode infections of cattle are generally targeted at first-year grazing calves. On farms where new leys or aftermaths are available, worming and grazing management can be integrated as a means of worm control. In this respect, 'clean grazing' systems can be designed, and function well for control of parasitic gastroenteritis. These should be encouraged, but offer little protection for the control of lungworm disease, because of its unpredictable nature.

By providing 'low risk' grazing at the start of the grazing season in the form of new leys, or grass previously grazed by sheep, anthelmintic treatments can generally be avoided or reduced. Where only 'medium' or 'high' risk pastures exist, then anthelmintic treatment(s) will be required at some point during the grazing season. These could be avoided by moving calves to 'low risk' pasture in the form of aftermaths (hay or silage fields) from mid-July onwards.

Where re-seeded pastures (new leys) are available, a rotational grazing system should be followed. This can take the form of either a 'leader-follower' system, in which first year heifers graze a series of paddocks ahead of older heifers, or a '1-2-3' system, in which heifers graze one paddock while the other two are cut for silage. Later in the season, the heifers graze the two silage paddocks, while the previously grazed block is cut for silage or hay.

The 'dose and move' strategy, in which calves were dosed and then moved to safe pasture mid-season, is now generally considered to be highly selective for anthelmintic resistance, and consideration should be given to the use of targeted selective treatments of cattle to be moved.

Knowledge of the epidemiology of parasitic gastroenteritis has led to the creation of a number of parasite control programs based on the use of early season anthelmintic prophylaxis. The basic rationale for these parasite control programmes is that suppression of faecal egg output by grazing calves over the first few months of turnout, through the strategic use of anthelmintics, will prevent the subsequent build-up of infective larvae on pasture. During the early part of the grazing season, the loss of over-wintered larvae on pasture proceeds until negligible numbers of these over-wintering larvae are present by mid-summer. As a consequence of the control of faecal egg output by strategic anthelmintic treatment, and the natural loss of over-wintering infective larvae, the threat of gastro-intestinal parasitism should be much reduced.

Thus, for many farms where provision of low or medium risk grazing is impracticable, worm control can be achieved by worming in the early part of the grazing season (sometimes referred to as 'poor man's clean grazing systems'). Examples of this include the 3-8-13 strategy for ivermectin (Ivomec), the 0, 8 dosing strategy for doramectin (Dectomax), or the use of boluses. Calves dosed strategically in this manner should remain set-stocked on the same fields for maximum benefits. Alternatively, calves should be moved to 'low risk' pasture when these become available, allowing sufficient time after the 'dose' to reduce selection pressure for anthelmintic resistance.

Some degree of control of parasitic bronchitis in calves can be achieved by early season suppression of pasture contamination, in much the same way as for the control of gastrointestinal nematodes. However, the epidemiology of lungworm infection is complex and still not fully understood, and vaccination of calves with an irradiated larval vaccine (Huskvac™) is the most reliable form of prevention in countries with endemic or high-risk areas of lungworm infections. For spring calving and all-year-round calving herds there may be practicality issues for use.

Control programmes for liver fluke must take into account the farm history, topography, geographical location and the prevailing weather conditions local to the area. Most programmes rely heavily on treatments with flukicidal drugs. The choice of product and frequency of use will depend on the level of fluke challenge, the time of year and prevailing weather conditions, as well as the management and husbandry systems on the farm.

Fluke burdens can be monitored in cattle herds by post-mortem examinations when the opportunity arises, with FECs, and by use of serological assays or a bulk tank milk ELISA. Herds should be monitored before a flukicide is used, unless there is a history of fluke infection on the farm. Continued monitoring can help determine the need for repeated treatments. Grazing cattle wintered outdoors can be treated with any of the flukicides effective against both adult and immature stages. In-wintered cattle need to be treated after housing, the timing of treatment depending on the flukicide used and its activity against immature stages.

Triclabendazole, which is effective against immature fluke less than six weeks old, can be used to treat cattle on housing; other products (containing rafoxanide or closantel) should be used 4–6 weeks post-housing. Dairy cows can be treated at drying-off. In high-risk years, out-wintered cattle should also be treated in spring to remove fluke burdens and reduce contamination of pastures with fluke eggs. Flukicides with adult activity only can be used at this time, thus reducing the selection pressure associated with products containing triclabendazole.

Combination fluke and worm products should only be used when both groups of parasites are present, as their use could potentially lead to off-target selection for resistance.

Where fluke infection is present, identification and exclusion of snail habitats from livestock offers some measure of control. Drainage eliminates the snail and offers an effective means of control, but the proliferation of environmental schemes to protect wetland areas has reduced the opportunities for this to be implemented. Simply keeping stock off the wettest fields in the autumn and the winter, when the incidence of disease is at its highest, can reduce the risk from fluke.

Although not currently widespread there is increasing concern with regards to anthelmintic usage and resistance. Evidence-based strategies to minimise the development are described in Taylor (2010). This endoparasite control programme, entitled 'Control of Worms Sustainably' (COWS), designed to minimise the development of anthelmintic resistance, is now being recommended for adoption in the UK. This approach includes: administering the anthelmintic effectively by ensuring the correct dosage is delivered effectively; using anthelmintic only when necessary following monitoring of faecal egg counts; using appropriate single narrow spectrum products where possible and avoiding combination products; rotating the class of anthelmintic used; and preserving susceptible worms on the pasture by not treating adults cows or a small percentage of the healthy youngstock.

Controlling coccidiosis is a balance between controlling and preventing disease while, at the same time, allowing the development of protective immunity through parasite exposure. Treatment should aim to prevent parasite replication in sufficient numbers to cause pathological damage and symptoms of disease but, at the same time, allow protective immunity to develop through adequate exposure of the hosts' immune systems to the parasite stages. It should also be borne in mind that immunity is species-specific and dependent on continual exposure to oocysts. Exposure to too few oocysts, or to oocysts of non-pathogenic species, may not be sufficient to prevent clinical or sub-clinical symptoms during future infections. The timing of treatment interventions should be based on epidemiological evidence and knowledge of anticipated disease outbreaks on farms.

Outbreaks of clinical coccidiosis can appear suddenly and may prove troublesome to resolve, as they often occur on heavily stocked farms, particularly where good husbandry and management are lacking. If deaths are occurring, early confirmation of the diagnosis is vital and should be based on the history, post-mortem examination and examination of smears. Affected animals should be medicated and moved to a cleaner environment or uncontaminated pasture as soon as possible.

In calves, coccidiosis usually occurs between three weeks and six months of age, but has been reported in cattle aged one year or more. The disease is usually associated with a previous stressful situation, such as weaning, crowding, shipping, overcrowding, food changes, nutritional deficiencies, severe weather or concurrent infections. Calves can become infected shortly after birth, with coccidiosis often appearing from 3–4 weeks old and oocyst shedding reaching a maximum between 3–6 weeks old. Thereafter, the incidence of disease decreases unless susceptibility is increased through impaired immune response or overwhelming levels of oocyst challenge.

Animals particularly at risk from coccidiosis are young calves kept indoors on damp bedding, or those on contaminated heavily stocked pasture, especially during cold, wet weather. The incidence of disease can be reduced through avoidance of overcrowding and stress. Other measures that can be taken include reducing stocking densities, batch rearing of animals, and avoidance of mixing different age groups. It also helps to provide plenty of clean bedding in birthing and rearing pens, and to keep young animals off heavily contaminated pastures when they are most susceptible. Good feeding of dams prior to parturition, and creep feeding of their progeny, will also help to boost resistance to coccidiosis.

Hygiene plays a major part in the control of coccidiosis and, to achieve effective control, good management and hygiene is vital. Regularly moving food and water troughs, and raising or covering them to prevent faecal contamination, can help to reduce the levels of infection. It is good practice to clean and disinfect all buildings between groups of animals. Steam cleaning helps remove faecal debris, and it is important to use a disinfectant that claims activity against coccidia oocysts, as not all disinfectants will kill oocysts. Ammonia-based disinfectants are normally used, although other disinfectants containing chlorophenol (chloro-m-cresole) are also effective.

Good hygiene and management are important in preventing disease from cryptosporidiosis. Feed and water containers should be high enough to prevent faecal contamination. Young animals should be given colostrum within the first 24 hours after birth, and overstocking and overcrowding should be avoided. Dairy calves should be either isolated in individual pens, or kept in similar age groups and cleaned out daily. On calf-rearing farms with recurrent problems, the prophylactic use of halofuginone can be considered by treating for seven consecutive days, commencing 24–48 hours after birth.

Ectoparasites

Flies can present a considerable nuisance to cattle, particularly in warmer climates or in the spring and summer months in more temperate countries in Europe. Control methods include removing all manure and organic material, in which many fly species breed, as often as possible and at least weekly in warm weather. Manure should be stacked so as to ferment, turned regularly, or treated with an insecticide. Buildings should be kept as clean as possible, sprayed with insecticides or fitted with insect traps, insecticidal strips or UV electrocutors.

The timing and frequency of treatments depends very much on individual circumstances. In many cases, treatment in late autumn or early winter will give adequate control of cattle lice. In Europe, louse control is usually undertaken when cattle are housed for the winter. Because a wide variety of products are effective, louse control is not difficult to achieve. Treatment of all stock on farm, and subsequent initial quarantine and treatment of all newly introduced animals, will allow a good degree of louse control to be maintained.

Cattle may be infected by a number of mange mites. Products containing macrocyclic lactones that include injectable and pour-on formulations of ivermectin, doramectin, eprinomectin, milbemycin and moxidectin are generally effective against *Chorioptes* and *Sarcoptes* mange mites. Some products containing doramectin and moxidectin have claims in controlling psoroptic mange mites, although activities and claims for individual products vary. In general, treated animals should be isolated for 2–3 weeks post-treatment to prevent re-infestation. Most treatments are not licensed for use in milking cattle. Eprinomectin is available as a pour-on formulation, and is the only macrocyclic lactone that may be used in dairy cattle. Pour-on products containing permethrin are also effective against mange mites in cattle.

For tick control, pasture improvement, where possible, should be practised, but is not always practicable. Traditional control methods, such as burning of cattle pastures, are still used in some areas, and are generally practised during a dry period before rain, when ticks are inactive. This technique is still a most useful one in extensive range conditions and, provided it is used after seeding of the grasses has taken place, regeneration of the pastures will rapidly occur following the onset of rain. Cultivation of land and, in some areas, improved drainage, help to reduce the prevalence of tick populations and can be used where more intensive systems of agriculture prevail. Few products have licensed claims for tick control in cattle and, as such, where ticks are a problem, little or no treatment may be given. Off-licence product use may occur and has been reported in some countries, with pour-on or spray synthetic pyrethroids and injectable or pour-on macrocyclic lactone products.

Summary

Cattle are affected by a range of parasites, the control of which requires detailed knowledge of the interplay between all the factors that may precipitate disease and what steps need to be taken to prevent or limit disease from occurring. Parasite control should aim to avoid, or reduce, the risk of parasite exposure by preventing parasites from coming on to a farm, and by implementing good management practices aimed at reducing levels of parasite contamination, through both disease monitoring and the use of strategic interventions to limit or reduce parasite exposure. Control measures need to take into account the systems of production and farm management, farm location and local prevailing climatic conditions, linked to knowledge of parasite incidence and epidemiology.

The range, standard and availability of diagnostic tests used in monitoring parasite infections will vary from country to country, and specialist laboratories may not exist in some localities. As a consequence, monitoring of on-farm parasite levels will often entail a combination of clinical evaluation, responses to therapy, and use of available support tests, where appropriate. Finally, the choice of the most appropriate treatments for use in parasite treatment and strategic control plans will vary, depending on their local availabilities, efficacies (including potential resistance issues) and, for farmers, their preferences and cost issues.

References and further reading

Charlier, J., Claerebout, E., Duchateau, L. and Vercruysse, J. (2005). A survey to determine relationships between bulk tank milk antibodies against *Ostertagia ostertagi* and milk production parameters. *Veterinary Parasitology* **129**, 67–75.

Duncan, J.L., Armour, J., Bairden, K., Urquhart, G.M. and Jorgensen, R.J. (1979). Studies on the epidemiology of bovine parasitic bronchitis. *Veterinary Record* **104**, pp. 274–278.

Eysker, M. and Ploeger, H.W. (2000). Value of present diagnostic methods for gastrointestinal nematode infections in ruminants. *Parasitology* **120**, S109–S119.

Taylor, M.A. (2004). Chapter 60: Bovine Antiparasitics. In: Andrews, A.H. (ed). *Bovine Medicine, Diseases and Husbandry of Cattle*, 2nd edition, pp. 1019–1034. Blackwell Scientific Publications.

Taylor, M.A. (2004). *Chemotherapeutics of Ectoparasiticides: Large Animals*, 9th Edition, pp. 2158–2168. Merck Veterinary Manual, Merial Whitehouse Station, NJ, USA.

Taylor, M.A. (2010). Sustainable worm control strategies for Cattle. *A Technical Manual for Veterinary Surgeons and Advisors*. COWS, EBLEX and Dairy Co. www.eblex.org.uk and www.dairyco.org.uk

Taylor, M.A. (2012). *Strategic control of ruminant eimeriosis (SCORES)*. A Technical Manual for Veterinary Surgeons and Advisors. www.takingcareofcoccidosis.com.

Taylor, M.A., Coop, R.M. and Wall, R. (2007). *Veterinary Parasitology*, 3rd Edition. Blackwell Publishing, Oxford.

Taylor, S.M., Hunter, A.G. and Andrews, A.H. (2004). Chapter 45: Ectoparasites, Tick and Arthropod Diseases. In: Andrews, AH (ed). *Bovine Medicine, Diseases and Husbandry of Cattle*, 2nd edition, pp. 740–777. Blackwell Scientific Publications.

CHAPTER 22

Cattle Poisoning: Principles of Toxicological Investigations

Jo Payne, Chris Livesey and Alan Murphy

Learning objectives

- Understand the epidemiology of poisoning in cattle.
- Be aware of the public health implications.
- Understand the range of sources of poisons.
- Understand the clinical syndromes that may be associated with poisoning.
- Be able to investigate and take appropriate samples when poisoning is suspected.
- Be aware of the common causes of poisoning in cattle.

Introduction

The cornerstone of modern toxicology is that most substances, including essential nutrients, are potential poisons if the dose is sufficiently large, although most potentially toxic substances do not cause poisoning as the dose is below the toxic threshold. Paracelsus (1493–1541) was the first person to report that effects are determined by dose.

Epidemiology of poisoning in cattle

The terms 'acute' and 'chronic' are generally applied to exposure/dose (i.e. short term or long term and higher or lower doses) and to the type and severity of effects. Some poisons are rapidly metabolised and/or excreted, resulting in immediate (acute or sub-acute) effects following (acute or sub-acute) exposure. Such effects are usually immediately apparent. However, the expression of immediate effects, such as DNA disruption, are delayed and can lead to chronic disease such as cancer. Poisons which are slowly excreted tend to accumulate and exert adverse effects following persistent (chronic) exposure and accumulation. Alternatively, they may persist at subclinical levels, which may have long-term consequences for food safety.

Poisons are usually acquired from the environment, diet, water supply, ambient air, or as a result of medicine overdose. Cattle are inquisitive and ingest materials that they encounter, especially if these are palatable. Therefore, most poisoning incidents occur as a result of ingested substances, although some can be absorbed through the skin or inhaled, as seen with toxic gases accumulating in buildings, slurry pits and silos. Environmental contamination is never homogeneous, while feed contamination is only homogeneous if the poison has been incorporated into a mixed feed. Nutritional deficiencies can cause pica, which increases the risk of ingesting poisons, as may boredom. Malicious poisoning of cattle is unusual, but they sometimes pick up baits laid for other species.

Acute exposure poisoning is typically sudden in onset, contrasting with the bell-shaped epidemic curve typical of infectious disease. Withdrawal from acute exposure may achieve equally sudden alleviation of symptoms. Chronic or delayed poisoning incidents are unlikely to present abruptly or with simultaneous onset and recovery, and are therefore harder to identify and investigate. Toxic teratogenesis can occur at levels of exposure that cause no other adverse effects in the dam and are not apparent until the calf is born or aborted. Chemical carcinogenesis could theoretically occur following a single exposure, but the effects are always delayed, and pathogenesis usually involves additional risk factors.

Most poisonings are diagnosed because adverse effects are severe, distinguishable from infectious diseases and can be associated with an immediately recognisable source of contamination. Poisoning tends to be overlooked if effects are subclinical, delayed, do not affect a group simultaneously, cause syndromes indistinguishable from infectious diseases, or cause insidious adverse effects such as suppressed immune function.

Bovine Medicine, Third Edition. Edited by Peter D. Cockcroft.

Public health

Food safety hazards arise from chemical residues transferred into tissues and milk. Contamination of animal produce does not occur in all poisoning incidents, but the possibility should always be considered. Also, it is important to remember that significant accumulation of residues in animal products can be entirely subclinical (e.g. lead). When poisoning or exposure to chemicals has occurred, relevant food safety authorities (the Food Standards Agency in the UK) should be consulted immediately for risk assessment and advice on potential withdrawal of produce from the food chain. Farmers should report incidents to their customers. Farmers need to demonstrate freedom from contamination as quickly as possible, especially when produce is leaving the farm frequently, such as milk. Precautionary withdrawal periods may be recommended by regulatory authorities, or imposed by dairies and supermarkets.

The use of unlicensed medicines as antidotes can engender long, even permanent, withdrawal intervals in food animals. Suspected adverse reactions can have implications for public health and should be reported.

Environmental toxicants, for example toxic gases in farm buildings, can be a direct risk to humans as well as livestock. Relevant authorities may need to be informed of such poisoning incidents.

Relevant legislation

Animal welfare regulations (UK Animal Welfare Regulations 2007) and welfare codes of practice (UK code of recommendations for welfare of livestock: cattle) are similar in most countries, and they require farmers to provide a wholesome diet, with implications for environments known to cause livestock poisoning.

Food safety regulations are also similar internationally. Food businesses, including farms, must take due diligence to avoid contaminating the food chain (The Food Safety Act 1990). Maximum levels for a range of contaminants are prescribed (Maximum levels for contaminants in food). Farmers are responsible for managing hazards expected to occur on their farms (Food and Feed Hygiene Regulations 2006; Official Feed and Food Controls (England) Regulations 2009).

Pathogenesis and pathology of poisoning in cattle

Poisons can affect all body systems and cause a range of syndromes, many of which are indistinguishable clinically from infectious and nutritional diseases. Poisons (either parent compound and/or metabolites) alter the metabolism. Low doses, causing minor metabolic changes, may be accommodated with no adverse effects or may cause subclinical biochemical changes, detectable only by clinical chemistry. Toxic doses vary, because individual animals have differences in genotype, nutrition and production, which all impact on susceptibility.

The pathology of poisoning is very diverse, but some general principles apply. Intracellular effects include binding, displacement or oxidation, which may be subclinical or cause functional abnormalities and structural changes. Extracellular effects cause secondary or indirect cell injury by restricting supplies of oxygen or nutrients, electrolyte balance and excretion of waste products, or by adversely affecting metabolic regulators, especially nervous, endocrine and immune systems. Allergic reactions are regarded as toxic processes. Structural changes may be absent, especially if functional changes are acutely fatal or levels of accumulation of chronic poisons are below the adverse effect threshold or delayed (e.g. development of cancer).

Cellular responses to poisoning include proliferation of intracellular organelles or degeneration, which may resolve or cause cell death. Tissues may proliferate (hyperplasia, metaplasia or neoplasia) or degenerate, causing inflammation, repaired by regeneration or fibrosis. Short-term exposures typically cause acute inflammation, whereas persistent exposures cause chronic inflammation.

Classification of poisons

There are many possible classifications. Table 22.1 classifies poisons according to source, while Table 22.2 describes common syndromes. Categories overlap because some poisons have multiple sources or cause multiple syndromes, and some clinical signs present in multiple syndromes.

Common clinical syndromes associated with poisoning

The first step in diagnosing infectious, nutritional or toxic diseases is to describe the syndrome. Syndromes range in severity, prevalence and incidence, and may overlap (e.g. dysentery and melaena fit in both alimentary and blood syndromes). The presenting syndrome does not necessarily indicate the affected organ or tissue – for instance, nervous syndrome can be caused by encephalopathy, metabolic disease (ketosis), hepatopathy or nephropathy. The mechanisms of action of some poisons are uncertain.

Table 22.1 Common sources of potentially toxic substances.

Source	Precipitating factors	Poison examples
Contamination of crops and soil: *Industrial pollution* Approximately 100 000 chemicals are produced on an industrial scale, with new chemicals introduced continuously *Natural phenomena* Mineral deposits on farms, volcanic eruptions	• Poor containment of emissions from industry, power generation, combustion, incinerators, waste disposal, fires. Illegal waste disposal. • Agricultural land: Aerial deposition, natural erosion, floods, landslips, historic mining and smelting of mineral deposits. • Proximity of farm animals to contaminated crops and soil. • Soil ingestion, crop contamination by soil splash and dust, wet weather or drought, overgrazing, pica.	• Brickworks, aluminium smelters (fluoride). • Nuclear accidents (caesium, iodine). • Combustion products (dioxins). • Fire retardants (surfactants) • Wastes (pesticides, PCBs, dioxins industrial solvents, substrates and by products) • Mineral deposits (lead, arsenic molybdenum) • Volcanoes (fluoride, sulphur)
Point source contamination in housing or on pasture	• Poor containment of hazardous materials. • Livestock access to workshops, stored feed, agrochemicals, fertiliser or waste. • Poor maintenance of ditches, pastures, buildings. • Negligent waste disposal • Fly tipping	• Toxic paints (lead) • Building materials (lead, arsenic), Batteries (lead) • Recycled wood as bedding (lead, arsenic) • Bonfire ash (lead, arsenic) • Feeds (acidosis, urea, mineral supplements, medicated feeds) • Fertilisers (fluoride, nitrate, ammonia salts, urea) • Pesticides (metaldehyde, rodenticides) • Fuel and lubricating oils (fuel oil poisoning, PCB, lead) • Ditch maintenance (water dropwort) • Fly tipping, garden waste, burned out vehicles (yew, rhododendrons, laurel, lead)
Surface water (Surface water should be assumed to be at risk of contamination)	• Eutrophication and run-off from farms. • Aerial contamination or run-off from active or abandoned industrial, waste or recycling sites, fires, accidents or environmental incidents.	• Blue-green algae • Agrochemicals and pesticides. • Industrial pollution. • Metals (lead, arsenic) • Combustion products (dioxins) • Fire retardants (surfactants) • Wastes, recycling (pesticides, persistent organic pollutants, lead, arsenic)
Ground water	• Contamination levels can increase in droughts. • Mining activities.	• Salt, • Fluoride • Arsenic • Nitrate
Poisonous plants	• Wide range of toxic doses and toxic mechanisms. • Usually eaten when pasture is inadequate. • Some become more palatable when dry or ensiled. • Incorporation into hay or silage. • Depraved appetite (e.g. pica) may predispose. • Plant toxins levels are unpredictable, unevenly distributed and affected by maturity and environmental factors. • May be related to feed crops, over-feeding, crop husbandry and storage	• Ragwort • Bracken • Hemlock • Hemlock, water dropwort • Laurel • Yew • Rhododendron • Nightshades • St John's Wort or Bog asphodel (photosensitisation) • Coumarin-containing plants (sweet clover, sweet vernal grass) • Brassicas, beets, potatoes
Misguided over-supplementation	• Over supplementation with normal diet. • Supplements with relatively small therapeutic indices. • Failure to take account of all sources of supplements. • Poor control of dose.	• Concentrate feeds (acidosis, sub-acute rumen acidosis) • Supplements (copper, selenium, urea, sulphur)

(continued overleaf)

Table 22.1 (*continued*)

Source	Precipitating factors	Poison examples
Contamination of feed crops during growth and harvest	• Mycotoxicoses which develop during growth of crops. Fungal invasion predisposed by adverse weather and crop diseases. • Contamination with *Aspergillus* and *Penicillium* fungi which release mycotoxins during storage. • Accumulation of chemicals in pasture. • Incorporation of poisonous plants, carcases or chemicals into hay and silage.	• Fusarium mycotoxins (trichothecenes, zearalenone, fumonisins). • Temorgenic mycotoxins (penetrem). • Ergots. • Tryptophan (3-methyl indole) (fog fever) • Poisonous plants (ragwort) • Carcases (*C. botulinum*) • Lead batteries.
Contamination of crops, feed ingredients and straights during processing, storage or transport	• Mycotoxicoses which develop in storage conditions. • Contamination with wastes, agrochemicals, carcases or carryover of previously stored or transported materials. • Malicious adulteration. • Contamination may occur prior to or after compounding into feedstuffs, or on the farm.	• *Aspergillus* and *Penicillium* mycotoxins (aflatoxins, ochratoxin, cyclopiazonic acid, citrinin). • Spoiled sweet potato (4-ipomeanol). • Carcases (botulism). • Paint, batteries (lead). • Pesticides (rodenticides). • Minerals, medicines or chemicals carried over from previous consignment. • Ammoniated forages, urea-molasses feeds (substituted imidazoles). • Malicious adulterants (melamine)
Contamination of compounded feeds at feed mills. Samples of feed are routinely retained for retrospective investigation.	• Errors in formulation, mixing and poor quality control. • Excess levels of normal ingredients • Carryover between batches, usually antibiotics. • Labelling errors. • Use of contaminated ingredients.	• Medicines (antibiotics, ionophores) • Supplements (salt, vitamins, minerals)
Contaminated bedding	• Sawdust or shavings from recycled painted or tanalised wood. • Fungal contamination.	• lead • arsenic
Fertilisers *Nitrates* *Ammoniacal compounds* *Phosphatic* *Broiler litter*	• Insufficient withdrawal time following application. • Ingestion of stored fertilisers. Poor containment of animals and fertilisers. • Long term application can cause soil contamination with stable elements.	• Nitrogenous fertilisers (nitrate, urea, ammonium salts) • Phosphatic fertilisers (fluoride, cadmium) • Broiler litter (carcases (botulism)) • Soil contamination (cadmium in phosphates or sewage sludge)
Medicines	• Overdose. • Inappropriate vehicle/ formulation. • Use of expired products. • Interaction between medicines.	Systemic, oral and topical preparations including pour-on products; see data sheets. Interactions (macrolides and ionophores)
Pesticides/rodenticides	• Spillage, contamination of feed, soil, bedding, pasture or general environment. • Withdrawn products which still cause poisoning.	• Slug bait (metaldehyde), anticoagulant rodenticides, calciferol, zinc phosphide, alphachloralose • Strychnine, copper chrome arsenate (CCA)
Toxic gases on farms	• Poor ventilation. • Inadequate detectors. • Lack of precaution when emptying silos or slurry pits. • Fires. • Volcanic eruptions.	• Exhaust and combustion gases (carbon monoxide, carbon dioxide) • Slurry (hydrogen sulphide) • Silos (nitrogen dioxide) • Smoke inhalation • Ash inhalation (silicosis)
Malicious poisoning	Not usually targeted at cattle but cattle may ingest baits	• Pesticides (alphachloralose) • Banned chemicals (strychnine)

(*continued overleaf*)

Table 22.2 Common syndromes associated with poisoning.

	Presenting signs	Examples
Sudden death syndrome	• Sudden death is a common presentation of poisoning. • Affected animals are found dead. • 'Sudden death' in grazing animals may have occurred over a 24 hour period depending on management and inspection times.	• Apnoea (hydrogen sulphide), • Convulsants (lead, water dropwort, strychnine), • Cardiomyopathy (ionophores), • Hypocalcaemia and circulatory shock (oxalates), hypercalcaemia (calciferol), • Cytochrome oxidase inhibition (hydrogen sulphide, cyanide), • Oxygen exclusion (carbon dioxide), • Oxygen displacement (carbon monoxide), • Haemoglobin oxidation and haemolysis (nitrate, copper), • Haemorrhage (anticoagulants), • Cardiotoxins (yew,) • Narcotics (alphachloralose), Anticholinergic (deadly nightshade), Paralysis, neuromuscular block (hemlock, botulism),
Tooth abnormalities	Staining, pitting, stunting of teeth. Excessive wear. Very severe lesions can depress feed intake, grazing and production.	Fluoride
Alimentary syndrome	• Feed refusal, colic, eating disorders, salivation, frothing, champing, grinding teeth, regurgitation (cudding) abnormalities, constipation, diarrhoea, melaena, dysentery, mucus in faeces. • Feed refusal alone can precipitate metabolic disease, especially in pregnant and high-yielding dairy cows.	• Agents affecting gut motility (botulism), • Digesta volume (acidosis), • Metabolism (molybdenum). • Destruction of rumen flora (antibiotics, detergents). • Hepatopathy (ragwort) • Irritants: Metals (arsenic, lead). Supplements (salt, urea) Plants (solanaceae, oak, beet, brassicas) • Agrochemicals: Corrosives (acids, alkalis). Oils (diesel) Detergents Fertilisers (nitrates, sulphur, fluoride)
Blood syndrome	• Increased respiratory rate, tachycardia, weakness, discoloration, haemorrhage, haematomas, dysentery, melaena, haemorrhage. • The blood may appear cyanotic, cherry red, bright red, brown (methaemoglobin). • There may be intravascular haemolysis and anaemia. • Radiomimetic (radiation exposure)	• Anticoagulants (rodenticides, spoiled sweet clover and sweet vernal grass) • Hypersensitivity (bleeding calf syndrome, haemolytic anaemia of newborn) • Carbon dioxide, • Hydrogen sulphide • Carbon monoxide • Cyanide (laurel, prunus) • Oxidising agents (copper, nitrates, chlorates, onions, brassicas, T2) • Bracken • Lead • Selenium • Chronic hepatopathy • Ionising radiation • Benzene • Trichloroethylene
Skeletal muscle syndrome	• Ataxia, lameness, paralysis, sometimes deformity. • Convulsions leading to spastic paralysis. • Flaccid paralysis.	• Myodegeneration (fluoracetate, propionic acid preservation, high PUFA diets, ionophores, selenium, gossypol) • Agents affecting innervation (organophosphates, organochlorines, carbamates, lead) • Convulsant poisons (strychnine, water dropwort) • Botulism

(*continued overleaf*)

Table 22.2 (*continued*)

	Presenting signs	Examples
Circulatory syndrome	• Sudden death: cardiac arrest. • Cardiac arrhythmias. • Oedema, anasarca, pale mucous membranes, weakness, circulatory shock: dyspnoea, collapse, anuria. • Necrosis/gangrene of extremities.	• Hypocalcaemia (fluorosis, oxalates) • Hypercalcaemia, myocardial degeneration (cholecalciferol) • Myodegeneration (fluoracetate, propionic acid preservation, high PUFA diets, ionophores, gossypol) • Cardiotoxic plants (yew, rhododendron, foxglove, hellebores, lily of the valley, monkshood) • Cardiotoxic metals (lead) • Cardiotoxic chemicals (alcohols, aldehydes) • Ergot
Respiratory syndrome	• Dyspnoea, rapid respiratory rate, coughing, • Nasal discharge • Pulmonary fibrosis. • Respiratory paralysis.	• Agents causing blood abnormalities • Inhaled irritants (nitrogen dioxide, inhaled regurgitated digesta) • Selenium toxicity • Paraquat, • Fog fever • 4-ipomeanol • Hypersensitivity to moulds • Hemlock • Water dropwort • Strychnine • Botulism
Illthrift syndrome	• Weight loss • Poor production, including decreased weight gains, decreased milk production, infertility, lameness.	• Chronic hepatopathy (ragwort) • Nephropathy (copper) • Alimentary disease (acidosis, type B botulism toxicoinfection) • Neuropathy or metabolic poisons (lead, arsenic, molybdenum) • Lameness (fluoride, selenium, ergot, acidosis)
Kidney syndromes	• Urolithiasis: oliguria, anuria, severe pain, kicking at abdomen, attempted urination, grunting and teeth grinding. Bladder or urethral rupture causes local necrosis, uraemia, death. • Uraemia can cause CNS signs (renal encephalopathy). • Acute nephropathy: oliguria, feed refusal, colic, depression, collapse, coma and death. • Chronic nephropathy: polyuria, feed refusal, depression, colic, weight loss, weakness, tremors, increased respiration and pulse rates. Uraemic encephalopathy or osteodystrophy may occur. Recumbency and coma terminally.	• Urolithiasis (melamine, mineral imbalance (high magnesium and phosphate), high concentrate rations, plants high in silica or oxalates, ethylene glycol antifreeze) **Nephrosis** • Microbiological toxins (endotoxaemias, blue green algae, citrinin, Pyrexia, pruritis, haemorrhage syndrome (PPH)) • Plants (beets [oxalate], oak [tannin] and onions [haemolysins]) • Pesticides (calciferol, paraquat, cholecalciferol) • Heavy metals (lead, mercury, cadmium, arsenic) • Supplements (copper, selenium, vitamins A and D) • Medicines (neomycin, sulphonamide)
Liver syndrome	• Acute and sub-acute hepatopathy: anorexia, constipation or diarrhoea, colic, depression or excitation, head pressing, blindness, clotting abnormalities, icterus, oedema and ascites, weakness, secondary convulsions and coma, photosensitisation. • CNS signs (hepatic encephalopathy). • Chronic hepatopathy: Similar signs to sub-acute hepatopathy but more long-term effects such as illthrift, photosensitisation, anaemia.	• Supplements (vitamin A, iron, copper, selenium) • Plants (ragwort, oak (tannins), gossypol) • Industrial and agrochemicals (paraquat, diquat, chlorinated hydrocarbons) • Environmental (heavy metals, especially arsenic)

(*continued overleaf*)

Table 22.2 *(continued)*

	Presenting signs	Examples
Bones and joints	• Lameness (pain or abnormal function in bones/joints /feet). • Bones and joints: • Joint/long bone deformity: • Exostoses and osteoporosis: • Pedal bone fracture, periosteal calcification, bridging around joints, osteoporosis. • Laminitis.	• Molybdenum/copper • Vitamin A • Fluoride • Chronic selenosis • Ruminal acidosis • Bacterial toxaemias
Nervous syndromes	• Depression, wandering, ataxia, head pressing, teeth grinding, blindness, recumbency, coma, paralysis. • Hyperaesthesia, excitation, mania, head pressing, teeth grinding, blindness, tremors, convulsions, paralysis, coma. • The two syndromes can sometimes be produced by the same poison, depending on dose and physiological factors such as age.	• Polioencephalomalacia (thiaminase, sulphur, molassed urea, ammoniated forage, salt, lead) • Enzyme inhibition (lead, methyl mercury) • Ammonia accumulation (urea, hepatic or renal encephalopathy) • Neurotransmission (strychnine, organophosphates, carbamates, organochlorines, metaldehyde, atropine, tremorgenic mycotoxins, blue-green algal toxins, tetanus, botulism, lead, alphachloralose)
Reproductive syndrome	• Abnormalities in reproductive cycle, decreased fertility. • Gestational abnormalities: embryo resorption, terratogenesis, abortions, mummification, prolonged gestation, dystocias, increased neonatal losses, low neonatal viability. • Loss of libido. Reduced sperm count, sperm abnormalities.	• Zearalenone (cereals but also pasture grass) • Teratogens (lupins, broom [quinolizidine alkaloids], hemlock [piperidine alkaloids]) • Abortion (nitrates)
Skin, horn and hair syndrome	• Reddened skin, haemorrhages, skin oedema, eruptions, pruritis (evidence of rubbing), ulcers, thickened or folded skin. • Hair discoloration, hair loss, lack of hair growth, brittle hair or wool, loss of normal hair structure, loss of crimp in wool. • Abnormal rate of hoof or horn growth, discoloured horn, hoof or horn deformity, soft horn, brittle horn, hoof (sole) ulcers.	• Pyrexia, pruritus, haemorrhage syndrome (PPH) • Molybdenumosis (copper deficiency) • Selenium, acidosis (laminitis)
Hypersensitivity syndrome *Reaction to ingested, inhaled or injected antigens*	• Sensitisation to allergens, usually proteins. Adverse reactions to vaccines, medicines, supplements. • Respiratory: rhinitis, dyspnoea, shivering. • Alimentary: salivation, bloat, diarrhoea. • Skin: contact dermatitis, local swelling. • General systemic: urticaria, oedema, anasarca, muscle tremors. • Haemorrhagic syndromes.	• Urticaria or respiratory distress at drying off • Hypersensitivity to inhaled moulds, haemolytic anaemia of newborn calves • PPH may be a hypersensitivity
Immune suppression syndrome	• Unusually high incidence of infectious diseases. • Unusual severity of usually mild endemic diseases, e.g. ringworm	• Some mycotoxins • Bracken • Ionising radiation • Radiomimetic chemicals (benzene) • Bleeding calf syndrome

Identifying harmful exposure

A toxic incident may be suspected immediately from knowledge of contamination of the environment or diet with a toxic substance, or from the observed syndrome and epidemiological presentation. Alternatively, suspicion may arise as a disease investigation progresses. Differentiation of poisoning from infectious and nutritional disease is a crucial part of the disease investigation.

Criteria for suspecting intoxication or chemical contamination:

- Presenting signs suggesting a specific intoxication.
- Sudden onset of abnormalities throughout a group of animals, unlike the typical pattern for infectious disease.
- Known release of chemicals into the environment (fire, flood, road accident, volcanic eruption, etc).
- Suspected contamination of feed, water, bedding or air.

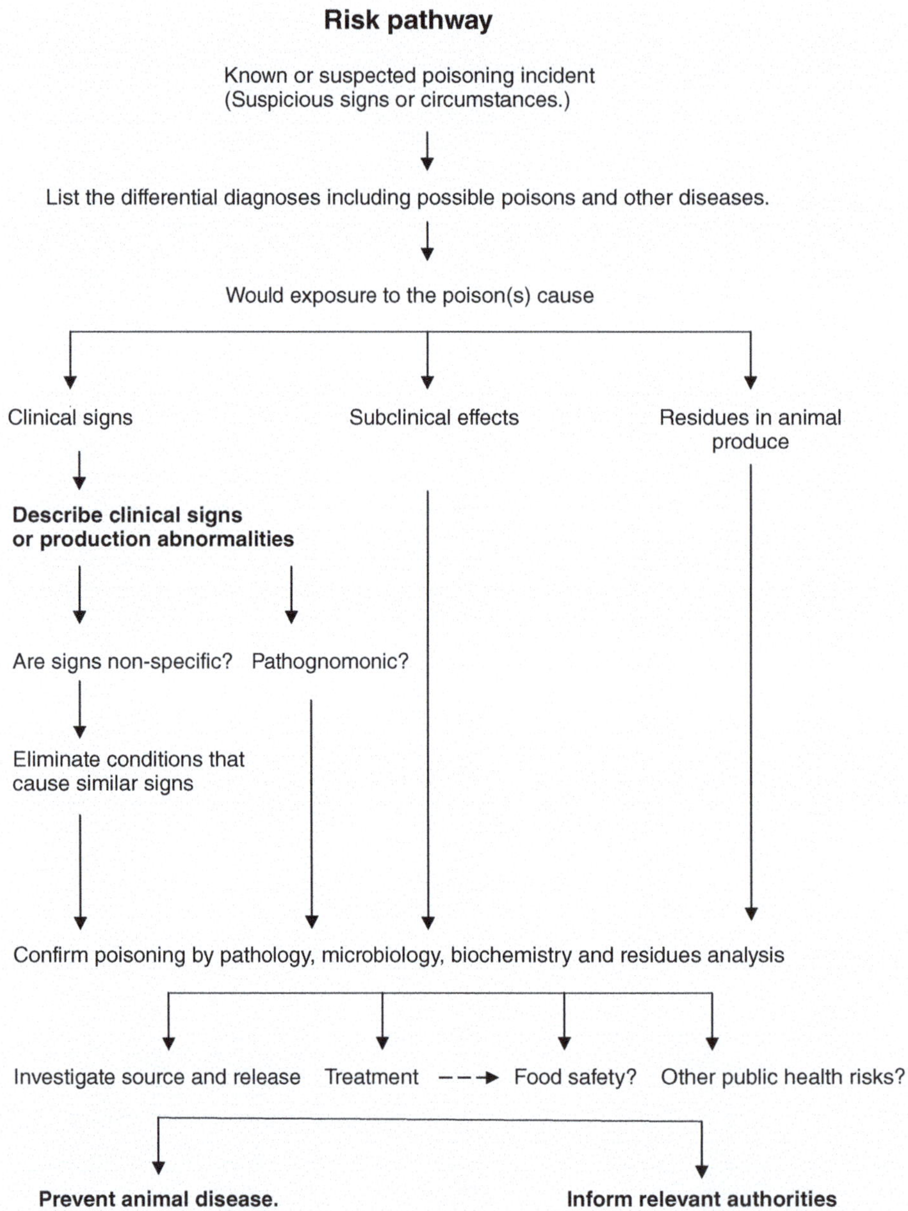

Figure 22.1 Investigation, diagnosis and control of suspected poisoning incidents.

- Suspected adverse reaction to feed, water, supplements, medicines, new deliveries or replacement feeds, new pasture or environment.
- Incidents that could be associated with environment, diet, water – especially recurrent disease or adverse effects which do not appear to be accounted for by infectious disease.
- Suspected infectious disease incidents in which the abnormalities are not entirely explained by the pathogens identified.
- Any incident for which no diagnosis is obtained.

Investigating suspected exposure to toxic substances

Disease investigation should be similar, irrespective of the cause (Figure 22.1):

- Describe the clinical syndrome (Table 22.2).
- Relate the clinical syndrome to possible sources of toxins/chemicals (Table 22.1) and to other factors. In addition to those listed above, other subjects for concern include the season, husbandry interventions and medications.
- Eliminate other (infectious and nutritional) diseases with similar clinical signs by biochemical, microbiological and pathological investigations. Toxic and nutritional diseases can present with similar epidemiology.
- The association of a clinical syndrome with evidence of contamination may be sufficient for diagnosis. Definitive confirmation requires pathology, chemical analyses and response to control measures.
- Investigate source, levels of contamination and exposure. Either eliminate or reduce contamination and/or exposure to acceptable levels. Monitored withdrawal from suspected contamination may be useful for suspected, but unknown, poisons.
- Confirmation of poisoning, especially chemical analyses, may be impractical or prohibitively expensive. If litigation is likely, retain samples so that confirmatory investigations are possible retrospectively.

Options for treatment, control and prevention of contamination

Metals can be chelated, usually using EDTA or penicillamine, and there are specific antidotes to opioids. Penalties for using unlicensed antidotes can be severe. Ammonium thiomolybdate (ATTM) is efficacious for treating copper poisoning, but ATTM is not a licensed medicine, so therefore has no MRL and, in the UK, treated cattle should never enter the food chain.

For most poisons, there is no specific antidote, and treatment should be symptomatic (e.g. controlling excitation, maintaining fluid balance) and rely on withdrawal from the source and prevention of further absorption. Laxatives and adsorbents may be indicated. For poisons that cause hyperaesthesia, treatments should not exacerbate the condition, and sedation may be indicated.

For point source poisons, elimination of the source should be possible. Many of these can be avoided using suitable protocols and appropriate disposal of waste. For natural, environmental contaminants, elimination is not usually possible, and controls are needed to reduce exposure to levels which protect animal and public health. Monitoring may be necessary to determine

Table 22.3 Sample collection for laboratory diagnosis.

	Tissue/sample	Amount	Preservation
Chemical analysis	liver	100 g	Freeze −30°C
	kidney	100 g	Freeze −30°C
	stomach contents	500 g	Freeze −30°C
	intestinal contents	200 g	Freeze −30°C
	fat	100 g	Freeze −30°C
	milk *(produce for food safety)*	200 g	Preserve with formalin
	muscle *(food produce for food safety)*	100 g	Freeze −30°C
Histopathology	liver	5 mm thick slice	Buffered formal saline
	kidney	5 mm thick slice	Buffered formal saline
	lung	5 mm thick slice	Buffered formal saline
	any tissue with visible lesions	5 mm thick slice through a lesion	Buffered formal saline
Clinical chemistry profile	serum and plasma	5 ml of each	
Haematology	EDTA blood	5 ml	
	blood smears collected as fresh as possible, preferably at the farm	Minimum of three	Air dry then heat fix
If clotting disorders suspected	citrated blood	5 ml	

Table 22.4 Common cattle poisons diagnosed in the UK.

Poison	Typical source or association	Clinical signs	Diagnostic samples required for investigation
Toxic elements			
Lead (Pb)	Manufactured materials: Batteries, paint, building materials, sump oil, fire ash. Environmental (mineral deposits): soil and feed crop contamination.	Acute: Nervous syndrome (hyperaesthesia), (typical calf syndrome). Chronic: Nervous syndrome (depression), (typical adult syndrome).	Lead analysis: liver and kidney. Brain: polioencephalomalacia Kidney: Nephrosis with acid fast inclusions.
Arsenic (As)	Wood preservatives (now withdrawn). Recycled wood products, building sites and bonfire ash. Soil contamination: former mining and smelting sites.	Acute: Gastroenteritis, colic, convulsions, circulatory shock. Chronic: Skin lesions illthrift and dullness.	Arsenic analysis; liver and kidney
Copper (Cu)	Feed supplements. Parenteral supplements. Narrow margin between requirement and toxic level. Biocide, e.g. foot baths; fungicide, molluscicide.	Sudden death Liver degeneration. Nephrosis Haemolysis, haemoglobinuria, jaundice Haemolysis and liver degeneration are frequently less apparent than in sheep.	Clinical chemistry: liver profile. Copper analysis: liver and kidney. Histology: liver and kidney degeneration. Monitor copper accumulation in supplemented animals.
Molybdenum (Mo)	Soil and herbage. Background Mo exposure reduces copper uptake. Severe molybdenumosis occurs in Somerset (teart pastures) and Caithness.	Chronic diarrhoea, illthrift. Other signs consistent with copper deficiency.	Feed analysis: Mo, Cu and S. Plasma and liver analysis: confirm raised Mo and Cu deficiency. Response to copper supplementation.
Selenium (Se)	Excess supplementation. Narrow safety margin between requirement and toxicity Natural: Selenium accumulator plants.	Acute: pulmonary oedema, gastroenteric syndrome, fever, ataxia, collapse and death. Chronic: rough coat, hair loss, hoof deformity, laminitis, lameness.	Selenium analysis: Diet, blood, kidney and liver. GSHPx is unsuitable to assess toxicity.
Farm chemical hazards			
Silo gases	Hydrogen sulphide gas from slurry	Sudden death	High sulphur PEM: analysis for sulphur. Environmental monitoring
Fertilizers *Nitrates,* *fluorides in phosphate fertilizers,* *urea,* *ammonia compounds*	Spillage and stored fertilizers.	Nitrates: Alimentary syndrome. Methaemoglobinaemia: cyanosis, brown blood, dyspnoea. Nervous syndrome. Protracted sub-lethal exposure causes abortion. Acute fluorosis: alimentary syndrome, circulatory syndrome, metabolic collapse.	Blood, urine, rumen contents analysis: nitrate and nitrite. Clinical signs occur when methaemoglobin exceeds 30%; lethal at 80–90%. Foetal ocular fluid: nitrate. Blood or urinary fluoride
Urea and ammonia compounds	Stored fertilizers or feed additives. Spillage.	Sudden death syndrome (hyperaesthesia).	Ammonia analysis: rumen contents
Salt	Excess salt, especially if drinking water is restricted Piles of salt for de-icing roads	Diarrhoea and colic. Weakness, dehydration, knuckling fetlocks (hind legs). PEM may occur when water is introduced.	Rumen contents and blood analysis: salt
Fuel oils, kerosene, diesel, petrol, sump oil (may contain lead).	Stored materials, wastes and workshops on farms. Poor containment of livestock. Sump oil.	Inhalation pneumonia. Nervous syndrome (depression). Chronic alimentary syndrome. Lead poisoning. Nervous syndrome.	Oil persists many weeks in intestinal contents. Odour: rumen and intestinal contents. Analysis for oil products. Lead analysis: liver and kidney.

(continued overleaf)

Table 22.4 *(continued)*

Poison	Typical source or association	Clinical signs	Diagnostic samples required for investigation
Ethylene glycol antifreeze	Drained vehicle radiators. Poor containment of livestock.	Neurological signs caused by oxalate poisoning	Urinalysis: (oxalate crystals) Smears and histopathology; brain and kidneys (oxalate crystals)
Pesticides			
Metaldehyde slug bait	Spillage. Animal access to stored pellets.	Nervous syndrome (hyperaesthesia)	Metaldehyde pellets in stomach contents. Liver analysis: metaldehyde
Organo-phosphates (OP)	Insecticidal sprays and washes. Pesticides for arable crops. Industrial chemicals.	Acute: Nervous syndrome (hyperaesthesia) Chronic: Relatively uncommon. Delayed onset ataxia and ascending paralysis.	Acute: Depressed acetyl cholinesterase activity in blood and brain. Analysis for OP residues: blood, stomach content, urine. Chronic: Histology of CNS: axonal degeneration.
Anticoagulant rodenticides. Second generation products (e.g. difenacoum, bromodialone) are very toxic for cattle.	Point sources in buildings, feed stores, stored grain etc Accidental access to stored baits. Poor containment of livestock.	Antagonists to vitamin K Haemorrhagic syndrome. Haemorrhages at critical sites cause other signs such as sudden death, bruising and haematomas, dyspnoea, lameness, ataxia, CNS signs and abortion.	Citrated blood: prothrombin time. Liver analysis: anticoagulants
Strychnine	Bait for moles. Withdrawn but still used illegally. May be malicious use.	Nervous syndrome (convulsions), extreme rigidity developing within 0.5–2 hours of exposure. No specific lesions	Analysis of bait or tissues
Feed imbalance			
Acute acidosis	Cereal engorgement Stored cereals and feeds. Poor containment of livestock.	Alimentary syndrome with nervous signs (ataxia, recumbency) Laminitis	Rumen pH < 5
SARA	Low fibre, high fermentable carbohydrate diets	Mild alimentary syndrome, milk fat depression, reduced feed intakes, reduced production, weight loss, laminitis.	Rumen pH < 5.5 Diet analysis
Low fibre, high fermentable carbohydrate diets predispose to polioencephalomalacia (PEM)	Cerebrocortical necrosis (CCN): thiaminase production in the rumen	Nervous syndrome.	Typical gross and histopathology. Association with diet. Measure thiamine dependent enzyme activities Response to thiamine.
Urea-molasses and ammoniated forages	Sudden introduction of novel feed Imbalance	Sudden death Hyperexcitability, grinding teeth, tremor, opisthotonus, convulsions, dyspnoea	Analysis for ammonia
Microbiological toxins			
Cl. botulinum *Types C and D cause typical botulism.* *Type B associated with atypical botulism.*	Putrid feed materials. Putrid materials in fertilizers (poultry litter) stored feeds and forages and in the environment.	Flaccid paralysis; clinically similar to hypocalcaemia and some encephalitides. Atypical botulism (alimentary syndrome) not yet identified in UK.	Eliminate other causes of flaccid paralysis. Analysis of gut contents: *C. botulinum* toxins.

(continued overleaf)

Table 22.4 (*continued*)

Poison	Typical source or association	Clinical signs	Diagnostic samples required for investigation
Mycotoxins	Feed materials spoiled during growth or during storage.	Ergot: necrosis of extremities Tremorgenic mycotoxins: tremors in cattle at pasture. T2 toxin: blood dyscrasias and haemorrhages. Citrinin: associated with PPH Zearalenone: reproductive syndrome. Aflatoxins: hepatopathy, imported feeds only.	Relate onset of disease or production problem to introduction to new feed or pasture. Relate signs and pathology to specific mycotoxins. Identify probable spoiled feed materials. Feed analysis for mycotoxins.
Blue-green algae Multiple toxins: *neurotoxins hepatotoxins nephrotoxins enterotoxins*	Blooms on surface water sources used for drinking. Toxins not invariably present. Toxins released from bloom as the algae start to die.	Types of toxins determine signs. Sudden death syndrome, nervous syndrome, liver syndrome, kidney syndrome, alimentary syndrome.	Presence of blue green algae in gut contents. Confirmation of toxins by chemical analysis of contaminated water.
Poisonous plants			
Lush grass, especially aftermath *High levels of D,L-tryptophan*	3-methylindole produced in the rumen	Fog fever. Acute respiratory syndrome. Acute respiratory distress.	Clinical syndrome. Enlarged firm lungs, emphysema, consolidation, fibrosis. Levels of D,L-tryptophan or 3-methylindole are not reliable for diagnosis.
Ragwort *Pyrollizidine alkaloids*	Unpalatable when growing. Dying or cut plants are palatable and toxic. Ragwort in hay and silage is palatable. Toxins are partially inactivated by ensilage although ragwort contaminated silage has caused herd outbreaks of poisoning in cattle.	Weight loss, oedema, straining, diarrhoea.	Liver cirrhosis with typical histology. Examine representative samples of hay or silage for ragwort.
Bracken *Ptaquilosides*	Eaten if grazing sparse and when new growth appears in the spring. Dried bracken has been used as bedding.	Depression, weakness, anorexia, haemorrhagic syndrome. Individuals develop clinical signs when an entire group is sub-clinically affected.	Access to bracken. Pancytopoenia with agranulocytosis leucopoenia and thrombopaenia.
Oak *Simple phenols and tannins*	Acorns, leaves.	Alimentary syndrome: Colic, anorexia, weight loss, ascites, oedema, constipation replaced by black tarry faeces. Haematuria.	Gastrointestinal ulceration and haemorrhage. Nephrosis, raised urea and creatinine. Liver degeneration. Clinical chemistry: liver profile.
Brassicas: Kale, rape and rape seed meal, turnips S-methylcysteine sulfoxide (SMCO) *Goitrogens* *Nitrates*	Feed varieties genetically improved to reduce content of toxins. SMCO destroyed in silage. High fertilizer applications and adverse weather increase nitrate levels	Blood syndrome: SMCO causes haemolysis, anaemia, haemoglobinuria, pallor, jaundice, tachycardia. Nitrates cause methaemoglobinaemia and abortions. Respiratory syndrome: Acute respiratory distress (similar to fog fever), Nervous syndrome: Depression, PEM and (reversible) blindness. Hypothyroidism, goitre.	Haematology. RBC inclusions on blood smears. Haemolysis, haemoglobinuria (brown urine). Methaemoglobinaemia (brown blood). Aborted foetus: nitrate levels in ocular fluids Goitre.
Hemlock *Cicutoxin, coniine, cyanapine*	Grows in damp regions and hedgerows. Exposed tubers.	Sudden death and nervous syndromes: Convulsions. Reproductive syndrome: teratogenic	Presence of plant in rumen

(*continued overleaf*)

Table 22.4 (*continued*)

Poison	Typical source or association	Clinical signs	Diagnostic samples required for investigation
Hemlock, water dropwort *Oenanthetoxin*	Grows in ditches. Exposed tubers.	Sudden death and nervous syndromes: Convulsions.	Presence of plant in rumen
Deadly Nightshade *Atropine, L-hyoscyamine*	Hedgerow plant	Nervous syndrome: Mydriasis, dryness and scaling of skin, thirst, hyperthermia, ataxia, death	Presence of plant in rumen
Yew *Taxine*	Access to trees and to tree and hedge prunings	Sudden death and Circulatory syndromes: Cardiotoxic. Tremor, dyspnoea, collapse, excitation, death in 1–3 days.	Presence of yew in rumen
Cyanide containing plants Laurel, prunus species, apple pips. *Cyanogenic glycosides*	Access to trees and to tree and hedge prunings. Unusual by-product feeds, e.g. apple pomace.	Sudden death. Blood syndrome: Bright red fully oxygenated blood.	Confirm cyanide in feed, blood, rumen contents, liver. Freeze samples immediately.
Primary photosensitivity St John's wort (*hypericin*)	Hypericin is photoactive. Fresh plant is more toxic, drying partially inactivates the toxin.	Skin and hair syndrome:	Sunburn on hairless and unpigmented skin, especially dorsal aspect. Presence of St John's wort. Pure ryegrass sward is low risk.
Secondary photosensitivity (*hepatotoxins*). *Ragwort, bog asphodel, swede rape (brassica napus), red clover, blue-green algae*	Secondary to diffuse liver disease. Usually pasture or forage crop associated. Cause rarely confirmed.	Liver syndrome: Evidence of chronic liver dysfunction such as jaundice.	GGT, AST, GLDH elevation. Jaundice. Histology: cholestasis, periportal fibrosis, bile duct proliferation. Presence of high risk forages or hepatotoxins.
Veterinary products			
Antimicrobials	Medicated feed. Usually accidental contamination, carryover or mislabelling at the feed mill.	Feed contamination: indigestion and production drop.	Immediate effect usually with recovery following feed replacement. Identify antimicrobial activity in the suspected source.
e.g. *Ionophore*	Unintended medication: Overdose of permitted ionophore. Interactions with other medication, e.g. tiamulin. Intended use: adverse reaction, or overdosage.	Sudden death syndrome: cardiomyopathy. Skeletal muscle syndrome: lameness, ataxia. See datasheets	Feed audit and analysis. Post mortem and histology: myodegeneration Heart and skeletal muscles. Feed analysis. Use of other medicines.
Other veterinary medicines	Unlicensed use	Implications for food safety	

the effectiveness of these measures and to identify when animal products are fit to enter the food chain. It may take several changes in husbandry to successfully control environmental contaminants.

Food safety, public health, suspected adverse reactions

Consultation with regulators is essential to avoid pitfalls. Report suspected adverse reactions, feed contamination or use of unlicensed medicines to food safety and medicines authorities. Food safety authorities can provide risk assessment and advice on withdrawal intervals for produce. Inform relevant other authorities if there are implications for public health for humans living or working in or close to a contaminated environment.

Laboratory investigations

To investigate any disease of uncertain aetiology, a comprehensive disease investigation is required, which could include autopsy, clinical chemistry, virology, microbiology, parasitology and histopathology. A concurrent nutritional investigation may also be required.

Chemical analysis confirms the presence of specific chemicals, but their presence has to be suspected before laboratories conduct specific analyses. Large-scale chemical screening is usually too expensive and too slow to be practical. A shortlist of possible chemicals should be determined from clinical presentation, pathology and associations with environment, feed, supplements, husbandry and medicines. Analytical methods are not routinely available for many natural toxins, including most plant toxins. Precise interpretation of levels of chemicals and toxins may not be available.

Routine samples for confirming a poisoning incident

Samples should be collected and stored in anticipation of possible need for laboratory investigations. These are presented in Table 22.3.

Common cattle poisons

The common cattle poisons diagnosed in the UK are presented in Table 22.4. The precise incidence of poisoning is unknown, because poisoning is not notifiable. Acidosis and SARA are probably the most common causes of poisoning in UK cattle. Most poisoning incidents are avoidable. Inadequate livestock containment, secure storage of materials, waste disposal, building inspection or maintenance, and grazing and nutritional management usually contribute to poisoning.

Sources of additional information

Plumlee, K.H. (ed., 2004). *Clinical Veterinary Toxicology*. Mosby Inc., an affiliate of Elsevier.

Klaassen, C.D. (ed., 2001). *Casarett and Doull's Toxicology; The Basic Science of poisons*, 6th Edition. McGraw Hill Professional.

Timbrell, J.A. (1991). *Principles of Biochemical Toxicology*, 2nd Edition. Taylor & Francis, London.

Nordberg, G.F., Fowler B.A., Nordberg, M., Friberg, L. (eds.,2007). *Handbook on the Toxicology of Metals*, 3rd Edition. Elsevier.

Seiler, H.G., Sigel, H. and Sigel, A. (eds., 1988). *Handbook on the Toxicity of Inorganic Compounds*. Marcel Dekker; New York and Basel.

The UK Animal Welfare Regulations 2007:
http://www.opsi.gov.uk/si/si2007/uksi_20072078_en_1

UK Code of recommendations for welfare of livestock: cattle
http://www.defra.gov.uk/publications/2011/04/18/pb7949-cattle/

Food and Feed Hygiene Regulations 2006:
http://www.legislation.gov.uk/uksi/2006/14/contents/made

Official Feed and food controls (England) Regulations 2009:
http://www.legislation.gov.uk/uksi/2009/3255/contents/made

Maximum levels for contaminants in food:
http://europa.eu/legislation_summaries/food_safety/contamination_environmental_factors/l21290_en.htm

The Food Safety Act 1990:
http://www.opsi.gov.uk/acts/acts1990/ukpga_19900016_en_1.htm

CHAPTER 23

Antimicrobial Selection in Cattle Practice

Peter D. Cockcroft

Learning objectives

- Understand the roles and responsibilities of the veterinarian with regards to the selection and use of antimicrobials.
- Be aware of the legal requirements with regarding to labelling, prescribing and record keeping
- Have a working knowledge of antimicrobial group sensitivities and characteristics
- Understand the criteria for the appropriate selection of antimicrobials
- Appreciate the strategies to maximise therapeutic efficiency of and minimise usage.
- Appreciate the need to reduce the risk of the development of resistance

Introduction

Antimicrobials are compounds that destroy or inhibit the growth of microorganisms. They can be used therapeutically (treatment of clinical cases), prophylactically (treatment prior to risk) and metaphylactically (treatment following exposure to pathogens). In the past, they have also be used for growth promotion, but this application is now in rapid decline due to increasing regulation. Antimicrobial therapy can be very effective in reducing the duration of infection, reducing the pain of disease, limiting further spread of the disease and lowering the severity of the disease.

The veterinarian has an important part to play in ensuring that meat and milk are as free as possible from antibiotic residues, resistant zoonotic bacteria and resistant bacteria which may transfer resistance to human bacteria. Organisations such as the British Veterinary Association (BVA), the American Veterinary Medical Association (AVMA) and the Association of American Bovine Practitioners (AABP) have developed general guidelines for antibiotic usage. These have been adapted by organisations such as the Responsible Use of Medicines in Agriculture Alliance (RUMA) in the UK, and the National Cattleman's Beef Association in the United States, specifically for cattle producers and cattle veterinarians. Examples are shown in Table 23.1 and Table 23.2. Alternative control and prevention strategies have been emphasised by RUMA to minimise the need for antimicrobials. These include improved biosecurity, appropriate vaccination, in-parlour hygiene and optimised husbandry protocols.

When the decision is made to use antimicrobial therapy, the veterinarian should strive to optimise therapeutic efficiency and minimise resistance to antimicrobials in order to protect public and animal health. Antimicrobials should not be used to replace other methods of reducing the risk of disease, such as nutrition, housing, hygiene, management and vaccination. The aim is to minimise antibiotic usage without compromising animal welfare, to maximise therapeutic efficiency and to minimise the selection of resistant organisms.

Therapy may fail because: the owner or keeper of the animals did not comply with the instructions (poor compliance); the diagnosis was incorrect; the dose prescribed was insufficient; the dose was given for too short a period of time to be effective; the pathogen was not sensitive to the antibiotic; the antibiotic failed to reach therapeutic levels in the organ/site of infection; immunosuppression reduced the host response; or the antibiotic was stored incorrectly and was no longer effective. Food residues may result as a consequence of: using incorrect dose rates, treating the wrong animals, using inappropriate withdrawal times and keeping inaccurate records of treatment.

Knowledge of the national regulations regarding which antimicrobials can be used in cattle, and the data sheet information regarding the specific conditions the product is licensed to treat, the dosage, the contraindications, the route of administration and the withdrawal times, is essential. Appropriate storage in terms of legal and temperature requirements should be implemented. If an antimicrobial is used to treat another

Bovine Medicine, Third Edition. Edited by Peter D. Cockcroft.

Table 23.1 Responsible use of antimicrobials in veterinary proactive (adapted and modified from BVA (2009)).

1 Work with clients to avoid the need for antimicrobials.	• Integrated disease control programs • Animal health and welfare planning • Isolate infected animals wherever possible
2 Avoid inappropriate use.	• Only use antibiotics when appropriate for the condition • Limit use to sick and at-risk animals • Advise clients on correct route of administration, dosages, frequency and duration
3 Choose the right drug for the identified/presumed pathogen.	• Identify likely target organisms and predict their susceptibility • Understand their actions, tissue distributions and pharmacodynamic properties • Use antimicrobials with a spectrum as narrow as possible
4 Monitor antimicrobial sensitivity.	• Culture and microbial sensitivity will enable a more informed selection of antimicrobial agent
5 Minimise prophylactic use.	• Use only when animals are at risk and there is evidence that usage reduces morbidity and/or mortality • Regularly reassess prophylactic use • Monitor antimicrobial sensitivity
6 Minimise use perioperatively.	• Only use when necessary • Aseptic techniques will reduce the risk • This may not be an option with on-farm surgery
7 Record and justify deviations from data sheet protocols.	• Be able to justify the choice of antibiotic and dosage recommended • Keep accurate records of treatments
8 Report suspected treatment failure to the relevant authorities.	• This may indicate resistance • Suspected adverse reactions should be reported to the relevant authorities
9 Flouroquinolones and third-/fourth-generation cephalosporins.	• Reserve these antimicrobials for clinical conditions that respond poorly to other classes of antimicrobial, and where antibiotic sensitivity has been performed • Do not administer systematically to groups of animals unless a risk assessment indicates justification • Avoid off-label use whenever possible
10 Resistance and responsible use.	• Antimicrobials are essential for the treatment and prevention of infectious and zoonotic diseases in animals and humans • The frequent use of antibiotics increases the risk of development of microbial resistance • Responsible use optimises the therapeutic effects and minimises the development of resistance

condition other than that appearing on the data sheet, then this is off known as off-label, and longer standard withdrawal times usually apply.

Drug selection, labelling, prescribing and record keeping

In the UK, the Cascade indicates the sequence with which the decision-making should proceed, and is as follows. The Veterinary Medicines Directorate (VMD) (2013) provides the following information regarding the Cascade:

1. Use a product that is authorised to treat the condition in that food-producing species.
2. Use a product that is licensed to treat another condition in that species, or a drug that is authorised in another food-producing animal species.

Food-producing animals may only be treated under the Cascade with medicines that contain pharmacologically active substances listed in the Table of Allowed Substances in Commission Regulation EU (European Union) No 37/2010. A veterinary surgeon prescribing for, or administering a medicine to, food-producing animals under the Cascade is required to specify an appropriate withdrawal period to the animal produce. When setting the withdrawal period, a veterinary surgeon must take into account known information about the use of the product on the authorised species when prescribing to another species under the Cascade. Unless the medicine indicates a withdrawal period for the species concerned, this should not be less than seven days for milk and 28 days for meat from mammals. The VMD provides additional information which is beyond the scope of this book.

Table 23.2 A producers guide for judicious use of antimicrobials (adapted and modified from Beef USA National Cattleman's Beef Association).

	Guideline	Comment
1	Prevent problems	Emphasise appropriate husbandry and hygiene, routine health examinations and vaccinations.
2	Select and use antibiotics carefully.	Consult with your veterinarian on the selection and use of antibiotics. Have a valid reason to use an antibiotic.
3	Avoid using antibiotics important in human medicine as first line therapy.	Avoid using as the first antibiotic, those medications that are important to treating strategic human or animal Infections.
4	Use the laboratory to help you select antibiotics.	Cultures and susceptibility test results should be used to aid in the selection of antimicrobials, whenever possible.
5	Avoid using broad spectrum.	Use narrow spectrum antimicrobials whenever possible.
6	Avoid inappropriate antibiotic use.	Confine therapeutic antimicrobial use to proven clinical.
7	Treatment programs should reflect best use principles.	Regimens for therapeutic antimicrobial use should be optimised using current pharmacological information and principles.
8	Treat the fewest number of animals possible.	Limit antibiotic use to sick or at-risk animals.
9	Treat for the recommended time period.	To minimise the potential for bacteria to become resistant to antimicrobials.
10	Avoid environmental contamination with antibiotics.	Steps should be taken to minimise antimicrobials reaching the environment through spillage, contaminated ground run-off or aerosolisation.
11	Keep records of antibiotic use.	Accurate records of treatment and outcome should be used to evaluate therapeutic regimens; always follow proper withdrawal times.
12	Follow label directions.	Follow label instructions and never use antibiotics other than as labelled without a valid veterinary prescription.
13	Off-label antibiotic use must follow FDA regulations.	Prescriptions, including off-label use of medications, must meet the Animal Medicinal Drug Use Clarification Act (AMDUCA) amendments to the Food, Drug, and Cosmetic Act and its regulations. This includes having a valid Veterinary-Client relationship.
14	Sub-therapeutic antibiotic use is discouraged.	Antibiotic use should be limited to preventing or controlling disease, and should not be used if the principal intent is to improve performance.

The relevant legislation and best practice needs to be observed with regards to record-keeping, prescribing and labelling of dispensed medicines.

Antimicrobials

Sensitivities

Antibiotics should only be used when it is known or suspected that an infectious agent is present that will respond to antibiotic therapy. Ideally, the sensitivity of the causal organism should been ascertained before therapy is started. In cases where the disease is severe and/or the spread is rapid, treatment should be started with an antibiotic with predicted sensitivity to the clinical diagnosis. Samples should be taken, and the sensitivity *in vitro* of isolates from outbreak of disease established, in case of an incorrect presumptive diagnosis or poor response to the chosen antibiotics.

There is much debate about the translation of *in vitro* sensitivity and *in vivo* clinical efficiency, but it is generally accepted to be of value. The response to antibiotic therapy should be monitored. *In vivo* factors affecting the response include: the ability to reach the site of infection and attain high enough concentrations; persistence at the site of infection; the nature of the pathological process; and the immune response of the host. It is useful to know the pharmokinetics and tissue distribution of the drug. Pharmokinetic parameters such as bioavailability, the tissue distribution, half-life and MIC 50 and MIC 90, can be used to compare different drugs. The route of administration should be considered. Prolonged oral use may raise concerns about the selection of resistant bacteria that inhabit the gut.

Antimicrobial group characteristics

Sulphonamides

- Good oral bioavailability.
- Good distribution throughout the body, including CNS and joints.
- Low concentrations in milk.
- Hepatic acetylation followed by renal excretion.
- Crystalluria may occur with overdose or water deprivation.
- Necrotic tissue and pus reduce efficacy.
- Bacteriostatic; combined with trimethoprim (potentiated sulphonamides), bactericidal.
- Environmental contamination may occur due to excretion in faeces and urine.
- Susceptible: *Streptoccocus* spp, *Staphyloccoccus* spp, *E. coli*, *Histophilus* spp.
- Highly resistant: *Mycoplasma* spp, Rickettsia.

Penicillins

- Bactericidal.
- Penicillin G and phenoxymethyl penicillin mainly gram-positive activity.
- Penicillin G and phenoxymethyl penicillin; gram-positive; drug of choice for infections with *Clostridia* spp, *Streptococcus* spp; some anaerobic gram-negative activity.
- Phenoxymethyl penicillin ampicillin, amoxicillin can be given orally.
- Ampicillin, amoxicillin have a wide range of gram-positive and gram-negative activity, including *Salmonella* spp and *E. coli*.
- Well distributed, with the exception of the CNS and joints.
- Low concentrations in milk.
- Hypersensitivity reactions may occur.
- Bactericidal with noted anaerobic capability.
- Penicillin, ampicillin and amoxicillin are susceptible to staphylococcus penicillinases.
- Cloxacillin and amoxicillin/clavulanic combinations are resistant to penicillinases.

Tetracyclines

- Well absorbed following parenteral administration.
- Bacteriostatic.
- Significant activity against gram positive-and gram-negative bacteria.
- Well distributed in tissues.
- Eliminated through bile and kidneys.
- Susceptible: *Histophilus* spp, *Mannhaemia* spp, *Pasteurella* spp, *Streptococcus*.
- Variable susceptibility: *Staphylococcus* spp, *E. coli*, *Salmonella* spp, *Clostridium* spp, *Mycoplasma* spp.

Macrolides (tylosin, erythromycin, tilmicosin)

- Erythromycin and tylosin are well distributed in tissues, particularly milk, with the exception of variable CNS.
- Tilmicosin and tulathromycin are found in neutrophils and macrophages at sites of inflammation.
- They are bacteriostatic.
- Elimination mainly by liver, some by kidney.
- Spectrum of activity mainly gram-positive with some gram-negative activity
- Sensitive organisms include *Staphylococcus* spp, *Streptococcus* spp, *Leptospira* spp, *Histophilus spp*, *Mannhaemia* spp, *Pasteurella* spp, Mycoplasmas.
- Erythromycin has limited activity against mycoplamas.

Aminoglycosides (spectinomycin and apramycin)

- Bactericidal.
- Excreted by kidneys.
- Poor CNS penetration.
- Spectinomycin: good gram-negative activity.

Cephalosporins (e.g. Ceftiofur and cephalexine)

- Bactericidal.
- Given parenterally.
- Eliminated through kidneys.
- Activity: Gram-negative, Gram-positive.

Lincosamides (Lincomycin)

- Good tissue distribution (with the exception of CNS).
- Eliminated mainly through liver.
- Bacteriostatic.
- Activity: Gram-positive – *Staphylococcus* spp, *Streptococcus*.
- Anaerobic bacteria: *Clostridium* spp., *Fusobacterium* spp, Mycoplasmas.

Table 23.3 indicates the characteristics of a selection of cattle pathogens which are important when considering their antimicrobial sensitivities. Table 23.4 provides information about the likely sensitivities of the major antimicrobial groups relative to the characteristics listed in Table 23.3.

Selecting an antimicrobial

Accurate diagnosis indicating a bacterial infection with susceptibility testing is important. Treating affected individuals only is the ideal. Clinical efficiency requires that the pathogen is susceptible, and that the drug can penetrate and retain activity at the site of infection. Ideally, the antibiotic will only target the causal pathogen and have minimal effect on other micro-organisms. Generally, broad spectrum antibiotics lead to the development of resistance in non-target microorganisms more rapidly than narrow spectrum, due to increased selection pressure. Therefore, where an appropriate narrow spectrum antibiotic is available, this may be preferable. Some antimicrobials are recognised as having important roles in human medicine, and should be used very selectively for acute severe individual cases only. Cephalosporins and fluoroquinolones fall into this category.

Bacteriostatic antimicrobials require a competent immune response to work effectively; therefore, bactericidal antibiotics may be preferred in immuno-suppressed or severely ill animals. Combinations of antimicrobials should be avoided in most cases, the exception being sulphonamide combinations with diaminopyrimidines, which are synergistic. Bactericidal and bacteriostatic antimicrobials are antagonistic, and reduce the clinical efficiency if used in combination. Parenteral administration is preferable to the oral route, to reduce the impact on gut flora.

Appropriate dosage regimes, based upon data sheet recommendations with regard to dose rate, interval between treatments and duration of treatment, should be applied, and

Table 23.3 Characteristics of some cattle bacterial pathogens which are important when considering their antimicrobial sensitivities.

Bacteria	Location	Gram stain	Oxygen affinity
Actinobacillus	Extracellular	Gram-negative	Facultative anaerobe
Campylobacter	Extracellular	Gram-negative	Aerobic
Clostridia	Extracellular	Gram-positive	Anaerobic
Trueperella	Facultative intracellular	Gram-positive	Facultative anaerobe
E. coli	Extracellular	Gram-negative	Facultative anaerobe
Fusobacterium	Extracellular	Gram-negative	Anaerobic
Histophilus	Extracellular	Gram-negative	Facultative anaerobe
Klebsiella	Extracellular	Gram-negative	Facultative anaerobe
Leptospira	Extracellular	N/A	Aerobic
Mycobacterium	Facultative intracellular	Acid-fast	Aerobic
Mycoplasma	Attached to cell membrane	N/A	N/A
Pasteurella	Extra-cellular	Gram-negative	Facultative anaerobe
Mannhaemia	Extra-cellular	Gram-negative	Facultative
Salmonella	Facultative intracellular or extracellular	Gram-negative	Facultative anaerobe
Staphylococcus	Extracellular or facultative intracellular	Gram-positive	Facultative anaerobe
Streptococcus	Extracellular	Gram-positive	Facultative anaerobe

data sheet recommendations with regards to withdrawal times and storage should be closely adhered to. Identification and re-evaluation of a case which fails to respond and improve is important. This assessment can be difficult, but a persistent pyrexia and a general decline in health over 2–5 days may indicate the need to consider switching to an antibiotic with a different, and possibly broader, spectral range of activity, if additional culture and sensitivity information is not available.

Data sheet instructions regarding species, disease indications, contraindications, dosage regimes, withdrawal periods and storage conditions should be understood. The dosage regime and duration of treatment should be carefully considered, to avoid the administration of sub-therapeutic doses and sub-optimal time exposure, leading to therapeutic failure and chronic disease. Group medication will be necessary in some cases, to treat clinically affected animals within the group, reduce the spread and prevent clinical disease developing in incubating/subclinical animals. Strategic medication to healthy animals should be justified by a risk assessment indicating that the animals are at high risk, and that other methods of reducing risk have been implemented or considered. Questions you should ask when considering antimicrobial therapy are:

- Does the diagnosis warrant antibiotic therapy?
- What pathogenic organism is involved?
- What is the *in vitro* antibiotic sensitivity of the organism?
- What organ(s) are involved?
- Will the antibiotic penetrate these tissues?
- Is there likely to be secondary infection as well as the primary pathogen?
- Is the organism extracellular or intracellular?
- Can I use an antibiotic with a targeted narrow range of activity?
- What dose, frequency and length of course will be required?
- Are there any side-effects to consider?
- What route of administration is appropriate?
- Which animals should be treated (clinical cases only, or at-risk animals as well?)
- What are the withdrawal times and residue implications?
- Is it the most cost-effective therapy?

Figures 23.1 and 23.2 indicate some common bacterial infections in calves and adult cattle respectively. Table 23.5 provides some guidelines and suggestions for the treatment of some selected common conditions in cattle.

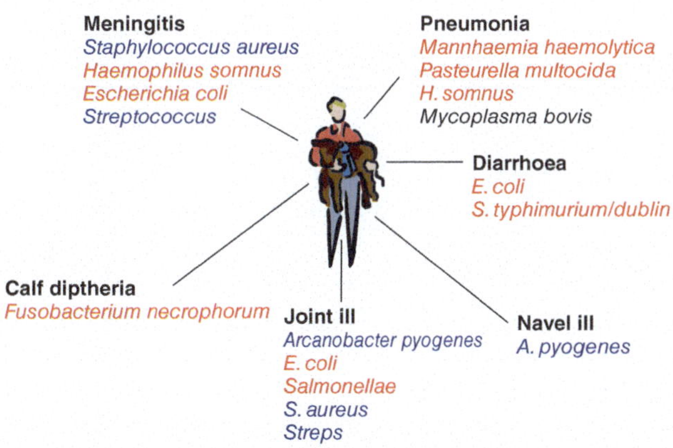

Figure 23.1 Common bacterial disease in calves: red indicates gram-positive organisms and blue indicates gram-negative organisms. Adapted from BVA 2009.

Pneumonia

Respiratory disease in growing cattle is associated with one or more of a number of pathogens, including: bovine respiratory

Table 23.4 General antimicrobial group sensitivities.

Antibiotic group	Antibiotic	Action	Activity spectrum	Aerobic		Anaerobic		Mycoplasma	Tissue penetration
				Gram +	Gram −	Gram +	Gram −		
Aminoglycosides	dihydrostreptomycin apramycin	Cidal	Narrow	Limited	Good	Poor	Poor	Poor	ECF, synovial, peritoneal and pleural fluid Kidneys Poor other tissues
Lincosamines	lincomycin	Static	Narrow	Good	Poor	Good	Moderate	Good	Lung, liver, spleen, reproductive tract, skin and bone
Macrolides	tylosin milmycosin tulatharomycin erythromycin spiramycin	Static	Narrow	Good	Limited	Good	Moderate	Good	Lung, liver, spleen, reproductive tract, skin and bone
Sulphonamides	sulphadimidine	Static	Narrow	Good	Good	Poor	Poor	Poor	Diffuse well into body tissues
Potentiated sulphonamides	sulphadimidine trimethoprim	Cidal	Narrow	Good	Good	Good	Good	Poor	Pleural, peritoneal, synovial, ocular fluids, CSF
Penicillin		Cidal	Narrow	Good	Poor	Good	Moderate	Poor	Soft tissue, bone, bile, urine peritoneum
Aminocyclitol	spectinomycin	Static	Narrow	Good	Good	Poor	Limited	Good	ECF Kidneys Poor other tissues
Tetracyclines	chlortetracycline tetracycline oxytetracycline doxycycline	Static	Intermediate	Moderate	Moderate	Moderate	Moderate	Good	Lung, liver, spleen, kidney, urine, milk
Penicillins (Semisynthetic)	ampicillin amoxicillin	Cidal	Intermediate	Good	Limited	Good	Moderate	Poor	Soft tissue, bone, bile, urine peritoneum
	amoxycillin potentiated with clavulanate	Cidal	Intermediate	Good	Good	Good	Moderate	Poor	Soft tissue, bone, bile, urine peritoneum
Chloaamphenicols	florfenicol	Static	Intermediate	Good	Good	Moderate	Moderate	Poor	CSF Most tissues
Quinolones Third generation	enrofloxacin danofloxacin marbofloxacin	Cidal	Broad	Good	Good	Good	Good	Good	Lung, liver, kidneys
Cephalopsporins third generation and fourth generation	cefquinone ceftiofur	Cidal	Broad	Good	Good	Good	Moderate	Poor	Soft tissue, bone, synovial, pleural, pericardial fluids, CSF, urine and bile

syncytial virus; parainfluenza 3 virus; bovine viral diarrhoea virus; bovine herpes virus-1; *Mannheimia haemolytica*; *Pasteurella multocida*; *Histophilus somnus*; *Trueperella pyogenes*; and *Mycoplasma bovis*. Everyone involved in prescribing for cattle with respiratory disease should be striving to improve the accuracy of their diagnosis, the efficacy of their treatment, and the efficiency of disease control measures on farms (Barrett, 2000).

Florfenicol, cefiofur, tilmicosin, tulathromycin and fluoroquinolones can penetrate the lung tissue to achieve MIC for *M. haemolytica*, *Pastuerella multocida* and *Histophilus somni*. Penicillin, ampicillin, amoxicillin, erythromycin and tylosin are much less effective in their lung penetration with less clinical efficiency. Factors to consider are: cost; volume; route of administration; frequency; withdrawal times; length of action; and safety (e.g. tilmicosin can cause severe health problems if self-injected). Cusack *et al.* (2003) reviewed the literature and found that oxytetracycline, trimethoprim potentiated sulphonamides, fluorfenicol, tilmicosin, enrofloxacine and ceftiofur had all been shown to significantly reduce the severity of clinical signs of BRD, and to reduce the case fatality rate in feedlot cattle. Further information is provided in Chapter 52 on bovine respiratory disease.

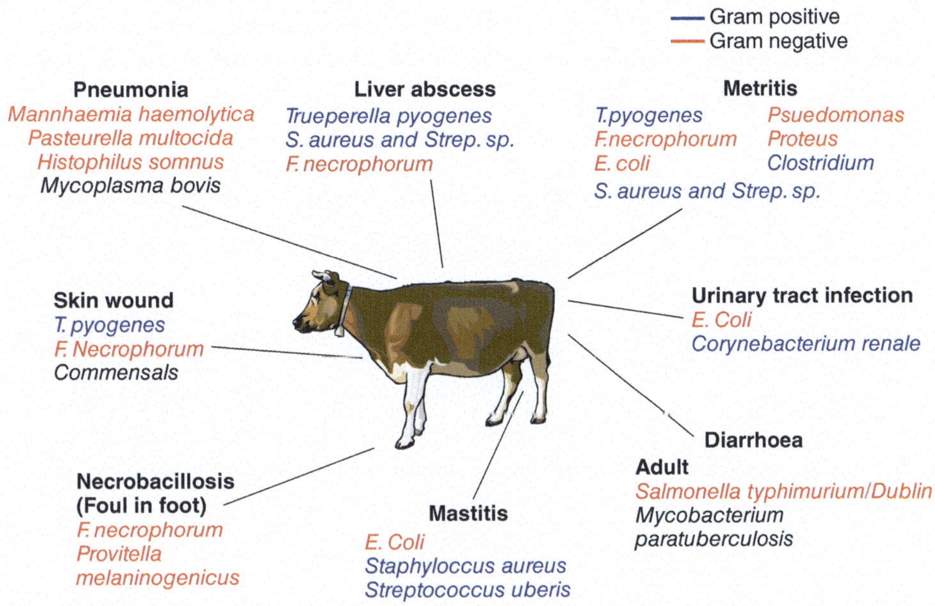

Figure 23.2 Common bacterial disease in adult cattle: red indicates gram-positive organisms and blue indicates gram-negative organisms. Adapted from National Cattleman's Beef Association.

Table 23.5 Antimicrobial selection guidelines for common conditions in cattle (adapted from Constable *et al*. (2008) and Apley (2013)).

Condition	Associated bacterial pathogen	Comments	First choice	Second choice	Third choice
Actinobacillosis (Wooden tongue)	*A. lignieresi*		oxytetracycline amoxycillin potentiated sulphonamides +/– sodium iodide i/v		
Actinomyces bovis (Lumpy jaw)	*A. bovis*		amoxycillin amoxycillin plus clavulanic acid potentiated sulphonamides oxytetracycline penicillin g +/– i.v. sodium iodide		
Anaplasmosis	*A. centrale*		oxytetracyclines imidocarb		
Arthritis Mycoplama	*Mycoplasma bovis*		oxytetracycline,	florfenicol, spectinomycin	fluoroquinolones
Arthritis -Septic arthritis Gram negative pathogen	*Histophilus somni*		oxytetracycline,	third or fourth generation cephalosporins, tilmicosin,	
Arthritis-Septic (undifferentiated)	Untargeted: Gram-positive (e.g. *A. pyogenes, S. aureus* and haemolytic streptococci) Gram-negative (e.g. *E. coli*)		potentiated suphonamides (pus may inactivate) oxytetracyclines, ampicillin and amoxicillin	third or fourth generation cephalosporin	fluoroquinolones

(continued overleaf)

Table 23.5 (*continued*)

Condition	Associated bacterial pathogen	Comments	First choice	Second choice	Third choice
Arthritis-septic Gram positive	*Trueperellaium pyogenes*		penicillins		
Arthritis-Septic Gram positive	*Streptococcus* spp.		penicillins	cephalosporins	
Arthritis-Septic Gram positive	*Staphylococcus aureus*		cephalosporins, tilmicosin, lincomycin,	fluoroquinolones	
Arthritis-Septic Gram negative pathogens	*E. coli*		aminoglycosides, potentiated sulfonamides	third or fourth generation cephalosporins	fluoroquinolones
Arthritis-Septic Gram negative pathogen	*Salmonella* spp.		aminoglycosides, potentiated sulfonamides	third or fourth generation cephalosporins	fluoroquinolones
Babseiosis	*B. bigemina* *B. bovis*		imidocarb diminazene		
Bull seminal vesiculitis	Various, including *Trueperella pyogenes*		potentiated sulphonamides	ceftiofur	
Calf diphtheria	*Fusobacterium necropherum*		oxytetracylcine	ampicillin, cefitofur, florfenicol penicillin g, potentiated sulphonamides, tulathromycin	
Clostridial diseases (Black leg Malignant oedema Tetanus Bacillary haemaglobinuria Black disease Abomasitis)	**Black leg** *C. chauvei* **Malignant oedema** *C. sordelli* *C. septicum* **Tetanus** *C. septicum* **Bacillary haemaglobinuria** *C. haemolyticum* **Black disease** *C. norvyi* **Abomasitis** *C. sordelli*		penicillin G amoycillin amoxycillin plus clavulanic acid tylosin		
Clostridial enter-toxaemia	*Clostridium perfringens* type C, D	Prognosis poor	amoxicillin, ampicillin, penicillin G		
Coccidoisis	*Eimeria bovis, E. zeurnii* and *E. alabamensis*	Metaphylaxis should be considered	decocquinate toltrazuril sulphaquinoxaline sulphamethazine amprolium		
Cryptosporidiosis	*Cryptosporidium parvum*	Accurate dose important	halofuginone lactate		
Cystitis	*Corynebacterium renale* *Arcanabacterium pyogenes* *E. coli*		penicillin G	amoxycillin and clavulanic acid	ceftiofur
Dermatophilosis	*Dermatophilus congolensis*		penicillin G oxytetracycline	erythromycin ampicillin amoxycillin	

(*continued overleaf*)

Table 23.5 (*continued*)

Condition	Associated bacterial pathogen	Comments	First choice	Second choice	Third choice
Digital dermatitis	*Sprochete-Treponema*	Topical application	oxytetracycline lincomycin and spectinomycin valnemulin erythromycin		
Digital dermatitis	*Sprochete-Treponema*	Injection	ceftofur (third generation) cefquinome (fourth generation)		
Endocarditis (gram positive)	*Trueperella pyogenes* *Streptococcus* spp.	Most common	penicillin G		
Endocarditis (gram negative or undifferentiated)	Undifferentiated *E. coli* and other organisms		ampicillin amoxycillin	ceftiofur	
Endometritis	*E. coli, Trueperella pyogenes, bacteroides* *Fusobacterium necrophorum* *Staphyloccocus* *Streptococcus* *Pseudomonas aeruginosa* Proteus	Intra-uterine	oxytetracycline ceftiofur		
Foul in the foot	*Fusobacterium necropherum* and *Provitella melaninogenica*		ampicillin oxytetracycline potentiated sulphonamides	florfenicol	third generation cephalosporin
Heartwater	*Cowdria ruminantium*		oxytetracycline		
Infectious keratoconjunctivitis (New Forest eye, pink eye))	*Morexella bovis*		oxytetracycline cloxacillin	florfenicol tilmicosin	
Leptospirosis	*Leptospira* spp.		ampicillin dihydrostreptomycin		
Listeriosis	*Listeria monocytogenes*		procaine penicillin dihydrosteptomycin		
Meningitis	Various, including *E. coli*		procaine penicillin dihydrosteptomycin	ceftiofur fluoquinolones potentiated sulphonamides	
Metritis	*E.coli, Arcanabacterium pyogenes, bacteroides* *Fusobacterium necrophorum* *Staphyloccocus* *Streptococcus* *Pseudomonas aeruginosa* Proteus +/– clostridia	Injection Intra-uterine	ampicillin procaine penicillin oxytetracycline (good action E.coli poor Trueperella pyogenes use within first seven days) oxytetracycline ceftiofur	ceftiofur	
Omphalitis	*Trueperella pyogenes* *Streptococcus* spp. *E. coli*		amoxycillin and clavulanic acid penicillin/dihydostreptomycin		

(*continued overleaf*)

Table 23.5 (*continued*)

Condition	Associated bacterial pathogen	Comments	First choice	Second choice	Third choice
Peritonitis	Multiple gram-positive and -negative anaerobes and aerobes.		third- or fourth- generation cephalosporin	fluoroquinolones	
Pneumonia	**Pneumonia (Shipping fever)** *Mannheimia haemolytica* *Pasteurella multocida* **Pneumonia (Histophilus)** *Histophilus somnii* *Pneumonia* **Enzootic pneumonia** *Pasteurella multocida* *+/– Mycoplasma bovis* *Pneumonia* **Chronic pneumonia** *Trueperella pyogenes*	Many antimicrobials are licensed for this condition	Oxytetracycline spectinomycin	florphenicol, tilmicosin tulathromycin	third (ceftiofur) and fourth (cefquinome) cephalosporins fluoroquinolones (enrofloxacin, danofloxacin, marbofloxacin)
Pneumonia Mycoplama bovis (EU)		Range of sensitivities	danofloxacin (limited sensitivity florfenicol, oxytetracycline and spectinimycn)		
Pneumonia Mycoplasma bovis (USA)		Range of sensitivities	fluorfenicol, oxytetracycline and spectonomycin (limited sensitivity tilmicosin)		
Pyelonephritis	*Corynebacterium renale* *Arcanabacterium pyogenes*		penicillin G	amoxycillin and clavulanic acid	ceftiofur
Ringworm	*Trichophyton metagrophytes*		iodine		
Septicaemia (adult)	Gram-negative, e.g. *E. coli* *Salmonella* Gram-positive, e.g. Staphs and streps	Broad spectrum recommended. Urgent treatment required. Identification of pathogen usually unknown	oxytetracyclines and potentiated sulphonamide amoxicillin +/- clavulanate	third or fourth generation cephalosporin	aminoglycosides fluoroquinolones
Septicaemia (calf)	Usually gram-negative *E. coli* *Klebsiella* spp *Salmonella* spp	Bacteriocidal recommended	potententiated sulphonamides	third or fourth generation cephalosporin	aminoglycosides fluoroquinolones
Thelieriosis	Multiple –regional		tetracyclines		
Thromboembolic meningoencphalitis (TEME)	*Histophilus somni*		oxytetracycline	florfenicol	
Toxic metritis		Intra-uterine Infusions β-lactam-resistant antimicrobial should be used	oxytetracycline ceftiofur		
Trypanosomiasis	Multiple – regional		diminizine		

The information contained within the table is provided as a guide, but the author cannot be held responsible for errors and omissions.

Table 23.6 Antimicrobial sensitivities of common selected mastitis pathogens.

Group	Antibiotics	β-lactamase *Staphyloccocus aureus*	Gram-positive *Streptococcus aureus* *Strepetococcus agalactiae* *Streptococcus dygalactae* *Streptococcus uberis* *Trueperella pyogenes*	Gram-negative Enterbacteriacae (E.coli)	Pseudomonas	*Mycoplasma bovis* (mastitis)
penicillins	penicillin G	–	++++	–	+	–
	penethamate (benzyl penicillin)					
	ampicillin		+++	+		
	amapicillin + clavulanic acid	+++	+++	+++	–	–
	cloxacillin	++	++	–		
amino-glycosides	framycetin neomycin	+++		++		–
1st generation cephalosporin	cephaprin	+++	+++	+/–	–	–
2nd generation cephalosporin	cefuroxine	+++	+++	+	–	–
3rd generation cephalosporin	cefoperazone ceftiofur	+++	++	+++	–	–
4th generation	cefquinome	+++	+++	+++	–	–
tetracyclines	oxytetracycline	++	++	++++	+	–
macrolides	erythromycin tylosin	+++	+++	–	–	–
lincosamide	pirilimycin		+++	–		–
aminocoumarin novobiocin	novobiocin penicillin + novobiocin	++ +++	++ +++	–	–	–

Barrett (2000) suggested that the selection of an anti-microbial product should be based, in part, on answers to the following questions:

- Are the probable bacterial pathogens likely to be sensitive to the product *in vitro*?
- Can the product be expected to reach therapeutic concentrations in the infected tissues for a sufficient period of time?
- Is the antimicrobial available in a preparation which is licensed for use in this class of animal?
- Is the route of administration appropriate, and does the dosing interval suit the current management system?
- What are the required minimum withdrawal periods, and are meat and/or milk residues likely to be a problem?
- Are there any risks to human health in the use of this product?
- Have you had previous success when using the product?
- Have animals on the same farm previously shown a good clinical response to treatment with the product?
- What is the cost of the product?
- What is the likely cost-benefit of using the product?

Mastitis

Antimicrobials are used extensively to treat and prevent clinical and subclinical mastitis infections. The antimicrobial sensitivities of common selected mastitis pathogens are shown in Table 23.6. The relative distribution in the mammary gland of selected antimicrobials administered by intra-mammary infusion and parenterally are shown in Tables 23.7 and 23.8 respectively. However, some mastitis pathogens are refractory to treatment with antibiotics. These include *Mycoplasma bovis*, *Pasteurella* spp, *Pseudomonas* spp, yeasts and algae (prototheca).

Systemic and intra-mammary routes are used. The beneficial effects of systemic antibiotics over intra-mammary preparations are limited to the treatment of severe acute mastitis and early treatment of *Staphyloccocus aureus* infections before the pathogen becomes chronic and persistent.

Antibiotics are used to treat infections during lactation, and are used to treat and prevent new intra-mammary infections during the dry period. Inert dry cow intra-mammary preparations are now frequently used, either independently or in combination with antimicrobial preparations, to prevent new intra-mammary infections during the dry period.

Clinical mastitis with systemic signs is often treated with a combination of systemic antibiotics and intra-mammary preparations. Due regard to licensed products for this combined usage should be observed, and appropriate withdrawal times applied. Other combinations should be considered off-label and standard withdrawal times applied.

Severe toxic mastitis is usually caused by either *E. coli* or *Staphylococcus aureus* infections. Bacteremia is a relatively common occurrence following *E. coli* infections. It is often stated that mammary gland *E. coli* numbers are already in decline once the clinical signs of disease are recognised. Systemic antibiotics and, in some cases, intra-mammary antibiotics, are administered. A survey of 264 cases of toxic mastitis pathogens isolated in Northern Ireland (Menzies *et al.*, 2000) indicated the following *in vitro* sensitivities to the 253 isolates: enrofloxacin (98%), amoxicillin/clavulanic acid (91%), apramycin (80%), spectinomycin (72%), sulphamethoxazole/trimethoprim (69%), ampicillin (65%) and tetracycline (59%). There were 179 gram-negative isolates, of which 93% were *E. coli*.

Clinical mastitis without systemic signs is normally treated with intra-mammary antibiotics supplied to the farmer by the farmer's veterinarian. If *Staphylococcus aureus* is suspected in an animal for the first time and there are no signs of chronicity, a short course of systemic antibiotics may increase the rate of a successful cure. This strategy has also been used at the point of drying off, in combination with dry cow antibiotic intra-mammary tubes, in an effort to increase the chances of a cure especially, with *Staphyloccoccus aureus* infections.

A useful protocol is to take a milk sample from the affected quarter before treatment and store it in the freezer. The addition of a small amount of glycerol will enhance the successful culture rate following prolonged storage. Once a useful batch number has been collected and stored, they can be dispatched for culture and bacterial sensitivity at a discounted cost. This profile of mastitis pathogens and antimicrobial sensitivities will be useful in shaping the selection of the first choice and the second choice intra-mammary product for routine use on farm. It will also inform the dry cow therapy decisions which need to target the pre-existing mammary infections at drying off in order to facilitate a cure.

Sub-clinical mastitis is recognised by an increase in the somatic cell count and the isolation of a recognised pathogen. The somatic cell count results returned from routine milk testing of composite samples will identify the affected cows. A useful procedure is to identify the infected quarters by using a Rapid Milk Test (CMT), and to collect a milk sample for culture. These can be sent as a batch to the veterinary laboratory for culture and sensitivity. This will also shape the selection of the first choice and the second choice intra-mammary product for routine use on farm. It will also inform the dry cow therapy decisions which need to target the pre-existing mammary infections at drying off in order to facilitate a cure.

Success rates of dry cow therapies are far greater than lactating cow tubes, due to their persistency. The dry period is the best time to address sub-clinical mastitis control.

The aim of the dry cow therapy is to eliminate pre-existing intra-mammary infections and prevent new intra-mammary infections occurring during the dry period by environmental pathogens such as *E. coli* or *Streptococcus uberis*. The control of the pre-existing intra-mammary infections is achieved by using appropriate long acting dry cow intra-mammary antibiotics (Tables 23.7 and 23.8). They will also reduce the new intra-mammary infection rate, while the antimicrobial persists at an effective concentration in the mammary gland.

Table 23.7 Distribution of drugs throughout the mammary gland after intra-mammary administration.

Good distribution	Limited distribution	Poor distribution
aminopenicillins	cephalosporins	dihydrostreptomycin
erythromycin	tetracyclines	framycetin
novobiocin	cloxacillin	neomycin
penethemate	naficillin	streptomycin
	penicillin G	

Table 23.8 Diffusion into the udder after parenteral administration.

Good	Moderate	Poor
potentiated	penethamate	aminoglycosides
sulphonamide	penicillin	cephalexin
erythromycin	ampicillin	ceftiofur
tylosin	amoxicillin	
cefquinome	oxytetracycline	

New infections can also be prevented by the use of a licensed inert intra-mammary infusion, which acts as a physical barrier in the teat canal and avoids new infections of the mammary gland. Its effectiveness supersedes that of the antibiotic alone at preventing new intra-mammary infections during the dry period. Routine milk testing enables cows to be treated selectively, based upon their somatic cell counts over the last three months prior to drying off. Cows with low somatic cell counts may require only the inert intra-mammary barrier, whereas a cow with a high somatic cell count, indicating an infection, would require a long-acting appropriate antibiotic intra-mammary preparation. The addition of an inert intra-mammary product would reduce the new infection rate still further.

The success of the dry cow therapy regime can be evaluated by comparing the individual composite somatic cell count just prior to drying off with the somatic cell count at the first milk recording, after joining the lactating herd post-calving. Deductions can then be made from the changes in the somatic cell counts.

Future availability of antimicrobials

The decision to use, and the selection of, appropriate antimicrobials in cattle practice is challenging in a cost-sensitive environment. However, their continued availability will be enhanced if we, as a profession, can demonstrate the application of best evidence-based judgment in the qualitative and quantitative use of anti-microbial on farm.

References and further reading

Apley, M.A. and Coetzee, J.F. (2013). Antimicrobial Drug Use in Cattle. In: Giguère, S., Prescott, J.F., Dowling, P., Praticia, M. (eds). *Antimicrobial Therapy in Veterinary Medicine*, fifth edition, pp. 495–518. Wiley Blackwell.

Barrett, D.C. (2000). Cost-effective antimicrobial drug selection for the management and control of respiratory disease in European cattle. *Veterinary Record* **146**, 545–550.

BVA (2009). *Responsible use of antibiotics in veterinary practice: the 8 point plan*. Poster, British Veterinary Association.

Constable, P., Pyörälä, S. and Smith, W.G. (2008). Guidelines for Antimicrobial Use in Cattle. In: Guardabassi, L., Jensen, L.B. and Kruse, H. (eds). *Antimicrobial Use in Animals*. Blackwell Publishing, Oxford.

Cusack, P.M.V., McMeniman, N. and Lean, I.J. (2003). The medicine and epidemiology of bovine respiratory disease in feedlots. *Australian Veterinary Journal* **81**(8), 480–487.

Malmo, J., Vermunt, J.J. and Parkinson, T. (2010). Practical therapeutics for the Cattle Veterinarian. In: Vermunt, J.J. and Malmo, J. (eds). *Disease of cattle in Australasia*, 1st edition, pp. 835–848. Vet Learn, New Zealand Veterinary Association for Continuing Education, Wellington.

Menzies, F.D., McBride, S.H.S., McDowell, W.J. *et al.* (2000). Clinical and laboratory findings in cases of toxic mastitis in cows in Northern Ireland. *Veterinary Record* **147**, 123–128.

Wagner, S. and Erskine, R. (2013). Antimicrobial Drug Use. In: Giguère, S., Prescott, J.F., Dowling, P., Praticia, M. (eds). *Antimicrobial Therapy in Veterinary Medicine*, fifth edition, pp. 519–528. Wiley Blackwell.

Veterinary Medicines Directorate (2013). Veterinary Medicines Guidance Note No 13: *Guidance on the use of the cascade*. Veterinary Medicines Directorate.

CHAPTER 24

Pain Management in Cattle Practice

Peter D. Cockcroft

Learning objectives

- Understand how to recognise pain in cattle.
- Be awareness of painful conditions and procedures in cattle practice.
- Be aware of the different methods of analgesia and pain management in cattle practice.
- Appreciate the analgesic drugs that can be used in pain management.
- Understand how improvements in pain management can be achieved on farm.
- Appreciate the roles and responsibilities of the veterinarian in pain management.

Introduction

Surveys performed in a number of developed countries indicate there is general agreement from people associated with the livestock sector that it is wrong to cause farm animals any pain, injury or stress. In spite of this sentiment, the adoption of proven methods of analgesia for routine husbandry procedures, elective procedures and painful conditions is incomplete. Castration, dehorning and disbudding without analgesia, and untreated chronic lameness and post-operative pain, are examples. In a stoical prey species such as cattle, behavioural signs of pain in mild to moderate cases may not be evident. If an insult that is likely to cause pain, has occurred, or will occur, then it is safe to assume that the animal will suffer a degree of pain. Avoidance of pain by adopting low stress-handling techniques instead of using electric prods, the use of chemical sedation instead of electro-immobilisation techniques, the implementation of disease prevention protocols, and early disease detection and treatment, are frequently neglected strategies which can reduce pain.

Recent review articles on analgesia in cattle, Hudson *et al.* (2012) and Coetzee (2013a), have highlighted that the veterinarian has a key role and an ethical responsibility to ensure the welfare of cattle with regards to pain. A knowledge of current legislation in a given country or state is important to ensure that owners are aware of their responsibilities, and that procedures are performed in accordance with the law. For example, in the UK, disbudding or dehorning at any age requires that an anaesthetic be used, with the exception of chemical cautery, which is permitted in the first week of life. The limited range of licensed drugs is an ongoing concern, with opioids largely unavailable. In addition, in some countries, the legislation does not reflect current scientific evidence with regards to certain routine procedures which are associated with pain. Calf disbudding and calf castration are two examples. Veterinarians also have a duty to educate their clients and to ensure that they are aware of all the therapeutic options, irrespective of the cost and the previous protocols employed.

There is a wide range of conditions, routine husbandry procedures and elective procedures in calves, growing cattle and adult cattle that are painful. Examples are given in Table 24.1.

The pain experienced will vary in severity and duration, depending upon the condition or procedure. Huxley & Whay (2006) surveyed UK cattle practitioners, using a prescribed list of painful procedures and conditions in cattle. The veterinarians were requested to indicate the severity of pain they thought was associated with the condition or procedure without any form of analgesia. Not surprisingly, invasive surgical procedures, such as claw amputation and LDA laparotomy surgery, and conditions such as fractures, were given a severe pain score, but there was a wide range of opinions regarding the degree of anticipated pain within a given condition. A further farmer survey with regards to the cost of providing analgesia revealed that, although cost was a consideration, a significant number of farmers were

Bovine Medicine, Third Edition. Edited by Peter D. Cockcroft.

Table 24.1 Examples of painful conditions and procedures in cattle.

Husbandry procedures	Elective procedures	Investigative procedures	Conditions
Disbudding/dehorning	Caesarean section	Liver biopsy	Fractures
Castration (rubber rings, burdizzo, surgical)	Laparotomy	Pericardio-centesis	Pneumonia
Heifer spaying	Claw amputation	Skin biopsy	Lameness
Hot iron branding	Joint flushing		Mastitis
Intra-muscular injections			Joint ill
Bull ring insertion			Dystocia
Supernumerary teat removal			Prolapsed uterus
			Peritonitis

prepared to pay a reasonable cost to provide analgesia (Huxley & Whay, 2007).

The aim of this chapter is to indicate the analgesic agents and methods available for pain management and reduction in cattle.

Pain

Pain is caused by excessive chemical, mechanical or thermal stimulation. Chronic pain results in a reduction in the pain threshold, with a heightened response to a painful stimulus (hyperalgesia), or a pain response to a previously non-painful stimulus (allodynia). It is important to recognise that the perception of pain may increase, even though the stimulus remains the same. Chronic lameness is an example in which hyperalgesia and allodynia are often present but overlooked.

Assessment and recognition of pain

As a prey species, cattle are stoical in order to minimise the risk of being selected by a predator, and pain may not be explicit to the casual observer unless it is severe. A variety of experimental methods have been used to try and measure pain objectively and subjectively. These have included behavioural observations, biochemical markers of inflammation (acute phase proteins), thermography and stress responses (cortisol). These are not generally available to the veterinary practitioner.

Prior knowledge of the association between the pain and a procedure or a diagnosed condition should assist the veterinarian in predicting the pre-existing pain or anticipated pain. Recognition of the behaviours and clinical signs associated with pain will enable the location and severity of pain to be identified during the clinical examination.

Huxley *et al.* (2012) have suggested that an evaluation of the following clinical signs, associated with pain, should be included in a standard clinical examination:

- Decreased movement/locomotion.
- Decreased interaction with other animals in the group.
- Decreased feed intake (e.g. 'hollow' left flank caused by an empty rumen).
- Changes relevant to the source of the pain being experienced (e.g. altered locomotion, flank watching or kicking, or ear twitching).
- Level of mental activity/responsiveness (animals in severe pain often show reduced responsiveness to stimuli).
- Changes in normal postures associated with pain (e.g. lateral recumbency, standing motionless or drooping of the ears).
- Easily measurable indicators of physiological stress (e.g. increased heart rate, increased pupil size, altered rate and depth of respiration or trembling).
- Bruxism (tooth grinding).
- Poor coat condition (e.g. rough, dusty or unkempt), caused by decreased grooming.

Useful additions could be:

- Inspiratory grunting (thoracic pain).
- Expiratory pain (abdominal pain).
- Inspiratory and expiratory pain (severe pneumonia/thoracic pain).
- A positive abdominal pain test.
- Flexing of a limb (and kicking) when a painful foot lesion is palpated.
- Sudden movement when a painful area is palpated.

Authorisation and regulation of analgesic drugs

Food safety is of paramount importance, and generally takes precedence over the unlicensed use of analgesic drugs. Regulations differ between countries, and the range of available drugs is likely to be different. Under EU regulations, the agents available for use as analgesics are limited to NSAIDS, xylazine, detomidine and procaine (local anaesthetic) (Huxley *et al.*, 2012). Phenylbutazone is not available for food animal administration. All the NSAIDS in cattle are currently administered by injection in cattle. In the UK, using the prescribing Cascade, a product licensed for the specific condition in the particular species should be used. If there are no products licensed for a particular condition, then a product that is licensed for another condition in the same species can be used off-label.

Pain and euthanasia

Long-term analgesic therapy is often unrealistic in conditions where a cure is unlikely and chronic pain persists (e.g. chronic lameness). In these cases, euthanasia is likely to be the best option. Euthanasia should also be considered in cases where acute severe pain is prolonged, and a poor prognosis is likely (e.g. fracture of the femur, generalised peritonitis, septic pericarditis).

Reducing pain in cattle practice

Preventing or reducing pain

Disease prevention strategies and early intervention will eliminate or reduce the severity and the length of time in pain. Reduced walking distances to the milking parlour, and minimising competition for food and water, will bring some relief in lame cows or post-operative patients. Support dressings, splints and casts will minimise the trauma and pain following a fracture. Hoof blocks, which lift a painful claw off the ground so that it is no longer weight-bearing, are commonly used and are a very cost-effective method of reducing pain. Pressure bandages can be used to reduce pain (e.g. following joint flushing). Restricting the use of electro-mobilisation and ensuring electro-ejaculation is performed correctly, with an appropriately designed annular rectal probe, will minimise the discomfort associated with the procedure.

Pain and analgesic drugs

It is important not to overlook the principle that any noxious mechanical, chemical or thermal insult will result in pain from direct stimulation of nerve endings, or from the induced inflammatory response. The precautionary principle should apply, and analgesics should be used, if pain is suspected or expected

General anaesthesia

Ketamine and xylazine are the only drugs licensed in cattle in the UK for this purpose. They can be used in combination to induce anaesthesia. Maintenance is achieved by using incremental doses of ketamine and, if prolonged, an additional increment of xylazine. Endotracheal intubation is recommended. The depth of anaesthesia required for an invasive procedure can be reduced by using appropriate regional anaesthesia.

Alternative standing procedures are usually preferable, provided suitable restraint facilities are available.

Optimising analgesia: timing and multimodal combinations

Pre-emptive administration before the exciting cause of pain should be possible in most elective procedures. In other situations, administration as soon as possible after the onset of pain is advisable, to reduce the severity and time period of discomfort. Using a combination of analgesic drugs, which act on different pathways, it is sometimes possible to increase and optimise the pain control. This is called multimodal analgesia. An example is the combined use of a systemic NSAID and a local anaesthetic line block in a caesarean section.

There is often a time delay between the administration of the analgesic drug and analgesic effect (Table 24.2). This is especially important when local anaesthetics are being used for invasive procedures. A good example is the use of a cornual block for hot iron disbudding of a group of dairy calves, when double handling to ensure time is allowed for analgesia may cause a protest by handlers and helpers. A test for analgesia should be performed before beginning the procedure, to ensure that analgesia is complete.

Table 24.2 The expected time delay between administration and analgesic effect.

Analgesia	Procedure	Time required for effect
NSAIDS	Pre-operative	10–30 minutes
Line block	Caesarean section	5–15 minutes
Paravertebral	Laparotomy	5–10 minutes
Intravenous regional anaesthesia	Claw amputation	10–15 minutes
Cornual block	Disbudding/dehorning	3–10 minutes

Systemic analgesics

Systemic analgesics which are licensed for cattle in the UK include NSAIDs (Carprofen, Meloxicam, Flunixen, Ketoprofen and tolfenamic) and α_2 agonists (xylazine and detomidine).

Non-steroidal anti-inflammatory drugs

Barrett (2004) reviewed the use of NSAIDs in cattle practice. They inhibit inflammatory mediators, which reduces inflammation and pain. NSAIDs are commonly used in animals to reduce inflammation (anti-inflammatory), to reduce pain (analgesic), to reduce pain sensitivity (anti-hyperalgesic), and to decrease overall body temperature (anti-pyretic). These drugs act by inhibiting cyclooxygenase enzymes (COX-1 and COX-2) which, in turn, prevents prostaglandin synthesis. They are effective for mild to moderate levels of pain with a duration of action between 24 and 72 hours depending on the half-life of the NSAID used. If the duration of administration exceeds the data sheet schedule, it will be off-label, and standard withdrawal times apply. On-label uses, which vary between products, include respiratory disease, mastitis, udder oedema and fog fever, although their potential off-label for inflammatory pain control is much greater.

α_2 Agonists

The α_2 agonists (xylazine and detomidine) reduce the release of noradrenalin by acting on the central and peripheral autonomic systems. Dependent upon the dose rate, this can provide different levels of sedation and analgesia for moderate pain. As the two effects occur together, their analgesic properties are usually used during elective procedures requiring sedation and analgesia.

Opioids

No opioids are licensed for use in cattle in the EU, although they are potent analgesics in cattle. Opioids include morphine, buprenorphine, pethidine and butorphanol. Butorphanol has been used most frequently in cattle practice, where allowed.

Regional and local analgesia

Epidural

A low epidural injection of local anaesthetic without adrenaline is administered at either the sacro-coccigeal space or the first inter-coccygeal space. The inclusion of adrenaline will cause vasoconstriction, and can cause spinal cord necrosis with hind-leg neurological deficits. This procedure will anaesthetise the genital tract, rectum and perineum, and mitigate any tenesmus. Xylazine can be used in combined with the local anaesthetic to provide an extended duration of analgesia. The use of xylazine for this purpose is off-label. A xylazine dose rate of 0.05mg/kg (1.25 ml of a two percent solution per 500 kg), made up to 5 ml with the local anaesthetic, has been suggested (Huxley *et al.*, 2012). Persistency of analgesia is 12–24 hours.

Intravenous regional anaesthesia

Intravenous regional anaesthesia can be used to desensitise the distal limb. It is particularly useful for invasive investigative and therapeutic procedures of the foot. In this procedure, a tourniquet is applied around the lower limb, usually just above the hock or carpus. 20–30 ml of a lidocaine, lignocaine or procaine local anaesthetic is administered intravenously, using a superficial vein distal to the tourniquet. The administered local anaesthetic should not contain adrenaline, as the vasoconstriction induced can be detrimental. Complete anaesthesia of the distal limb usually takes 10–12 minutes. Testing of the interdigital skin for desenatisation is recommended before any invasive procedure is performed. With the tourniquet in place, anaesthesia persists for at least an hour, although earlier release is desirable due to blood supply restriction.

Local nerve blocks

Local nerve blocks require the administration of a local anaesthetic around a peripheral nerve This results in analgesia of the region supplied by the sensory nerves of the peripheral nerve. Local nerve blocks include: paravertebral (flank); cornual (horn/hornbud and surrounding skin); retrobulbar and Peterson block (eyeball and adnexa); Auriculo-palpebral (eyelids: motor only); internal pudendal (prepuce and penis); and infra-orbital (nares). Lower limb nerve blocks have also been described in cattle, but are technically more challenging in cattle with a less cooperative patient.

Line and ring blocks

Line blocks can be used to anaesthetise the peripheral nerve supply to a region (e.g. inverted L-block on the flank), or to anaesthetise the nerve endings in the tissue at the procedural site. Ring blocks are used to anesthetise the teat and, sometimes, a distal limb. A ring block is achieved by interlinking multiple injections encircling the area to be anaesthetised.

Topical analgesia

Unfortunately, the use of topical ophthalmic local anaesthetics, such as amethocaine, is no longer permitted as there is no licensed product. Topical application onto the cornea prior to examination was extremely useful, enabling a thorough search for foreign bodies and a detailed examination of the eye. This included the evaluation for uveitis or corneal ulceration. In blockages of the teat canal requiring intervention, a local anaesthetic can be instilled into the teat canal to anaesthetise the mucosal surface. A rubber band tourniquet is applied to the base of the teat to facilitate this procedure.

Electro-immobilisation and surgical procedures

The use of electro-immobilisation in extensive fractious animals for restraint and surgical procedures is controversial. Additional local anaesthetic is required to ensure analgesia of the surgical site in heifer spaying or any other invasive procedure, if this method of restraint is used.

Analgesic protocol examples for condition and procedures

Table 24.3 provides examples of analgesic options for various conditions.

Evidence for the effectiveness of analgesic drugs in reducing pain during and after castration and dehorning

Castration and analgesia

Coetzee (2013b) reviewed the evidence in the primary literature and concluded the following: administration of a local anaesthetic alone effectively mitigates acute distress associated with castration, but the integrated cortisol response is only modestly reduced. NSAID administration alone is not effective in reducing acute distress associated with castration; however, the reduction in overall integrated cortisol response is greater in NSAID-treated calves, compared with calves receiving only local anaesthesia. The combination of local anaesthesia and an NSAID achieved the greatest reduction in cortisol response in published reports. This suggests that a multimodal analgesic approach is more effective in mitigating the pain associated with castration than the use of a single analgesic agent.

Dehorning, disbudding and analgesia

Stock *et al.* (2013) have reviewed the literature regarding the analgesia and de-horning procedures (chemical cautery, hot iron disbudding and chemical cautery). Their conclusions were

Table 24.3 Examples of analgesic options for selected conditions.

Procedure/condition	Systemic NSAID	Systemic α_2 agonists (xylazine and detomidine)	Epidural (+/–α_2 agonists)	Local nerve block	line block/ ring block/ local tissue infiltration	Intravenous regional anaesthesia	Limit movement
Caesarean section	+ (BP)	+/– (MS)	+	+	+		+
Calf castration	+ (BP)				+		
Calf disbudding	+ (BP)			+			
Claw amputation	+ (BP)	+ (MS)				+	+
Dystocia	+ (BP)	+/– (MS)	+				
Uterine prolapse	+ (BP)	+/– (MS)	+				
Pneumonia	+						
Mastitis	+						
Joint ill	+						+
Metacarpal fracture	+	+					+
Solar ulcer	+					+/–	+
Eye enucleation	Before surgery	+ (MS)			Retrobulbar Auriculo-palperbral Palpebral ring block		

BP: before procedure.
MS: Standing mild sedation.

as follows: dehorning causes behavioural, physiologic, and neuroendocrine changes, indicating a stressful or painful response in cattle. Following dehorning, an acute painful response is observed within the first 30 minutes, followed by a period of suggested inflammatory pain lasting up to eight hours. Local anaesthetics provide analgesia for the initial acute pain response, but a delayed cortisol response is observed, presumably once sensitivity returns to the anesthetised area. Acute pain following dehorning is mitigated using local anaesthetics, non-steroidal anti-inflammatory drugs (NSAIDs), and sedatives providing analgesia. NSAIDs help to attenuate the inflammatory mediated pain response following dehorning. They recommended a multimodal approach using local anaesthetics, NSAIDs and, when possible, sedative analgesics.

Analgesia and performance

Newton & Conner (2013) performed a critical appraisal of the evidence that pain for castration and dehorning in cattle is associated with improved production. They concluded that there was little evidence that pain management is associated with increased production outcomes, such as average daily gain, feed intake, or feed to gain. However, they indicated that most studies are too short to assess production outcomes meaningfully, and few approaches to pain mitigation have been assessed multiple times. They recommended that, if assessing production outcomes is important, studies specially designed to assess this outcome are needed.

The incentive to use analgesics for these commonly used husbandry procedures should be focused upon the welfare aspects of pain control and the legislative requirements, rather than increased performance based upon the current level of evidence provided by inadequate studies.

Mastitis

Moderate and severe mastitis are associated with pain in cattle. Studies by Fitzpatrick *et al.* (2002) and Kemp *et al.* (2008) found that animals with cases of moderate clinical mastitis had significantly greater heart rates, rectal temperatures and respiratory rates, when compared to cows with cases of mild clinical mastitis and normal cows. Cortisol levels were also significantly increased in cows with mastitis, compared to normal cows. Cows with both mild and moderate mastitis cases had significantly larger hock-to-hock distances compared to normal cows, thereby indicating an altered stance. The mechanical threshold to pain of the cows with mild and moderate mastitis was significantly lower than that of the control cows. (Fitzpatrick *et al.*, 2002; Kemp *et al.* 2008). Acute toxic mastitis is associated with pain in cattle (Fitzpatrick, 2011).

Surveys of the use of analgesia in cattle practice

All of these surveys included common conditions and procedures that were considered to have varying degrees of pain associated with them.

There have been a number of UK surveys regarding the use of analgesic drugs in cattle practice (Watts (2000); Fitzpatrick *et al.* (2002); and Huxley & Whay (2007).

Some of the results from Huxley and Whay (2007) are presented in Table 24.4. There were 641 respondents from a survey of 2 391 cattle veterinarians listed in a pharmaceutical company's database. The authors concluded that '*The proportions of cases in which analgesics were used varied widely, depending on the condition and the agent. The use of analgesic agents for the conditions and procedures considered in the survey was widespread, although there were wide variations in the agents used and the proportions of cases in which they were administered. However, it is surprising that only 61 per cent, 68 per cent and 60 per cent of the respondents used NSAIDs to control pain after the major surgical procedures of claw amputation, caesarean section and surgery to repair an umbilical hernia, respectively, and even then they were not administered to all the cases seen.*'

The outcomes from survey questionnaires regarding the use of analgesia in selected procedures and conditions in cattle in Canada and the United States have been reported (Hewson *et al.*, 2007a; Fajt *et al.*, 2011). In the study by Fajt *et al.* (2011), US members of the American Association of Bovine Practitioners (AABP) were surveyed. There were 666 respondents. Respondents reported not providing analgesic drugs to approximately 70% of calves castrated at less than six months old. The most commonly administered analgesics were NSAIDs, local anaesthetics, and α2-adrenergic receptor agonists out of the following options: none, NSAIDs (e.g. flunixin meglumine), opioids (e.g. butorphanol), dissociative anesthetics (e.g. ketamine), α_2-adrenergic receptor agonist (e.g. xylazine), local anesthetics (e.g. lidocaine), and other. The details of this survey are presented in Table 24.5.

Some of the outcomes for cattle from the study by Hewson *et al.* (2007a) in Canada are presented in Table 24.6 (dairy) and Table 24.7 (beef). The authors concluded that '90% of veterinarians used analgesic drugs for caesarean section in cows, for bovine claw amputation and for left displaced omentopexy. However, in these and other categories, the analgesics used were often inadequate, and many veterinarians did not give analgesics to young animals. Analgesia was only used in the following proportions of castrations: 6.9% of beef calves and 18.7% of dairy calves $\leq$ 6 months old, 19.9% of beef calves and 33.2% of dairy calves $\geq$ 6 months old. The results indicate an urgent need for veterinarians to manage pain in livestock better.

Several surveys have reported on the pain scores that veterinarians associate with different conditions and procedures (Hewson *et al.*, 2007b; Huxley & Whay, 2007) and how this relates to their use of analgesics. It is clear that there is a wide variation in perceptions of pain in cattle conditions, the frequency of administration and choice of analgesic agents.

An agreed list of conditions and procedures with pain management guidelines should be given a high priority to ensure that appropriate analgesia is achieved in cattle practice.

References and further reading

Barrett, D.C. (2004). Non-steroidal anti-inflammatory drugs in cattle – Should we use them more? *Cattle Practice* **12**, 69–73.

Coetzee, J. (2013a). Pain Management. *Veterinary Clinics of North America: Food Animal Practice* **29**(1), 1–266.

Coetzee, J. (2013b). Assessment and Management of Pain Associated with Castration in Cattle. *Veterinary Clinics of North America: Food Animal Practice* **29**, 75–101.

Fajt, V.R., Wagner, S.A. and Norby, B. (2011). Analgesic drug administration and attitudes about analgesia in cattle among bovine practitioners in the United States. *American Veterinary Medical Association* **238**, 755–767.

Fitzpatrick, C. (2011). *Assessing and Mediating Pain in Dairy Cows with Experimentally-Induced Clinical Mastitis.* MSc., University of Guelph.

Fitzpatrick, J.L., Nolan, A.M., Scott, E.M., Harkins, L.S. and Barrett, D.C. (2002). Observers' perceptions of pain in cattle. *Cattle Practice* **10**, 209–212.

Hewson, C.J., Dohoo, I.R., Lemke, K.A. *et al.* (2007a). Canadian veterinarians' use of analgesics in cattle, pigs and horses in 2004 and 2005. *Canadian Veterinary Journal* **48**, 155–164.

Hewson, C.J., Dohoo, I.R., Lemke, K.A., *et al.* (2007b). Factors affecting Canadian veterinarians' use of analgesics when dehorning beef and dairy calves. *Canadian Veterinary Journal* **48**, 1129–1136.

Hudson, C., Whay, H.R. and Huxley, H. (2012). Recognition and management of pain in cattle *In Practice* **30**, 126–134.

Huxley, J.N. and Whay, H.R. (2006). Current attitudes of cattle practitioners to pain and the use of analgesics in cattle. *Veterinary Record* **159**, 662–668.

Huxley, J.N. and Whay, H.R. (2007). Attitudes of UK veterinary surgeons and cattle farmers to pain and the use of analgesics in cattle. *Cattle Practice* **15**, 189–193.

Kemp, M.H., Nolan, A.M. Cripps, P.J. and Fitzpatrick, J.L. (2008). Animal-based measurements of the severity of mastitis in dairy cows. *Veterinary Record* **163**(6), 175–179.

Newton, H.P. and O'Connor, A.M. (2013). The Economics of Pain Management. *Veterinary Clinics of North America: Food Animal Practice* **29**, 229–250.

Stock, M.L., Baldridge, S.L., Griffin, D. and Coetzee, J.F. (2013). Bovine Dehorning Assessing Pain and Providing Analgesic Management. *Veterinary Clinics of North America: Food Animal Practice* **29**, 103–133.

Watts, S.A. and Clarke, K.W. (2000). A survey of bovine practitioners' attitudes to pain and analgesia in cattle. *Cattle Practice* **8**, 361–362.

Whay, H.R. and Huxley, J.N. (2005). Pain relief in cattle: A practitioner's perspective. *Cattle Practice* **13**, 81–85.

Table 24.4 Proportions of respondents who stated that they used analgesic agents for a number of procedures/conditions, and their frequency of use in adult cattle and calves (adapted from Huxley & Whay, 2007).

		% of respondents using the analgesic agents (% of respondents using analgesic agent in > 50% of cases)		
Procedure/condition	**None used**	**NSAID**	**α_2 agonist**	**Local anaesthetic respondents**
Adult cattle				
Treatment of a sole ulcer	43.2	42.7 (32.9)	9.5 (21.3)	23.3 (20.4)
Claw amputation	0.3	61.2 (86.6)	55.8 (66.7)	96.4 (99.1)
Caesarean section	0.3	68.1 (70.3)	60.3 (41.8)	98.4 (99.3)
Dystocia (traction)	23.0	66.0 (39.3)	11.8 (3.0)	37.1 (18.4)
Dehorning (>8 cm long)	1.0	2.6 (33.3)	26.1 (23.7)	99.0 (99.3)
Uveitis	44.3	46.4 (47.0)	2.3 (26.4)	13.6 (50)
Debriding a digital dermatitis lesion	43.6	18.5 (44.1)	16.9 (36.6)	41.4 (49.8)
Calves				
Surgical castration	25.1	4.6 (25.9)	17.4 (16.8)	73.9 (80.1)
Joint ill	21.7	77.0 (59.0)	2.2 (38.5)	2.2 (45.5)
Umbilical hernia (surgery)	1.3	60.1 (84.9)	81.4 (96.8)	80.0 (97.0)
Disbudding	1.2	1.7 (27.3)	8.8 (32.0)	98.7 (99.8)
Distal limb fracture	10.7	77.1 (84.8)	39.8 (70.9)	4.34 (5.8)
Following a dystocia (traction)	59.6	39.0 (12.0)	0.7 (0)	1.5 (22.2)

Table 24.5 Responses obtained from veterinarians in bovine practice to questions concerning analgesic drug administration for common procedures and medical conditions in cattle (adapted from Fajt *et al.*, 2011).

			Percentage of respondents using these drugs and drug combinations some of the time. Percentages less than 10% are not reported in the table.						
Procedure and condition	**'No analgesia' respondents %**	**Median range of cattle treated by 'Yes analgesia' respondents**	**NSAID %**	**Local %**	**α_2**	**α_2 + Local %**	**NSAID + Local %**	**NSAID + Local + α_2 %**	**NSAID + Local + α_2 + Opiods %**
Acute lameness in adult beef cattle	15.7	51–75	56.0				12.4		
Acute lameness in dairy cows	7.6	51–75	60.9				14.8		
Acute Lameness in feedlot cattle	46.1		40.8						
Chronic lameness Adult beef	14.7	51–75	57.3				11.2		
Chronic lameness Dairy	10.9	26–50	64.1				10.3		
Chronic lameness feedlot cattle	43.0	51–75	42.2						
Caesarean section in beef cows	6.4	100		27.6		10.3	18.1	13.4	
Caesarean in dairy cows	3.7			14.9			28.7	14.4	12.8
Castration of beef calves < 6 months	69.8	10–25							
Castration of dairy calves < 6 months	70.1	1–10							
Castration of beef calves > 6 months	54.9	51–75		11.2	11.4				
Dehorning beef calves < 6 months	50.9	90–99		30.3					
Dehorning dairy calves < 6 months	37.3	75–90							
Dehorning beef calves > 6 months	35.9	100		34.2		18.2			
Dehorning Dairy calves > 6 months	26.5	100		37.4					
Toxic mastitis in dairy cows	4.4	100	93.1						

Table 24.6 Analgesic usage by veterinarians in selected surgeries and medical conditions in dairy cattle (adapted from Hewson *et al.*, 2007a).

Condition	Respondents who attended condition	% of respondents using analgesia in some or all cases	% of cases receiving analgesia	Most common analgesic drugs used in treated cases (% of treated cases given drug)
Castration up to age 6 months	167	19.1	18.7	Xylazine (54) Lidocaine (29)
Castration over age 6 months	105	48.1	33.2	Xylazine (62) Lidocaine (25)
Umbilical hernia repair up to age 3 months	214	94.2	96.0	Ketamine (36.4) Lidocaine (29.2)
Dehorning up to age 6 months	236	85.0	90.2	Lidocaine (67) Xylazine (29)
Dehorning over age 6 months	211	84.7	84.8	Lidocaine (58) Xylazine (36)
Caesarean section	321	97.1	98.5	Lidocaine (60) Ketoprofen (13)
Displaced abomasum (omentopexy)	314	96.8	96.9	Lidocaine (59) Xylazine (13)
Claw amputation	96	98.0	97.1	Lidocaine (44) Xylazine (28)
Acute toxic mastitis	309	93.3	95.7	Ketoprofen (40) Flunixin (32)
Acute lameness (cows)	258	52.1	33.3	Ketoprofen (42) Aspirin (16)
Chronic lameness (cows)	269	39.9	29.7	Ketoprofen (29) Aspirin (23)
Dystocia	334	33.9	26.5	Lidocaine (33) Ketoprofen (27)
Corneal ulcer	191	33.5	28.4	Ketoprofen (25) Lidocaine (20)

Table 24.7 Analgesic usage in selected surgeries and medical conditions in beef cattle (adapted from Hewson *et al.*, 2007a).

Condition	Respondents who attended condition	% of respondents using analgesia in some or all cases	% of cases receiving analgesia	Most common analgesic drugs used in treated cases (% of treated cases given drug)
Castration up to 6 months old	285	15.4	6.9	Xylazine (54) Lidocaine (27
Castration over 6 months old	306	35.1	19.9	Xylazine (52) Lidocaine (35
Umbilical hernia repair in calves up to 3 months old	159	96.9	97.2	Xylazine (30) Lidocaine (27)
Dehorning up to 6 months old	209	60.5	57.5	Lidocaine (73) Xylazine (25)
Dehorning over 6 months old	267	72.3	68.7	Lidocaine (67) Xylazine (28)
Caesarean section	369	95.9	95.6	Lidocaine (62) Xylazine (10)
Dystocia	388	38.2	33.8	Lidocaine (48) Ketoprofen (18
Corneal ulcer	231	43.0	38.9	Lidocaine (34) Xylazine (15)

CHAPTER 25

Bull Health and Breeding Soundness

Peter Chenoweth

Learning objectives

- Understand the principles of biosecurity and general health of the bull.
- Understand the important components of bull selection, evaluation and breeding management.
- Understand the principles and conduct of the bull breeding soundness evaluation (BBSE).
- Understand the interpretation of the bull breeding soundness evaluation (BBSE).
- Understand the factors which can compromise bull reproductive capabilities.

Introduction

Despite the growing use of artificial insemination (AI) in both beef and dairy cattle, natural mating is the most common breeding system used for beef and dairy cattle throughout the world. Natural-mating or breeding bulls differ markedly in their reproductive capabilities, and it is not uncommon for individuals to be sub-fertile or even infertile.

Bull health and breeding soundness are topics which are inseparable, as so many health issues affect bull reproduction. Therefore, this chapter will focus on the reproductive function of bulls with attention to relevant issues of health.

Bull reproduction can be compromised by many factors which include genetic, traumatic, nutritional, toxic or infectious considerations. Although problems may emerge at different stages of the bull's reproductive career, it makes sense to identify problems prior to breeding by applying a bull breeding soundness evaluation (BBSE). The BBSE procedures used to examine bulls are effective in identifying sub-fertile and infertile bulls and are very similar in different parts of the world. For example, in North America, the Society for Theriogenology recommends a standardised approach (Chenoweth *et al.*, 1992, 2010) which is used in a number of countries. Bull evaluation protocols have also been developed in Australia, New Zealand, Canada and Brazil. In the UK, a bull pre-breeding examination certificate was recently introduced by the British Cattle Veterinary Association (Penny, 2010). The Australian Cattle Veterinarians recently published a comprehensive manual on the conduct and interpretation of BBSEs (Beggs, 2013), which represents a valuable resource for those undertaking this task. This publication has been used as a template for much of the information provided herein.

Today, the BBSE is regarded as a relatively rapid and economic screening procedure for bulls (Chenoweth, 2000) which is advantageous for fertility, genetic and economic outcomes (Fitzpatrick *et al.*, 2002; Chenoweth, 2005). However, although the BBSE has been refined and promoted for over 50 years, its overall acceptance has been less than desired by beef producers, particularly when cattle prices are depressed (Chenoweth, 2005) and disappointingly low by those dairy producers who employ natural breeding.

Bull selection and purchase

Biosecurity considerations are very important when bulls are purchased or moved to and from home base (e.g. for shows and exhibitions). Purchase from a source with a known effective health program is the first line of defence, followed by immunisation against relevant diseases and a period of monitored quarantine before admission to the main herd. The process of quarantine can also help to acclimatise bulls to their new environment, which can include new feed, water, climate and microorganisms. A recommended period for quarantine is at least 28 days (Givens & Marley, 2008), during which appropriate tests and immunisations can be achieved.

Bovine Medicine, Third Edition. Edited by Peter D. Cockcroft.

Although breeders and producers must consider a number of desirable genetic traits when selecting a breeding bull, the transmission of these traits to his offspring is dependent upon his reproductive capabilities (i.e. he must produce and deliver sufficient viable sperm to females at the opportune time for optimal fertility to occur). Thus, he should be physically 'fit' and have the motivation (sex-drive, serving capacity or libido) to do this repeatedly and consistently. Prospective breeding bulls should thus be subject to a BBSE prior to purchase and/or use.

The BBSE, as detailed below, aims to provide an assessment of as many of the relevant criteria as possible within the constraints of logistics and economics.

The Bull Breeding Soundness Evaluation (BBSE)

The major elements of the BBSE are:

1 Physical examination.
2 Reproductive evaluation (including measurement of testicular or scrotal size).
3 Semen collection and evaluation.
4 Report.

Other tests may be included, such as those for male libido/serving ability, or to detect reproductive pathogens such as *Campylobacter foetus* or *Tritrichomonas foetus* in bulls. However, these are not generally regarded as being automatically integral to the BBSE.

In 2013, the Australian Cattle Veterinarians (ACV) updated its standards for the evaluation of bulls, which includes a BBSE accreditation system for veterinarians. A computer program, *Bull Reporter*, has been developed, which allows participating ACV members and accredited sperm morphologists to combine information and prepare reports on bull tests.

Other systems in use throughout the world (e.g. in Canada, South Africa, and Australia) have commonalities with the approach adopted by the Society for Theriogenology (Chenoweth *et al.*, 1992, 2010), in which thresholds for sperm motility and normal sperm morphology were established as 30% and 70%, respectively. The main differences between BBSE systems occur with the minimum thresholds adopted for scrotal circumference (SC), sperm motility, and sperm morphology and also in the reporting of results.

For example, the guidelines developed by the Western Canadian Association of Bovine Practitioners contain specific breed/age recommendations for minimum SC and a minimum sperm motility threshold of 60%. Moreover, bulls can be classified as satisfactory, unsatisfactory, as questionable potential breeders or as 'decision deferred' (Barth, 1994). The South African Veterinary Association guidelines (Irons *et al.*, 2007) agree with those of the SFT with respect to minimum thresholds for SC, although they differ in those for motile and morphologically normal sperm (70% and 75%, respectively). The Australian Cattle Veterinarian (ACV) guidelines provide thresholds for sperm motility and normal morphology of ≥30%, ≥50%, ≥60% and ≥70%, respectively for bulls used for natural breeding and those for which semen is to be frozen for A.I. Here, it is considered important that the examining veterinarian makes the final determination as to whether a bull should be categorised as a satisfactory potential breeder or not, using established standards for physical soundness, SC, sperm motility, and sperm morphology as important considerations (Fordyce *et al.*, 2006), in conjunction with factors such as individual bull, herd and client histories.

BBSE conduct and criteria

Timing

Although it is recommended to conduct a BBSE on all bulls prior to breeding, it is most commonly employed prior to sale and/or first breeding of young bulls. In principle, the BBSE should occur as close to breeding as possible. However, as adequate time should be allowed for treatments, retesting or replacement before breeding, it is common to schedule the initial BBSE within 4–6 weeks of sale or introduction to the breeding herd.

The physical examination

Whenever possible, bulls should be observed prior to restraint, as this helps to detect physical and conformational problems (as below). When restraint is applied, it should be secure, with due regard for the safety of both the examiner and the bull. Permanent, unambiguous identification of the bull should be recorded.

The physical exam, although not a full clinical exam, should include a systematic assessment of external appearance, conformation, feet and leg status, body condition, vision, overall health, and the relative location of reproductive organs. Where breed associations have established physical, conformational and pigment standards for their respective breeds, this should be acknowledged. However, the traits required for a bull to be an effective breeder do not necessarily coincide with those phenotypic characteristics which are valued by different breed organisations.

The physical exam includes per-rectal assessment of the more accessible parts of the male tract (pelvic urethra, vesicular glands, ampullae and vasa deferentia). In addition, the scrotum should be palpated for both presence and normality of its internal structures (testicle, epididymides and scrotal neck structures). Both the 'tone' (or resiliency) and 'firmness' (or degree of hardness) of the testicles should be recorded, especially if either are considered to be abnormal. The sigmoid flexure should also be palpated, and the penis exteriorised and

Table 25.1 Checklist for bull reproductive problems.

Conformation	Locomotion	Physical	Scrotum	Sheath	Penis	Genital tract & Accessory genital organs
Symmetry, muscle wasting, hoof wear, joint swellings.	*Ease and fluidity of movement, placement of feet, hoof conformation*	Movement, *conformation, symmetry, claws, swellings, body condition, eyes.*	*Circumference, shape, epithelial status* **Testes** *Size, shape, symmetry, position, mobility*	*Size, angle, volume, distance from ground, eversion*	*Erection, protrusion, external swelling, nerve damage*	*Symmetry, size, tone, pain on palpation, swellings.*
Problems Post-leg Sickle-hock Interdigital corn(s) Wart(s) Foot abscess Trauma/foreign body Laminitis	**Problems** Lameness Step short Step long Spastic paresis Spastic syndrome Muscle weakness	**Problems** Hernia (inguinal/scrotal) Pink-eye Eye cancer Facial paralysis Wooden tongue/jaw. Mouth/tooth problems Muscle wasting/weakness Respiratory disease	**Problems** *Scrotum:* Trauma Dermatitis Abnormal carriage Varicocoele *Testes:* Cryptorchid Hypoplasia Enlarged Orchitis Degeneration Incomplete descent Adhesions	**Problems** Prolapse Trauma Penile haematoma	**Problems** Phimosis Paraphimosis Adhesions Deviations Hair ring Persistent frenulum Fibro-papilloma Haematoma Hypospadia Congenitally short penis Short retractor penis muscle CCP shunts Urolithiasis Insensitivity	**Problems** Aplasia/hypoplasia Inflammation/ infection Thickened/ firm epididymis Sperm granuloma Inguinal hernia

examined. Scrotal circumference measurement is usually made at this point, using an approved method. A checklist of bull problems that the examiner should be aware of when conducting a physical examination of bulls for breeding soundness is provided in Table 25.1.

Testicle size (scrotal circumference)

Assessment of testicular size is usually accomplished by measuring scrotal circumference (SC) with an approved measuring tape. SC is an important aspect of the BBSE, particularly in younger bulls, as it closely reflects the volume of productive testicular parenchyma which, in turn, is related to sperm production and, to some extent, to semen quality and natural mating fertility. In addition, SC is moderately heritable and related to age at puberty of female offspring (Brinks *et al.*, 1978). This means that larger SCs are associated with earlier ages at puberty in female progeny. Here, an estimate has been made that for every 1 cm above herd average, a bull will sire heifers that get to puberty four days earlier. The scrotal circumference also provides a reliable estimate of bull puberty (i.e. at approximately 27–29 cm) which is remarkably consistent across genotypes and environments. An important caveat, however, is that the measurement of SC is made in the prescribed manner (Figure 25.1).

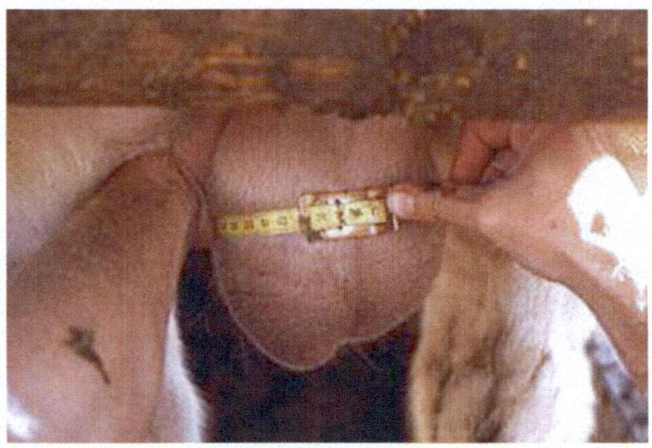

Figure 25.1 Correct placement of hands and scrotal tape for measurement of scrotal circumference in bulls.

The recommended thresholds for bull scrotal circumference in Australia are shown in Table 25.2.

Semen collection

Bull semen can be collected using an artificial vagina (AV), electro-ejaculator (EEJ), or by massage of internal reproductive

Table 25.2 Recommended thresholds for bull scrotal circumference*.

Age	*Bos taurus* (cm)	*Bos indicus* (cm)
12–15 months	30	–
18 months	32	28
2 years plus	34	30

*Bulls must be puberal for these thresholds to be valid.

structures (vesicular glands, ampullae and pelvic urethrae), with each method having advantages and disadvantages (see Beggs, 2013). Regardless of the method used, however, the most important consideration is that a representative semen sample is obtained; in this respect, the AV method has advantages over the others, in that it more reliably results in a complete ejaculate.

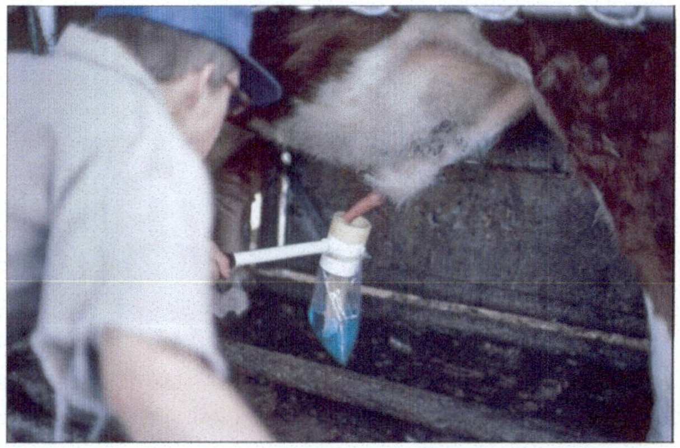

Figure 25.2 Electro-ejaculation of a bull. Note that the operator is focused on the bull's reaction to stimuli and that the semen collecting tube is enclosed in a plastic water bath for temperature control.

Welfare considerations

Welfare concerns exist for the BBSE in relation to the use of the EEJ to obtain semen. The introduction of effective electro-ejaculation in the 1950s allowed routine testing procedures to be conducted on unhandled range beef bulls. Such bulls cannot be safely collected with an artificial vagina (AV), while collection via per-rectal massage can be inconsistent. Semen collected via proper use of EEJ is comparable with that obtained with an AV. In addition to its advantages with range-type bulls, EEJ also allows semen to be collected from bulls in which physical problems rule out AV collection. However, EEJ does cause some discomfort in individual bulls, although improvement in probe design and machine circuitry over the years have led to a marked reduction of this side-effect. In one study, it was reported that bull heart rates were lowered when an epidural was given prior to EEJ, although no comparison was made with other activities, either painful or pleasurable. Other work showed that, whereas blood cortisol levels were elevated with bull EEJ, these were not as high as those due either to restraint alone, or per-rectal palpation.

However, it is still valid to ask whether or not EEJ should be regarded as a useful routine managerial procedure. If so, does it cause more distress than other accepted routine procedures, and does it inflict unnecessary pain or harm? The form of this discussion may differ with context. For example, in regions in which cattle are largely run under relatively extensive conditions and natural breeding is common (e.g. the Americas and Australasia), EEJ is probably more acceptable than in regions in which AI predominates (e.g. Europe). Although male fertility is important for all systems, there are important differences with regard to bull handling and safety.

In range-type/more extensive environments, bulls are often unhandled and fractious, whereas AI bulls are generally more used to handling and AV collection. For unhandled bulls, the choice is either to employ a method of semen collection which poses minimal danger to both man and animal (e.g. EEJ), or to avoid semen assessment altogether – an option that would lead to decreased fertility in breeding herds, add to the economic burdens of producers and increase strains on natural resources. If EEJ is acceptable as a useful managerial tool, then we could ask whether or not the 'gain' outweighs the 'pain'. Here, although objective studies are lacking, observations indicate that this procedure, when conducted properly (Figure 25.2), is no more stressful to bulls than other routine managerial procedures such as vaccination and lateral restraint.

Semen/sperm evaluation

The semen/sperm characteristics most commonly assessed are sperm motility and sperm morphology, with methodologies being discussed in the 2013 ACV publication. Initial examination of the collected semen sample, particularly for sperm motility, should be conducted expeditiously to avoid adverse environmental effects.

Levels of acceptability for sperm motility and morphology differ slightly among different BBSE evaluation systems used throughout the world. Here, the threshold levels recommended by the ACV (Beggs, 2013) are shown in Table 25.3.

Table 25.3 Sperm Motility and Morphology Thresholds (ACV, 2013). Reproduced with permission of ACV.

Trait/status	Pass (qualified)* %	acceptable %
Initial motility (progressive)	30	60
Morphology (normal sperm)	50–69	70

*This category is applied to bulls used for natural service under range conditions.

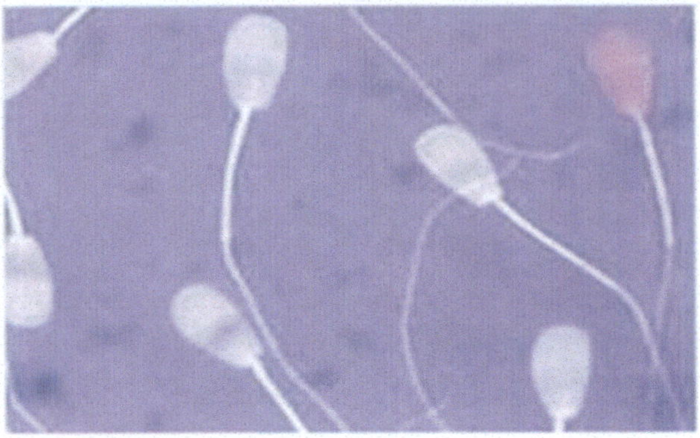

Figure 25.3 Eosin-nigrosin ('live-dead' stain of bull sperm at 1000× (oil immersion objective).

Qualifications

Initial sperm motility

The description applies to progressively motile sperm – that is, those which are purposefully moving forward. The 'pass' threshold for motility (i.e. 30% progressive motility) recognises that sperm motility assessment in the field can be more subjective, and more subject to adverse environmental influences, than it is under controlled conditions.

Sperm morphology

The microscopic evaluation of sperm morphology should entail counting at least 100 sperm per sample, using 1000× microscopy wherever possible. In the field, practitioners can achieve this level of magnification using a bright-field microscope with an oil immersion lens (or objective), and employ this satisfactorily with eosin-nigrosin stained semen smears (Figure 25.3). For optimal results, however, it is preferable to use either phase or differential-interference-contrast (DIC) phase microscopy with a sample of semen which is 'fixed' as a wet preparation. Appropriate fixatives include buffered formal saline (BFS) or PBS-gluteraldehyde. For interpretation of bovine sperm morphology, readers are referred to the following sources: Barth & Oko, 1989; Chenoweth, 2006; Beggs, 2013.

Rule-outs

Even if an otherwise satisfactory semen sample is obtained, bulls should not pass the BBSE if any of the following are detected:

- A heritable fault (e.g. inguinal hernia).
- Unacceptably small testicle size (usually measured as scrotal circumference).
- One testicle (even if very large!).
- Frank pus or blood in semen.
- Active accessory genital disease ('seminal vesiculitis').
- Significant loss of vision.
- Positive tests for campylobacteriosis or trichomonosis.
- Lameness.

Some of these conditions will be discussed in the ensuing pages.

The bottom line

The BBSE aims to provide a rapid and reasonably priced screening process which removes much of the doubt associated with bull purchase and/or use. To achieve this, the process used by veterinarians should be consistent and comprehensive, and the ensuing report should be relatively simple and unambiguous. Although this seems like a tall order, the employment of procedures and protocols, such as those promoted via the ACV (Beggs, 2013), will help to minimise risk for both the bull buyer/owner and veterinarian.

Risk, however, still exists in making any prediction of bull health and performance, and clients should be made aware of this fact. Risk also occurs in that not every possible factor that might adversely affect bull performance is evaluated as part of the routine BBSE. Notable exceptions might include an assessment of serving ability/libido, as well as tests for disease. Again, clients should be made aware of the limitations of the BBSE. The final outcome is the ultimate responsibility of the examining veterinarian, and its acceptance is integral to the veterinarian/client relationship, in which good communications are essential.

In all BBSE schemes, the findings are placed into certain categories following the BBSE. In the ACV scheme (Beggs, 2013), these are based on each component of the evaluation, namely, general physical and reproductive evaluation, scrotal circumference, serving ability (if done), initial semen assessment and sperm morphology.

Each of these elements are placed into one of four categories:

- **Satisfactory**. All attributes for this component are consistent with ACV standards. No risk factors for reduced fertility were identified in this category.
- **Unsatisfactory**. Some attributes for this component are not consistent with ACV standards. This bull has a significant risk of reduced fertility, in the short term at least. Because some conditions may be temporary, the client should seek advice from the cattle veterinarian.
- **Qualified**. Not all attributes for this component are consistent with ACV standards, but these abnormalities may not preclude the bull's use. The client should seek advice from their cattle veterinarian regarding the suitability of this bull for a particular purpose. Retesting may be recommended.
- **Not tested**. This component was not evaluated, or adequately evaluated, for reasons indicated.

BBSE outcomes

In general, approximately 65–85% of beef bulls are classified as satisfactory prospective breeders, based on BBSEs (Carroll *et al.*, 1963; Vale-Filho *et al.*, 1980; Carson & Wenzel, 1997; Spitzer & Hopkins, 1997; Chacon *et al.*, 1999; Barth & Waldner, 2002; Godfrey & Dodson, 2005; Sylla *et al.*, 2007). However, the proportion of bulls in a given population that pass the BBSE, at least on initial exam, will vary, depending on bull ages, genotypes, genetics, environment, management, prior selection and the particular BBSE criteria employed (Vale-Filho *et al.*, 1980; Fields *et al.*, 1982; Larsen *et al.*, 1990). It is not uncommon for the percentage of satisfactory bulls to increase over time following initial implementation of a bull testing programme.

Such variables also influence the types and numbers of different physical abnormalities encountered in a given bull population. For example, in the USA, the prevalence of bull physical abnormalities in bulls has varied between 1.5% and 9.5 %, along with the most common abnormalities encountered, e.g. *viz* eye lesions, feet and leg problems (Carson & Wenzel, 1997), penile problems (fibropapilloma, persistent frenulum) (Bruner *et al.*, 1995) and vesicular adenitis (Spitzer *et al.*, 1988; Kennedy *et al.*, 2002). In Italy, 4.3% of Italian beef bulls (i.e. purebred Chianina, Romagliola and Marchigiana) had physical problems which most commonly involved the testes (hypoplasia, orchitis, cryptorchidism) (Sylla *et al.*, 2007). In Western Canada, a relatively high prevalence of physical abnormalities (24.3%) was reported in beef bulls, with the most common being scrotal frostbite, as well as feet and leg problems (Barth & Waldner., 2002).

In a survey of pre-breeding BBSEs in mainly beef bulls ($n = 443$) in the UK (Walters, 2012), the overall 'pass' was 69.1% ($n = 306$), whereby the animal was deemed suitable for breeding. Pass rates were highest in bulls less than 37 months, being 74.3% ($n = 78$), 77.3% ($n = 51$) and 71.3% ($n = 57$) in the =18 months, 19–24 months and 25–36 months categories respectively. The pass rate then declined with increasing bull age, being 63.6% ($n = 42$) in 37–48 months category, 57.1% ($n = 20$) within the 49–60 months group, and 44.1% ($n = 26$) in bulls older than 60 months. This author concluded that pre-breeding BBSEs are at least as important for older bulls as they are for younger.

In another recent survey of BBSEs conducted on both beef and dairy bulls in the U.K. (Williams, 2013), 65% of bulls were passed as fertile, whereas 35% were failed. Of those bulls examined because of suspect sub-fertility, 44% failed the BBSE compared with 25% of bulls undergoing a routine pre-breeding examination ($P = 0.041$). Of those bulls which failed, 72% could have been identified on clinical examination alone, without the need for semen evaluation. For beef bulls, the main reason for failure was testicular abnormalities, combined with abnormal sperm morphology; for dairy bulls, the main reason was lameness.

In a recent survey of dairy herd bulls in Tasmania (Dwyer, 2013), it was found that 23.5% of the bulls were not suitable for use in the ensuing mating period. A further 26.2% were given qualified passes and regarded as suitable for use in multiple sire matings and/or with specific stipulations only. The majority of the problems encountered in these bulls were only apparent after semen collection and analysis. In this survey, the semen analysis was critical, with over 70% of the problems identified relating to semen motility and morphology.

In large US dairies in which natural breeding bulls are widely employed, approximately 23% of bulls had lameness problems, of which more than 50% were severely lame (Chenoweth, 2003). Other problems included seminal vesiculitis (17%) and penile inflammation/ injury (7%).

Fertility and economic considerations

The positive effects on herd fertility of employing BBSE screened bulls are evident in a number of studies (Chenoweth, 2000).

For example, an earlier study in the US estimated that fertility problems increased significantly when sperm motility was less than 37% and normal sperm morphology was less than 65%. Another showed that single-sire bulls classified as satisfactory, questionable, and unsatisfactory obtained average pregnancy rates of 75%, 52% and 12% respectively. In Texas, bulls having 70% or 80% normal sperm obtained at least 6% better pregnancy rates than did bulls unselected for semen quality. Florida studies indicated that percentage normal sperm ($p < 0.01$), proximal droplets ($p < 0.01$), and 'primary' abnormalities ($p < 0.01$) significantly influenced fertility.

In Northern Australia, a large-scale study employed DNA parentage technology to determine major fertility influences in *Bos indicus*-derived bulls. Here, highest calf crops were obtained from bulls with >70% normal sperm, while bulls with <50% normal sperm sired relatively few calves (Fitzpatrick *et al.*, 2002). The conclusion from this study was that 'semen quality, particularly percent normal spermatozoa, was consistently related to calf output'. In addition, factors such as bull dominance, sex-drive and scrotal circumference were also important for bull fertility. The summation was that 'these results confirm that semen examination, including sperm morphology, should be standard procedure when assessing bulls for reproductive soundness' (Holroyd *et al.*, 2002).

A more recent study by Menegassi *et al.*, (2011) examined the bio-economic impact of breeding soundness evaluations on beef cattle production in southern Brazil. Two similar beef production systems comprising large herds (approximately 5000 breeding females each), with and without bull BSEs, were compared over four years (1998–2001), starting with the introduction of the BSE procedure on one of the properties. Over the study period, it was estimated that performing bull BSEs increased calf production by 31%, or 13.8 calves/bull/year and 24 kg calf/cow/year. The benefit/cost ratio of the investment in BSEs was approximately 36 : 1.

Similar benefits were observed in a dairy context in Southern Australia (Dwyer, 2013). Here, it was estimated that a herd with infertile bulls would experience a 5.5% decrease in in-calf rate. Based on 2013 economic returns, in which herds benefited by approximately $A550 per 100 cows/year for every 1% increase in in-calf rate, this decrease could cost a dairy farm $A3025 per 100 cows/year. If all bull mating was employed, this would result in an annual loss of approximately $A12 000 for a 400-cow herd employing 14 bulls. Eliminating this cause of lowered fertility by implementing bull breeding soundness evaluations (estimated at approximately $A100 each) prior to breeding, represents an economic return of approximately 14 : 1 on the amount invested in bull testing.

Genetic considerations

There are both positive and negative genetic considerations with regard to bull fertility. Space constraints prevent a detailed discussion here of the use of Estimated Breeding Values (EBVs), on which subject readers are referred to material supplied by Meat and Livestock Australia, such as the publication *Buying Better Bulls* (MLA, 2009). One caveat, however, is that it is always wise to consider the possibility of genetic/environmental interactions – for example, when traits assessed in temperate genotypes and environments are being applied in the tropics.

On the positive side, a number of advantages are associated with the use of BBSE selected bulls. For example, bull scrotal circumference is moderately to highly heritable in beef bulls (approximately 50%), and it is favourably related to both quantitative and qualitative seminal traits (Brinks, 1994). In addition, scrotal circumference in young bulls is associated with age at puberty in related females (Brinks, 1994), with favourable relationships also occurring with other female reproductive traits (Brinks, 1994; Vargas *et al.*, 1998). Heterosis also benefits both bull scrotal circumference and heifer age at puberty. Bull scrotal circumference is an accurate predictor of bull puberty, with remarkable agreement between breeds in pubertal scrotal circumference. With beef females, earlier age at puberty is linked with improved lifetime fertility and pounds of calf produced. Thus, use of BBSE criteria to select bulls for scrotal circumference (and associated improved semen traits) can improve both immediate and future herd fertility and production.

On the negative side, there is a long and growing list of inherited faults which can adversely affect bull reproduction. Here, caution is urged whenever the term 'genetic' is applied within a livestock breeding context, and this is particularly important in relation to breeding bulls. The term 'genetic', in relation to a phenotypic condition, means that it is caused by factors directly associated with genes or chromosomes. Thus, genetic disorders may be transmitted via parental genes, as well as being a result of DNA changes or mutations which are not necessarily heritable. Congenital disorders are those existing at birth, even though they may not become first evident at that time.

In turn, these may be due to a variety of causes, which can include genetic disorders, as above, but also developmental anomalies, infections, uterine environments and metabolic, nutritional and toxic factors, in addition to genetic-environmental and epigenetic influences. Those that are proven heritable (or inherited) may be transmitted via single gene (or Mendelian) inheritance, or via complex mechanisms that may involve multiple genes as well as environmental effects. For examples of conditions subject to the former mode of inheritance in cattle, readers are referred to the website: http://www.angis.org.au/Databases/BIRX/omia

Although a full description of inherited disorders of cattle is considered beyond the scope of this chapter, a listing is provided in Table 25.4 of some of the more relevant conditions in breeding bulls, as well as current understanding of their mode of inheritance. An example of a sperm abnormality that may be heritable (i.e. the knobbed acrosome defect) is shown in Figure 25.4.

Bull libido or sex drive

Interest in bull sex-drive, or libido, arose from early work in Sweden which showed that this trait had a strong genetic component. Since then, a number of methods have been developed for measuring bull sex-drive (Chenoweth, 1983, 1997).

Libido, or sex-drive is an important, if sometimes overlooked, consideration with regard to bull reproductive performance (Chenoweth, 1981), especially as it has genetic implications (Chenoweth & Landaeta-Hernandez, 1998). Using bulls of high sex-drive can benefit pregnancy rates, time of conception, length of calving season, homogeneity of weaned calves and efficient use of labour (Blockey, 1978, 1989; Godfrey & Lunstra, 1989). However, although such relationships might be expected, other studies have shown poor or inconclusive relationships between bull libido/serving capacity assessments and herd fertility. This anomaly has occurred even when bulls of superior libido completed more services, and serviced more females, than did lower libido bulls.

Such mixed findings should be anticipated whenever attempts are made to demonstrate the effects of a single male trait, such as libido, on herd fertility. This is because other male traits, as well as those associated with females and social interactions, can also influence fertility. Although bulls may be superior in one or more traits, their fertility can be compromised by deficiencies in others. This was illustrated in one study in which differences in bull libido (and sexual activity) were confounded by differences in BBSE parameters (Farin *et al.*, 1989). Another qualification of bull libido/sex-drive assessments is that a learning component is often recognised in young, inexperienced, bulls. Thus, in one study, which compared multiple libido/serving capacity tests in young (two years old) *Bos taurus* bulls, showed that at least 6–8 tests were required to adequately predict the sex drive of all bulls tested (Landaeta-Hernandez *et al.*, 2001), although bulls which initially performed well were consistently ranked highly.

Table 25.4 Genetic conditions that can adversely affect bull reproductive capability. Data source: McNitt 1965.

Problem	Heritable (H) Congenital (C) Acquired (A)	Type of inheritance	Other Factors?
1/29 Translocation (Robertsonian)	H	Chromosomal	No
Androgen Insensitivity Syndrome	H	Single locus, sex linked	Yes
Aplasia/hypoplasia of the Wolffian duct	C	n.a.	No
Corpus cavernosal shunts	H, A	?	Yes
Cryptorchidism	H?	Recessive, sex linked?	Yes
Double muscling	H	Autosomal recessive	No
Epididymal aplasia	H?	Autosomal recessive	No
Freemartinism	C	n.a.	No
Gonadal hypoplasia (GH)	H	Autosomal recessive	Yes
Hip dysplasia	H, A	Autosomal recessive	Yes
Hypoplastic seminal vesicles (HASV)	H	Autosomal recessive	No
Hypospadia	C	n.a.	Yes
Inguinal (scrotal) hernia	H?, A	?	Yes
Lack of retractor prepuce muscle	H	Recessive, Poll link	?
Lameness	H, A	Multi-factorial*	Yes
Leg defects (structural)	H	Mendelian*	?
Muscle contraction	H	Autosomal recessive	?
Ovo-testicular disorder	H, A	Single locus, sex linked?	?
Patellar luxation	H, A	?	Yes
Penile hypoplasia (short penis)	H	?	No
Persistent frenulum	H	?	No
Post legs	H?	Mendelian*	?
Preputial prolapse	H?, A	?	Yes
Short retractor penis muscle	C	n.a.	No
Sickle hocks	H	Mendelian*	No
Spastic paresis	H	Autosomal recessive	No
Spastic syndrome	H	Autosomal dominant?	No
Spiral penile deviation	H?, A	?	Yes
Syndactyly	H	Autosomal recessive	No
Testicular feminisation (TSF)	H	Chromosomal	Yes
Testicular hypoplasia (TH)	H?, A	?	Yes
Undescended testes	C	n.a.	Yes

n.a. = non-applicable

*Feet and leg conformation, in general, were assessed as of medium heritability, whereas persistent penile frenulum was of high heritability in a study with inbred lines of beef bulls at the San Juan Basin Research Center, Colorado State University (McNitt, 1965).

In summary, tests to determine bull libido or sex-drive can be useful in differentiating bulls on the basis of breeding (or mating) activity, as well as in detecting faults in mating ability (such as spiral deviation of the penis). However, the results of such tests do not necessarily predict fertility, except when severe mating disability is apparent.

Special considerations

Young bulls

There is considerable pressure to assess relatively young bulls for sale or initial breeding. This occurs for several reasons, including:

(a) it can provide the breeder with a more rapid return on investment;

(b) the end-user can achieve faster genetic gain by using young, genetically superior bulls.

In considering BBSE outcomes, it is important to consider all factors and their interactions, including age and genotype of the bulls and the environment in which they have been raised. This is particularly important when young bulls are being assessed, as commonly occurs prior to sale and/or first breeding. It is not uncommon for young bulls to have not fully achieved puberty, and this is reflected in an immature spermiogram which can persist for some months following the onset of puberty (Coulter, 1986; Persson & Söderquist, 2005) – a process which may be prolonged in young bulls raised on high-energy diets.

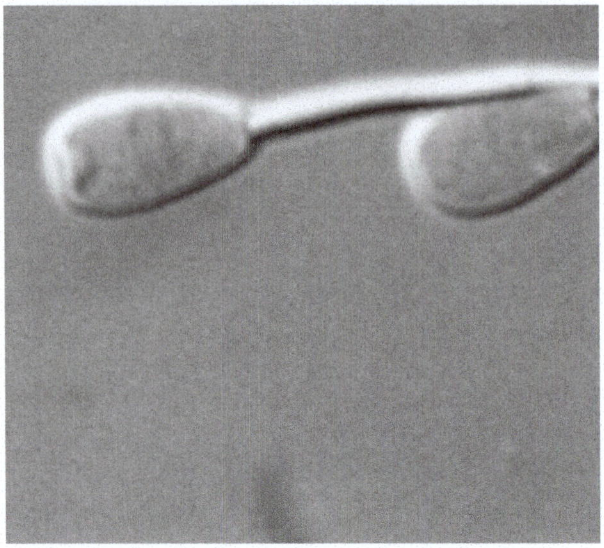

Figure 25.4 Knobbed acrosome defect in bull sperm (differential interference contrast, 1000×). In bulls, this defect is most commonly encountered as a flattened anterior aspect of the sperm head above a folded and thickened acrosomal ridge.

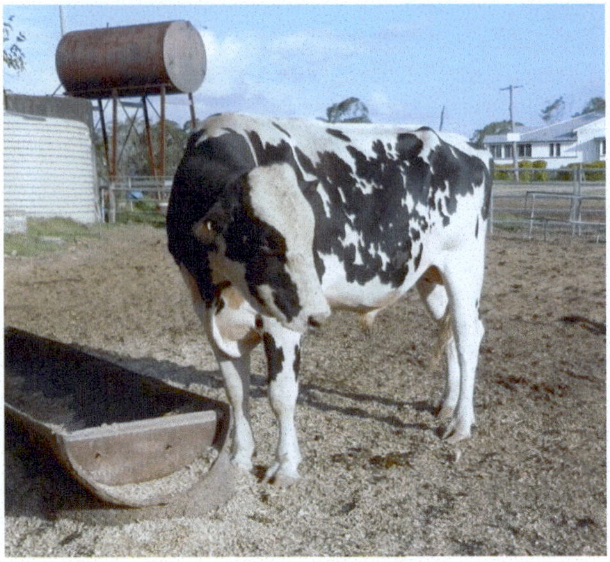

Figure 25.5 Bull used for natural breeding on a dairy farm in Queensland.

For example, the proportion of well-fed yearling *Bos taurus* beef bulls in the USA which were classified as satisfactory potential breeders changed from 55% to 72% and then 78% at 10, 11 and 12 months of age, respectively (Higdon *et al.*, 2000; Kennedy *et al.*, 2002). Here differences occur between breeds in which sexual development occurs earlier and those in which it occurs later. Thus, in tropically-adapted Senepol bulls, which are regarded as being in the latter group, less than 50% were classified as satisfactory as yearlings, although this increased to 70–85% at approximately two years of age (Chenoweth *et al.*,. 1996). BBSE outcomes can also decline with older bulls (>5–6 years of age), due to development of age-related physical and reproductive problems (Carson & Wenzel, 1997; Barth *et al.*, 2002).

In addition, young bulls probably need higher levels of management and monitoring during breeding than do older bulls. For example, in a Nebraska study with yearling bulls ($n = 74$) used for multi-sire pasture-breeding at a BFR of 1 : 20 over 60 days, all lost considerable body weight (73 kg) as well as scrotal circumference (1.4 cm), and the majority (75%) incurred some form of injury (Ellis *et al.*, 2005).

Dairy bulls

Although there is little doubt that effective genetic (and economic) progress in dairy cattle requires the exploitation of assisted reproductive technologies such as AI, it is still relatively common for natural breeding bulls to be employed on dairies (Figure 25.5). This occurs for a number of reasons, and there is also a variety of management strategies which are used with natural breeding bulls on dairy farms (Chenoweth, 2003).

In general, however, it is apparent that dairy bulls are not subject to the same degree of scrutiny and monitoring as are their beef counterparts. It is evident that appropriate selection and management of natural breeding bulls has been a relatively neglected aspect of dairy management, and this has allowed a number of preventable problems to arise (Chenoweth & Larsen, 1992; Chenoweth, 2003). Current efforts to improve the selection, evaluation, management and monitoring of natural breeding bulls on dairies include the recommendations of the Dairy Australia In-Calf program (http://www.dairyaustralia.com.au/Animals-feed-and-environment/Fertility/Bulls-power-up.aspx), in concert with those below;

Recommendations for natural breeding bulls on dairies

1. Appropriate quarantine and biosecurity measures should be strictly followed for all bulls being brought onto the farm.
2. All virgin bulls should be subjected to a breeding soundness evaluation (BSE) before being admitted to the female herd.
3. All bulls should be given a physical exam every six months and a full breeding soundness exam every 12 months.
4. Adequate handling facilities should be provided for the working and handling of bulls, to reduce the risk of injury to both animals and personnel.
5. Bulls in free stall-type housing should be given access to dirt lots.
6. All working bulls should be monitored daily. Particular attention should be paid to recognising early signs of lameness and/or injury. Lame or otherwise injured bulls should be treated and/or replaced as soon as possible.

7 Bulls ideally should be less than 2.5 years old. Aggressive, older and large, heavy bulls should not be retained on the dairy.
8 A suitable bull to female ratio is approximately one bull to 15–25 open cows (this should be modified for synchronised groups).
9 If a dairy has large pens, it may be beneficial to distribute open cows over more pens to reduce the number of bulls in any given pen.
10 Avoid drastic changes in diets fed to bulls. Do not put bulls abruptly onto the same diets as lactating cows without slowly increasing intake and energy in steps.
11 Minimise the effects of heat stress by providing shade and cooling systems.
12 In general, subject bulls to the same vaccination and preventive health programme as the cows, with the exception of vaccinations for brucellosis, trichomoniasis and modified live virus IBR, where applicable.

Pathological conditions

Lameness

Lameness represents a significant cause of bull infertility, especially in intensively managed dairies (Chenoweth, 2003). To identify and diagnose lameness, it is useful to have the bull moving in the paddock or pen prior to a close-up examination in the race or crush. The bull should move freely and easily; problems in gait can signal problems, as can uni- or bi-lateral muscle wasting, particularly in the lumbo-sacral region. Asymmetrical or overgrown claws and swellings over lower limb joints are common abnormalities, and may reflect poor conformation, pathological conditions, or both.

Conditions such as chronic lameness, sole abscesses, arthritis, severe quarter cracks, interdigital fibromas, hairy warts and foot rot can adversely affect mobility, mating ability and libido, as well as contribute to testicular degeneration particularly if the bull is recumbent for protracted periods. High body temperatures, associated with foot rot (or pyrexia from any other cause), can also cause semen/sperm problems. As the hind limbs are most important in supporting bulls during service, they should be examined most critically. Poor conformation (e.g. 'post legs' or 'cow hocks') is highly heritable in bulls (McNitt, 1965), and increases the chance of bull attrition. Spondylosis/spondyloarthrosis in the lumbo-sacral region is not uncommonly encountered in bulls, and this may contribute to service disability and related loss of libido. Young bulls fed on a high grain diet may develop particular problems, including laminitis and 'weak' fetlocks.

It is not uncommon for bulls to suffer injury or disease process during the breeding season, which can adversely affect breeding performance. For example, Ellis *et al.*, (2005) recorded a 75% total injury rate in yearling bulls used for breeding in Nebraska, which included a lameness rate of 63%, a reproductive injury rate of 12% and an overall attrition rate of 22%. At the end of the breeding season, only 45% of the bulls used for breeding were physically sound.

Common injuries to breeding bulls include preputial prolapse and laceration, 'broken penis' and feet and leg injuries. Disease entities include Bovine Ephemeral Fever, pink-eye and cancer eye. Monitoring the breeding herd at regular intervals helps to detect problems early, and thus minimise costly losses.

Vesicular adenitis (seminal vesiculitis)

Although the term 'seminal vesiculitis' is commonly employed, this condition should more appropriately be termed 'accessory genital disease', as it is rare for the problem to be confined to the vesicular glands alone. However, inflammation of the ampullae, prostate or bulbourethral glands are not readily recognised clinically. The condition is most often encountered in young post-pubertal bulls housed together and fed high energy diets, although it can be encountered in aged bulls also, with reported prevalence rates varying from 0.9% up to 49% (Linhart & Parker, 1988). Detection generally occurs via trans-rectal examination of internal reproductive organs, where physical findings often include enlargement and thickening of the gland, in conjunction with loss of lobulation, increased firmness, heat and pain on palpation. Bulls with active seminal vesiculitis often exhibit pain or discomfort on EEJ. Diagnostically, any of these signs, in conjunction with purulent material (often in clumps) and/or blood in the ejaculate, can indicate active seminal vesiculitis. Sequelae can include fibrosis, adhesions and fistulation, as well as progression of infection to the epididymis and testicle. Active seminal vesiculitis is generally associated with depressed semen quality.

The pathogenesis and aetiology are still unclear, with ascending, descending and hematogenous routes of infection all being mooted. Some evidence suggests that reflux of semen and urine into the vesicular glands may be a contributing factor, perhaps associated with maldevelopment or dysfunction of the duct systems involved (Linhart & Parker, 1988). Grain-fed young bulls raised together in pens tend to ride each other, which may lead to ascending infections via the urethra.

The condition can resolve spontaneously in young bulls, especially when they are dispersed and placed on a lower energy diet. However, it is not possible to determine which individuals will undergo spontaneous recovery. A culture sample, obtained by passing a catheter up the urethra and massaging the glands, may be useful in deciding treatment. Causal organisms, either proven or suggestive, have included *Aeromonas hydrophila*, *Actinomyces pyogenes*, *Brucella abortus*, *Chlamydia psittaci*, *Mycoplasma bovigenitalium*, *Mycoplasma mycoides subsp mycoides SC*, *Hemophilus somnus*, *Ureaplasma diversum* and IBR-like viruses. However, organisms are often not isolated.

Treatment options can be frustratingly inconsistent. The treatment of choice would be a long-term antibiotic to which

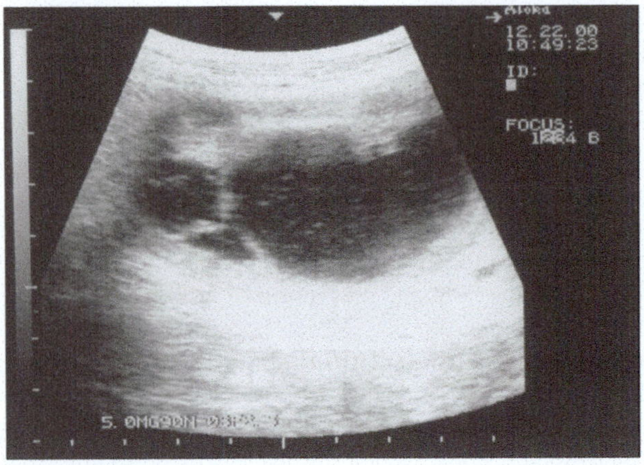

Figure 25.6 Real-time ultrasound image of a varicocoele in a two-year-old bull.

the causative organism is susceptible. To determine this requires collecting an uncontaminated sample from the vesicular glands, using a urethral catheter. Non-targeted options have included 1–2 week regimes of parenterally administered penicillin or tetracycline, with a number of more recent reports using Micotil® or Naxcel®. More adventurous treatments have included intra-glandular injection of antibiotics or sclerosing agents, surgical removal of the glands and laser stimulation. A prevalent opinion appears to be that treatment of seminal vesiculitis in older bulls is often less successful than in younger bulls.

When encountered in groups of young, grain-fed bulls, recommended control measures have included lowering both the energy level of feed and the population density of pens, as well as feeding antibiotics such as erythromycin or tetracycline.

Varicocoele

Varicocoele is an abnormal dilatation of the venous return from the testes, and may be uni- or bi-lateral. Although rarely diagnosed, it should be considered when other tests have failed to reveal the cause of sperm/semen irregularities. It can sometimes be palpable as a cystic dilatation in the area of the pampiniform plexus, just above the head of the epididymis. However, real-time ultrasound is the preferred tool for diagnosis (Figure 25.6).

Testicular hypoplasia

The term 'testicular hypoplasia' refers to a relative lack of development of the spermatogenic epithelium. As such, it has a range of manifestations and can be difficult to accurately diagnose. However, as it can sometimes have a heritable basis, care should be taken to ensure proper diagnosis, which should be made histologically. Clinical diagnosis should not be attempted until bulls are well past puberty. Testicular hypoplasia is relatively rare (<1%), often unilateral (left) and often misdiagnosed as cryptorchidism (which is much more rare in bulls; <0.1%). It should be noted that bull testicles often differ in size (with up to 25% difference being 'acceptable') and also in conformation.

Testicular degeneration

Testicular degeneration may be temporary or permanent, depending on the type and duration of the particular stressor which has caused the problem. Although the causes are multiple, the spermatogenic epithelium usually reacts in a very predictable way. A normal degree of testicular degeneration is associated with ageing. Orchitis (swelling of the testicle proper) is a common precursor, and this may be due to trauma or infection (Figure 25.7). Orchitis should be differentiated from other causes of swelling within the scrotum, which can include scrotal hernia, haematoma and fluid accumulation within the tunics. Any swelling of the testicle is potentially damaging to sperm production, as the tunica albuginea is relatively inflexible, allowing pressure to rapidly build up within the testicle.

Aetiological factors associated with testicular degeneration include:

- Elevation of testicular temperature (directly or indirectly).
- Increase in intra-testicular pressure.
- Scrotal frostbite (supercooling plus adhesions).
- Ischemia.
- Congenital or inflammatory occlusion of excurrent ducts.
- Toxins.
- Infection.

Testicular degeneration can often be detected clinically, and it usually progresses as follows:

1. Increased 'tone', size and heat.
2. Loss of testicular tone.
3. Loss of size, accompanied by increased firmness (fibrosis, calcification).

Seminal indicators also occur, depending on the cause, duration and severity (see scrotal insulation study below). A progression can often be seen in the ejaculate as follows:

1. Loss in sperm motility associated with increased 'secondary' abnormalities.
2. Increased morphologic defects ('primary' defects).
3. Increased spermatogenic precursors (spermatocytes, spermatogonia).
4. Azoospermia.

Libido and mating (service) ability

Libido in bulls has a strong genetic component. It is best determined in younger bulls, as older bulls may have superimposed learning patterns, pathological conditions and inhibitions. Young bulls, particularly those group-raised, may show

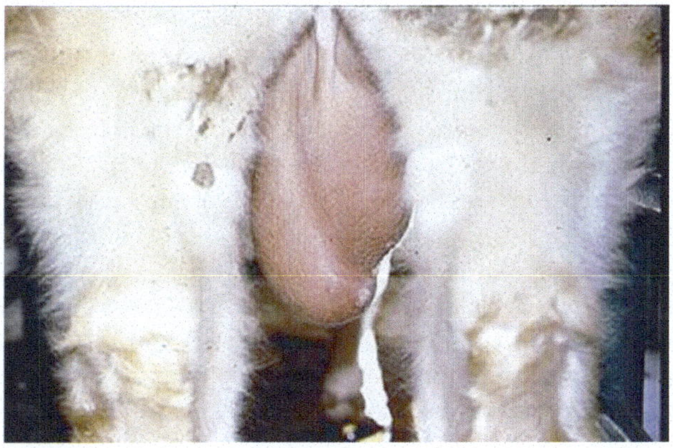

Figure 25.7 Unilateral orchitis in a Charolais bull.

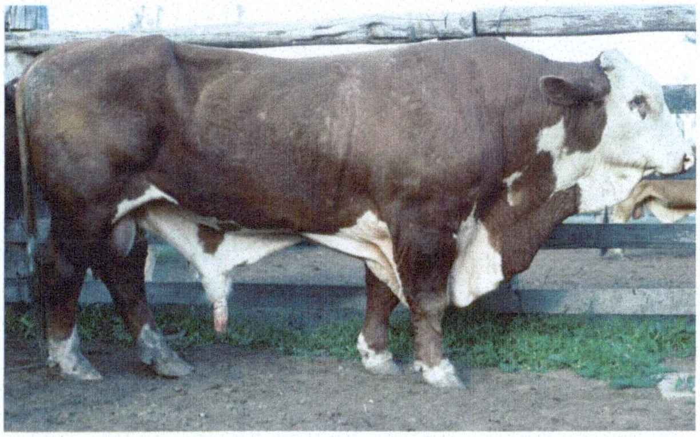

Figure 25.8 Mature Braford bull, showing signs of muscle wasting in the rear, semi-chronic preputial eversion and rear-limb toe dragging. These signs are suggestive of a back problem, probably in the lumbo-sacral region.

inexperience and delayed development of competent service behaviour. High-gain bulls may also show depressed libido, as may bulls in very poor condition and those suffering from disease and/or pain.

Service disability associated with back problems

This condition, most commonly observed in older bulls, is often due to progressive deterioration of articular surfaces, with spondylosis deformans often being present. Younger bulls, particularly fast-growing ones, may also develop similar problems. Affected bulls often step 'short' with their hind legs, and may show some muscle wasting in the gluteal region as, well as chronic eversion of the preputial epithelium (Figure 25.8).

Service disability associated with feet and leg problems

Careful observation of claw growth and symmetry can often help to identify pathological or conformational problems of the feet and legs of bulls. Similarly, swellings of the lower joints are indicators of potential problems. Checks should always be made for

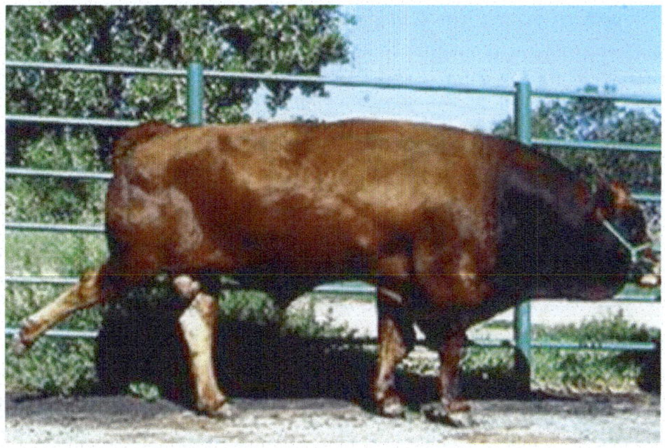

Figure 25.9 Spastic paresis in a mature Tarentaise bull showing permanent contraction of the gastocnemius muscle in the right rear limb.

contributing causes such as interdigital corns or necrobacillosis, bruised sole, foot abscesses or laminitis.

Spastic syndrome ('crampy' or 'stretches') is usually first seen as abnormal flexion and extension of one hind limb, where it is sometimes colloquially termed 'stringhalt'. If allowed to progress, it will subsequently involve both hind limbs. This condition is generally first seen as animals approach mature weight, especially in heavier breeds. It has a genetic basis, and has been associated with arthritis, 'post' legs and weak hocks.

Spastic paresis, on the other hand, may initially be observed in animals as young as 3–6 months. Here, the condition is represented by spastic contraction of hindlimb muscles, in particular the gastrocnemius and superficial flexor muscles and tendons, and extension of the stifle and tarsal joints. It is heritable (see Table 25.4), progressive and can be unilateral (more common) or bilateral. Extreme hyperextension can occur, in which the gastrocnemius muscle is quite firm and the affected animal cannot place the foot on the ground (Figure 25.9). The disorder has been associated with overstimulation of the myotatic (stretch) reflex. Although options exist to alleviate this condition by medical or surgical means, this should be discouraged, due to its heritable nature.

Service disability associated with penile and preputial problems

Penile and preputial problems are not an insignificant cause of service disability. Consequently, every effort should be made to adequately examine the bull's penis and prepuce at the time of the breeding soundness examination.

Inability to protrude the penis may be due to phimosis, or to congenitally short penis or retractor penis muscle. The last two conditions may be confused with delayed penile development or separation in young, over-fat bulls. Phimosis may be due to adhesions caused by injury (traumatic, physical, chemical), non-specific and specific balanoposthitis.

Persistent frenulum (otherwise known as a 'tied penis', or a persistent fibrous raphe) is not uncommonly encountered, particularly in some breeds and lines. At present, most of these are surgically separated when detected, even though there is strong evidence for a genetic basis (see Table 25.4). Some breeders cull bulls with this problem.

Paraphimosis occurs when the penis cannot be retracted into the prepuce, and is most commonly associated with penile hematoma or traumatic damage to the penis and/or prepuce.

Preputial prolapse can be a serious condition in bulls, as it can adversely affect breeding and be difficult to repair. Breed differences have been reported for this condition. Although not regarded as a heritable condition *per se* (see Table 25.4), it is apparent that there are predisposing factors, some of which are heritable. Implicating factors include;

1 Excess amounts of parietal preputial epithelium.
2 Absence or lack of development of the caudal prepuce muscle; a condition which is genetically linked with the poll gene in cattle.

Penile deviation (phallocampsis) is observed in several forms, with the most common being spiral or corkscrew. The deviations may occur secondarily to trauma, such as with penile lacerations, and some evidence of the predisposing injury is often apparent. However, spontaneous deviations also occur, and are often observed in three- or four-year-old bulls that have already completed at least one breeding season. Deviations are best diagnosed at natural service, as use of EEJ can induce misleading results. Heritability of deviations is reported as low (Table 25.4), although a genetic link has been suggested in Poll Hereford bulls in Australia. Surgical correction (several options available) often provides some relief and can even allow normal service to resume, although this is usually temporary.

Penile analgesia, due to peripheral nerve degeneration, should be considered when bulls show excessive (seeking), or fail to achieve either intromission or to complete the ejaculatory thrust. Here, damage often occurs to the dorsal peripheral nerves of the penis which are essential for the ejaculatory reflex. Common causes of damage to these nerves include rupture of the tunica albuginea (penile haematoma or 'broken penis') or damage to the penile surface when removing fibropapillomas or separating persistent penile frenulums. Care should be taken to ensure that surgical interventions close to the surface of the penis cause minimal damage to the integrity of the penile membrane and its nervous supply.

Failure of the bull to achieve a full erection can occur due to defects in the vascular erectile mechanism. Bulls have a fibro-elastic penis, which relies upon vascular mechanisms to greatly increase rigidity on erection. Vascular shunts between the corpus cavernosum penis and either the corpus spongiosum or the superficial vasculature, as well as occlusions, can compromise this mechanism. Both shunts and occlusions may be congenital, or may be acquired through penile injury, inflammation or infection. Full diagnosis might require contrast radiography of the corpus cavernosum penis.

Bull health and reproductive biosecurity

Infectious disease

A number of diseases affect cattle reproduction, with some acting in the male, or the female, or both. This discussion will focus on those that are most relevant for the male, and will include diseases that may be transmitted in semen, as well as those that are currently regarded as venereal in cattle. Table 25.5 indicates the infectious agents that can be transmitted in bull semen.

Table 25.5 Infectious agents that can be transmitted in bull semen.

Bacteria	Viruses	Protozoa
Brucella abortus (H)	Bluetongue (BTV) (L)	*Tritrichomonas foetus* (H)
Chlamydia pscitiscii (L)	Bovine virus diarrhoea/pestivirus (H)	*Neosporum caninum* (?)
Histophilus somnus (L)	FMDV (H)	
Leptospira hardjo-prajitna (H)	BHV1 (IBR) (H)	
Campylobacter fetus (H)	Maedi-visna (?)	
Bovine TB (L)	Bovine leukosis (L)	
Chlamydia (L)	Bovine ephemeral fever (?)	
Mycoplasma mycoides ssp. Mycoides	Rinderpest (L)	
Mycoplasma avian subsp Para TB	Bovine vesicular stomatitis	
Ureaplasma diversum (?)	Epizootic haemorrhagic disease	
Mycobacterium bovis (?)	Bovine immunodeficiency-like virus (L)	
Coxiella burnetti (L)	Bovine paratuberculosis	
	Contagious bovine pleuropneumonia	
	Akabane/Aino/Schmallenburg (?)	
	Lumpy skin disease (M)	

Low risk (L); High risk (H); Unproven transmission in semen (?).
After Eaglesome & Garcia (1997) and Givens & Marley (2008).

It is recognised that bull semen is a contaminated product which often contains many organisms. Some of these are innocuous contaminants, others may directly affect semen quality and yet others may be transmitted in semen to females, in which they can become established and cause problems. The last category is the one of greatest concern in terms of herd health and biosecurity and, as such, it has received much attention from organisations that address AI health concerns, such as the World Organisation for Animal health (OIE), which provides standards for disease control with respect to animal semen (see Appendix 3.2.1 of the OIE Terrestrial Animal Health Code). Such standards can also provide biosecurity guidelines for animal quarantine and introduction to the herd (Givens & Marley, 2008).

Venereal diseases

Venereal diseases are contagious diseases transmitted during coitus (or mating). In cattle, the list of accepted venereal diseases is much shorter than the list of disease entities that may be transmitted via semen, and consists of trichmonosis (or trichomoniasis) and campylobacteriosis (or vibriosis). Others, such as ureaplasmosis, are potential candidates.

Trichomonosis and campylobacteriosis

These two disease entities are grouped together because, despite being caused by markedly different organisms, they are similar in effect and, not uncommonly, will exist side by side. Both replicate in a micro-aerophilic environment within the bull's preputial crypts, and result in no discernable pathology in the bull. Both are transmitted in bull semen (both fresh and frozen) causing infertility and/or abortion in susceptible females. Differences do occur in some aspects. For example, trichomonosis is more associated with early abortion and occasional pyometra, whereas campylobacterosis is more associated with infertility (although it can cause abortions), despite regular cyclicity. A convalescent humoral immunity in females develops for both disease entities after approximately 3–6 months, although this is not absolute. This has allowed the development of a killed-organism vaccine for *Campylobacter foetus var venerealis*, which has a finite effective duration of protection (≤ 6 months). A vaccine for trichomonosis which offers limited protection is available in the USA.

Ureaplamosis

Ureaplasmas (formerly T-strain mycoplasmas) belong to the Mycoplasmataceae family of cell-wall deficient bacteria, which includes *Mycoplasma*. They are antigenetically diverse and species-specific.

Ureaplasmosis in cattle is caused by *Ureaplasma diversum*, which has been implicated in a number of reproductive tract disorders, including granular vulvovaginitis, infertility, early embryonic loss, mid-to-late term abortion and birth of low-viability calves. *U. diversum* strains differ in pathogenicity, as does female susceptibility, with heifers being particularly susceptible. Although *U. diversum* may be cultured from prepubertal heifers, breeding activity appears to disseminate it more rapidly, suggesting that venereal transmission may occur (Rae *et al.*, 1993).

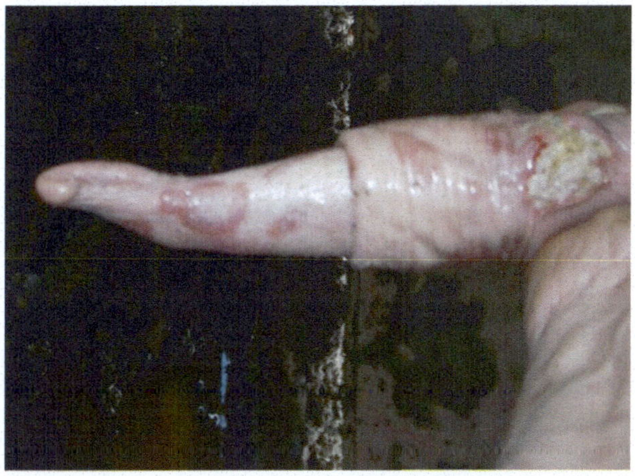

Figure 25.10 Penile lesions associated with Murray Valley Balanitis. Image courtesy of Dr David Hall, Walwa Veterinary Practice.

U. diversum is commonly isolated from the reproductive tract of apparently normal female cattle (60–70%), particularly from the vulva and vestibular regions. Breeding age beef heifers tend to have the highest prevalence (70–80%). It is also a common inhabitant of the bull reproductive tract (5 ≥ 70%), particularly within the prepuce and distal urethra. The high prevalence rates of *U. diversum* in otherwise healthy cattle does not explain why problems may occur under certain unspecified conditions, which are probably multi-factorial.

Clinical signs in females include granular vulvovaginitis, hyperaemia of the vulval and vaginal mucosa, raised red to grey nodules and occasionally, a mild to marked mucopurulent discharge.

In bulls, *U. diversum* has been associated with granular balanoposthitis and possibly seminal vesiculitis. *U. diversum* was recently isolated from beef cattle in Australia as part of an investigation into a syndrome, locally termed 'Murray Valley Balanitis', which was first recognised as severe penile lesions in beef bulls in south-eastern New South Wales (Argue *et al.*, 2013; Figure 25.10).

Summary

The health and reproductive capabilities of bulls are closely interrelated. The bull breeding soundness evaluation (BBSE) is an effective tool to reduce the risk of poor bull reproductive performance. Although the BBSE does not usually include a full clinical examination, it does provide a framework which allows detection of many problems which might adversely affect reproduction. This capability is enhanced by improvements in methodology and interpretation which are, in turn, driven by advances in relevant knowledge. This chapter attempts to address a number of topics which can enhance this process.

References

Argue, B., Chousalker, K.K. and Chenoweth, P.J. (2013). Presence of *Ureaplasma diversum* in the Australian cattle population. *Australian Veterinary Journal* **91**(3), 99–101.

Barth, A.D. (1994). *Bull Breeding Soundness Evaluation Manual*. Saskatoon: The Western Canadian Association of Bovine Practitioners.

Barth, A.D. and Oko, R.J. (1989). *Abnormal Morphology of Bovine Spermatozoa*. Iowa State University Press, Ames, Iowa. 285 pp.

Barth, A.D. and Waldner, C.L. (2002). Factors affecting breeding soundness classification of beef bulls examined at the Western College of Veterinary Medicine. *Canadian Veterinary Journal* **43**, 274–284.

Beggs, D. (2013). Ed. Australian. *Veterinary Bull Breeding Soundness Evaluation*. Australian Cattle Veterinarians, Eight-Mile Plains, Qld 4113. ISBN: 978-9807.

Blockey, M.A. deB. (1978). The influence of serving capacity of bulls on herd fertility. *Journal of Animal Science* **46**, 589–595.

Blockey, M.A. deB. (1989). Relationship between serving capacity of beef bulls as predicted by the yard test and their fertility during paddock mating. *Australian Veterinary Journal* **66**, 348.

Brinks, J.S. (1994). Relationships of scrotal circumference to puberty and subsequent reproductive performance in male and female offspring. In: Fields, M.J. and Sand, R.S. (eds). *Factors Affecting Calf Crop*, pp. 363–370. Boca Raton, CRC Press.

Brinks, J.S., Mclnerney, M.J. and Chenoweth, P.J. (1978). Relationship of age at puberty in heifers to reproductive traits in young bulls. *Proceedings, Western Section, American Society of Animal Science* **29**, 28.

Bruner, K.A., McCraw, R.L., Whitacre, M.D. and Van Camp, S.D. (1995). Breeding soundness examination of 1,952 yearling beef bulls in North Carolina. *Theriogenology* **44**, 129–145.

Carroll, E.J., Ball, L. and Scott, J.A. (1963). Breeding soundness in bulls – a summary of 10,940 examinations. *Journal of the American Veterinary Medical Association* **142**, 1105 –1111.

Carson, R.L. and Wenzel, J.G. (1997). Observations using the new bull-breeding soundness evaluation forms in adult and young bulls. *Veterinary Clinics of North America: Food Animal Practice* **13**, 305–311.

Chacón, J., Pérez, E., Müller, E., Söderquist, L. and Rodríguez-Martínez, H. (1999). Breeding soundness evaluation of extensively managed bulls in Costa Rica. *Theriogenology* **52**, 221–231.

Chenoweth, P.J. (1981). Libido and mating behaviour in bulls, boars and rams. A review. *Theriogenology* **16**(2), 155–177.

Chenoweth, P.J. (1983). Examination of bulls for libido and breeding ability. In: *Veterinary Clinics of North America; Large Animal Practice* **5**, 59–74.

Chenoweth, P.J. (1997). Bull Libido/Serving Capacity. *Veterinary Clinics of North America: Food Animal Practice* **13**(2), 331–344.

Chenoweth, P.J. (2000). The breeding soundness evaluation of bulls: A rationale. *Compendium on Continuing Education for the Practising Veterinarian* **22**, S48–55.

Chenoweth, P.J. (2003). *Management of Breeding Bulls on Dairies*. Proc. 6th Annual Western Dairy Management Conference, Las Vegas, pp 107–117.

Chenoweth, P.J. (2005). Breeding Bull Assessment and Management. In: Chenoweth, P.J. and Sanderson, M.W. (eds). *Beef Practice: Cow-Calf Production Medicine*. Blackwell Publishing, Ames, Iowa. ISBN 13, 978-0-8138-0402-6.

Chenoweth, P.J. (2006). *The Pathogenesis of Sperm Problems*. Proc. Australian Cattle Veterinarians, Hobart.

Chenoweth, P.J. and Landaeta-Hernandez, A. (1998). Influence of genetics on maternal and reproductive behaviour of livestock. In Grandin, T. (ed). *Genetics and Behaviour of Domestic Animals*. Academic Press, San Diego, CA.

Chenoweth, P.J. and Larsen, R.E. (1992) Selection, Use and Management of Natural Service Bulls. In: Van Horn, H.H. and Wilcox, C.J. (eds). *Large Dairy Herd Management*, pp. 209–218. American Dairy Science Association, Champaign, Illinois.

Chenoweth, P.J., Spitzer, J.C. and Hopkins, F.M. (1992). *A new bull breeding soundness evaluation form*. Proc. Society for Theriogenology AGM, pp 63–70.

Chenoweth, P.J., Chase, C.C. Jr.,, Thatcher, M.-J.D., Wilcox, C.J. and Larsen, R.E. (1996). Breed and other effects on semen traits and breeding soundness categorization in beef bulls in Florida. *Theriogenology* **46**, 1159–1170.

Chenoweth, P.J., Hopkins, F.M., Spitzer, J.C. and Larsen, R.E. (2010). Guidelines for using the bull breeding soundness evaluation form. *Clinical Theriogenology* **2**(1), 43–50.

Coulter, G.H. (1986). Puberty and postpuberal development of beef bulls. Ch in Ed D Morrow, *Current Therapy in Theriogenology*, 2nd Edition, pp. 142–148. WB Saunders, Philadephia.

Coulter, G.H. and Kozub, G.C. (1989). Efficacy of methods to test fertility of beef bulls used for multiple-sire breeding under range conditions. *Journal of Animal Science* **67**, 1757–1766.

Dwyer, C. (2013). *Results of an investigation into dairy herd bull fertility and management in Tasmania*. Proc Australian Cattle Veterinarians, Darwin, pp. 123–126.

Eaglesome, M.D. and Garcia, M.M. (1997). Disease risks to animal health from artificial insemination with bovine semen. *Revue Scientifique et Technique de l'Office International des Epizooties* **16**(1), 215–225.

Ellis, R., Rupp, G.P., Chenoweth, P.J., Cundiff, L.V. and Lunstra, D.D. (2005). Fertility of yearling beef bulls during mating. *Theriogenology* **64**(3), 657–78.

Elmore, R.G., Bierschwal, C.J., Martin, C.E. and Youngquist, R.S. (1975). A summary of 1,127 breeding soundness examinations in beef bulls. *Theriogenology* **3**, 209–218.

Farin, P.W., Chenoweth, P.J., Tomky, D.F., Ball, L. and Pexton, J.E. (1989). Breeding soundness, libido and performance of beef bulls mated to estrus synchronized heifers. *Theriogenology* **32**, 717.

Fields, M.J., Hentges, J.F. Jr., and Cornelisse, K.W. (1982). Aspects of the sexual development of Brahman versus Angus bulls in Florida. *Theriogenology* **18**, 17–31.

Fitzpatrick, L.A., Fordyce, G., McGowan, M.R., Bertram, J.D., Doogan, V.J., DeFavieri, J., Miller, R.G. and Holroyd, R.G. (2002). Bull selection and use in Northern Australia. Part 2. Semen Traits. *Animal Reproduction Science* **71**, 39–49.

Fordyce, G., Entwistle, K., Norman, S., Perry, V., Gardiner, B. and Fordyce, P. (2006). Standardising bull breeding soundness evaluations and reporting in Australia. *Theriogenology* **66**, 1140–1148.

Givens, M.D. and Marley, M.S.D. (2008). Pathogens that cause infertility of bulls or transmission via semen. *Theriogenology* **70**, 504–507.

Godfrey, R.W. and Dodson, R.E. (2005). Breeding soundness evaluations of Senepol bulls in the US Virgin Islands *Theriogenology* **63**, 831–840.

Godfrey, R.W. and Lunstra, D.D. (1989). Influence of single or multiple sires and serving capacity on mating behaviour of beef bulls. *Journal of Animal Science* **67**, 2897–2903.

Higdon, H.L. 3rd,, Spitzer, J.C., Hopkins, F.M. and Bridges, W.C. Jr., (2000). Outcomes of breeding soundness evaluation of 2,898 yearling bulls subjected to different classification systems. *Theriogenology* **53**, 1321–1332.

Irons, P.C., Nothling, J.O. and Bertschinger, H.J. (2007). Bull breeding soundness evaluation in southern Africa. *Theriogenology* **68**, 842–847.

Holroyd, R.G., Doogan, V.J., De Faveri, J., Fordyce, G., McGowan, M.R., Bertram, J.D., Vankan, D.M., Fitzpatrick, L.A., Jayawardhana, G.A. and Miller, R.G. (2002). Bull selection in northern Australia. 4. Calf output and predictors of fertility of bulls in multiple-sire herds. *Animal Reproduction Science* **71**, 67–69.

Kennedy, S.P., Spitzer, J.C., Hopkins, F.M., Higdon, H.L. and Bridges, W.C., Jr., (2002). Breeding soundness evaluations of 3,648 yearling beef bulls using the (1993 Society for Theriogenology guidelines. *Theriogenology* **58**, 947–961.

Landaeta-Hernandez, A.J., Chenoweth, P.J. and Berndtson, W.E. (2001). Assessing sex-drive in young *Bos taurus* bulls. *Animal Reproduction Science* **66**, 151–160.

Larsen, R.E., Littell, R., Rooks, E., Adams, E.L., Falcon, C. and Warnick, A.C. (1990). Bull influences on conception percentage and calving date in Angus Hereford, Brahman and Senepol single-sire herds. *Theriogenology* **34**, 549–568.

Linhart, R.D. and Parker, W.G. (1988). Seminal vesiculitis in bulls. *Compendium on Continuing Education for the Practising Veterinarian* **10**(12), 1428–1433.

McNitt, J.I. (1965). *Genetic aspects of estimated breeding soundness of bulls.* MSc Thesis, Department of Animal Science, Colorado State University.

MLA (Meat and Livestock Australia) (2009). *Buying better bulls.* http://www.mla.com.au/General/Search-results-publications?keyword=bull+ebv%26iw_field_in_publicationscategory%3d. (accessed Feb. 26, 2014).

Menegassi, S.R.O., Barcellos, J.O.J., Lampert, V.doN., Borges, J.B.S. and Peripolli, V. (2011). Bioeconomic impact of bull breeding soundness examination in cow-calf systems. *Revista Brasileira de Zootecnia* **40**(2), 441–447.

OIE Terrestrial Code Terrestrial Animal Health Code. (2007). *Bovine and small ruminant semen*, 16th Edition, World Organisation for Animal Health.

Penny, C. (2010). The BCVA's bull pre-breeding examination certificate. *Veterinary Record* **167**, 551–554. doi: 10.1136/vr.c5216. (accessed Feb 26 2014).

Persson, Y. and Söderquist, L. (2005). The proportion of beef bulls in Sweden with mature spermiograms at 11–13 months of age. *Reproduction in Domestic Animals* **40**, 131–135.

Rae, D.O., Chenoweth, P.J., Brown, M.B., Genho, S.A., Moore, S.A. and Jacobsen, K.E. (1993). Reproductive performance of beef heifers: Effects of vulvo-vaginitis, *Ureaplasma diversum* and prebeeding antibiotic administration. *Theriogenology* **40**, 497–508.

Risco, C.A., Chenoweth, P.J., Smith, B.I., Velez, J.S. and Barker, R. (1998). Management and economics of natural service bulls in dairy herds. *Compendium on Continuing Education for the Practising Veterinarian* **20**, 385–390.

Spitzer, J.C. and Hopkins, F.M. (1997). Breeding soundness evaluation of yearling bulls. *Veterinary Clinics of North America: Food Animal Practice* **13**, 295–304.

Spitzer, J.C., Hopkins, F.M., Webster, H.W., Kirkpatrick, F.D. and Hill, H.S. (1988). Breeding soundness examination of yearling beef bulls. *Journal of the American veterinary medical association* **193**, 1075–1079.

Sylla, L., Stradaioli, G., Borgami, S. and Monaci, M. (2007) Breeding soundness examination of Chianina, Marchigiana, and Romagnola yearling bulls in performance tests over a 10-year period. *Theriogenology* **67**, 1351–1358.

Vale Filho, V.R., Pinto, P.A., Megale, F., Fonseca, J. and Soares, L.C.O. (1980). *Fertility of the bull in Brazil. A survey of 1088 bulls and 17945 ejaculations from* Bos taurus *and* Bos indicus *and crosses under tropical conditions.* Proc. 9th Internat Cong Animal Reprod and A.I., Madrid, Spain, Vol **VI**, pp 545–548.

Vargas, C.A., Elzo, M.A., Chase, C.C. Jr., Chenoweth, P.J. and Olson, T.A. (1998). Estimation of genetic parameters for scrotal circumference, age at puberty in heifers, and hip height in Brahman cattle. *Journal of Animal Science* **76**, 2536–2541.

Walters, J.A. (2012). *Influence of age on outcomes of 443 bull pre-breeding examinations performed in the United Kingdom.* Proc 27th World Buiatrics Congress, Lisbon, Portugal. Abst OC:87, p.65, http://www.ivis.org/proceedings/wbc/2012/toc.asp.

Williams, J.H. (2013). *Results of bull breeding soundness examinations from a UK farm practice.* Proc 27th World Buiatrics Congress, Lisbon, Portugal. Abst OC:886, p.65, http://www.ivis.org/proceedings/wbc/2012/toc.asp.

CHAPTER 26

Euthanasia of Cattle

Karin Mueller

Learning objectives

- Understand the various aspects that must be addressed for successful euthanasia.
- Be aware of associated legal matters.
- Understand the advantages, disadvantages, procedures and technicalities of methods available.
- Appreciate health and safety aspects.
- Be aware of potential complications and know how to react.
- Have an outline understanding of large-scale euthanasia.

Introduction

Euthanasia is a common and important activity of veterinarians. The reasons for performing euthanasia in cattle include: acutely injured animals; unfeasible treatment options; national or regional disease control measures; and neonates in cases of unresolved dystocia requiring fetotomy.

Aside from technical, logistical and welfare considerations, effects on attending people have to be carefully considered. These include emotional response, and the potential danger posed by both the patient and the euthanasia method.

Euthanasia derives from the Greek words 'eu', meaning 'good' or 'well', and 'thanatos', meaning 'death'. Its use for 'mercy killing' appears in the English language in the late 19th century (Harper, 2012).

Euthanasia of animals is legally allowed in many countries, subject to animal welfare laws and regulations. Obligations include avoidance of any undue pain or distress during the *entire* procedure. In some countries and communities, euthanasia is rarely utilised because of religious or moral beliefs.

Planning stage

Considering the following aspects will facilitate the successful performance of the procedure:

1 Consent
2 Timing (when)
3 Place (where)
4 Persons present (who)
5 Method (how)
6 Back-up options
7 Safety considerations
8 Emotional impact
9 Disposal

Legal aspects encroach on almost every aspect of the process – for example, the qualifications of the person allowed to perform euthanasia, the legal aspects of gun ownership, animal welfare regulations, controlled drug regulations, and health and safety regulations.

Owner's consent

Obtaining the owner's or agent's written consent is often neglected in cattle practice, because of the typically close relationship between veterinarians and their farm clients. It is highly advisable in every case, and not just because the owner is not well known. Consent should include animal type and ID, date, location and owner's or agent's signature.

Where the owner requests euthanasia, but is not going to be present during the procedure, the animal in question needs to be positively identified by an unambiguous permanent or temporary mark. The attending veterinarian should also ascertain that the request was for euthanasia, especially when receiving the request via a third party (e.g. a receptionist).

Bovine Medicine, Third Edition. Edited by Peter D. Cockcroft.

It should be confirmed that the owner clearly understands the procedure involves death and that it is irreversible. Colloquial language, such as 'put to sleep' may appear more fitting in emotionally charged situations, but it carries the risk of misunderstandings. The term 'euthanasia' is understood by most owners. One indirect way to check that the owner fully understands the implications is to ask what they intend to do with the body.

Where the owner is not known or present, for example a road traffic accident, the welfare of the animal is the overriding governing factor and, if indicated, euthanasia must be carried out without delay. However, where the animal can be made comfortable with reasonable means to gain some time to locate the owner, this option should be given consideration. Relevant details about the animal, the clinical decision process, and any attending authority (such as police) should be recorded in case of a subsequent challenge.

Where a valuable animal is involved, for example at an agricultural show, the second opinion of a veterinary colleague is advisable. Prior to officiating at such events, consideration should be given as to how owner's consent can be obtained if necessary, and whether indemnity insurance is sufficient in case of allegations of wrongful destruction. Where livestock insurance exists, the company's wishes must be ascertained. Death insurance may be conditional on the company being informed prior to euthanasia. For a claim under 'loss of use', destruction of the animal may not be required.

Timing

Euthanasia must not be delayed where this would compromise the patient's welfare. Otherwise, factors such as availability of assistance, collection of the cadaver, exposure of herd mates to the dead animal or blockage of facilities can be taken into account, and the procedure timed accordingly.

Place

Severely injured or diseased cattle should be killed where found. For mobile young stock and adult patients, restraint and access to remove the cadaver are the two main factors to consider. If mobility is good, and the animal is unlikely to go down, then the animal may be restrained within a crush. If the crush has lateral gates and no obstructive vertical bars, it may be possible to euthanise the animal *in situ* and retrieve the cadaver. Where handling facilities are not conducive for the removal of the cadaver, heavy sedation, leading to recumbency in an open space, may be employed when using firearms. If it is not possible for the animal to be euthanised in and collected from the handling facility, a risk assessment should be performed to ensure that there is a safe, viable, option.

For lethal injection, an intravenous catheter should be placed into a suitable vein (e.g. jugular) while the animal is restrained in a handling facility, for example a crush. If the crush does not allow the retrieval of the cadaver following euthanasia, then sedation may first be required, so that the animal can be safely moved to a preferred location. This would, ideally, be an adjacent secure pen or yard. In placid or heavily sedated animals, restraint at the collection point may be achieved using a halter; or a temporary pen made from hurdles. An extension tube affixed to the catheter and secured near the withers reduces stress induced by any head and neck shyness, and allows the veterinarian to stand at a distance from the falling animal when the animal is euthanised. Where lethal injection is required in a trailer or vehicle, an intravenous catheter is also invaluable. The injection is administered via an extension tube passed through a ventilation gap, thus avoiding the operator becoming trapped.

If collection is delayed, the cadaver should be moved to a site that accommodates the increase in size caused by bloating and which carries little risk of disease transfer.

The logistics of large-scale euthanasia are considered later.

Persons involved

Euthanasia is typically not an act of veterinary surgery, but may be carried out by any person capable of performing it in a humane way. Equally, in many countries, veterinarians do not have statutory powers to destroy animals, but are allowed to do so under the instruction of an owner, an authority (police, ministry), or under animal welfare and protection acts. Standard operating procedures for euthanasia should form part of a client's herd health plan, with the veterinarian providing adequate training to farm staff.

Lethal injection is usually restricted to veterinarians, as the solutions are subject to veterinary medicine regulations.

Assistants are often needed for restraint and cadaver removal. To ensure that the process can be carried out safely and efficiently, euthanasia should not be attempted without such assistance in place.

Methods

Firearms and lethal injection are the two main methods available (Table 26.1). One means of euthanasia should always be carried for unexpected cases requiring destruction. For planned euthanasia visits, two different options should be taken.

The choice of method is governed by accessibility and restraining facilities, operator's preference, cadaver disposal route, post-mortem diagnostic requirements, and aesthetic concerns.

It should be remembered that on-farm casualty slaughter for human consumption requires stunning, followed by exsanguination, and that lethal injection renders the cadaver unsuitable for use as pet food.

Prior sedation is useful when using firearms, in fractious patients or where suitable restraining facilities are lacking. The effect of sedation on the uptake of euthanasia solutions

Table 26.1 Overview of available methods of euthanasia for cattle.

Method	Details	Suitable for	Advantages	Disadvantages	Special considerations
Captive bolt	Penetrating 0.22 calibre	All types of cattle. May fail to stun mature bulls.	Low risk of human injury.	Exsanguination or pithing required to achieve kill	Hold in firm contact with head. Use correct or heaviest power charge.
Pistol	0.32 calibre Round-nose lead ammunition	All types of cattle. May fail in mature bulls.	Outright kill.	Risks created by free bullet	Unless specially adapted ('humane killer'), keep 5–10 cm from head
Rifle	0.22 rim-fire (for close-range)	All types of cattle. May fail in mature bulls.	Good for distance kill.	Risks created by free bullet; good marksmanship required	Standing elevated useful.
Shotgun	12, 16 or 20 bore; 4, 5 or 6 birdshot pellets	All types of cattle. May fail in mature bulls.	Commonly available. Pellets rarely leave body (i.e. safer than pistol or rifle).	Cumbersome to carry and store	Hold 5–20 cm from head. Standing elevated useful.
	0.410 calibre	Calves and youngstock			
Barbiturates	Pentobarbital sodium 20% to 40% solution 60–120 mg/kg BW	All types of cattle.	Effective. Relatively safe and cheap.	Intravenous access required. Excitement phase and involuntary movements common. Controlled drug regulations in some countries.	Give as fast bolus.
Somulose® (Dechra)	Quinalbarbitone and cinchocaine 1 ml/10 kg BW	All types of cattle.	Smooth transition into unconsciousness and recumbency. Low volume.	Intravenous access required. Expensive. Occasional failure of efficacy	Inject steadily over minimum time.

BW: Body weight.

must be considered, particularly with α_2-agonists (xylazine, detomidine) and their profound effect on cardiac output when used at high doses.

Lethal injection

General considerations

The intravenous route is used whenever possible for barbiturates, and always for combination drugs, to allow controlled administration. Suitable veins include the jugular vein in all types of cattle, cephalic and saphenous veins in calves, ear vein in adult cattle, and milk vein in lactating cows. In calves, intraperitoneal administration may be used where venous access is difficult. In adult cattle, the uptake after intraperitoneal injection is too slow to result in efficient euthanasia. The intracardial route must only be used under deep sedation. Spinal needles with a stylet are commonly used. A 7.5 cm needle for calves, or a 12.5 cm for adult cattle, is introduced into the 5th intercostal space at the level of the elbow.

An intravenous catheter avoids perivascular injection and its associated pain and inefficacy. Venous access is often lost during change-over of syringes, or during the excitement phase commonly induced by barbiturates. A cheap brand of catheter, held in place using superglue, makes catheter placement a quick and affordable procedure.

Precautions to avoid self-injection or skin and mucous membrane contact include: thorough restraint of the patient by physical means or sedation; disposable gloves; eye protection; and discarding the needle used to draw up the solution. Spillage onto skin, or into mouth or eyes, is washed off immediately with copious amounts of water. Medical advice should be sought after either spillage or self-injection. Driving is inadvisable because of potential sedatory effects.

Barbiturates

Given as an overdose, this class of drugs leads to unconsciousness followed by cardiac and respiratory arrest. A compound licensed for euthanasia is pentobarbital sodium, available as 20% to 40% solutions. A guide dose rate for cattle is 60–120 mg/kg body weight (BW), equating to 150 to 300 ml of a 20% solution for a 500–600 kg animal.

Barbiturates should be given as a fast bolus, using a large-gauge needle or catheter (12–14 gauge for adult cattle, 16–18 gauge for calves). Some variation in effectiveness appears to exist between brands based on field reports. Common intervals between start of injection and reaction are shown in Table 26.2.

Table 26.2 Time intervals between start of intravenous barbiturate injection and reaction of 263 calves, young cattle and adult cows (Data Source: Blank, 2005).

Event	Common interval (70–80% of patients)	Maximum interval
Recumbency	20 seconds	45 seconds
Respiratory arrest	30–60 seconds	4.25 minutes
Heartbeat cessation	2 minutes	8.25 minutes
Palpebral reflex absent	40 seconds	2 minutes
Corneal reflex absent	2 minutes	5 minutes
Pupil dilation (maximal)	4 minutes	9 minutes

For administration via an ear vein, 30% or 40% solutions are diluted 1 : 1 with isotonic sodium chloride to reduce pain sensation during injection.

Combination drugs

Somulose® (Dechra) contains 400 mg/ml quinalbarbitone (hypnotic effect) and 25 mg/ml cinchocaine hydrochloride (cardiotoxic). A guide dose rate is 1 ml/10 kg body weight. It is important to adhere to the maximum injection rate stated in the datasheet to avoid cardiac arrest prior to unconsciousness. According to field reports, this drug has occasionally been ineffective in cattle.

T 61™ (MSD Animal Health) contains 5 mg/ml tetracainhydrochlorid (cardiac and CNS depressant), 50 mg/ml mebezoniumiodid (skeletal and respiratory muscle relaxant) and 200 mg/ml embutramid (general anaesthetic and brainstem paralytic). Its use is restricted to unconscious animals under anaesthesia at a dose rate of 4–6 ml/50 kg BW, injected steadily. Cardiac arrest may take 10–15 minutes.

Firearms

General considerations

Veterinarians must remember that they are subject to legal regulations when purchasing, storing, carrying and operating firearms. Detailed recording of ammunition use may be required. In some countries, the captive bolt is exempt from firearms regulations when used for non-commercial purposes.

Firearms must be treated with respect and handled under the assumption that they are loaded at all times. This includes pointing the barrel to the floor until ready to discharge, only arming the gun immediately before discharge, and disarming it should an unexpected delay occur. Before handling the gun for any purpose, ascertain whether a cartridge is loaded or not. In the event of a misfire, allow 30 seconds to lapse before opening the breech in case of delayed ignition. Veterinarians unfamiliar with firearms should spend a day at a shooting range to gain practice in the safe handling, arming, disarming and discharging of guns.

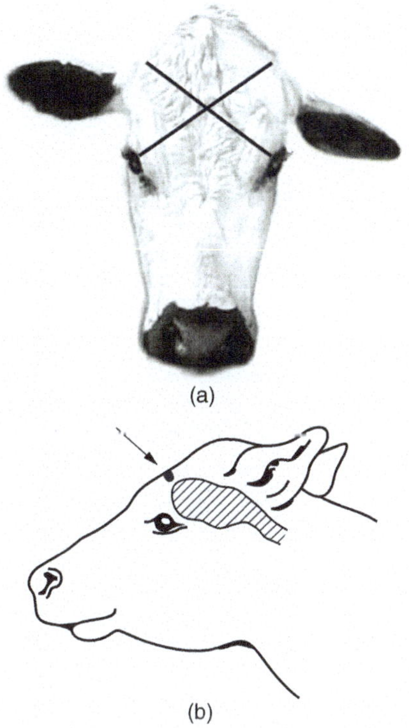

Figure 26.1 a/b: In cattle, the ideal shooting or stunning point is on the central forehead, at the crossing point of two imaginary lines drawn between the centre of the eye and the centre of the opposite horn base. In polled cattle, the line is drawn to above the ear where the horn base would be. The gun is held at a right angle to the skull in order to achieve the target line along the brainstem and neck into the body. Standing elevated to non-recumbent cattle aids achieving this target line.
In calves, the aiming point is slightly lower and, from an initial right angle position, the barrel is slightly tilted upwards.

Ricocheting is a danger with free-bullet weapons, especially in enclosed spaces (e.g. milking parlour, calving box, transport vehicle), when the patient is on a solid floor, and in calves. Only those people required should be present, with all standing level with or behind the person operating the gun, never at a forward point. A captive bolt, while not posing a risk of ricochet, has a typical range of 12 centimetres, and any body part held in front of the gun is at risk. Impact injury may result when discharging in close proximity to a solid object, such as a wall.

Regardless of type of firearm, an impact energy of at least 200 Joules is required (HSA, 1999). Especially in mature cattle, an effective stun or kill may not be obtained on the first attempt. The operator should be mentally prepared for this, and should be ready to reload promptly and re-fire away from the immediate area of the first shot. Where the first shot was off-target, this should be as close to the optimum position as possible. Where the first shot was on-target, this should be above and to one side of the first shot. Figure 26.1 shows the correct shooting and stunning position.

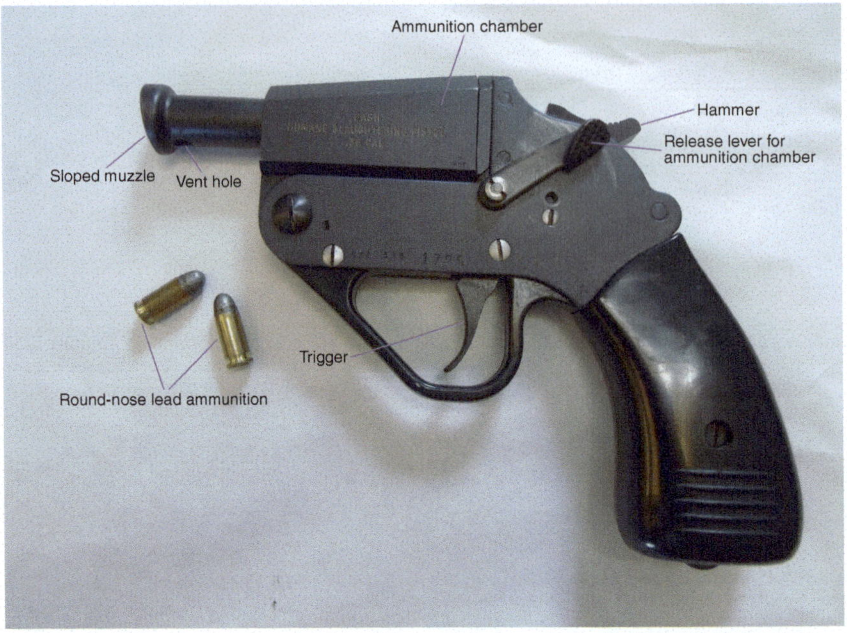

Figure 26.2 A single-shot, 0.32 calibre pistol, adapted for veterinary euthanasia, to be used with round-nose lead ammunition. Note the muzzle slope and vent hole in the barrel.

Free-bullet weapons

A suitable firearm for a veterinary practice is a 'humane killer' – an adapted 0.32 calibre, single-shot pistol. The muzzle slope is designed to aid correct angulation onto the head of a horse. The vent hole in the barrel allows the gun to be held in contact with the head when firing. Where the animal resents contact, or a vent hole is absent, the gun should be held 5–10 cm from the head. Round-nose lead ammunition is required, to ensure skull penetration and an effective kill, while reducing the risk of the bullet leaving the animal (Figure 26.2).

Rifles are useful when the animal has to be shot from a distance, but they require good marksmanship. For close-range operation, a 0.22 rim-fire rifle is used, as other types are too powerful.

A shotgun provides effective means for emergency euthanasia, is commonly present on farms, and is safer than rifles and pistols, as shot pellets rarely leave the animal's body. A 12, 16 or 20 bore shotgun, using 4, 5 or 6 birdshot, is suitable for all types of cattle. A 0.410 calibre shotgun can only be relied upon in calves and youngstock. A shotgun should be held close to (5–25 cm), but never in direct contact with, the skull (HSA, 1999).

Captive bolt

Penetrating captive bolts are effective and, for veterinary purposes, the 0.22 calibre trigger-fired type is suitable (Figure 26.3). Outright death cannot be relied upon, so either exsanguination or pithing of the unconscious animal must follow immediately. Non-penetrating captive bolts are not reliable in cattle, and must not be used.

Cartridges for captive bolts come in different power charges (from 1.25 grain for calves, to 4.0 grain for heavy and mature cattle). For a veterinary practice, only the most powerful charge available for the particular gun is required. Some excessive wear will result from using a heavy charge on smaller cattle, but the infrequent use in veterinary practice makes this aspect negligible.

In contrast to free-bullet firearms, the captive bolt gun must be in firm contact with the head when firing, so good restraint is required.

Exsanguination is achieved with a 15 cm long blade inserted into the proximal neck and cutting deeply from one side to the other, severing both carotid arteries and jugular veins. While a reliable method to follow stunning, blood is often classed as hazardous waste, and its collection and appropriate disposal is a problem on farm. Pithing is an alternative: a 5–7 mm diameter flexible plastic, metal or wooden rod of about one metre length is inserted into the skull through the hole created by the bolt and is fully advanced through the fore- and hindbrain into the spinal canal. The pithing rod is left inside the cadaver to avoid dissemination of pathogens.

The captive bolt must be dissembled after every use and blood, tissue and carbon residues cleaned off all parts. After drying out, lubrication is applied. The reverberating discs are replaced in a different order to even out wear and tear. Captive bolts used infrequently should be dissembled, cleaned and lubricated every six month. Velocity, and therefore kinetic energy, can be substantially reduced in poorly maintained guns, resulting in ineffective stuns and compromised patient welfare.

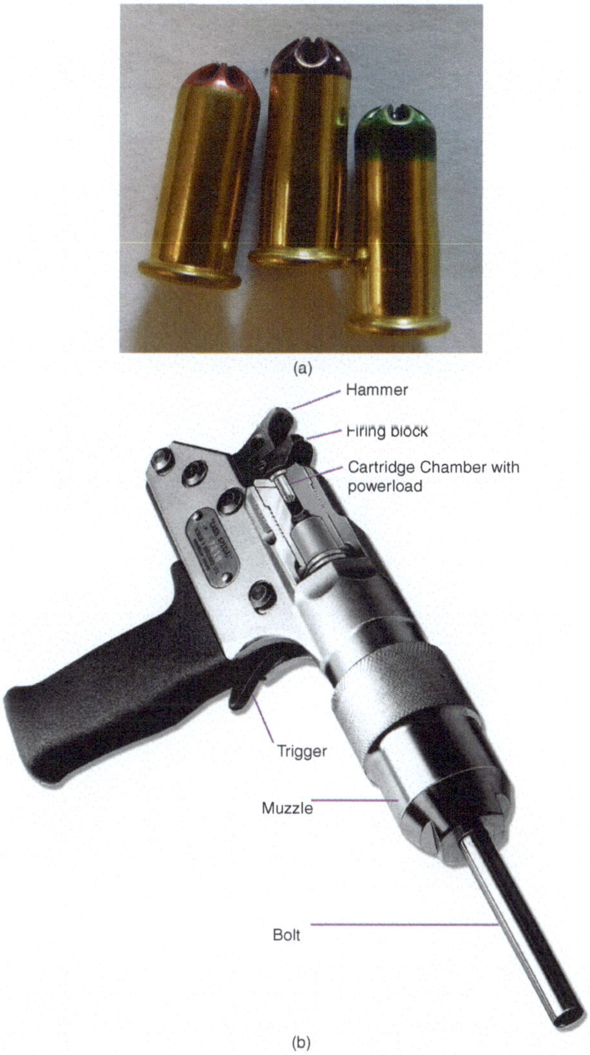

Figure 26.3 A CASH Special captive bolt gun (Reproduced courtesy of Accles & Shelvoke). (b) The bolt is shown extended for demonstration purposes. The inset (a) shows captive bolt cartridges in three power charges (from left to right: pink for calves, purple for heavy animals, green for bulls and very heavy animals).

Alternative methods

Table 26.3 shows conditionally acceptable methods. They must only be used in cattle rendered unconscious by heavy sedation or general anaesthesia.

Unacceptable methods

Concussion from a heavy strike against the head is not an acceptable method of stunning any type of cattle, including calves. Other unacceptable methods include oral or external exposure to chemicals, thermal burning, hypothermia, decompression, drowning and smothering. While chloroform is likely to achieve loss of consciousness and death effectively, it is hazardous to the handler (AVMA, 2013).

Euthanasia of calves *in utero*

A live foetus requires euthanasia prior to fetotomy to manage dystocia. The jugular or cephalic veins can be used in anterior presentations. For posterior presentations, the saphenous vein is available or barbiturates can be given intra-abdominally. Where the chest is exposed (e.g. in hip-lock), intracardial injection may be considered. 30 ml of a 20% barbiturate solution is usually sufficient. The effect on the dam is negligible, because of the low dose rate and limited reverse uptake through the placenta.

Signs of effective stun and death

Table 26.4 shows signs of an effective stun or death, and signs that consciousness is returning (HSA, 1999 and 2001). Always check the animal over a period of 15–20 minutes to ensure it does not regain consciousness. This applies to both lethal injection and firearms.

The animal's reaction to the euthanasia method should be explained to attending lay people, as it can appear distressing to the untrained observer.

Safety considerations

Physical injury risks arise from the method used and the patient. The risks associated with particular methods are highlighted under their respective paragraphs.

Risks from the conscious animal include aggression and panic movements. Thorough consideration must be given to the risk of becoming trapped by the falling animal. The application of ropes and halters may give some influence over the direction of fall, but this cannot be guaranteed. Involuntary movements of the unconscious animal can be severe and sudden, and the operator should always position themselves along the spine of the animal, never between their legs.

Extreme care must be exercised when dealing with road traffic accidents. No attempt to approach a trapped or injured animal must be undertaken until the crash site is secured and the vehicle is stabilised.

Safety considerations have to be balanced with welfare considerations and, where necessary, the animal moved prior to death, even if this results in stress.

Emotional impact

Although commonly performed, euthanasia can place a considerable burden on the veterinary surgeon. The situation is often emotionally charged, and the practitioner may themselves have formed a close connection with the animal. Subconsciously, resorting to euthanasia may be perceived as a failure to offer effective treatment, or as capitulation to economic considerations. The killing of healthy animals during disease control measures may feel contradictory to the Hippocratic oath. One

Table 26.3 Conditionally acceptable methods of euthanasia in cattle. Must only be used in cattle rendered unconscious by heavy sedation or general anaesthesia (data source: AVMA, 2013).

Method	Details	Indications	Contra-indication in conscious animal
T 61™ (MSD Animal Health)	Tetracain hydrochloride and mebezoniumiodid and embutramid. 4–6 ml/50 kg BW	Destruction during surgery. Low volume injection.	Excitation and cardiac or respiratory arrest prior to loss of consciousness.
Severing caudal aorta	Trans-rectal.	When head or neck cannot be reached.	Hypovolaemia causes marked anxiety
Potassium chloride	1–2 meq/kg BW, intravenous or intracardial	Destruction during surgery.	Cardiac arrest prior to loss of consciousness.
Magnesium sulphate	Intravenous overdose	Euthanasia solution fails to induce cardiac arrest.	Cardiac and respiratory arrest prior to loss of consciousness.
Air embolism	Intravenous	Destruction during surgery.	Convulsions, opisthotonus, vocalisation

Table 26.4 Signs of effective stun or death, and signs of returning consciousness (HSA, 1999 and 2001).

	Sign	Comment
Firearms	Collapse	
	Tonic activity for 10–20 seconds, then involuntary kicking	Immediate paddling or kicking indicates *ineffective* stun
	Rhythmic breathing is absent	
	Fixed, glazed expression	
	Corneal reflex absent	Sign of deep unconsciousness and death
	Jaw relaxation, tongue protrusion	
Lethal injection	Collapse	
	Breathing ceases	Ascertain by watching flank. Irregular or shallow breathing can make assessment difficult
	Heartbeat ceases	Easiest to determine by starting auscultation while heartbeat still present. Background noises and muscle fasciculation can make assessment difficult
	Palpebral reflex absent	Sign of unconsciousness
	Corneal reflex absent	Sign of deep unconsciousness and death
	Pupillary dilation (maximal)	Sign of death
Consciousness returning	Rhythmic breathing	
	Blinking and blinking reflex	
	Righting reflex	
	Vocalisation	
	Nystagmus	

should not hesitate to address these thoughts with persons of trust, such as a colleague, mentor, doctor, or professional support group.

Disposal

The onus of correct disposal lies with the owner, but the veterinarian may be asked for advice, and should know the basic regulations pertinent to the area. Whether the professional fee includes disposal of the cadaver should be made clear.

With cattle owners, disposal can typically be discussed in an open and direct way. The preferred route of disposal will influence the choice of method and site.

Cadaver disposal is subject to human and animal health and safety regulations and environmental protection (especially those pertaining to hazardous waste, and ground water and water courses). Air quality regulations govern the burning of cadavers. Special regulations may come into force during national or regional disease outbreaks. Disposal rules may also differ depending on the type and age of the animal. Equally, different juridical regions may impose different rules, and it is advisable to check regulations when moving to a new practice area.

Where burial is allowed, general guidelines are to have at least one metre of subsoil beneath the cadaver, to cover with at least one metre of topsoil to prevent access by wild carnivores or scavengers (to avoid pathogen transfer and exposure to drug residues), and to keep distances of 250 metres from drinking water sources, ten metres from field drains, and 50 metres from other water courses. Sites at risk of flooding or erosion must be avoided.

Clients must not feed cadavers euthanised by lethal injection to farm dogs, as the drug residues will cause adverse effects.

Large-scale euthanasia

Farm animal practitioners may become involved in large-scale euthanasia for disease control as advisors or team leaders. Careful planning of the task, especially of restraint and flow of the animals, is worth the effort, and will aid a smooth operation, while safeguarding animal welfare. Health and safety considerations include a full understanding by all people involved of the risks posed by the euthanasia method and the animals, and provision of appropriate protective equipment. With large-scale euthanasia, there is a risk of ineffective stuns, compromising welfare, caused by operator haste and fatigue, overheating of guns, etc.

Accommodating typical cattle behaviour traits will support a smooth and stress-free operation. This includes taking account of their tendency to move towards light and being 'spooked' by shadows and objects in their path; acknowledging their herd instinct by keeping several animals together; avoiding excitement and fighting by keeping social groups apart; and using silencers on guns to take account of their sensitivity to noise.

Depending on the individual farm, the following options for handling and killing are suggested (DEFRA, 2003). Wherever possible, routes familiar to the cattle should be used, for example through the collecting yard and milking parlour for dairy cattle.

(a) Up to six cattle restrained in pens with 1.8 metre high sides, followed by stunning and pithing pen by pen.

(b) Sedation, followed by stunning and pithing. Where it allows cadaver removal, killing can be carried out in a crush after sedation in the race. Alternatively, animals can be moved through a race or milking parlour for sedation, and allowed to settle in a yard. Sedation of dairy cows may be possible in their cubicle house or straw yard. Where a race is erected for the task, it should ideally be curved to shield forward activities from following cattle and to aid flow.

(c) Shot unrestrained by a marksman. For this, a large pen can be created from straw bales, providing an elevated platform for the marksman. Straw bales absorb any ricocheting bullet and screen activities from public view.

Generally, young animals are more easily stressed than older cattle, and should be euthanised first. Unweaned calves should not be moved through restraining facilities with their dams, to prevent crushing injuries, but should be separated shortly before euthanasia. Wherever possible, the owner's preferences should be accommodated, and one should be prepared for the owner not wishing to be present.

References

AVMA (2013). *Guidelines on Euthanasia.* https://www.avma.org/KB/Policies/Documents/euthanasia.pdf

Blank, C.M. (2005). *Studies on euthanasia of cattle using pentobarbital* (Untersuchungen zur Euthanasie des Rindes mit Pentobarbital). Thesis, University of Munich.

DEFRA (Department for Environment, Food & Rural Affairs) (2003). *Getting it right, first time, every time* (practical guidance on the management and operation of large scale humane killing of livestock during emergencies). Crown copyright, The National Archives, UK.

Harper, D. (2012). *Online etymology dictionary.* www.etymonline.com

HSA (Humane Slaughter Association) (1999). *Guidance notes no. 3: Humane killing of livestock using firearms.* Wheathampstead, UK.

HSA (Humane Slaughter Association) (2001). *Guidance notes no. 2: Captive-bolt stunning of livestock.* Wheathampstead, UK.

Further reading

Svendsen, O., Jensen, S.K., Karlsen, L.V., Svalastoga, E. and Jensen, H.E. (2008). Observations on newborn calves rendered unconscious with a captive bolt gun. *Veterinary Record* **162**, 90–92.

SECTION IV

Herd Health

CHAPTER 27

Important National and International Diseases of Cattle

Michael P Reichel and Charles G B Caraguel

Learning objectives

To have a understanding of:
- the important 'old diseases';
- diseases which are increasing in importance; and
- emerging diseases.

The 'old diseases'

Rinderpest ('cattle plague')

Rinderpest (caused by a bovine morbillivirus in the family Paramyxoviridae) was a most devastating disease of cattle, with mortalities often exceeding 70%. It has now been eradicated, and was only the second infectious disease (after smallpox) to be declared eradicated (Roeder, 2011). This was achieved in 2011, after a concerted global effort by veterinary health officials. Historically, Rinderpest provided not only the impetus for the foundation of the first veterinary school in the Western world, some 250 years ago in Lyon (France), and thereafter in countries across Europe (Vallat, 2012; Yamanouchi, 2012), but also for the establishment of the World Organisation for Animal Health, the OIE (Office International des Epizooties) itself, after a particularly devastating Rinderpest epidemic was imported from India into Belgium in 1924 (Yamanouchi, 2012).

Foot-and-mouth disease

Foot-and-mouth disease (FMD), however, is still affecting, amongst others, cattle populations around the world, with enormous and devastating economic and social impacts. The epidemic in the United Kingdom (2001) was estimated to have cost the UK economy a total of GBP 9 billion (Thompson *et al.*, 2002). There has also been a recent epidemic in Japan (Muroga *et al.*, 2012).

Historically, control strategies involved the culling of infected and neighbouring herds. The numbers involved are high. In 2012, in Japan, an estimated 290,000 animals were culled (Muroga *et al.*, 2012) and, in 2001, in the Netherlands and the UK, 260,000 (Backer *et al.*, 2012) and 10 million animals were culled respectively.

The resultant losses in the animal populations due to the authorities' efforts to 'stamp out' the epidemics are increasingly difficult to justify from an animal welfare perspective, and it is a strategy that is becoming politically unacceptable due to the growing public concern. Alternative control strategies are now being explored, using modelling to evaluate the utility of more and earlier vaccination (Backer *et al.*, 2012). The DIVA ('Differentiating Infected from Vaccinated Animals') vaccination approach is likely to be an increasingly used option in future outbreaks, if marker vaccines can be produced (Pastoret & Mackay, 2003).

Bovine brucellosis

Bovine brucellosis, caused by *Brucella abortus*, is an important disease of cattle, mainly causing abortions, but it is also an important zoonosis. Largely now eradicated from many developed countries, such as Australia (Chamberlin, 1985), New Zealand (O'Neil, 1995) and large parts of Europe and the United States, it is still present (and possibly neglected) in many countries around the world (Godfroid *et al.*, 2011), particularly in Africa, the Middle East and parts of Asia. Vaccination, at least in the early stages of any control program, has been the cornerstone of successful eradication efforts, and it invariably relies on attenuated live vaccines such as strain 19 and RB 51 (Godfroid *et al.*, 2011) to reduce clinical disease in cattle and transmission to humans. Complicating eradication efforts can be wildlife reservoirs that are largely uncontrolled, or uncontrollable, such as bison and elk in Yellowstone National Park in the US (Van Campen and Rhyan, 2010).

Bovine Medicine, Third Edition. Edited by Peter D. Cockcroft.

Bovine tuberculosis

Bovine tuberculosis, caused by *Mycobacterium bovis*, is another important zoonosis that still afflicts cattle populations around the world, and it also presents a significant zoonotic risk to humans. While eradicated from countries such as Australia (Cousins and Roberts, 2001), considerable challenges persist in countries where wildlife populations have been infected, such as possums in New Zealand (Nugent *et al.*, 2012), badgers in the United Kingdom (Green *et al.*, 2012; Smith *et al.*, 2012) and a variety of wild ruminant species in the United States (Van Campen and Rhyan, 2010). A very recent report that co-infection with liver fluke (*Fasciola hepatica*) may interfere with the sensitivity of diagnostic tests for bovine tuberculosis, and reduce it by a third, is very concerning (Claridge *et al.*, 2012), and increases the challenge that the application of diagnostic tests to mycobacterial diseases already present.

Still there, and increasing in importance

Bovine Viral Diarrhoea

In most cattle industries around the world where control programs are not in place, *Bovine Viral Diarrhoea* (BVD) is the most prevalent viral cattle disease. Yet, possibly because it is so widespread and endemic, it is, paradoxically, the one pathogen that is most often ignored. BVD virus is subject to control programs in a number of countries and regions, and the disease has been successfully eradicated, most notably from Scandinavia (Moennig *et al.*, 2005; Sandvik, 2004) and also, in recent times, probably from the Swiss dairy industry.

In Switzerland, BVD has been the subject of a very intense, short, test-and-cull campaign (Presi *et al.*, 2011). Testing occurred over a two-year period. During this period, a virtual national 'stand-still' was enforced, with movement of cattle only allowed to a slaughterhouse. During the first year, all adult cattle were tested for the presence of the virus, as an indication of their status as 'persistently-infected' virus carrier. In the following year, all newly born calves were tested (a total of 2.85 million cattle). The prevalence of PIs decreased from initially 1.8% to below 0.2% in new-born calves over the period.

BVD virus is a pestivirus, of the family of Flaviridae and related to viruses such as border disease virus and classical swine fever (CSF). The BVD virus occurs in two main genotypes – BVDV-1 and BVDV-2 – which are both capable of causing serious disease, especially when introduced for the first time to BVD-naïve cattle. BVDV-2 is reputed to cause more severe disease, and is absent from Australia and New Zealand (Littlejohns and Horner, 1990; Vilcek *et al.*, 1998).

It is the timing of infection in a pregnant cow that is critical to the production of 'persistently infected' (PI) animals. If exposure of the dam occurs between 40–110 days of gestation, the formation of a PI calf might occur (Schweizer *et al.*, 2006).

The creation of a PI animal relies on infection with the non-cytopathogenic biotype of the BVD virus (Orban *et al.*, 1983), and superinfection with the homologous cytopathogenic strain results in the creation of mucosal disease (Brownlie *et al.*, 1984).

Johne's disease and Crohn's

Bovine paratuberculosis (or Johne's disease), caused by *Mycobacterium avium* spp. *paratuberculosis* (MAP), has risen in prominence in recent years because of its putative causal link to Crohn's disease in humans (Collins, 2011; Davis and Masen-Bouterse, 2012; Pierce, 2011). Both diseases share a remarkably similar pathology, and MAP have been identified in some patients with Crohn's disease (Dell'Isola *et al.*, 1994). More recently, there has also been increased focus on the possible contamination of the food chain for humans, particularly meat and milk, by MAP (Alonso-Hearn *et al.*, 2009, Gill *et al.*, 2011; Smith *et al.*, 2011), and its subsequent ability to survive commonly employed pasteurisation processes and cooking (Stabel and Lambertz, 2004). As Johne's disease is quite common in many cattle-producing countries in the world (Carter, 2012; Kennedy, 2011; Larsen *et al.*, 2012; Norton *et al.*, 2009; Stevenson *et al.*, 2009; Wilson *et al.*, 2010), the hypothesised link with Crohn's disease, and the concern about the safety of the food chain, is likely to bring pressure to bear on the cattle industries – be they beef or dairy – to control Johne's disease.

Bovine neosporosis

Neospora caninum was first recognised as a pathogen of dogs in Norway in the mid-1980s (Bjerkås *et al.*, 1984). *N. caninum* is a protozoon, apicomplexan parasite, closely related to *Toxoplasma gondii* and *Hammondia heydorni* (Dubey *et al.*, 2002; Dubey *et al.*, 2007). Not long after its first description came the realisation that *N. caninum* was also a significant pathogen of cattle, causing embryonic loss, abortion, stillbirths and 'dummy calves' (Dubey, 1989; Thilsted and Dubey, 1989). The organism and disease is reported virtually from every corner of the globe. Most of the reports in recent times have focused on abortion events in cattle, which can reach epidemic proportions, while clinical cases in dogs appear rarely reported (Barber and Trees, 1996; Gasser *et al.*, 1993; Reichel *et al.*, 1998; Ruehlmann *et al.*, 1995). While sheep and goats can be infected with *N. caninum* (Barr *et al.*, 1992; Dubey *et al.*, 1995), and sheep in particular often been used as experimental models for neosporosis (McAllister *et al.*, 1996b), it is only recently that reports have emerged that suggest that *N. caninum* may be a significant pathogen of sheep *per se*, causing abortions and CNS signs (Bishop *et al.*, 2010; West *et al.*, 2006). Fortunately, in contrast to *T. gondii*, neosporosis does not appear to have any zoonotic potential (McCann *et al.*, 2008; Petersen *et al.*, 1999).

About ten years after the original reports of the disease, the life cycle was elucidated by McAllister *et al.* (1998) and was shown to involve dogs in the sexual part of its life cycle as definitive hosts. Since then, other canids have been added to the list of definitive hosts, and this now extends to American coyotes (Gondim *et al.*, 2004), grey wolves (Dubey *et al.*, 2011) and Australian dingoes (King *et al.*, 2010). Despite some serological evidence that foxes can be infected with *N. caninum* (Barber *et al.*, 1997), there is no evidence (yet) (Schares *et al.*, 2002) that they can also act as definitive hosts of the parasite and complete the sexual replication within them (Schares *et al.*, 2001).

N. caninum abortions can reach epidemic proportions (McAllister *et al.*, 1996a; Pfeiffer *et al.*, 2000; Thornton *et al.*, 1994), and the large number of mid-term abortions that are the hallmark of neosporosis can be very costly to the primary producer. *N. caninum* abortions have been reported from beef and dairy cattle, although it is generally assumed that they are economically more devastating in the dairy industry (Reichel and Ellis, 2006, 2008; Trees *et al.*, 1999). Costs are incurred through the loss of the calf and subsequent loss in milk yield, and veterinary diagnostic and treatment costs, as a minimum, and are estimated to be in excess of a billion dollars in total, worldwide (Reichel *et al.*, 2013).

Almost thirty years after its first discovery, control options are still surprisingly limited (Reichel *et al.* 2014). They are also complicated by the propensity of the parasite not only to be passed from canids to cattle, but also to be able to be vertically transmitted with high efficiency, from dam to offspring. Vertical transmission rates of 75–95% have been reported (Hall *et al.*, 1995; Pare *et al.*, 1996; Schares *et al.*, 1998). Large numbers of cattle are thus born already congenitally infected and, apart from testing, identifying and then eliminating them from the herd, there appear to be no other management options.

Neospora-infected cattle are generally accepted to be at a three times higher risk of abortion than their uninfected cohorts (Wouda *et al.*, 1998), and repeat abortions do occur (Thurmond and Hietala, 1997). A vaccine (Neoguard) that prevented some abortions in cattle (Weston *et al.*, 2012) has now been withdrawn from worldwide sales. A live vaccine has been demonstrated to be efficacious in preventing abortions (Williams *et al.*, 2007), but it has not yet been commercialised. Alternative vaccination options have recently been reviewed (Reichel *et al.*, 2014). Treatment with a coccidiostat (Toltrazuril®) has only been shown to be efficacious for the treatment of experimentally-induced tachyzoite infection (Kritzner *et al.*, 2002), but would be expensive in adult cows and would raise concerns about milk and meat withdrawal periods.

Emerging diseases

Schmallenberg virus (SBV)

The most recent prominent emergence of a novel disease in cattle was caused by the so-called *Schmallenberg virus*, named after a town in North-Rhine Westphalia in western Germany, where it was first described in the northern autumn of 2011 (Hoffmann *et al.*, 2012). The clinical signs reported included fever, decreased milk yield and diarrhoea, but also abortions and stillbirths in cattle, sheep and goats. Lesions were reported to be localised in the muscolo-skeletal system (arthrogryposis, various malformations of the spine (torticollis, scoliosis)) as well as in the brain (hydrocephalus and cerebellar hypoplasia) (Herder *et al.*, 2012).

The diagnosis and demonstration of the virus shows the power, and potential for contribution to veterinary science, of modern molecular tools. The presence of the causal agent was originally hypothesised and identified by metagenomic methods only, rather than by classical virus isolation techniques (Hoffmann *et al.*, 2012). It has since been identified as belonging to the Simbu serogroup of Orthobunyaviridae, being closely related to the Shamonda virus. Other viruses in that group are the Akabane and Simbu viruses (Hoffmann *et al.*, 2012).

The virus was quickly found at and beyond the Dutch border, and cases in cattle, sheep and goats were then also reported in Belgium, the Netherlands and the United Kingdom, as well as Italy, Spain and Luxembourg (Peperkamp *et al.*, 2012; Steinbach *et al.*, 2012). Recent serological surveys suggest infection to be widespread in the Netherlands (>70%) (Elbers *et al.*, 2012) and also in Belgium (>90%, Garigliany (2012)), but there is no evidence that it infects humans (Ducomble *et al.*, 2012). Culicoides insects (midges) are thought to be responsible as vectors and have been found to contain virus genetic material as far north as Denmark (Rasmussen *et al.*, 2012).

Because of the high sero-prevalence observed in areas with recent outbreaks, there are some suggestions that SBV might quickly disappear again – say, after a two-years cycle – as the epidemic runs out of naïve individuals to infect. There is now an inactivated, commercially available vaccine available for cattle.

Bluetongue (BTV)

Bluetongue virus, serotype 8 (BTV-8), suddenly emerged as a significant pathogen in north-western Europe (Belgium, Germany, Luxembourg and the Netherlands) in 2006, where it had not previously been recorded.

In cattle, clinical signs included 'ulcerations and/or erosions of oral mucosa or erosions of lips/crusts in or around nostrils or oedema of the nose or hyperaemic/purple coloration of tongue, tongue protrusion or coronitis or apathy/tiredness or muscle necrosis, stiffness of limbs or loathing or refusal to move, prostration or torticollis or anoestrus' (Elbers *et al.*, 2008). Culicoides species (midges) were again thought to be vectors, but not those species usually associated with transmission in Mediterranean countries, where BTV is endemic (Meiswinkel *et al.*, 2008).

Control measures relying on vaccination were not instituted until 2008 (Caporale and Giovannini, 2010), due to concerns about the use of live vaccines and safety (Gethmann *et al.*, 2009; Probst *et al.*, 2011), and resulted in significant delays in bringing the epidemic under control. An inactivated vaccine is commercially available.

Besnoitia besnoiti

Besnoitiosis has emerged as a significant pathogen of cattle in Europe in the 21st century (Fernandez-Garcia *et al.*, 2009a; Fernandez-Garcia *et al.*, 2009b; Jacquiet *et al.*, 2010; Lienard *et al.*, 2011; Rostaher *et al.*, 2010; Schares *et al.*, 2009), when previously it had been thought confined to Africa and the Middle East (Dubey *et al.*, 2003; Mehlhorn *et al.*, 2009). Clinical signs in the acute phase include anorexia, dyspnoea and pyrexia, and skin lesions (lichenification and hypotrichosis) in the chronic phase (Rostaher *et al.*, 2010). Significant morbidity (70%) and also mortality (10%) have been reported. The life cycle of *Besnoitia* is still poorly understood and, while it is thought that a carnivorous host is involved in the sexual part of the life cycle, this host has hitherto not been identified. Post-natal transmission by direct contact between cattle or biting insects (culicoides or tabanids, or stable flies) have been hypothesised. These are as yet largely unproven (although physical separation by distance from infected animals appears to prevent transmission to uninfected ones) and, hence, suggestions regarding control options are still limited.

Bibliography

Alonso-Hearn, M., Molina, E., Geijo, M., Vazquez, P., Sevilla, I., Garrido, J.M., Juste, R.A. (2009). Isolation of *Mycobacterium avium* subsp. *paratuberculosis* from muscle tissue of naturally infected cattle. *Foodborne Pathogens and Disease* **6**, 513–518.

Backer, J.A., Hagenaars, T.J., Nodelijk, G., van Roermund, H.J. (2012). Vaccination against foot-and-mouth disease I: Epidemiological consequences. *Preventive Veterinary Medicine* **107**(1–2), 27–40.

Barber, J.S., Gasser, R.B., Ellis, J., Reichel, M.P., McMillan, D., Trees, A.J. (1997). Prevalence of antibodies to *Neospora caninum* in different canid populations. *Journal of Parasitology* **83**, 1056–1058.

Barber, J.S., Trees, A.J. (1996). Clinical aspects of 27 cases of neosporosis in dogs. *Veterinary Record* **139**, 439–443.

Barr, B.C., Anderson, M.L., Woods, L.W., Dubey, J.P., Conrad, P.A. (1992). Neospora-like protozoal infections associated with abortion in goats. *Journal of Veterinary Diagnostic Investigation* **4**, 365–367.

Bishop, S., King, J., Windsor, P., Reichel, M.P., Ellis, J., Slapeta, J. (2010). The first report of ovine cerebral neosporosis and evaluation of *Neospora caninum* prevalence in sheep in New South Wales. *Veterinary Parasitology* **170**, 137–142.

Bjerkås, I., Mohn, S.F., Presthus, J. (1984). Unidentified cyst-forming sporozoon causing encephalomyelitis and myositis in dogs. *Zeitschrift fur Parasitenkunde* **70**, 271–274.

Brownlie, J., Clarke, M.C., Howard, C.J. (1984). Experimental production of fatal mucosal disease in cattle. *Veterinary Record* **114**, 535–536.

Caporale, V., Giovannini, A. (2010). Bluetongue control strategy, including recourse to vaccine: a critical review. *Revue Scientifique et Technique* **29**, 573–591.

Carter, M.A. (2012). Prevalence and prevention of paratuberculosis in North America. *The Japanese Journal of Veterinary Research* **60** Suppl, S9–18.

Chamberlin, W.E. (1985). Early history of bovine brucellosis eradication in Australia. *Australian Veterinary Journal* **62**, 289–292.

Claridge, J., Diggle, P., McCann, C.M., Mulcahy, G., Flynn, R., McNair, J., Strain, S., Welsh, M., Baylis, M., Williams, D.J. (2012). *Fasciola hepatica* is associated with the failure to detect bovine tuberculosis in dairy cattle. *Nature Communications* **3**, 853.

Collins, M.T. (2011). Food safety concerns regarding paratuberculosis. The Veterinary clinics of North America. *Food Animal Practice* **27**, 631–636, vii–viii.

Cousins, D.V., Roberts, J.L. (2001). Australia's campaign to eradicate bovine tuberculosis: the battle for freedom and beyond. *Tuberculosis* **81**, 5–15.

Davis, W.C., Madsen-Bouterse, S.A. (2012). Crohn's disease and *Mycobacterium avium* subsp. *paratuberculosis*: the need for a study is long overdue. *Veterinary Immunology and Immunopathology* **145**, 1–6.

Dell'Isola, B., Poyart, C., Goulet, O., Mougenot, J.F., Sadoun-Journo, E., Brousse, N., Schmitz, J., Ricour, C., Berche, P. (1994). Detection of *Mycobacterium paratuberculosis* by polymerase chain reaction in children with Crohn's disease. *The Journal of Infectious Diseases* **169**, 449–451.

Dubey, J.P. (1989). Congenital neosporosis in a calf. *Veterinary Record* **125**, 486.

Dubey, J.P., Hartley, W.J., Lindsay, D.S., Topper, M.J. (1990). Fatal congenital Neospora caninum infection in a lamb. *Journal of Parasitology* **76**, 127–130.

Dubey, J.P., Hill, D.E., Lindsay, D.S., Jenkins, M.C., Uggla, A., Speer, C.A. (2002). *Neospora caninum* and *Hammondia heydorni* are separate species/organisms. *Trends in Parasitology* **18**, 66–69.

Dubey, J.P., Jenkins, M.C., Rajendran, C., Miska, K., Ferreira, L.R., Martins, J., Kwok, O.C., Choudhary, S. (2011). Gray wolf (*Canis lupus*) is a natural definitive host for *Neospora caninum*. *Veterinary Parasitology* **181**, 382–387.

Dubey, J.P., Schares, G., Ortega-Mora, L.M. (2007). Epidemiology and control of neosporosis and *Neospora caninum*. *Clinical Microbiology Reviews* **20**, 323–367.

Dubey, J.P., Shkap, V., Pipano, E., Fish, L., Fritz, D.L. (2003). Ultrastructure of *Besnoitia besnoiti* tissue cysts and bradyzoites. *The Journal of Eukaryotic Microbiology* **50**, 240–244.

Ducomble, T., Wilking, H., Stark, K., Takla, A., Askar, M., Schaade, L., Nitsche, A., Kurth, A. (2012). Lack of evidence for schmallenberg virus infection in highly exposed persons, Germany (2012). *Emerging Infectious Diseases* **18**, 1333–1335.

Elbers, A.R., Backx, A., Ekker, H.M., van der Spek, A.N., van Rijn, P.A. (2008). Performance of clinical signs to detect bluetongue virus serotype 8 outbreaks in cattle and sheep during the 2006-epidemic in The Netherlands. *Veterinary Microbiology* **129**, 156–162.

Elbers, A.R., Loeffen, W.L., Quak, S., de Boer-Luijtze, E., van der Spek, A.N., Bouwstra, R., Maas, R., Spierenburg, M.A., de Kluijver, E.P., van Schaik, G., van der Poel, W.H. (2012). Seroprevalence of Schmallenberg Virus Antibodies among Dairy Cattle, the Netherlands, Winter 2011–2012. *Emerging Infectious Diseases* **18**, 1065–1071.

Fernandez-Garcia, A., Alvarez-Garcia, G., Risco-Castillo, V., Aguado-Martinez, A., Marugan-Hernandez, V., Ortega-Mora, L.M. (2009a). Pattern of recognition of *Besnoitia besnoiti* tachyzoite and bradyzoite antigens by naturally infected cattle. *Veterinary Parasitology* **164**, 104–110.

Fernandez-Garcia, A., Risco-Castillo, V., Pedraza-Diaz, S., Aguado-Martinez, A., Alvarez-Garcia, G., Gomez-Bautista, M., Collantes-Fernandez, E., Ortega-Mora, L.M. (2009b). First isolation of *Besnoitia besnoiti* from a chronically infected cow in Spain. *The Journal of Parasitology* **95**, 474–476.

Garigliany, M.M., Hoffmann, B., Dive, M., Sartelet, A., Bayrou, C., Cassart, D., Beer, M., Desmecht, D. (2012). Schmallenberg virus in calf born at term with porencephaly, Belgium. *Emerging Infectious Diseases* **18**, 1005–1006.

Gasser, R.B., Edwards, G., Cole, R.A. (1993). Neosporosis in a dog. *Australian Veterinary Practitioner* **23**, 190–193.

Gethmann, J., Huttner, K., Heyne, H., Probst, C., Ziller, M., Beer, M., Hoffmann, B., Mettenleiter, T.C., Conraths, F.J. (2009). Comparative safety study of three inactivated BTV-8 vaccines in sheep and cattle under field conditions. *Vaccine* **27**, 4118–4126.

Gill, C.O., Saucier, L., Meadus, W.J. (2011). *Mycobacterium avium* subsp. *paratuberculosis* in dairy products, meat, and drinking water. *Journal of Food Protection* **74**, 480–499.

Godfroid, J., Scholz, H.C., Barbier, T., Nicolas, C., Wattiau, P., Fretin, D., Whatmore, A.M., Cloeckaert, A., Blasco, J.M., Moriyon, I., Saegerman, C., Muma, J.B., Al Dahouk, S., Neubauer, H., Letesson, J.J. (2011). Brucellosis at the animal/ecosystem/human interface at the beginning of the 21st century. *Preventive Veterinary Medicine* **102**, 118–131.

Gondim, L.F., McAllister, M.M., Pitt, W.C., Zemlicka, D.E. (2004). Coyotes (*Canis latrans*) are definitive hosts of *Neospora caninum*. *International Journal of Parasitology* **34**, 159–161.

Green, L.E., Carrique-Mas, J.J., Mason, S.A., Medley, G.F. (2012). Patterns of delayed detection and persistence of bovine tuberculosis in confirmed and unconfirmed herd breakdowns in cattle and cattle herds in Great Britain. *Preventive Veterinary Medicine* **106** (3–4), 266–274.

Hall, C.A., Reichel, M.P., Ellis, J.T. (2005). *Neospora caninum, Options for control downunder*. In: 20th International Conference of the World Association for the Advancement of Veterinary Parasitology, Christchurch, p. 204.

Herder, V., Wohlsein, P., Peters, M., Hansmann, F., Baumgartner, W. (2012). Salient Lesions in Domestic Ruminants Infected With the Emerging So-called Schmallenberg Virus in Germany. *Veterinary Pathology* **49**, 588–591.

Hoffmann, B., Scheuch, M., Hoper, D., Jungblut, R., Holsteg, M., Schirrmeier, H., Eschbaumer, M., Goller, K.V., Wernike, K., Fischer, M., Breithaupt, A., Mettenleiter, T.C., Beer, M. (2012). Novel orthobunyavirus in Cattle, Europe, 2011. *Emerging Infectious Diseases* **18**, 469–472.

Jacquiet, P., Lienard, E., Franc, M. (2010). Bovine besnoitiosis: epidemiological and clinical aspects. *Veterinary Parasitology* **174**, 30–36.

Kennedy, D. (2011). International efforts at paratuberculosis control. The Veterinary clinics of North America. *Food Animal Practice* **27**, 647–654, viii.

King, J.S., Šlapeta, J., Jenkins, D.J., Al-Qassab, S.E., Ellis, J.T., Windsor, P.A. (2010). Australian dingoes are definitive hosts of *Neospora caninum*. *International Journal of Parasitology* **40**, 945–950.

Kritzner, S., Sager, H., Blum, J., Krebber, R., Greif, G., Gottstein, B. (2002). An explorative study to assess the efficacy of Toltrazuril-sulfone (Ponazuril) in calves experimentally infected with *Neospora caninum*. *Annals of Clinical Microbiology and Antimicrobials* **1**, 4.

Larsen, J.W., Webb Ware, J.K., Kluver, P. (2012). Epidemiology of bovine Johne's disease (BJD) in beef cattle herds in Australia. *Australian Veterinary Journal* **90**, 6–13.

Lienard, E., Salem, A., Grisez, C., Prevot, F., Bergeaud, J.P., Franc, M., Gottstein, B., Alzieu, J.P., Lagalisse, Y., Jacquiet, P. (2011). A longitudinal study of *Besnoitia besnoiti* infections and seasonal abundance of *Stomoxys calcitrans* in a dairy cattle farm of southwest France. *Veterinary parasitology* **177**, 20 27.

Littlejohns, I.R., Horner, G.W. (1990). Incidence, epidemiology and control of bovine pestivirus infections in Australia and New Zealand. *Revue Scientifique et Technique de l'Office International des Épizooties* **9**, 195–205.

McAllister, M.M., Dubey, J.P., Lindsay, D.S., Jolley, W.R., Wills, R.A., McGuire, A.M. (1998). Dogs are definitive hosts of *Neospora caninum*. *International Journal of Parasitology* **28**, 1473–1478.

McAllister, M.M., Huffman, E.M., Hietala, S.K., Conrad, P.A., Anderson, M.L., Salman, M.D. (1996a). Evidence suggesting a point source exposure in an outbreak of bovine abortion due to neosporosis. *Journal of Veterinary Diagnostic Investigation* **8**, 355–357.

McAllister, M.M., McGuire, A.M., Jolley, W.R., Lindsay, D.S., Trees, A.J., Stobart, R.H. (1996b). Experimental neosporosis in pregnant ewes and their offspring. *Veterinary Pathology* **33**, 647–655.

McCann, C.M., Vyse, A.J., Salmon, R.L., Thomas, D., Williams, D.J., McGarry, J.W., Pebody, R., Trees, A.J. (2008). Lack of Serologic Evidence of *Neospora caninum* in Humans, England. *Emerging Infectious Diseases* **14**, 978–980.

Mehlhorn, H., Klimpel, S., Schein, E., Heydorn, A.O., Al-Quraishy, S., Selmair, J. (2009). Another African disease in Central Europe: Besnoitiosis of cattle. I. Light and electron microscopical study. *Parasitology Research* **104**, 861–868.

Meiswinkel, R., Baldet, T., de Deken, R., Takken, W., Delecolle, J.C., Mellor, P.S. (2008). The 2006 outbreak of bluetongue in northern Europe – the entomological perspective. *Preventive Veterinary Medicine* **87**, 55–63.

Moennig, V., Houe, H., Lindberg, A. (2005). BVD control in Europe: current status and perspectives. *Animal Health Research Reviews* **6**, 63–74.

Muroga, N., Hayama, Y., Yamamoto, T., Kurogi, A., Tsuda, T., Tsutsui, T. (2012). The 2010 foot-and-mouth disease epidemic in Japan. *Journal of Veterinary Medical Science/Japanese Society of Veterinary Science* **74**, 399–404.

Norton, S., Heuer, C., Jackson, R. (2009). A questionnaire-based cross-sectional study of clinical Johne's disease on dairy farms in New Zealand. *New Zealand Veterinary Journal* **57**, 34–43.

Nugent, G., Whitford, J., Yockney, I.J., Cross, M.L. (2012). Reduced spillover transmission of *Mycobacterium bovis* to feral pigs (*Sus scofa*) following population control of brushtail possums (*Trichosurus vulpecula*). *Epidemiology and Infection* **140**, 1036–1047.

O'Neil, B. (1995). Brucellosis eradication scheme successfully completed. *The New Zealand Medical Journal* **108**, 393.

Orban, S., Liess, B., Hafez, S.M., Frey, H.R., Blindow, H., Sasse-Patzer, B. (1983). Studies on transplacental transmissibility of a Bovine Virus Diarrhoea (BVD) vaccine virus. I. Inoculation of pregnant cows 15 to 90 days before parturition (190th to 265th day of gestation). *Zentralblatt für Veterinärmedizin B* **30**, 619–634.

Paré, J., Thurmond, M.C., Hietala, S.K. (1996). Congenital *Neospora caninum* infection in dairy cattle and associated calfhood mortality. *Canadian Journal of Veterinary Research* **60**, 133–139.

Pastoret, P.P., Mackay, D. (2003). Regulatory considerations for emergency use of vaccines in the European Union. *Developments in Biologicals* **114**, 53–58.

Peperkamp, K., Dijkman, R., van Maanen, C., Vos, J., Wouda, W., Holzhauer, M., van Wuijckhuise, L., Junker, K., Greijdanus, S., Roumen, M. (2012). Polioencephalo-myelitis in a calf due to infection with Schmallenberg virus. *The Veterinary Record* **170**, 570.

Petersen, E., Lebech, M., Jensen, L., Lind, P., Rask, M., Bagger, P., Björkman, C., Uggla, A. (1999). *Neospora caninum* infection and repeated abortions in humans. *Emerging Infectious Diseases* **5**, 278–280.

Pfeiffer, D.U., Williamson, N.B., Reichel, M.P. (2000). *Long-term Serological Monitoring as a Tool for Epidemiological Investigation of Neospora caninum Infection in a New Zealand Dairy Herd.* In: IX Symposium, Breckenridge, USA, p. 524.

Pierce, E.S. (2010). Ulcerative colitis and Crohn's disease: is *Mycobacterium avium* subspecies *paratuberculosis* the common villain? *Gut Pathogens* **2**, 21.

Presi, P., Struchen, R., Knight-Jones, T., Scholl, S., Heim, D. (2011). Bovine viral diarrhea (BVD) eradication in Switzerland – experiences of the first two years. *Preventive Veterinary Medicine* **99**, 112–121.

Probst, C., Gethmann, J.M., Horeth-Bontgen, D., Cussler, K., Conraths, F.J. (2011). Lack of evidence for claims of farmers in south-eastern Germany regarding adverse reactions ascribed to BTV-8 vaccines. *Berliner und Munchener tierarztliche Wochenschrift* **124**, 282–287.

Rasmussen, L.D., Kristensen, B., Kirkeby, C., Rasmussen, T.B., Belsham, G.J., Bodker, R., Botner, A. (2012). Culicoids as vectors of schmallenberg virus. *Emerging Infectious Diseases* **18**, 1204–1206.

Reichel, M.P., Ellis, J.T. (2006). If control of *Neospora caninum* infection is technically feasible does it make economic sense? *Veterinary Parasitology* **142**, 23–34.

Reichel, M.P., Ellis, J.T. (2008). Re-evaluating the economics of neosporosis control. *Veterinary Parasitology* **156**, 361–362.

Reichel, M.P., Ellis, J.T. (2009). *Neospora caninum* – how close are we to development of an efficacious vaccine that prevents abortion in cattle? *International Journal of Parasitology* **39**, 1173–1187.

Reichel, M.P., Thornton, R.N., Morgan, P.L., Mills, R.J., Schares, G. (1998). Neosporosis in a pup. *New Zealand Veterinary Journal* **46**, 106–110.

Reichel, M.P., Alejandra Ayanegui-Alcerreca, M., Gondim, L.F., Ellis, J.T. (2013). What is the global economic impact of *Neospora caninum* in cattle – the billion dollar question. *International Journal of Parasitology* **43**, 133–142.

Reichel, M.P., McAllister, M.M., Pomroy, W.E., Campero, C., Ortega-Mora, L.M. and Ellis, J.T. (2014) Control option for Neospora caninum – is there anything new or are we going backwards? *Parasitology* **141**, 1455–1470; http://dx.doi.org/10.1017/S0031182014000158

Roeder, P.L. (2011). Rinderpest: the end of cattle plague. *Preventive Veterinary Medicine* **102**, 98–106.

Rostaher, A., Mueller, R.S., Majzoub, M., Schares, G., Gollnick, N.S. (2010). Bovine besnoitiosis in Germany. *Veterinary Dermatology* **21**, 329–334.

Ruehlmann, D., Podell, M., Oglesbee, M., Dubey, J.P. (1995). Canine neosporosis: a case report and literature review. *Journal of the American Animal Hospital Association* **31**, 174–183.

Sandvik, T. (2004). Progress of control and prevention programs for bovine viral diarrhea virus in Europe. *Veterinary Clinics of North America: Food Animal Practice* **20**, 151–169.

Schares, G., Basso, W., Majzoub, M., Cortes, H.C., Rostaher, A., Selmair, J., Hermanns, W., Conraths, F.J., Gollnick, N.S. (2009). First in vitro isolation of Besnoitia besnoiti from chronically infected cattle in Germany. *Veterinary Parasitology* **163**, 315–322.

Schares, G., Heydorn, A.O., Cuppers, A., Mehlhorn, H., Geue, L., Peters, M., Conraths, F.J. (2002). In contrast to dogs, red foxes (*Vulpes vulpes*) did not shed *Neospora caninum* upon feeding of intermediate host tissues. *Parasitology Research* **88**, 44–52.

Schares, G., Peters, M., Wurm, R., Barwald, A., Conraths, F.J. (1998). The efficiency of vertical transmission of *Neospora caninum* in dairy cattle analysed by serological techniques. *Veterinary Parasitology* **80**, 87–98.

Schares, G., Wenzel, U., Muller, T., Conraths, F.J. (2001). Serological evidence for naturally occurring transmission of *Neospora caninum* among foxes (*Vulpes vulpes*). *International Journal of Parasitology* **31**, 418–423.

Schweizer, M., Matzener, P., Pfaffen, G., Stalder, H., Peterhans, E. (2006). 'Self' and 'nonself' manipulation of interferon defense during persistent infection: bovine viral diarrhea virus resists alpha/beta interferon without blocking antiviral activity against unrelated viruses replicating in its host cells. *Journal of Virology* **80**, 6926–6935.

Smith, G.C., McDonald, R.A., Wilkinson, D. (2012). Comparing Badger (*Meles meles*) Management Strategies for Reducing Tuberculosis Incidence in Cattle. *PloS One* **7**, e39250.

Smith, S.I., West, D.M., Wilson, P.R., de Lisle, G.W., Collett, M.G., Heuer, C., Chambers, J.P. (2011). Detection of Mycobacterium avium subsp. paratuberculosis in skeletal muscle and blood of ewes from a sheep farm in New Zealand. *New Zealand Veterinary Journal* **59**, 240–243.

Stabel, J.R., Lambertz, A. (2004). Efficacy of pasteurization conditions for the inactivation of *Mycobacterium avium* subsp. *paratuberculosis* in milk. *Journal of Food Protection* **67**, 2719–2726.

Steinbach, F., Dastjerdi, A., Drew, T., Cook, A., Davies, I. (2012). Continued presentation of cases of Schmallenberg virus in sheep in England. *Veterinary Record* **170**, 547.

Stevenson, K., Alvarez, J., Bakker, D., Biet, F., de Juan, L., Denham, S., Dimareli, Z., Dohmann, K., Gerlach, G.F., Heron, I., Kopecna, M., May, L., Pavlik, I., Sharp, J.M., Thibault, V.C., Willemsen, P., Zadoks, R.N., Greig, A. (2009). Occurrence of Mycobacterium avium subspecies paratuberculosis across host species and European countries with evidence for transmission between wildlife and domestic ruminants. *BMC Microbiology* **9**, 212.

Thilsted, J.P., Dubey, J.P. (1989). Neosporosis-like abortions in a herd of dairy cattle. *Journal of Veterinary Diagnostic Investigation* **1**, 205–209.

Thompson, D., Muriel, P., Russell, D., Osborne, P., Bromley, A., Rowland, M., Creigh-Tyte, S., Brown, C. (2002). Economic costs of the foot and mouth disease outbreak in the United Kingdom in 2001). *Revue Scientifique et Technique* **21**, 675–687.

Thornton, R.N., Gajadhar, A., Evans, J. (1994). *Neospora* abortion epidemic in a dairy herd. *New Zealand Veterinary Journal* **42**, 190–191.

Thurmond, M.C., Hietala, S.K. (1997). Effect of congenitally acquired *Neospora caninum* infection on risk of abortion and subsequent abortions in dairy cattle. *American Journal of Veterinary Research* **58**, 1381–1385.

Trees, A.J., Davison, H.C., Innes, E.A., Wastling, J.M. (1999). Towards evaluating the economic impact of bovine neosporosis. *International Journal of Parasitology* **29**, 1195–1200.

Vallat, F. (2012). An outbreak in France in the XVIIIth Century: Rinderpest. *Comptes Rendus Biologies* **335**, 343–349.

Van Campen, H., Rhyan, J. (2010). The role of wildlife in diseases of cattle. The Veterinary clinics of North America. *Food Animal Practice* **26**, 147–161, table of contents.

Vilcek, S., Bjorklund, H.V., Horner, G.W., Meers, J., Belak, S. (1998). Genetic typing of pestiviruses from New Zealand. *New Zealand Veterinary Journal* **46**, 35–37.

West, D.M., Pomroy, W.E., Collett, M.G., Hill, F.I., Ridler, A.L., Kenyon, P.R., Morris, S.T., Pattison, R.S. (2006). A possible role for *Neospora caninum* in ovine abortion in New Zealand. *Small Ruminant Research* **62**, 135–138.

Weston, J.F., Heuer, C., Williamson, N.B. (2012). Efficacy of a *Neospora caninum* killed tachyzoite vaccine in preventing abortion and vertical transmission in dairy cattle. *Preventive Veterinary Medicine* **103**, 136–144.

Williams, D.J., Guy, C.S., Smith, R.F., Ellis, J., Björkman, C., Reichel, M.P., Trees, A.J. (2007). Immunization of cattle with live tachyzoites of *Neospora caninum* confers protection against fetal death. *Infection and Immunity* **75**, 1343–1348.

Wilson, D.J., Rood, K., Biswas, P., Byrem, T.M. (2010). Herd-level prevalence of Johne's disease in Utah and adjacent areas of the intermountain west as detected by a bulk-tank milk surveillance project. *Journal of Dairy Science* **93**, 5792–5797.

Wouda, W., Moen, A.R., Schukken, Y.H. (1998). Abortion risk in progeny of cows after a *Neospora caninum* epidemic. *Theriogenology* **49**, 1311–1316.

Yamanouchi, K. (2012). Scientific background to the global eradication of rinderpest. *Veterinary Immunology and Immunopathology* **148**, 12–15.

CHAPTER 28

Population Medicine and Herd Health Planning

Nigel B. Cook

Learning objectives

- Appreciate the three different types of models of veterinary practice: the 'physicians model', the 'consultative model' and the 'facilitator model'.
- Appreciate the different types of model that are used for fundamental and auxiliary records for 'top level' and 'drill down' analysis.
- Recognise the value of benchmarking herds.
- Recognise the importance of records, herd performance indicators for monitoring production , reproduction, milk quality health and welfare.
- Appreciate the importance of herd economics and partial budgets when changes are made.

Introduction

In recent times, the dairy industry in many parts of the world has consolidated, and herd size has increased. With this consolidation has come a shift in the requirements for veterinary care, and a change in the skill set required to better serve our new clientele. Those that have failed to make this change increasingly find themselves doing the work of a paid technician, and become passengers in the management decisions of the herd, while those that have succeeded find themselves aligned with the interests of the herd owner, serving as a confidante, someone who can filter advice for the herd manager, implement recommendations and monitor outcomes.

This chapter will discuss the training and tools that a successful herd veterinarian needs to acquire if they are to adapt to the changing needs of the dairy industry and provide sought-after population medicine and herd health services.

Models of veterinary practice

Veterinary schools train veterinarians to treat a single patient, take a history, make observations of the abnormal, gather other information from imaging and biochemical testing, and match the data with an appropriate diagnosis. This 'physicians model', when implemented on the farm with the successful treatment of an individual sick patient, is the reason why veterinarians have largely been viewed with trust and respect by our clients. However, in larger herds, where farm personnel act as the caregivers, this type of relationship with the individual animal is challenged, and the 'physicians model' breaks down.

The failure of the old 'physicians model' of veterinary practice in large herds warrants a new approach, and some have switched to a 'consultative model' for supplying veterinary services, where the herd veterinarian receives payment for the delivery of herd health advice, usually on an hourly rate or on a per-head basis. There are notable examples of success using this model, where the veterinarian visiting the herd regularly may be called upon to be the sole purveyor of advice, and this is likely to continue in smaller to medium-sized herds, where there is less competition for time and access to the herd owner.

However, provision of the 'consultative model' in larger herds can be very challenging. Managers and owners of these large herds receive advice in a myriad of forms from multiple sources, most of it without direct payment. These herds are well served by the industry, with consultants from feed and breeding companies, technical service veterinarians from pharmaceutical companies, and advisors from universities, extension services and even grocery chains, all delivering advice on every aspect of production and management. It is easy for the veterinarian to feel threatened in this environment, and frustrated that it is difficult to get paid for their consultative services.

Bovine Medicine, Third Edition. Edited by Peter D. Cockcroft.

For large herds, I believe that another model of practice is needed – I call it the 'facilitator model'. In it, veterinarians must seize the opportunity to align themselves with management and become an enterprise partner – someone with an intimate knowledge of how the herd functions, entrusted to seek out referral from experts when a problem arises, filter the recommendations provided, create the action plan to be followed, implement it with appropriate training of the farm employees and set up a monitoring system to determine success or failure.

To make this change, the veterinarian needs a new skill set that incorporates the clinical skills we have at the foundation of our training, but adds computer, epidemiology, economics, statistical and communication skill sets. The 'facilitator model' must be billed in an entirely different way: the success of the veterinarian must be intertwined with the success of the herd. Some veterinarians become an employee, or even part-owner of the herd, others are paid on a retainer for their services, while others aim to receive a percentage of the milk shipment receipts or live-weight gain. The approach, when implemented successfully, will ensure that the herd veterinarian becomes an integral part of the management team on the farm, and not a passenger in the decision-making process.

The successful veterinarian may practice all three types of service model to meet the needs of different clients, but this type of veterinarian must 'own the records' on the farm. This chapter will continue with a discussion of the use and implementation of benchmarking and monitoring systems for milk production, reproduction, milk quality, health and welfare in dairy herds, to facilitate the delivery of the 'facilitator model' of practice.

Fundamental and auxiliary records for 'top level' and 'drill down' analysis

Some records are essential to the management of the day-to-day operations of the herd, while other records enhance our ability to investigate problems and fine-tune the operations of the dairy. I call these 'fundamental' and 'auxiliary' records.

'Fundamental records' answer simple questions such as: "*Is milk production increasing or decreasing*"; "*Do I need to feed the cows more or less*"; and "*Is the milk being shipped safe and free of drug residues*". These fundamental records provide for a 'top-level' monitor of performance, for which there should be set herd goals or benchmarks.

Departure from these goals would initiate a more in-depth analysis of the problem, for which we need 'auxiliary' records. These records are usually attached to the permanent individual cow record on the farm, and are accessible via an on-farm software program. 'Auxiliary' records, when used appropriately, can be used to develop a 'drill-down' analysis of a problem, flagged from a failure to meet a herd goal from one or more of the 'top-level' monitors. To achieve this purpose, the records must be able to be sorted into different sub-groups such as by parity, stage of lactation or by pen, and their use requires a skilled veterinarian with an understanding of epidemiology and statistics.

Benchmarking

Herds should be managed so that the veterinarian can easily monitor departures from goal in their 'top-level' monitors. These departures may be changes detected when comparing the herd's current performance with its historical record. Data analytics, such as statistical process control, have been used to flag when these departures become statistically significant (Reneau & Lukas, 2006), but simple relative risk or odds ratio calculations and z-test or t-tests may suffice when coupled with other herd management information and the veterinarians' clinical knowledge (Slenning, 2006).

Benchmarking has been used in business practice for several decades to promote the adoption of best practices (Camp, 1989), and there is a trend to benchmark performance between dairy herds in a similar manner. In this situation, the herd performance is ranked and compared in percentiles to other similar herds in the industry – matched for size or management style. This approach values the competition created by telling a herd where they rank compared to their competitors and facilitates a culture of continuous improvement. An example of a Dairy Herd Improvement (DHI) herd benchmark report is shown in Figure 28.1, where each 'top-level' monitor in each management category is compared to a scale showing the 10th, 50th and 90th percentile performance of other, similar herds. In a separate report, herds are able to track the change in their percentile ranking in each monitor over time, helping the veterinarian to identify management areas that require attention and improvement. This type of reporting is also very useful in determining the success or failure of a herd intervention.

Herd performance indicators

Production monitors

Production records are essential for providing the herd adequate nutrition and calculating herd profitability, and are fundamental for monitoring the success or failure of herd interventions. Monitoring the bulk tank milk pick-up data that includes milk volume (kg or litres), milk fat percentage, milk protein percentage and somatic cell count (SCC) is an essential practice for all dairy herds. In some countries, the focus is on weight of solids shipped (e.g. kg fat plus protein). For these data to be optimally used, an

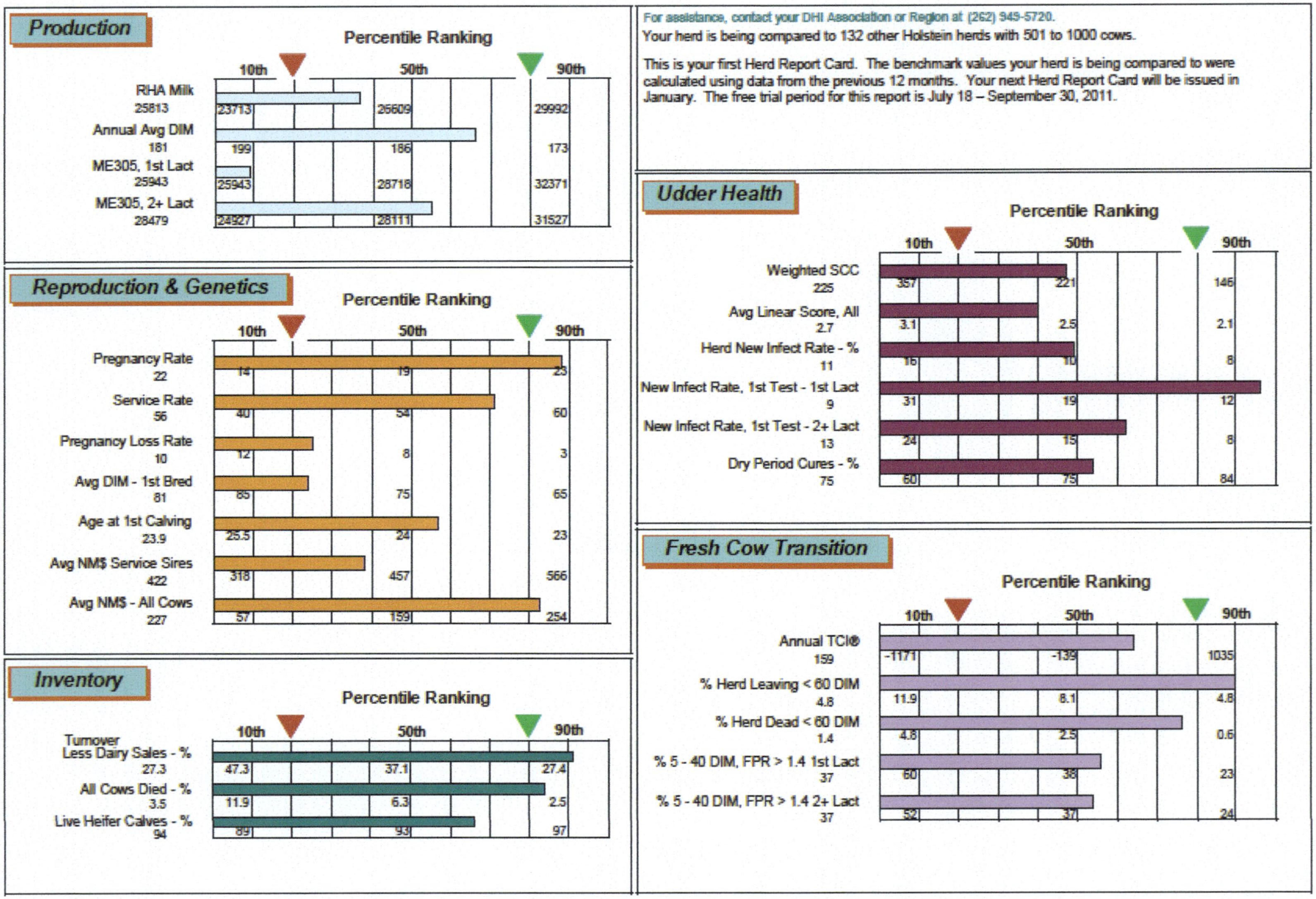

Figure 28.1 A herd benchmark report for a 600-cow dairy herd compared against 132 herds with between 500 and 1,000 cows. Reproduced with permission of AgSource Cooperative Services.

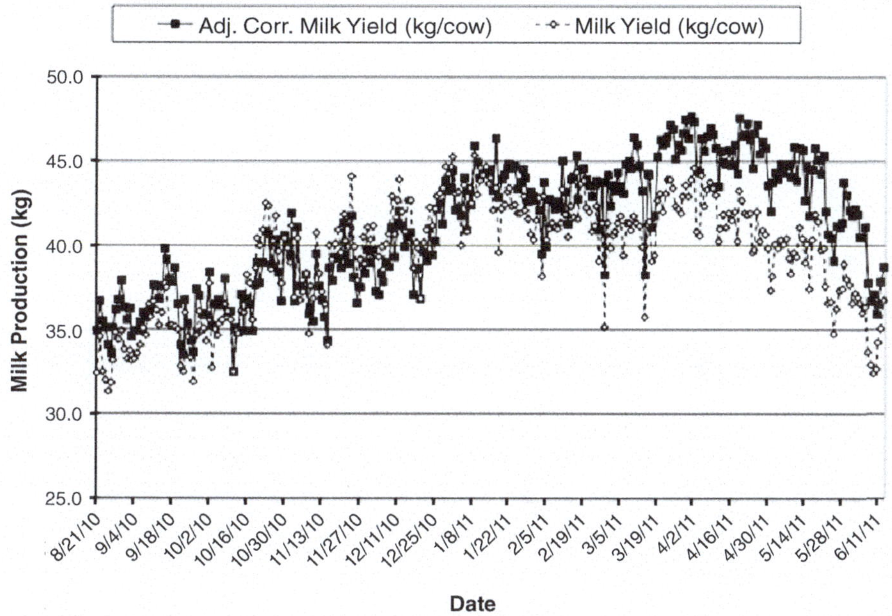

Figure 28.2 A graphic presentation of milk production change over time, using raw milk yield and adjusted corrected milk yield. Note the increase in production following a switch from component feeding to total mixed ration (TMR) feeding in October 2010, and the reduction in milk production the following spring, as herd average days in milk increased and summer heat stress occurred.

accurate count of the number of cows in milk contributing to the bulk tank must be kept alongside the herd.

From these basic data, a simple spreadsheet can be used to calculate daily milk yield per cow, along with yields of fat and protein. Herd managers respond well to visual presentation of these data in the form of line graphs and/or histograms, and such information can be used to drive changes in herd management and to identify the approximate timing of positive or negative interventions. An example is shown in Figure 28.2.

The record can be enhanced with a breakdown of the number of primiparous and multiparous cows, and the herd average days in milk can be used to calculate a yield monitor that controls for different stages of the calving season, group parity profile changes and differences in milk quality. Various calculations exist, with adjusted corrected milk (ACM) being the most basic approach taken in non-seasonal herds in North America and used in Figure 28.2 (the formula for calculation is included in Appendix 1, Nordlund, 1987). ACM may be useful in circumstances where, for example, the daily milk production is dropping because a lot of cows are in late lactation, which may signal a breeding problem rather than a nutritional problem, thereby assisting the veterinarian and herd owner to make the right management change.

Production records are frequently made available through individual cow-based test day interval sampling through various organisations (typically administered monthly); through individual daily milk weight recording (via advanced milking machine monitoring equipment); and through robotic systems that are now becoming more commonplace, where data may be accessed not only from the individual cow, but from each quarter within each cow.

These types of data do not replace the need for bulk tank monitoring, but do supply additional individual cow (or quarter) information that may prove useful. It is, therefore, essential that the herd veterinarian be well versed in the interpretation of these records, which may be provided in paper form (see Figure 28.3 for an example of a Dairy Herd Information Association (DHIA) Herd Summary Report), or may be made available through an on-farm software program or via the web, through cloud-based services. Much of these types of data go beyond the 'fundamental' record set required by every herd each and every day, but they can be useful if a problem arises, to 'drill-down' and investigate problems in more detail at a sub-group level by parity grouping, stage of lactation, season or pen type. These monitors would include peak milk production, management level milk, mature equivalent 305-day milk production, and monitoring of percentage fat and percentage protein and their ratios.

Reproductive monitoring

Traditionally, the veterinarian has had an important role to play in the provision of the herd reproductive program. However, this role has been challenged by new technologies that provide alternatives for pregnancy diagnosis. Where veterinarians can continue to remain unchallenged is in their understanding of

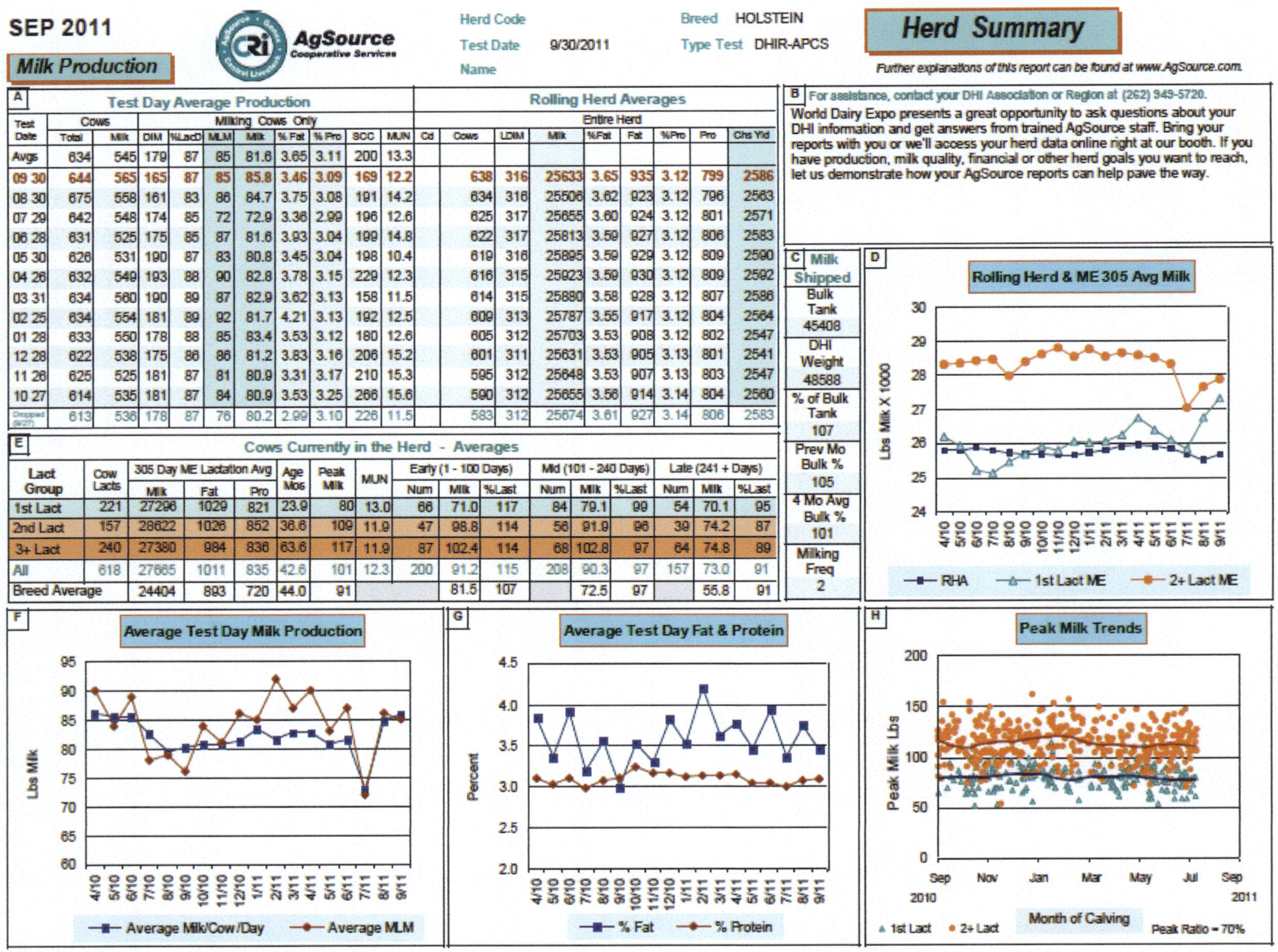

SEP 2011

Milk Production

AgSource Cooperative Services

Herd Code

Test Date 9/30/2011

Name

Breed HOLSTEIN

Type Test DHIR-APCS

Herd Summary

Further explanations of this report can be found at www.AgSource.com

A — Test Day Average Production / Rolling Herd Averages

Test Date	Cows Total	Cows Milk	DIM	%LactD	MLM	Milk	% Fat	% Pro	SCC	MUN	Cd	Cows	LDIM	Milk	%Fat	Fat	%Pro	Pro	Chs Yld
Avgs	634	545	179	87	85	81.6	3.65	3.11	200	13.3									
09 30	644	565	165	87	85	85.8	3.46	3.09	169	12.2		638	316	25633	3.65	935	3.12	799	2586
08 30	675	558	161	83	86	84.7	3.75	3.08	191	14.2		634	316	25506	3.62	923	3.12	796	2563
07 29	642	548	174	85	72	72.9	3.36	2.99	196	12.6		625	317	25655	3.60	924	3.12	801	2571
06 28	631	525	175	85	87	81.6	3.93	3.04	199	14.8		622	317	25813	3.59	927	3.12	806	2583
05 30	626	531	190	87	83	80.8	3.45	3.04	198	10.4		619	316	25895	3.59	929	3.12	809	2590
04 26	632	549	193	88	90	82.8	3.78	3.15	229	12.3		616	315	25923	3.59	930	3.12	809	2592
03 31	634	560	190	89	87	82.9	3.62	3.13	158	11.5		614	315	25880	3.58	928	3.12	807	2586
02 25	634	554	181	89	92	81.7	4.21	3.13	192	12.5		609	313	25787	3.55	917	3.12	804	2564
01 28	633	550	178	88	85	83.4	3.53	3.12	180	12.6		605	312	25703	3.53	908	3.12	802	2547
12 28	622	538	175	86	86	81.2	3.83	3.16	206	15.2		601	311	25631	3.53	905	3.13	801	2541
11 26	625	525	181	87	81	80.9	3.31	3.17	210	15.3		595	312	25648	3.53	907	3.13	803	2547
10 27	614	535	181	87	84	80.9	3.53	3.25	266	15.6		590	312	25655	3.56	914	3.14	804	2560
Dropped (9/27)	613	536	178	87	76	80.2	2.99	3.10	226	11.5		583	312	25674	3.61	927	3.14	806	2583

B — For assistance, contact your DHI Association or Region at (262) 949-5720.

World Dairy Expo presents a great opportunity to ask questions about your DHI information and get answers from trained AgSource staff. Bring your reports with you or we'll access your herd data online right at our booth. If you have production, milk quality, financial or other herd goals you want to reach, let us demonstrate how your AgSource reports can help pave the way.

C — Milk Shipped

Bulk Tank	45408
DHI Weight	48588
% of Bulk Tank	107
Prev Mo Bulk %	105
4 Mo Avg Bulk %	101
Milking Freq	2

E — Cows Currently in the Herd - Averages

Lact Group	Cow Lacts	305 Day ME Lactation Avg Milk	Fat	Pro	Age Mos	Peak Milk	MUN	Early (1 - 100 Days) Num	Milk	%Last	Mid (101 - 240 Days) Num	Milk	%Last	Late (241 + Days) Num	Milk	%Last
1st Lact	221	27296	1029	821	23.9	80	13.0	66	71.0	117	84	79.1	99	54	70.1	95
2nd Lact	157	28622	1026	852	36.6	109	11.9	47	98.8	114	56	91.9	96	39	74.2	87
3+ Lact	240	27380	984	836	63.6	117	11.9	87	102.4	114	68	102.8	97	64	74.8	89
All	618	27665	1011	835	42.6	101	12.3	200	91.2	115	208	90.3	97	157	73.0	91
Breed Average		24404	893	720	44.0	91			81.5	107		72.5	97		55.8	91

Figure 28.3 An example DHIA herd summary record detailing monthly test information for a 634 cow dairy. Reproduced with permission of AgSource Cooperative Services.

Table 28.1 Top-level reproductive monitors of efficiency used in all-year-round calving herds in North America, with benchmarks from DHIA recorded herds (500–1,000 cow herd size) (see Caraviello *et al*. (2006) and Schefers *et al*. (2010) for definitions)

Monitor	Percentile		
	10th	50th	90th
Service rate	40	54	60
Pregnancy rate	14	19	23
Conception rate	25	35	45
Pregnancy loss	12	8	3
% Herd pregnant by 150 DIM	50	65	80

breeding records and their ability to analyse problems, when this is coupled with their intimate knowledge of the individual cow. Table 28.1 shows the top-level monitors frequently used in North America to assess reproductive efficiency with benchmarks appropriate for high-yielding freestall-housed Holstein dairy cows. Obviously, benchmarks must be reflective of the breed and management type under review.

Historical measures of calving interval, and calving to conception interval, that may still have some value in seasonal breeding herds, have largely been replaced by monitors of breeding effort and conception success – service rate, conception rate, pregnancy loss, pregnancy rate (or risk), and proportion of the herd pregnant by 150 days in milk.

Recent work has examined risk factors for failure to meet goals in these herd level monitors (Caraviello *et al.*, 2006; Schefers *et al.*, 2010), to assist the herd veterinarian troubleshoot herd reproductive problems. Failure to reach target in any or all of these categories may trigger a 'drill-down' analysis, which should consider AI technician performance and conception rate differences between standing heat breeding and timed AI synchronisation. Injection compliance must be considered where complex synchronisation programs are utilised, while seasonal influences due to feed access and heat stress may also be important considerations – not to mention infectious causes of infertility, and the effect of health conditions such as lameness and mastitis.

Milk quality

Somatic cell count (SCC) in the bulk milk tank must be monitored for each milk shipment, along with whatever industry measure of bacterial contamination of milk is being used (e.g. standard plate count, Bactoscan). Departures from the herd goal at this 'top-level' monitor should trigger immediate investigation into the possible causes as, in many markets, quality premiums are paid to promote the shipment of high-quality milk.

Interval milk component testing provides SCC at the individual cow level that may be used for 'drill-down' assessment. Most

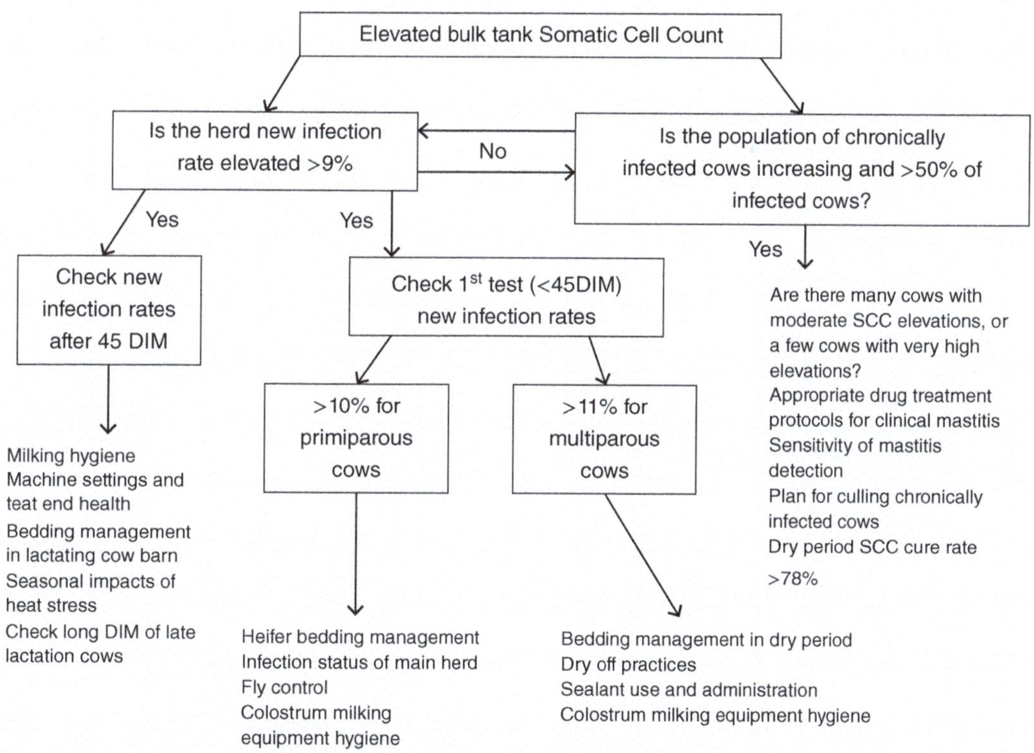

Figure 28.4 A decision tree analysis for investigating a high bulk tank somatic cell count (SCC) problem.

commonly, a threshold of around 200 000/ml has been used to identify infected cows with approximately 80% sensitivity and specificity (Dohoo, 2001), and this definition of infection may be used at the herd level to calculate various monitors that may gauge infection pressure. Among the most useful measures are the new infection rate, the infection rate at first test for primiparous and multiparous cows, the dry period cure rate and the proportion of infected cows that are chronic – testing above the threshold for at least the last two tests (see Cook *et al.*, 2002 for definitions). These measures allow some understanding of infection dynamics operating within the herd, and allow the veterinarian to focus on the population of animals at risk. Figure 28.4 shows a simple trouble-shooting decision tree which, when coupled with bacteriology of infected quarters, will assist the herd response to udder health challenges.

Health recording and management

Concerns over the use of pharmaceuticals in food supply animals in most countries make basic records of drug use on the farm fundamental to the safe production of meat and milk. The fundamental record must itemise the drugs administered to each animal on the day(s) they were treated, alongside the appropriate milk and meat withdrawal periods. These records often take the form of a written notation in a log book, usually in date order. Such fundamental records meet the needs of food safety, where drug withdrawal periods may be checked and drug use oversight achieved. Such records can also be used to monitor protocol drift, which is common unless caregivers are regularly supervised and their activities assessed by the herd veterinarian. When identified, the reasons can be obtained, and an investigation launched if necessary.

For more detailed supervision, the drug use record must be transferred to an individual cow's permanent record, and the veterinarian must be involved in the set-up of these records to allow for appropriate oversight. This essential step requires appropriate disease definitions (see Table 28.2), and the veterinarian must train the individuals responsible for recording to identify these diseases accurately and consistently.

Table 28.2 Case definitions for common health conditions along with targets for acceptable levels of incidence (adapted from Kelton *et al.*, 1998; Nordlund & Cook, 2004)

Disease condition	Case definition	New case definition	Goal herd incidence rate (%)
Milk fever	Clinical signs consistent with stage 1 (mild excitement, nervousness, weakness, rapid heart rate), stage 2 (sternal recumbency depression, muscle tremors, rapid heart rate, cold ears, decreased rumen movements, pupils dilated and low rectal temperature (<37.8°C) or stage 3 (lateral recumbency, bloat, rapid heart rate and weak pulse) of the disease, within 72 hours of calving.	Limit to one per lactation.	2
Retained placenta	Foetal membranes visible at the vulva or identified within the vagina or uterus by examination more than 24 hours after calving.	Limit to one per lactation.	5
Metritis	An abnormal uterine, cervical, vaginal or vulval discharge observed within 21 days of calving.	Usually limit to one per lactation.	15
Ketosis	Defined as a reduction in DMI in association with elevated blood, milk, urine or breath ketones.	New case if no signs within last 30 days.	20
Displaced abomasum	An audible high-pitched tympanic resonance (ping) produced by percussion of the left (LDA) or right (RDA) abdominal wall between the 9th and 12th ribs, in association with reduced DMI.	Usually limit to one per lactation.	3
Pneumonia	Presence of at least two out of three signs among fever, nasal discharge, cough, and increased respiratory rate.	New case if no signs within last 30 days.	3
Mastitis	A cow with one or more quarters with visually abnormal milk (clots, flakes or watery) with or without other local (heat, swelling or discoloration) or systemic (fever or signs of toxic shock) signs.	New case if no abnormal milk in previously infected quarter for previous 14 days, or no abnormal milk in new quarter.	20
Lameness	An abnormal gait determined by locomotion (mobility) score attributable to a focus of pain or disease in one or more limbs.	New case if not clinically lame in previous 30 days in affected limb, or not lame in new limb.	15

A cow-side record must be developed that allows for the recording of information from day to day and reflects the changes in the course of treatment needed to communicate the status of the cow accurately between care-givers. The cow-side record is frequently completed on paper but, in the future, it is likely that, with the growth of tablet computers, a touch-screen data entry device may streamline the entry of information and facilitate its summarisation without the need for a paper record. These fundamental records are useful day to day, but only certain aspects of the information need to be transferred to the cow's auxiliary record. This auxiliary record might include: the disease diagnosed; its severity; the drug protocol used, with details of individual drug use (dose and frequency); the days to clinical cure; and the days that the milk was withheld from the bulk milk tank.

None of these steps occur by accident, and good records require significant effort in their set-up if they are to prove useful. The veterinarian can examine the information in a variety of different ways. Simple incidence rates may be monitored over time as a 'top-level' assessment of performance. A simple relative risk calculation may be used to identify significant changes over time, or between risk groups, that may warrant further 'drill-down' analysis.

I frequently find it useful to track the timing (days in milk) of the first disease event and remove the noise created by recurrent events. Such an approach has been commonly used for conditions such as mastitis and lameness, which are prone to recurrence. Re-treatments and recurrent disease events may be tracked separately as an indicator of treatment failure, along with protocol compliance.

Because of the importance of the transition period, fresh cow health monitoring has almost become a special sub-set of overall health management on the farm. Obviously, early lactation is a critical period, during which periparturient diseases occur, and monitoring the incidence of milk fever, metritis, retained placenta, displaced abomasum and ketosis can be useful. However, because of the difficulties in case definition and comparison of these types of records between farms, other monitors have been used to track the effectiveness of the transition program. The commonly used 'top-level' transition monitors are listed in Table 28.3.

Herd-based biological testing, using strategic sampling of at-risk cows for BHBA, NEFA and serum calcium, may be used in response to changes in performance to the 'top-level' transition monitors in Table 28.3. The approach has been fully described (see Oetzel, 2004), and the alarm levels, cut-points and populations at risk have been updated in Table 28.4.

However, with the increasing availability of cheaper cow-side tests, the approach to biological testing has switched in recent years to regular routine monitoring of all cows at-risk by the caregivers on farm, rather than a single point in time assessment. The approach may be particularly beneficial for BHBA testing in high-yielding herds where two tests between 3 and 10 DIM, coupled with propylene glycol treatment, is economically justifiable and beneficial to the cow (McArt *et al.*, personal communication).

Table 28.3 Transition cow performance monitors with benchmarks from DHIA recorded herds (500–1,000 cow herd size).

Monitor	Percentile		
	90th	50th	10th
Turnover less than 60 DIM	12	8	5
Death rate less than 60 DIM	5	3	1
Transition cow index®	−1200	−100	1035
Stillbirth rate	11	7	3
Fat protein ratio percentage greater than 1.4			
Multiparous cows	60	38	23
Primiparous cows	52	37	24

Table 28.4 Herd-based biological tests with cut-points, alarm levels and at-risk group that should be sampled (from Oetzel (2004), with updates from Chapinal *et al.* (2012) and Roberts *et al.* (2012)).

Test	Cut-point	Alarm level proportion	At-risk group
BHBA	≥ 1.2 mmol/L	>15%	Lactating cows 3–15 days in milk
NEFA	≥ 0.40 mmol/L	>10%	Pre-fresh dry cows 2–14 days before actual calving
Serum calcium	≤ 2.1 mmol/L	>30%	Lactating multiparous cows at 1–7 days in milk

Objective welfare monitoring

Dairy herds of all sizes are increasingly being scrutinised for the quality of animal care and well-being. Welfare audits and assessments often employ objective outcomes, and veterinarians should be involved in their measurement and monitoring; indeed, the primary focus of welfare assessments should be on the outcome, not the process.

For replacement heifers, monitoring of failure of passive immunity transfer through the regular monitoring of serum total protein concentration or direct immunoglobulin testing is a prerequisite assessment (McGuirk & Collins, 2004).

For adult cattle, locomotion or mobility scoring, hock or other injury scoring, hygiene scoring and body condition scoring are performed, to objectively assess the physical well-being of the herd. These methods utilise categorical scores, usually on

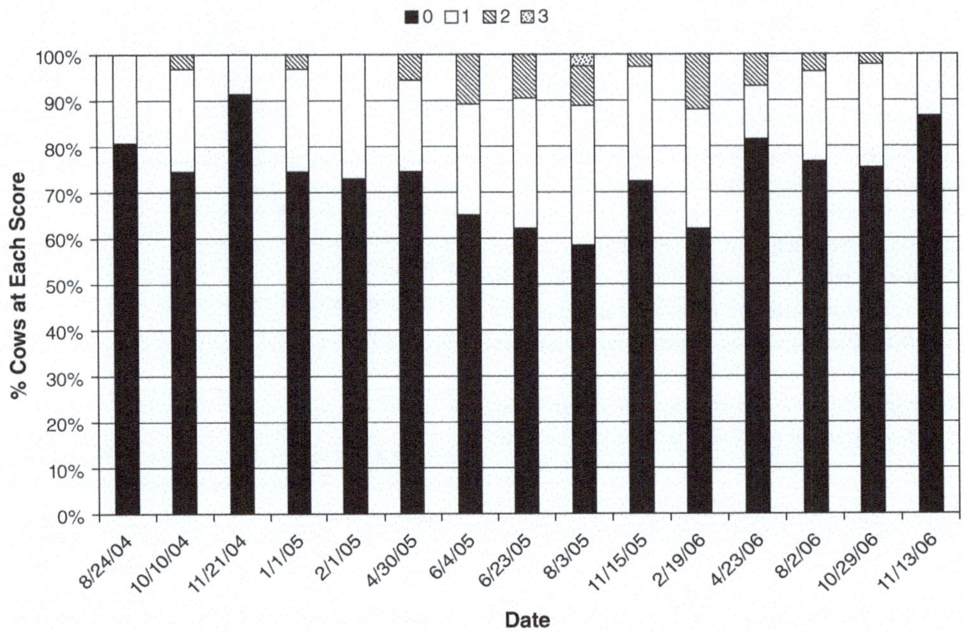

Figure 28.5 Proportion of cows at each locomotion (mobility) score (0–3) over time for a 50-cow dairy. Note the change in scores during the summer of 2005, the subsequent improvement through 2006 following an intervention in the autumn of 2005 which involved a change from rubber mats to sand bedding.

a 1–4 or 1–5 basis, to identify the affected population. These scores may be compared with a goal, often provided by the auditing company as a pass/fail threshold. However, I prefer the benchmarking approach, where herds are compared with their competition regularly over time and with their prior history. The herd veterinarian is in an excellent position to perform these measures, summarise them and bring departures from the norm to the attention of the herd owner, along with a plan to resolve them. Figure 28.5 gives an example of the use of regular locomotion (mobility) scoring over time in a small 50-cow dairy herd.

Herd economics and partial budgets

The veterinarian, working alongside herd ownership and management, must be aware of the economics of dairy production systems. In particular, use of a partial budget is a particularly useful skill. A partial budget is an estimation of the financial impact of a single change to a system over a fixed period of time (usually one year) without the need to examine the overall business situation. Constructing these budgets allows for a detailed examination of the processes or facilities that may need to be changed on a dairy, with assessment of the estimated cost and an examination of the likely benefits. An example budget is shown in Figure 28.6.

The veterinarian is ideally situated to examine the strengths and weaknesses of any proposal, and a well-constructed partial budget can be used to perform a sensitivity analysis to examine which variables carry the biggest impact on the outcome, and a breakeven analysis to measure the minimum required outcome to cover the cost of the intervention. Such an analysis can be extremely useful to a herd owner trying to make a difficult decision, and its use by the herd veterinarian can make them a valuable asset to the herd management team.

Conclusions

In this chapter, I have attempted to create a vision of a new 'facilitator model' for veterinary practice, adapted to the situation found in larger dairy herds. The reality is that, in many parts of the world, veterinarians may continue to make a living providing the 'physicians model', while others provide the 'consultative model' and, in many practices, individuals may be able to provide all three models to clients requiring different levels of service. However, it is also clear that our traditional veterinary training needs to be supplemented with new skill sets, detailed in this chapter, that make us invaluable to progressive dairy herd owners as we find a new role alongside them, assisting with the management decisions that need to be taken to optimise herd productivity and well-being.

Partial Budget - Mattress to Sand Conversion

Nigel B. Cook, MRCVS, Ken Nordlund, DVM, & Rebecca Brotzman, DVM

School of Veterinary Medicine, University of Wisconsin-Madison

To unprotect this sheet, click the Review tab above and select Unprotect sheet.

Fill in the BLUE cells in the Assumptions table below

Dairyland Initiative
UNIVERSITY OF WISCONSIN–MADISON

POSITIVE IMPACTS		
Increased Income		
Improved milk production	$	401,500
Improved SCC premium	$	55,845
Total Increased Incomes	$	457,345
Reduced Costs		
Reduced number clinical mastitis cases	$	21,450
Reduced number of lameness treatments	$	18,200
Reduced cost of replacement heifers	$	90,000
Reduced cost of bedding on mattresses	$	273,750
Total Reduced Costs	$	403,400
Total Positive Impacts	$	860,745

NEGATIVE ECONOMIC IMPACTS		
Increased Costs		
Increased feed costs	$	200,750
Amortized cost of stall modifications	$	92,390
Amortized cost of manure system modifications	$	138,585
Cost of sand bedding	$	91,250
Total Increased Costs	$	522,975
Reduced Incomes		
Reduction in cull cow sales	$	54,000
Total Reduced Incomes	$	54,000
Total Negative Impacts	$	576,075
NET ANNUAL IMPACT	$	283,770

Herd Assumptions			Units	Instructions or reference values
Herd size		1,000	# cows	*Enter herd size*
Number of stalls		1,000	# stalls	*Enter # stalls*
Current bedding usage		10	lbs/stall/day	*Estimate organic bedding use at 5-15 lb per stall per day*
Cost of current bedding		150	$/ton	*Typical range $50-250 per ton*
Anticipated sand usage per stall per day		50	lbs/stall/day	*Typical range 30-80 lb per stall per day*
Cost of sand bedding		10	$/ton	*Typical range $7-14 per ton*
Milk price ($ per lb)	$	0.22	$ per lb milk	*Typical range $0.12-0.18*
Lbs TMR dry matter per lb of milk	$	0.55	lb DM/lb milk	*Expected range 0.5-0.6*
Cost per lb of TMR dry matter		0.20	$ per lb DM	*Typical range $0.1 to 0.2 per lb of TMR dry matter*
Lbs of milk per cow per day, past yr		80	lbs	*Enter lbs milk per cow per day, past year*
Projected change in milk per cow per day		5	lbs	*Usual response 5-9 lbs per cow per day*
		85	lbs	*Projected milk yield per cow per day*
Milk production			1679	lbs, estimated change in milk yield per cow per year
SCC premium per 1,000 SCC reduction	$	0.003	$/cwt	*Estimate from creamery rates, usually $0.002-.004/cwt per 1,000 SCC*
Current annual bulk tank average SCC		300,000	scc/ml	*Enter annual average bulk tank SCC*
Estimated % reduction in SCC		20	%	*Expected reduction of 15-25%*
		240,000	scc/ml	*Projected SCC after change*
Bulk tank SCC			60,000	reduction in herd average SCC
Direct cost of a case of clinical mastitis	$	110	$ per case	*Enter average cost of treatment*
Current clinical mastitis rate, %		65	cases/100 cows	*Enter average # of clinical cases per 100 cows per year*
Estimated reduction in clinical mastitis rate		30	%	*Expected reduction of ~25-35%*
		46	cases/100 cows	*Projected clinical mastitis rate after change*
Clinical mastitis			195	reduced cases of mastitis in herd per year
Direct cost of a case of lameness ($ per case)	$	70	$ per case	*Enter average cost to treat lameness*
Current lameness rate, %		65	cases/100 cows	*Enter average # of lameness treatments per 100 cows per year*
Estimated reduction in lameness treatment rate		40	%	*Expected reduction of clinical lameness by 25-50%*
		39	cases/100 cows	*Projected clinical lameness rate after change*
Clinical lameness			260	reduced cases of lameness in herd per year
Cost of replacement heifer ($)	$	1,500	$ per heifer	*Enter estimate for heifer purchase*
Cull price per cow ($)	$	900	$ per cull	*Enter average cull price*
Turnover rate before change (%)		46	%	*Enter annual herd turnover rate*
Expected reduction in annual turnover rate		6	%	*Enter expected reduction of 5-8 points*
		40	%	*Projected annual turnover rate after change*
Culling			60	reduced culls from herd per year
Financial Assumptions				
Cost of stall changes ($)	$	400,000		*Enter cost of proposed stall changes*
Cost of manure handling system change ($)	$	600,000		*Enter cost of proposed manure handling changes*
			$1,000,000	*Total cost of conversion*
Repayment Period (years)		5	yr	*Suggest 3-7 years*
Interest Rate of Loan		0.05	interest rate	

Figure 28.6 An example partial budget for switching a freestall facility from mattresses to sand bedding (available at www.thedairylandinitiative.vetmed.wisc.edu).

References

Camp, R. (1989). Benchmarking: the search for industry best practices that lead to superior performance. ASQC Quality Press, Milwaukee, WI.

Caraviello, D.Z., Weigel, K.A., Craven, M., Gianola, D., Cook, N.B., Nordlund, K.V., Fricke, P.M. and Wiltbank, M.C. (2006). Analysis of reproductive performance of lactating cows on large dairy farms using machine learning algorithms. *Journal of Dairy Science* **89**, 4703–4722,

Chapinal, N., Carson, M.E., LeBlanc, S.J., Leslie, K.E., Godden, S., Capel, M., Santos, J.E.P., Overton, M.W. and Duffield, T.F. (2012). The association of serum metabolites in the transition period with milk production and early-lactation reproductive performance. *Journal of Dairy Science* **95**, 1301–1309.

Cook, N.B., Bennett, T.B., Emery, K.M., and Nordlund, K.V. (2002). Monitoring nonlactating cow intramammary infection dynamics using DHI somatic cell count data. *Journal of Dairy Science* **85**, 1119–1126.

Dohoo, I. (2001). *Setting SCC cut-points for cow and herd interpretation.* In: Proc. 40th Ann. Meeting of the National Mastitis Council, Reno, NV. February 11–14, 2001. Madison, WI, p. 10–18.

Kelton, D.F., Lissmore, K.D., Martin, R.E. (1998). Recommendations for recording and calculating the incidence of selected clinical diseases of dairy cattle. *Journal of Dairy Science* **81**, 2502–2509.

McGuirk, S.M. and Collins,M. (2004) Managing the production, storage, and delivery of colostrum. McGuirk and Collins (2004) Managing the production, storage, and delivery of colostrum. *Veterinary Clinics of North America: Food Animal Practice* **20**, 593–603.

Nordlund, K.V. (1986). *Adjusted corrected milk*, pp 87–89 in Proceedings of 19th Annual Convention of the American Association of Bovine Practitioners, Louisville, KY.

Nordlund, K.V. and Cook, N.B. (2004): Using herd records to monitor transition cow survival, productivity, and health. *Veterinary Clinics of North America* **20**, 627–649.

Oetzel, G.R. (2004). Monitoring and testing dairy herds for metabolic disease *Veterinary Clinics of North America* **20**, 651–674.

Østergaard, S. and Grohn, Y.T. (1999). Effects of diseases on test day milk yield and body weight of dairy cows from Danish research herds. *Journal of Dairy Science* **82**, 1188–1201.

Reneau, J.K. and Lukas, J. (2006). Using statistical process control methods to improve herd performance. *Veterinary Clinics of North America* **22**, 171–193.

Roberts, T., Chapinal, N., LeBlanc, S.J., Kelton, D.F., Dubuc, J., and Duffield, T.F. (2012). Metabolic parameters in transition cows as indicators for early-lactation culling risk. *Journal of Dairy Science* **95**, 3057–3063.

Schefers, J.M., Weigel, K.A., Rawson, C.L., Zwald, N.R., and Cook, N.B. (2010). Management practices associated with conception rate and service rate of lactating Holstein cows in large, commercial dairy herds. *Journal of Dairy Science* **93**, 1459–1467.

Slenning, B.D. (2006). Hood of the truck statistics for food animal practitioners *Veterinary Clinics of North America* **22**, 149–170.

Appendix I (From Nordlund (1986))

Adjusted corrected milk (ACM) is calculated on a herd basis and corrects for proportion of first lactation heifers, current days in milk and milk components. It is not applicable for seasonal calving herds. It assumes that primiparous cows produce 80% of the milk of multiparous cows, milk production declines at a rate of 0.29% per day from 80 days to 225 days in milk, and milk fat is corrected to 3.5% and is calculated using the following formulae in a spreadsheet:

(a) (1+ (1– (((cows/(heifers+cows)) + (0.8 × (heifers/(heifers + cows))))/0.93)))

(b) (0.432 × (lbs milk + (((average DIM-150) × 0.0029) × lbs milk)))

(c) (16.23 × ((lbs milk + (((average DIM-150) × 0.0029) × lbs milk)) × % fat/100))

Where

ACM = a × (b + c)
Lbs milk = bulk tank milk per cow per day
Average DIM = average days in milk of the cows contributing to the tank
% fat = % fat of the bulk tank milk tested.

CHAPTER 29
Welfare and Cattle Behaviour

Clive Phillips

Learning objectives

- Understand the principle concepts of the welfare of cattle.
- Be able to compare the advantages and disadvantages of different methods of welfare assessment.
- Understand the difference between normal and abnormal behaviour of cattle.
- Know the time required for the major normal behaviours .
- Be able to identify the major welfare problems in dairy and beef cattle farming systems.
- Be able to identify the major welfare problems in cattle transport and slaughter and the constraints imposed by religious slaughter.
- Provide recommendations for improving welfare in the different production systems and during transport and slaughter.

This chapter indicates how cattle welfare can be measured and highlights major concerns and solutions in cattle farming systems and in transport and slaughter. It includes time budgets for important parameters of for cow behaviour, and enables welfare assessors and veterinarians to be able to identify inadequacies and their possible causes.

Introduction

Good welfare of cattle in any system of production is important in ensuring public and, particularly, consumer support, as well as being an important contributor to job satisfaction for those working in the system. Cattle evolved in a warm, humid climate as prey animals, able to digest fibrous plants, grasses, forbs and browse material. These were harvested rapidly during daylight and held in a rumen, where microbial fermentation was used to commence the digestion process. Reverse peristalsis during rumination enabled cattle to re-masticate their food, assisting with the physical breakdown of fibre and adding alkaline saliva to buffer volatile fatty acids produced during the rumen fermentation. Domestic cattle differ little in these fundamentals from their progenitors, *Bos aurochs*, but have developed as two distinct subtypes. *Bos taurus* are more productive and intolerant of heat stress than the other subtype, *Bos indicus* cattle. As domesticated animals, cattle tolerate the presence of humans well, and as prey animals they give few overt signals of welfare problems, making mistreatment difficult to detect from the animals themselves.

Anthropomorphic assessment of cattle welfare carries with it the risk of misreading their very different sensory and cognitive apparatus, compared to our own. They are more responsive to the covert signals provided by odours and pheromones, and are less vocal than ourselves. The smell of blood is particularly potent. Their vision is mostly monocular, with their eyes positioned at the sides of their heads, giving them a 330° field of view. The possession of a tapetum and preponderance of rods provides good vision in low light conditions, and their dual cone reception limits colour vision, compared with our own trichromatic vision. Their hearing is acute, especially at high frequencies that we cannot hear, and they are also sensitive to stray electric current that we cannot feel. They have sensitive skin to remove flies, and need to engage in mutual grooming. Coat maintenance can be assisted by the provision of rubbing posts and brushes.

Cattle adjust slowly to change in their management system, including their feed type – hence, maintaining consistent conditions is important for their welfare. Veterinarians should be armed with a good understanding of the different sensory, behavioural and physiological characteristics of cattle, before attempting welfare assessment.

Welfare measurement

The optimum welfare measurement technique depends on the purpose of the assessment. Although welfare can be variously considered to relate primarily to the animal's ability to cope with

Bovine Medicine, Third Edition. Edited by Peter D. Cockcroft.

its environment, its feelings, experiences or ability to express natural behaviour, it is important to remember that welfare is primarily a state of both physical and mental good health. This is indicated by several parameters, and it is advisable to use a combination of these to gain an understanding of the animals' welfare.

Behaviour

Behaviour is usually the indicator that is most accessible to the farmer, herdsperson or veterinarian. However, with herd sizes increasing, it may be hard to discern individuals with behaviour problems, especially if regular contact with the herd is limited, as in the case of robotically-milked cows or rangeland cattle. Using behaviour to assess welfare requires knowledge of both normal and abnormal behaviour in the situation in which the cattle are kept. They are a social species that is highly gregarious, and they become stressed when isolated. They develop a social hierarchy which governs their movement patterns. Mutual grooming performs an important social function, helping to maintain bonds between individuals, as well as cleaning the coat. If allowed, calves naturally remain with their mothers until maturity, and as juveniles 'hide' in crèches when their mothers are grazing with them.

Ruminant cattle typically spend about 8–10 hours per day grazing, declining to about six hours per day if they are fed conserved feeds, such as a total mixed ration (TMR), which can be eaten faster. Fly control is important for grazing cattle, which use their tail to assist in fly removal. About 6–8 hours each day will be spent regurgitating boluses of feed into their mouth and chewing them before returning them to the rumen, a process known as rumination. Most rumination occurs while the cattle are lying down. Chewing while eating or ruminating is reduced if the fibre content of the diet is low and, in this situation, cattle may develop abnormal oral behaviours, such as stereotyped tonguing or tongue rolling. Sick cows also spend little time ruminating.

High-yielding dairy cows readily tire and need to lie down for about 12 hours per day. They will not get adequate rest if they are offered bare concrete (Figure 29.1) or free stalls (cubicles) that are overcrowded or not designed well for the comfort of the cow, or if they are removed from their housing or pasture for milking for long periods each day.

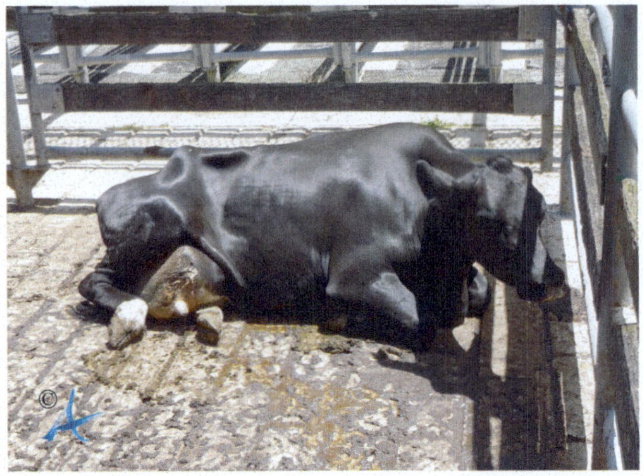

Figure 29.1 Cows should have access to a comfortable, soft, absorbent bed, not bare concrete. Reproduced with permission of Animal Angels.

Physiology

The most commonly used physiological indicators of cattle welfare are those that indicate stress – in particular, cortisol and adrenocorticotropic hormone, heart rate and its variability (the former increasing and the latter decreasing with stress). Cattle invoke homeostatic mechanisms to regulate their major functions, such as nutrition and reproduction, using hormones to moderate the relevant physiological processes. Concentrations of these hormones, for example ghrelin and leptin in undernutrition, can indicate welfare status. However, our knowledge of the normal range of concentrations is often scant, and they remain largely a research tool.

Other physiological indicators indicate the metabolic processes that are taking place, such as mobilisation of non-esterified fatty acids and β-hydroxybutyrate during undernutrition. Since its inception in the 1970s, metabolic profiling has been facilitated by more automated analytical methods, but that alone does not justify its routine use in cattle herds, unless we have a clear understanding of how to interpret the indicators. The dynamic nature of many welfare challenges and the body's response systems makes identification of the most appropriate welfare indicator important. For example, cortisol is a good indicator of medium-term stress in cattle, but in the short term may be affected by handling the animals to obtain samples and, in the long term, will give variable results, depending on the animal's capacity for maintaining the stress responses.

Emotions

There are few tools to directly measure emotions in cattle, although it is generally acknowledged that these are central to understanding their welfare. We can infer emotions in cattle from their behavioural and physiological responses to stimuli, for example their exuberant response on gaining access to food, which is accompanied by elevated heart rate, and presumably indicates pleasure (Hagen & Broom, 2004). We can also infer emotions when cattle show preferences, for example to avoid walking in slurry.

Longevity

Cattle are usually culled from a herd when they are infertile or diseased, either acutely or, more commonly, chronically, with disorders such as lameness or mastitis. Their endurance in the herd is a measure of their ability to resist disease. High-producing dairy cows typically last only 2–3 years, after entering at two years of age, which demonstrates the major challenges to their welfare when one considers that the natural lifespan of cattle can exceed 25 years.

Disease state

Most diseases are intrinsically painful to cattle, and also may predispose them to other diseases. Disease risk is affected by local conditions, but dairy cows are particularly susceptible to mastitis, lameness and metabolic diseases, and beef cattle to parasites. As well as providing treatment, veterinarians should assist in monitoring disease prevalence and recommending control measures.

Production

Milk production and cattle growth are reduced by disease, by abnormal behaviour, such as having to walk long distances to get water, and by negative emotions, experienced when herdspeople treat cattle badly. Hence, low productivity can imply poor welfare. However, this does not mean that high-yielding dairy cows or rapidly growing beef bulls are necessarily in good welfare, because high production may be associated with significant metabolic challenges.

Major welfare concerns

Dairy cattle

Genetic potential for milk production has increased considerably, without commensurately increasing the ability to provide additional nutrients. Hence, high-yielding cows enter a prolonged energy deficit in early lactation, predisposing them to diseases, including ketosis, mastitis, abomasal displacement and infertility.

Housing cows on concrete covered with their excreta, with free stalls for rest and conserved feeds offered behind a barrier, increases lameness, especially laminitis. Grazing cattle suffer less lameness, but punctured soles can be a problem. Cow excreta in the passageways frequently contaminates their tails when they lie down, encouraging farmers to dock them. This prevents the tail from performing its vital functions of fly removal and signalling to other cattle.

Poorly designed free stalls, or an insufficient number, prevents cows getting adequate rest. Cows prefer barns bedded with deep straw, and there is less lameness. The ease of managing cows, providing their feed and milking them in a barn is encouraging farmers not to allow cows access to pasture. Cows at pasture are able to feed, walk and lie comfortably, in a natural manner and synchronised within the herd whereas, in housing, natural behaviour may be constrained by poor building design or high stocking densities, and cows behave more independently. At pasture, however, cows should be given shade, either artificial or natural (Figure 29.2), to protect them from heat stress.

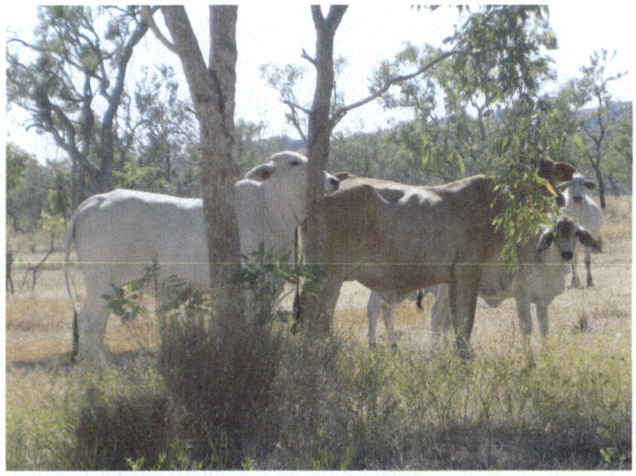

Figure 29.2 Natural shade prevents heat stress and provides grooming opportunities. Reproduced with permission of AP Phillips.

Dairy bulls are usually kept alone, often near the cows so that they encourage them to come into oestrus. Their small pens and limited human and animal contact restricts their social contact, making them aggressive and dangerous to handle.

Beef cattle

Beef cattle are commonly raised at pasture and may then be transferred to feedlots before slaughter, where they are fed a highly nutritious diet to make them grow quickly. Feedlots bring cattle into unnaturally close proximity, which may encourage aggressive interactions if conditions are poor. Mounting of subordinate steers by dominant animals is one of the biggest problems (buller steer syndrome), occurring most commonly in large pens with many cattle. It can only be solved by relocating the ridden animal. The cattle are held on loose dirt, which has the potential to become dusty in dry conditions, or boggy in wet ones. Either may cause welfare problems; dusty conditions predispose cattle to respiratory problems, and wet soil gives them foot rot.

Suitable siting and good design of the feedlot, including the right soil type and good drainage, will help to control these problems, as will water spraying during dry conditions. Feedlot cattle are prone to heat stress because of their high intake and rapid growth rate; the use of heat-tolerant *Bos indicus* cattle and provision of shade will help to limit this problem (Blackshaw & Blackshaw, 1994). Growth promoters have been linked to both heat stress susceptibility and the buller steer syndrome.

Beef cattle kept on extensive pasture are handled infrequently, and there is less opportunity to manage them or the pasture because of the large distances over which they range. Nevertheless, improved management can increase cattle growth and welfare by provision of better feed and water supplies. Increasing the number of watering points will encourage more even pasture utilisation. Rangelands are usually marginal lands which

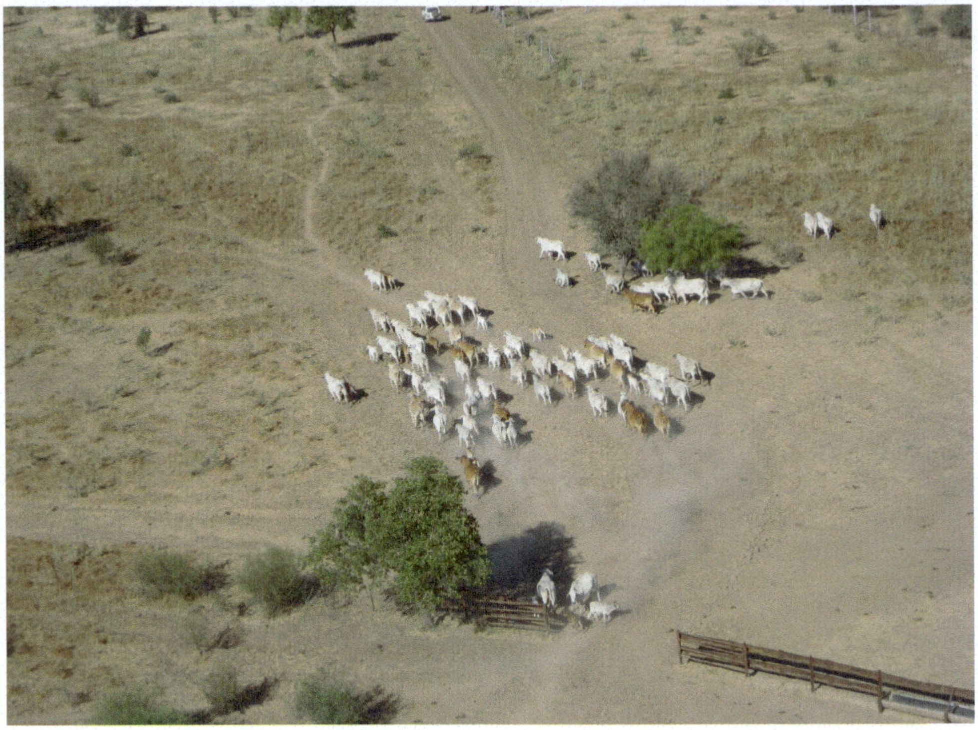

Figure 29.3 Cattle should not be hurried during mustering by helicopter, especially close to the yards. Reproduced with permission of AP Phillips.

are prone to weather extremes – in particular, drought. Mineral deficiencies, such as phosphorus, are common. Reducing stock numbers on rangeland allows feed stocks to build up and reduces susceptibility to drought. However, if necessary, cattle should be offered supplements, agisted to another region, or sold. All imply additional cost, and under-nutrition, particularly in times of drought, is a major issue for rangeland cattle.

Rangeland cattle are mustered from their paddocks by plane, helicopter (Figure 29.3), vehicle or on horseback. This can stress the cattle, especially if they are not allowed to slow down before entering handling facilities.

Operations deemed necessary are then performed, usually without anaesthetic:

(a) spaying young females, either per vagina or following a flank incision, to prevent breeding;
(b) dehorning by knife or cutters, to prevent cattle damaging themselves (Figure 29.4) or humans, or becoming stuck in fences and hedges;
(c) castration of males by knife or burdizzo to improve temperament; and
(d) identification by hot iron branding or ear marking.

All of these techniques stress cattle, but are necessary if they are to be kept on extensive rangelands.

Rangeland cattle are particularly prone to ectoparasites, especially flies, ticks and lice, which can reduce their welfare by disruption of grazing and resting behaviour and irritation of the skin. Control using parasiticides is hampered by the development of resistance in the parasites, and similar problems may eventually render parasiticides of little value. Selection for tick and disease resistance in livestock, and using of breeds with proven resistance, such as N'Dama and West African Shorthorn, offer a solution, even though they have lower productivity than breeds currently used.

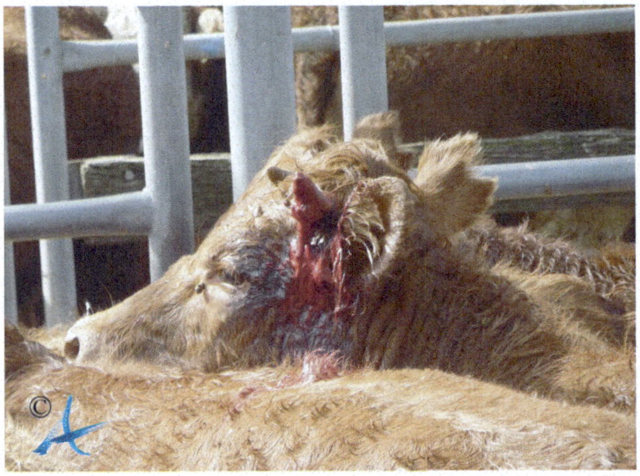

Figure 29.4 Dehorning with an anaesthetic at an early age is important to avoid pain and distress later. Reproduced with permission of Animal Angels.

Smallholder systems

Smallholdings are important systems of cattle management worldwide, particularly because so many people rely on them in developing countries. The public image of the welfare of the cattle is not as negative as it is for cattle in intensive management systems, but there are still welfare problems of significance. Provision of adequate pasture can be hindered by inadequate land resources, particularly in developing countries. In developing countries the ability to purchase veterinary medicines and feed supplements may be limited, but labour availability per animal is likely to be better than for intensive systems. Smallholders may be reluctant to sell cattle during drought, because they represent a capital asset. Smallholders often use oxen for field work or traction, and there is a constant risk of overwork or underfeeding. Working cattle have special nutritional requirements, such as increased sodium to replenish the salts lost during sweating. In developed countries, smallholders and hobby farmers may have limited knowledge and, sometimes, time, to deal with cattle welfare requirements.

Calves

Removal of the calf from the cow will result in separation distress unless it is done soon after birth (Flower & Weary, 2001), but ensuring that the calf suckles soon after birth is important for it to acquire the passive immunity needed to counteract infections. After removal, dairy calves may be kept in groups or individually, with normal interactions between calves supported only in groups. Infections are, however, spread more easily in groups. A good housing environment is important to prevent diarrhoea and pneumonia, both common diseases in poorly-ventilated, dirty sheds that are highly stocked with calves. Natural feeding behaviour is best promoted by offering a milk replacer via an artificial teat rather than a bucket.

In parts of the world where the dairy and beef industries use separate genetic stock, highly selected for their purpose, there is no use for male (bobby) calves born to dairy cows, and these are usually sent to slaughter within a week. Although, to many, this is primarily an ethical problem, the welfare of calves transported for perhaps a day without food or water causes concern. Hunger begins a few hours after their last feed, and will be acute by the time of slaughter. As they have not yet developed a herding behaviour, they can be difficult to move, and it is particularly important to avoid rough handling or the use of electric goads.

In extensive systems, beef calves are usually separated from their mothers at about six months, which results in stress to both for several days. Dairy calves used for meat production are mostly raised on artificial milk for periods of about six weeks, followed by forage feeding for up to 2–3 years. However, veal calves will remain on artificial milk for 3–6 months and will receive limited or no roughage, preventing the development of a functional rumen. Iron supply may be limited, and they are often housed in individual crates in dark conditions to restrict movement, in order to produce a pale meat that consumers like. Veal calves commonly develop stereotyped licking behaviour in response to the limited roughage supply. The European Union has introduced regulations to prevent the rearing of veal calves in this way.

Handling and transport

Electronic goads are frequently used to move cattle, but they cause a stress response and should only be used in emergencies, not routinely. Repeated use at critical points in a loading procedure (e.g. onto a ship) will result in animals arriving highly stressed and poorly prepared for their journey.

Good handling techniques require extensive training of stock people, using the animal's natural centre of balance at the shoulder to move them quietly and with minimum stress (Grandin & Deesing, 2008). Allowing them to move at their own pace is likely to prove the most efficient method in the long term.

Transport is often over long distances if cattle have been reared on rangelands far from their intended market. Loading and unloading are the most stressful times, and it is unwise to break the journey unless sufficient time is available for them to be adequately fed, watered and rested in clean, safe conditions. Maximum journey times vary considerably between jurisdictions, but may allow adult stock to be off water for transporting purposes for up to 48 hours, which includes mustering and holding in yards. Such long periods of transport result in animals that are stressed, tired and hungry at the end of their journey. Overcrowding of transport vehicles will increase the stress to the animals, which need space around them to get an adequate footing to avoid slipping during the movement of the vehicle (Figure 29.5).

Animals that are too thin should not be transported (Figure 29.6). Transport over long distances by ship is increasingly common, and involves potential stressors of ship movement during high seas, excessive heat and accumulation of ammonia from excreta. International transport of animals has the added risk of sending cattle to countries with different management standards from those of the country of origin.

Slaughter

Slaughtering cattle requires them to be effectively restrained, which is not possible unless there are adequate handling facilities. Cattle from rangelands that are not used to regular handling, and cattle that have been stressed by long journeys, will be more difficult to restrain. The final process in what is often a long and stressful journey is the stunning by a captive bolt, fired into the head to end brain function. The animal loses consciousness and is then shackled by a chain, hoisted up by its hind leg and its throat is cut with a sharp knife. The resulting exsanguination causes the heart to stop beating. There are occasions when sticking is not completed soon enough and

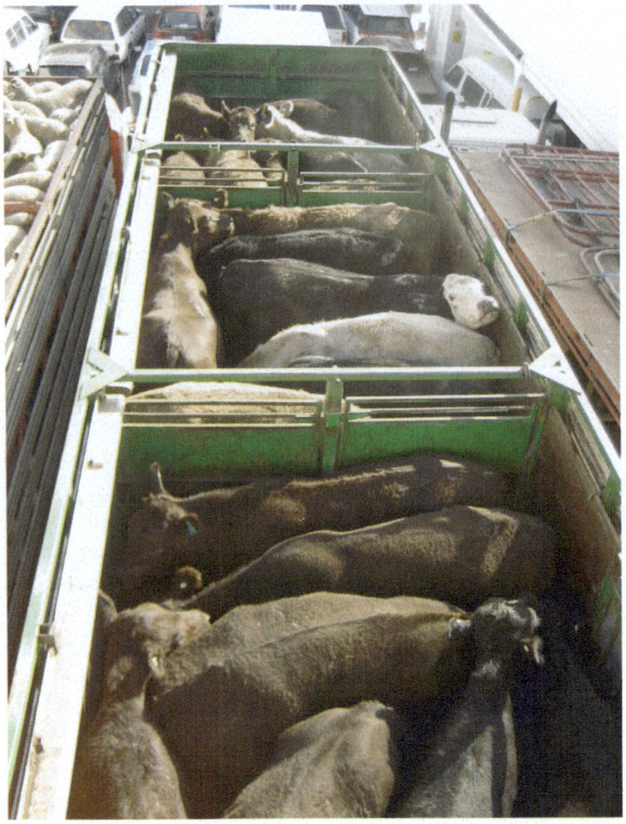

Figure 29.5 Overstocking of cattle vehicles should be avoided.

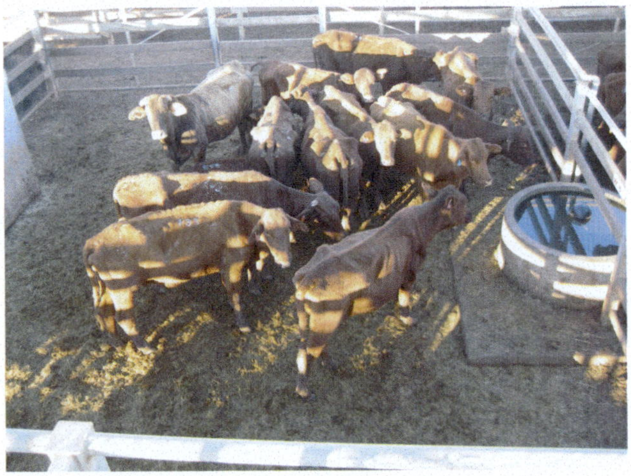

Figure 29.6 Excessively thin cattle at sale yard during drought period.

cattle, especially calves, may regain consciousness, or clots at the severed ends of the carotid arteries delay exsanguination and maintain brain function.

Religious slaughter for the Muslim and Jewish faiths usually prevents the use of stunning, requiring the animal to die by the knife cut to the throat. This usually requires the cattle to be cast beforehand, which is a cause of significant stress. Because a blood supply to the brain is maintained by the vertebral arteries after the throat is cut, the animal remains conscious for typically about one minute afterwards, and sometimes for several minutes.

Conclusions

Cattle have been domesticated as one of our major animal protein providers, but the farming systems utilised in many parts of the world are causing serious concern for the welfare of the animals. Veterinarians should play a vital role in supporting the welfare of livestock by treating disease, monitoring their health and supporting management improvements to meet welfare standards that consumers are increasingly requiring.

References

Blackshaw, J.K. and Blackshaw, A.W. (1994). Heat stress in cattle and the effect of shade on production and behaviour: a review. *Australian Journal of Experimental Agriculture* **34**, 285–295.

Flower, F.C. and Weary, D.M. (2001). Effects of early separation on the dairy cow and calf: 2. Separation at 1 day and 2 weeks after birth. *Applied Animal Behaviour Science* **70**, 275–284.

Grandin, T. and Deesing, M. (2008). *Humane Livestock Handling*. Storey Publishing, North Adams, MA, USA.

Hagen, K. and Broom, D.M. (2004). Emotional reactions to learning in cattle. *Applied Animal Behaviour Science* **85**, 203–213.

Useful sources of information

Broom, D.M and Fraser, A.F. (2007). *Domestic Animal Behaviour and Welfare*, 4th edition. CAB International, Wallingford, UK.

Grandin, T. (2007). *Livestock Handling and Transport*. 3rd edition. CAB International, Wallingford, UK.

Phillips, C.J.C. (2002). *Cattle Behaviour and Welfare*. Blackwell's Scientific, Oxford, UK.

Phillips, C.J.C. (2010). *Principles of Cattle Production*. 2nd edition. CAB International, Wallingford, UK.

Rushen, J., de Passille, A.M., von Keyserlingk, M.A.G. and Weary. D.M. (2008). *The Welfare of Cattle*. Springer, Dordrecht, the Netherlands.

CHAPTER 30

Rumen Health in the Dairy Cow

Dai Grove-White

Learning objectives

- Understand the basic physiology of rumen fermentation.
- Understand pathogenesis and the differences between acute, chronic and sub-acute ruminal acidosis.
- Be able to recognise the clinical signs of sub-acute ruminal acidosis.
- Understand how to monitor for SARA using rumen fluid samples from targeted groups of at-risk cows.
- Understand how to prevent and control SARA.

Introduction

Herbivorous animals enlist microorganisms to aid in the digestion of plant materials such as cellulose and hemi-celluloses. The ruminant forestomachs, namely the rumen and reticulum, have evolved to allow fermentation of foodstuffs, with the end products being: volatile fatty acids (VFAs), which are absorbed across the rumen wall; microbial protein, which undergoes further digestion in the abomasum and small intestine; together with certain vitamins, chiefly of the B group, which are absorbed further downstream.

A limited amount of digestion and absorption of short chain carbohydrates, proteins and lipids occurs in the small intestine. Hind-gut fermentation is of relatively minor importance in ruminants (unlike the horse), and essentially deals with carbohydrates that have 'escaped' ruminal fermentation or small intestinal digestion. Thus, over-exuberant colonic fermentation may occur, associated with sub-optimal rumen fermentation, thereby contributing to the clinical picture seen in sub-acute ruminal acidosis (SARA).

The rumen microflora is a complex ecosystem comprising archaea, bacteria, protozoa and fungi. While the bacteria are chiefly concerned with breakdown of carbohydrates and proteins, the archaea are the main contributors to methane production, utilising hydrogen produced by bacteria and protozoa for the reduction of CO_2 to CH_4, with protozoa involved in digestion of carbohydrates and proteins as well as phagocytosis of bacteria. It must be appreciated that the ecosystem is dynamic, and will change in response to dietary constituents fed. In essence, the maintenance of rumen health may be thought of as ensuring the health and suitability of the microflora for the presented diet.

Rumen acidosis

It must be appreciated that the fate of all ingested carbohydrates is fermentation to volatile fatty acids; thus, the rumen may be thought of as a vat of weak acids. Maintaining the rumen fluid pH at the optimal level, between 6.0–6.4, is a considerable challenge in the high-producing ruminant, due to the massive amounts of acid being produced. At this point, it is worth bearing in mind that the high yielding dairy cow may have energy requirements in excess of four times maintenance requirements.

Rumen acidosis is generally recognised to occur when the pH falls below a threshold of 5.5. Rumen VFAs have a pK_a value of about 4.9 meaning that the VFAs will shift towards the undissociated form at pH values below 5.5, thereby removing protons from the fluid. Furthermore, since VFAs are absorbed in the undissociated form, absorption will be encouraged at this pH. These phenomena are key components of the homeostatic mechanisms operating in the rumen. However, these efforts at homeostasis may be offset by the production of lactic acid by *Streptococcus bovis* and *Lactobacilli* spp. if high levels of starch and sugars are present.

Lactic acid, a strong acid with a pK_a of 3.9, will be considerably less dissociated at pH 5.0 than other VFAs and will contribute to a downward spiral in rumen pH, since it cannot be removed by absorption (by virtue of being dissociated). Furthermore, growth of lactate-utilising bacteria such as *Megasphaera*

Bovine Medicine, Third Edition. Edited by Peter D. Cockcroft.

elsdenii and *Selemonasruminatium* is impaired as pH falls, thus further reducing lactate removal. The end result is a failure to maintain a stable optimal pH, the most common manifestation of sub-optimal rumen health.

Ruminal acidosis is generally categorised into three clinical entities although there is considerable overlap

Acute rumen acidosis or grain overload

This occurs when animals have sudden access to large amounts of highly fermentable sugars or carbohydrates resulting in consumption of large amounts. Rumen pH falls rapidly to ≈ 5.2, with the development of concurrent metabolic acidosis, dehydration and endotoxaemia (due to leakage of bacterial endotoxins across the damaged rumen epithelium). Lactic acid-producing bacteria such as *Streptococcus bovis* and *Lactobacilli* spp. proliferate, while there is a reduction in the populations of lactate-metabolising bacteria such as *Selenomonas ruminantium*, with the net result being the production and accumulation of large amounts of lactic acid. Affected animals are depressed and ataxic, with ruminal bloat and diarrhoea. Recumbency ensues, and this may be followed by death.

In the event of an outbreak, it is advisable to triage the animals, with severe cases undergoing rumenotomy to remove all rumen contents, accompanied by intravenous therapy with five litres of 5% sodium bicarbonate, followed by balanced isotonic fluids such as Hartmann's solution. Less severe cases should receive intravenous alkalinising therapy, together with a ruminal antacid such as 500 g of aluminium hydroxide or magnesium oxide. All animals should be fed good quality hay. There is considerable debate about the advisability or otherwise of restricting water intake in cases of acute rumen acidosis, on the grounds that giving water will increase the systemic absorption of lactic acid.

Chronic acidosis

This is seen in feedlot cattle fed high grain low forage diets. Cases of acute acidosis will also be seen often following a change or disruption of feeding regime. Chronic acidosis in feedlot situations is associated with a high incidence of liver abcessation, associated with haematogenous spread of *Fusiformis necrophorum* via the portal vein.

Sub-acute ruminal acidosis (SARA)

The amount of dietary energy required by the modern dairy cow to support increased milk yield has necessitated feeding higher and higher levels of carbohydrates. This may be achieved in two ways: first, by increasing the amount of food consumed by the cow (i.e. increasing her Dry Matter Intake (DMI), thereby increasing the total amount of carbohydrate consumed), and second by increasing the energy density (M/D) in the diet while DMI remains the same. This latter approach dramatically increases the risk of SARA, due to the increasing concentration of VFAs which will be present in the rumen. The concentrations of VFAs in the rumen at any given time point will depend on the balance between three processes:

- Rate of production of VFAs. This will depend on the dietary carbohydrate make-up, with short-chain starches and sugars being fermented more rapidly than long-chain starches, celluloses and hemi-celluloses. Traditionally, short-chain starches and sugars are often referred to as the Fermentable Metabolisable Energy (FME) fraction of the diet.
- Rate of absorption of VFAs across the rumen wall. This will depend on the integrity of the wall and papillary size and health. It must be borne in mind that low ruminal pH will damage the wall, thereby inducing the potential of a positive feedback loop with respect to future episodes of SARA.
- Buffering of rumen VFAs. Copious amounts of saliva are produced by the cow during rumination (chewing the cud), and the salivary sodium bicarbonate and phosphate act to buffer the rumen. A healthy cudding cow will produce up to 3.5 kg of sodium bicarbonate daily, which represents considerable buffering capacity. However, rumination is consequent of the amount of long fibre in the diet.

Lactic acid acidosis is not a marked feature of SARA, with the acidosis primarily being due to high VFA concentrations, unlike acute ruminal acidosis.

Case definition and clinical signs of SARA

SARA is a herd diagnosis and should not usually be used to describe the condition of an individual cow. In fact, in any herd, there will always be a small proportion of cows whose rumen pH is below the threshold taken to indicate a diagnosis of SARA (this may be thought of as a consequence of the normal distribution of any parameter where a few values are in the 'tail' areas). A case definition of SARA adopted by many (Nordlund, 2001) is one-third of animals in the at-risk group having rumen pH values less than 5.5 at a given point in time.

Generally, at-risk animals are considered to be those in early lactation (within 21 days of calving) and cows at peak Dry Matter Intake (DMI) (10–14 weeks post-calving). The former group is at risk due to lack of ruminal adaption to the high energy lactating diet and, possibly, reduced absorption of VFAs across the rumen wall, due to poor dry cow management. The latter group is at risk due to the sheer amount of VFAs produced at peak intake overwhelming the buffering and absorptive capacity of the rumen.

The clinical signs associated with SARA are vague and on many farms are likely to be accepted as being 'normal'. The key signs, which are rarely recognised are *decreased DMI and reduced feed conversion efficiency (FCE)* (Garrett *et al.*, 1999), associated with sub-optimal rumen function. It should be borne in mind that a healthy Holstein cow fed a TMR should be able to consume up to 4% of her body weight daily (DMI) at peak milk production. Thus, for a group of high-yielding Holstein cows in the first half of lactation, average DMI should be in the region of 26 kg daily.

In SARA, fibre digestion by the rumen falls due to the change in microflora thereby reducing FCE. Other signs are:

- *Variable faecal consistency* among the group, with many cows having loose faeces. This is likely a consequence of colonic fermentation of undigested foodstuffs and subsequent osmotic diarrhoea. It may be accompanied by the passing of fibrin casts, indicative of severe colonic inflammation due to a colonic acidosis (2° to the ruminal acidosis).
- *Cows are excessively dirty*, often with soiling of the rump due to tail swishing consequent to irritation of the perineal area by acidic faeces and urine. However, there are many other causes of dirty cows, and these should be investigated (e.g. housing conditions).
- *Frequent cases of 'cows off their food'* with no other clear presenting signs. These usually resolve in 48 hours as rumen pH normalises.
- *High incidence of digestive disease*, including displacement of the abomasum.
- *Liver abcessation, endocarditis and pulmonary thromboembolism* are common sequelae to rumen wall damage associated with SARA.
- *Lameness.* There is increased evidence that bacterial endotoxin (LPS), histamine and other inflammatory mediators may be released into (or enter) the circulation (Plazier *et al*, 2009), and these are thought to play an important role in general ill health and immuno-suppression in affected herds. This may in part be the mechanism whereby SARA is associated with laminitis, leading to a high prevalence of foot lameness, although there is often a time lag between the episode of SARA and subsequent lameness.
- *Excessive weight loss in early lactation* as a consequence of the reduced DMI and FCE. This is often accompanied by ketosis (sub-clinical and possibly clinical), with poor reproductive performance being an inevitable consequence of this chain of events.
- *Milk yield and composition.* Milk yield is likely to be reduced, although this is often not recognised on affected farms as being associated with SARA; rather, it is what the farmer expects on his farm (!). Butterfat content of milk is usually reduced in SARA and, traditionally, this has been thought to be due to reduced production of acetate from fibre digestion in the rumen. However, recent work suggests this may not be the complete picture, with interference with ruminal biohydrogenation of fatty acids also playing a role (Bauman & Griinari, 2001). With the increased popularity of on-line milk component recording, the milk fat : protein ratio has been used for herd level diagnosis of ketosis, with high fats in early lactation cows suggestive of ketosis. In a similar vein, some consultants have suggested that inversion of this ratio can be used for herd-level diagnosis of SARA, indicating low butterfat content. This is unwise, since the effect, if any, of SARA on milk protein is unknown.
- *Environmental mastitis.* This is a consequence of the increased faecal soiling associated with loose faeces, coupled with immune-suppression associated with both SARA and negative energy balance.

Risk factors for sub-acute ruminal acidosis

The condition of SARA is the most frequently diagnosed nutritional disorder of dairy cows. It is chiefly recognised as a problem associated with housed cattle and relatively high levels of concentrate feeding, classically affecting cattle in the first 150 days of lactation. However, it is now recognised in pasture grazed animals (Westwood, 2003) associated with high levels of fermentable sugars and low levels of physically effective fibre in lush pastures.

Risk factors for SARA may be grouped as follows:

1. *Factors leading to excessive intake of rapidly fermentable carbohydrates*, allowing VFA production to occur at an excessive rate, such that concentrations build up, leading to a change in flora and a fall in rumen fluid pH.
2. *Factors leading to inadequate intake of sufficient physically effective fibre* for stimulation of cudding and formation of an adequate rumen fibre mat.
3. *Factors resulting in sub-optimal rates of absorption of VFAs* across the rumen wall.
4. *Factors resulting in a sub-optimal rumen flora* for the diet currently fed.

Diet formulation, in terms of concentrate-to-forage ratio, is absolutely critical in ensuring both that adequate physically effective long fibre is fed, and that excessive short-chain carbohydrates are not fed. In part, diet formulation is a consequence of known (or anticipated) dry matter intake since, for a given milk yield, a certain amount of dietary energy is required. The greater the DMI of the animals, then the lower the energy density of the supplied diet can be, thus reducing the likelihood of SARA.

In this context, dry period nutrition is of critical importance. It is increasingly recognised that even moderate over-feeding in the dry period, in particular during the last 2–3 weeks pre-calving, can have dramatic effects in terms of fat deposition and reduced DMI post-calving. Energy intake in the late dry period should not be greater than about 110 MJ per cow per day. A particular problem relates to cows gaining weight in late lactation. While this is not immediately recognised as a risk factor for SARA, it results in reduced DMI during both the dry period and early lactation, both of which serve to increase the risk of SARA.

Similarly, adaption to the lactating diet in the first 14–21 days after calving is of critical importance. Introduction of freshly calved cows to a high-energy lactating diet, for example formulated at an energy density of M/D 12.3 MJ/Kg DMI (as might be fed to cows yielding up to 50+ litres daily) carries a high likelihood of inducing an episode of SARA, due to the cow's lack of prior ruminal adaption to the diet. An episode of SARA at this time will have a deleterious effect on her rumen flora and wall, thus inducing a vicious cycle, characterised by further bouts of SARA. It is advisable to feed a diet of lower energy density during this period (e.g. M/D 11.2–11.5). This may be achieved easily by diluting the lactating diet with straw or hay for the first 14–21 after calving. The nutritional objective at this stage of the production cycle should be to stimulate the cow's DMI, rather than keep up with her energy requirements for production *per se*.

Incorrect feeding and management during the dry period is a major risk factor for SARA, due to the impact of incorrect feeding on rumen papillar development and functionality. Optimal development and functionality is associated with feeding diets that will produce propionate and butyrate in the last few weeks. This is the basis of transition diets, whereby moderate amounts of starches or sugars are fed in the last three weeks of the dry period, to encourage both development of a rumen flora suitable for the lactation diet and ensure papillar development. However, it is critical that energy is not over-fed at this time, due to its deleterious effect on subsequent DMI, as mentioned previously.

Rumen microflora health and suitability for a given diet will be adversely impacted by numerous factors, including frequent, large changes in dietary composition which, by their nature, may induce SARA, thereby severely damaging the integrity of the microflora. As a general rule, it takes three weeks for the microflora to adapt to a dietary change. Certain mycotoxins may have an adverse effect on the microflora and thus be implicated in SARA, although confirmation of their presence and impact is notoriously hard to demonstrate.

Influence of feeding systems on risk of SARA

As well as diet formulation and preparation, the method of presentation of the diet is critical. Three feeding systems will be considered:

- *Component-based systems*, whereby fodder and concentrates are fed separately. Fodder may be grazed grass or silage (or a mix of silages), fed at a feed barrier if cows are housed with concentrates fed as boluses often in the milking parlour. This practice of twice-daily concentrate feeding is not without risk, since the ingestion of large 'slugs' of short-chain carbohydrates (concentrates) will inevitably be followed by a rapid fall in rumen pH. If this fall is excessive, then SARA will result. Thus, it is advisable not to feed more than 2–3 kg of concentrate at any time. This will limit the use of such management systems in high-yielding herds, where greater intakes of energy are required. An increasingly popular system in the UK is 'out of parlour concentrate feeders', in which the cows visit such feeders and are fed pre-programmed amounts of concentrates throughout the day. Such systems can be programmed to deliver, for example, 10 kg of concentrate in boluses no greater than 1 kg, with cows not allowed to be fed more than a certain amount during a given time. Such systems will minimise the risk of SARA, while allowing individual feeding of cows according to milk yield or other criteria. This system has considerable attraction for the smaller herd, where Total Mixed Ration feeding may be problematic.
- *Total Mixed Rations (TMR).* As herd sizes have increased, there has been a shift from individual cow feeding, as exemplified by the component-based systems, to group feeding of lactating cows, whereby all components are fed together as a complete diet. In theory, if not always in practice, it should be possible to feed all lactating cows, apart from the freshly calved cows which are still transitioning from the dry cow diet to the lactating diet (see earlier), on one diet. This should be possible, since cows will self-regulate in that DMI is dependant in part on milk yield; thus, as cows yield more, they will eat more, and *vice versa*. However, in reality, this is often not the case, with late-lactation cows becoming excessively fat, so many farmers will group cows by yield or stage of lactation, and feed diets of differing energy densities. The TMR feeding, if carried out correctly, will increase dry matter intakes and minimise pH fluctuations, thereby ensuring a stable microflora and reducing the risk of SARA. However, success of TMR feeding depends critically not only on formulation and delivery of the diet, with particular attention being paid to fibre length and the risk of sorting, but also on all other aspects of the cow's environment, such as space, comfort, social grouping and time budgeting, all of which impact on DMI and thus SARA risk (Figures 30.1 and 30.2).
- *Hybrid systems.* Such systems revolve around feeding a TMR for a given production level at the feed barrier, and feeding extra concentrate in the milking parlour if the cow produces above this production level. Such systems are theoretically flawed, and represent a considerable risk in terms of SARA (Figure 30.3). First, dietary substitution will occur, in that cows fed extra concentrate in the milking parlour will consume less at the feed barrier, thus consuming more short-chain carbohydrate and less forage. Second, even relatively small slugs of concentrate will depress rumen pH when fed alongside a diet of high M/D. Finally, it may be argued that such a system is incompatible with maximising

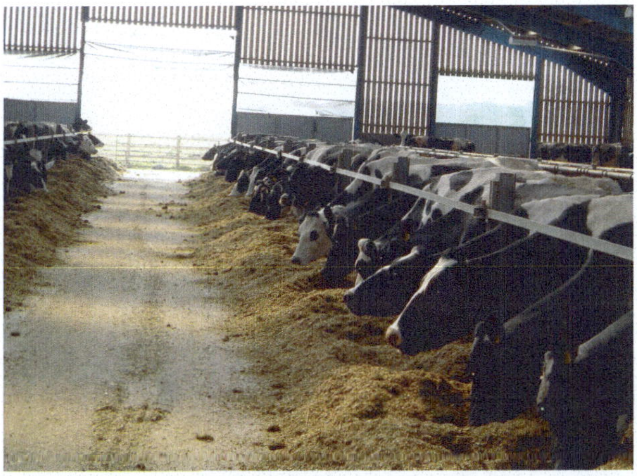

Figure 30.1 Feeding a suitable TMR ration at a well designed feed barrier minimises perturbations in rumen pH.

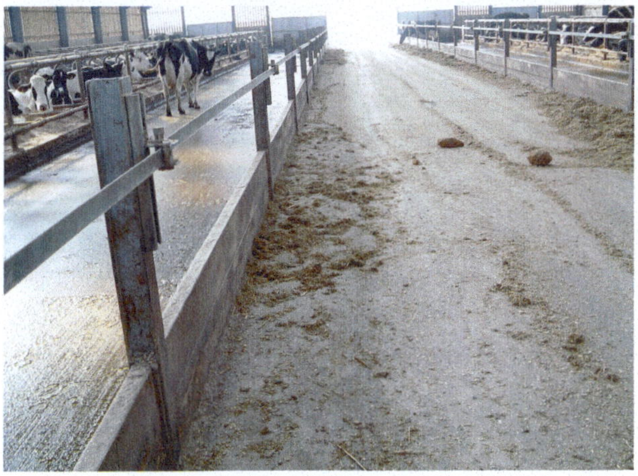

Figure 30.2 Food must be available at all times. Food deprivation, even for short periods, impacts adversely on the rumen microflora.

DMI, which should be the primary objective of all feeding strategies in early lactation.

Diagnosis of SARA

As should be apparent, the signs associated with SARA are largely non-specific, but may offer clues as to the likelihood of SARA. Key steps in arriving at a diagnosis are:

1 *Assessment of diet, environment and management practices.* This must include all stages of the production cycle, especially the dry cows – not only the production group where SARA is suspected. Diets must be evaluated for peNDF and quality of mixing as well as composition. Evaluation of the diet collected at differing times through the day will demonstrate whether sorting is occurring, although careful observation of cows eating will also show this.

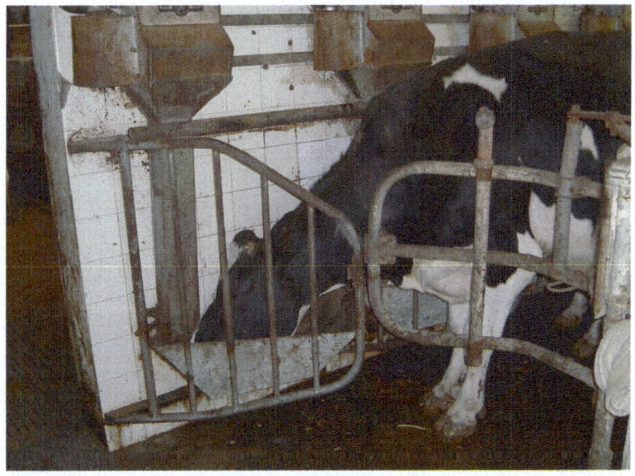

Figure 30.3 Twice-daily feeding of large amounts of concentrates in the milking parlour is a major risk factor for SARA, especially if combined with TMR feeding (hybrid TMR feeding).

2 *Assessment of cows.* The following should be assessed:
   a. Condition score (CS) and changes in CS throughout lactation.
   b. Rumen fill.
   c. Rumination. At least 60% of cows should be cudding if not eating or sleeping.
   d. Dirt scores (Hughes, 2001), indicating the pattern of faecal soiling.
   e. Overall appearance of cows. Dull, staring coats are often associated with SARA, although this is often only appreciated retrospectively.
   f. Milk production and quality records.
   g. Health records, including locomotion scoring if carried out.
   h. Examination of faeces. This is a two-stage process. First, assessing faecal score on as many pats as possible; variability in score is suggestive of SARA. Second, faecal pats (ideally 20–30) should be collected and sieved under running water. The presence of long fibre (>2.0 cm) and large amounts of undigested grains are suggestive of SARA (Figures 30.4a, 30.4b and 30.4c). However, care is required in interpretation of sieve results, since the presence of some grains is normal in faeces from high yielding cows. It must also be borne in mind that poor processing of preserved crops may result in the passage of undigested grains (e.g. poor 'cracking' of maize grains during ensiling).

Rumenocentesis

The gold standard for diagnosis of SARA is rumenocentesis on a random selection of cows in the at-risk group (Garrett *et al.*, 1999). It is a herd-based test, and correct animal selection is

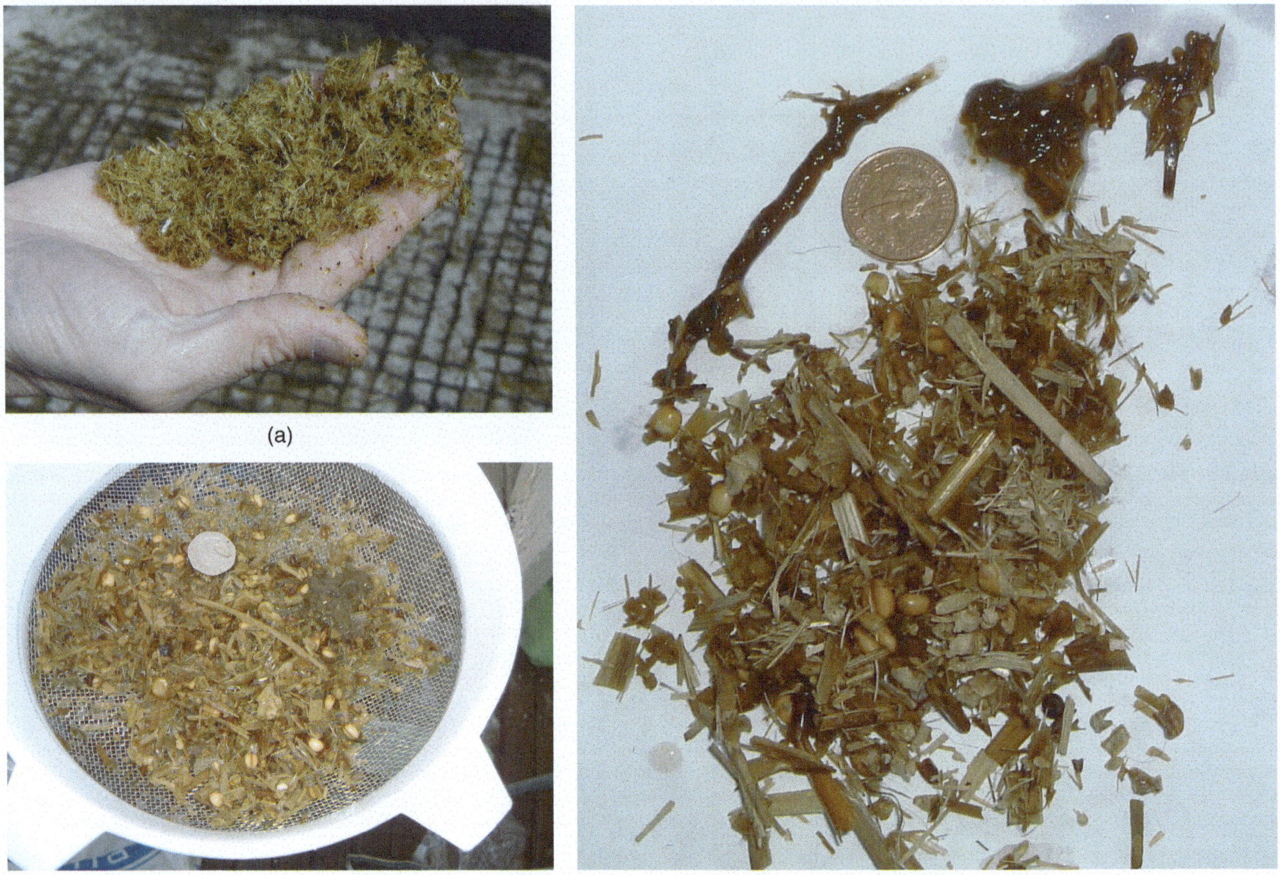

(a) (b) (c)

Figure 30.4 Faecal sieving.
(a) Short fibre length and almost complete absence of grains in faeces indicate good rumen function.
(b) Presence of long fibre, undigested grains are indicative of SARA.
(c) Presence of mucin casts suggest excessive colonic fermentation secondary to SARA.

key to achieving a correct diagnosis. The timing of sampling is critical, with the intention being to sample when pH is at its nadir. In the case of cows fed a TMR only, this is about 6–10 hours after feeding while, in the case of cows fed concentrates separately (e.g. parlour feeding), they should be sampled 2–3 hours after feeding.

A minimum of 12 cows should be sampled, although sampling more animals may be advantageous in both arriving at a diagnosis and determining the cause; for example, if 12 fresh calved cows and 12 cows at peak lactation are sampled, it may give insight as to whether the problem is due to diet formulation or due to poor transitioning in early lactation. Cook *et al.* (2006) suggest that whilst a definitive diagnosis may be arrived at if five out of 12 cows sampled have a rumen pH less than 5.5, a herd should be considered borderline if two out of 12 cows have a pH less than 5.5. Other workers have suggested that pH < 5.8 may be suggestive of SARA (O'Grady *et al.*, 2008).

Prevention and treatment of SARA

In essence, this involves attending to the risk factors identified on any particular farm. While many factors are relatively straightforward to rectify, such as dietary composition (providing suitable dietary components are available), others, such as prevention of sorting, may require considerable ingenuity, such as adding water or molasses to the TMR diet to ensure that constituents do not separate. Addition of alfalfa hay to the diet is almost 'first aid', in that it can offer dramatic improvements in outbreaks associated with lack of peNDF.

Sodium bicarbonate (100–400 g per head daily) is often fed in TMR diets to minimise SARA, but it is relatively unpalatable and may reduce DMI at higher levels of feeding. Similarly, yeast-based additives may be fed in an attempt to minimise SARA. However, such methods are often palliative in nature, and response may be variable.

Box 30.1 Dietary long fibre

With the requirement to feed high levels of starches and sugars to ruminants in order to satisfy energy requirements for production, the issue of adequacy of long fibre has become increasingly important. To ensure optimal rumen health, the diet must contain sufficient long fibre to stimulate rumination, in order to produce sufficient saliva for buffering. In addition, there must be adequate long fibre to ensure the presence of an adequate fibre mat floating on the top of the liquid rumen contents. This mat serves both as a 'home' for much of the microflora, and as a trap for food particles, allowing their breakdown by the rumen microflora.

Long fibre is generally defined as fibre greater that 2.5 cm (1'') in length. While structural carbohydrates (fibre) in the diet has traditionally been described in terms of 'neutral detergent fibre' (NDF) and 'acid detergent fibre' (ADF), such measures, as presented in a dietary analysis, offer no information as to the physical composition of the fibre source. Consequently the concept of 'physically effective fibre' (peNDF) has been introduced to account for the physical structure of NDF. However, peNDF is hard to quantify, and estimation of peNDF of a forage is carried out by visual inspection of fibre length, or by sieving dietary component – for example, a silage, or the complete Total Mixed Ration (TMR) diet using a Penn State Forage Particle Separator (Pennsylvania State University).

Guidelines are available for diets fed in the USA (http://extension.psu.edu/animals/dairy/health/nutrition/forages/forage-quality-physical/separator), but caution must be taken in interpreting these guidelines for other diets, especially those based on grass silages. Analysis of such diets with the Penn State Forage Particle Separator may be problematic due to 'balling' of the forage if it is relatively wet, stopping it passing through the sieve holes. Air drying of the sample for 12–24 hours can aid in preventing this balling. However, if air drying of rations is carried out, the change in dry matter content must be accounted for in any dietary calculations performed after analysis.

Silage making involves anaerobic fermentation of forages with optimal fermentation and preservation occurring with small forage chop lengths. Thus, there is a tendency for silages to be cut short, thereby reducing the peNDF. This is particularly so in the case of maize silage, which is cut short and pulverised to ensure grain cracking. This dramatically reduces the effectiveness of maize silage as a fibre source, thus increasing the risk of SARA if high levels are included in diets. In the UK, many farmers will aim for a longer chop length for second and third cut grass silages, thereby increasing their value as a source of peNDF, albeit at the expense of energy yield, while retaining a shorter chop length for the first cut silage, thereby maximising its energy yield, albeit at the expense of peNDF. Increasingly, hay or straw is included in TMR diets, in amounts ranging from 0.5–2.0 kg per head, as a means of ensuring optimal rumen health. Alfalfa hay is of particular value in this respect, acting both as a long fibre source and as a ruminal buffer by virtue of its ability to bind protons.

Box 30.2 The four diets fed to cows

Classically it is said that there are four diets a cow may be fed. The art of feeding dairy cows is in ensuring all four diets are the same. This is highly pertinent in the case of SARA.

1. *Diet formulated by the nutritionist.* There are numerous guidelines regarding NDF, starch, and sugar levels that should be fed to the cow and software programs allowing diet formulation according to various systems (e.g. Nett Energy (NE), Metabolisable Energy (ME), Feed into Milk (FiM), etc). Diets are formulated based on a given DMI which often is not known but rather is assumed. This can lead to major 'errors' in diet formulation, for example, if the cows eat more/less than what has been assumed. Furthermore, in formulating diets, many assumptions are made regarding the nutritional composition of dietary constituents (e.g. the dry matter (% DM) and energy content (MJ/kg DM of ME)). The impact of errors in estimating these basic values can be vast; for example, if the nutritionist assumes the dry matter of a silage content to be 30%, when in reality it is 25%, this would result in gross underfeeding by 16% of that silage. Such an error would imbalance the fodder : concentrate ratio and likely increase the risk of SARA. Constant regular evaluation of nutritional content and dry matter content of fodder crops throughout the feeding period is advisable.
2. *Diet fed by the farmer to the cows.* Of particular importance here is the issue of mixing of TMR rations in a mixer wagon, both in terms of accuracy of weighing of the quantity of ingredients to be added to the food mix and in terms of the mixing process itself. Insufficient mixing will lead to diets which are amenable to sorting by the cows, whereby cows select certain constituents to ingest (as a rule, these will be the high-energy concentrate fractions). Sorting of diets is a major risk factor for SARA. Over-mixing of the ration will destroy the integrity of the fibre components, thereby reducing the physically effective fibre in the diet, and so increasing the risk of SARA.
3. *Diet the cows actually receive.* Major issues to consider here are the availability of the food to the cows. Key factors are the space available at the feed barrier or bunk. Cows are social eaters, in that they will eat together at the same time, thus sufficient space should be available for all cows to eat at the same time, and it is recommended that 0.6–0.7 m of barrier space per cow is available. Positioning of the actual feed barrier is also critical for ensuring maximal DMI. The barrier should be at least 1.3 m high and offset 20–30 cm forward. Food must be pushed up to the feed barrier, such that it is available at all times; thus, ideally it should be pushed up 6–8 times daily. Anecdotally, the act of pushing the food up to the barrier will encourage increased feeding activity in its own right, so increasing DMI and rumen health. Most farmers feed once daily, although evidence suggests that twice daily feeding may increase DMI. Irrespective of this, there should always be food in front of the cows, such that 5% is remaining prior to the next feed. This should be removed and either disposed off or fed to other classes of stock (e.g. fattening animals); it must not be fed to dry cows or growing heifers, since it is unsuitable for these in terms of energy content. Food deprivation, even for a few hours, has a deleterious effect on the rumen flora, reducing the population of lactate-consuming microbes and thus increasing the risk of SARA.
4. *Diet the cows actually need.* While this is impossible to truly know, the impact of the diet can be assessed in terms of health and productivity. Monitoring of condition score changes during lactation, faecal consistency and rumen fill, milk quality, yield and health events, will help in this judgement.

Box 30.3 Rumenocentesis

Technique for rumenocentesis (Grove-White, 2004):

Samples of rumen fluid may easily be collected from the ventral sac of the rumen using a 4–5 inch 16G or 18G needle (e.g. Air-Tite Products, 565 Central Drive, Virginia Beach, VA 23454, USA), or a 3.5'' 18G spinal needle. The collection site is at the level of the stifle joint 4–5 inches caudal to the last rib. The site should be clipped and prepared with chlorhexidine or povidone-iodine solution prior to collection. Adequate restraint is essential, and it is advisable to have one person lift the tail, while another person holds the nose. Administration of local anaesthetic is advisable but not essential. The needle is thrust through the skin and abdominal wall into the rumen, and a small (2–4 ml) amount of rumen fluid withdrawn (Figure 30.5). If the needle becomes clogged, it may be cleared by pushing air through it into the rumen (N.B. negative pressure should not be applied, since this may produce false readings). Rumen pH is best determined using a portable pH meter (e.g. Cardy Twin pH meter: Spectrum Technologies, Plainfield, Illinois 60544, USA). The use of pH indicator papers is not recommended, due to difficulties in interpreting colour changes.

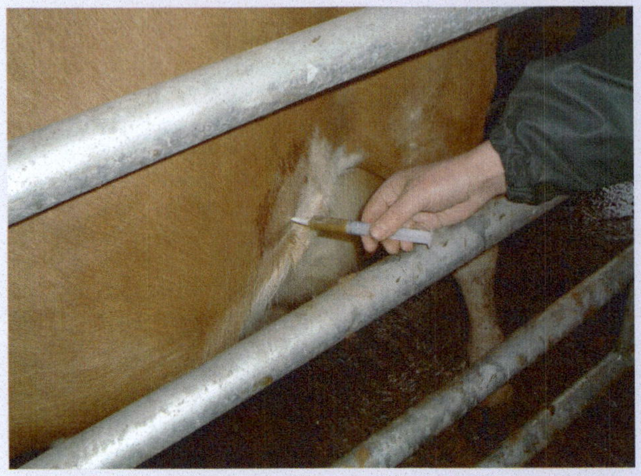

Figure 30.5 Site for performing rumenocentesis.

Key to successful prevention is regular reviewing of diets and constituents, ideally with regular analyses of components. Farmer education in recognition of signs and in use of simple tools, such as faecal scoring and sieving, can pay dividends in prevention. There is considerable research interest in indwelling ruminal pH monitors that would allow continuous monitoring, but these are not yet available commercially.

References

Bauman, D.E. and Griinari, J.M. (2001). Regulation and nutritional manipulation of milk fat: low fat milk syndrome. *Livestock Production Science* **17**, 15–29.

Cook, N., Oetzel, G. and Nordlund, K. (2006). Modern techniques for monitoring high-producing dairy cows 2. Practical applications. *In Practice* **28**, 598–603.

Garrett, E.F., Pereira, M.N., Nordlund, K.V., Armentano, W.J., Goodger, W.J. and Oetzel, G.R. (1999). Diagnostic methods for the detection of subacute ruminal acidosis in dairy cows. *Journal of Dairy Science* **82**, 1170–1178.

Grove-White, D. (2004). Rumen healthcare in the dairy cow. *In Practice* **26**, 88–95.

Hughes, J. (2001). A system for assessing cow cleanliness. *In Practice* **23**, 517–524.

Nordlund, K.V. (2001). *Herd Based diagnosis of subacute ruminal acidosis.* Pre-Convention Seminar B: Dairy Herd Problem Investigations. 34th Annual Convention of the American Association of Bovine Practitioners, Vancouver, Canada.

O'Grady, L., Doherty, M.L. and Mulligan, F.J. (2008). Subacute ruminal acidosis (SARA) in grazing Irish dairy cows. *The Veterinary Journal* **176**, 44–49.

Plazier J.C., Krause, D.O., Gozho, G.N. and McBride, B.W. (2009). Subacute ruminal acidosis in dairy cows: The physiological causes, incidence and consequences. *The Veterinary Journal* **176**, 23–31.

Westwood C,T., Bramley, E. and Lean, I.L. (2003). Review of the relationship between nutrition and lameness in pasture-fed dairy cattle. *New Zealand Veterinary Journal* **51**, 145–156.

CHAPTER 31

Genetics for the Bovine Practitioner

Nicholas N. Jonsson and Emily K. Piper

Learning objectives

- To understand the genetic basis of modern cattle breeds.
- To understand the principles of parentage testing.
- To recognise the range of inherited diseases in cattle.
- To appreciate the heritability of and markers for production traits.
- To be aware of disease resistance and genetics.
- To have an understanding of chromosomal anomalies in cattle.
- To be aware of the samples required for genetic testing.

Genome and genomic organisation

The bovine genome consists of about 22 000 protein-coding genes, coded by about three billion base pairs (2.87 Gbp), organised into 30 chromosomes (29 autosomes plus X, Y), giving a diploid number ($2n$) of 60 chromosomes. Most cattle chromosomes correspond well with human chromosomes, the main differences being due to multiple re-arrangements within chromosomal blocks.

Origin of cattle – bovine phylogenetics and domestication

Cattle are members of the Pecoran group, which includes antelopes, through sheep and cattle, to giraffes. The group, which was originally represented on all continents except Oceania and South America, is believed to have emerged and rapidly radiated (branched out into different forms adapted to specific environments) in the middle of the Eocene period (56–34 million years ago). Because there was such rapid radiation of the group during this period, their evolutionary relationships are now quite difficult to resolve.

Recent developments in genotyping technologies have enabled researchers to make deeper insights into the evolution of cattle, including domestication and the origins of the modern breed groups. The theories regarding evolution and domestication of cattle are not universally accepted, but there is general agreement that there were several foci of domestication of modern cattle during the period 5000 to 10 000 years ago. Animals that were domesticated in southern and eastern Asia were *Bos taurus indicus* (indicine) cattle, whereas those domesticated in central Asia and Africa were *Bos taurus taurus* (taurine) cattle. These two major groups are believed to have diverged from each other some 500 000 to 800 000 years ago and evolved with quite different biogeographical challenges.

Genetic basis of modern cattle breeds

Several recent papers have reported similar findings about the genetic basis of the existing breeds. Figure 31.1 shows a phylogenetic network of common ancestry for 48 breeds of cattle, based on analysis of 50 000 polymorphic loci (SNP) in 372 animals. The figure clearly shows the distinctiveness of the *Bos taurus indicus* cattle and the African *Bos taurus taurus* cattle (N'dama).

Domestication, formation of breeds, and selection of animals within breed for milk production or other traits, has caused tight genetic bottlenecks and relatively low effective population sizes (the number of breeding individuals in an idealised population that would explain the observed level of allelic diversity) in most modern breeds. Recent estimates suggest that the effective population size in most breeds is small, being less than 100 in all of the dairy breeds and many beef breeds, and that most of the restriction in diversity arose pre-domestication and during initial domestication events. N'dama and Brahman

Bovine Medicine, Third Edition. Edited by Peter D. Cockcroft.

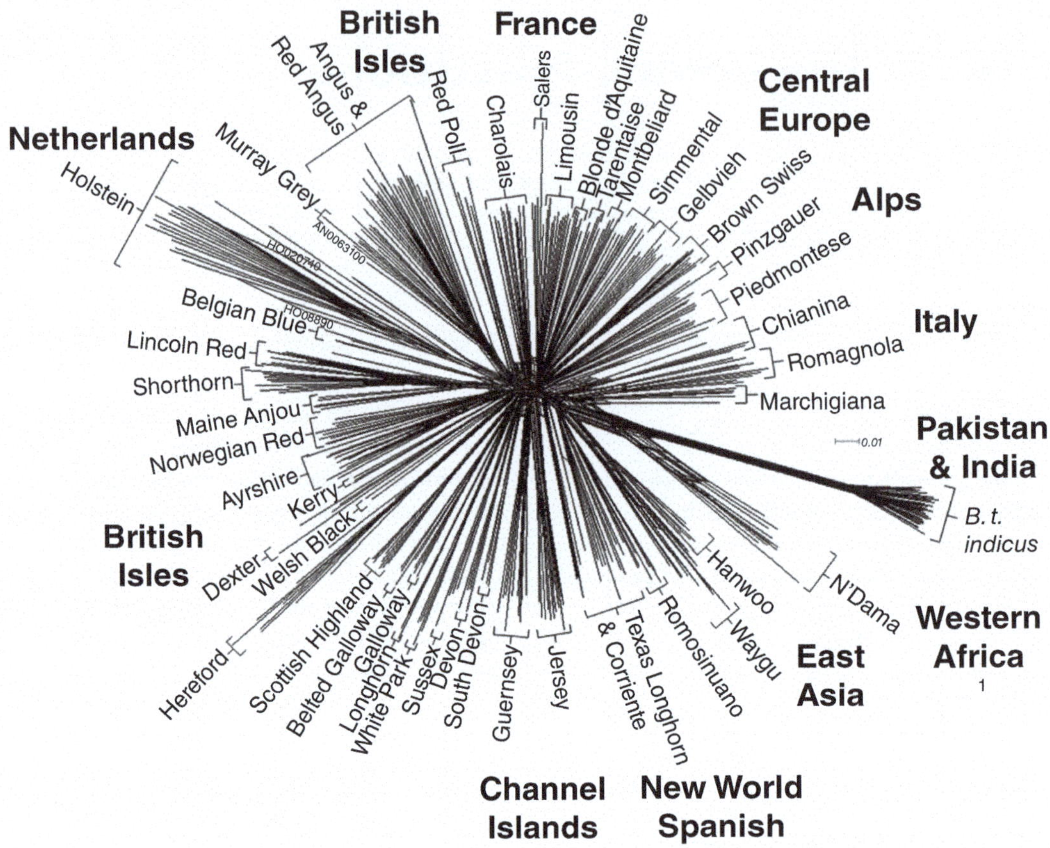

Figure 31.1 Phylogenetic network showing common ancestry for 48 breeds of cattle, based on analysis of 50,000 polymorphic loci in 372 animals. The figure clearly shows the distinctiveness of the *Bos taurus indicus* cattle and the African *Bos taurus taurus* cattle (N'dama). Reproduced with permission of Decker 2009.

cattle appear to have been derived from wild populations of greater diversity than taurine cattle. It is possible to infer from signs of selection across the genome that domestication and subsequent selection has resulted in strong pressure on milk and meat production, growth, feed efficiency, temperament or behaviour and immunity.

Parentage testing

Parentage testing of cattle has long been employed by breed societies to maintain the reliability of their pedigree records and, hence, the 'purity' of their breeds, which in turn helps to speed genetic progress in breeding programs, and increases confidence for buyers. The accuracy of parentage tests is important to stud producers and commercial cattle producers who wish to use multiple-sire mating systems in their herds and allocate calves to their correct sires. This enables producers to trace the calf-getting ability of their bulls, and to identify those bulls producing superior calves and the sire lines producing superior carcasses.

Basic principles of parentage testing

Parentage and paternity tests are performed using genetic (DNA) markers, which have superseded blood typing methods in recent years. A genetic marker is any unique DNA sequence that has a known chromosome location. In all animals, there are two copies of every gene, one of which is inherited from its dam and the other from its sire. Therefore, if a marker is present in a calf but absent from both alleged parents, the calf must be excluded as the offspring of that mating. No matter how it is performed, parentage and paternity testing always work by exclusion, since no test can *positively* identify an animal with 100% certainty.

The accuracy of a DNA-based parentage test is influenced by the degree of variability in the DNA markers used and the number of markers used. The greater the variability of the marker panel, the better the chance of the panel excluding an incorrect sire (known as the exclusion probability). Accuracy is reduced in those breeds of cattle with lower diversity, such as Poll Herefords, and is improved in those breeds with higher diversity, such as Brahmans. Also, the greater the number of markers used, the more accurate the test but the greater the cost, so a compromise must be reached to achieve reasonable accuracy at an affordable price.

The most widely used DNA markers for parentage testing have been microsatellite (or Short Tandem Repeat) markers. Microsatellites are repeated motifs in the non-coding DNA of organisms and are highly polymorphic (many alleles present at each marker locus in the population). Single nucleotide polymorphisms (SNP) have now replaced microsatellites for parentage verification in many parts of the world, driven by the uptake of SNP genotyping to predict animal performance in marker assisted selection programs. Although many more SNP are needed to achieve powers of exclusion in a similar range to microsatellite panels, low- and medium-density panels of SNP markers (3000 to 50 000 SNP) are now being used routinely in marker assisted selection programs, yielding plenty of data with which to perform parentage verification.

Most laboratories use between 10 and 20 microsatellite markers for a standard DNA test, and there is an internationally recognised and standardised panel of 12 markers for cattle. There is similarly an internationally recognised panel of around 100 SNP markers that commercial genotyping laboratories employ for parentage verification purposes, which was developed by the US Department of Agriculture (Heatly). The combined results of all markers produce a DNA profile for each animal, and the chances of any two animals having the same profile lies somewhere between one in ten million to one in 100 billion, depending on the breed and number of markers.

Inherited diseases of cattle

Many inherited diseases caused by single autosomal genes can now be detected by PCR targeting the causal mutation responsible for the disorder – usually a SNP or insertion/deletion mutation. A useful resource for information on inherited diseases in cattle is Online Mendelian Inheritance in Animals (OMIA – found at http://omia.angis.org.au/home/). At the time of writing, OMIA lists 399 diseases (or, more generally, conditions, as the database also includes coat colour) of cattle, the causative mutation of which is known in 78. Diagnostic tests for many of these conditions are offered by a variety of laboratories around the world. Some of the more widely recognised or topical conditions are listed in Table 31.1.

Production traits

Markers for performance traits

Quantitative trait loci (QTL) are regions of the genome that contain, or are linked to, genes that influence quantitative traits. Quantitative traits are continuous traits (measured quantitatively, not discrete), such as feed efficiency, carcass weight and milk yield, and are under the control of two or more genes. It is desirable to identify the causative genes and their variants that underlie quantitative traits for use in marker-assisted selection and breeding programs. Identification of QTL is most commonly achieved by genotyping individuals that are recorded for the trait of interest with DNA markers scattered throughout the genome. This was previously performed with microsatellite or STR markers, but is now more commonly undertaken with SNP. Associations are then identified between the genotype and the phenotype to reveal regions of the genome that contain genes which influence the trait of interest, a process known as a genome-wide association study (GWAS).

The QTL identified from mapping studies can be very large and may contain many genes that might influence the trait of interest. Fine mapping studies (utilising a denser panel of markers scattered throughout the region of the QTL) can narrow the region further, in an attempt to identify the gene(s) responsible for causing variation in the trait. The causative gene may be identified from this fine-mapping process, or a 'candidate gene' may be chosen for further investigation, based on prior knowledge of the gene's functional role and suspicion of its involvement in influencing the trait. It is desirable to elucidate the causative variants responsible for influencing quantitative traits of economic importance but, often, this is not possible and, instead, marker-assisted selection programs employ 'linked markers'. Linked DNA markers are generally located close by to the gene influencing the trait of interest, and the informative allele at the marker locus will almost always be inherited with the same allele at the causative locus.

An example of linked markers employed to predict performance traits are the tests currently on the market for predicting poll status in beef cattle. The poll locus has been mapped to bovine chromosome 1 (BTA1) but, at the time of writing, the causative gene is yet to be identified. Thus, currently available tests for predicting poll status (determining whether a polled animal is carrying two copies of the poll allele or carrying the recessive horn allele) rely on a group of linked markers to predict the true genotype at the poll locus.

Genomic selection schemes are employed for predicting performance of both beef and dairy cattle around the world. Genomic selection typically uses information from thousands of SNP markers scattered across the genome to identify regions associated with economically important traits, and assumes that the causative genes affecting the trait will be linked to the markers. Each SNP is given a weighting of relative importance with regards to influencing the trait of interest, and a Direct Breeding Value (DBV), based purely on the animal's genotype, can be predicted. Many genomic selection schemes blend the DBV with phenotypic and pedigree information to increase the accuracy of the prediction.

Table 31.1 List of some well known conditions of cattle from the website database Online Mendelian Inheritance in Animals (http://omia.angis.org.au/home/). Data source: Nicholas 2004.

Condition	Breeds affected	Abnormality	Major signs
Complex vertebral malformation (CVM)	Holstein	Mutation of a G to T nucleotide in position 559 of the bovine solute carrier family 35 (UDP-N-acetylglucosamine (UDP-GlcNAc) transporter) gene (SLC35A3).	Abortion, neonatal death, shortened neck, symmetrical arthrogryphosis of front and sometimes hind limbs.
α-mannosidosis	Angus, Murray Grey, Galloway	Several mutations have been described in the gene coding α-mannosidase, which lead to accumulation of mannose-rich compounds.	Lysosomal storage disease causing still birth through to progressive neurological signs with death at 3–4 months.
β-mannosidosis	Saler	A single nucleotide substitution in the gene coding β-mannosidase which leads to accumulation of mannose-rich compounds.	Still birth through intention tremor, neurological signs to craniofacial deformity.
Glycogen storage disease II (Pompes disease)	Brahman, Shorthorn	Deficiency of acidic a-glucosidase.	Poor growth, muscle weakness, incoordination, death.
Citrullinaemia	Holstein	Nonsense mutation in the fifth of nine exons of the argininosuccinate synthase gene, results in accumulation of ammonium and subsequent toxicity.	Normal at birth but rapid development of progressive central nervous signs, including depression, head pressing and death by 3–5 days of age.
Maple syrup urine disease (MSUD)	Poll Hereford, Poll Shorthorn	Two distinct nonsense mutations in the branched chain keto acid dehydrogenase gene have been reported in the two breeds.	Normal at birth but development of progressive neurological signs associated with cerebellar and cerebral vacuolation.
Leukocyte adhesion deficiency type I (BLAD)	Holstein	Deficiency of functional leukocyte integrin beta-2 subunit (ITGB2 or CD18) prevents normal neutrophil function.	Chronic, recurrent infection and early mortality in calves.
Protoporphyria	Limousin	Single base substitution in stop codon of ferrochelatase gene causes extra 27 nucleotides and results in no activity. Causes accumulation of protoporhyrin and other porphyrins, some of which are photoreactive. Aminolevulinic acid accumulation may contribute to neurological signs.	Photosensitisation, seizures.
Factor XI	Holstein and Japanese black cattle	Two loss of function inducing insertions into the F11 gene coding for factor XI (serine protease) have been indentified.	Severe haemorrhage.
DUMPS	Holstein	Deficiency of uridine monophosphate synthase, which is caused by a single nucleotide substitution, preventing binding of an essential restriction enzyme.	Failure of growth and development of foetus, causing embryonic loss.
Factor XIII	Wagyu	Insertion mutation in F13 gene.	Severe haemorrhage.
Xanthinuria	Wagyu	Autosomal recessive, deletion mutation in *MCSU*.	Renal problems, elevated xanthine secretion in the urine, growth retardation.
Neuropathic hydrocephalus	Angus, Murray Grey	[a] Simple autosomal recessive.	Enlargement of the head due to accumulation of fluid. Dead at birth.
Arthrogryposis multiplex congenita (curly calf syndrome)	Angus	[a] Simple autosomal recessive.	Small calves with little muscle mass, twisted spine, rigid legs (either hyperextended or contracted). Dead at birth.
Contractural arachnodactyly (fawn calf syndrome)	Angus, Murray Grey	[a] Simple autosomal recessive.	Upwards arching of the spine, hyperextension of the fetlock, muscle contracture. Around 20% of affected calves die in the neonatal period without intervention. Affected animals can recover from these symptoms and affected animals can be more difficult to diagnose when older.
Hypotrichosis	Hereford, Holstein	[a] Simple autosomal recessive.	Abnormal hair development. Holstein calves are either born dead or die soon after birth. Hereford calves are born alive (semi-hairless) but do not tend to perform well.

Table 31.1 (*continued*)

Condition	Breeds affected	Abnormality	Major signs
Pulmonary hypoplasia with anasarca	Dexter, Belted Galloway, Shorthorn	[a] Autosomal recessive.	Affected calves are born dead with swollen, under-developed lungs caused by excessive fluid retention.
Idiopathic epilepsy	Hereford	[a] Autosomal recessive.	Affected animals experience seizures that can be triggered by environmental stressors and the age of onset can be variable.
Spherocytosis	Wagyu	Autosomal dominant due to a missense mutation in SLC4A1.	Anaemia and retarded growth.
Chediak-Higashi syndrome	Wagyu	Missense mutation in lysosomal trafficking regulator gene LYST.	Prolonged bleeding, partial albinism.
Renal tubular dysplasia	Wagyu	Autosomal recessive mapped to CLDN16.	Renal failure, growth retardation.
Multiple ocular defects	Wagyu	Autosomal recessive caused by insertion mutation in WFDC1.	Microphthalmia, lens dysplasia, retinal detachment.
DUMPS	Holstein	Uridine monophosphate synthase.	Failure of growth and development of foetus, causing embryonic loss.

[a]Although the causal mutation is known, details are not publicly available. Commercial laboratories offer testing for these conditions.

Most reproductive traits can be considered to be controlled by QTL. Heritability estimates of reproductive performance of beef and dairy cattle are measured in terms of pregnancy rates, intercalving interval and submission rate. These tend to be relatively low – generally less than 0.15 – although measures such as age of puberty in heifers and bulls, scrotal circumference in bulls and interval from calving to first ovulation, all tend to be moderate to high (0.3–0.6). As a result, there are a number of SNP and other markers for reproductive traits that are useful in specific breed groups. As with other production traits, the greatest challenge is to identify markers that have a high predictive value across breeds.

Disease resistance

In recent years, there has been considerable interest in selecting animals that have high levels of resistance to infectious diseases. Susceptibility or resistance to most diseases is incomplete, and is usually due to many intrinsic factors. Therefore, disease resistance can mostly be considered as a quantitative trait, even more so than with QTL for production traits, and understanding the genetic basis of the known variability in disease resistance is complicated by the difficulty in obtaining useful disease phenotypes. Phenotype is difficult to define in many cases, because the infectious challenge is variable under field conditions, and the performance of diagnostic tests varies.

Apart from the inherited autosomal recessive disorders listed above, there are a few examples in pigs, poultry and sheep of diseases which are essentially under the control of a single gene. These include susceptibility of sheep to scrapie, susceptibility of chickens to some subgroups of avian leucosis virus, and susceptibility of pigs to *E. coli* F18 and F4. High levels of genetic control might be expected where infection and subsequent disease is dependent on the infectious agent binding a specific host cell surface receptor. Mutation of the receptor can prevent binding of the pathogen, rendering the host resistant to that pathogen. This is the case with *E. coli* F18 and F4 in pigs. In other diseases, including malignant catarrhal fever virus MCFV infection of buffalo, variation in the major histocompatibility complex (MHC) leads to variation in the ability of the host to detect and deal with infection.

Specific viral bovine diseases for which there is evidence of genetically controlled variation in susceptibility include MCFV (likely due to variation in MHC), bovine herpes virus 1 (BHV-1 – apparently due to variation in type I interferons) and bovine leukaemia virus (BLV – also likely due to variation in MHC). This knowledge has not, however, led to any commercially available diagnostic tests for susceptibility to these diseases.

Among bacterial diseases, the susceptibility to paratuberculosis or Johne's disease is estimated to have a heritability lying between 0.03 and 0.1, the low heritability likely being partly as a result of the well known problems with diagnosis of the disease. Despite this, recent work has identified specific SNP that are claimed should be useful for genomic selection for resistance.

Perhaps reflecting experimental logistics rather than biology, heritability estimates for bovine tuberculosis are higher, ranging from 0.1 to 0.2. Mastitis is arguably the most important predominantly bacterial disease in dairy cattle, and some progress has been made in the selection of animals that are less susceptible to mastitis. Because of the variety of microorganisms involved and the complex, polygenic nature of resistance to mastitis, selection has been on the basis of milk somatic cell count (SCC), for which heritability estimates are in the order of 0.05–0.15, and on the incidence of clinical mastitis (CM), which has a low heritability of less than 0.05. Norway, which began selecting cattle on the basis of CM incidence, has seen a slow reduction in the incidence of CM of 0.15–0.27% per year. SNPs associated with resistance have been identified, and will be incorporated into genomic selection strategies for dairy sires.

Resistance to helminths and ectoparasites is known to have moderate to high heritability, and considerable research has been invested in the identification of the molecular basis of this resistance, which is certainly controlled by many genes. Molecular diagnostic tests are currently being offered commercially for resistance to nematode infection of sheep, and some studies have identified panels of SNP that should be useful for genomic prediction of resistance.

In contrast to the situation of resistance to scrapie in sheep, resistance to bovine spongiform encephalopathy (BSE) in cattle is less clearly under genetic control. None of the PrP alleles have been shown to be associated with resistance to BSE, although there is some evidence to suggest that polymorphisms in the promoter might be associated with susceptibility. Several production diseases are known to be genetically controlled. Susceptibility to pasture bloat, driven by variation in salivary protein composition, has a heritability of 0.44, while resistance to copper deficiency has a heritability of about 0.2, and ketosis and milk fever are both in the range 0.05–0.1. Recent work has shown that left-displaced abomasum has a heritability between 0.2–0.5 and, in German Holsteins at least, there is a strong association with a mutation in the *motilin* gene, which influences its expression and, likely, the motility of the abomasums.

Chromosomal anomalies

Chromosomal anomalies occur in cattle, although the frequency of occurrence is somewhat difficult to determine. Because most chromosomal anomalies result in failure of development, the frequency of anomalies decreases with increasing embryonic age, and most anomalies are simply seen as reproductive failure. Each bovine should have two of each of 29 autosomes and a pair of sex chromosomes, to make a full diploid complement of 60 chromosomes.

Aneuploidy is an abnormal number of chromosomes and results from non-disjunction during meiotic division in the gonad, with the result that gametes have either no chromosome or two, instead of the one that is required to result in diploid zygotes. Monosomy is the condition where the zygote has only a single chromosome, and trisomy is where the zygote has three chromosomes instead of two. Clinical manifestations of chromosomal anomalies include infertility in the case of sex chromosome aneuploidy, or congenital malformations in other cases. Cytogenetic analyses, including karyotyping, are required to confirm chromosomal anomalies, and these are more readily available through human medical laboratories.

Chromosomal translocation occurs when a fragment of a chromosome breaks during gametogenesis and joins onto another chromosome. There is no loss or duplication of genetic material, but alterations at the sites of the break and junction with the new chromosome can lead to specific problems. Most commonly, however, the main effect of translocation is to prevent normal meiotic division, causing infertility. A related anomaly is inversion, in which the broken fragment rejoins the original chromosome, but after inverting. Depending on the break-point of the inversion, the consequences of an inversion can be minimal. There are many examples of inversions becoming incorporated into a normal genome.

Samples for genetic testing of cattle

DNA is present in all nucleated cells and can be extracted from many tissue types, although hair follicles are most commonly submitted for commercial DNA testing applications. Other commonly used tissues submitted for DNA extraction and analysis include semen, blood (whole blood tube or blood spot on paper), nasal swabs and ear punch biopsies. Recently, there have been several products commercialised for DNA sample collection from livestock, and considerations on the most suitable method should include:

- cost and ease of collection and transportation to the laboratory;
- cost and ease of DNA extraction;
- intended end use application for the DNA.

The latter two points are considerations for the laboratory, and genotyping service providers will advise on the best sample type for the intended application. Tail hair samples are generally favoured, as they are easy to collect, transport and store, and are suitable for the vast majority of laboratory applications. When collecting tail hair samples for DNA analysis, it is crucial that the hairs are plucked from the tail with the hair root attached, as the DNA is contained in the root of the hair (not the hair shaft). It is also important that the hairs are clean and dry when they are collected, as wet samples can grow mould that will destroy the sample. Tubes of blood can yield a large amount of high-quality DNA but must be kept cool (4°C) after collection, and transport can consequently be an issue. The potential for twin animals to carry their twin's DNA type in their blood (chimerism) is also an important consideration when submitting blood for DNA analysis.

References

Bishop, S.C., Axford, R.F.E., Nicholas, F.W. and Owen, J.B. (eds, 2010). *Breeding for disease resistance in farm animals*, 3rd edition. CAB International.

The Bovine Genome Sequencing and Analysis Consortium, Elsik, C.G., Tellam, R.L., Worley and K.C. (2009). The genome sequence of taurine cattle: A window to ruminant biology and evolution. *Science* **324**, 522–528.

The Bovine HapMap Consortium, *et al.* (2009). Genome-wide survey of SNP variation uncovers the genetic structure of cattle breeds. *Science* **324**, 528–532.

Chan, E.K.F., Nagaraj, S.H. and Reverter, A. (2010). The evolution of tropical adaptation: comparing taurine and zebu cattle. *Animal Genetics*, doi10.1111/j.1365–20522010.02053.x.

Charlier, C., Coppieters, W., Rollin, F. *et al.* (2008). Highly effective SNP-based association mapping and management of recessive defects in livestock. *Nature Genetics* **40**, 449–454.

Decker, J.E., Pires, J.C., Conant, G.C. *et al.*, (2009). Resolving the evolution of extant and extinct ruminants with high-throughput phylogenomics. *Proceedings of the National Academy of Sciences of the USA* **106**, 18644–18649.

Haynurst, C., Bradley, A., Forbes, A.B., Hunter, K. and Royal, M.D. (2010). Genetic and nongenetic factors influencing *Ostertagia ostertagi* antibodies in UK Holstein-Friesian cattle. *Journal of Dairy Science* **93**, 2239–2243.

Kirkpatrick, B.W., Shi, X., Shook, G.E. and Collins, M.T. (2010). Whole-genome association analysis of susceptibility to paratuberculosis in Holstein cattle. *Animal Genetics* **42**, 149–160.

Mömke, S., Sickinger, M., Rehage, J., Doll, K. and Distl, O. (2012). Transcription factor binding site polymorphism in the motilin gene associated with left-sided displacement of the abomasums in German Holstein cattle. *PLoS One* **7**(4): e35562. doi: 10.1371/journal.pone.0035562.

CHAPTER 32

Abortion and Perinatal Mortality in Cattle

Richard D. Murray

Learning objectives

- Understand the pregnancy loses that can occur at different ages and growth phases of the foeto-maternal placental unit and the mechanisms that may be involved.
- Appreciate the important infectious and non-infectious causes of abortion.
- Understand the samples that may be useful in abortion investigations.
- Appreciate the gross pathological changes that may occur in different causes of abortion.
- Appreciate the diagnostic methods that may be useful in an investigation.

Introduction

The word 'abortion' is derived from the Latin prefix *ab*– (reverse the meaning) and *oriri*– to rise. It is defined generally as anything that fails in the course of coming into being: in medical terms, it is the premature expulsion of an embryo or foetus, or the procurement of this outcome especially in the first three months of pregnancy. As an adjective, it means born untimely, unsuccessful, in imperfect condition, checked in development; hence, the phrase 'perinatal mortality' is used more widely to define the unsuccessful outcome of a confirmed pregnancy – specifically, the birth of an unviable foetus.

Within the veterinary literature, cattle abortion, 'picking' or 'slinking', has been recognised as a difficult problem to manage. At the beginning of the 19th century, it was considered to be 'a contagion', the infection density being related to the intensity of smell of the associated retained placenta that was conveyed in the air. Abortions could affect all the small herds located in a rural village. At that time, country folk frequently consulted a witch doctor, following an abortion episode occurring in their herd: this local worthy would invent spurious stories of why a neighbour should wish to invoke bad luck on the luckless farmer. In 1858, a paper in the *Edinburgh Veterinary Review* described the effect of late pregnant cattle eating ergot as a cause of abortion, and the Scottish Metropolitan Veterinary Medical Society, at its June, 1870 meeting held in Edinburgh, discussed the high incidence of premature births in sheep and cattle in Selkirk and the considerable financial losses that accompanied it.

As microbiological science developed, specific infections were identified that caused abortion in cattle: *Brucella abortus*, related to Bang's Disease, and *Trichmonas foetus* were both described by Marek (1937). In the United Kingdom, the economic losses associated with contagious abortion in cattle were considered to be second only to tuberculosis (Buxton, 1934). Surprisingly, it was not until 1946 that other infectious causes of bovine abortion were recognised and accepted universally, such as *Vibrio foetus* (now *Campylobacter foetus* vars.), *Bacterium pyogenes* (formerly *Arcanobecterium pyogenes,* now *Truperella pyogenes*), *Streptococcus* spp. and *Mycobacterium* spp. (Manninger, 1946). Nowadays, around 40 microorganisms have been isolated from, and attributed as a cause of, bovine abortions.

It is difficult to give a precise estimate of the incidence and cost of bovine abortions in different global regions, purely because the monetary value of cattle themselves, a dairy replacement heifer or a litre of milk varies from one country to another. For example, the cost of an abortion has been estimated at $143 in Chile, while in North America it was $500–900. In the large intensively-managed dairy herds of California, 3–10% of pregnancies can be lost in cattle known to be pregnant (Thurmond *et al.*, 1990), and the annual loss to that state's economy may be as high as $200 million (Hansen *et al.*, 2003). In Denmark, the risk for abortion increases with herd size with a median estimate of five cases per herd per year at a cost of $500 per cow aborting (Carpenter *et al.*, 2001).

Another factor is the relative infection pressure for a specific abortifacient. For example, in New Zealand, with a dairy cow

Bovine Medicine, Third Edition. Edited by Peter D. Cockcroft.

population of around 3.5 million, the abortion rate attributable to bovine viral diarrhoea virus (BVDv) infection is around 2.6%, which contributes 95% of the annual cost of NZ$44.5 million associated with loss of productivity due to lowered fertility in the national dairy herd (Heuer *et al.*, 2007). In the United Kingdom, an estimated 48,000 cattle abort annually out of a population of just over 2.7 million, at a cost of £31.2 million, and 12% of which may be related to neosporosis (Davison *et al.*, 1999).

Generally, in animal reproduction 2–4% of confirmed early pregnancies will not survive, as a result of faulty chromosomal assembly at fertilisation. This is a natural process for early elimination of a potentially lethal genotype in the conceptus, thereby attempting to improve reproductive efficiency within a species by reducing the intervals between births of viable offspring to the same mother.

In cattle, particularly dairy cows, pregnancy is confirmed in three ways: milk progesterone estimation 19–22 days after service, and *per rectum* examination off the uterus and its contents from 32 days gestation onwards, using either ultrasound or manual palpation, which is used commonly in beef suckler cows. At these stages of early pregnancy, placental attachment through trophectodermal (chorionic epithelia cell) invasion of the endometrium is occurring as the late embryo is developing and the products of fertilisation are detectable. The factors controlling this process are under the influence of the thousands of genes imprinted within the trophectoderm and present in endometrial epithelia. This process is independent of the mechanism for early maternal recognition of the bovine embryo, through the synthesis of interferon-*tau* by trophectodermal cells 15–21 days after service. Therefore, we should not consider early embryonic loss that occurs before within 16 days after service in this chapter, since the term 'abortion' should relate only to pregnancies that are confirmed.

Stages of pregnancy

We will consider pregnancy losses at four stages of pregnancy, each of which comprises different development and growth phases of the foeto-maternal unit – the functional placenta.

Late embryonic and early foetal loss: days 25–70 of gestation

This first trimester of pregnancy is characterised mostly by growth of the foeto-maternal unit, which is under the control of approximately 35 000 genes imprinted in trophectodermal cells, and the same number expressed in the endometrium. Although the foundations of the bovine syndesmoepithelio-chorial placenta are created at around 19–21 days gestation, the foeto-maternal unit is complete by day 60 in terms of numbers of functional placentomes, and the area of the foeto-maternal interface continues to grow to around day 270.

For such rapid placental growth to occur, there is considerable crosstalk between foetal and maternal compartments controlled by both endocrine, paracrine and autocrine interactions. Our detailed knowledge of this process is in its infancy, but several paracrine and autocrine growth factors have been identified, such as platelet-derived growth factors and the integrins that are associated with inter-cellular adhesion and stability. It is vascular growth and angiogenesis, particularly in the maternal compartment, that is crucial (Grazul-Bilska *et al.*, 2010). Another important group of cell growth and adhesion molecules are the galectins. At this stage of pregnancy, they are highly expressed in carunular epithelia and inter-cotyledonary maternal *lamina propria*, their role being to regulate trophoblast invasion of the endometrium (Froelich *et al.*, 2012).

The risk factors for abortion at this stage of pregnancy are all associated with disruption of these crosstalk mechanisms, particularly within the maternal compartment. Three infectious diseases have been identified: *Tritrichmonas foetus, Leptospira interrogans* var *hardjo*, and bovine viral diarrhoea virus (BVDv) (BonDurant, 2007). All cause endometrial epithelial degeneration or necrosis, with an associated inflammatory response that may have a direct effect on two early pregnancy regulators – pregnancy-associated plasma protein A and macrophage inhibitory cytokine-1.

Some years ago, nine veterinary surgeons in the UK, specialising in cattle fertility, wished to investigate the risk factors for cows confirmed as pregnant between 36–56 days after service returning to service within 30 days of the pregnancy diagnosis *per rectum*. By comparing serological results obtained from individual cows that had lost their pregnancy with a contemporaneous bulk milk sample, the infectious disease status of those now-barren cows was investigated, and the results are summarised in Table 32.1.

These results ($p \leq 0.01$) suggest that acute active infection involving BVDv within a herd, vaccinated or unvaccinated, is a significant risk factor for abortion at this stage of pregnancy.

However, a number of non-infectious factors probably have an even greater impact on early pregnancy loss, because they are mostly husbandry-related. For example, in-calf heifers have a lower risk of early pregnancy loss than first lactation cows, probably because the latter are exposed to changes in husbandry related to joining the adult milking herd; a further increased risk is present when the milking herd is newly housed at the beginning of winter. Also, the risk is higher with twin pregnancies, and there is a significant sire effect (Markusfeld-Nir 1997).

Some other risks have been identified in humans, such as impaired thyroid function and production of reactive oxygen species (ROS). In cattle, low bio-availability of iodine and/or selenium in the ration may create similar risks. Recently, in a 350-cow dairy herd where a low bioavailability of selenium/vitamin E had been confirmed by soil analysis, the calving

Table 32.1 Numbers of cows who lost their pregnancies around 40–65 days gestation in herds vaccinated and unvaccinated for bovine viral diarrhoea virus and were always seronegative for the virus (Murray, 2006).

Herd disease category for BVDv	Vaccinated herds		Unvaccinated herds	
	Number of herds	Number of cows seronegative	Number of herds	Number of cows seronegative
Negative (OD units < 0.2)	0	0	2	2
Low positive (OD units 0.2–0.4)	0	0	5	5
Moderate positive (OD units > 0.4–0.7)	2	1	8	4
High positive (OD units > 0.7)	8	7	8	11

interval was reduced from 452 days to 411 within a year of dietary supplementation being implemented.

Another risk factor, poorly understood in cattle but better defined in pig and equine reproduction, is contamination by *Fusarium* moulds of cereals fed to cows around the time of service. The pharmacologically-active compound, common to many mycotoxins, is zearalenone, which is converted to α-zearalenol in the liver, and this has oestrogenic effects, which affects normal folliculogenesis. In very low dietary concentrations, its effects on cattle fertility are purely conjecture, but there are concerns that it may increase early and late embryonic mortality rates.

At this age of pregnancy, the *corpus luteum* (CL) is the predominant source of progesterone. Unless there is inflammation and release of prostaglandins, particularly $PGF_2\alpha$ from the endometrium, the CL persists, and it is not until its endocrine support is lost – (e.g. the early pregnancy regulators, because the foetus has died) that it regresses and the cow returns into season. Rarely are placental remnants seen – often, only a mild haemorrhagic mucus discharge after the cow has returned to service.

Evidence of this form of lowered fertility is usually obtained following analysis of herd breeding records or herd manager observations.

70–130 days gestation

This stage of pregnancy is characterised by a fully-formed placental unit being present with the *corpus luteum* secreting progesterone to maintain pregnancy. Some placental steroid hormones are secreted from binucleate trophoblast cells, primarily progesterone, which is luteotrophic. At the same time, the immune-competence of the foetus is developing so that, by around days 120–130 gestation, it can recognise foreign antigen as a prerequisite to mounting a humoral immune response to *in utero* infectious agents.

Foetal losses at this stage are around 2%, characterised by incomplete lysis of the CL of pregnancy and related anoestrus, resorption of fluids from the amniotic and allantoic sacs, and dehydration of foetal tissues as water passes through its immature, porous skin and membranes. The resulting mummified foetus remains *in utero*, often for several weeks or even months, and a diagnosis is made by *per rectum* palpation or ultrasound at a routine herd fertility visit. Progression to a macerated foetus occurs in less than half of cases. On palpation, the foetus is compact and immobile within a distended pregnant uterine horn that has contracted around the foetal remnants. Ultrasound pictures confirm that neither placental fluids nor placentomes are present.

Infections such BVDv, *L. interrogans* var. *hardjo* and fungal infections have been implicated commonly as risk factors. To confirm their true aetiological role in a clinical diagnosis, it is impractical to use any aborted foetal tissues, since none are suitable for pathological or laboratory examinations. Within a research context, such material may be useful. Also, because foetal death has occurred long before the foetus is delivered, maternal serology offers little except to confirm that the pregnant cow had met an infectious challenge sometime previously.

Non-infectious causes have been identified, such as anatomical abnormalities within the foeto-maternal unit and genetic/chromosomal defects. In the United States, it has been estimated that around 2% of pregnancy losses at this time originate from genetic abnormalities – for example, the autosomal recessive gene disorder for a deficiency in the enzyme uridine monophosphate synthase (DUMPS) and an X-chromosome deletion locus have been investigated recently (Lefebrve *et al.*, 2009).

Treatment is designed to remove the foetal tissue remnants, either using $PGF_2\alpha$ or surgery. In European countries, the ancillary use of oestrogens with $PGF_2\alpha$ for this purpose is not allowed in food producing animals, but elsewhere it may be acceptable, and the success rate of this combined treatment appears to be higher than using prostaglandins alone. The physiological explanation of this: that exogenous oestrogen stimulates oxytocin receptors within the endometrium that trigger synthesis and release of $PGF_2\alpha$, which is luteolytic. At the same time, oestrogen is itself luteolytic and initiates myometrial contractures, which assist in expelling any foetal fragments. Lefebrve *et al.* (2009) described a surgical method for removing mummified foetuses whose crown-rump length varied between 20–40 cm, the mean pregnancy rate being 36% at the following service.

130–270 days gestation

At this stage, the foeto-maternal unit controls pregnancy from endocrine, immunological and biochemical standpoints. At the start of this period, the end-point of placental steroidogenesis is progesterone, which continues to support and maintain the CL of pregnancy. As the foetus develops, secretion of cortisol from its adrenal gland controls the expression of enzymes present in binucleate trophoblast cells that direct the steroidogenic pathway towards oestradiol-17α synthesis, with a corresponding reduction in progesterone secretion. In their biologically-active forms, both these steroid hormones are essential for preparing the dam for parturition.

One of the target organs for oestradiol is the myometrium, where changes to its Calcium ion flux create ordered smooth muscle contractures, associated with first- and second-stage labour, that emerge from the uncoordinated random contractures that occur throughout pregnancy. In the absence of these placental steroids, an inevitable outcome of degeneration and necrosis of trophoblast following uterine infection, these initial stages of normal labour are absent prior to abortion. The cervix relaxes partially, a result of matrix metallo-proteinase (MMPs) activity on cervical collagen, controlled through enzymes delivered by macrophages to the reproductive tract, and any concomitant myometrial contractures have low amplitude and frequency. Pelvic ligaments do not relax fully, and some degree of mammary gland hyperplasia and hypertrophy occurs, but premature birth in cattle is often an apparently sudden, passive event in the absence of obvious organised myometrial contractures and behavioural changes observed with normal first- and second-stage labour.

Understanding of the immunological aspects related to late abortion is scant, because it is difficult to separate and investigate independently foetal and maternal tissues within the placentome. However, some aspects of the innate immune system within the endometrium have been elucidated. Epithelial, endothelial and leukocyte cells all detect pathogen-associated molecular patterns (PAMPs), presented by foreign antigen, which stimulate local inflammatory responses and cytokine production. Toll-like cellular receptors (TLRs), such as C-type lectin receptors (CLRs), recognise antigenic lipopolysaccharides, lipoproteins, and flagellins, and nucleotide-binding oligomerisation domain receptors (NLRs) are intracellular sensors of PAMPs.

Different TLR sub-classes recognise various specific antigenic molecules – TLR 1, 2, and 6 bacterial lipids, TLR 4 lipopolysaccharides, and TLR 5 flagellins. Their differential expression varies with the stage of pregnancy and uterine location. For example, TLR 4 and 5 are prominent in the last third of gestation, inter-cotyledonary endometrium expresses TLRs more than in placentomes, and there is greater expression of TLR 2 and 4 in endometrial epithelium than trophoblast. Specific bacteria trigger release of pro-inflammatory cytokines in the pregnant cow; for example, *Brucella abortus* and *Aspergillus fumigatus* have been associated with interleukin-8 (IL8) and IL6 respectively, and *Salmonella* Dublin and *Listeria monocytogenes* upregulate synthesis of both (Silva *et al.*, 2012). These cytokines are involved in the cross-talk within the foeto-maternal unit. While this explains partially the interaction of obligate and opportunistic pathogens – particularly Gram-negative organisms – with the endometrial epithelium in the pregnant uterus, it does not describe how a primary abortifacient infects a foetus trans-placentally.

This was investigated for *B. abortus*, using a goat model, by Anderson *et al.* (1986). The pathogen was carried into the foetal compartment of the placentome via erthyrophagocytic trophoblast, where it spread to chorioallantoic trophoblast and replicated in its rough endoplasmic reticulum. Subsequent necrosis of this trophoblast then released large numbers of bacteria into the uterine lumen, from where the infection spread to produce a severe intercotyledonary placentitis and vasculitis. Bacteria then infected the foetus via the transplacental route, following contaminated amniotic fluid being ingested and inhaled. This model is one example of how a primary infectious abortive agent must behave to cross from the maternal endometrial septae in the placentome to the foetal chorionic villi.

Other bacteria causing foetal infection by this route include *Coxiella burnetti, Campylobacter foetus*, var. *venerealis* and *Listeria moncytogenes.* There are other mechanisms: for example, maternal infection with *A. fumigatus* or *Bacillus licheniformis* can lead to formation of thrombo-emboli in the septal blood capillary network, which causes necrosis of dependant foeto-maternal tissues. Some viruses, such as bovine herpes virus-1 (bovHV-1) and bovHV-4, infect the caruncular epithelium, and foetal infection occurs via the haematogenous route. Also, there are cell surface receptors – CD46 – for BVDv present on these same epithelial cells. This virus induces apoptosis, which creates a breach in the foeto-maternal barrier, but rarely is the resulting foetal infection fatal. However, such a disruption allows a large number of opportunistic pathogens to colonise the chorio-amnion and infect the foetus via the transplacental route (see Table 32.2).

An abortion investigation must focus on identifying probable primary abortifacients that disrupt the foeto-maternal barrier and can be controlled, rather than the multitude of opportunistic microorganisms that actually cause foetal death. At a workshop on bovine abortion held in Edinburgh during 1996, this topic was discussed at length. The best, but not necessarily the most cost-effective, strategy was an investigation based on gross foetal and placental pathology (see Table 32.3) and histological examination of soft tissues, with support provided by microbiological and serological evidence. Alternatively, the contribution of abortion to wider issues of loss of productivity can be investigated

Table 32.2 Opportunistic bacteria isolated from aborted bovine foetuses.

Gram-positive bacteria	*Corynebacterium ulcerans* *Listeria monocytogenes* *Nocardia farcinica* *Propronibacterium acnes* *Staphylococcus aureus* *Staphylococcus warner* β-haemolytic *Streptococci* *Truperella pyogenes* (formerly *Arcanobacterium pyogenes*)
Gram-negative bacteria	*Aeromonas* sp. *Campylobacter jejuni* *Enterbacter* sp. *Eschericia coli* *Fusobacterium necrophorum* *Histophilus somni* *Mannhaemia haemolytica* *Moraxella* sp. *Pasteurella multocida* *Proteus* *Pseudomonas aeruginosa* *Salmonella* Dublin *Salmonella* Typhimurium *Yersinia pseudotuberculosis*
Others	*Anaplasma marginale* *Mycoplasma bovigenitalium* *Ureaplasma diversum*

and, more importantly, the risks controlled using vaccination. Other risks that have health and safety implications for farm workers or associated with specific herd management practices can also be investigated.

Primary infectious risk factors

Production-related infectious disease

Besides abortion, viral infections such as parainfluenza virus-3 (PI3) and bovHV-1 are primary pathogens associated with bovine respiratory disease. Concurrent active BVDv infection in young calves is an immunosuppressant that increases their susceptibility to these viruses. Occasionally, in adult milking cattle, bovHV-1 causes clinical signs of upper respiratory tract infection and a sudden drop in milk yield. In both of these examples, an abortion investigation could focus only on the involvement of these specific pathogens and their control. In a dairy herd, evidence of recent infection in a cow that has aborted is problematical; the entire investigation is historical and, therefore, serology offers evidence only of previous exposure.

Usually, two blood samples are obtained: the first at the time of abortion occurring, and the second not less than four weeks later. Serum is removed from the first sample, labelled correctly, and stored at −20°C. When the second serum sample has been collected, the two samples should be submitted for serological investigation together, as this ensures that both titres can be estimated using the same daily laboratory protocol. These titres can then be compared with recent bulk milk antibody titres in dairy herds or, in a beef suckler herd, sera obtained from around 15 pregnant cows and in-calf heifers three months before the start of the calving period (say, at the time of housing, screening cattle for tuberculosis or brucellosis, or when dosing cattle). Infection can be confirmed using several methods, all of which involve obtaining foetal samples (see Table 32.4).

Public health issues

Of concern in the United Kingdom are three pathogens: *Salmonella* Dublin and *Salmonella* Typhimurium, which are both reportable diseases in cattle, and *L. interrogans* var. *hardjo*. In 2011, there were 712 incidents involving salmonellosis in cattle; in 2010, the latest year where epidemiological data is available, there were 6120 cases in humans, excluding typhoidal serotypes and *Salmonella* Enteritidis. In 2010, 42 human cases of leptospirosis were recorded, of which six involved farm or abattoir workers. In Europe during 2009, per 100 000 of the population, 23.6 cases were recorded of non-typhoidal *Salmonella* serotypes, and 0.14 cases involving leptospirosis that were mostly occupation-related.

Dairy farmers, in particular, should reduce the risks of their families and staff acquiring these zoonotic infections, and an abortion investigation could be directed specifically at these pathogens. Bacterial examination of foetal stomach contents should identify any *Salmonella* spp. present, and microscopic agglutination antibody (MAT) titres of >1/400, or optical density (OD) units > 0.6, in dams' serum obtained at the time of abortion, are suggestive of recent acute infection with leptospires. Two of these infections can be controlled by cattle vaccination to some degree.

Use of bulls and venereal infection

While natural service is not a favoured method for breeding replacement dairy heifers in modern intensively-managed herds, a variety of terminal beef sires are used in suckler herds. A young bull, purchased from a pedigree breeder at auction, has a low risk for introducing infection into a herd; it will have had its fertility proven by mating with only one or two of the vendor's cows, and the purchaser should introduce him to a small number of mature cows at the start of the mating period. However, sharing mature bulls between herds, hiring them for a season, or simply borrowing a bull in the short term to overcome the temporary loss of a bull, all carry a high risk for introducing venereal disease associated with *Ureaplasma diversum*, *Mycoplasma bovigenitalium*, *Campylobacter foetus* var. *venerealis* or var. *foetus*, and bovHV-1. Other infectious diseases, such as BVDv and *L. interrogans* var. *hardjo*, may also be introduced into naïve herds when the health status of such a

Table 32.3 Summary of foetal gross pathological lesions, without autolysis present, that suggest further aids to diagnosis would be valuable when investigating primary risk factors for abortion in cattle.

Gross foetal pathology	
crown-rump length (CRL)	estimate gestational age using the formula: $\text{foetal age at death (days)} = \frac{\text{CRL(mm)} + 297.1}{4.7}$
skin	white/grey plaques attached to hair over head, shoulders or abdomen – foetal fungal infection brown/yellow meconium on hind limbs – foetal hypoxia or 'foetal distress syndrome'
eyes	cataracts – BVDv infection
cerebrum and cerebellum	cerebellar hypoplasia – BVDv infection ecchymotic meningeal haemorrhages – 'foetal distress syndrome'
thyroid gland	to assess degree of thyroid hyperplasia, use the formula: $\frac{\textit{max/min range weight of normal}}{\textit{foetal thyroid gland (g)}} = \frac{\text{weight of foetus}}{\text{2 (max) or 3(min)}}$ enlargement – maternal dietary iodine deficiency
pleura	ecchymotic haemorrhages – 'foetal distress syndrome'. adhesions– foetal bacteraemia
lung	inter-lobular oedema – possible circulatory failure: solidification/congestion – broncho- or interstitial pneumonia
heart and pericardium	epicardial ecchymotic haemorrhages – 'foetal distress syndrome' myocardial pallor – vitamin E/selenium deficiency pericardial adhesions to epicardium – foetal bacteraemia
liver	congestion – circulatory failure with 'foetal distress syndrome' and bovine herpesvirus-1 infection rupture with abdominal haemorrhage – severe foetal trauma at parturition
adrenal gland	haemorrhage on cut surface, cortex/medulla boundary – 'foetal distress syndrome'
placentome	congestion on cut surface – bacterial placentitis chorionic villous necrosis – placentitis
inter-cotyledonary	congestion/oedema – placentitis; vasculitis focal epithelial plaques – significance unknown
chorio-amnion	thickening with red/brown discolouration – fungal infection

bull is unknown. An abortion investigation carried out in a herd with such a history could focus on the three infectious diseases named above, together with microbiological examination of foetal stomach contents for *C. foetus*.

Neosporosis

Over the last 15 years, there has been an increasing awareness of the potential link between abortion and neosporosis. For cattle worldwide, there is huge variation in seroprevalence, varying from 1–91%, depending on the different serological methods used: in the UK, it is 7–13% and in Spain, 7–26%. The natural cycle of infection with this protozoan parasite in cattle is vertical transmission, from infected dam to foetus. The proportion of aborted foetuses presenting evidence of infection also varies widely from 4–57%, also depending on the method used to confirm foetal parasitic infection (Dubey & Schares, 2011).

There have been attempts in some countries to eradicate this infection from dairy herds, but the cost-benefit of such an approach is far from proven. Indeed, the risk factors for neosporosis causing abortion and lower productivity in a herd are similar to those associated with BVDv, although not necessarily related (Tiwan *et al.*, 2007). Nevertheless, if the impact of this infection is of concern, diagnosis may be confirmed only after identifying tachyzoites in foetal cerebrum and/or myocardium, or high antibody titres to *N. caninum* present in foetal thoracic/pericardial fluid.

270 days to full term

It is at this stage of pregnancy when it is most unhelpful to separate perinatal mortality attributable to abortion from that associated with stillbirth at full term. It is accepted widely that non-infectious primary risk factors play a significant role,

Table 32.4 Foetal samples, diagnostic methods and outcomes suitable for investigating risk factors associated with bovine abortion episodes.

Foetal sample	Appropriate diagnostic method	Interpretation
Thoracic/pericardial fluid: Antigen	RT-PCR: for BVDv, bovHV-1, PI3 virus, PCR – RFLP: specific pathogenic leptospires	Identifies viral RNA and DNA, cost-effective, useful in autolysed foetuses. Identifies bacterial DNA.
Antibody	direct ELISA: for BVDv, bovHV-1, PI3 virus, *L. interrogans* var. *hardjo, N. caninum*	Identifies specific antibody in foetus after 120–170 days gestation which should be absent in a healthy foetus.
Total protein	biochemistry: values > 25 mg/L suggest immunoglobulin and/or acute phase proteins and/or enzymes present.	Non-specific indicator of either up-regulated foetal immune response, or cardiomyopathy associated with selenium/vitamin E deficiency or foetal hypoxia.
Liver/kidney homogenate	IFAT: for *L. interrogans* var. *hardjo*	Confirms foetal leptospira infection.
Stomach contents	Routine microbiological investigation	Identifies specific primary and opportunistic pathogens present in foetus at time of death
Tissues for examination:		
Myocardium and cerebrum	Immunohistochemistry: for *N. caninum*	Confirms foetus infected with *N. caninum* at time of death
Eyelid/conjunctiva	Routine histology	Pathognomic lesion associated with *U. diversum* infection (Figure 32.1)
Thyroid gland	Routine histology	Confirms thyroid hyperplasia associated with low availability of iodine in cow's diet
Left ventricle	Routine histology	Non-specific focal myocarditis associated with BVDv, *N. caninum* and other opportunistic infections. Myocardial degeneration associated with selenium/vitamin E deficiency in cow's diet (Figure 32.2).
Lung	Routine histology	Transplacental bacterial infections characterised by broncho-pneumonia. Viral infections spread via the haematogenous route characterised by interstitial pneumonia (Figure 32.3). Meconium/epithelial cells in airway confirm foetal hypoxia at time of death.
Liver	Immunohistochemistry: for bovHV-1 antigen Routine histology	Confirms bovHV-1 primary cause of abortion together with hepatic centrilobular necrosis (Figure 32.4). Non-specific hepatitis associated with bacterial infections
Kidney	Routine histology	Amyloid in proximal tubules suggestive of 'foetal distress syndrome'.
Adrenal	Routine histology	Congestion associated with foetal hypoxia;
Tibia	Radiology	Estimate gestational age at time of foetal death $=114 + (0.91 \times \text{tibial length (mm)})$ (Figure 32.5)

RT-PCR: real time polymerase chain reaction.
IFAT: indirect immunofluorescence.
ELISA: enzyme linked immune-assay.
RFLP: restriction fragment length polymorphism.

such as low bioavailability of selenium/vitamin E and iodine in the rations fed to late pregnant cattle. Should the foetal and maternal tissue components within the foeto-maternal unit grow disproportionally, the integrity of the placentome is destroyed, which allows opportunistic pathogens to invade the foetus via the transplacental route to cause its death. The general physiological relationships between poor maternal nutrition, foetal health and growth, and eventual outcomes of pregnancy are summarised in Figure 32.6.

Across all farm animal species, essential macronutrients must be supplied in the pregnant dam's diet for placental and foetal growth. Glucose is the primary source for adenosine

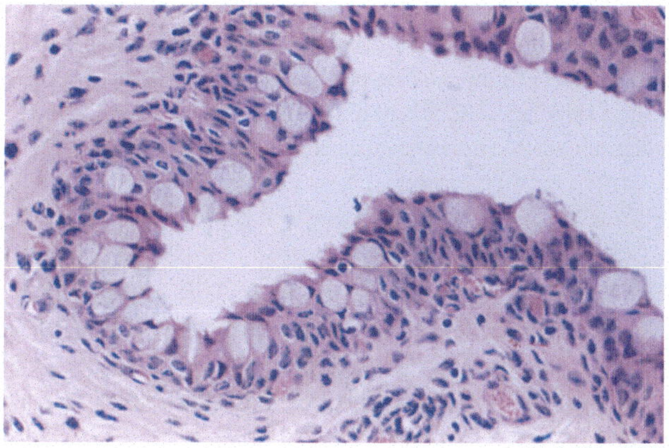
(H & E: x 540)

Figure 32.1 Hypersensitivity type 3 response in conjunctiva of aborted Holstein-Friesian bovine foetus presenting epithelial pseudo-stratification, goblet cell formation and epithelial hyperplasia with mild sub-epithelial mixed inflammatory cell infiltration associated with *U. diversum* infection. Courtesy of Murray RD.

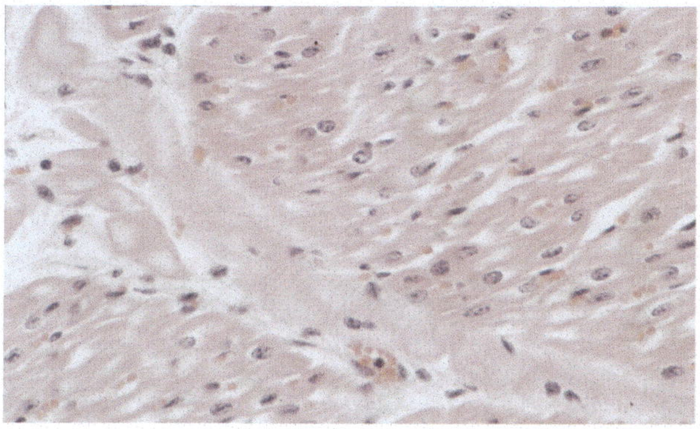
(H & E: x 540)

Figure 32.2 Myocardium of left ventricle from a stillborn Belgian-Blue bovine foetus presenting subepithelial rhabdomyolysis with entangled myoblasts and colliquative myocytolysis characterised by intracellular oedema. Some vacuolated Purkinje fibres are evident.

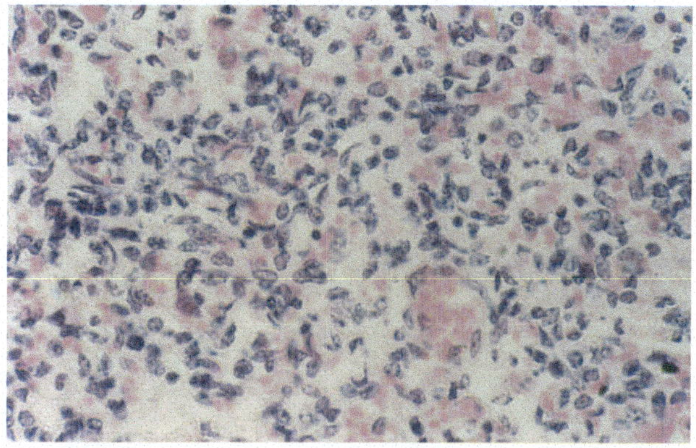
(H & E: x 540)

Figure 32.3 Lung of aborted Holstein-Friesian bovine foetus presenting severe congestion, a mixed inflammatory cell infiltration in parenchyma with some mast cells present, associated with concurrent bovHV-1 and β-haemolytic *Streptococcal* infections.

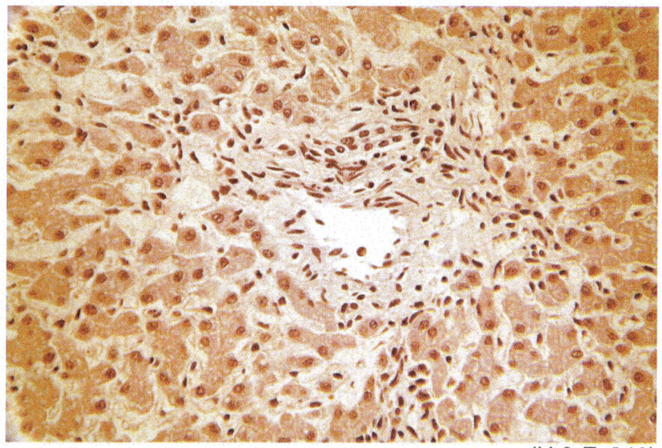
(H & E: 340)

Figure 32.4 Centrilobular hepatic necrosis with mixed/predominantly mononuclear inflammatory cell infiltration in aborted Friesian bovine foetus, associated with bovHV-1 infection.

triphosphate (ATP) synthesis in foetal red blood cells, brain, retina and kidneys. Together with lactate, it is essential for optimal myocardial function. It is within foetal intestinal epithelia where oxidation of amino acids, glutamate, glutamine and aspartate occurs, which provides energy for growth of the gastro-intestinal tract itself.

The effect of feeding a low-energy density ration to pregnant ruminants, especially in the middle and late stages of pregnancy, is most commonly recognised as 'twin lamb disease' in ewes carrying twins or triplets, but is also found in spring calving beef suckler cows wintering outside on hill grazing. However, the threat to foetal growth and development occurs long before clinical signs in the pregnant dam are obvious, since lowered peripheral blood glucose concentrations found in the pregnant dam in the first trimester of pregnancy are reflected in the foetus, leading to impaired foetal growth, particularly of the CNS. If this trend extends into the second trimester, placental growth relative to that of the foetus is compromised; prolonged foetal hypoglycaemia is an important risk factor for dysfunction within the foeto-maternal unit and subsequent perinatal mortality.

Three micronutrients are essential for placental and foetal growth: iodine, selenium/vitamin E, and zinc. Iodine is essential for growth hormone synthesis in the foetal thyroid, and deficiency is correlated with thyroid hyperplasia (see Figure 32.7). Growth hormones regulate placental growth through differential gene expression within trophoblast, and also growth of the foetal central nervous system and development of its hypothalamic-pituitary-thyroid axis, and control of energy metabolism *in utero* and as a neonate.

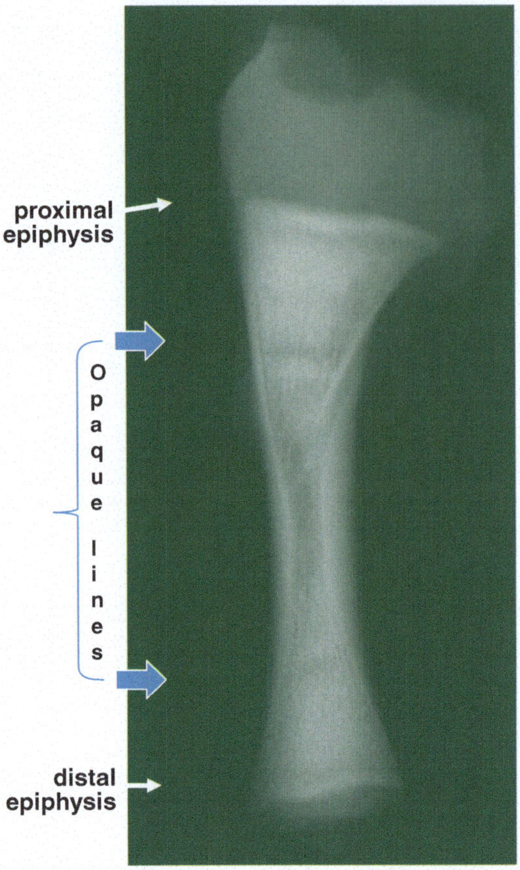

Figure 32.5 Foetal tibia from aborted bovine foetus: the distance between proximal and distal epiphysis was 160 mm, and between proximal and distal radio-opaque lines 58 mm.

In all mammalian species, deficiency carries a high risk for stillbirth. Selenium is a co-factor for antioxidant enzymes present in all mammalian cells that is protective against oxidative stress. Low bioavailability of selenium/vitamin E in the diet of cattle during mid- and late pregnancy carries a high risk of myocardial dysfunction (Murray *et al.*, 2008; see Figure 32.2), as it does in all other mammals investigated. Finally, zinc is a co-factor for cytosolic Zn/Cu superoxide dismutase involved in cell-to-cell signalling through regulation of gene expression, especially within the immune regulatory system. It is essential for foetal organogenesis and growth (Wu *et al.*, 2012).

However, the most common diagnosis associated with bovine perinatal mortality at term is foetal hypoxia or 'foetal distress syndrome' (FDS). The risk factors for this are extended first and second stage labour, which initiate a series of pathophysiological changes within the foetus; lowered blood partial pressure (pp O_2); elevated (pp CO_2); higher lactate concentration and lowered pH; reduced cardiac output in response to increasing frequency; and amplitude of maternal uterine contractures, with corresponding reduction in foetal blood pressure.

The circumstances leading up to FDS will have impacted on the foetus for up to 12 hours before the stockman has recognised dystocia in the calving cow, and relate directly to the gross findings (see Table 32.3) and histological lesions (see Table 32.4). Hypoxia leads to increased muscular excitability in the live foetus which, in turn, causes the rectum to void meconium into the amniotic cavity, with consequential yellow-brown staining of the perineum and hind limb hairs prior to birth. Also, increased diaphragmatic and inter-costal muscle activity causes inhalation of amniotic fluid and its contents, and meconuin and epithelial cell debris present in the foetal upper airway stimulates a predominantly peribronchiolar mononuclear inflammatory cell infiltration (see Figure 32.8) which, even if the foetus is born alive, compromises lung function in the neonate. More general foetal lesions associated with cardiac and circulatory failure are often present (see Table 32.3).

Diagnosis is made by examination of the foetus post-mortem, which should identify the predominant risk factors associated with stillbirth that can be controlled at herd level:

- allowing cows/heifers to calve down in familiar surroundings and not in complete isolation;
- allowing parturition to proceed and assessing its progression without repeated internal examinations *per vagina*;
- correct selection of suitable sires to breed individual cows/heifers with, thereby reducing the risk of relative foetal oversize occurring;
- feeding a suitable transition ration to late pregnant cows, to reduce the risk of hypocalcaemia and preventing cows calving down with too high a body condition score;
- ensuring adequate provision of essential micro-nutrients during late lactation/dry period.

Chapter summary

Placental animals are born in a more advanced state of development than non-placental species; the placenta adds to reproductive efficiency in a species, it does not compromise it. The synepitheliochorial placenta of ruminants has contributed significantly to the evolutionary success of this diverse group, by reason of its robust anatomical construction. In wild herds or flocks, such as Chillingham cattle in Northumberland, breed survival depends on a successful outcome of mating with the birth of a healthy viable foetus, following a successful pregnancy. In modern farming systems, an artificial breeding system has evolved; neither bull nor cow/heifer need invest in an achievable reproduction strategy, since their breeding and relate decisions have been taken over entirely by humans – farmers! Hence, most of the problems related to perinatal mortality in cattle result from human interference.

It is within this context that a strategy for reducing ruminant abortion and stillbirth rates should be considered. Mitigate the effects of poor husbandry and nutrition in late pregnant and calving animals, and put into place effective infectious disease

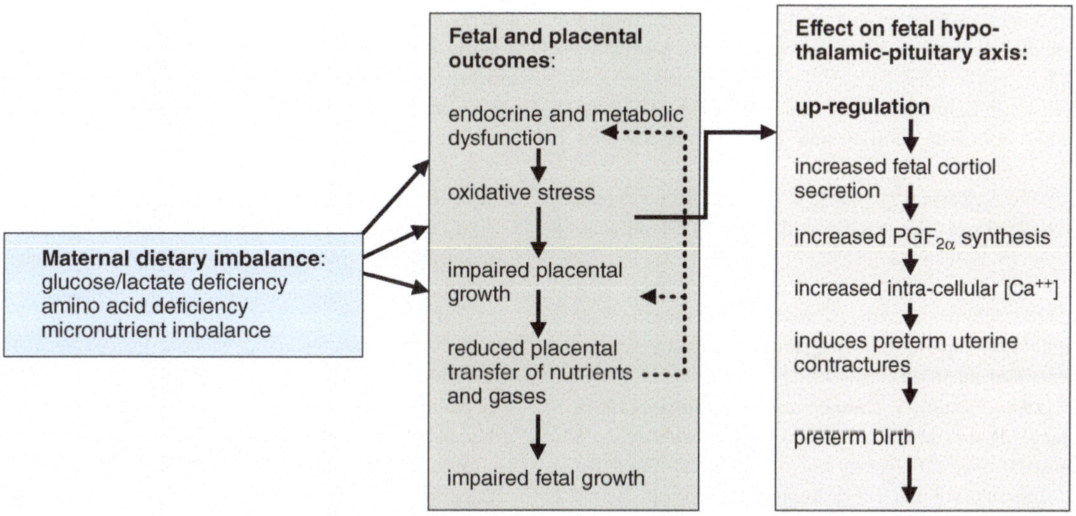

Figure 32.6 Summary inter-relationships between poor maternal nutrition and effect on placental and fetal growth, and perinatal mortality.

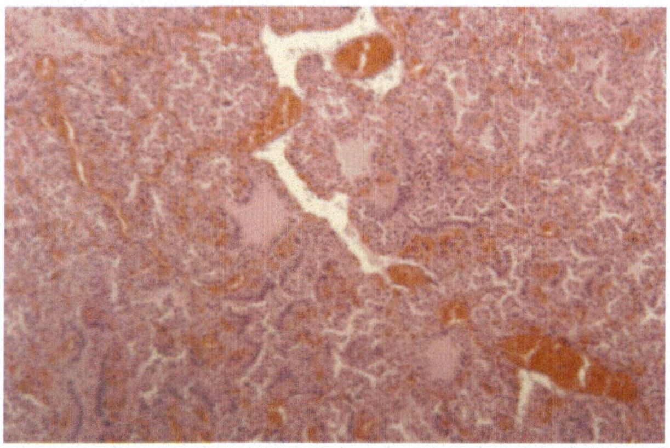

Figure 32.7 Diffuse hyperplasic goitre in a stillborn Holstein-Friesian calf, characterised by irregular shape and size of follicles lined by columnar epithelial cells with hyperchromatic nuclei in their basal parts.

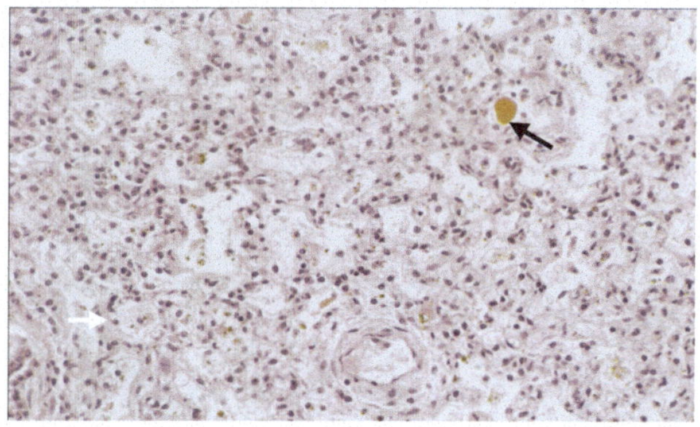

Figure 32.8 Lung from a stillborn Holstein bull calf presenting with meconium (black arrow) and epithelial cells (white arrow) in airways and moderate mononuclear inflammatory cell infiltration of interstitial tissue.

control measures for a relatively small number of primary pathogens associated with abortion. This is easier said than done!

References

Anderson, T. D., Cheville, N. F. and Meador, V. P. (1986). Pathogenesis of placentitis in the goat inoculated with *Brucella abortus*. II. Ultra-structural studies. *Veterinary Pathology* **23**, 227–239.

BonDurant, R.H. (2007). Selected diseases and conditions associated with bovine conceptus loss in the first trimester. *Theriogenology* **68**, 461–73.

Buxton, J.B. (1934). Contagious abortion. In: Wooldridge, G.H. (ed). *Encyclopaedia of Veterinary Medicine, Surgery and Obstetrics*, 2nd edition, pp 106–111. Oxford University Press, London.

Carpenter, T.E., Chriel, M. and Greiner, M. (2001). An analysis of an early-warning system to reduce abortions in dairy cattle in Denmark incorporating both financial and epidemiologic aspects. *Preventive Veterinary Medicine* **78**, 1–11.

Davison, H.C., Otter, A. and Trees, A.J. (1999). Significance of *Neospora caninum* in British dairy cattle determined by estimation of sero-prevalence in normally-calving and aborting cattle. *International Journal of Parasitology* **29**, 1189–1194.

Dubey, J.P. and Schares, G. (2011). Neosporosis in animals – the last five years. *Veterinary Parasitology* **180**, 90–108.

Froelich, R., Humbruch, N., Haeger, J-D., Dilly, M., Kaltner, H., Gabius H-J. and Pfarrer, C. (2012). Galectin fingerprinting detects differences in expression profiles between bovine endometrium and placentomes as well as early and late gestational ages. *Placenta* **33**, 195–201.

Grazul-Bilska, A.T., Borowicz, P.P., Johnson, M.L., Minten, M.A., Bilska, J.J., Wroblewski, R., Redmer, D.A. and Reynolds, L.P. (2010). Placental development during early pregnancy in sheep: vascular growth and expression of angiogenic factors in maternal placenta. *Reproduction* **140**, 165–174.

Hansen, T., Bedrick, E.T., Johnson, W.O. and Thurmond, M.C. (2003). A mixed model of bovine abortion and fetal survival. *Statistics in Medicine* **22**, 1725–1735.

Heuer, C., Healy and A., Zerbini, C. (2007). Economic effect of exposure to bovine viral diarrhoea virus in dairy herds in New Zealand. *Journal of Dairy Science* **90**, 5428–5438.

Lefebrve, R.C., Saint-Hilaire, E., Morin, I., Cuto, G.B., Francoz, D. and Babkine, M. (2009). Retropsective case study of fetal mummification in cows that did not respond to prostaglandin $F_2\alpha$ treatment. *Canadian Veterinary Journal* **50**, 71–76.

Manninger, R. (1946). Section V: Chronic infectious diseases 10. Brucellosis (contagious abortion). In: Russell Grieg, J., Mohler, J.R. and Eichhorn, A. (eds). *Special Pathology and Therapeutics of the Diseases of Domestic Animals*, Volume 1, 5th English edition, pp. 793–827. Bailliere, Tindall and Cox, London.

Marek, J. (1937). Geschlechtsorgane. In: *Lehrbuch der Klinischen Diagnostic der Inneren Krankheiten der Haustiere*, 2nd edition, pp 393–422. Jena, Germany.

Markusfeld-Nir, O. (1997). Epidemiology of bovine abortion in Israeli dairy herds. *Preventive Veterinary Medicine* **31**, 245–255.

Murray, R.D. (2006). A practical approach to infectious abortion diagnosis. *Proceedings 24th World Buiatrics Congress, Nice*, pp. 260–268.

Murray, R.D., Williams, A.J. and Sheldon, I.M. (2008). Field investigation of perinatal mortality in Friesian cattle associated with myocardial degeneration and necrosis. *Reproduction in Domestic Animals* **43**, 339–345.

Silva, A.P.C., Costa, E.E., Macêdo, A.A., Martins, T da M., Borges, A.M., Paixão, T.A. and Santos, R.L. (2012). Transcription of pattern recognition receptors and abortive agent induced chemokines in the bovine pregnant uterus. *Veterinary Immunology and Immunopathology* **145**, 248–256.

Tiwan, A., VanHeeuwen, J.A., Dohoo, I.R., Keefe, G.P., Haddad, J.P., Tremblay, R., Scott, H.M. and Whiting, T. (2007). Production effects of pathogens causing bovine leucosis, bovine viral diarrhoea, paratuberculosis and neosporosis. *Journal of Dairy Science* **90**, 659–669.

Thurmond, M.C., Picanso, J.P. and Jameson, C.M. (1990). Considerations for use of descriptive epidemiology to investigate fetal loss in dairy cows. *Journal of American Veterinary Medical Association* **197**, 1305–1312.

Wu, G., Imhoff-Kunsch, B. and Girard, A.W. (2012). Biological mechanisms for nutritional regulation of maternal health and fetal development. *Paediatric and Perinatal Epidemiology* **26** (Suppl. 1), 4–26.

SECTION V

Dairy Cattle Herd Health

CHAPTER 33

The Prevalence and Cost of Important Endemic Diseases and Fertility in Dairy Herds in the UK

Alastar Macrae and Richard Esslemont

Learning objectives

- Assess the prevalence of the common endemic diseases in UK dairy herds in comparison to average figures and targets.
- Be able to indicate appropriate values for Key Performance Indicators.
- Understand the basis for deriving disease costs.
- Be able to perform an economic cost analysis for the common endemic diseases.
- Be able to identify the main health issues influencing profitability of dairy herds.
- Be able to target areas for improvement in dairy herd health, fertility and productivity.

Introduction

Currently, the average costs of milk production for UK dairy herds are higher than the DEFRA average farmgate milk price, and some 40% of milk is produced at a loss (Colman & Harvey, 2004). With margins so tight, wastage due to culling and disease in UK dairy herds can make the difference between profit and loss. Veterinary services and medicine costs are a relatively small proportion of the overall costs of milk production (Figure 33.1), yet, all too often, these are the costs that concern farmers and their financial advisers. Such a short-term view overlooks the waste from disease and infertility that represents such a significant drain on marginal incomes in many dairy herds.

Recent trends in increasing herd size, increasing milk yield per cow and more cows per staff, in order to reduce fixed costs per litre, have resulted in less individual animal attention, which was the norm in smaller dairy herds previously (Figure 33.2). Increased mechanisation and automation can help, but cannot completely replace the stockmanship critical for managing modern high-yielding dairy cows to optimise fertility, cow health and welfare. There is therefore potential for disease problems to increase and to spread more rapidly in modern larger dairy herds, especially those that are housed all year round. All of this means that it is more important than ever for modern dairy herds to monitor and manage levels of wastage due to culling and disease, to maximise profitability.

The incidence and prevalence of the major diseases in UK dairy herds is surprisingly difficult to determine, due to the lack of a centralised database for disease recording (unlike Scandinavian countries, for example), and a lack of joined-up communication between the disparate systems that might be used for disease recording on-farm. Milk recording information is often very basic, with poor reliability. The recent advent of modern computer programs such as *Interherd Plus* and *TotalVet* enables analysis of data from different sources, which should help. However, all of our knowledge of disease rates on UK dairy farms is based on surveys of small groups of herds, which cannot be assumed to be fully representative of the national herd.

Costs of disease are usually broken down into two parts: direct and indirect costs (Table 33.1). Direct costs are those that are obvious to the farmer such as discarded milk due to antibiotic residues, or veterinary time and treatments. However due to the close inter-relationships of many of these diseases, the indirect costs (such as an increased risk of culling or reduced fertility) often exceed the direct costs.

Another way of categorising the cost of disease is to consider these traditional direct and indirect costs as 'failure costs', which have occurred because preventative measures have not worked. This balance between incurring some 'failure costs', while spending sufficient money on effective 'preventative costs', describes the 'ideal' optimal costs for disease control. The aim is to spend as little as possible to achieve the level of control of disease that maximises profits (Hogeveen *et al.*, 2011).

Bovine Medicine, Third Edition. Edited by Peter D. Cockcroft.

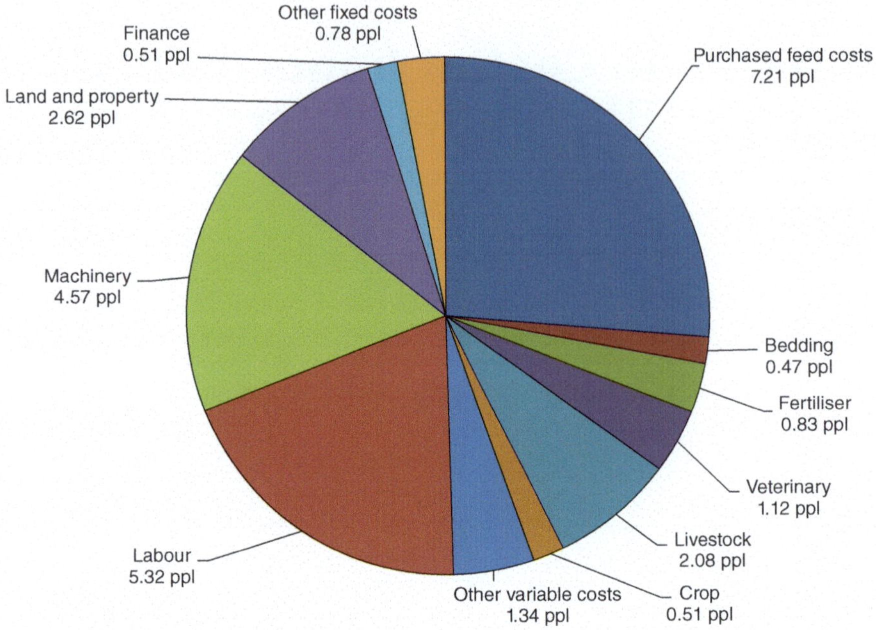

Figure 33.1 Breakdown of costs of milk production for UK dairy herds in 2009–2010 in pence per litre (ppl) (NFU, 2010). The average cost of milk production was 27.4 ppl, and the average farmgate milk price was 25.9 ppl in November 2010. Courtesy of Murray RD.

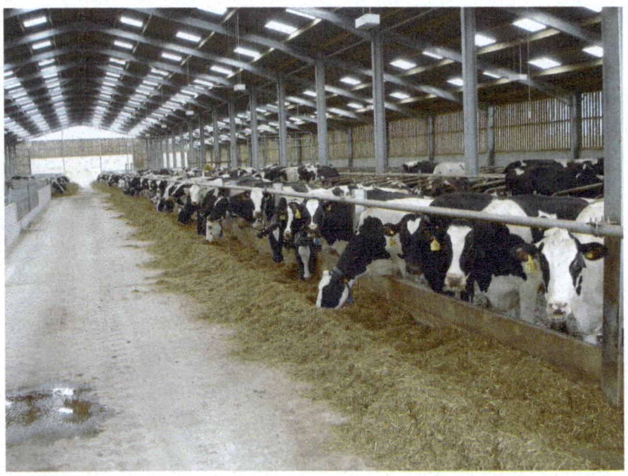

Figure 33.2 Increasing herd size and reduced staffing can spread fixed costs, but it is critical to ensure that health and fertility does not compromise farm profitability.

Table 33.1 Costs of production diseases in dairy cows. Data source: Esslemont and Kossaibati 2002.

Direct costs	Indirect costs
Treatment cost (drugs)	Increased culling rate
Veterinary costs (vet's time)	Possible risk of fatality
Labour costs (herdsman's time)	Susceptibility to other disease
Discarded milk (antibiotic withdrawal)	Extended calving interval
Reduction in milk yield	Extra services per conception
Other direct costs (e.g. Calf mortality)	

Preventive costs have been described. For example, in Dutch herds, preventive costs of mastitis were €88 (£70) per average cow on the farm per year (ranging from €43–€131), and predominantly consisted of labour costs (Hogeveen, 2012). The 'failure costs', as detailed in this chapter, necessarily apply to average cases under specific conditions (e.g. 8000 litre cows with a milk price of 27 ppl), but such an approach argues that costs of disease and preventative medicine must be applied to specific situations on individual farms. This is where the veterinary surgeon, with his/her local knowledge, has a key role in determining the costs of disease specific to the individual farm, and the cost benefit of potential 'preventative costs'.

All of these strategies look at the economic cost of disease for dairy farmers. However, in the wider context, there are also costs associated with animal welfare and greenhouse gas emissions that are difficult to quantify. Improving production efficiency by reducing disease losses and improved reproduction will reduce greenhouse gas emissions per unit of milk (Place & Mitloehner, 2010), so reducing wastage in dairy herds will not only improve economic output for the farm but will also have wider benefits for the dairy industry.

Table 33.2 Disposal rates in DHHPS dairy herds (566 herds, April 2007 to March 2012).

		Average	Median (25%–75%)	Suggested target
Percent of herd sold due to:	*Average herd size*	155 cows	140 cows (96–192 cows)	
	Infertility or FTC	4.9%	4.5% (2.4–6.8)	Below 6%
	Mastitis	3.5%	2.8% (1.2–4.9)	Below 6%
	Lameness	2.2%	1.7% (0–3.1)	Below 6%
	Age	3.6%	2.6% (0.8–5.1)	–
	Yield	0.9%	0% (0–1.3)	–
	Other (including death)	6.3%	5.1% (2.4–8.4)	–
	Total	21.4%	21.2% (16.1–25.9)	Below 20%

Culling

Most studies suggest that the overall culling rate has remained relatively constant at around 20–24%, which means that a fifth of the dairy herd is replaced annually (Table 33.2; Whitaker *et al.*, 2004; Orpin & Esslemont, 2010). The current average lifespan of National Milk Records (NMR) recorded dairy cows in the UK is around 3.9 lactations (Hanks & Kossaibati, 2011), while a recent UK study showed that 22% of heifers born failed to calve for the first time, and only 55% of replacement heifers made it to their third calving (Brickell & Wathes, 2011). Measures such as percentage of days milking during lifetime and Lifetime Daily Yield (LDY–the total amount of milk a cow gives in her lifetime, divided by her age) are good indicators of overall performance, in that they reflect heifer rearing, nutrition, health and welfare. It is generally desirable to keep cows in the herd for longer, as this spreads rearing costs, results in more milk produced per day over their lifetime, and saves on replacement costs.

Cows are culled for two main reasons:

- *'Forced' or involuntary culls*. These are animals that must be culled due to death, disease or poor reproductive performance, and they represent over half of all cows culled (Table 33.2). The three most common reasons are infertility (cows not back in calf when the farmer wants them to be – also known as Failure to Conceive (FTC)), mastitis and lameness.
- *'Selected' or voluntary culls*. These are animals that the farmer chooses to cull for reasons such as poor milk yield, old age, poor conformation, temperament, and management reasons.

The ideal situation for the dairy farmer is to minimise culling through involuntary reasons, and thus have control over which cows are culled. By choosing which cows to cull, the farmer can improve the genetics of the herd by bringing in replacements that are of higher quality than the cows being culled. Management, nutrition and stockmanship all play a key role in reducing the number of involuntary culls, and correct veterinary advice is central to this.

Recent attention has focused on involuntary culls in early lactation and on-farm deaths, which represent a significant cost to the farm and have been used as a proxy measure of cow welfare (as they imply serious issues with health and production diseases). Orpin & Esslemont (2010) found that 5.3% of the cows were culled due to sickness, death, recumbency or casualty, with 2.5% due to deaths. Comparable figures from the USA show around a 10% death rate. Another way of looking at this is the number of cows culled in the first 30 or 60 days of lactation, and the aim is to keep this figure below 2%. Values higher than this would suggest issues with transition cow management and diseases in early lactation, such as milk fevers and LDAs.

Especially in North America, some argue that high culling rates are not necessarily of concern, provided that most of the culling is voluntary, and that replacement costs are low and cull cow prices high (Bethard & Nunes, 2011). It will result in more rapid genetic improvement of the herd, provided that sufficient high genetic merit replacement heifers are available. Such a scenario is most commonly seen in UK herds that sell surplus freshly calved cows, which provide a valuable income stream for the farm but will result in high apparent culling rates. Recording accurate reasons for culling or sale is therefore critical for the proper interpretation of culling records.

Using an average milk yield of 8000 litres per lactation and a milk price of 25 ppl, Orpin & Esslemont (2010) calculated that the cost of a cull ranged from £1,238 for a cull cow sold live at the end of her lactation and £2,744 for a fatality in late lactation losing 90 days of milk margin, to £3,499 for a fatality in early lactation. Figures in 2012 using updated cull cow prices put these figures at £1,328 for a live cull at the end of lactation and £3,307 for a fatality in early lactation.

Mastitis

Most of the surveys on clinical mastitis in UK dairy herds put the clinical case rate at around 40 cases per 100 cows per year (Table 33.3; Esslemont & Kossaibati, 2002; Whitaker *et al.*, 2004; Bradley *et al.*, 2007), and it appears to have changed little in the last decade (Figure 33.3). NMR milk recording data would suggest that the prevalence of subclinical mastitis (based on cows with individual cow somatic cell count (ICSCC) over

Table 33.3 Disease treatment rates in DHHPS dairy herds (566 herds, April 2007–March 2012), given as number of cases per 100 cows per year.

	Average	Median (25%–75%)
Fertility	26.1	11.1 (0–35)
Assisted calving	7.2	5.9 (2.1–9.9)
Mastitis	37.5	32.5 (20.6–48.7)
Digestive disease (including LDAs)	1.1	0 (0–1.4)
Hypomagnesaemia	0.2	0 (0–0)
Hypocalcaemia	4.9	4.1 (0.8–7.5)
Ketosis	0.6	0 (0–0.6)
Lameness	22.3	17 (9.3–29.9)
Injury	0.8	0.8 (0–1.2)
Other	2.6	0.6 (0–2.6)

200 000 cells/ml) is 23%, with 13% of cows having chronically elevated somatic cell counts (Table 33.4). With the top 25% of herds having clinical mastitis case rates of 20 cases per 100 cows per year. and only 18% of cows with elevated ICSCC, there is plenty of scope for improvement in udder health in UK dairy herds using developments such as the DairyCo Mastitis Control Plan.

Reworking of the Esslemont & Kossaibati (2002) costs for clinical mastitis in 2012, using a milk price of 27 ppl, gives a total cost of clinical mastitis per affected cow of £276.77 for a mild case, £761.49 for a severe case and £3,525.61 for a fatal case. Using a prevalence of 90% mild, 9.8% severe and 0.2% fatal cases, this gives the cost of an average case of clinical mastitis per affected cow to be £179.74 in direct costs, and £330.73 in total (Figure 33.4). These costs are similar to those reported in a review by Hogeveen *et al.* in 2011 who reported direct costs of mastitis of £49–78 per average cow in the herd per year (converted from €61–97), which would give direct costs of £122.50–£195.00 for an average herd with a clinical mastitis case rate of 40 cases per 100 cows per year.

Lameness

It is well recognised that lameness in dairy cows is under-recorded on UK dairy farms (Leach *et al.*, 2010). Most figures for treatment rates as recorded by farmers estimate a lameness incidence around 20–24 cases per 100 cows per year (Table 33.3; Esslemont & Kossaibati, 2002; Whitaker *et al.*, 2004). This rate appears to have changed little in the last decade (Figure 33.5). However, more recent detailed analysis in 205 UK dairy herds, using mobility scoring, gave a mean lameness prevalence of 36.8% (range 0–79.2%) (Barker *et al.*, 2010), implying that the actual lameness rate in UK herds is likely to be significantly higher.

Original costs of lameness in UK dairy herds (Esslemont & Kossaibati, 2002) were reviewed by Willshire & Bell (2009), describing costs in an average 112 cow herd giving 6885 litres of milk per cow per year (Table 33.5). The majority of the costs of lameness are due to fertility costs, reduced yield and culling

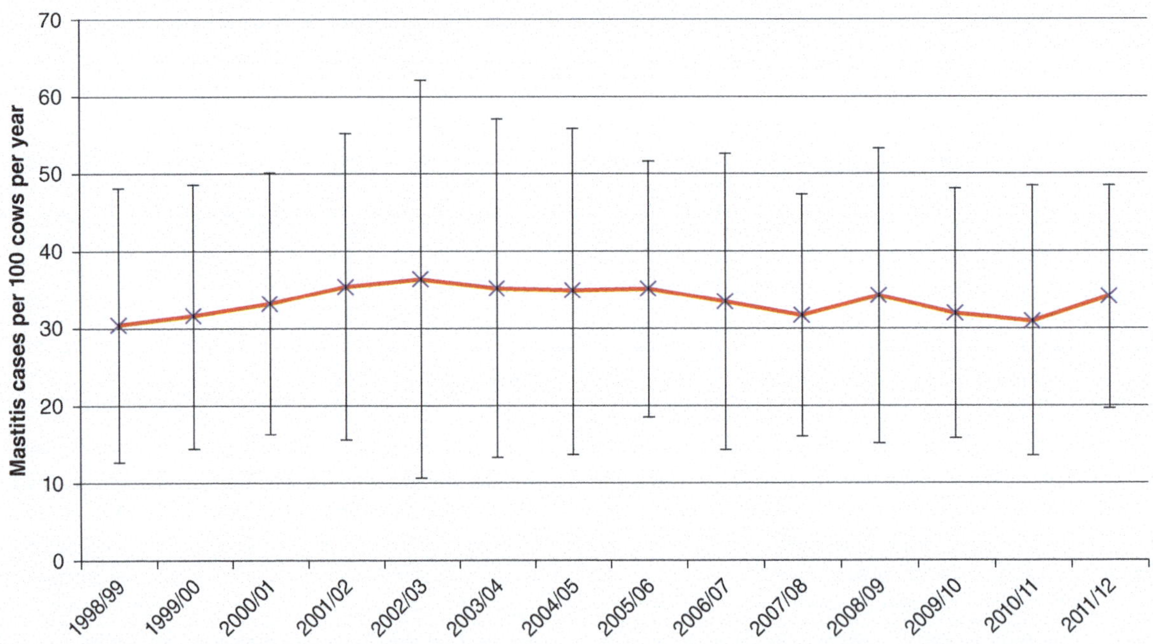

Figure 33.3 Clinical mastitis treatment trends in DHHPS recorded herds from 1998–2012. Line shows median values ± interquartile range.

Table 33.4 Summary of UK udder health parameters and targets. Clinical mastitis figures taken from DHHPS (Table 33.3), with cell count information from Hanks & Kossaibati (2011). Data source: Hanks 2011, Bradley 2005.

	Lower 25% of herds	Median	Upper 25% of herds	Suggested target
Clinical mastitis (cases per 100 cows per year)	20.6	32.5	48.7	Less than 30
Average Somatic Cell Count ('000 cells/ml)	158	203	249	150–200 (dependant on milk contract)
Percentage of cows with chronic infections (i.e. ICSCC greater than 200 000 cells/ml)	9%	13%	17%	Less than 5%
Percentage of cows with ICSCC above 200 000 cells/ml in any one recording.	18%	23%	29%	Less than 10%
Percentage of cows with ICSCC above 200 000 cells/ml at first milk recording of lactation.	15%	19%	24%	15%

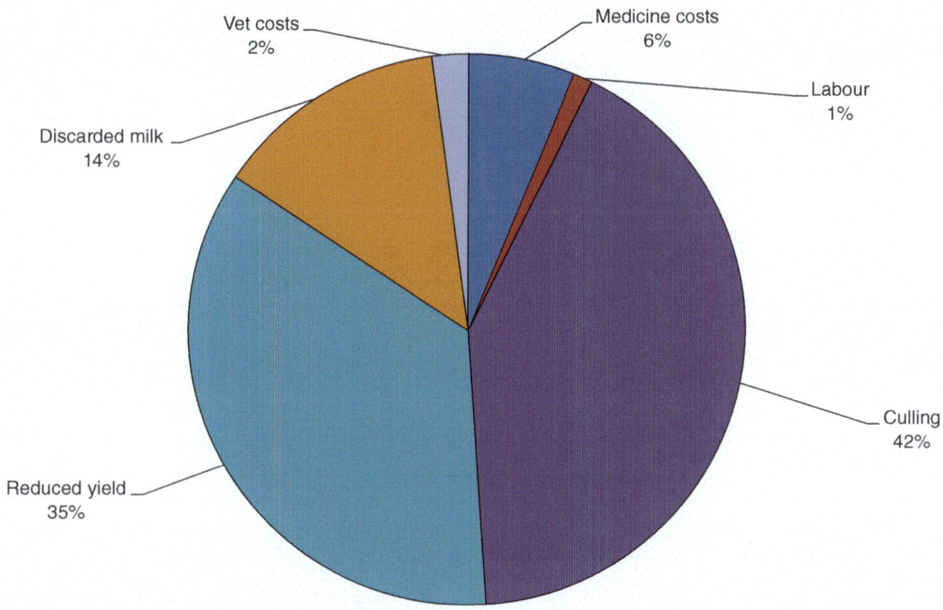

Figure 33.4 Lameness treatment trends in DHHPS recorded herds from 1998–2012. Line shows median values ± interquartile range.

(Figure 33.6). Extrapolating these figures to the national herd, the authors estimated that clinical lameness costs the typical UK dairy herd 0.97 ppl, with lameness in dairy herds costing the UK dairy industry over £127 million per annum.

Fertility

Poor fertility performance is a major constraint on dairy herd profitability in the UK. However, our current knowledge of the status of fertility performance in UK dairy herds is inadequate, and even the quality of the available information is questionable. It is of note that one recent study of fertility data gathered from UK farms rejected over half the datasets due to poor recording of service events (Hudson *et al.*, 2010). However, the three most recent UK studies on dairy cow fertility have come up with similar headline figures: calving intervals of 404–421 days, all service conception rates of 31–38% and heat detection rates of 29–36% (Table 33.6; Hanks & Kossaibati, 2011; Hudson *et al.*, 2010; Kerby, 2009). These figures, compared to targets in Table 33.6, suggest that there is significant scope for improvement in UK dairy fertility performance.

Various costings models are applied to fertility performance, with the majority looking at the effects of extended lactations

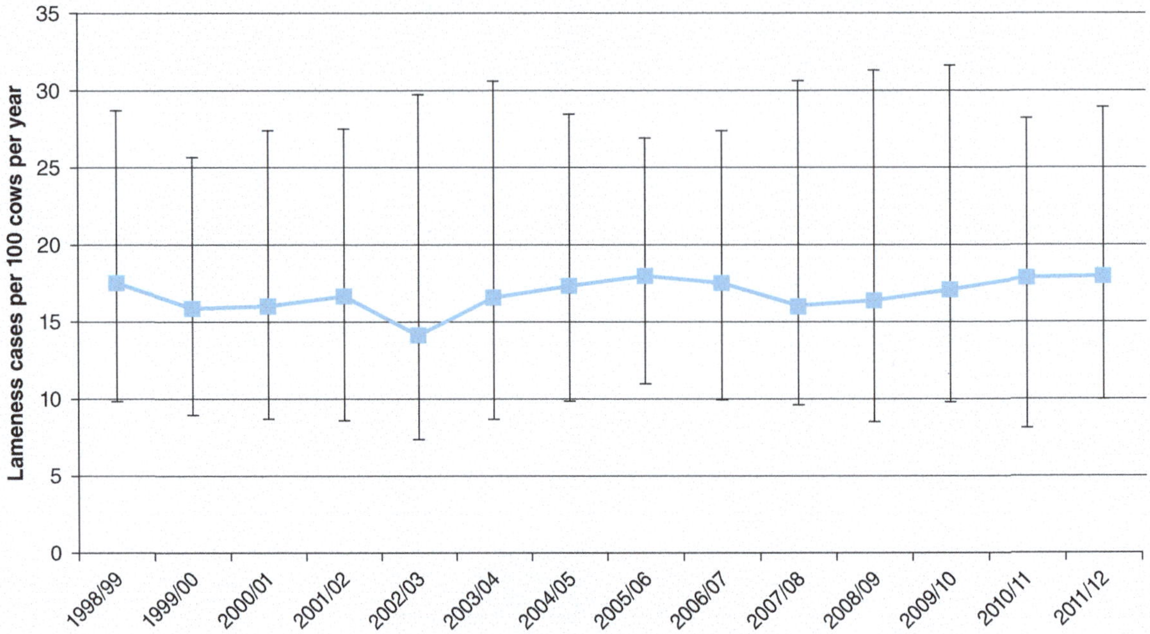

Figure 33.5 Breakdown of mastitis costs in UK dairy herds. Data source: Esslemont and Kossaibati 2002.

Table 33.5 Costs of lameness in dairy cows per case by lesion. Data source: Willshire 2009.

	Incidence (cases/100 cows/year)	Cost per case
Digital dermatitis	1.7	£75.57
Digital dermatitis (not white line disease)	6.2	£185.83
Interdigital lameness	–	£154.31
Sole ulcer	7.2	£518.73
White line disease	5.6	£300.05

on milk yield, which results in costs based on days over target calving intervals (Table 33.7). It is of note that the majority of the costs of poor fertility are due to reduction in milk yield due to extended lactations, when these cows could be in early lactation with higher levels of milk production (Figure 33.7). Instead of the focus on milk produced per lactation (which can be manipulated by extended lactations), the focus should be on milk produced per cow per year.

Comparison of these figures often reveals the losses associated with poor fertility, which will not compensate for any reduction in transition cow diseases, as is often argued (Table 33.7). However culling for failure to conceive (FTC) also needs to be accounted for when assessing costs, due to extended calving intervals, and this is the basis of the FERTEX score as described by Esslemont & Kossaibati (2002). This takes into account calving interval, number of services per conception and FTC culling rate. Reworking of these figures in 2012, compared to standard figures, gives a cost of poor fertility in the average UK dairy herd of £443 per cow or 5.54 ppl (Table 33.9).

While the 2012 costs of reproductive related disorders can be calculated for individual conditions (Table 33.8), the key is looking at overall herd fertility performance. Table 33.9 summarises the effect of the five key indices required to achieve target outcomes in terms of calving interval and FTC culling rate, and their associated costs:

- Percentage served of calved (target over 93%)
- Calving to 1st service interval (target 65 days)
- Voluntary Waiting Period (50 days)
- Heat Detection Rate (target 58% or above)
- Conception rates (target 47% or above)

Table 33.9 can be used to derive the costs of poor fertility in dairy herds, but illustrates the importance of not focusing on limited indices such as conception rates (Figure 33.8) in isolation.

Production disease

The production diseases listed in Table 33.10 are relatively uncommon in comparison to mastitis and lameness – hence, the minor gains seen in Table 33.7 due to extended calving intervals. Diseases such as milk fever and ketosis are often seen

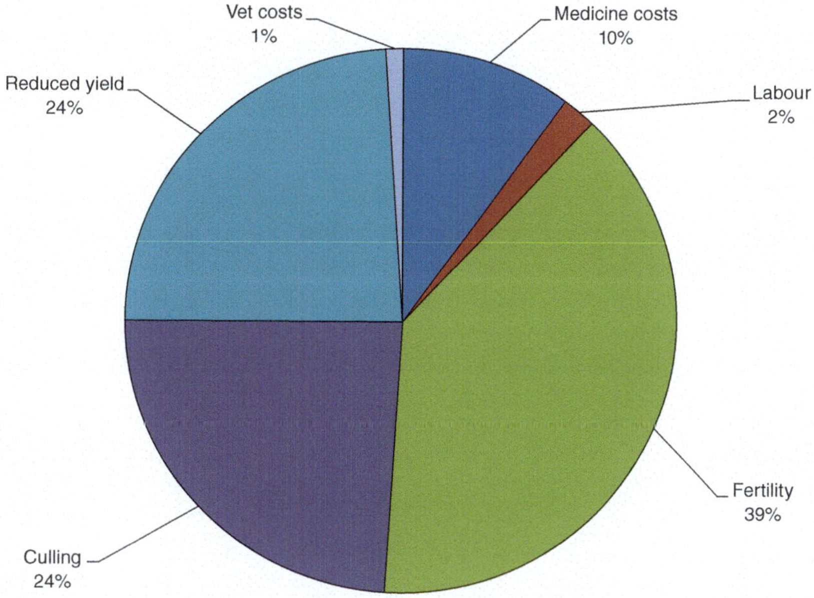

Figure 33.6 Breakdown of lameness costs in UK dairy herds. Data source: Willshire and Bell 2009.

Table 33.6 Summary of UK fertility parameters and targets. Data source: Kossaibati 2011.

	Lower 25% of herds	Median	Upper 25% of herds	Suggested targets
Lifetime Daily Yield (litres of milk per cow per day of life)	10	12	13	Over 14 litres
Actual calving interval (days)	408	421	436	365 days if block calving 365–400 days if all year round
Calving to 1st service interval (days)	82	98	119	65 days
Percentage served by 80 days after calving	33%	47%	59%	Over 65%
100 day in-calf rate (%)	16%	25%	33%	Over 45% if calving all year round, 75% if block calving
200 day not-in-calf rate (%)	–	–	–	Less than 10%
Conception rate (%)	24%	31%	37%	Over 45%
Heat Detection Rate (%)	20%	29%	40%	Over 55%
Pregnancy rate (%) – also known as Reproduction Efficiency *or* Fertility Factor *or* Pregnancy Risk	5%	9%	13%	Over 20%

as minor by farmers, as clinical cases are frequently treated successfully without veterinary intervention. However, their costs are relatively high, due to indirect costs associated with lost milk production, reduced fertility and increased susceptibility to other diseases. In farms with 'outbreaks' of LDAs, or milk fever cases associated with poor transition cow management, these costs will soon mount up and illustrate the benefit of preventative action.

Endemic infectious disease

A 2007 bulk milk sample survey of 400 dairy herds in Scotland, prior to the BVD eradication scheme, reported that only 22% of farms were bulk tank seronegative, and that 42% of study farms showed high antibody titres (indicative of recent BVD exposure or vaccination). Similar figures have been reported for UK national bulk tank serological surveys (Paton *et al.*, 1998),

Table 33.7 Breakdown of the costs of an extra day on the calving interval for a herd with a calving index of 396–425 days. Data souce: Hudson 2009. Note that these costs do not include culling for failure to conceive.

	Cost
Lost production from next lactation (litres/day)	29.51 litres
Gained production in this lactation (litres/day)	12.96 litres
Net loss of milk production (litres/day)	16.54 litres
Cost of lost milk production @ 26 ppl	£4.30
Gain due to concentrate saved feeding for lost production	+ £0.94
Cost of reduced calf crop	£0.27
Cost of extra days dry	£0.30
Cost of extra services and vet treatments	£0.70
Gain due to reduction in calving-associated disease	+ £0.43
Gain in milk yield in barren cows	+ £0.13
Overall net loss per day	**£4.07**

Table 33.8 Summary of costs of reproductive related diseases in dairy herds. Methodology from Esslemont & Kossaibati (2002), updated in 2012 for an average lactation yield of 8000 litres and milk price of 27 ppl.

	Direct costs	Indirect costs	Total costs
Oestrus not observed	£18.17 for 1.5 treatments per cow	None	£18.17
Endometritis	£98.86 for 1.5 treatments per cow	£114.10	£212.96
Twinning	Gain of £84.77 due to extra calf	£316.09	£231.31
Calf mortality	£147.44	£273.26	£420.70

and it is estimated that 1% of cattle in the UK are persistently infected with BVD virus. Cost estimates for BVD infection vary, depending on whether an acute outbreak occurs in a naïve herd (£217.79 per cow) or the herd is endemically infected (£90.65 per cow) (Bennett *et al.*, 2007; Table 33.11).

Paton *et al.* (1998) also found that 69% of UK dairy herds were seropositive for IBR. This virus has been shown to result in milk drop, abortions, reduced fertility and deaths in dairy herds. Cost estimates for IBR infection in dairy herds have not been published; a loss of 0.92 kg of milk per cow per day during a period of nine weeks has been modelled in Dutch herds (van Schaik *et al.*, 1999), giving a loss of £16 per cow in milk yield loss alone at 2012 prices. Including two cow deaths (not uncommon in IBR outbreaks) would increase the cost markedly, by £66 per cow in the herd, and this does not include any losses associated with reduced fertility and abortions.

Leptospirosis is also endemic in UK dairy herds, with serological surveys suggesting that approximately 75% of cattle have been exposed. Costs arise due to abortions, infertility and loss of milk yield, and were calculated to be £68–£106 per cow in an affected herd (Owen, 2003).

Paratuberculosis (Johne's Disease) is endemic in UK dairy herds, and a recent survey has suggested that approximately one-third of UK dairy herds are infected (DEFRA, 2009). Calculations of the cost of Johne's disease take into account the associated mortality, increase in replacement costs, veterinary testing and reduction in milk yield from affected cattle. Using recent cost calculators (Bennett *et al.*, 2007), these costs are calculated to be £103.66 per cow in an endemically infected herd with no control measures in place, with other estimated costs in UK herds ranging from £94–£170 per cow per year.

Lungworm infection of adult cows is also a growing issue in UK dairy herds, and a recent Dutch study estimated the total costs to be €159 and €167 per cow on the farm, mostly as a result of lost milk production and cow deaths (Holzhauer *et al.*, 2011).

Youngstock disease

The major losses in youngstock have been recently highlighted by a study of 1097 calvings on 19 dairy farms in England (Brickell *et al.*, 2009). On average, 7.9% of calves died or were stillborn (range 2.7% to 14.3%), a figure similar to that reported by Esslemont & Kossaibati (2002). This figure was significantly higher if assistance was required at calving, and in twins. In total, 14.5% of live born heifer calves failed to make it to their first calving: 6.8% of heifers died or were culled between one day and six months old, and 7.7% of heifers died or were culled between six months old and their first calving (mostly due to infectious disease, accidents or infertility).

The majority of infectious disease issues in calves arise due to calf diarrhoea or pneumonia. Recent costings for these diseases are not available: Stott & Gunn (1995) calculated that a case of calf diarrhoea costed £44 per calf affected, and Andrews (2000) calculated that pneumonia in dairy calves costed £43 per sick animal and £30 per animal in the group. Of interest is more recent work from AFBI Hillsborough that showed that calves that had multiple episodes of pneumonia as calves produced approximately 5% less milk in their first lactation, and 10% less milk in their second lactation (a financial cost of £297 over the two lactations) (Morrison, SJ, Personal Communication).

Table 33.9 Effect of poor fertility on financial performance in dairy herds based on five grades of fertility (A+ to D). Figures based on Esslemont & Kossaibati (2002), updated for 2012 using yield of 8,000 litres and milk price of 27 ppl.

	Fertility Management Assessment Grades (Target A or A+)	A+	A	B	C	D	UK
		Excellent	Adequate	Slight Problem	Moderate Problem	Severe Problem	Average
Crucial Factors	*Per Cent Served of Calved (%)*	94+	90 to 93	87–89	84–86	< 83	88
	Voluntary Waiting Period	50	55	60	65	70	68
	Calving to First Service (days)	55–65	65 to 75	75 to 80	80 to 85	> 85	87
	Average Calving to First Service Interval	65	75	80	83	96	90
	1st Service 24 Day Submission Rate (%)	69+	59 to 68	48-58	33–47	< 32	50
	16 to 28 day Returns Service Heat Detection rate (%)	68	59 to 68	53–59	40–52	< 39	40
	Average Heat Detection Rate %	68	64	56	46	40	43
	80 Day Submission Rate (%)	77	67	52	35	25	40
	Inter Service Interval (days)	31	33	38	46	53	44
	1st Service Pregnancy Rate (%)	58	52 to 57	47-51	42-46	< 41	40
	All Services Pregnancy Rate (%)	58+	52 to 57	47-51	42-46	< 41	38
	FERTILITY FACTOR (%)*	40+	32 to 39	28-31	21-27	< 21	21
	Services per Conception	1.72	1.82	2.04	2.33	2.63	2.63
Outcomes	100 Day In Calf Rate	73	55	44	34	28	31
	Per Conceiving of Served (%)	96+	92 to 95	89-91	85-88	< 84	80
	Per Cent Conceiving of Calved (%)	88+	82 to 87	79-81	74–78	< 73	70
	Average Calving to Conception (days)	85	93	100	133	157	129
	Calving Interval (days)	365	373	380	413	437	424
	Days Open	86–109	110 to 120	121–133	134–154	> 154	170
	200 Day Not In Calf Rate	4	6	14	20	33	23
	Failure to Conceive Culling Rate (%)	6	*9*	*12*	*17*	*28*	*18*
	All Other Culling Rate	10	11.5	13.5	16	14	12
	Total Culling Rate (%)	16.0	20.5	25.5	33.0	42.0	30.0
	Calving Interval Adjusted Conceiving Rate (%)	95	85	82	69	63	71
FERTEX	Calving Interval	£0	£1,200	£2,250	£19,200	£32,400	£26,550
	Services per Conception	£0	£200	£640	£1,220	£1,820	£1,823
	FTC Culling Rate	£0	£3,984	£7,968	£14,608	£29,216	£15,936
	FERTEX Score (£/100 cows)	£0	£5,384	£10,858	£35,028	£63,436	£44,309
	FERTEX Score Pence per Litre	0.00	0.67	1.36	4.38	7.93	5.54
			Loss	Loss	Loss	Loss	Loss
	Cost of day Extended Calving Interval	0.0	1.5	2.0	4.0	4.5	4.5

Yield	8000

Target Calving Interval (days)	365	Cost per day's delay-ave (£)	3.10
Target Services per Conception	1.72	Cost per extra Service (£)	20
Target FTC Culling (%)	6	Cost per Extra FTC Cull (£)	1328

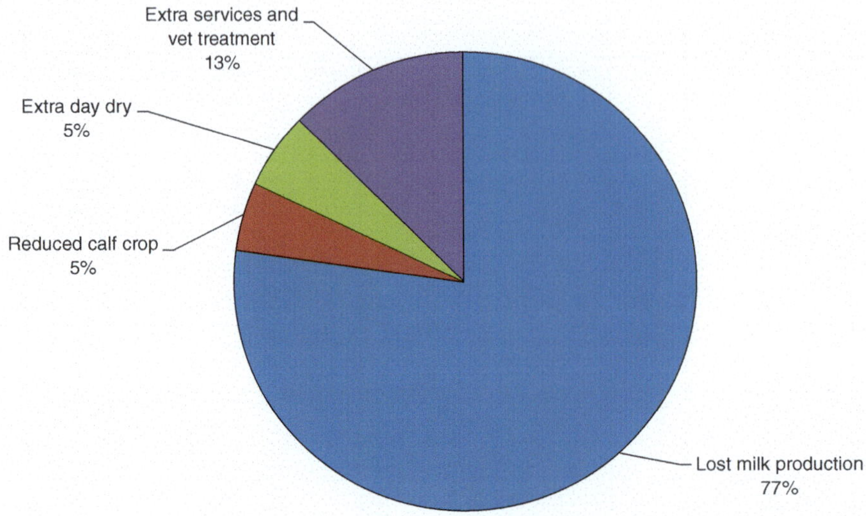

Figure 33.7 Breakdown of fertility costs in UK dairy herds. Data source: Hudson 2009.

Table 33.10 Summary of production disease rates, targets and associated costs. Methodology from Esslemont & Kossaibati (2002), updated for 2012 for an average lactation yield of 8000 litres and milk price of 27 ppl.

	Current UK rate	Target	Direct costs	Average cost per case
Hypocalcaemia	5%	Under 5%	£130.89	£420.63
Clinical ketosis	1%	Under 1%	£109.56	£823 per clinical case
Left displaced abomasum	1–2%	Under 1%	£220.58	£689.23
Retained placenta	4%	Under 3%	£109.69	£470.04

Table 33.11 Endemic infectious disease costs in UK dairy herds.

	UK Herd Prevalence	Annual cost per cow in herd	Reference
Bovine virus diarrhoea (BVD)	42–90%	£90.65	Bennett *et al.* (2007)
Leptospirosis	75%	£68–£106	Owen (2003)
Infectious bovine rhinotracheitis (IBR)	69%	£82 associated with reduced milk production and two deaths	–
Paratuberculosis (Johne's disease)	34.7% (95% CI: 27.6–42.5%)	£103.66	Bennett *et al.* (2007)

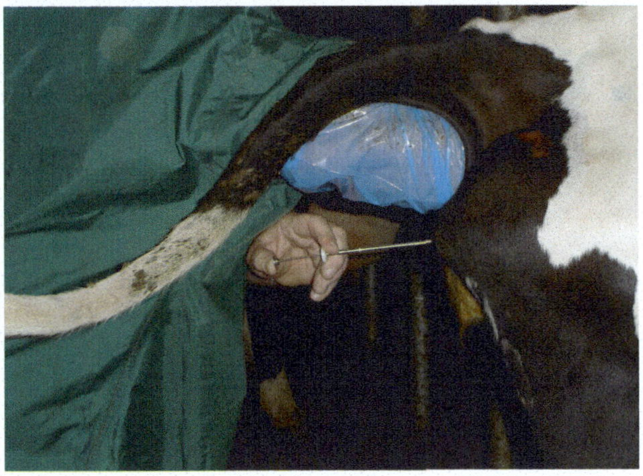

Figure 33.8 Conception rates are only one of five key components for optimum herd fertility performance.

This serves to illustrate both the complexity and long-term nature of disease problems in youngstock.

The farm audit

By analysing key performance indicators and comparing the outcomes on farm to realistic target values, it is possible to identify strengths and weaknesses and quantify the losses in economic terms. This will enable prioritised targeted investigations of management practices to be made, and recommendations to be made with a cost benefit estimation. An example of the

Question:
What are the economic losses associated with poor youngstock management in a dairy herd?
Best practice/gold standard:
- 10% losses from birth to first calving.
- Age at First Calving (AFC): 24–25 months old.

Data collection:
Use calving or BCMS records to identify birth dates of all the heifers born in a 12-month period at least 36 months ago.
- How many were born: dead, alive?
- How many were lost: date, reason, age, and destination.
- Rough income if sold.
  - Dead or alive?
  - How many were barren or pregnant?

Data-analysis
- Total and percentage that did not calve.
- Percentage that died.
- Distribution of age at calving – < 22 months too soon, > 20 months too late.

Key performance indicator values and target values
- 98% of heifers born alive, 2% stillborn/died within 24 hours: Satisfactory
- 95% of heifers weaned at 7 weeks, 3% died due to scour: Satisfactory
- 85% of heifers bred by 18 months of age, 10% died: Mortality high
- Most lost due to pneumonia at 10–14 weeks of age, 40% of heifers treated for pneumonia.
- 83% of heifers born reached first calving.
- Median age at first calving: 26 months, with 15% over 28 months.

Comments:
- High mortality rate in heifers from weaning to breeding .
- Treatment records suggest that post-weaning pneumonia is the main issue.
- 15% AFC too high, most likely due to reduced growth rates as a result of pneumonia.
- Investigate pneumonia problems: ventilation, pathogen involvement, mixing of age groups, etc.

Costs:
- Cost to rear a heifer about £1400 = £1.92 per day.
- Heifer culled or dying in rearing loses about £500 per animal lost.
- 17% mortality for 25% replacement rate in herd = £2,125 per 100 cows in herd.

Associated KPI:
Target growth rates for heifers for 24 month AFC: 0.7 kg per head per day for Holsteins.
Potential and actual impact on profitability: High

Figure 33.9 The farm audit: the application of prevalence and cost information for youngstock management.

application of prevalence and cost information for youngstock management in the audit process is presented in Figure 33.9.

Conclusions

With the current tight margins in dairy production in the UK, it is even more essential to minimise losses due to poor health and productivity, in order to maximise herd profitability. However, with a UK average clinical mastitis case rate of 40 cases per 100 cows per year, a lameness prevalence of 37%, calving intervals over 420 days, and major infectious diseases such as BVD and IBR endemic in UK dairy herds, there is plenty of scope for improvement in reducing the financial impact of these production diseases. Indeed, reworking of the Health Index (HEALEX) for the average UK dairy herd (Esslemont & Kossabati, 2002) suggests that such disease issues are currently costing £284 per cow, or 3.56 ppl (Table 33.12) (i.e. 15% of the 2012 farmgate milk price).

While diseases such as mastitis and lameness cannot be eradicated from dairy herds, appropriate control measures can be put in place to reduce their prevalence and impact on overall herd viability. The modern farm animal veterinary surgeon therefore has a key role in identifying constraints on farm profitability, assessing the economic losses involved, with the aim of applying cost benefit analysis of potential strategies to improve herd health, cow welfare and farm profitability.

Table 33.12 Summary of the effect of health problems on financial performance in a dairy herd based on four grades (A to D). Figures based on Esslemont & Kossaibati (2002), updated for 2012 using yield of 8000 litres and milk price of 27 ppl.

Diseases		A TARGET	B OK	C POOR	D VERY POOR	UK Average	Direct Cost £/case
Health Problem							
Twins-Cases per 100 Cows		1	4	5.5	6	6	
Cost £/100 cows		−85	−339	−466	−509	−509	−84.77
Calf Mortality - cases per 100 Calves Born		3	7	9	10	9	
Cost £/100 cows		442	1032	1327	1474	1327	147.44
Aid at Calving - cases per 100 Cows		2	7	11.5	15	10	
Cost £/100 cows		77	269	441	575	384	38.36
Retained Foetal Membranes - cases per 100 Cows		1.5	3	4.5	5	6	
Cost £/100 cows		165	329	494	548	658	109.69
Milk Fever - cases per 100 Cows		1.5	6	9.5	11	9	
Cost £/100 cows		196	785	1243	1440	1178	130.89
Displaced Abomasum	LDA	1.5	4	6	8	5	
Cost £/100 cows		447	1193	1790	2387	1492	298.33
Oestrus Not Observed - % of Herd Affected		21	28.5	38.5	45	40	12.11
cases per 100 cows		30	42	55	68	60	
repeat cases per 100 cows		9	13.5	16.5	23	20	12.11
Cost £/100 cows		363	509	666	823	727	
Vulval Discharge - % of herd affected		6	11	17.5	21	14	84.47
cases per 100 cows		8	17	26.5	31	22	
repeat cases per 100 cows		2	6	9	10	8	28.79
Cost £/100 cows		564	1102	1737	2062	1413	
Clinical Mastitis - % of herd affected		10	20	25	27	40	139.8
cases per 100 cows		16	30	45	51	61	
repeat cases per 100 cows		6	10	20	24	21	66.37
Cost £/100 cows		1796	3460	4822	5367	6986	
Sub Clinical mastitis Yield Reduction		90000	175000	270000	325000	230000	
8000 litres % Loss		0	0.0075	0.0270	0.00325	0.0130	
Herd Loss Cost £/100 cows	0.17	0	1020	3672	4420	1768	
Months Penalty Paid High SCC		0	1	2	4	3	
0.015 p/litre 66667 £1,000	litres per month	0	1000	2000	4000	3000	1000
Lameness-% of herd affected		6	12	20	24	45	128.77
cases per 100 cows		8	17	28	36	60	
repeat cases per 100 cows		2	5	8	12	15	65.9
Cost £/100 cows		904	1875	3103	3881	6783	
Dairy Youngstock Losses (2 days to calving) %		4	9	16	25	14	
Number of Dairy Heifers lost: Number born	42	1.68	3.78	6.72	10.5	5.88	550
Cost £/100 cows		924	2079	3696	5775	3234	
Total C cost £/100 cows		**5795**	**14313**	**24525**	**32245**	**28440**	
Cost in ppl 800000		0.72	1.79	3.07	4.03	3.56	
HEALEX (Cost Above The Target) £/100 Cow herd		0	8518	18730	26450	22645	

References

Andrews, A.H. (2000). Calf pneumonia costs. *Cattle Practice* **8**, 109–114.

Barker, Z.E., Leach, K.A., Whay, H.R., Bell, N.J. and Main, D.C. (2010). Assessment of lameness prevalence and associated risk factors in dairy herds in England and Wales. *Journal of Dairy Science* **93**, 932–41.

Bennett, R.M., McFarlane, I. and McClement, I. (2007). Demonstration Models of the Cost and Benefits of BVD and Johne's Control on Cattle Farms. *Cattle Practice* **15**, 175–177.

Bethard, G. and Nunes, A.L. (2011). *Are You Efficiently Replacing Your Herd?* Proceedings from the Western Dairy Management Conference, March 9–11th Reno, Nevada. p53–65. Accessed 22nd June, 2012 http://www.wdmc.org/.

Bradley, A.J. and Green, M.J. (2005). Use and interpretation of somatic cell count data in dairy cows. *In Practice* **27**, 310–315.

Bradley A.J., Leach, K.A., Breen, J.E., Green, L.E and Green, M.J. (2007). Survey of the incidence and aetiology of mastitis on dairy farms in England and Wales. *Veterinary Record* **160**, 253–7.

Brickell, J.S. and Wathes, D.C. (2011). A descriptive study of the survival of Holstein-Friesian heifers through to third calving on English dairy farms. *Journal of Dairy Science* **94**, 1831–8.

Brickell, J.S., McGowan, M.M., Pfeiffer, D.U. and Wathes, D.C. (2009). Mortality in Holstein-Friesian calves and replacement heifers, in relation to body weight and IGF-I concentration, on 19 farms in England. *Animal* **3**, 1175–82.

Coleman, D. and Harvey, D. (2004). *The future of UK dairy farming.* Accessed 22nd June, 2012 http://archive.defra.gov.uk/foodfarm/food/industry/sectors/milk/pdf/colman-harveyreport.pdf.

DEFRA (2009). *SB4022: An Integrated Strategy to Determine the Herd Level Prevalence of Johne's Disease in the UK Dairy Herd.* Accessed 22nd June, 2012 http://archive.defra.gov.uk/foodfarm/farmanimal/diseases/atoz/documents/johnes-report0911.pdf.

Esslemont, R.J. and Kossaibati, M. (2002). DAISY Research Report Number 5. *The costs of poor fertility and disease in UK dairy herds. Trends in DAISY herds over 10 seasons.* Copies available from dick@dickesslemont.co.uk.

Hanks, J. and Kossaibati, M. (2011). *Key Performance Indicators for the UK national dairy herd: A study of herd performance in 500 Holstein/Friesian herds for the year ending 30th September 2011.* Accessed 22nd June, 2012. http://www.veeru.rdg.ac.uk/documents/HolsteinFriesian500HerdsSept2011.pdf.

Hogeveen, H., Huijps, K. and Lam, T.J. (2011). Economic aspects of mastitis: new developments. *New Zealand Veterinary Journal* **59**, 16–23.

Hogeveen, H. (2012). *Cost of production diseases.* 27th World Buiatrics Congress 2012, Lisbon, Portugal. Keynote lectures and round tables proceeding, pp. **36–42**.

Holzhauer, M., van Schaik, G., Saatkamp, H.W. and Ploeger, H.W. (2011). Lungworm outbreaks in adult dairy cows: estimating economic losses and lessons to be learned. *Veterinary Record* **169**, 494, doi: 10.1136/vr.d4736.

Hudson, C.D., Breen, J.E., Bradley, A.J. and Green, M.J. (2010). Fertility in UK Dairy Herds: Preliminary findings of a large-scale study. *Cattle Practice* **18**, 89–94.

Hudson, C.D. (2009). Fruitful findings on fertility; in article by Phil Christopher. *Veterinary Times* **39**(4), 6–7.

Kerby, M. (2009). The reproductive performance of 42 commercial dairy herds in the South-West of England in 2006/07. Observations, lessons learnt and thoughts for the future. *Cattle Practice* **17**, 26–32.

Leach, K.A., Whay, H.R., Maggs, C.M., Barker, Z.E., Paul, E.S., Bell, A.K. and Main, D.C. (2010). Working towards a reduction in cattle lameness: 1. Understanding barriers to lameness control on dairy farms. *Research in Veterinary Science* **89**, 311–7.

NFU (2010). *NFU Cost of Milk Production Report.* Accessed 22nd June, 2012. http://www.nfuonline.com/News/COP-Report-February-2011.

Orpin, P.G. and Esslemont, R.J. (2010). Culling and wastage in dairy herds: an update on incidence and economic impact in dairy herds in the UK. *Cattle Practice* **18**, 163–172.

Owen, G. (2003). Bovine leptospirosis. *The Moredun Foundation Newssheet* **3**(20).

Paton, D.J., Christiansen, K.H., Alenius, S., Cranwell, M.P., Pritchard, G.C. and Drew, T.W. (1998). Prevalence of antibodies to bovine virus diarrhoea virus and other viruses in bulk tank milk in England and Wales. *Veterinary Record* **142**, 385–91.

Place, S.E. and Mitloehner, F.M. (2010). Contemporary environmental issues: a review of the dairy industry's role in climate change and air quality and the potential of mitigation through improved production efficiency. *Journal of Dairy Science* **93**, 3407–16.

Stott, A.W. and Gunn, G.J. (1995). The costs of bovine enteritis in suckled calves. *Scottish. Agricultural Economics Review* **8**, 83–88.

Van Schaik, G., Shoukri, M., Martin, S.W., Schukken, Y.H., Nielen, M., Hage, J.J. and Dijkhuizen, A.A. (1999). Modeling the effect of an outbreak of bovine herpesvirus type 1 on herd-level milk production of Dutch dairy farms. *Journal of Dairy Science* **82**, 944–952.

Willshire, J.A. and Bell, N.J. (2009). An economic review of cattle lameness. *Cattle Practice* **17**, 136–141.

Whitaker, D.A., Macrae, A.I. and Burrough, E. (2004). Disposal and disease rates in British dairy herds between April 1998 and March, 2002. *Veterinary Record* **155**, 43–7.

Useful sources of Information

www.rdg.ac.uk/fhpmodels	Cost calculators for Johne's and BVD.
www.mastitiscontrolplan.co.uk	DairyCo Mastitis Control Plan.
www.farm-cost.co.uk	Merial Mastitis Cost Calculator.
www.dairyco.org.uk	DairyCo website.

CHAPTER 34

Dairy Cow Housing Audit

Chris Watson

Learning objectives

The scope of this chapter is limited to outlining basic principles and helping to source and utilise accurate detailed concepts of housing for particular production systems.

- Be able to reference diseases and conditions of a particular livestock system that would affect design features.
- Be able to reference values for housing designs and layout details.
- Understand the principles of building design and use systems of physical and animal measures as key performance indicators.
- Be able to compile a farm audit questionnaire and perform an audit.
- Be able to indicate appropriate values for key performance indicators and benchmark against industry standards or previous farm performance.

Introduction

Cattle are robust animals that are quite capable of surviving in a wide variety of environmental conditions, and do so in many parts of the world. They have evolved minor differences to manage everything from the heat of the tropics to the cold, frozen wastes of the tundra. However, to manage cattle within a controlled production system in temperate climates, there is a distinct requirement to supply housing for a variety of reasons:

- Protect the grazing area from damage during heavy rainfall or winter periods.
- Protect the animal from extreme adverse conditions that may occur.
- Enable better management of the cattle production system – everything from proper control of feeding, health examination and attention, to producing improved results with routine tasks such as heat detection and disease control.

Commercial modern agriculture means that stock have to be confined and managed within a building for a major part of the year and this must fulfil the basic requirements which can be summarised by the welfare of the animal to express the 'Five Freedoms' (Farm Animals Welfare Council - FAWC - 1997 report).

- *Freedom from hunger and thirst* – by ready access to fresh water and a diet to maintain full health and vigour.
- *Freedom from discomfort* – by providing an appropriate environment including shelter and a comfortable resting area.
- *Freedom from pain, injury or disease* – by prevention or rapid diagnosis and treatment.
- *Freedom to express normal behaviour* – by providing sufficient space, proper facilities and company of the animal's own kind.
- *Freedom from fear and distress* – by ensuring conditions and treatment which avoid mental suffering.

In the UK we are only just emerging from an era when the majority of cattle buildings have been adapted from older existing structures. The inherent faults within them mean they do not meet the modern requirements for livestock, especially an increase in stocking density, different size of animals, and the different approaches to feeding cattle. For instance, many older buildings have the space requirement but lack the ventilation characteristics so, with modern high-moisture diets (e.g. silages) and the need for increased stocking densities, they fail to perform adequately. Many cubicle systems for dairy cows have not taken account of the increase in physical size and udder capacity of the animals now needing to be accommodated.

Building design based on economics will always try and produce designs or constructions that are 'multi-purpose', or 'Design and Build', as they are known. This may be cost-effective, but it often compromises the finer specific details and requirements of the animal that will eventually use the building. In most farm situations, there will be a need for a variety of different housing environments to suit different classes of stock (based on age or size), as well as the specific management characteristics

Bovine Medicine, Third Edition. Edited by Peter D. Cockcroft.

needed for these animals (e.g. dry cows or lactating, calves, youngstock, etc.).

Dairy cows present the biggest housing challenge, as their health and welfare is very significantly affected by building design and function, and these needs change with the various stages of their lactation cycle. The basic underlying principles of housing are the same for all types of cattle, and it is only the detail that differs. The veterinarian and adviser will need to have a detailed knowledge of the health risks, as well as production requirements, in order to understand the implications that both have for housing each class of stock.

It is also important to remember that any housing structure is simply that – a construction to accommodate animals – and often, the key features for the successful performance of the housing are the way that is managed and used for the cattle occupying it. Good design and function are heavily reliant on good management techniques and stockperson skills. Poor management can make a good design function badly, and yet excellent stockmanship can produce miracles out of appalling buildings. It is this vital interaction between management and housing that effects the success, or otherwise, of the outcome. An important consideration in the modern working place is the safety and working comfort of the staff managing the building.

A useful methodology when performing an housing audit is to consider the following three approaches:

- *Standard Specifications.* Start with accepted standard specifications for building design that have been set down for the particular stock age group or management purpose. These guidelines need to allow for the scale of the enterprise.
- *Measurables.* Use techniques to assess and monitor the physical building performance based on measurements or observations that can easily be carried out in practice.
- *Animal Measurables.* Observe the animal's behaviour, health and response to the building environment once the house is occupied. This obviously cannot be done in the design phase.

Standard specifications

First, there needs to be a decision about what type of housing is required for the management system to be used:

- All year round housing for full indoor management control with zero grazing systems.
- Seasonal housing to balance access to grass with housing at key times of the year.
- The class of stock being housed – adults, fattening, calves or rearing.

Animal welfare and legislation

There is animal welfare legislation in place which governs some aspects of building design. Examples of these for the United Kingdom are listed below:

- Animal Welfare Act of 2006.
- Various regulations extracted from The Welfare of Farmed Animals (England) Regulations 2007, Scotland (2000), Wales (2007). These appear in various editions of the 'Code of Recommendations for the Welfare of Livestock', as an interpretation of the various regulations.
- Dairy Products (Hygiene) Regulations 1996.
- Control of Pollution (Silage, Slurry and Agricultural Fuel Oil) regulations 1991, SI No 324, as amended 1997 (SI No547).

The interpretation of these through codes of practice and welfare guidelines is what makes them realistic and enforces the legal aspects of them.

Although the Five Freedoms are a basic part of welfare codes and guidelines they are, by themselves, perhaps not quite enough. FAWC, in 2011, introduced an extension to these Freedoms in terms of 'a life worth living'. This is going beyond minimal welfare requirement to actually trying to define a 'good life', where the animal is content and has the opportunity to have 'positive experiences' of being in a production system. This is a difficult concept to define but, nevertheless, it needs to be considered with building design.

Various assurance schemes have been devised which embrace the current legislation and the various codes of practice. They may be industry-wide, such as the UK 'Red Tractor' labelling, or they may be specific to a milk buyer or supermarket outlet to lift the perceived value of their product or their commitment to the industry and animal welfare. The scope of the assurance schemes vary but often include welfare, management, hygiene, disease status, environmental conditions and product quality.

There is now a European initiative for the development of welfare assessment, known as 'Welfare Quality'.

Safety for personnel working in the housing area must also be addressed, and design considerations put in place to minimise risks – for example, the provision of escape routes for staff working with dangerous stock such as bulls. The UK Health and Safety Executive (Design and Management) Regulations 2007 (CDM) cover many aspects of building safety and will need to be consulted, especially during the initial design and building process.

Finally, there needs to be knowledge and assessment of the impact of the housing and the way it is managed on the environment, to control pollution and protect water, soil and air quality.

There are many references for set standards for space, bedding and feeding available – important design characteristics that should be incorporated. A brief summary of some of the more important issues is given below.

Moisture

Moisture is an important, common problem in buildings. Adult cows produce around 50 litres of fluid a day in urine and faeces, and most forage-based feeds use silages with very high moisture content. Wet conditions increase the risk of high humidity, which supports increased pathogen loads in the air. Wet bedding and high levels of standing slurry increases the risk of slurry gas accumulation, digital dermatitis infections and environmental mastitis pathogens, and increases the dirty cow scores. The following measures can be used to reduce moisture levels:

- Good drainage.
- Keep the feed out of the building area with a separate external feed face.
- Water troughs should not be in the bedded area and, preferably, should be either on the outside or in areas that can be well drained or scraped (Figure 34.1).
- Slurry scraping areas around feeding passages so faeces can be removed easily and frequently (Figure 34.2).

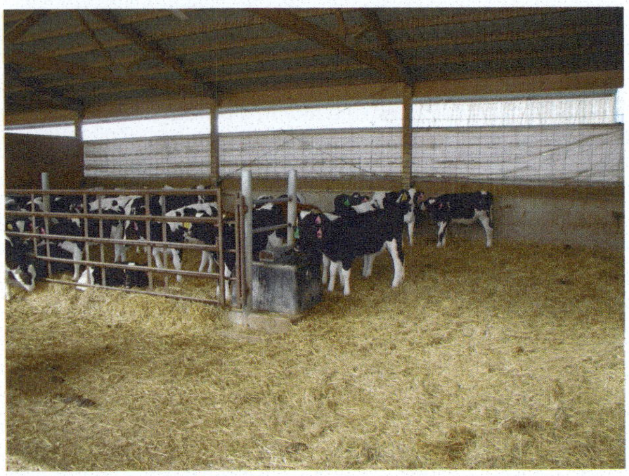

Figure 34.1 Putting a water trough in the bedded area is certain to increase moisture levels in the surrounding bedding and result in increased ammonia, poor ventilation and poor hygiene.

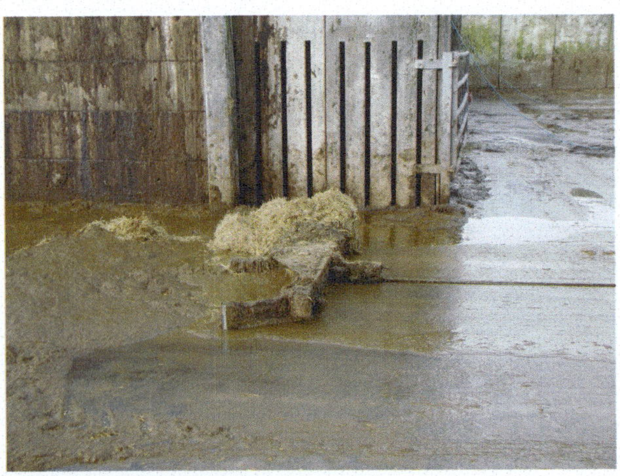

Figure 34.2 Automatic scraping systems can keep cattle clean but must prevent pooling of slurry in the housing where the cows can stand in it. Systems should draw the slurry clear of the housing.

Ventilation

Many aspects of building specification are not linear. Ventilation based on the ability of fresh air to enter and stale air to be removed will usually be dependent on the external area of the building, inlet through side walls and outlet through the roof ridge. As the building size increases, the external size does not keep step with the internal volume and, thus, ventilation could become limiting.

Ventilation removes excess heat and moisture and airborne infectious agents, as well as noxious gases that build up from bedding and faeces. It should do this effectively without producing a cooling draught directly over the animal itself. There are two basic systems used to achieve this:

- The stack effect, where heat rising from the livestock and bedding rises and exits from the ridge, drawing fresh air in from the side inlets by convection.
- Natural ventilation, due to external wind movement drawing gases out of the ridge and thus pulling fresh air through the side inlets.

It is difficult to have a flexible arrangement to suit various outside environmental conditions, but there are a few systems that can accommodate this. Using flexible curtain sides to a building can mean that the inlet is variable with the outside temperature. This design feature is becoming increasingly common in dairy cow systems, where housing has to accommodate huge temperature fluctuations when cattle are housed for longer periods, or even all year round.

The other option is to use forced ventilation, with either ducted air introduced through roof inlet systems, or fans to move or extract air in a controlled fashion, based on external/internal temperatures or moisture levels (Figures 34.3 and 34.4)

There are calculations for ventilation requirements listed in many publications (DairyCo). However, key calculations are:

- First calculate outlet area required for the building. Allow 5 cm of ridge width opening for every 3 m of building width.
- Then calculate the inlet area to support this by natural ventilation.

As a guide, every calf weighing up to 125 kg needs 0.04 m^2 of ventilation outlet in the roof, while growing and adult cattle typically need at least a 200 mm gap along the full length of the ridge. Most dairy cow housing will need a complete air change at least ten times every hour to meet ventilation requirements in summer, and five times every hour in winter.

Space requirements

When calculating requirements such as bedding area and feeding area, these are again, as with ventilation, not linear, and increase with the number of animals. Specifications must account for increasing stock numbers in very large cattle units. A cow cubicle shed designed to house 50 cows will need to make allowances for the behavioural characteristics of cattle. For

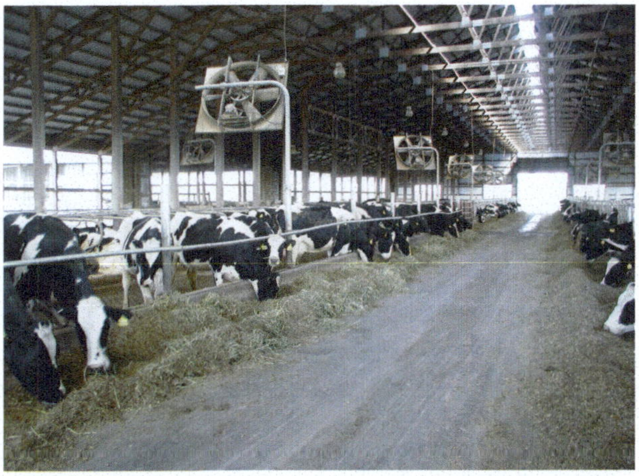

Figure 34.3 A well-designed building used to house dairy cattle all year round. Good ventilation from open sides and the option to increase cooling in hot weather.

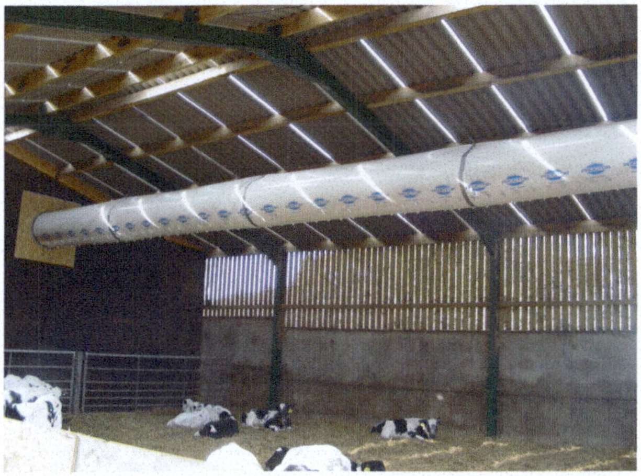

Figure 34.4 Forced air systems such as this can hugely improve ventilation especially for young stock.

example, the vast majority of the animals could be either feeding or lying down at any one time, so the feed fence allocation per animal and the number of cubicles perhaps needs to allow for 5% under-occupation (5% oversupply). In a modern unit housing with over 200 cows, some reduction of this allowance is possible, as it is improbable that the cattle will be either feeding or lying down at the same time. The building can, therefore, be quite typically 'overstocked', to allow for different functions being undertaken at the same time by different sub-groups of animals. Quite frequently in the USA, a cubicle building will be technically 20% 'overstocked' when the numbers in it are high, but will function perfectly adequately. This is, at present, at odds with the welfare requirements of some countries, such as the UK, that still have accreditation limits of one cubicle unit per animal.

Calculations for space can be based upon:

- Cow body weight.
- Milk yield.
- Bedding area and loafing area, separately or together.
- Cubicle dimensions and layout.

Space requirements are fully described in many publications but, without reproducing the many tables in them, as a simple basic summary they are:

Straw yards

- Keep the area rectangular with no more than 10 metres from the back wall to the feed face.
- Allocate separate space for bedding and for loafing/feeding.
- As a single figure, an adult 700 kg cow needs 7.5 m^2/cow for bedding and an allowance of 3.0 m^2 for loafing. Total: 10.5 m^2/cow
- The DairyCo mastitis plan indicates a bedded area for lactating cows of 1.25 m^2 per 1000 litres of milk production, which gives a figure 25% higher than the above. Total: 13 m^2 for a cow giving 8000 litres
- Straw requirements are around 20 kg per adult cow per day

Cubicles or stalls

Design is important in order to offer the right width for comfort (without risking damage to the cow by becoming trapped due to turning), the right length for lying down and for getting up, the correct features of the structure to restrict the cow in the cubicle area without injury from neighbouring cows, and to keep the cubicle clean (Figure 34.5):

- Cubicle dimensions should be based on an adult dairy cow of 700 kg requiring:
  - 2.55 m length when there is a closed front to the cubicle;
  - 300 mm less if there is an open or 'head to head' front.
- Cubicle width should be at least 1.8 times the hip pin bone width of the cow (distance between tuber ischii). In practice, this means a cubicle width of 1.125–1.2 m, depending on the type of cubicle partition.
- Use partitions that do not intrude into the lying area by adopting freely suspended dividers at least 400 mm above the bedding.
- Head rails position the cow for lying down, to optimise comfort and cleanliness, and should be 1.3 m above the bedded area and 2.2 m diagonally from the kerb.
- Once lying down, position the cow primarily with the brisket board set at 1.8 m from the rear kerb.
- Details of slope and kerb will depend on the bedding used.
- Bedding requirements are a lot less than loose housed, and apart from sand ranges from 1–2 kg per adult cow unit per day (sand is 15 kg per day).

This basic outline for space can be varied by reference to published tables for different weights and sizes of cattle.

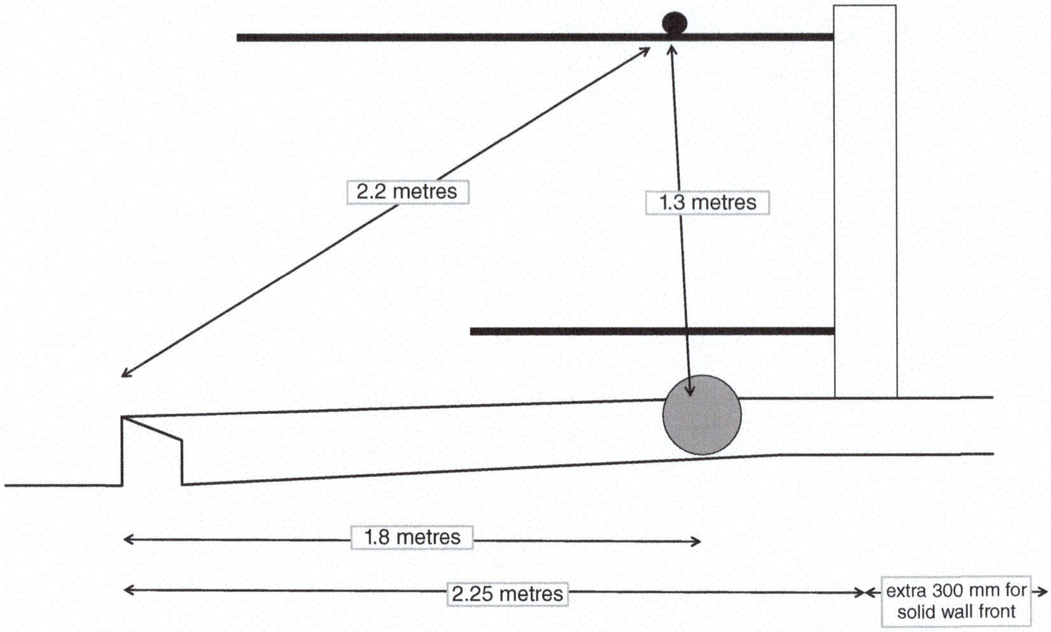

Figure 34.5 Basic dimensions for a 700 kg cow cubicle. The details will depend on the partitions and bedding material.

Movement and handling

Building design needs to manage the movement of animals either as part of the daily routine of the milking parlour or the more occasional movements for handling, scraping out areas, bedding and possibly feeding. Cows need adequate access logically planned down passage ways and easy means of being held back in areas for daily management as well as specific requirements for being parted, restrained and handled safely for husbandry processes such as treatment or weighing.

Floor surfaces

Cattle need to be housed partly, or even wholly, on concrete surfaces for loafing areas, feeding areas, movement passages, and handling. Only the lying area will comprise a bedded area. Concrete is a necessity for hygiene and removal of fluids, even though it presents huge physical problems. There are many design elements that can improve the floor surfaces in areas dedicated to different functions within the building. Below are some important design elements in relation to function that should be considered:

- Scraping areas should have a slight fall to stop fluids pooling and to keep large areas of it dry to maintain hygiene and improve foot health.
- Prevent slippage at feed faces or transit passages, by using grooving techniques or concrete profiling methods for new floors. The design of the groove or floor pattern will depend on whether the cow movement direction is known or not.
- Slats are useful to prevent slurry and fluid pooling, but the design must prevent abrasion or foot damage, and care must be taken to prevent gases coming back into the housing area from the slurry store.
- Automatic scraping which does not produce excessive pooling in front of the scrapers, with slats placed at intervals or drawing completely outside the building at the end of the run.
- The use of rubber matting is still controversial, with results often showing little or no benefit. The main variable may be the type of rubber used, as the different types are not all equivalent.

Calves

The young bovine animal is quite adaptable to a range of housing conditions. The problem is when movement is restricted (e.g. Individual calf pens) due to feeding systems and disease concerns; then, it is unable to select its own 'microenvironment' within the housing. This is probably the basic principle for housing calves well. Given a range of options for warmth, bedding and ventilation, the calf will choose the area it is most comfortable with. Also, sharing with other animals allows communal warmth in very cold conditions when cattle lie together. Preventing draughts on or at the animal level is of key importance. If calves are individually penned to allow a traditional twice-daily bucket feeding system, then proper insulation is needed to prevent condensation and temperature extremes, and to produce adequate ventilation, as the calf cannot move around to accommodate changes by itself.

There are also disease considerations when deciding on group size with loose-housed calves. Many systems show that loose housing in small groups has distinct benefits for calf health

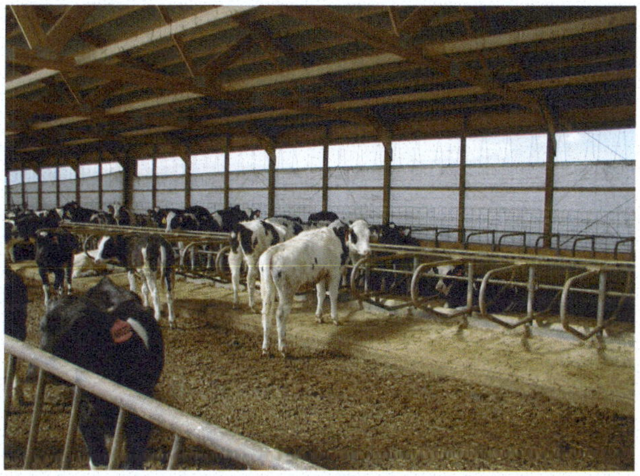

Figure 34.6 Monopitch building for young stock, with curtain sides that can be raised or lowered to improve ventilation, depending on the weather.

and growth, especially when the pen size can expand as the animals grow. Typical systems that suit a flexible approach for youngstock are monopitch buildings which produce a range of environments from the back to the front, and can grow with the animal's requirements (Figure 34.6).

The same is true with calf hutches and 'igloos'; the calf has the option of choosing its own environment, with outside options and a closed-off inside bedded area. Ventilation is particularly important with calves, to reduce the risk of pneumonia, and care has to be taken to get good ventilation without draughts on the animal itself. Forced ventilation options often work well with youngstock.

More specific requirements

- Lighting: good lighting is necessary for animals to express normal behaviour, such as oestrous, and can affect milk production in some climates
- Emergency procedures and contingency plans for power failures affecting lights, ventilation and muck scraping are essential in large building design. Protocols for fires should also be developed and well understood by all.
- Biosecurity: good building design should aim to minimise the risk of introducing or spreading disease. Many aspects, such as access of stockpersons to key areas and the flow pattern of daily routines, are important for disease transmission. Allowing off-site locations for visitor parking, and animal isolation facilities for reducing disease risks when cattle are introduced, should be catered for.

Measurables

An initial good general observation will indicate if there is a need to collect other specific measurable data. Visible evidence of poor ventilation can be useful, such as condensation (tiger stripes on beams), cobwebs forming in the roof structure, and the level of dust. Smelling the air in various parts of the building should give a good idea as to the levels of gases such as ammonia and hydrogen sulphide. Oxygen and carbon dioxide levels will not be easily detectable although, with large-volume buildings, this is rarely an issue. Manually checking the bedding material to detect moisture and heat build-up is simple to do. After this preliminary scan, specific physical data can be collected if there is a need for additional information. This may include:

- Ammonia levels – target 10 ppm (guidelines are usually around 25 ppm (20 ppm for the EU)).
- Hydrogen sulphide levels (10 ppm maximum).
- Oxygen/carbon dioxide levels at different parts of the building.
- Bedding depth, temperature, moisture content.
- Ventilation rates.
- Temperature (maximum and minimum thermometer).
- Humidity (use a psychrometer – a wet and dry bulb thermometer).
- Lighting levels (use a light meter).
- Bacterial counts in the air space – direct measurement.
- Smoke testing for ventilation characteristics (use a 'smoke bomb').

Animal measurables

Farm records may give good background health information, but they are often erratically recorded and incomplete. It is much better, where possible, to use actual measurements and observations on the cows themselves for a health and welfare assessment. The way the animal interacts with both the building and the management system used is the final arbiter of success for design and function. The end result of successful design and management should be that this results in effective welfare and a healthy environment for the cattle being housed. This can be measured from the way the animal relates and interacts with it. The main problem with this approach is that the relationship between animal and housing is often not specific, and animal measurements, in many instances, simply indicate that the system is lacking in design and function, and not precisely what features are at fault. Deficiencies in animal measurables will require a more thorough investigation to uncover specific design faults.

For an audit of actual animal measurables, we need to look at the following:

- Time budget for behaviour patterns.
- Hygiene scoring legs, flanks, udders.
- Specific injury scores.
- Body condition score (BCS).
- Lying times and comfort measurements.
- Lameness (mobility score).
- Observing major cattle movements (partial time budget).

This should be supplemented with evidence from the farm records about disease levels such as mastitis, pneumonia and lameness.

Time budget

Looking at what the animal is doing, at what time and for how long, will show how the animal is interacting with the building dynamically over a typical 24-hour period. The use of closed circuit television cameras (CCTV) has made this much simpler, but it still requires quite a lot of human input spent observing the animals over a typical 24-hour period to produce the detail required. Target periods for each function should indicate whether these are being achieved, and any deficiencies may indicate shortfalls in design or management and have health and welfare consequences (Figure 34.7).

Hygiene scoring

Several workers have devised simple hygiene scoring systems for cattle based on a 1 to 5 grade of the amount of faecal contamination on the flanks, udder and legs of cattle. The hygiene score is directly related to the level of bedding being used, cubicle use, stocking rate, and slurry handling. The overall score also relates directly to disease levels, such as lameness and mastitis in the herd. There is a good visual description of the various hygiene scores and their interpretation, devised by N.B. Cook at the University of Wisconsin, at: http://www.vetmed.wisc.edu/dms/fapm/fapmtools/4hygiene/hygiene.pdf.

Hughes (2001) provides an alternative scoring system, with excellent photographs.

Injury scoring

Superficial injuries are often a good indicator of the lying area design and overall comfort level. A cow lying down comes into contact with the bedded surface of the cubicle or loose housing system, and typical lesions can be observed as evidence as to whether this is satisfactory or not. Any sign of injury or damage is a sign of poor design, or problems with the bedded surface and cubicle area directly causing trauma. It can also be a sign that the cow is spending too long lying down, due to lameness or other illness, allowing pressure necrosis or abrasion more time to produce lesions. Cubicle housing is most often associated with comfort or lying injuries, but poorly bedded loose housing can produce similar lesions. Typical injuries observed are:

- Hock damage – this can range from simply losing hair over the lateral tarsal protrusion on the hock, to granulation tissue being formed which swells, presenting as a hock hygroma. Often, the overlying skin is broken and abscesses or open sores are seen. This type of lesion will only cause lameness in the extreme, but is a clear sign of interaction with the bedding surface and the amount of time the cow spends lying down in contact with it. A more severe injury is a capped hock, infection of the tendon sheath over the tuber calcis, often associated with poor cubicle design at the kerb.
- Skin ulceration. Again, the same principle applies that the lying time and surface texture can produce pressure necrosis and ulceration of the skin, especially over the lateral aspect of the hindlimb, and this is usually associated with lame cows lying down for too long in poor conditions (Figure 34.8).
- Knee damage – abrasion or problems getting up and lying down in cubicles, due to difficulties with space requirements or badly positioned cubicle partitions.
- Brisket hygroma – pressure sores due to bedding surface or increased lying time.
- Rib injuries from cubicle partitions intruding into the lying comfort area.

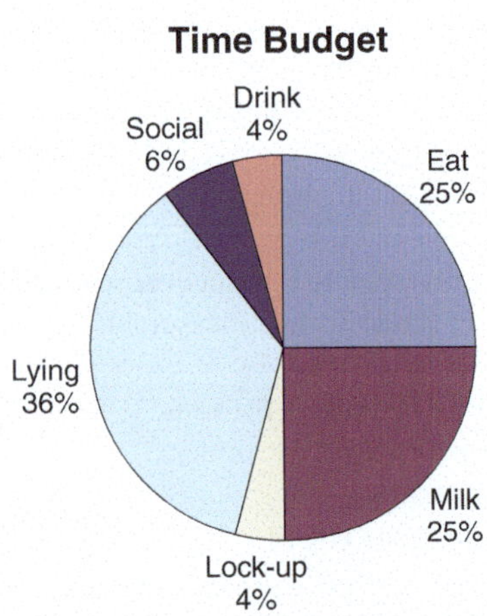

Figure 34.7 Time Budget – a typical time budget for an adult lactating cow.

Body Condition Score (BCS)

The nutrition of the animals is a combination of the management system, the feed quality, and many aspects of building design and function that allow the animal to feed such as the amount of feed face size of trough, design of trough, and a suitable time budget to allow the animal to feed. Many aspects of management diseases, such as lameness, will also have an impact on body condition. The BCS can be easily assessed by reference to many simple guides that are available pictorially describing a standardised system (DairyCo is one of the best). With this, any operator can produce their own comparative system, though it will probably only apply to their own observations, so may not be an exact comparative farm benchmark system between herds. In a dairy herd, take a representative sample of animals from each key stage of lactation:

- Fresh calved cows.
- Mid-lactation (breeding stage).
- Late lactation.
- Dry cows.

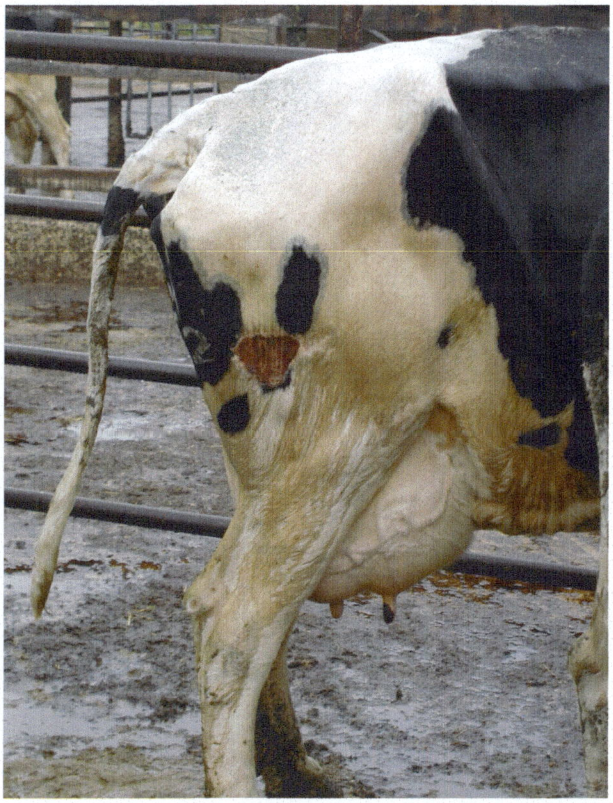

Figure 34.8 Skin ulceration on the hind limb muscles means that this cow is lying down for too long, has insufficient bedding material, or cubicle comfort. Perhaps all are involved.

Similar systems can be used for beef animals and youngstock, to assess body condition relative to benchmarks for the age, breed, and stage of production they are at. However, often weighing the stock regularly is a simpler option for these cattle.

Having set benchmarks in place means that, in practice, the animals can be easily assessed against them. Start by investigating the ration being fed, but a time budget will be needed to check feeding times and feed access by the stock.

Comfort scoring

A good time budget score for housed dairy cattle is that we should aim for 12 hours lying time. However, a quick assessment of comfort can be achieved by looking at the 'prevalence' of comfort scores at any one time or, more accurately, at specific times during the cow cycle:

- Cow Comfort Index (CCI, the number of cows *lying in a cubicle* divided by the number of cows *touching a cubicle surface* (e.g. standing in a cubicle)), gives a numerical expression for the proportion of cows in cubicles that are actually lying down. Eighty five percent or more of the cows should be lying in a cubicle two hours before morning milking. The CCI describes actual physical cow comfort.
- Proportion Eligible Lying (PEL, the number of cows *lying in cubicles* divided by number of cows *in the pen not eating*) shows how many of the cows in the pen that are eligible to lie down in the cubicles (i.e. they are not eating) are doing so. One hour after returning from morning milking, 75% or more of the cows should be lying in a cubicle (this depends on feeding time, as well). PEL describes cubicle acceptance.

Mobility scoring

The principle is that cows are examined for lameness by visually assessing their gait and posture as they individually move past the observer. Most scoring systems are carried out by checking the cows as they walk back from the milking parlour after milking (see DairyCo guidelines). Lameness measurements are often associated with many aspects of building design, such as lying area comfort, flooring quality, standing times and movement patterns, as well as slurry handling and moisture levels.

Cattle movements

Simply observing cattle being moved in the housing (e.g. collected for milking and returning from the parlour) will provide useful information about cattle flow, walking surface quality and the way the cattle are managed when moving. Record the number of animals seen:

- slipping down;
- losing footing;
- flow times for set functions (e.g. moving out of the cubicles).

It is worth carrying out a 'round trip' of typical cow movements from housing to parlour and back again to check on all these aspects. Observations should be made of the feeding practices and the way the manger, trough or floor is managed for feeding. When food is put out observe:

- how many come up to feed;
- the percentage manger space use at this 'peak time';
- the manger clean-up before feeding;
- the level of competition at feeding.

Audit summary

A simple scoring system of direct measurement of critical control points of a building can be designed, which can then be monitored for change, when buildings are altered, or benchmarked against industry standards for the design or farming system. Any audit design should look for critical control points (CCP). The key performance indicators should have the following characteristics:

- It should be a key performance indicator which is an outcome of important components of management and building design. For example, a hygiene score is a single measurement, but is a good indicator of many aspects of the building and the way it is managed.
- It is specific in its interpretation – counting the percentage of cows using the cubicles is a precise single piece of data.

Table 34.1 A basic housing audit.

Parameter	Comments
Hygiene score.	Cleanliness of flanks, feet and udders reflects many aspects of building function, and is significantly related to welfare and disease. It reflects on slurry handling, bedding, stocking rate, and animal comfort.
Hock and other superficial damage visible.	Hock damage is easy to score and record, and is the most obvious sign to use for animal injuries due to interaction with bedding surface and housing design (cubicle) and levels of lameness.
Comfort indices	Simple prevalence measurements for cow comfort parameters accurately reflect acceptance and actual comfort of the bedding area.
Body condition score	Body condition score is a quick method of assessing the overall wellbeing of the stock. It is not specific to building design, but reflects interaction of layout with feeding management, comfort, and diseases such as lameness – but it needs to be in context with the farm production system.
Mobility score	Done at key times and, preferably, once a month, this accurately describes overall lameness, which is a key issue with many aspects of the housing.
An observation of a full movement cycle for the animals, including feeding	A full observation of a typical management cycle for the cattle, such as the milking and feeding routine, will allow the dynamics of how animals move through the daily management cycle. Many aspects of building design and use impact on this.

- It can be used to benchmark for improvement or deterioration and is a repeatable index for the farm in question, to monitor changes over time and allows comparison between farms.

Audit planning

- A knowledge of the diseases and production characteristics of the class of stock and how this will specifically affect the needs of the housing is required.
- Training of assessors to carry out an audit visit may be needed.
- The legal and contractual requirements for the type of housing need to be understood.
- The standard specifications for size and layout detail relating this to size, animal capacity, and the function of the building, need to be defined.
- A preliminary visit and planning phase may be required to decide what measurable variables need to be recorded and what will be included in the audit.
- A knowledge of specific measurement techniques and how to use them is required (e.g. visual observation for ventilation, specified gas assessments, analysis of bedding moisture, heat, and depth).
- Use simple animal measurements and observations. A basic list is presented in Table 34.1.

References

Hughes J. (2001). Farm Animal Practice: A system for assessing cow cleanliness. *In Practice* **23**(9), 517–524.

Further sources of information

ADAS (2005). Action on Animal Welfare publication on *Housing the Modern Dairy Cow.*

British Standard for Agricultural Buildings and Structures, BS5502-40 (2005).

Cook, N, Oetzel, G and Nordlun, K – University of Wisconsin, Madison. They have an excellent website which you can access all their papers and work: www.vetmed.wisc.ed, www.cals.wisc.edu and www.cias.wisc.edu.

Dairy Housing (DairyCo) (2012). They also produce excellent publications on body condition scoring and lameness assessment. Many publications are available online at: www.dairyco.org.uk.

Grandin, Temple – many good cattle handling designs at www.grandin.com.

SAC publications on the costs of agricultural buildings:

Tucker, C. and Weary, D., University of British Columbia, Canada. They are doing some excellent work on cow behaviour and lameness. Look at: http://www.agsci.ubc.ca/animalwelfare/

CHAPTER 35

Cattle Signs

Kiro Petrovski

Learning objectives

- To appreciate which signs are normal and which are abnormal.
- To understand how cattle signs can indicate suboptimal health, welfare and production.
- To understand how cow signs can provide diagnostic information
- To understand how cattle signs can be used to monitor the 'health' of the farm and management

Introduction

Cattle signs are parameters that can be observed and measured. They include behavioural (particularly attitude and body language), physiological (particularly body condition, and condition of skin and hair coat) and management parameters (particularly comfort and husbandry). Unfortunately, many signs do not have agreed units of measure or standards. An understanding of conditions which may cause a sign is crucial for their correct interpretation. For example, cattle walking uncomfortably, with arched backs, is unusual walking behaviour and may indicate lameness. However, the same signs may be observed with abdominal pain or bad design of the walking surfaces. The prevalence of a given sign or set of signs needs to be established, as well as the 'qualitative' severity of the sign.

The concept of auditing a farm, by observing and measuring cattle signs to identify problem areas in the facility or management, is growing in popularity. High performance requires optimal conditions. The farmer needs to create welfare friendly environments if they expect cattle to deliver a high performance. Low stressed cattle are healthier and more productive; stressed cattle have increased concentrations of cortisol, which can potentially reduce metabolic efficiency and, in turn, productivity. Cow sign audits can provide the consumer with increased assurance that, on that farm, welfare standards are being maintained or improved.

The assessment of cattle signs starts with observation from a distance, followed by a closer, more detailed examination of high-risk cattle and environments. It does not include a detailed topographical or system physical clinical examination by body systems or regions. Observing cattle involves the individual, as well as the herd/group, and associating the findings with husbandry processes.

A common problem when assessing cattle signs is the number of animals to assess. As a rule of thumb, when the group of cattle is smaller than 100, it is best to assess them all. For larger groups, it is best to assess a minimum of 80–100 cattle at random, or 20%, whichever number is larger. These numbers can change depending on the size of cattle facility, the group in question and the prevalence of the sign. If some of cattle signs are detected in more than 3–5 cattle, it may be necessary to assess briefly each animal in the group. A sign detected on a single animal is usually not indicative of a group problem.

Time management

An important prerequisite in understanding cattle signs is a basic knowledge of normal time management and the basic needs of cattle. The time management of cattle encompasses negotiable and non-negotiable elements. The non-negotiable elements dictate the amount of remaining time that can be spent on negotiable elements. Unfortunately, little information is available, except for time management of lactating dairy cows. Time management of housed dairy cows in a day should include the elements listed in Table 35.1. The time management per day differs between housed and grazing cattle. Grazing cattle need more time for grazing (usually double 6.0–10.0 hours per day) and, due to longer walking distances (usually 3–5 hours per day), their resting time is significantly shortened.

Bovine Medicine, Third Edition. Edited by Peter D. Cockcroft.

Table 35.1 Normal time management of dairy cow in a day.

Activity	Type of activity	Average time devoted to activity per day (in hours)
Eating	Non-negotiable	3.0–5.0
Drinking	Non-negotiable	0.5
Walking (compulsory,	Non-negotiable	1.5–3.0
i.e. to milking shed)	Non-negotiable	1.0–2.0
Milking	Semi-negotiable	7.0–10.0
Ruminating	Negotiable	12.0–14.0
Resting	Negotiable	1.0–3.0
Socialising		

Design and maintenance of cattle facilities

The design of the cattle facility should allow for normal behaviour. The layout of the farm should ensure that cattle are protected from the negative effects of inclement weather (e.g. through use of sunshade, natural or artificial shelter, and sprinklers). Cattle should be allowed access to water and food, space for resting (e.g. lying down, stretching), socialising with group-mates (e.g. grooming, exhibiting oestrous behaviour) and exercise. Mistakes in design, layout and maintenance of the facility may interfere with cattle behaviour and comfort (Table 35.2). The design (e.g. presence of sharp corners), type and maintenance of floors, and walking surfaces on a farm and in facilities, are of high importance for normal behaviour and health of cattle, and hygiene. These areas, in addition to the stalls, are in regular and closest contact with cattle.

Cattle usually rest longer when provided with good quality soft bedding (e.g. sand). They prefer soft, deep, clean and dry bedding over hard concrete and mattress (Haley *et al.*, 2001; Tucker *et al.*, 2003; Tucker & Weary, 2004; Camiloti *et al.*, 2012). Lame cattle prefer sand over mattress bedding, probably due to the softer feeling and better grip when raising up. Poorly maintained bedding results in decreased lying times (Drissler *et al.*, 2005; Fregonesi *et al.*, 2007).

Observations of walking patterns, presence of skin lesion and foreign material suggest that the quality of floors and walking surfaces should be examined. Foot placement, length of stride, step and walking speed provide indicators for the health of cattle and the quality of the environment (Table 35.2). Healthy cattle on pasture place their rear foot into the position vacated by the front foot on the same side.

Another simple observation is scoring the condition of the hocks and knees of cattle. Hock lesions, and knee swelling and lesions are good indicators of the comfort of the stalls and the abrasiveness of the flooring and bedding (Weary & Taszkun, 2000). The incidence of hock and knee lesions is increased on mattresses (Wechsler *et al.*, 2000; Fulwider *et al.*, 2007) and concrete stalls (Rushen *et al.*, 2007).

Floors and walking surfaces should also be assessed for evidence of foreign material (stones, nails) and sharp corners. If foreign material is identified, the source should be found and removed. Sharp corners should be corrected. As a temporary measure, a rubber mat may be used to cover any damaged flooring and sharp corners.

To check for slippery floors and walking surfaces, the so-called 'ballerina test' can be carried out. The assessor stands on the surface to be evaluated and twists around on one foot. A slippery surface results in more than half a turn. To check the comfort of the walking surfaces, the assessor should wear thin-soled moccasins. The floor and walking surface should be comfortable. Discomfort that will be felt by the assessor will be felt by cattle as well.

Dirty cows indicate a dirty environment and/or inappropriate lying places (e.g. in the passage way instead of cubicles). The degree of hygiene of a cattle facility can be assessed by the amount of dirt on the animals (Figure 35.1). Cattle scoring three and above indicate a problem and the assessor should try to find out the reason and propose appropriate changes.

Social interactions

Cattle are herd animals, social interactions are part of natural herd behaviour, and they become highly stressed when separated from the rest of their group. The clear signs of stress when isolated are vocalisation, increased heart rate, and defecation and urination (Rushen *et al.*, 1999). They are accustomed to doing things in groups. When dominant cattle start feeding or walking towards the exit, the others will follow, and it is a common picture to see the whole group of cattle doing the same thing at the same moment. Therefore, to accurately assess cattle signs, the assessment must be carried out at group, not individual level (Table 35.3).

Each herd has a social hierarchy. Dominant (larger, older, cattle with more seniority in the group, horned over dehorned) cattle push and bunt the submissive (recently calved or introduced to the group, younger) cattle. Submissive cattle usually avoid contact with dominant cattle. In a group of female cattle, the most dominant cow (referred to as the 'bull cow'), when approached, comes towards the approaching person, while all other cows walk away.

Group composition influences the type and intensity of social interactions. The more similar the cattle are within a group, the fewer the negative social interactions. Replacements raised together tend to be less aggressive and associate together more. Additionally, the level of social interaction may be affected through the design of cattle facilities. The lack of escape routes for submissive cattle results in more negative interactions. To prevent problems associated with no escape route in a facility with stalls, removing a few dividers from a row opens up a cross-passageway.

Table 35.2 Common problems in the environment associated with changes in cattle behaviour and health.

Problem with the environment	Cattle signs associated with the problem
Uncomfortable walking surface; slippery floors	Cattle walking with short steps and wide open rear legs Placement of the rear foot outside the track of the front foot Altered stride, step length and walking speed Prolonged queuing Increased incidence of injuries and lameness
Dirty floors	Dirty cattle Increased incidence of skin disorders
Too abrasive floors	Cattle walking carefully Increased risk of lameness and hock and knee lesions
Presence of dump walking surfaces	Hooves absorbing water Cattle avoiding areas with 'bird-baths' Increased incidence of lameness, infectious disorders of the feet, skin disorders and mastitis
Presence of foreign material on the walking surfaces	Cattle walking carefully Increased risk of claw and other foot lameness
Sharp corners	Altered walking speed Cattle queuing altered placement of rear foot Increased incidence of lameness, particularly in outer claw of one foot in many cattle in the group
Improper ventilation	Excessive condensation and moisture damage, especially on the roof, cobwebs, air that smells of ammonia; excessive coughing, nasal discharge, open-mouthed breathing by cattle in the facility or changes in behaviour and non-uniform usage of the facilities; running the fingers through the hair coat of cattle finds moisture
Draft	Non-uniform usage of the facilities Congregation of cattle to keep warm
Dark environment	Cattle walking with short steps and wide open rear legs Cattle walking carefully
Suboptimal hygiene	Increased incidence of hoof, udder, skin infections and changes in normal behaviour Decreased cattle comfort
Uncomfortable stalls	Cattle avoiding to use stalls and lie down in walking areas Increased incidence of hock and knee lesions and other injuries; short laying bouts
Poorly designed stalls	Cattle avoiding to use stalls, decreased lying down times, insufficient rest; Increased risk of lameness
Unpleasant odours around the feeding facilities	Cleaning not regular; build-up of waste food, mud and manure; growth of moulds Feeding surfaces of low quality (e.g. presence of grooves and holes)
Presence of uncomfortable matter	*See Uncomfortable stalls* Cattle suddenly abort attempts to lie down Cattle take longer time to lie down (more than one minute)
Nech rail too far back	Cattle standing half-in half-out of the stalls Lameness; Slower recovery of lame cows
Brisket board too far back Neck rail too far forward	Cattle laying half-in half-out of the stalls Increased dirtiness of hind quarters Increased risk of mastitis, hock and skin lesions

The social hierarchy in group of cattle is not permanent, and management practices often contribute to the shifting dynamic. When dominant cattle become older, or sick, or are moved from the mob, some of the subordinate cattle will take over. Shifting of cattle between groups on a farm result in disturbance of the normal social hierarchy. After movement of cattle between the groups on a farm, it takes usually 2–7 days for the hierarchy to be re-established. However, for heifers and freshly calved cows, this period extends to more than ten days (Grant & Albright, 1995). Any disturbance to the social hierarchy caused by moving cattle around may result in stress and, consequently, suboptimal productivity and health (Phillips & Rind, 2001).

Social interactions, and particularly social problems, can impact on feeding time, ruminating time, water intake and resting time. Dominant cattle set the pace for all these activities. Subordinate cattle are likely to keep clear of dominant cattle, to whom they will inevitably lose any competition. Dominant cattle may inhibit submissive animals, particularly younger

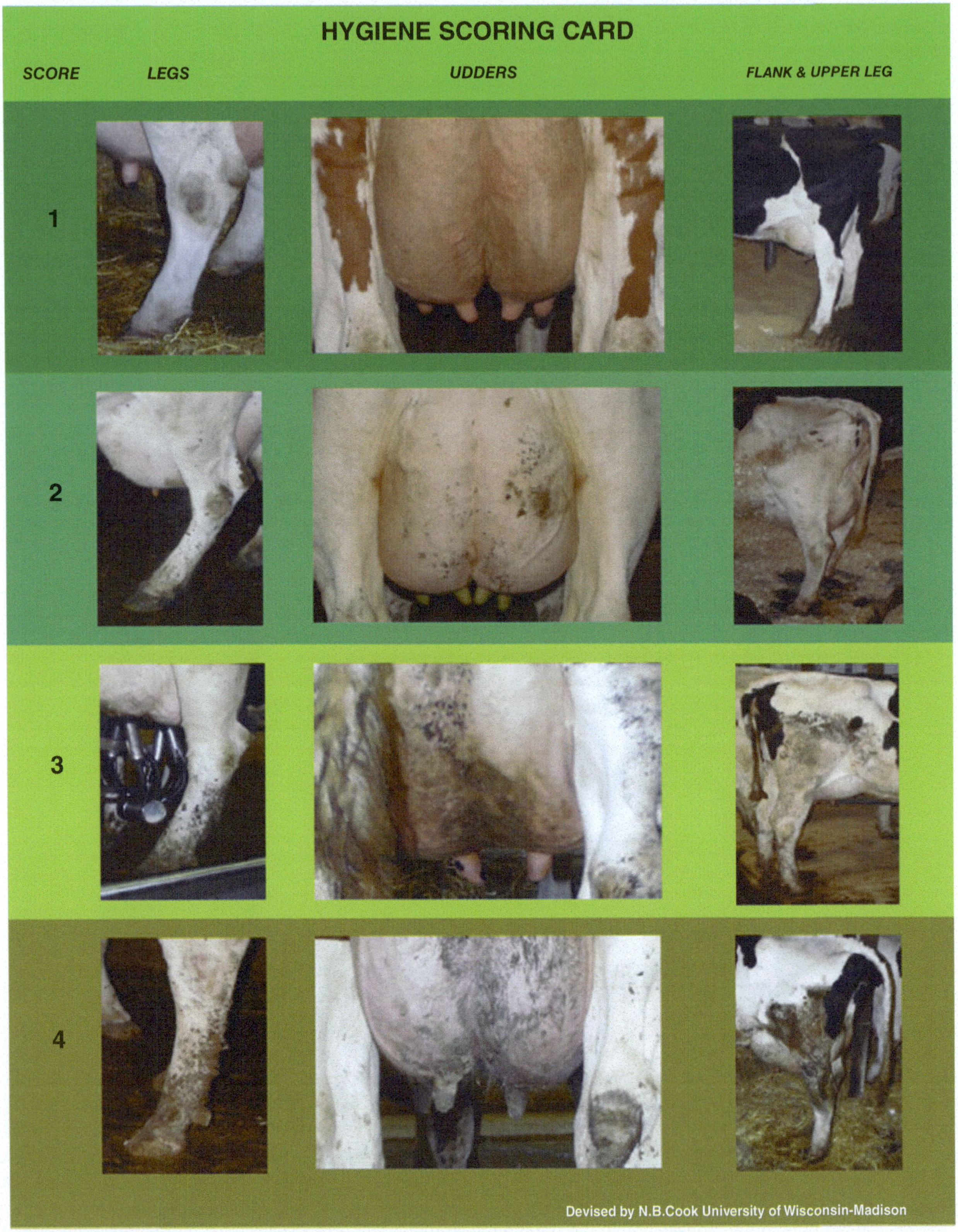

Figure 35.1 Hygiene scoring chart. Reproduced with permission of American Dairy Science Association.

Table 35.3 Common cattle signs and causes associated with social behaviour.

Description	Reasons
Cattle beast isolated from the rest of the group or not participating in the activity that others do	• ill • injured • oestrus
Cattle beast doing what the rest of the group does but at a slower pace	• ill • injured
Cattle beast without licking marks	• ill • injured
Increased incidence of fights within a group	• recent re-grouping • presence of dead ends in the facilities • presence of areas with no escape route • overcrowding
Aberrant behaviour	• overcrowding • ill • injured
Increased incidence of lameness	• overcrowding • unbalanced nutrition favouring acidic rumen environment • problems with walking surfaces
Increased incidence of trauma	• problems with walking surfaces • walls and stalls • overcrowding
Short lying down bouts	• uncomfortable stalls • lower ranking cattle being displaced by higher ranking cattle • overcrowding
Decreased lying down times	• overcrowding • uncomfortable stalls • lower ranking cattle being displaced by higher ranking cattle
Cattle depositing the faeces on the bedding and inside the stalls, rather than in the walkways	• overcrowding • stalls too short • recent re-grouping
Buller-steer syndrome	• overcrowding • use of androgen hormones for increased productivity
Eating poisonous plants and grazing browse in pasture systems	• overcrowding • insufficient availability of feedstuffs
Increased aggressiveness	• overcrowding • close contact • lack of shade in hot, sunny days • narrow passageways • invading the 'personal space' • uncastrated males • new group members

Table 35.3 (*continued*)

Description	Reasons
Gathering around water troughs	• not enough troughs or drinking water • not enough drinking/trough spaces • hot weather
Decreased use of stalls	• uncomfortable stalls • overcrowding • improper stall design (e.g. not enough launch and bob space, no escape route) • presence of harmful material
Changes in getting-up behaviour	• improper stall design (e.g. not enough launch and bob space) • neck rail too far back • lameness
Dirty hind quarters	• suboptimal hygiene • neck rail too far forward

ones, from eating, drinking, or resting. This will result in loss of body condition, decreased productivity and increased risk of lameness in submissive cattle.

Changes in social behaviour may be physiological or due to disorders. A common reason for changed social behaviour is oestrus. Oestrus behaviour and the formation of so-called sexually active groups is out of the scope of this text.

Cattle have their own 'personal space'. The size of the zone depends on the character (calm animals need a smaller personal space than a nervous one), age (heifers need a larger personal space than older cattle) and contact with people. As cattle age, they frequently become higher in rank, so they are no longer afraid of other cattle in the group.

A normal, affiliative behaviour of cattle is grooming by licking. Social licking is often directed at the neck and shoulder regions. All cattle in a group are licked, but not all of the animals lick. Social grooming behaviour is usually, but not restricted, to cattle of similar ranks. They often form grooming partners with specific individuals within the group. Social licking seems to have a calming effect and usually happens around times of changes of activities, such as after feeding and before rest.

Feeding

Feed quality, quantity and delivery method may influence the feed intake. The position of the body of cattle when they eat should be as similar to grazing grass as possible. To maximise the intake of dry matter of cattle, access to the feed at all times is essential. Feedstuffs should be prepared, stored, mixed and delivered to the feeding area in ways that prevent contamination and spoilage. However, just providing food does not ensure good intake; the design and maintenance of the feeding facilities are also important. Feeding may be affected by available feeding space, social interactions, quality of the feed bunk surfaces and hygiene.

On pasture, cattle show distinct diurnal feeding behaviour. They spend more time grazing during the day, with a laying bout around midday. The diurnal feeding behaviour in housed cattle is less distinct, or may be completely absent (DeVries & von Keyserlingk, 2008). Cattle kept on pasture-based systems should be allowed longer grazing periods in late afternoons and early mornings. Extended grazing periods around midday indicate incorrect milking management or insufficient pasture availability. Shorter grazing periods around midday are recommended, particularly during hot days.

Best practice recommends the feeding areas to be shaded or covered to provide cattle with protection from the sun and other weather elements, and to increase the life of the feeding facilities. The standing area around the feeding facilities is best covered with a rubber mat. This provides a cushion for the feet and legs of cattle, allowing for longer periods of time spent around the feeding facilities and, hopefully, feeding.

Ideal feeding facilities should provide 60–85 centimetres of space per cattle-head (Grant & Albright, 1995). The dimensions vary, depending on age, breed, size and category of cattle, and climate. Farms in hotter climates should provide a larger feeding space because of the reduced evaporation of heat produced by the body in crowded conditions. For good food utilisation and better production, there should be enough room for all cattle to feed at the same time (Grant & Albright, 1995). This is important, as cattle are social animals and eat at the same time. Feeding is affected by social ranking, with younger cattle, particularly heifers, being left aside if there is not enough feeding space. A good 'rule of thumb' is to provide 120% feeding spaces of the number of cattle.

The length of each feeding session varies with the type and availability of feed, social ranking and age of cattle. Heifers tend to eat less at a feeding and prefer to visit the feeding facilities more frequently (DeVries *et al.*, 2005), probably due to their smaller rumen capacity.

Competition at the feeding platform is highest when cattle return from milking and when fresh food is offered (Grant & Albright, 1995). At these times, dominant cattle demand priority in feeding and attempt to pick the good quality food. Less dominant and particularly submissive cattle may have limited access to food at these times. Consequently, these cattle eat less, or choose to eat at times when there is less competition at the feeding platform, which is associated with lower quality feed being available. Aggression around feeding on pasture is less common than in feeding barns, as grass is spatially distributed over large areas, and all cattle can feed at one time.

Cattle eating with their heads down produce more saliva, increasing the buffering ability of the feed. The feed bunk should be 10–15 centimetres higher than the floor where cattle stand to feed, mimicking grazing conditions. The feeding facilities should prevent cattle getting down on their knees, or having to step up to access the food. The feeding rail should be positioned high enough, and possibly 10° forward, to prevent rubbing and the formation of calloused area on the cattle necks.

Availability of food is assessed by observing the residual food in the feeding bunker after each feeding period. The availability of feedstuffs to the cattle is affected by the frequency of feeding and access. During feeding, cattle push a proportion of the feed beyond reach. This needs to be pushed back regularly to maintain access and to minimise overstretching and possible trauma (DeVries & von Keyserlingk, 2005). Pushing the feedstuffs back into the bank may, sometimes, be enough to trick cattle into thinking that fresh feed has been offered again, and stimulate feeding activity anew.

The proportion of residual food in the feed bank should be no more than 3% to 4% at the end of the prescribed feeding period, just before a new batch of feed is deposited. For female cattle in the transition period, the proportion of residual food may be as high as 15%. The forage material that is less palatable, spoiled, or of a poorer quality than the rest will be sorted out by cattle during feeding and left behind. This feed is of a lower digestibility. If consumed, it will likely reduce the feed intake and, ultimately, lead to lowered productivity. Cattle that are being forced to eat the residual feed left in the bunk are underfed. The residual feedstuffs should be removed regularly, particularly when feeding high-moisture feeds such as silage and potatoes. Regular removal will minimise the risk of spoiling.

Water

Cattle like to drink quickly, up to 20 litres of water per minute. They prefer to drink from a large, calm surface rather than from flowing water. Water intake is better when drinking quickly, and without stress. Lactating cows like to drink when they eat and just after milking; therefore, it would be beneficial to have water available at the exit of the milking shed, as well as the feeding area, although this may disrupt the cow flow. The natural drinking behaviour promotes further eating, which is particularly important for dairy cows.

Water intake may be reduced significantly when there is limited access to enough water of a good quality. Cattle are sensitive to water quality, and they will reject or reduce their intake if the quality is poor. Access to the water supply must be available at all times, especially during periods of heat or bitter cold. The water flow should supply at least ten litres per minute. Water depth should be a minimum of eight centimetres, to allow cattle to submerge their muzzle 2–5 centimetres.

To avoid the risk of environmental pollution (i.e. manure), water troughs should be installed a minimum of 1.3 m from the ground to the edge of the trough. Watering facilities should be at least 3–4 metres from the nearest obstacle, so accessibility is good. At least two sources of water in each facility/paddock are recommended, to provide an option to avoid social conflict.

Rumination

Rumination is a normal and important function essential to maintain and support rumen health. Time spent on rumination in cattle (Table 35.1) depends on feed quality and quantity, particularly the adequacy of fibre content and length, and the availability and quality of space for rest in a stress-free environment. Cattle lying down in a stress-free environment ruminate longer, associated with improved digestibility of the feedstuffs, feed conversion efficiency and, in turn, productivity. Approximately 70%–85% of cattle not eating, drinking or sleeping at any one point in time should be ruminating. Cattle not ruminating when resting may have problems that should be investigated. Chewing movements stimulate production of saliva, lowering the risk of sub-acute ruminal acidosis (SARA) and lameness. The length of each bout of rumination varies with the type, availability and digestibility of feedstuffs, and social ranking and interactions within a group. The number of movements of the jaw required to chew a cud is indicative of the food quality (Table 35.4).

Table 35.4 Problems associated with changes in rumination.

Observation	Associated problem
Less than 50 chewing movements per cud	Insufficient or non-effective fibre in the diet
More than 60 chewing movements per cud	Excessive fibre in the diet
50 to 60 chewing movements per cud	Food of acceptable fibre content and quality
Less than 60% cattle lying down, and not sleeping, chewing the cud	Subacute ruminal acidosis
Disturbed rest and rumination	Presence of sexually active group

Milking

Efficient milking requires appropriate settings of regularly serviced equipment, trained milkers and a consistent milking routine, carried out in a comfortable and safe milking shed. Behavioural responses during entry and exit of the dairy parlour, and during milking, can be used to indicate potential problems (Table 35.5).

Rest

Cattle should spend up to 14 hours per day lying down (rumination, rest, grooming, sleeping) in 6–14 lying sessions. Therefore, the comfort of the stalls or pasture is important for normal cattle behaviour. Laying times and the number of laying sessions can be affected by the quality of the lying surfaces (Cook *et al.*, 2004; Ito *et al.*, 2009).

Comfort

Comfort describes the relationship between the wellbeing of cattle, housing facilities or pasture conditions, and management. Poor comfort of cattle is likely to be associated with higher involuntary culling, low longevity in the group, and lowered lifetime production. Several comfort indices have been devised with target values. Lying time should be about 50% of the cows' total time budget.

The Cow Comfort Index (CCI) is the proportion of cows touching a stall surface that are actually lying down. The assessment should be performed at least two hours prior to milking, before the cows anticipate the event and begin standing. A high percentage is desirable. The target value is 85%. Low values indicate that comfort is suboptimal.

The Proportion Eligible Lying Time (PEL) is the number of cows lying in cubicles divided by the number of cows in the pen

Table 35.5 Behavioural assessment during entry and exit of the dairy parlour and during milking.

Behaviour	Reason
Unwilling to enter the milking shed	Milking as non-enjoyable experience; wrong attitude of milkers; stray voltage; floors of bad design; slippery floors; improper ventilation; improper lighting; small bales; wrong design of milking facility
Stamping	Stressed cows; wrong attitude of milkers; floor of bad design; small bales
Kicking (at application of cups, mid milking, late milking, at removal of cups or throughout milking)	Stressed cows; pain; high vacuum; improper pulsation: faulty milking machine; wrong attitude of milkers; stray voltage; flies
Delayed or completely aborted milk let-down	Stressed cows; pain; high vacuum: faulty milking machine; wrong attitude of milkers
Excessive defecation	Stressed cows; wrong attitude of milkers; stray voltage; flies
Excessive urination	Stressed cows; wrong attitude of milkers; stray voltage; flies
Flicking the tails	Stressed cows; improper pulsation; faulty milking machine; wrong attitude of milkers; stray voltage; flies
Chewing the cud	Relaxed cows: milking is enjoyable experience
High speed of exiting the shed	Stressed cows; wrong attitude of milkers; stray voltage; floors of bad design; slippery floors; improper lighting; small bales; flies; wrong design of milking facility (e.g. not enough exit space)

not eating. This shows how many cows in the pen that are eligible to lie down in the cubicles are doing so. The assessment is made at least an hour post-milking, to ensure that the cows have once more settled. A high value is desirable. The target value is 75%.

The Stall Standing Index (SSI) is the number of cows standing with two or four feet in a stall, divided by the number of cows touching a stall surface (it is the inverse of the CCI), and shows the proportion of cows in cubicles that are standing. The assessment should be performed at least two hours prior to milking, before the cows anticipate the event and begin standing. A low percentage is desirable. The target value is 15%.

The availability of shade at pasture in warmer climates may provide a conflict between encouraging grazing and cow comfort as the provision of shade results in cattle seeking shade in preference to feed during the day in hot weather (Kendall *et al.*, 2006).

Stall design, dimensions, lying surface material, management and layout are important in cow comfort. This is covered in more detail in Chapter 34 (Dairy Cow Housing Audit). Cross-lying in stalls, lying in passageways, frictional lesions on hocks, tails head and pelvis, cows unable to get up (cannot lunge) (Ito *et al.*, 2010) and high dirty cow scores are indicative of poor comfort related to stall design. The comfort of the stalls for housed cattle may be tested implementing the so-called 'knee-drop' test. The farm attendant is asked to drop to his/hers knees in the stall, stays in this position for 30 seconds, then describes how comfortable he/she feels.

Lying down and raising up

During quieter periods (approximately two hours after milking), most cattle from a group should be lying down, with less than 30% not resting. In lactating cows, the laying behaviour shows a diurnal pattern influenced by milking. In housed cattle, laying behaviour is often affected by feeding management (Overton *et al.*, 2002; DeVries & von Keyserlingk, 2005). Laying behaviour of cattle is also affected by stall availability, stall location and pen layout (Wagner-Storch *et al.*, 2003), stall size and configuration (Tucker & Weary, 2004; Tucker *et al.*, 2006), social ranking (Galindo & Broom, 2000), production and health status (Fregonesi & Leaver, 2001; Walker *et al.*, 2008). The number of stalls should be approximately 120% of the number of cattle in the facility. This allows even the submissive cattle to find a stall where they can rest.

The requirement for rest is likely a threshold event. All cattle, regardless of type, age and production level require a minimum period of rest. Failure to achieve the minimum rest time or increased standing behaviour results in increased prevalence of lameness and stress (Leonard *et al.*, 1994; Galindo & Broom, 2000; Cook *et al.*, 2004). Uncomfortable or unsafe resting surfaces result in reduced resting time and stress. In such cases, cattle stay on their feet for extended periods. Once these cattle are finally down, they stay down for prolonged periods. Lameness has significant impacts on production and involuntary culling (Monti *et al.*, 1999). Cattle with decreased time of rest have demonstrated changes in the growth hormone and ACTH concentrations, and the response of cortisol to ACTH stimulation. Additionally, in lactating cows, there is decreased blood supply to the udder. This, in turn, may lead to reduced feed and water consumption, and reduced production.

The lying periods of cattle fit in between the periods of feeding and standing. Under ideal conditions, cows lie down for approximately 12.0–14.0 hours per day. During that time, they sleep for only 30 minutes. The lying time and the number of lying periods depend on the age, heat cycle and state of health of cattle. Factors that also influence the lying time and the number of lying periods are the environment (e.g. weather), design of stalls, type, quality and quantity of bedding, type of housing, and cattle number per square metre. A lying period typically lasts from one-half to three hours, so cattle stand up and lie down many times per day (usually 10–16). During the long lying periods in the middle of the day or during the night, the animal rises, stretches, defecates, urinates and lies down again immediately, usually on the contra-lateral side.

Behaviour of cattle while laying down and getting up may also be indicative of discomfort or hazards. Cattle lie down in four steps: bend the front limbs; fall onto the front knees; the rest of the body falls backward; and the body rolls on the side that the first front limb was bent.

Cattle should get up the same way in a stall as they would outside on pasture. To facilitate rising, they need to take a full stride forward. Cattle on pasture rise and end up standing 60 to 90 cm in front of where they were lying. Cattle need to bob their heads down and forward, so that they can shift their weight from their hind limbs. In a stall, cattle can either bob forward or to the side. The horizontal area in front of the resting space is referred to as the lunge space, and the vertical area at the end of the lunge as the bob zone. Providing inadequate lunge and bob space may result in a dramatic reduction in stall occupancy or, more commonly, alter the way that cattle use the stalls. If adequate lunge and bob spaces are not available, cattle will have difficulty in rising up, and may eventually stop using the stalls. They can sometimes find it impossible to rise due to the inadequate lunge space, and have to require manual assistance.

Cattle rise up in five steps: roll the body to lie on the sternum; lunge the head forward (or a side); rise the body onto the knees and sternum; extend the head and neck upward; and lastly, straighten up one front limb, immediately followed by the other.

Physiological parameters

Locomotion or mobility scoring

Locomotion scoring (on a 1–5 scale) uses the signs of impaired mobility and pain which include walking at a slower speed, a shortened stride length, an arched back and diminished weight bearing of affected limbs. Locomotion scoring is a relatively quick and simple qualitative assessment of the ability of cattle to walk normally. It is described in detail in Chapter 41 (The Farm Audit: Foot Health, Lameness and Foot Care). A locomotion score of 3.0 or higher indicates that affected cattle should be examined to determine the reason for the lameness. A reasonable goal is to have more than 65% of cattle in a group scoring 1.0, and less than 3% scoring 4.0 and above. Cattle with a locomotion score of 5.0 should be immediately removed from the main group and treated.

Body condition scoring

The body condition scoring (BCS) is an indicator of the past nutritional status of cattle. The most common body condition scoring system ranks cattle from 1 to 5, with a score of 1 being thin and a score of 5 being obese. It is important that the BCS is matched to each stage of the cycle of production (calving, early, mid, and late lactation, early dry period, late dry period and transition period), to ensure that the lactational and reproductive performance is optimised. Body condition scoring on a cattle enterprise should be carried out monthly. Monthly changes in body condition tend to correlate better with health, productivity and reproduction than the actual BCS on any particular day or single-day recording of body weight. Monthly scoring allows for management or nutritional changes to be made on time and prevent serious problem arising.

Each feeding group should have the average BCS determined separately. The uniformity of the BCS within a feeding group is another important measure. Cattle from a feeding group should be fairly uniform. Less than 20% of cattle should be outliers in lactating cows, and less than 15% for beef. Groups with non-uniform distribution of BCS for longer than a month are an indication that there is a problem, and corrective feeding is required.

Body condition should have the final word on the energy content of the diet, rather than the computer-predicted energy value of the ration. For example, thin cows in early lactation need an increase in the energy content of the diet and the dry matter intake. It is critical that cows do not exceed one point of BCS loss in the first month after calving. Cows with excessive loss in BCS usually have an irregular cycling pattern and a longer

Table 35.6 Scoring of quality of faeces.

Score	Description	Reasons
1	• Very liquid • Diarrhoea • Non-desired score	• Excess protein or starch • Lack of fibre • Excess urea • Some mineral excess or poisonings • Mouldy feed • Excess of an osmotic gradient in the intestine • Gastro-intestinal parasitism • Various disorders of digestive tract • Various generalised disorders
2	• Runny • Do not form a distinct pile • Splatters when hit the ground or concrete • Pat measures less than 2.5 cm in height • More watery than optimal	• Cattle on lush pasture • Gastro-intestinal parasitism • Low fibre • Lack of functional fibre
3	• Porridge-like appearance with several concentric rings, a small depression or dimple in the middle • Makes a plopping sound when hit concrete floors. • Faeces pat measures up 4–5 cm. • Sticks to the shoes when touched • Optimal score for lactating cows • Sticks to the shoes	• Cattle on lush pasture • Optimal level of total and functional fibre
4	• Thick • Faeces pat measures up over 5 cm • Firmly sticks to the shoes when touched • Optimal score for dry cows and heifers	• Dry stock, replacements • The level of total and functional fibre is high • Adding extra grain or protein to the diet can decrease the score.
5	• Appears as firm faecal balls • Resembles horse faeces • Not wanted score	• Straw-based diet • Dehydration • Blockage of digestive tract

post-partum anoestrus period, and they may fail to conceive. The low BCS at that time may be from an imbalanced diet, insufficient food, group hierarchy, metabolic problems, lameness and other health problems.

Faecal scoring

Assessment of the faeces may provide valuable information about general health, the state of rumen fermentation and the digestive function of cattle. Faecal scoring is a tool that can be used in assessing the digestibility of the food, particularly the balance of protein, fibre and digestible carbohydrates, and the water intake. Faecal pats are assessed while still fresh, by observation, by sliding the boot through the upper 1–2 cm of the pat, by palpation of a handful by gloved hand, and by sieve washing. These tests allow assessment of consistency (Table 35.6) and digestibility (Table 35.7).

Quality of faeces in cattle on pasture-based systems is more variable, dependent on the content of easily-digestible components and water. Faeces produced by cattle consuming immature (lush) pasture tend to fall to the ground in shapeless deposits of lower score (2 or even lower). Faeces produced by cattle eating mature pasture, with increased structural non-digestible fibre, appears more solid (score 3 to 4).

The presence of specific components in the faeces may indicate where the problem is in the feeding, or the type of disorder of the digestive tract (Table 35.8).

Finally, faeces may be screened by washing a cup of manure under running water through a sieve (0.2 to 0.3 mm) for approximately 30 seconds. The residual material is used to qualify the digestion of consumed food. There should be less than 10% of remaining starch, and less than 12.5% of the screened dry matter, in the residue in the sieve. The presence of grain with residual starch indicates an insufficient preparation of the feedstuffs or impaired digestion. The presence of feedstuffs longer than 15 mm usually reflects a lack of long fibre to maintain healthy rumen mat, a decrease in cud-chewing movements, and faster passage of ingesta through the digestive tract.

Adverse changes in faecal scores may indicate problems with the balance of nutrients in the ration, inadequate mixing, sorting of food at the feeding area, and unacceptable competition at feeding.

Table 35.7 Scoring of digestive function by squeezing faeces with gloved hand.

Score	Description	Reasons
1	• Creamy, homogenous emulsion • No visible undigested food particles • Shiny surface of fresh faeces	• Good passage of ingesta through the digestive tract • Good digestion • Good food quality • Good rumination • Ideal score for cattle
2	• Creamy, homogenous emulsion • Few undigested food particles of small size • Shiny surface of fresh faeces	• Lightly impaired passage of ingesta through the digestive tract • Lightly impaired digestion • Less than ideal food quality • Lightly impaired rumination • Common in lactating and dry cows
3	• Faeces not homogeneous. • Some undigested particles • On hand squeeze, some undigested fibres stick to the fingers • Dull to shiny surface of fresh faeces	• Higher then normal speed of passage of the ingesta through the digestive tract • Poor formation of rumen mat • Poor digestion • Problems with processing the grain (not broken) • Acceptable score for dry cows and heifers
4	• Bigger undigested food particles • On squeeze, a ball of undigested food remains in the hand • Particles sometimes > 2 cm • Dull surface of fresh faeces	• Higher then normal speed of passage of the ingesta through the digestive tract • Poor formation of rumen mat • Poor digestion • Forages of poor quality • Poor rumination
5	• Bigger food particles • Undigested components of the feed ration are clearly recognisable • Very dull surface of fresh faeces	• High speed of passage of the ingesta through the digestive tract • Poor formation of rumen mat • Poor digestion • Forages of very poor quality • Very poor rumination

Table 35.8 Admixtures and variability of faeces and common reasons.

Component in the faeces	Reasons
Undigested fibre	• Higher then normal speed of passage of the ingesta through the digestive tract • Poor formation of rumen mat • Poor digestion • Forages of poor quality • Poor rumination
Undigested grain	• Higher then normal speed of passage of the ingesta through the digestive tract • Poor formation of rumen mat • Poor digestion, particularly acidosis • Problems with processing the grain (not broken)
Mucin	• Acidosis • Increase in digestive role of caudal part of the intestines
Bubbly diarrhoea	• Excess in soluble protein, particularly compared to fibre content • Excess of urea, particularly compared to fibre and energy content
Variability within the group of cattle	• Feedstuffs not mixed well • Parts of food mouldy

Table 35.9 Scoring of rumen fill.

Score	Description	Reasons and category of cattle
1	• A deep dip in the left flank • More than one hand-width deep • Rectangular appearance • The skin under the lumbar vertebrae curves inwards • The skin fold from the hook bone goes vertically downwards	• Cattle have eaten little or nothing • Sudden illness • Insufficient food • Unpalatable food • Alarming situation
2	• The skin under the lumbar vertebrae curves inwards • Triangular appearance • The skin fold from the hook bone runs diagonally forward towards the last rib • The paralumbar fossa behind the last rib is one hand-width deep	• Common in cattle in the first week after calving • In other cattle is alarming situation • Later in lactation, sign of: ◦ insufficient food intake ◦ too fast passage of food.
3	• The skin under the lumbar vertebrae goes vertically down for one hand-width and then curves outward • The skin fold from the hook bone is not visible • The paralumbar fossa behind the last rib is still just visible	• Right score for lactating cows • Right score for beef cattle on pasture: ◦ Good food intake ◦ Good timing of passage of food
4	• The skin under the lumbar vertebrae curves outwards • No paralumbar fossa is visible behind the last rib	• Right score for cows in late lactation • Right score for beef cattle in feedlot • Right score for early dry cows
5	• The lumbar vertebrae are not visible as the rumen is very well filled • The skin over the whole belly is quite tight • There is no visible transition between the flank and ribs	• Right score for dry cows • Right score for heifers

Rumen scoring

Scoring of the rumen fill (Table 35.9) is used to assess the food intake and the speed at which food is moving through the digestive tract. It is a visual assessment, carried out from behind and slightly to the left of the animal. The rumen is assessed by observing the left flank. The degree of fill is a function of the feed intake, the fermentation speed and the rumen outflow rate.

Conclusion

The assessor should use a holistic approach to identify all problem areas, and combine the physical findings with an assessment of the behaviour and health of the cattle. Information gathered through assessment of cattle signs should be used as an advisory tool to assist producers in decision-making about their management practices and farm facilities. The assessment should be carried out in presence of the producer. All problematic areas should be listed and prioritised by the importance and the ease of implementing the corrective changes.

It is imperative that the assessor provides cost-effective solutions to all problem areas. The proposed solutions should assist the producer in achieving the set targets. Increasing the awareness of the producer to the value of auditing important cow signs will increase their participation and improved outcomes.

References

Camiloti, T.V., Fregonesi, J.A., von Keyserlingk, M.A.G. and Weary, D.M. (2012). Effects of bedding quality on the lying behavior of dairy calves. *Journal of Dairy Science* **95**(6), 3380–3383.

Cook, N.B., Bennett, T.B. and Nordlund, K.V. (2004). Effect of free stall surface on daily activity patterns in dairy cows with relevance to lameness prevalence. *Journal of Dairy Science* **87**(9), 2912–2922.

Cook, N. B., Bennett, T.B. and Nordlund, K.V. (2005). Monitoring indices of cow comfort in free-stall-housed dairy herds. *Journal of Dairy Science* **88**(11), 3876–3885.

DeVries, T.J. and von Keyserlingk, M.A.G. (2005). Time of feed delivery affects the feeding and lying patterns of dairy cows. *Journal of Dairy Science* **88**(2), 625–631.

DeVries, T.J. and von Keyserlingk, M.A.G. (2008). *Understanding cow behavior from a nutritional perspective*. Tri-State Dairy Nutrition Conference, **2008**.

DeVries, T.J., von Keyserlingk, M.A.G. and Beauchemin, K.A. (2005). Frequency of feed delivery affects the behavior of lactating dairy cows. *Journal of Dairy Science* **88**(10), 3553–3562.

Drissler, M., Gaworski, M., Tucker, C.B. and Weary, D.M. (2005). Freestall maintenance: effects on lying behavior of dairy cattle. *Journal of Dairy Science* **88**(7), 2381–2387.

Fregonesi, J.A. and Leaver, J.D. (2001). Behaviour, performance and health indicators of welfare for dairy cows housed in strawyard or cubicle systems. *Livestock Production Science* **68**(2/3), 205–216.

Fregonesi, J.A., Veira, D.M., von Keyserlingk, M.A.G. and Weary, D.M. (2007). Effects of bedding quality on lying behavior of dairy cows. *Journal of Dairy Science* **90**(12), 5468–5472.

Fulwider, W.K., Grandin, T., Garrick, D.J., Engle, T.E., Lamm, W.D., Dalsted, N.L. and Rollin, B.E. (2007). Influence of free-stall base on tarsal joint lesions and hygiene in dairy cows. *Journal of Dairy Science* **90**(7), 3559–3566.

Galindo, F. and Broom, D. M. (2000). The relationships between social behaviour of dairy cows and the occurrence of lameness in three herds. *Research in Veterinary Science* **69**(1), 75–79.

Grant, R.J. and Albright, J.L. (1995). Feeding behavior and management factors during the transition period in dairy cattle. *Journal of Animal Science* **73**(9), 2791–2803.

Haley, D.B., d., Passille, A.M. and Rushen, J. (2001). Assessing cow comfort: effects of two floor types and two tie stall designs on the behaviour of lactating dairy cows. *Applied Animal Behaviour Science* **71**(2), 105–117.

Ito, K., von Keyserlingk, M.A.G., LeBlanc, S.J. and Weary, D.M. (2010). Lying behavior as an indicator of lameness in dairy cows. *Journal of Dairy Science* **93**(8), 3553–3560.

Ito, K., Weary, D.M. and von Keyserlingk, M.A.G. (2009). Lying behavior: assessing within- and between-herd variation in free-stall-housed dairy cows. *Journal of Dairy Science* **92**(9), 4412–4420.

Kendall, P. E., Nielsen, P.P., Webster, J.R. Verkerk, G.A., Littlejohn R.P. and Matthews, L.R. (2006). The effects of providing shade to lactating dairy cows in a temperate climate. *Livestock Science* **103**(1/2), 148–157.

Leonard, F. C., O'Connell, J. and O'Farrell, K. (1994). Effect of different housing conditions on behaviour and foot lesions in Friesian heifers. *The Veterinary Record* **134**(19), 490–494.

Monti, G., Tenhagen, B.A. and Heuwieser, W. (1999). Culling policies in dairy herds. A review. *Journal of Veterinary Medicine. Series A* **46**(1), 1–11.

Overton, M.W., Sischo, W.M., Temple, G.D. and Moore, D.A. (2002). Using time-lapse video photography to assess dairy cattle lying behavior in a free-stall barn. *Journal of Dairy Science* **85**(9), 2407–2413.

Phillips, C.J.C. and Rind, M.I. (2001). The effects on production and behavior of mixing uniparous and multiparous cows. *Journal of Dairy Science* **84**(11), 2424–2429.

Rushen, J., Boissy, A., Terlouw, EM. and de Passillé, A.M. (1999). Opioid peptides and behavioral and physiological responses of dairy cows to social isolation in unfamiliar surroundings. *Journal of Animal Science* **77**(11), 2918–2924.

Rushen, J., Haley, D. and de Passillé, A.M. (2007). Effect of softer flooring in tie stalls on resting behavior and leg injuries of lactating cows. *Journal of Dairy Science* **90**(8), 3647–3651.

Tucker, C.B. and Weary, D.M. (2004). Bedding on geotextile mattresses: how much is needed to improve cow comfort? *Journal of Dairy Science* **87**(9), 2889–2895.

Tucker, C.B., Weary, D.M. and Fraser, D. (2003). Effects of three types of free-stall surfaces on preferences and stall usage by dairy cows. *Journal of Dairy Science* **86**(2), 521–529.

Tucker, C.B., Zdanowicz, G. and Weary, D.M. (2006). Brisket boards reduce freestall use. *Journal of Dairy Science* **89**(7), 2603–2607.

Wagner-Storch, A.M., Palmer, R.W. and Kammel, D.W. (2003). Factors affecting stall use for different freestall bases. *Journal of Dairy Science* **86**(6), 2253–2266.

Walker, S.L., Smith, R.F., Routly, J.E., Jones, D.N., Morris, M.J. and Dobson, H. (2008). Lameness, activity time-budgets, and estrus expression in dairy cattle. *Journal of Dairy Science* **91**(12), 4552–4559.

Weary, D. M. and Taszkun, I. (2000). Hock Lesions and Free-Stall Design. *Journal of Dairy Science* **83**(4), 697–702.

Wechsler, B., Schaub, J., Friedli, K. and Hauser, R. (2000). Behaviour and leg injuries in dairy cows kept in cubicle systems with straw bedding or soft lying mats. *Applied Animal Behaviour Science* **69**(3), 189–197.

CHAPTER 36

The Farm Audit: Health and Management of the Calf

Katrine Bazeley

Learning objectives

- Understand the important husbandry practices that impact on the productivity, welfare, health and hence profitability of the calf rearing unit.
- Understand the terms processes, key performance indicators and target values.
- Be able to compile a farm audit questionnaire and perform an audit.
- Be able to define 'best practice' for each process.
- Be able to set appropriate values for key performance indicators.
- Be able to communicate the important outcomes of the farm audit.
- Be able to select which records need to be kept.

Introduction: 'disease is just a failure of management'

Care of the calf is pivotal to profitable dairy farming, as the dairy heifer calf represents the future of the milking herd. Nevertheless, problems are common, costly and often intractable. This chapter explores how the clinician can evaluate calf performance and investigate problems when they occur.

A variety of management systems are used to meet the calf's needs for feed and shelter, any of which can be effective or, on a different unit, can go disastrously wrong. Attention to detail and stockmanship quality are the keys to success. The veterinarian who works with the farmer to improve calf management must collect evidence from as many sources as possible to monitor performance, since calf rearing records are often scanty, and their accuracy must be validated. However, enough data can usually be gathered to identify principal areas of loss. Thorough observation and questions to the farmer, the manager and the stockperson(s) are then required to investigate the causes of problems and to look for potential solutions.

Records

A recording system should allow regular analysis of herd performance and, ideally, should also provide graphic displays and interpretation of results. There is usually a trade-off between the sophistication of analysis and ease of use, so the priority should be to ensure that data recorded are timely, accurate and complete. This may mean simple, paper-based records, which may or may not be transferred to computer.

The success of the calf-rearing enterprise can be measured using Key Performance Indicators as follows:

1. Mortality rate is a blunt instrument, but it should be available on every unit. The target is less than 5%, and higher mortality rates represent significant economic loss. Calculation of age at death allows for the identification of possible causes and further investigations required (see Table 36.1). The minimum records required to calculate calf mortality rate are:
   - Number of calves born alive (and dates)
   - Number of calves born dead (and dates)
   - Calf deaths (and dates of death)

   It is useful to compare results on different units, and a practice survey can provide a valuable benchmark for clients. The farmer can monitor calf mortality over successive seasons, using a simple line graph.
2. Disease records enable the incidence of different diseases to be calculated, but are often not available. Ideally, disease records can be kept in conjunction with treatment records, including a summary of calf identity, condition treated and outcome after seven days.

Bovine Medicine, Third Edition. Edited by Peter D. Cockcroft.

Table 36.1 Calf mortality (adapted from Bazeley, 2007).

Age at death	Common causes	Investigations
Born dead or death within 24 hours	Lack of skilled supervision. Inadequate supervision at calving, especially heifers. Over-zealous, early intervention at calving.	Check quality of stockmanship (Table 36.6) and time to monitor calving cows, especially if they calve away from main buildings. Check overnight monitoring of calving cows.
	Dystocia, especially wrong choice of bull or small heifers (Mee *et al.*, 2008).	Post-mortem examination (PME) of calves born dead. Weigh. Check for signs of prolonged dystocia, sample for trace element deficiency and *in utero* infection (e.g. *neospora)*.
	Hypocalcaemia and associated problems.	Check calving records, treatment records and use of drugs for treatment of Hypocalcaemia.
	Cows too fat at calving (target 2.75-3 in a 1–5 scale) (Lorenz *et al.*, 2011a).	Monitor cow Body Condition Score (BCS) in transition group, early dry period and late lactation. Look for variation in BCS and its causes.
	Group size too big, or overcrowded housing, so cows unable to calve without disturbance.	Group size should be < 40. The calving cow in a straw yard requires 12 m^2 per animal.
	Trace element deficiency, particularly iodine and selenium/vitamin E.	Bloods from transition cows to investigate trace element status.
	Early calving – twins, neospora, BVD or other abortion agent.	Abortion investigation, including serology of cows.
	Early induction of parturition (not induction at term).	Check treatment records.
	Idiopathic stillbirth (causes unknown).	
1–7 days	Often neonatal septicaemia. Small or weak at birth, congenital defects.	PME as above. Check quality of stockmanship (Table 36.9).
	Inadequate colostrum intake or poor quality colostrum.	Check colostrum status (Table 36.6).
	Overwhelming infection: • Poor hygiene • Overcrowding • Build-up of disease organisms.	Observe environmental hygiene. Measure stocking density (Table 36.10).
7–28 days	Inadequate colostral protection as above. Most deaths due to: **1** diarrhoea – many causative agents. Nutritional scour may also occur in artificially reared calves; **2** respiratory disease – many causative agents.	PME Check: • colostrum status (Table 36.5); • quality of stockmanship (Table 36.9); • nutrition factors (Tables 36.7 and 36.8); • housing factors (Table 36.10).
More than 28 days	Chronic disease sequels Respiratory disease Post-weaning disease Accident	PME. Checks as above, and check for risks of injury.

3 Treatment used, batch number and expiry date, identity of animal treated and date should always be recorded, and can be used to monitor the numbers of animals treated and repeat treatments. In conjunction with performance records (mortality, weaning weight, heifer wastage and age at first calving), they can be used to estimate the impact of disease on calves. This then enables informed decisions to be made about the cost-effectiveness of disease control interventions. However, treatment records are often incomplete, the policy for utilising medical treatment varies (e.g. group treatment and prophylactic treatment) and disease may be missed, leading to a false impression of disease levels. A target of less than 10% requiring treatment by the age of weaning is often used, but the veterinarian and farmer should set realistic targets for the individual herd, to be achieved within a specified time-frame (e.g. four months), review progress and set new targets as progress is made.

4 Farm purchases of prescription-only medicines will be accurate, but must be interpreted with care, because many antibiotics are also used for treatment of other classes of stock as well as calves. These records can be used to check the accuracy of treatment records. Routine use of whole-group treatments

(e.g. antibiotic in milk powder, or anticoccidial agents in concentrate feed) should be reviewed.

5 Calf weights and growth rate can be monitored. Targets depend upon breed, but generally the calf should approximately double her birth weight by weaning. A scatter graph of weights of calves will show both the average and the variation (Figure 36.1). Growth rate can be calculated using an estimate of average calf birth weight for the breed (e.g. Holsteins, about 40 kg) if calves are not weighed at birth. Calves fed restricted milk (approximately 10% body weight daily) grow little for the first three weeks until concentrate feed intake increases. Calves fed *ad lib* milk may drink 20% of their body weight per day and growth rate may be more than 1 kg daily. Many other factors also affect the growth rate of calves up to weaning (Figure 36.2).

6 A weigh-band can be used to estimate calf weight, but accuracy and repeatability should be checked. Other measures such as withers height and nose-tail length have also been used to estimate calf growth (Wathes *et al.*, 2008).

Observations and investigations

Accurate and thoughtful observation is the key to understanding the calf unit, because many problems are the result of failure in management and lack of attention to detail. Interpretation of the observations is also important. The following questions should be asked (from Hulsen and Swormink, 2006):

- *What do I see?* Describe the situation objectively
- *Why has this happened?* Try to identify the cause
- *What does this mean?* Determine whether action is required

Calves – health and disease

Calf vigour at birth is associated with lower perinatal mortality and lower incidence of neonatal disease (Lorenz *et al.*, 2011a). It can be measured using a modified APGAR (Appearance, Pulse, Grimace, Activity, Respiration) score (Table 36.2) (Sorge *et al.*, 2009). Alternatively, time taken to achieve sternal recumbency and to stand provides an objective assessment of neonatal calf vigour (Table 36.3) (Schuijt and Taverne, 1994).

Observation of the calves provides the most direct evidence of the success of the unit, albeit only a snapshot. The animals should first be observed as a group, then individuals can be examined clinically. Some of the abnormalities that may be observed and detected during the examination are listed in Figure 36.3. A checklist of observations in the calf can be found in Table 36.4.

In outbreaks of disease, a systematic investigation is required to ensure that the all risk factors are identified. Examples for diarrhoea and pneumonia (Bovine Respiratory Disease BRD) are presented in Figures 36.4 and 36.5, respectively.

Colostrum and care of the newborn calf

Most disease in the pre-weaned calf is at least in part due to the failure of passive transfer (FPT) of maternal antibodies. The neonatal calf derives all its immediate humeral immunity against neonatal environmental antigenic challenge from colostrum, so it is vital to ensure that every calf receives at least

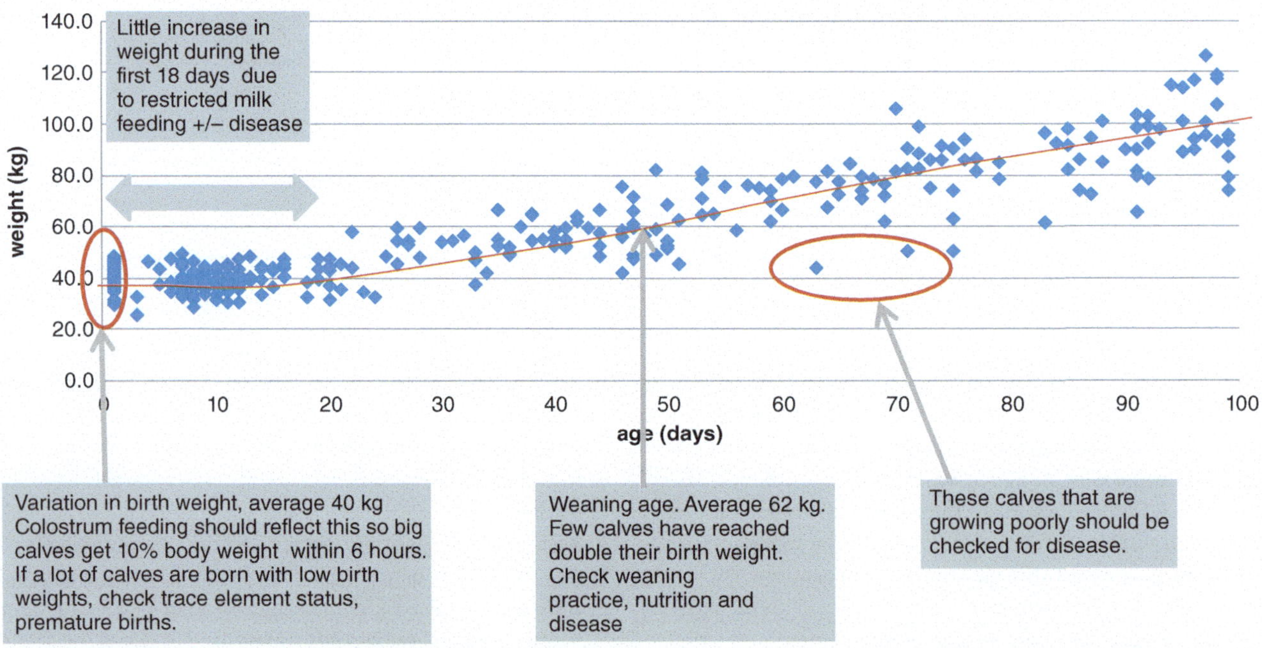

Figure 36.1 Scattergram of weight and age for heifer calves.

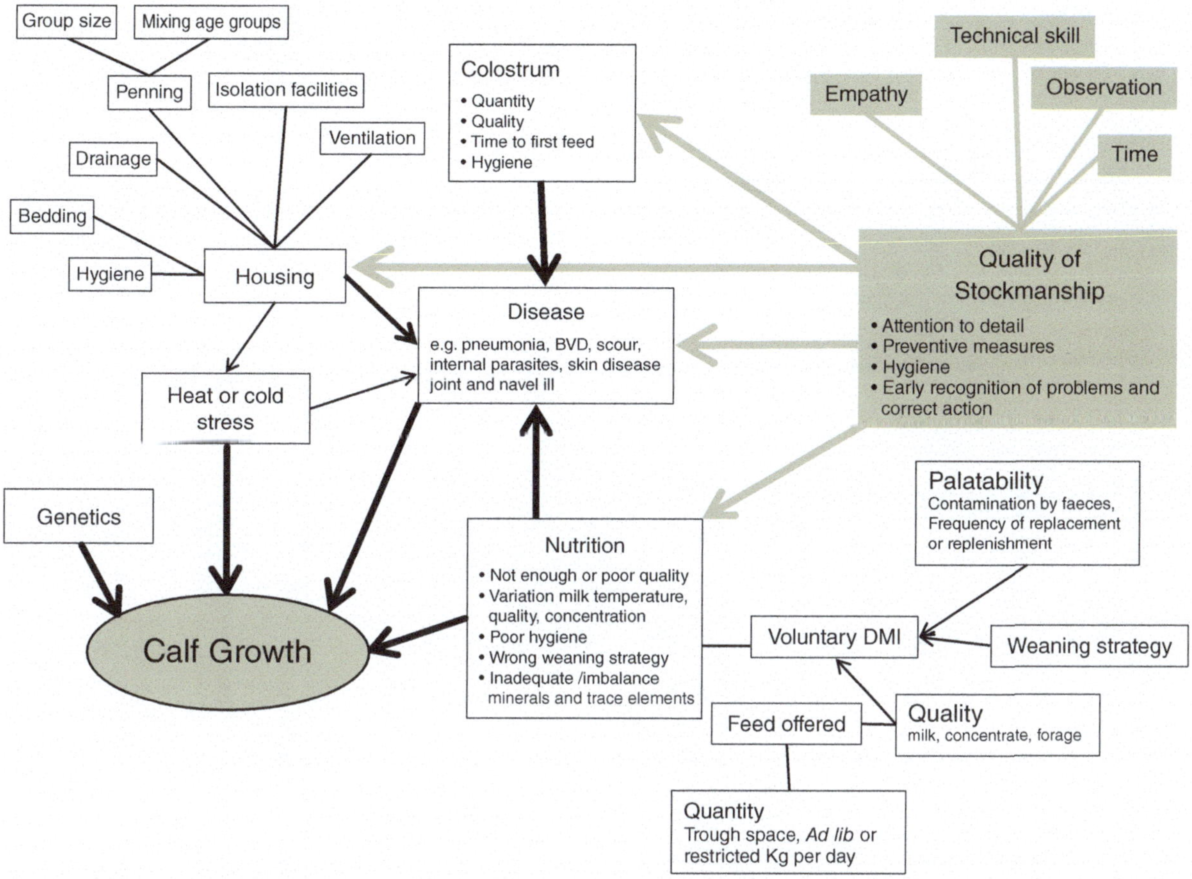

Figure 36.2 Factors affecting calf growth.

Table 36.2 Modified APGAR scores for calves (Adapted from Sorge *et al.*, 2009).

Parameter	Score 0	Score 1	Score 2
Reaction to cold water on head	No reaction	Reduced late reaction	Lifting, shaking head
Interdigital reflex	No reaction	Pulls away slowly, weak	Pulls back strongly immediately
Mucous membrane colour	White	Pale pink or cyanotic	Pink
Respiration	Absent	Irregular frequency and intensity	Regular frequency and intensity

Table 36.3 Target times to stand in the newborn calf (adapted from Schuijt and Taverne, 1994).

Measure of calf vigour	Target time after birth (mins)
Lift its head	3
Sternal recumbency	5
Attempt to stand	20
Stand spontaeously	60–90

four litres of good quality colostrum within six hours of birth. Continued colostrum feeding will boost antibody uptake for up to 24 hours, and colostrum feeding for two weeks provides local mucosal protection that reduces the incidence of diarrhoea (Berge *et al.*, 2009).

The dairy-bred calf may be removed early from its mother and rely mainly or entirely on the stockperson for colostrum milked from its mother or other fresh-calved cows, or artificial colostrum/colostrum substitute. Navels should be dipped soon after birth. Tincture of iodine or chlorhexidine is best practice, although some use tetracycline spray or navel clips. The calf's environment will also influence the risk of infectious disease.

The calf requires a clean, dry and draught-free bed. An investigative check list of calf colostrum management, status and neonatal care can be found in Table 36.5. Weaver *et al.*

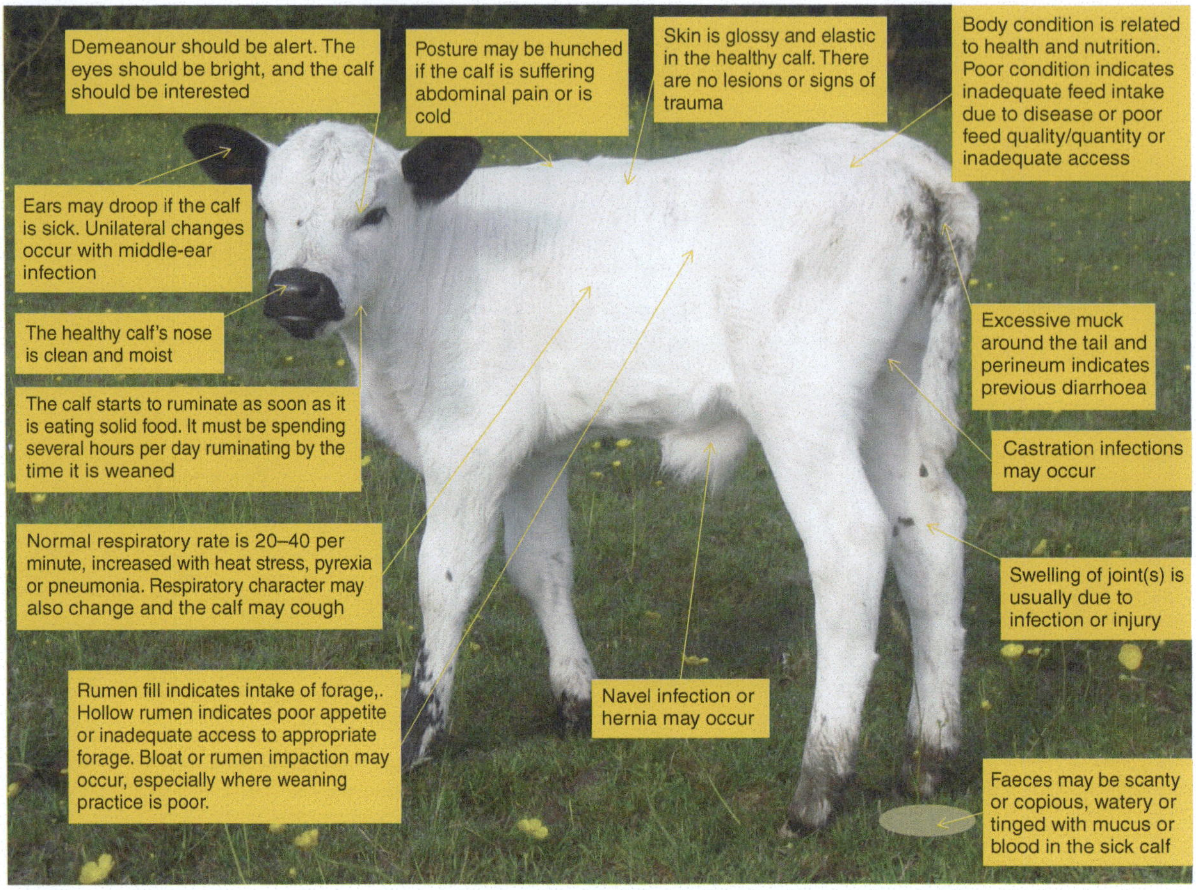

Figure 36.3 Observation of the calf.

Table 36.4 Observations of the calf.

Factor	Physical	Behavioural	None/little	Some	Most/ all
Indicators of excellent health and welfare.	Clean, glossy coat. No discharges from eyes or nose. Normal rumen fill. Good body condition.	Bright, alert demeanour. Playing. Good appetite. Normal locomotion. Ruminating at rest. Stretches after getting up.			
Indicators of health and welfare problems.	Injuries (including disbudding injuries, castration infections). Skin lesions (e.g. ringworm). Dull coat. Hair loss. Dirty limbs. Dirty flanks. Hoof lesions. Navel abscess.	Skin irritation (scratching and rubbing). Dull or apathetic. Collapsed. Lame. Reluctant to stand or move. Abnormal behaviours (navel-sucking, urine-drinking, bar-biting).			
Respiratory health (Potter and Aldritch, 2010).	Nasal discharge. Ocular discharge. Pyrexia.	Increased respiratory rate. Abnormal respiratory character. Cough (spontaneous or induced).			
Nutritional health (Whay *et al.*, 2003).	Body condition. Bloat. Empty/hollow rumen. Dirty perineum and tail. Diarrhoea. Dehydration.	Loss of appetite No rumination Hunched (painful) abdomen			

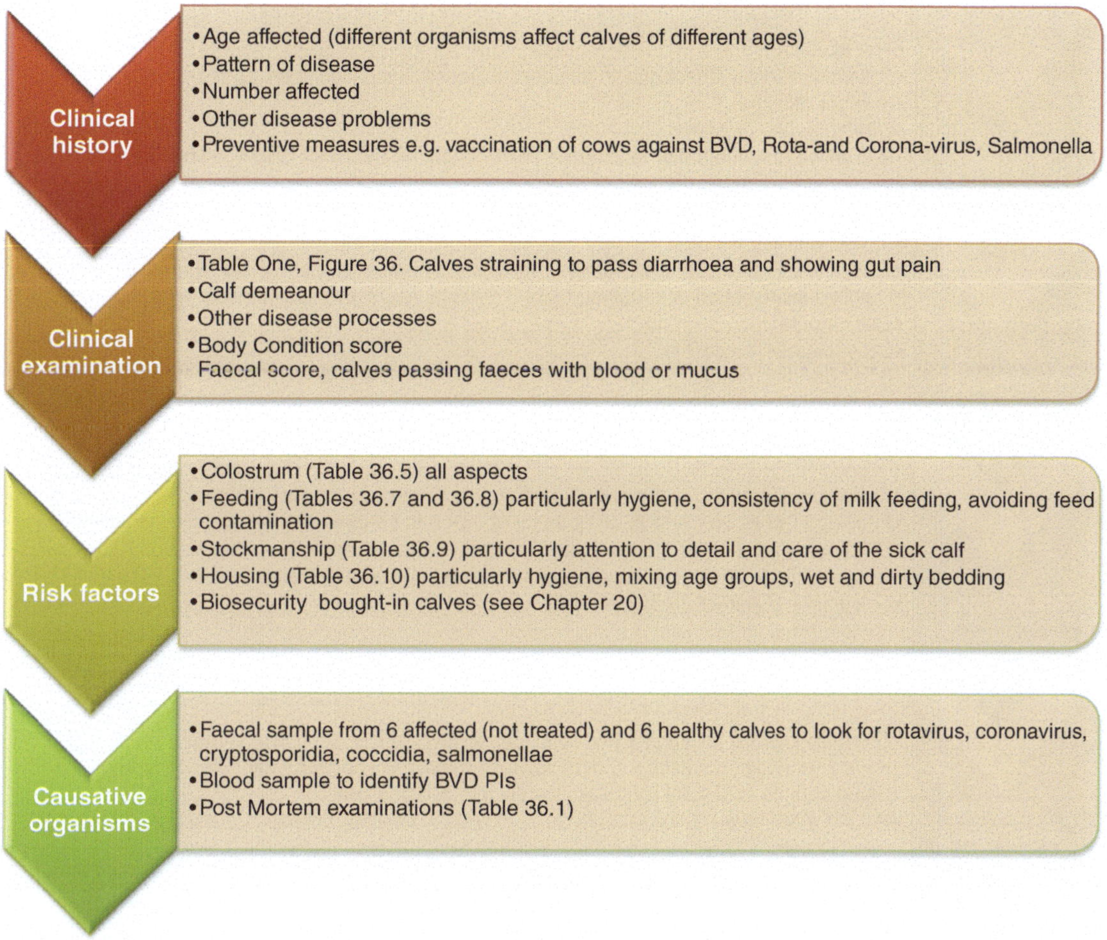

Figure 36.4 Investigation of calf diarrhoea.

(2000) review the passive transfer of colostral immunoglobulins in calves and the different methods used to measure passive transfer. Table 36.6 provides indicative values for the parameters used to assess the success or failure of the passive transfer of colostral immunoglobulins in the neonatal calf.

Nutrition

A number of artificial rearing systems are used to feed milk to the calf (summarised in Bazeley and Hayton, 2007), delivering whole milk or milk replacer, restricted or *ad lib*, warm or cold, via teat or bucket, fresh or pasteurised or cultured as yoghurt. The calf can thrive on any system, provided that hygiene is excellent, the milk is fed regularly and the same every time. A checklist for the milk-fed calf is shown in Table 36.7.

The calf fed a restricted quantity of milk must start eating solid feed from a few days old, or health and growth rate will be compromised. Palatable, high-quality concentrate should be offered fresh at least once a day, in troughs that are off the ground (to avoid faecal contamination). Fresh forage (hay or straw) should be provided daily in racks (not floor fed – calves will not eat forage that is dirty) (see also Table 36.8). Sufficient trough space must be available for calves to compete for forage and to avoid risk of injury. A clean supply of fresh water should always be available.

The calf may be weaned from about six weeks old, by which time it must be eating enough solid feed to continue to thrive as a functioning ruminant. The success of the calf's development is, therefore, dependent on feeding the calf correctly during the first weeks, and weaning the calf only when it is ready. A checklist for artificially reared calves is shown in Table 36.8.

Stockmanship

Stockmanship quality is probably the factor that most influences the calf's health and welfare. The good stockperson ensures that the needs of every calf are met, notices health problems early and takes immediate, appropriate action when things go wrong. This requires technical knowledge, observational skills, attention to detail, empathy with stock and enough time to do the job

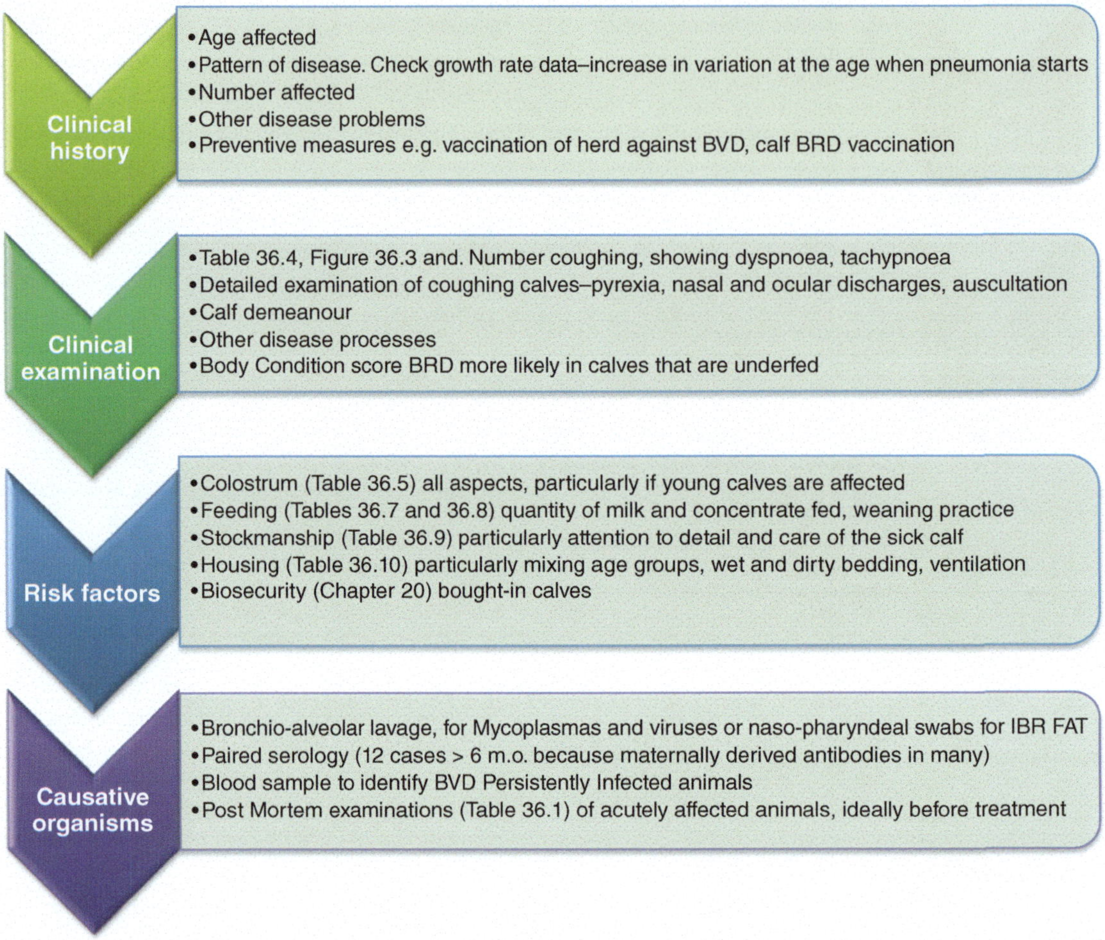

Figure 36.5 Investigation of calf pneumonia (BRD).

Table 36.5 Investigation of calf colostrum status and neonatal care.

Factor		Investigation and notes
Calf immunoglobulin status		Blood sample calves 2–8 day of age. Target is 12 calves. Investigate causes if results show that > 20% have failure of passive transfer (high risk category). Table 36.6 provides the interpretation of the parameter values.
Colostrum intake	Supervision.	Check protocol: Observe the calf sucking (takes 20 minutes to drink 1 L colostrum). Feed 4 L colostrum (at least 10% body weight) within six hours after birth (ideally as two feeds) by teat or stomach tube. Continue to feed colostrum for at least 24 hours.
	Overcrowding and mis-mothering.	Group size should be no more than 40. Down-calving cows are often particularly keen to mother a new calf, so ideally group < 10. Space allowance minimum 12 m^2 per cow. Individual calving pens probably best (16 m^2 per cow).
	Cows exhausted after prolonged calving.	Investigate prevalence of dystocia and diseases such as Hypocalcaemia. Check for skilled supervision of the calving cow.
	Heifers do not let calves suck, or cows with pendulous udders.	Observe calved animals with their calves. Check quality of stockmanship (Table 36.9) and time for care of the newborn calf.
	Calves small or weak.	Investigate incidence of twins, premature calvings, congenital abnormalities. Check trace element status (Vitamin E/selenium, iodine).

Table 36.5 (*continued*)

Factor		Investigation and notes
Colostrum quality		Measure using colostrometer, with colostrum at about 22°C temperature. Or weigh colostrum – quality is usually less in cows producing more than 8.5 kg colostrum (Weaver *et al.*, 2000).
	Cows in poor body condition.	BCS calving cows. Feed quality for late lactation/dry/transition animals.
	Trace element deficiency (selenium/vitamin E/iodine).	Blood sample transition cows. Liver sample from dead calves. Other trace element deficiency diseases.
	Low specific antibody protection (bought-in cows or heifers).	Check history of cows and heifers. N.B. heifer colostrum quality often better than average in high-yielding dairy herds.
	Cow vaccination.	Vaccination against BVD, Rotavirus + coronavirus and *E. Coli F5* provides calves with specific antibody protection which may reduce clinical incidence of disease (for review, see Lorenz *et al.*, 2011b).
	Cow factors.	Check records: Breed, yield potential, lactation number, pre-milking, running milk before calving or short dry period (less than three weeks). Colostrum from first-lactation heifers and high-yielding cows have reduced quality, 32% of Holstein cows produce poor quality colostrum (Lorenz et al., 2011a).
	First milking.	Check that every calf receives colostrum from the first milking because antibody levels in colostrum fall in subsequent milkings.
	Delay before first milking.	Check protocol. Dairy cows are often not milked for several hours after calving, and colostrum quality falls significantly over time (3.7% every hour after calving; Morin *et al.*, 2010).
	Storage of colostrum before feeding.	Check protocol. Observe stored colostrum. Bacterial contamination reduces uptake of antibodies by the calf. Colostrum should be collected into a clean container and fed immediately, or refrigerated and stored in a covered container. Heat treatment at 60°C for 30 minutes may reduce bacterial contamination and increase IgG absorption (Berge *et al.*, 2009), but routine pasteurisation may reduce IgG level in colostrum. Total colostrum bacterial counts > 100 000 cfu/ml or faecal coliform counts in excess of 10 000 cfu/ml are often associated with FPT.
	Frozen colostrum.	Check protocol. Freezing colostrum causes little alteration in antibody levels, but colostrum must be thawed slowly and not over-heated to prevent damage to proteins.
Johne's risk		Check test results for Johne's status of herd, and how infected cows are identified Check whether calves are fed pooled colostrum.
Hygiene	Calving environment and calf house, cow teats, calf feeding utensils.	Observe for wet and dirty bedding, cows with dirty teats and check protocol for cleaning calf feeding utensils. Bacterial contamination causes premature closure of the calf gut, so antibody uptake is reduced. Dirty environment will also increase the risk of infection via the navel or gut.
Navel dip		Check protocol. Observe navel cover in navel dressing for all young calves Check incidence of navel infections, joint infections and neonatal abscesses.

properly. Where more than one person looks after the calves, excellent communication is essential. Table 36.9 provides a checklist to evaluate the quality of stockmanship on farm.

Housing

The suitability of calf housing can be assessed in terms of animal comfort and performance, ease of use and level of housing-related disease, particularly pneumonia (Figure 36.6). Table 36.10 provides a basic checklist.

Biosecurity and biocontainment

This is covered in detail elsewhere, and many of the factors covered above relate to reducing exposure of the calf to infectious organisms. The farmer who buys calves, particularly from market (where they are stressed, hungry, exhausted from travel and introduced to a wide variety of pathogens), is at risk of buying in diseases such as BVD, respiratory viruses and Salmonella. If calves are to be bought, they should come directly from a single local farm whose disease status and vaccination history are

Table 36.6 Parameter values for assessing passive transfer using blood and serum samples.

Measure	Comments	High risk	Low risk
Total proteins	Refractometry. laboratory analysis.	<50 g/L	>60 g/L
Immunoglobulins	Radial immune-diffusion. ELISA.	<10 g/L Ig	>24 g/L Ig
IgG1	ELISA.	<8 g/L	>20 g/L
Zinc sulphate turbidity test (ZST)		<10 units	≥20 units
ϒGT	Declines rapidly with age. Reliability has been questioned.	<50 IU/L	>200 IU/L
Sodium sulphite test		18% (no precipitation)	18% (precipitation)
Gluteraldehyde test		No coagulation (five minutes)	Coagulation (five minutes)

Table 36.7 Milk feeding.

Factor	Investigation and notes
Calf health	See Table 36.4.
Calf body condition	Target <10% too thin.
Incidence of diarrhoea	<10% Disease records, treatment records, calf PME (see above).
Incidence of pre-weaning bloat	<2% Disease records, treatment records, calf PME.
Average calf growth rate and individual variation in growth rate	Many factors affect growth, but nutrition is one of the most important. The calf should double birth weight by weaning.
Environmental temperature	The calf whose environment is below Lower Critical Temperature (approx 15°C for neonatal calf, 0°C by 1 m.o.) requires extra feed to maintain body temperature.
Attention to detail	Check quality of stockmanship (Table 36.9)
Quantity milk fed per day	4 litres daily minimum for maintenance and minimal weight gain (Holstein calf) in thermo-neutral conditions. *Ad lib* and computerised milk feeder systems require enough teats – at least one per 20 calves.
Hygiene	Thorough cleaning of all utensils between uses. Communal teats used in automatic feeders may aid the spread of *Mycoplasma* agents (which cause pneumonia), and should be disinfected twice daily.
Milk replacer quality	Many products available for different feeding systems, including acidified milk that can be fed cold, high-protein-low-fat milk for enhanced growth, whey-based and skimmed-milk base. All can work well, provided they are used to manufacturer specifications.
Milk replacer storage	Dry, vermin-proof container.
Milk replacer mixing	Powder weighed every time. Water temperature measured using thermometer every time. Powder added to water and mixed thoroughly.
Computerised feeder	Calibrated daily. At least one teat per 20 calves. Adequate time to teach new calves to use the machine. No more than ten days age difference between oldest and youngest calves in group.
Whole fresh milk	No antibiotic milk used (may contribute to antibiotic resistance, may spread mastitis organisms). Fed at the same temperature every time. Exclude milk from known Johne's infected cows.
Yoghurt	Clean drums regularly (intake falls over time as the yoghurt becomes more acidic). Stir at least once per day. Add 5 ml of hydrogen peroxide/litre of milk to reduce spoilage in hot weather. No antibiotic milk used.

Table 36.8 Solid feed and weaning.

Factor	Investigation and notes
Calf health	Observations (see Table 36.2). Prevalence of disease in recently weaned animals. Thin calves. Empty rumen.
Growth rate	Check for reduced growth rate around weaning time and variation in growth rate within groups (often increases after weaning).
Prevalence of post-weaning problems	Scour, pot belly, Off-feed sufficient to require intervention. Target <5% calves affected.
Criteria for weaning	At least two criteria used: • age (minimum six weeks old); • quantity of concentrate consumed per day more than 1.5 kg per day; • weight; • chewing cud regularly; • no disease.
Weaning method	Gradual over several days
Concentrate feed	Introduced from seven days old. Available after milk feed. Fresh concentrate added daily. No stale feed in feeder. Adequate trough space for all (350–400 mm per head on restricted feed, 220 mm per head if fed *ad lib*). Check that calf concentrate is stored in dry, vermin-proof container.
Forage	Changed daily – always fresh available. Good quality straw or hay. Adequate access for all (in feeder).
Water	Check that fresh water is always available. Small automatic drinkers ideal (water may get stale, dirty in large troughs). Check that water troughs are at the correct height for calves to reach.
Time of disbudding	Should be more than ten days from weaning.
Calves ruminating	Resting calves should spend much of their time ruminating.

Table 36.9 Quality of stockmanship

Factor	Investigation and notes	
Number of people looking after calves	Number of people to be recorded. Best practice if one person in charge and usually cares for calves. Worst if many look after calves without clear strategy.	
Clear responsibility and job descriptions, SOPs	Each task precisely defined. Evidence of consistent approach. Good practice demonstrated for: • hygiene; • mixing milk powder; • feeding; • bedding up; • disinfection of pens; • care of the sick calf.	
Clear communication method between stockpersons	Whiteboard/computer/text.	
Time for calf care	Depends on feeding method: (Dairy Co Feeding + 2010, average figures)	Hours/calf/week
	Twice daily bucket milk	3.5
	Once daily bucket milk	2.5
	Group feeding	1.5
	Ad lib machine or computerised feeder	1.0

Table 36.9 *(continued)*

Factor	Investigation and notes
Agricultural training	Needs to take account of multiple stockpersons.
Specific training in calf care	Needs to take account of multiple stockpersons.
Evidence of stockmanship skills and empathy with stock	Examples: • Knowledge of individual animals. • Positive interactions with calves (stroking ears, talking to calves). • Extra time and care for the sick calf.
Logical treatment strategy for sick calves	Milk withhold and use of electrolytes for scouring calves. Use of therapeutic agents for sick calves. Heat lamp available and used. Equipment (stomach tube, thermometer) and drugs available, clean, suitably stored. Records kept.
Veterinary investigation of unexplained disease	Early intervention requested if calves become sick.

Table 36.10 Housing. Adapted from Lorenz *et al*., 2011c.

Factor	Target	Investigation of common risks
Calf health		See Table 36.1.
Incidence of pneumonia	<10%	Disease records, treatment records, calf PME.
Incidence of diarrhoea	<10%	Disease records, treatment records, calf PME.
Average calf growth rate and individual variation in growth rate	Doubling of weight over a six week period from birth.	Growth rate variation: • pneumonia treatments and clinical signs; • trough space; • variation in size and age in each group.
Mixing age groups	No mixing age groups. All-in, all-out policy.	More than one week's difference in age within one pen. Nose-to-nose contact between animals in different pens. Mixed age groups within one airspace.
Space allowance	1.1 m^2 per calf at 4 weeks old. 1.8 m^2 per calf at 12 weeks old.	Measurement of housing dimensions. Overcrowding.
Ventilation	six air changes per hour (higher in summer). Air smells clean and fresh. No draughts.	Ventilation inadequate in 50% calf housing (Caldow *et al*., 2011). Cobwebs in the roof. Ammonia smell. Damp air. Draughty at calf level. Smoke bomb test.
Airspace	0–12 weeks old require 5–12 m^3.	Airspace usually adequate for young calves 'Stack effect' does not work in high buildings housing young calves
Temperature	Keep calves within thermo-neutral zone: 15–25°C for neonate; 0–28°C at one month old for optimal performance and comfort.	Too cold: huddling, shivering, draughts at calf level, wet bedding, thin calves despite adequate feed, calves outside with no shelter or shade. Use of calf coats protect from cold. Too hot: tachypnoea, sweating.
Bedding	Dry, clean bed	Dirty, wet bedding. Dirty, wet calves. Ammonia smell. Pooled water (e.g. around milk feeder).
Feed troughs	350–400 mm per head on restricted feed, 220 mm per head if fed *ad lib*	Floor troughs (contamination likely). Inadequate space. Stale feed.
Water troughs	Easily cleaned. Fresh water always available.	Too high. Contaminated water. Not available 24/7 (e.g. buckets that must be manually filled for groups).
Forage	Fed fresh straw/hay daily in trough.	Floor fed forage. Poor quality or stale forage. No forage available.

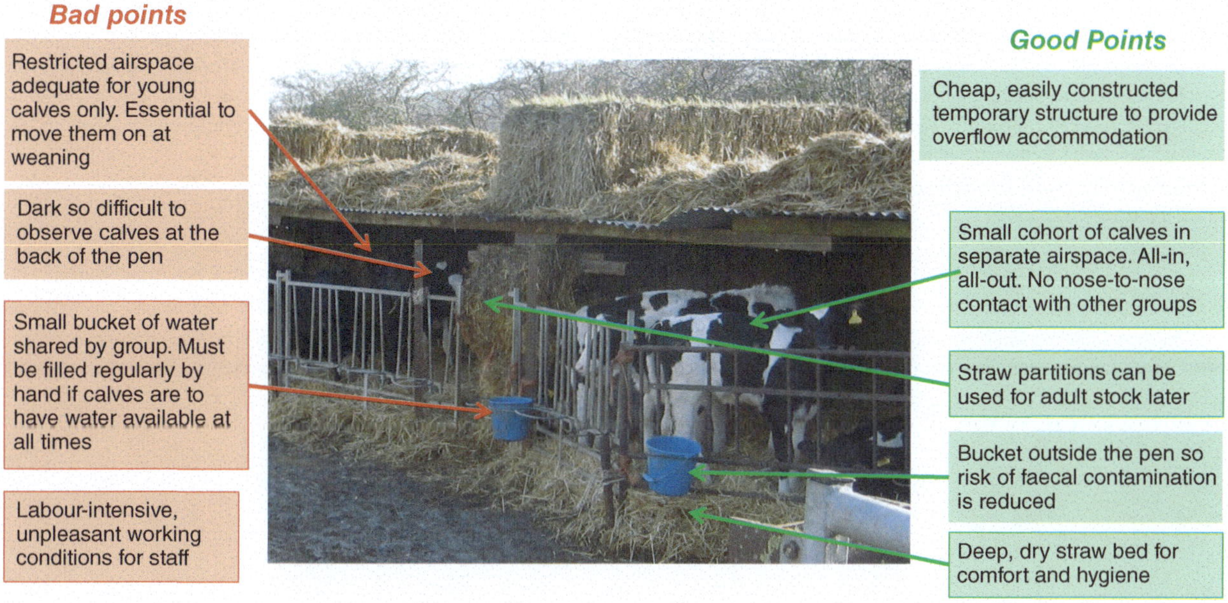
Bad points
Restricted airspace adequate for young calves only. Essential to move them on at weaning
Dark so difficult to observe calves at the back of the pen
Small bucket of water shared by group. Must be filled regularly by hand if calves are to have water available at all times
Labour-intensive, unpleasant working conditions for staff
Good Points
Cheap, easily constructed temporary structure to provide overflow accommodation
Small cohort of calves in separate airspace. All-in, all-out. No nose-to-nose contact with other groups
Straw partitions can be used for adult stock later
Bucket outside the pen so risk of faecal contamination is reduced
Deep, dry straw bed for comfort and hygiene

Figure 36.6 Make an objective assessment of calf housing by undertaking detailed observations and monitoring calf performance (courtesy of Chris Price).

known, and where calves are born into a clean environment and fed enough colostrum.

Young calves are peculiarly susceptible to infectious diseases carried by older cattle, so they should be kept in cohorts of animals the same age. Early removal of the calf from its dam (before 90 minutes) is advocated by some to prevent spread of disease (McGuirk, 2003), and calf housing should provide a separate airspace for groups of different ages and sufficient accommodation to allow for all-in, all-out groupings, with seven days for thorough cleaning, disinfection and drying between occupants.

References

Bazeley, K. (2007). Mortality in calves less than 7 days old in a beef suckler herd. *UK Vet* **12**(7), 36–40.

Bazeley, K. (2003). Investigation of diarrhoea in the neonatal calf. *In Practice* **25**, 152–159.

Bazeley K. and Hayton A. (2007). *Practical Cattle Farming*. Crowood Press, ISBN 978 186 126 975 1.

Berge, A.C., Besser, T.E., Moore, D.A. and Sischo, W.M. (2009). Evaluation of the effects of oral colostrum supplementation suring the first fourteen days on the health and performance of preweaned calves. *Journal of Dairy Science* **92**, 286–295.

Caldow G., Anderson R., Cutler K., Macfarlane J., Potter T. (2011). Clinical Forum: Control of the bovine respiratory disease complex. *UK Vet* **16**(1), 29–40.

Dairy Co (2010). Chapter 10 in: *Managing youngstock feeding in Feeding*. DairyCo Agriculture and Horticulture Development Board (AHDB), 10.1–10.15.

Hulsen, J. and Swormink, B.K. (2006). *From Calf to Heifer a practical guide for rearing young stock*, p.6. Kleinswormink, ISBN-90-75280-95-5.

Lorenz, I., Mee, J.F., Earley, B. and More, S.J. (2011a). General aspects of disease prevention *Irish Veterinary Journal* **64**(10), Calf health from birth to weaning I., 1–8.

Lorenz, I., Fagan, J. and More, S.J. (2011b). Calf health from birth to weaning II. *Irish Veterinary Journal* **64**(9), 1–6.

Lorenz, I., Earley, B., Gilmore J., Hogan, I., Kennedy, E. and More S.J. (2011c). Calf health from birth to weaning III. Housing and management of calf pneumonia Irish Veterinary Journal **64**(10), 1–9.

McGuirk, S. (200). *Solving calf morbidity and mortality problems*. American Association of Bovine Practitioners 36th Annual Conference, pp. 1–13.

Mee J.F., Berry D.P. and Cromie A.R. (2008). Prevalence of, and risk factors associated with, perinatal calf mortality in pasture-based Holstein-Friesian cows *Animal* **2**, 61–620.

Morin, D.E., Nelson, S.V., Reid, E.D., Nagy, D.W., Dahl, G.E. and Constable, P.D. (2010). Effect of colostral volume, interval between calving and first milking, and photoperiod on colostral IgG concentrations in dairy cows. *Journal of the American Veterinary Medical Association* **237**(4), 420–8.

Potter, T. and Aldritch, B. (2010). Systematic approach to calf pneumonia. *UK Vet* **15**(6), 31–34.

Schuijt, G. and Taverne, M.A. (1994). The interval between birth and sternal recumbency as an objective measure of the vitality of newborn calves. *Veterinary Record* **135**, 111–115.

Sorge, U. Kelton, D. and Staufenbiel, R. (2009). Neonatal blood lactate concentration and calf morbidity. *Veterinary Record* **164**, 533–534.

Wathes, D.C., Brickell, J.S., Bourne, N.E., Swali, A. and Cheng, Z. (2008). Factors influencing heifer survival and fertility on commercial dairy farms *Animal* **2**(8), 1135–1143.

Weaver, D.M., Tyler, J.W., VanMetre, D.C., Hostetler, D.E. and Barringgton, G.M. (2000). Passive transfer of colostral immunoglobulins in calves. *Journal of Veterinary Internal Medicine* **14**, 569–577.

Whay, H.R., Main, D.C.J., Green, L.E. and Webster, A.J.F. (2003). An animal based welfare assessment of group-housed calves on UK dairy farms. *Animal Welfare* **12**, 611–617.

CHAPTER 37

Heifer Rearing, Weaning to Second Calving: Optimising Health and Productivity

Peter D. Cockcroft

Learning objectives

- Understand the key elements in heifer rearing programmes.
- Be familiar with the measure, manage and monitor approach to the rearing of replacement heifers.
- Understand the importance of monitoring the growth rates of the heifers from weaning to calving by regular weighing; condition scoring and measuring the height of the withers to ensure recommended targets are met.
- Understand the need to plan the breeding program carefully with careful selection of the bull for genetic improvement and easy calving.
- Understand how to manage the heifers for longevity by reducing the competition with older cows for space, dominance and access to food.
- Appreciate the importance of transition management of the heifer into the lactating herd.
- Appreciate the importance of accurate records on heifer health and performance from birth.
- Be aware of the common and important diseases that can impact adversely on heifer health and welfare.
- Be able to devise a farm specific heifer health management plan.

The aim of this chapter is to highlight the key components of a heifer rearing programme to optimise health and productivity. The scope of the topic will be divided into nutrition and target growth rates, disease risk and health care programmes, breeding programmes and the transitional period, when the heifer is entering the herd, and getting the heifer back into calf.

Introduction

Ideally, we would like all heifers that are weaned and selected as herd replacements to calve down unaided at 24 months old, fulfil their genetic and physiological potential with regards to their first lactation yield and milk composition, and calve for a second time with an optimised calving-to-calving interval. This is rarely, if ever, achieved, with retention in the herd for a second calving often being poor. The cost of poor heifer rearing practices is high. Improvements are frequently cost-effective.

The advantages of calving at two years include a longer productive life, lower replacement rates, better fertility, faster genetic improvement, lower feed, capital and labour costs and more surplus heifers for sale. The use of sexed semen is still under-utilised as a strategic management tool in heifer replacement planning and enterprise profitability.

The need for heifer replacements is a function of the herd culling rate, the calf and heifer mortality rate and the calving age of the heifer. By reducing heifer mortality and calving down at two years of age, the number of replacements is reduced, with attendant cost savings. 'Heifer' is defined as any female calf up to the second calving. The Daisy Survey (2002) indicated that 22% of replacement heifers born are lost before they reach their first lactation, and a further 14% are culled during their first lactation, with fertility being the main reason (46%). Infertility, dystocia, mastitis and lameness are principal reasons why heifers are lost or culled. Annual herd mean culling rate is 25%, and at least 31 replacement heifers are needed per year to replace these cull cows. The mean age at first calving in this survey was 28 months, with a wide range of age at first calving. The current costs of rearing a heifer to calve down at two years old in the UK is approximately £1100–1200. A cull cow is worth £700–800.

The objectives of replacement rearing should be to increase the genetic merit of the herd, and rear heifers with the potential for a high lifetime productivity cost-effectively. In order to achieve these goals, health care and growth rates are important.

Auditing the farm to establish the current practices and performance is the starting point for all further investigations and consultations. This may reveal that insufficient records are kept,

Bovine Medicine, Third Edition. Edited by Peter D. Cockcroft.

or that the records are inaccurate. The concept of 'measure, manage and monitor' is applicable to heifer rearing.

Establishing the herd size, the number of replacements on farm, the cow culling rates, young stock mortality rates and culling rates, age and body size at first calving, retention rates to second calving, calving to conception interval of the first calving heifers, and cost of rearing replacements, is an important first step. The current values of the key performance indicators can then be compared with appropriate target values for the production system under investigation. The farm's strategic plan and requirements need to be identified. Seasonal calving herds will need to synchronise the target heifer calving dates with the cows – ideally with the heifers calving before the main herd, to enable the first calving heifers to conceive well within the established breeding season.

Heifer rearing in autumn calving herds in the northern hemisphere allows greater nutritional control over the pre-pubertal period, and two-year calving dates are more easily achieved. Spring calving herds may need to house their weaned heifer calves to achieve the desired weight gains required in the pre-pubertal period, although supplementary feeding at grass is also used. Analysis of the mean age at calving and the distribution of calving ages will provide some important insight into the current performance. In addition, the culling rate of the heifers up to second calving may be a revealing parameter.

Nutrition and growth rate targets

Rearing heifers is relatively expensive, and there is a substantial economic advantage if heifers calve down at two years of age. The growth rates need to be managed carefully to ensure that productivity and fertility are optimised to achieve the goal of two year calving. For example, Holstein-Frisian heifers will need to attain an average growth rate of 0.7 kg/day from birth to caving if they are going to achieve a post-calving weight of between 550–600 kg.

There are substantial differences in the mature body weight and withers height of different breeds, and appropriate withers weight and height for age charts need to be used. Alternatively, using charts which indicate the height or weight as a percentage of the mature values for these parameters have more universal application. Table 37.1 indicates target weights as a percentage of mature body weight. Mature body weight is attained by the third lactation, and members of the herd which have attained their third lactation can be used to establish this value, provided they are at body condition score 3.0 (1–5 scale). Care is required to distinguish between growth rates from weight gain by fattening rather than growth. Growth rates vary with time, rising to a maximum at puberty, then slowing down thereafter.

Puberty in heifers is a function of weight, rather than size, with puberty occurring at approximately 40% of mature body weight which, in well-fed heifers, usually occurs between 10 and 12 months old. In Holsteins, this occurs at weight of 270–300 kg. There is some controversy in the literature about high growth rates in the pre-pubertal period and the replacement of mammary gland milk-producing tissue with fat, resulting in reduction in lactational yield. Growth rates up to 0.85 kg/day seem to have no impact, in contrast to earlier advice regarding limiting the growth rates in this period to 0.7–0.8 kg/day. Higher growth rates in the 3–10 months pre-pubertal period have been shown to reduce subsequent lactation yields. Heavier heifers have higher first lactation yields, but the incremental gains are reduced above 570 kg (Keown and Everett, 1986). For example, a Holstein heifer weighing 590 kg post-calving will give 600 kg more milk in the first lactation than a heifer weighing 430 kg.

Table 37.1 Heifer growth targets (adapted from DairyCo 2005).

Age	Percentage of mature body weight (%)
6 months	30
9 months	40
Mating (15–16 months)	55–60
Immediately pre-calving	90
Immediately post-calving	85
Second calving	92

In order to attain conception by 16 months old, growth needs to be sufficient to allow puberty, and 2–3 cycles before the proposed mating. Fertility increases successively up to the third oestrus cycle.

Heifer growth can be measured in different ways, but height at the withers is a useful parameter, and easy to measure using measuring sticks. Breed-specific growth charts provide target height for age values, and should be used to monitor the progress of the rearing system. Measurement at six months old is pivotal to allow for corrective feeding for under-developed heifers to attain puberty by 12 months of age. Periodic weighing with intervals of 4–8 weeks is desirable. Table 37.2 gives heifer rearing targets for Holstein, Friesian and Jersey heifers.

Condition score is also important, as over-fat heifers have an increased incidence of dystocia and a condition score of 2.5–3.0 (scale 1 (thin) to 5 (fat)) is desirable. Table 37.3 indicates target condition scores and withers height in Friesians and Holsteins at service and calving There is a danger of over-conditioning in the last two months of pregnancy, and restriction of growth to 0.65 kg/day may be desirable. There is increased risk from udder oedema if the heifers calve on a diet high in protein, high in potash or on high-silage diets. To ensure adaptation of the rumen flora and rumen mucosa to the post-calving diet, a

Table 37.2 Heifer rearing targets for Holstein, Friesian and Jersey heifers (adapted from DairyCo 2005).

Age (months)	Holstein		Friesian		Jersey	
	Weight (kg)	Withers height (cm)	Weight (kg)	Withers height (cm)	Weight (kg)	Withers height (cm)
2	76	87	72	84	55	78
3	110	93	100	88	75	82
4	127	96	120	93	95	89
6	180	104	162	100	130	94
12	340	124	285	118	220	109
15 (mating)	420	129	350	122	265	114
16	440	131	370	126	280	117
18	490	133	405	130	305	119
21	545	137	470	132	355	120
22	586	138	490	133	362	121
24 (pre-calving)	636	140	535	134	395	122
24 (post-calving)	568	140	485	134	350	122

Table 37.3 Target conditions scores and withers height at service and calving.

Breed/type	Condition score		Height at withers (cm)	
	Service	Calving	Service	Calving
Friesian	2.0–2.5	2.5–3.0	120	130
Holstein	2.5–3.0	3.0–3.5	126	140

similar diet with an appropriate mineral composition should be introduced three weeks before calving.

Major diseases and health care programmes

In the UK, autumn-born growing heifers will have alternating periods of housing and grazing at pasture. In warmer climates, heifers may spend their entire growing period out of doors. The risk factors associated with specific diseases will, therefore, differ between localities and climates. Many of the diseases will be covered in detail in Chapter 54. Table 37.5 indicates the major diseases of concern in dairy heifers.

Vaccination and disease prevention

Vaccination is important in the prevention of disease in heifers. In addition, the strategic use of anthelmintics, ectoprasiticides, mineral and vitamin supplements (copper, cobalt, selenium, iodine, zinc) is important. Infectious kerato-conjunctivitis can be a particular concern in the fly season in certain areas, and insecticidal 'pour ons' and/or ear tags may be a wise prophylactic strategy.

Not all the vaccines listed are available in all countries, but consideration should be given to the risk, cost benefit and timing of the vaccination, to ensure that appropriate protection is provided. The vaccines include: BVD, PI3, IBR, RSV, Leptospirosis, *Mannheimia haemolytica*, Vibriosis (*Campylobacter fetus venerialis*), Trichmonosis, Bluetongue, Smollenberg, Salmonella (Typhimurium and Dublin), Clostridial diseases, Rota/corona, *E. coli*, Infectious kerato-conjunctivitis (New Forest Eye), Louping ill, Babesia (exotic), Anaplasma (exotic), Heart water (exotic) and Ephemeral fever (exotic).

Endoparasites

The risk of endoparasite infections should be considered – in particular, liver fluke *(Faciola hepatica*), lungworm (*Dictylocaulus viviparous*) and parasitic gastroenteritis (which includes *Ostertagia ostertagia* Type I and Type II).

With regards to parasitic gastroenteritis, strategic use of clean pastures may obviate the need for anthelmintic usage, but may result in a group of susceptible heifers the following season. Confining treatment to the first season at grass, and applying the principles of Control of Worms Sustainably (COWS) (Taylor, 2010) to minimise the development of anthelmintic resistance, is now being recommended. This approach includes: administering the anthelmintic effectively by ensuring the correct dosage is delivered effectively; using anthelmintic only when necessary following monitoring of faecal egg counts; using appropriate single narrow spectrum products where possible, and avoiding combination products; rotating the class of anthelmintic used; and preserving susceptible worms on the pasture by not treating adults cows or a small percentage of the healthy heifers.

The presence of liver fluke on the farm may be known, or a risk assessment can be performed. This may include active surveillance using strategic faecal egg counts, serological ELISA tests, post-mortem results or abattoir feedback. A control plan should be formulated if the risk is significant. Treatment with an effective larval flukicide at housing may be required.

Parasitic bronchitis, caused by the lungworm *Dictylocaulus viviparous*, is a common and important disease. Outbreaks usually occur towards the end of the first season at grass, although it may occur in older susceptible animals, and continued immunity requires repeated exposure. There is an effective vaccine which is commonly used in animals at risk. Alternatively timely and appropriate anthelmintic treatment is required.

Ectoparasites

Lice is a common problem in closely confined animals, and strategic treatment at housing of all the animals that will be confined together should be considered.

Breeding programmes

If a bull is being used, a fertility check prior to the breeding season to ensure potency is a wise precaution. The selection of an easy calving bull is advisable. Rotating bulls is desirable, if possible. Oestrus synchronisation can be achieved using prostaglandin injections – two injections 11 days apart, followed by a timed AI. Alternatively, intra-uterine progesterone devices are effective and are sometimes used in combination with prostaglandins.

Oestrus manipulation/synchronisation programmes enable AI to be used, with the advantages of allowing the selection of a bull with the required genetic merit and ease of calving.

Breeding should begin at 14–15 months, to ensure calving at about 24 months of age. The heifers should have attained 55–60% of their mature body weight. No major dietary changes should occur in the 4–6 weeks after mating, and weight gain should continue to avoid stress, which may cause embryonic losses. Protocols which involve handling or painful procedures should be avoided during this period. If the heifers are to be housed during the breeding period, it is best to house them six weeks prior to breeding, as the first oestrus after housing is often suppressed.

The transitional period: entering the dairy herd

There are many transitions that occur around calving for the heifer. During the rearing phase, the heifer will have been kept in a stable social group at pasture, or in bedded housing. There will have been little or no competition for food, and lying times would go undisturbed. This all suddenly changes as calving approaches. The post-calving diet will be introduced, and the heifer will go through the stress of calving for the first time. The heifers will then join the lactating herd, and will have multiple social interactions with the more dominant cows. The heifer may be housed on concrete for the first time, with unfamiliar cubicles. Her udder will be large and heavy, which may affect her gait. There is often competition for food and cubicle space, with disturbed lying times and frequent chasing. Twice a day, she will go through the milking parlour, with all the unfamiliar noises and procedures associated with the process.

The transitional period therefore needs careful management to ensure that lactation losses are minimised and fertility is maximised. Heifers being in competition with cows during this period can result in reduced food intake, excessive weight loss, reduced lactation yield and delayed conception. Lameness is also common amongst first calving heifers. The risk of heifer oedema should be minimised by diet management, and calving boxes should be clean, to minimise the risk of udder infections and the spread of Johne's disease to the calf in infected herds.

Ideally, the heifers would be kept in a separate heifer group until six weeks in calf. This may not be realistic in many herds. Introducing the pre-calving heifers to training cubicles and concrete floors, and putting the heifers through the milking parlour, can be beneficial. Ensuring unrestricted access to TMR rations or silage feeding is helpful in maintaining intake and reducing adverse weight loss. Cubicle numbers should be adequate to allow the newly joined lactating heifers to find sanctuary. Escape routes should be available within the row of cubicles. The introduction of the heifer to the lactating group should be delayed for 4–5 days post-calving, and then timed to occur at the end of the day, when the cows are less active.

Heifer rearing audit

The audit should reveal how the management and current protocols compare to best practice, and how the current performance compares to realistic target values for the key performance indicators (Table 37.4). Strengths and weaknesses in the management and protocols can then be identified. The cost

Table 37.4 Heifer key performance indicators and target values (adapted from Brand *et al*., 1996).

Key performance indicator	Target value
Age at first calving	≤24 months
Body weight post-calving	570 kg
Wither height post-calving	142 cm
% abortion in heifers	<4%
Mortality 3–24 months	<1%
Body weight gain 3–10 months	800g/day
Age at conception (months)	≤15 months
Conception rate first service	70%
Inseminations/pregnancy	1.3
% dystocias in heifers	<5%
Body condition score at calving	3.0–3.5

Table 37.5 Important conditions in dairy heifers.

Condition	Risk factors	Control and prevention	Monitoring
Abortion	Various.	Various.	Analysis of records.
Babesiosis (tick areas only)	Tick area.	Imidocarb. Tick control. Vaccinate.	Blood smear.
Blue tongue	Exposure to infected culicoides.	Vaccinate prior to pregnancy.	Serology if not vaccinated.
Bovine tuberculosis	Direct or indirect contact with infected badgers and cattle.	Testing. Manage badger interface.	Testing. Biosecurity.
Bovine viral diarrhoea	Persistently infected individuals in herd.	Indentify PIs and remove. Vaccinate heifers before breeding. Screen introduced animals.	Bulk milk.
Calcium, phosphorous and vitamin D deficiency	Dietary deficiency.		
Cocciodiosis	High stocking density. Contact with infected faeces. Housing or at grass.	Anti-coccidial drugs. Reduce environmental contamination. Destock.	Faecal sampling Faecal oocyte speciation
Copper deficiency	Dietary deficiency.	Supplement.	Blood levels
Dystocia	High condition score at calving. Narrow pelvic. Low calving weight.	Measure and manage condition and growth.	Records
Infectious bovine keratitis (*Moraxella bovis*)	Flies.	Prompt treatment.	Close daily observation
Iodine deficiency	Dietary deficiency.	Supplement.	Blood levels
Johnes disease	Endemic in herd.	Minimise risk of calf infection.	Biosecurity
Leptospirosis	Direct or indirect contact with infected cattle or sheep.	Vaccinate.	Serology if unvaccinated
Lice	Close contact housing.	Prophylactic treatment at housing. Monitor.	Clinical examination Pruritus
Liver fluke	Contaminated pastures.	Strategic treatment with flukicide.	Faecal oocyte analysis Post-mortem Abattoir report ELISA
Louping ill (Tick areas only)	Tick area.	Vaccinate.	Serology
Not pregnant	Free martin. Underweight. Infertile bull. Poor AI technique.	Pre-breeding check of heifers and bull. Ensure target weight. House six weeks before breeding.	Early pregnancy diagnosis post-breeding
Ostertagia type II	Hypo biotic larvae present (winter).	Effective anthelmintic at housing.	Pepsinogen levels
Over-conditioning	Over-feeding. Unbalanced diet.	Diet analysis. Corrective dietary management.	Condition score every two months
Parasitic gastroenteritis	Contaminated pastures.	Anthelmintics. Grazing management.	Faecal egg count
Poor growth rates	Under-feeding. Dietary deficiency. Disease.	Monitor. Diet analysis. Health monitoring.	Measure height and weight every two months

(continued overleaf)

Table 37.5 (*continued*)

Condition	Risk factors	Control and prevention	Monitoring
Respiratory disease (bacterial/mycoplasma/viral) IBR (BVD) PI3 RSV *Mannheimia haemolytica* *Histophilus somni*	Housing. Mixing. Stress. Poor ventilation. High humidity. Stocking density.	Vaccinate. Management. Improve ventilation. Reduce stocking density.	Check housing Review incidence Serological screen Post-mortem
Ringworm (*Trichphyton verrucosum*)	Close contact. Housing.	Vaccinate. Turnout. Treat.	Observation
Salmonellosis	Endemic. Brought-in animals.	Vaccination. Hygiene. Antibiotics.	Faecal swabs Serology Biosecurity
Schmallenberg	Exposure to infected culicoides.	Vaccinate prior to pregnancy.	Serology is not vaccinated
Summer mastitis	At grass. High fly population.		Close daily observation
Tick infestation	Tick area.	Tick control.	Observation
Tick-borne fever (*Cytoectes phagocytophilia*) (Tick areas only)	Tick area.	Tetracyclines.	Blood smear
Udder oedema	High cation-anion balance. High protein levels.	Modify diet in the transition period.	Appropriate transitional diet
Vitamin E/selenium deficiency (white muscle disease)	Dietary deficiency.	Supplement.	Blood levels
Warts on the teats	Flies. Presence in herd.	Fly-repellent impregnated ear tags.	Observation

Table 37.6 Heifer rearing audit template.

Housing
- Are the heifers housed during the winter period?
- Are the heifers mixed with older cows or share the same air space during the housing period?
- What is the stocking density and the airspace allowance?
- What is the trough space allowance?
- Is there adequate ventilation?

Growth rates
- Do you weigh and/or measure the height at the withers of your growing heifers?
- How frequently and at what ages do you perform this?
- Where do you record this information?
- How frequently do you analyse the growth rates?
- What target values do you compare the growth rates to?
- What are the weights of the current replacement heifers at:
  - 6 months
  - 9 months
  - Mating (15–16 months)
  - Immediately pre-calving
  - Immediately post-calving
  - At second calving
- What is your target age and weight for breeding?
- What was the age and weight of the first calving heifers at breeding in the last 12 months?

Endoparasites (Tx and monitoring)

Parasitic gastroenteritis
- What is your endoparasite control programme at grass?
- Do you routinely use anthelmintics?
- Do you perform faecal egg counts?
- Do you perform fecal egg reduction tests?
- Do you vaccinate for lung worm?
- Do you use anthelmintics at housing?

Lungworm
- Has lungworm been diagnosed on your farm
- When do you vaccinate for lungworm?
- Do you strategically use anthelmintics to control lungworm?

Liver fluke
- Have you a liver fluke problem on your farm?
- Do you routinely check for liver fluke infestation?
- What is your liver fluke control programme?
- Do your treat your heifers at housing in autumn?

Ectoparasites
- Do you have a problem with lice during the housing period?
- Do you routinely treat all the animals to be housed together during the housing period?
- Do you have a major fly problem?
- Do you have a problem of summer mastitis and/or infectious bovine keratitis (New Forest disease)?

Table 37.6 (*continued*)

Condition scoring?
- Do you condition score your growing heifers?
- At what ages do you condition score them?
- Where do you record this information?
- How frequently do you analyse this information?
- What are the condition scores of your current replacement heifers at:
  - six months old
  - two months pre-service
  - service
  - two months pre-calving
  - At calving

Age at calving
- What were the ages at first calving of the replacement heifers in the last 12 months?
- What was the calving-to-calving interval of the replacement second calving heifers in the last 12 months?

Breeding
- Do you use an oestrus synchronisation as part of your breeding programme?
- What is you oestrus synchronisation programme, and does it included a timed AI?
- Do you use AI?
- Who performs the AI?
- Do you use sexed semen?
- How do you select your semen for your heifers?
- Do you select semen from a bull with an easy calving EBV?
- Do you use a bull in your breeding programme?
- What is the breed of the bull, and has he an easy calving index?
- What has been the age, weight and withers height of the heifers at the point of breeding in the last 12 months?
- When is pregnancy diagnosis performed?
- Who performs the pregnancy diagnosis?
- Is the pregnancy diagnosis performed by manual palpation or ultrasonography?
- What is your 6 week in-calf rate?

Supplements
- Do you have the following deficiencies:
  - Copper
  - Iodine
  - Selenium
  - Vitamin E
- Have growing heifers ever been tested for the above deficiencies?
- Do you provide a mineral and vitamin supplement? If so, what?

Health
- What are your heifer mortality rates during the following periods?
  - weaning to mating
  - mating to first calving
- Do you keep records of disease outbreaks in you heifers?
- Which disease have you recognised in the last five years (reference to table)
- Do you routinely implement any preventative procedures for any specific diseases, excluding vaccinations?

Vaccinations
Which of the following vaccines do you use in your heifers?
- BVD
- PI3
- IBR
- RSV
- Leptospirosis
- Mannhaemia heamolytica
- Vibriosis (*Campylobacter fetus venerialis*)
- Bluetongue
- Smollenberg
- Salmonella (Typhimurium and Dublin)
- Clostridial diseases
- Rota/corona
- *E. coli*
- Louping ill
- Trichmonosis
- Infectious kerato-conjunctivitis (New Forest Eye)
- Babesia (exotic)
- Anaplasma (exotic)
- Heart water (exotic)
- Ephemeral fever (exotic)

What protocols are used?

benefit of prioritised changes can be computed and agreed with the farmer. Following the implementation of the action plan, improvements to the management and performance can be monitored. An audit template for rearing heifers is presented in Table 37.6.

In summary, the key points for successful heifer rearing are:

1 Adopt a *measure, manage and monitor* approach to the rearing of replacement heifers.
2 Monitor the *growth rates* of the heifers from weaning to calving by regular weighing, condition scoring, and measuring the height of the withers to ensure that recommended targets are met.
3 Plan the *breeding program* carefully, with careful selection of the bull for genetic improvement and easy calving. Check the six week pregnancy rate.
4 Manage the heifers for *longevity* by reducing the competition with older cows for space, dominance and access to food.
5 *Condition the pre-calving heifer* to the post-calving diet, concrete surfaces, cubicles and the milking parlour.
6 Keep *accurate records* on heifer health and performance from birth.
7 Adopt a *strategic approach to endoparasite control* that minimises the development of anthelmintic resistance and risk of disease.

8 Be aware of the *common and important diseases* that can impact adversely on heifer health and welfare and implement appropriate monitoring, preventative and control measures.

References and further reading

Breen, J., Down, P., Kerby, M. and Bradley, A. (2012). Chapter 3, Restoring the Dairy Herd. In: Green, M. (ed). *Rearing Young Stock and Replacing Cows in Dairy Herd Health*, pp. 35–67. CABI, Wallingford, UK.

Blowey, R.W (2000). Chapter 2, Rearing the Dairy Heifer. In: Andrews, A.H. (ed). *The Health of Dairy Cattle*, pp. 15–48. Blackwell Science Ltd, Oxford.

Brand, A., Noordhuizen, J.P.T.M. and Schukken, Y.H. (1996). Chapter 2, Monitoring replacement rearing. In: *Herd Health and Production Management in Dairy Practice*, pp 75-168, Wangeningen Pers, The Netherlands.

Boersema, J., Cannas da Silva, J., Mee, J. and Noordhuizen, J. (2010). *Farm Health and productivity management of dairy young stock*. Wageningen Academic Publishers, The Netherlands.

Keown, J.F. and Everett, R.W. (1986). Effect of days carried calf, days dry, and weight of first calf heifers on yield. *Journal of Dairy Science* **69**(7), 1891–6.

Taylor, M.A. (2010). *Control of Cows Worms Sustainably: A Technical Manual for Veterinary Surgeons and Advisors*. Agriculture and Horticulture Development, Kenilworth, UK.

CHAPTER 38

The Farm Audit: Health and Management of the Transition Cow

Ian J. Lean and Peter J. DeGaris

Learning objectives

- Perform an audit of the health and management of the transition cow.
- Identify and provide corrective advice for disorders of lipid metabolism.
- Identify and provide corrective advice for disorders of rumen health.
- Identify and provide corrective advice for disorders of macro-mineral metabolism.
- Identify and provide corrective advice for disorders associated with periparturient immune suppression.

Introduction

There is now an overwhelming body of evidence showing that the management of the transition period is pivotal to the successful management of dairy cattle. The intention of this chapter is to identify key performance indices and to provide suggested diagnostic aids and responses. A critical position in regards to these is that:

- a single static measures of metabolism such as blood metabolites provide, at best, measures that have only moderate diagnostic value;
- one needs to be extremely cautious in extrapolating to the whole herd from limited measures on animals presented for disease, or from very limited sample sizes of not to the population; consequently, the most critical measures are those of production and disease and monitoring these is vital;
- regular and repeated monitoring, often with the veterinarian acting as the external monitor for the herd, is more effective than occasional visits;
- monitoring that only evaluates the sick herd is not effective monitoring, an evaluation can easily be biased by a failure to evaluate whole population (e.g. body condition scores or ketone measures based on sick cows will likely be misleading for the population) (Tyler & Cullor, 1989).

These guidelines will provide assistance in the practical application of the principles outlined in Chapter 44 to manage reproductive performance, because transition nutrition can profoundly influence fertility (DeGaris *et al.*, 2010b (erratum)).

It is also important to note that monitoring disease is much more effective in larger herds, because many of the disorders are relatively rare, and the confidence intervals around changes in incidence are very large for small herds. However, when control measures are effective, the expectation of a low incidence rate can be used to advantage. Simply, the alarm threshold for discussion of some of the disorders can be set low – very low – and cases of disorder are a prompt to review management.

Step 1 Define achievable targets

Defining achievable targets for performance is the most important or essential step in establishing an audit. The targets for common peri-parturient disorders presented in Table 38.1 were established by Lean & DeGaris (2011), based on data from Morton (2004), Curtis (1997), Beckett (1997), Moss (2001) and Stevenson (1995).

Step 2 Understanding the pathogenesis

Lean *et al.* (2003) established a series of understandings of the metabolic conditions that influence the risks of many of the disorders identified in Table 38.1. These understandings are highlighted in Table 38.2.

Step 3 Provide an integrated approach to managing key risks based on the following areas:

1 Disorders of lipid metabolism
2 Rumen disruption
3 Macro-mineral disorders
4 Peri-parturient immunosuppression.

Bovine Medicine, Third Edition. Edited by Peter D. Cockcroft.

Table 38.1 Health Performance Indicators (expressed as percentage of cases of calving cows within 14 days of calving).

Indicator	Target performance	Alarm level
Milk fever	1% (old cows > 5 yrs 2%)	3%
Clinical ketosis	<1%	2%
Pregnancy toxaemia	0%	1 case
Abomasal displacements (left or right)	<1%	2%
Mastitis	1.8 cases/100 cows/ 30 days	2.5 cases/ 100cows/30 days
Lameness (Sprecher scale 1–5)	<2% > score 2	>4% > Score 2
Hypomagnesaemia	0%	1 case
Retained placenta > 12 hrs after calving	<3%	>6%
Metritis % infected after 21 days	<5%	>10%
Calving difficulty	<2%	>3%
Clinical acidosis	0%	1%

Table 38.2 Establishing four freedoms: the goals of transition are to avoid the conditions outlined in this table.

Condition	Detail
Disorders of lipid metabolism	Includes ketosis, fatty liver and pregnancy toxaemia – diseases that are largely influenced by a failure to provide sufficient or effective energy sources around calving.
Ruminal health	Cows are very vulnerable to grain overload resulting from higher energy intake and rapid introduction of grains. Sub-acute ruminal acidosis is common in dairy cows worldwide.
Macro-mineral deficiency	Mainly refers to calcium, magnesium and phosphorus. Milk fever and grass tetany (hypomagnesaemia) can result from a conditioned deficiency, where excess potassium reduces the capacity of the cow to maintain stable blood concentrations of calcium and magnesium.
Periparturient immunosuppression	Often associated with lack of energy or protein intake – micronutrients are often involved, including copper, selenium, zinc, vitamin E and vitamin D.

Disorders of lipid metabolism

A pivotal goal of managing the transition period is to maintain appetite. Inappetence will predispose to a large number of conditions including ketosis, hepatic lipidosis, pregnancy toxaemia and abomasal displacement. Be particularly alert to feeds that can disrupt rumen function, such as spoiled silages and hays. Note that acidosis and hypokalaemia, addressed below, can also cause inappetence, resulting in lipid mobilisation disorders. The following are useful in troubleshooting diseases that may result from disorders of lipid metabolism.

1 **Body Condition Score (BCS)**
  a. *Time to measure*: Peak lactation, day 150 of lactation, drying off and calving.
  b. *Trigger for action*: BCS > 3.5 (scale 1–5) (cows over-conditioned) or BCS < 3.25 (scale 1–5) (cows under-conditioned).
  c. *Impacts*: Cows that are too fat are at increased risk of excessive lipid mobilisation and inappetence, leading to a negative nutrient balance (NNB) as well as an increased risk of milk fever around calving. Cows that are too thin are slow to return to oestrus, and are at risk of poor reproductive performance.
  d. *Actions*: Cows too fat – change diets to ensure less lipid accumulation and avoid cows becoming over-fat, particularly in late lactation (most commonly, increase metabolisable protein by manipulating protein and energy components in the diet). Cows too thin – increase energy density of diet or more commonly increase dry matter (DM) availability. Ensure abundant feed in three weeks before calving and a positive energy and protein balance.

2 **Milk fat content and milk fat to protein ratio**
  a. *Time to measure*: In first two weeks after calving (most cows reduce mobilisation and dilute milk fat and protein content after this).
  b. *Trigger for action*: A high prevalence (20 % of eligible cows) of milk fat content > 4.75% for Holsteins, > 6.60% for Jerseys. A milk fat-to-protein ratio of > 1.5.
  c. *Impacts*: Cows mobilising excessive tissue have very high milk fat content, which is suggestive of inappetence. A high incidence of high milk fat-to-protein ratios may indicate either under nutrition or over-conditioning.
  d. *Actions*: Evaluate diet: i) is feed sufficiently available? May need to offer more feed and/or increase feed access; ii) is the energy density and non-fibre carbohydrate (NFC) concentration sufficient (36–38% of DM)? If energy density is low, but NFC ideal, consider using fats rather than concentrates to increase energy density to avoid acidosis (note: the total intake of dietary long chain fatty acids should not exceed the milk output).

3 **Milk protein content**
  a. *Time to measure*: Peak lactation (50–90 days).
  b. *Trigger for action*: High prevalence (20% of eligible cows) of milk protein content <2.9% for Holstein and <3.3% for Jerseys.
  c. *Impacts*: Low milk protein content is suggestive of a lack of dietary energy density. Cows are at risk of excessive mobilisation of body fat.

   d. *Actions*: Increase the energy and protein content of the diet to ensure adequate Metabolisable protein (MP) for production. Ensure adequate concentration of minerals involved in energy metabolism (e.g. cobalt and phosphorus).

4 **Monitor energy and protein content of transition diet**
   a. *Time to measure*: Test dietary feed components prior to commencing transition period and prior to any changes in diet ingredients occurring during transition period.
   b. *Trigger for action*: Any case of pregnancy toxaemia is a critical trigger for a full review of the transition diet and management. Excessive or rapid changes in BCS around calving. Blood NEFA > 0.400 mEq/l in 10% of cows in last two weeks of gestation (minimum sample size is 12 cows) (Oetzel, 2004).
   c. *Impacts*: NNB pre-calving will promote loss of body condition and increase the risk of hepatic lipidosis and pregnancy toxaemia.
   d. *Actions*: Aim for CP of 14–16%, NFC of ≤ 32%, NDF of > 36%, with a neutral or slightly positive MP and ME balance. In many cases, feed availability or access is the key limiting factor.

5 **Monitor energy and protein content of lactating diet**
   a. *Time to measure*: Analyse all feeds regularly during lactation, particularly with any change in feed. Particular attention needs to be paid to the early lactation diet.
   b. *Trigger for action*: Lower than expected production, excess or rapid changes in BCS. Blood BHB > 1000 μmol/L in 10 % of cows tested in first 30 days of lactation (minimum sample size of 12 cows). Note: assessed using the kinetic assay – the threshold is test specific (Rabiee *et al.*, in press).
   c. *Impacts*: NNB during lactation will impact on production and promote excess or rapid changes in BCS.
   d. *Actions*: Aim for CP of 16–18 %, NFC of 36–38 %, NDF of 32–34 % and a ME density of 11–12.5 MJ/kg DM. These are very rough rules of thumb. If the diet analyses are within guidelines, check for problems associated with feed availability (e.g. bunk access, grazing management).

6 **Monitor feeds for organoleptic defects (e.g. spoilage)**
   a. *Time to measure*: Every farm visit.
   b. *Trigger for action*: Suspicion of spoiled/contaminated feed.
   c. *Impacts*: Feed refusal, reduced production, loss of BCS, toxicities.
   d. *Actions*: Removal from ration. This may be achieved by avoiding spoiled areas in the silage or by excluding poor hays. Ultimately, facility design, hay storage and better harvest, management of silage to exclude oxygen, treatment of silages with inoculants and/or organic acids will help reduce spoilage. Particular care is needed if feeding by-products that may spoil quickly, especially in warm weather.

Rumen health

The diagnosis of ruminal (sub-acute/acute) acidosis is simpler at the herd level than at the individual cow level. A good indication of acidosis is a high simultaneous prevalence of scouring (especially bubbling and grain in the faeces), low milk fat, low pH in rumens tested (15% < 6.0 on ruminocentesis or < 6.5 stomach tube tested 2–4 hours after feeding) and, critically, diets > 38% NFC and < 19% physically effective neutral detergent fibre (peNDF).

Ensure that, if the diet appears valid, feeding systems enable good access to the feed for the group. Inconsistent feeding of a diet that appears valid on paper can easily result in outbreaks of acidosis. The condition acts as a continuum of risk associated with the need to dispose of hydrogen ions generated by fermentation. To a large degree, the artificial categories and misnomers used to describe the condition are a distraction for clinicians. The focus should be on identifying risk of disease caused by feeding highly fermentable diets.

1 **Scouring**
   a. *Time to measure*: Any time, but especially in the first 30 days of lactation. Stomach tube determination of rumen function should be part of any routine animal health monitoring program. The larger volume of fluid, speed of sampling and non-invasive technique makes this preferable to ruminocentesis. Visual and touch assessment should be used to exclude samples containing saliva.
   b. *Trigger for action*: High percentage of cows scouring (>20 %) – particularly sweet/sour-smelling faeces, with bubbling and undigested grain and or fibre. Moderate prevalence of scouring in conjunction with low rumen pH (<6.5 stomach tube or <6.0 ruminocentesis) in 25% of tested cows (a minimum of 12 cows from the group of interest – e.g. fresh cows <30 days in milk) (Golder *et al.*, 2012). More than 1% of milking cows with clinical acidosis.
   c. *Impacts*: May be relatively *minor* with moderate conditions, but likely predisposes cows to other health problems, and is likely reducing fat and protein yields. Note that herds with mild forms often have good milk yields.
   d. *Actions*: Differential diagnosis should include parasitism and enteric disorders (although these can co-exist and may mutually predispose). Evaluate fibre in the ration (greater than 19% peNDF) and control NFC (<38% of DM). Evaluate management for inconsistent feeding practices and 'extra' feed allocations (e.g. grain in the milking parlour).

2 **Lameness**
   a. *Time to measure*: Anytime.
   b. *Trigger for action*: High prevalence of lameness (>15 % of cows with a Sprecher lameness score > 2) (Sprecher *et al.*, 1997), with pathology consistent with acidosis-induced laminitis (hot swollen coronary bands, poverty lines, solar

paint brush haemorrhages, soft yellow waxy soles, white line disease). Note that, with the exception of swelling and inflammation of the coronary band, all the above indicators of laminitis and acidosis are chronic changes, often occurring months after the initial insult. It is important to note that not all pathologies of the hoof are necessarily associated with an increased lameness score, and acidosis is only one of many contributing factors to lameness.

c. *Impacts*: Economic losses associated with lameness are extensive through decreased DM intake (up to 16%), decreased milk production (up to 36%), increased culling, poor reproduction (15% increase in risk of not conceiving), high treatment and labour costs.

d. *Actions*: Evaluate herd for non-dietary risk factors (poor free stall design, overcrowding, poor track design and maintenance, human-cow interaction etc). If lameness is due to acidosis, review diet as above.

3 **Milk fat content and milk fat to protein ratio**

a. *Time to measure*: Any time. but especially in fresh cows. Bulk tank samples are often useful throughout lactation.

b. *Trigger for action*: Milk fat to protein ratio < 1.02. Note that fat to protein ratio has a poor sensitivity (0.54) for acidosis but a moderate specificity (0.81) (Golder *et al.*, 2012). Consequently, acidotic herds may have a fat to protein ratio above 1.02.

c. *Impacts*: Loss of income from reduced milk fat yields.

d. *Actions*: Rule out other causes of milk fat depression, such as high dietary intake of polyunsaturated C18:3 and C18:2 fats, that may increase the risk of conjugated linoleic acid formation. Review diet as above to limit risk of acidosis.

4 **Milk protein content**

a. *Time to measure*: Peak lactation (50–90 days).

b. *Trigger for action*: High prevalence (20% of eligible cows) of milk protein content < 2.9% for Holstein and < 3.3% for Jerseys.

c. *Impacts*: Low milk protein content is suggestive of a lack of dietary energy density. Milk protein may drop dramatically in acidotic cows and herds.

d. *Actions*: Review diet as above to limit risk of acidosis. Evaluate management of herd, with particular emphasis on key feeding risk areas such as adequate access to feed, poor presentation of feeds, including over-mixing (TMR), adverse social interaction, particularly with cows and heifers being mixed, and release cows to pasture before heifers and overcrowding (>105% cows to headlocks).

5 **Monitor energy and protein content of transition diet**

a. *Time to measure*: Feed test dietary components prior to commencing transition period, and if any changes in diet ingredients occur during transition period.

b. *Trigger for action*: Diagnosis of ruminal acidosis in fresh cows (up to 30 days in milk).

c. *Impacts*: May be profound with substantial disruption to DM intake, increased disease risk (e.g. ketosis, abomasal displacement, lameness). Increased risk of secondary culling.

d. *Actions*: Often due to inadequate adaptation of rumen to concentrates/lush forages during the transition period, and sudden introduction of such feeds in early lactation. Increase concentrates/lush forages in transition diet if planning to feed these in early lactation, but maintain NFC < 32% and peNDF > 24% to control the risk of acidosis in the transition period.

6 **Liver abscess, thrombo-embolic peneumonia (TEP), epistaxis**

a. *Time to measure*: Anytime – monitor incidence of liver abscess and TEP at slaughter to necropsy. Epistaxis often reported by farm personal.

b. *Trigger for action*: High incidence of any is a strong indication of historical ruminal acidosis.

c. *Impacts*: Substantial for individual cows, but difficult to assess on a herd basis unless significant numbers of individual animals are affected. In lot-fed beef cattle, severe liver abscessation has been shown to reduce DM intake and carcass weight at slaughter.

d. *Actions*: Review diet as above to limit risk of acidosis.

7 **Uncontrolled risk factors for ruminal acidosis**

a. *Time to measure*: Anytime.

b. *Trigger for action*: If there exist significant risk factors for acidosis that cannot be eliminated due to management constraints.

c. *Impacts*: Significant as acidosis will likely be endemic and ongoing.

d. *Actions*: Additional control of rumen fermentation is required, over and above dietary manipulation. This may include buffers (sodium bicarbonate, calcined seaweed), neutralising agents (NaOH, MgO), ionophores (monensin, lasalocid) and antibiotic rumen modifiers, where legal (tylosin, virginiamycin).

Macro-mineral disorders

Perhaps no condition exemplifies the need to think about integrated nutrition more than milk fever and the associated hypokalaemia. It is relatively easy to control milk fever, if cattle are significantly underfed before calving. Low energy and protein density diets reduce mammary development and milk production, but the consequences of this strategy are that risks of other disorders – especially lipid mobilisation disorders and reproductive failure – increase.

Monitoring is vital. While there is merit in measuring urine pH to identify whether strategies to lower dietary cation difference are effective, and monitoring blood calcium within 12–24 hours of calving to assess the incidence of sub-clinical hypokalaemia, it is far more important to analyse feeds and to assess the value of these, including macro-mineral values, in order to evaluate the adequacy of the diet. This emphasis is highlighted by the typical decrease in blood mineral concentrations around calving. Laboratory 'normal values' should be interpreted with care for samples obtained close to calving.

1 **Milk fever – after calving**
   a. *Time to measure*: Predominately within 48 hours of calving.
   b. *Trigger for action*: Milk fever incidence > 3% of calved animals (cows and heifers). Subclinical hypokalaemia may be monitored via blood calcium concentration 12 – 24 hours after calving. Total blood calcium < 1.8 mmol/L or ionised calcium < 0.9 mmol/L in > 20% of animals is cause for concern. Urine pH can be monitored in cows that have been exposed to the transition diet for at least three days, with a target of between 6.0 and 7.0 being appropriate (Oetzel, 2000). Note that the true incidence of milk fever or sub-clinical hypokalaemia may be masked by the routine treatment of all cows at calving with calcium products.
   c. *Impacts*: Milk fever and sub-clinical hypokalaemia are risk factors for many of the common diseases of early lactation, including displaced abomasum, RFM and metritis through decreased gastro-intestinal tract and uterine motility and possible negative impacts on immune function. Death and premature culling due to prolonged recumbency are not uncommon sequelae of milk fever.
   d. *Actions*: Laboratory analysis of feeds for mineral content using wet chemistry methods. Rules of thumb for formulate transition diet are DCAD < 0 mEq/kg of DM, calcium 0.4–0.6%, phosphorus < 0.4%, magnesium > 0.4%, potassium 1.1–1.6% and sodium 0.12% and sulphur < 0.4% of DM. Dietary chloride should be approximately 0.5% less than the potassium concentration. Check especially for feeds that can cause inappetence, especially spoiled silage. A high dietary protein (>18%) may increase the risk of milk fever. Check age of cattle calving – the risk of milk fever increases by 9% each calving.

2 **Milk fever – before calving**
   a. *Time to measure*: Constant monitoring.
   b. *Trigger for action*: Incidence > 1% before calving.
   c. *Impacts*: Probably low, as most cases are mild and readily respond to treatment. May indicate excessive exposure to low DCAD transition diet.
   d. *Actions*: Evaluate duration of exposure to low DCAD diet and aim for 21–28 days. Check for very low calcium concentration in transition diet and adequacy of calcium supplementation through lactation. Improve accuracy of calving date estimates through early pregnancy diagnosis. If cows are not on a low DCAD diet, investigate, as this may be a case of grossly inadequate calcium intake.

3 **Hypomagnesaemia**
   a. *Time to measure*: Constant monitoring, particularly during cold and wet weather and after a sudden drop in temperature.
   b. *Trigger for action*: Any cases require urgent review of diet.
   c. *Impacts*: Can be substantial, with high morbidity and mortality.
   d. *Actions*: Increase magnesium concentrations before and after calving. After calving > 0.2% of diet DM. Finely ground magnesium oxide is the source of choice. Check potassium and sodium concentration of diets – high potassium and low sodium are risk factors for hypomagnesaemia.

4 **Hypophosphataemia**
   a. *Time to measure*: Constant monitoring.
   b. *Trigger for action*: Any case requires urgent review of diet. Note that low blood phosphorus in a downer cow may be due to inappetence, and blood phosphorus also drops just after calving.
   c. *Impacts*: Minor. Hypophosphataemia is a rare disorder.
   d. *Actions*: Control phosphorus intake to between 0.2–0.4% of DM before calving. After calving, 0.4% of diet DM is a reasonable target.

5 **Hypokalaemia**
   a. *Time to measure*: Constant monitoring.
   b. *Trigger for action*: Any primary case requires review of diet and management of cows around calving.
   c. *Impacts*: Minor. Hypokalaemia is rare as a primary condition, and is associated with the use of long acting corticosteroids around calving, but it does have a high case mortality rate. Secondary cases are associated with enteric disorders.
   d. *Actions*: Review management of cows around calving – in particular, the use of corticosteroids in the treatment of ketosis. Ensure dietary potassium is not limiting.

6 **Hyponatraemia**
   a. *Time to measure*: Constant monitoring.
   b. *Trigger for action*: Any primary case requires review of diet.
   c. *Impacts*: Minor. Hyponatraemia is rare as a primary condition. Secondary cases are associated with enteric disorders.
   d. *Actions*: Ensure dietary sodium is not limiting (>0.12% of DM).

Periparturient immunosuppression

The immunological component is perhaps the most complex and least clear in terms of identifying the importance of a change in any particular component on animal health and production. There are some very clear effects of particular trace elements and vitamins, but the most important factors influencing immune competence are *the energy and protein nutrition of cattle*. Macro- and micro-nutrients also play a role in energy and protein metabolism that should not be ignored. In all cases of investigation below, ensure that the diet is adequate for DM intake, energy and protein content, as well as checking other nutrients.

1 **High incidence of retained foetal membranes (RFM)**
   a. *Time to measure*: 6–12 hours after calving. It is practical to measure at the first milkings after calving.
   b. *Trigger for action*: More than 6% RFM six hours after calving twelve hours.
   c. *Impacts*: Severe, morbidity, mortality (rare), health costs and reproductive failure.
   d. *Actions*: Check the energy and protein intake in the dry and transition period to ensure adequate energy and protein (see above). Check for milk fever incidence – if high, correct. Check for micro-nutrients, especially Se, Vitamin E, Vitamin A, beta-carotene. Review other micro-nutrient intake. Note that rates of RFM can increase under conditions of heat stress. Consider methods of reducing the impacts of climate on dry and transition cows.

2 **High incidence of metritis and endometritis**
   a. *Time to measure*: Constant monitoring.
   b. *Trigger for action*: Incidence > 10% of calving cows with purulent vaginal discharge at 14 days.
   c. *Impacts*: Metritis – can be severe, morbidity, mortality, health costs and reproductive failure; endometritis, similar, but unlikely to result in immediate mortality, but increased culling.
   d. *Actions*: Review calving environment for cleanliness. Avoid iatrogenic disease (e.g. insertion of hands into uterus in attempts to treat RFM). Corrective actions as per RFM.

3 **High incidence of clinical mastitis**
   a. *Time to measure*: Constant monitoring.
   b. *Trigger for action*: An incidence of more than 5 cows/100 cows in the first 30 days of lactation.
   c. *Impacts*: Can be substantial with very high morbidity and occasional mortality.
   d. *Actions*: Review milking machine function, actions of milkers, teat dipping and sanitation, check environmental conditions (i.e. where are cows lying and calving, check for specific organism involvement). Check especially Se, Vitamin E, Vitamin A, beta-carotene, zinc and copper. Review other micronutrient intakes.

4 **Increase other infectious disease – especially respiratory**
   a. *Time to measure*: Constant monitoring
   b. *Trigger for action*: A threefold increase in underlying incidence within a month.
   c. *Impacts*: These can be severe, but usually mild.
   d. *Actions*: Consider epidemiology of the outbreak and specific pathogens. Check for immunosuppressive disorders (e.g. Pestivirus and Herpes viruses). Also check for acidosis. Review micronutrient status. See review for beef cattle (Duff & Galyean, 2007).

5 **Poor calf survival**
   a. *Time to measure*: Constant monitoring, breakdown measures into immediate, < 2 weeks, 2–6 weeks and greater
   b. *Trigger for action*: Any primary case requires review of diet and management of cows around calving.
   c. *Impacts*: Immediate losses with slow calving. Later, check colostral transfer, environmental pressure and pathogen status (*E. coli*, *Salmonella* spp., Pestivirus, Rotavirus, Coronavirus, *Cryptosporidium* spp. and others).
   d. *Actions*: Check calcium, energy and protein nutrition and sire factors (large calves). Ensure an adequate volume of colostrum within four hours of birth (four litres of high quality colostrum). Review calving environment. Consider vaccination.

References

Beckett, S.D. (1997). *Epidemiological investigations in animal populations*. Masters thesis, University of Sydney, Australia.

Curtis, M.A. (1997). *Epidemiology of uterine infections in dairy cows. Antioxidant and metabolic investigations*. PhD thesis, University of Sydney, Australia.

DeGaris, P.J., Lean, I.J., Rabiee, A.R. and Heuer, C. (2010). Effects of Increasing Exposure to a Pre-partum diet Containing BioChlor®. 1 Effects of increasing days of exposure to prepartum transition diets on reproduction and health in dairy cows. *Australian Veterinary Journal* **88**, 84–92.

DeGaris, P.J., Lean, I.J., Rabiee, A.R. and Heuer, C. (2010b). Effects of Increasing Exposure to a Pre-partum diet Containing BioChlor®. 1 Effects of increasing days of exposure to prepartum transition diets on reproduction and health in dairy cows. *Australian Veterinary Journal* **88**, 189–190 (Erratum).

Duff, G.C. and Gaylean, M.L. (2007). Recent advances in management of highly stressed, newly received feedlot cattle. *Journal of Animal Science* **85**, 823–840.

Lean, I.J and DeGaris, P.J. (2011). Transition cow management: A review for nutritional professionals, veterinarians and farm advisors. *Dairy Australia*. Available at: http://www.dairyaustralia.com.au/

Golder, H.M., Bramley, E, Rabiee, A.R., Celi, P. and Lean, I.J. (2012). Validation of an Acidosis Model. Recent *Advances in Dairy Science*

Lean, I.J., DeGaris, P.J., Wade, L.K., and Rajczyk, Z.K. (2003). *Transition Management of Dairy Cows, 2003*. In: Australian & New Zealand combined Dairy Veterinarians' Conference. Foundation for Continuing Education of the N.Z. Veterinary Association, Taupo, New Zealand Pp. 221–248.

Morton, J. (2004). *Determinants of reproductive performance of dairy cows in commercial herds in Australia*. PhD thesis, University of Melbourne, Australia.

Moss, N. (2001). *The epidemiology of subfertility in Australian dairy cows*. PhD thesis, University of Sydney, Australia.

Oetzel, G.R. (2004). Monitoring and testing dairy herds for metabolic disease. *Veterinary Clinics of North America: Food Animal Practice* **20**, 651–674.

Sprecher, D.J., Hostetler, D.E. and Kaneene, J.B. (1997). A lameness scoring system that uses posture and gait to predict dairy cattle reproductive performance. *Theriogenology* **47**, 1179–1187.

Stevenson, M.A. (1995). *Risk factors for culling in dairy cattle*. Masters thesis, University of Sydney, Australia.

Tyler, J. and Cullor, J. (1989). Titres, tests and truisms. Rational interpretation of diagnostic serologic testing. *Journal of the American Veterinary Medical Association* **194**, 1550–1558.

Further reading

Disorders of lipid metabolism

Duffield, T.F. (2000). Subclinical ketosis in lactating dairy cattle. *Veterinary Clinics of North America: Food Animal Practice* **16**, 231–53, Review.

Grummer, R.R., Mashek, D.G. and Hayirili, A. (2004). Dry matter intake and energy balance in the transition period. *Veterinary Clinics of North America: Food Animal Practice* **20**, 447–470.

Lean, I.J., Bruss, M.L., Baldwin, R.L., and Trout, H.F. (1992). Bovine ketosis: A review. II. Biochemistry and prevention. *Veterinary Bulletin* **62**, 1–14.

Lean I.J. (2011). Ketosis. In: Rojinski, H. (ed). *Encyclopedia of Dairy Science*, 2nd edition. Elsevier Science Ltd.

Lean I.J. (2011). Pregnancy toxaemia. In: Rojinski, H. (ed). *Encyclopedia of Dairy Science*, 2nd edition. Elsevier Science Ltd.

Rumen health

Bramley E., Lean I.J., Fulkerson W.J., Stevenson M.A., Rabiee A.R. and Costa N.D. (2008). The definition of acidosis in dairy herds predominantly fed on pasture and concentrates. *Journal of Dairy Science* **91**, 308–321.

Enemark, J. Mn., Jorgensen R.J. and Enemark P.S. (2002). Rumen acidosis with special emphasis on diagnosis aspects of subclinical rumen acidosis: A review. *Veterinarija ir Zootechnika* **42**, 16–29.

Lean, I.J, Annison, E.F., Bramley, E., Browning, G., Cusack, P., Farquharson B., Little, S. and Nandapi, D. (2007). *Ruminal acidosis – aetiopathogenesis, prevention and treatment. A review for veterinarians and nutritional professionals*. Australian Veterinary Association.

O'Grady, L., Doherty, M.L. and Mulligan, F.J. (2008). Subacute ruminal acidosis (SARA) in grazing Irish dairy cows. *The Veterinary Journal* **176**, 44–49.

Plaizier, J.C., Krause, D.O., Gozho, G.N. and McBride, B.W. (2008). Subacute ruminal acidosis in dairy cows: The physiological causes, incidence and consequences. *The Veterinary Journal* **176**, 21–31.

Macro-mineral deficiency

Charbonneau, E., Pellerin, D. and Oetzel, G.R. (2006). Impact of lowering dietary cation–anion difference in nonlactating dairy cows: a meta-analysis. *Journal of Dairy Science* **89**, 537–548.

Constable, P.D. (1999). Clinical assessment of acid-base status: strong ion difference theory. *Veterinary Clinics of North America: Food Animal Practice* **15**, 447–471.

Curtis, C.R., Erb, E.H. and Sniffen, C.J. (1983), Association of parturient hypocalcemia with eight periparturinet disorders in Holstein cows. *Journal of the American Veterinary Medical Association* **183**, 559.

Curtis, C.R., Erb, E.H., Sniffen, C.J., Smith, R.D. and Kronfeld, D.S. (1985). Path analysis of dry period nutrition, postpartum metabolic and reproductive disorders, and mastitis in holstein cows. *Journal of Dairy Science* **68**, 2347–2360.

DeGaris, P.J. and Lean, I.J. (2008) Milk fever in dairy cows: A review of pathophysiology and control principles. *The Veterinary Journal* **176**, 58–69.

Goff, J.P. (2004). Macromineral disorders of the transition cow. *Veterinary Clinics of North America: Food Animal Practice* **20**, 471–494.

Goff, J. (2008). The monitoring, prevention, and treatment of milk fever. and subclinical hypocalcemia in dairy cows. *The Veterinary Journal* **176**, 50–57.

Lean, I.J., DeGaris, P.J., McNeil, D.M. and Block, E. (2006). Hypocalcemia in dairy cows: meta analysis and dietary cation anion difference theory revisited. *Journal of Dairy Science* **89**, 669–684.

Oetzel, G.R. (2000). Management of Dry Cows for the Prevention of Milk Fever and Other Mineral Disorders. *Veterinary Clinics of North America: Food Animal Practice* **16**, 369–386.

Periparturient immunosuppression

Gaylean, M.L., Perino L.J. and Duff, G.C. (1999). Interaction of cattle health/immunity and nutrition. *Journal of Animal Science* **77**, 1120–1134.

Nutrient requirements of dairy cattle, 7th revised edition. (2002). National Academy of Sciences, Washington, D.C.

CHAPTER 39

The Farm Audit: Clinical Dairy Cow Nutrition

Tom Chamberlain

Learning objectives

- Develop a rational and valid approach to performance record analysis.
- Be able to clinically assess how a recommended ration is delivered on farm.
- Appraise aspects of the cow's environment that might impact on her feeding and performance.
- Assess the cow herself to investigate any nutritional problems.

Introduction

Most dairy farms now benefit from rations formulated specifically for their farm, created using modern and comprehensive rationing software. From investigating farm problems, it is clear that many more on-farm issues arise due to the translation of the recommendations into the rations that the cows eat, rather than problems due to underlying flaws with the original formulation.

Sorting out problems with the on-farm delivery is a clinical task. As with any clinical examination, care must be taken not to over-interpret a single observation, a diagnosis should only be made once a range of results and observations have been combined to build up a picture. Where numerical assessments are made, then simple statistical tests must be used to determine the importance of any differences and variation seen.

Any audit should comprise four sections:

- Analysis and interpretation of all available farm records.
- The ration and feeds available.
- Assess the cow's environment, including the feeds available.
- Assess the cow.

Records

In a world with ever greater computerisation, there is often a wealth of records available to the clinician. Tools are being developed to process such data, but great care must be taken to avoid over-interpretation; the findings are merely 'an indication to investigate further', and are very rarely pathognomonic in their own right. When looking at such data, three comparisons can be made:

- Comparison with a target and intervention level – useful where these have been defined, especially where they have been assessed on a financial basis. However, often there are no definitive figures available, or they do not relate to the appropriate production systems.
- Comparison with others – usually achieved by 'benchmarking'. Care needs to be taken to identify the benchmarking group, so that comparisons are valid. Where the group is tightly defined and members know each other, this can be a powerful comparator and motivator.
- Comparisons over time – requires regular monitoring, but does allow changes to be seen quickly. Often combined with wider benchmarking or assessment against targets to determine what change is desired.

Milk records

Milk is the primary output of any dairy farm; in many situations volumes produced are paramount with composition (butter fat, protein) being of lesser financial value. As it is such a key income driver there is generally ample data available on farm relating to milk production.

Milk production

The most basic records are for daily collection volumes, and these are often aggregated over time, by month and annually. In addition, the majority of farms have regular (usually monthly) milk recording with a specialist company (such as NMR or CIS) and, finally, a growing number of modern parlours record milk volumes at every milking. When assessing such data, clinicians need to be clear about several points:

- Do the data relate to milk produced or milk sold? The latter can be 5–8% less.

Bovine Medicine, Third Edition. Edited by Peter D. Cockcroft.

- Do the data relate to annual milk production, which is related to annual income, or to milk production over 305 days (which allows metabolic loads to be compared), or lactational yields (which rise with worsening fertility and are of little value other than for 'bragging rights')?

Milk sold per cow per year and per cow per 305d lactation

These assessments give an indication of the metabolic stress that the herd is under, and the likely types and magnitude of problems that could be observed. For example, a herd averaging 5000 L/cow/year would expect a zero incidence of displaced abomasa, but a herd selling 10 000 L/cow/year may accept a 4% incidence as a realistic target.

Milk produced per cow per day

A widely quoted figure within the industry, but of very limited value unless the average stage of lactation is known – often expressed as the average days in milk (DIM). A herd with a tight spring calving block will have falling milk sales in the autumn, simply because average DIM is increasing, and any attempts to correct the decline would be very ill-judged. For such reasons, milk produced is usually assessed alongside average days in milk (Figure 39.1).

Interpretation of figure 39.1 shows that generally, over the past two years, the trend is that DIM has increased, while milk produced has fallen. Looking in more detail it can be seen that volumes produced from April 2012 onwards has fallen, even through the herd is fresher, with declining DIM. The reverse happened from October 2011 onwards where, although DIM increased, milk production rose. Such observations point to differences in adequacy of feeding from summer to winter.

Where 'milk recording' is carried out and all cows are recorded and sampled monthly, it can be very useful to plot daily milk production per cow by stage of lactation (DIM). Such a plot for a single recording gives an approximation of the lactation curve, but such data become more informative when plotted over successive months (Figure 39.2). The comparison then shows how the herd has milked at the two past recordings after the stage of lactation effect has been removed. In this example, at almost every stage of lactation, milk production in September was lower than in August and, overall (for the 98 cows where comparisons could be made), production was down by 3.8 L/cow/day ($p < 0.05$). Such a big (13%) and statistically significant change would warrant investigation, and may point towards over-dependence on autumn grazing.

Modern milking parlours allow such analyses to be carried out on a daily basis, allowing quicker response to changes. Our initial work with such data sources indicates that care must be taken not to over-react; if sufficient comparisons are made between enough subsets of the overall herd, you will find differences, but these may be due to random error or caused by effects such as differing cohort age profiles, etc. Careful data handling and a sound statistical basis is needed before such analyses are carried out routinely on farm data.

Milk yields in stale milkers

Analysis of yields in cows towards the end of the lactation is rarely carried out, but it can be very rewarding. A problem common in many herds is that poor fertility performance results in overly long calving intervals and, hence, lactation length. Many farms consistently produce good quality forages and group-feed cows, such that it is difficult to offer a balanced diet to a low yielder. Typically, cows yielding under 0.2% of their annual

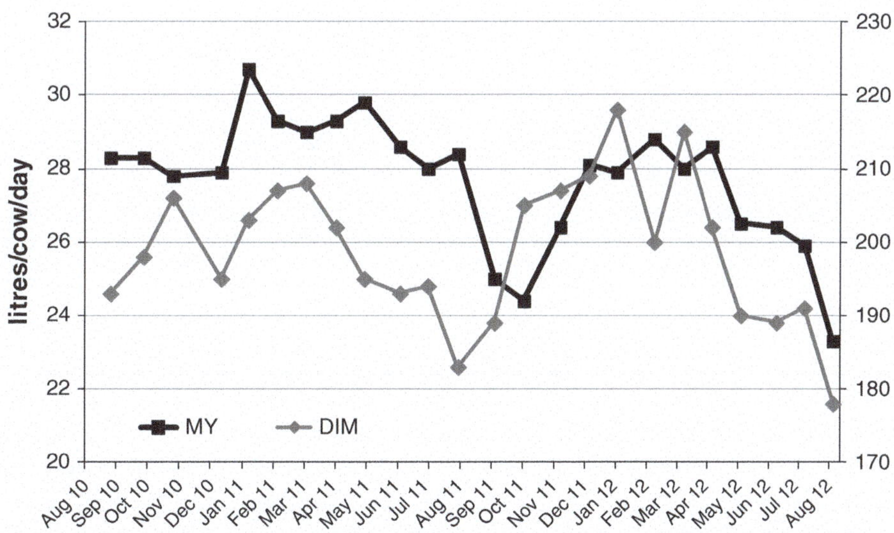

Figure 39.1 Plot of daily milk production (litres produced) and herd average 'days in milk' over a two year period (derived from NMR milk recording data).

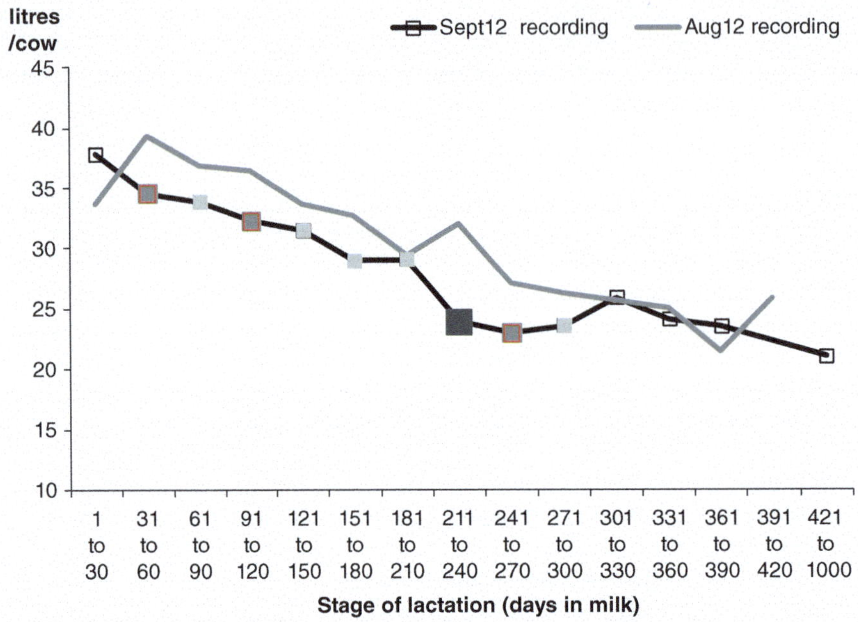

Figure 39.2 Daily milk production plotted against days in milk (stage of lactation) for two successive milk recordings (data derived from CIS milk recording data). The size and boldness of the line markers are related to the statistical significance between the two months.

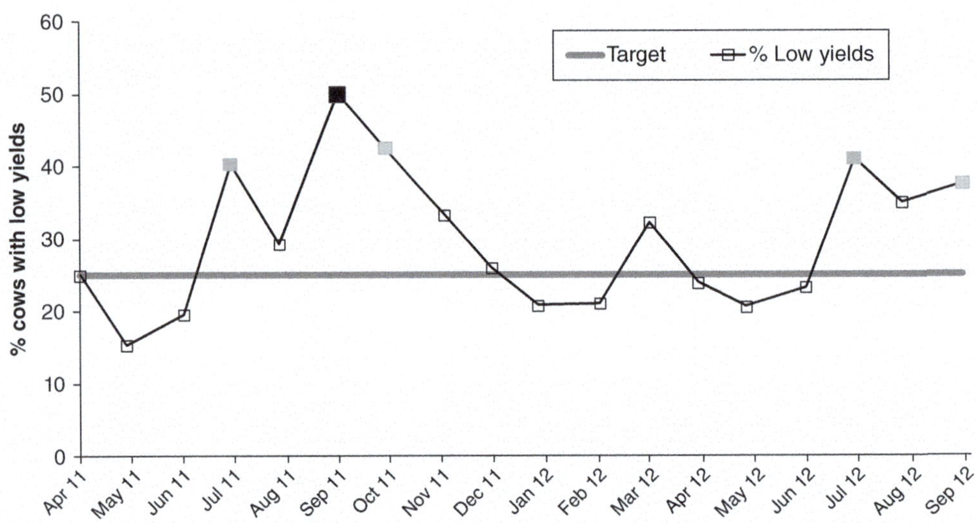

Figure 39.3 Percentage of stale milkers (over 300 days DIM) with low milk yields (under 15 L/day) at milk recording (derived from NMR milk recording records), compared to a target of 25%. The size and boldness of the line markers are related to the statistical significance of the difference between observed value and the target.

milk production (15 litres for 7500 L/cow/year) are difficult to feed correctly. The magnitude of the problem will vary with the feeding systems used but, often, such cows gain weight as stale milkers. The weight gain stays with them through the dry period, such that they calve in over-conditioned, have a higher risk of peri-parturient diseases, mobilise more body fat and eat less. This promotes excessive body condition and subsequent poor fertility, which perpetuates the problem.

A valuable monitoring exercise is to track how many stale milkers have low milk yields (Figure 39.3). In the example shown here, in autumn 2012 and autumn 2011, the percentage of stale milkers with low milk yields rose above the 25% target. In the herd represented here, the milkers were managed on two TMRs as 'highs' and 'lows', with the latter fed for 22 litres in the TMR, such that considerable numbers of cows were being incorrectly fed.

Such monitoring needs to be followed up by careful inspection of individual cow records. In this case, in September 2012, 20 out of 42 stale milkers were yielding less than 15 litres, and seven less than 10 litres. Some of these cows may be destined to be culled, in which case the economics of keeping them on a milker's ration needs to be assessed. A bigger concern is where such cows are destined to re-calve in the herd; these cows need inspecting for body condition score and dried off before they become fat, to help break the cycle outlined above.

Milk quality

In recent years, there has been considerable interest in monitoring aspects of milk quality. Associations between low butter fats and acidosis, and between low milk proteins and ketosis, have been promoted by various groups. While the underlying biological pathways look sensible and sound, the on-farm relationship between milk solids and disease is far less clear, and there is a grave risk of over-interpretation of such data. The reasons for such over-interpretation, especially of butter fats, can be:

- Precisely how the milk sample is extracted from the volume of milk produced, and how often this is done per recording (factoring), can have a considerable effect on milk composition
- Spring grass and dietary supplements, such as protected fats, fish oils and processed linseed oils, can affect milk butter fat content.

Low butter fats have been associated with acidosis but, in the author's experience, this is not common. The two assessments that are most useful are as follows.

High butter fats at first recording

This is generally defined as a butter fat over 5% at the first milk recording (less than 30 DIM). This seems to be linked to high levels of weight loss around calving, suggesting that fatty acids in the blood overflow into the milk. Excessive weight loss around calving, with raised blood NEFAs, has been shown to be an important risk factor for a wide range of peri-parturient diseases (Dyk *et al.*, 1995). However, the close temporal association makes high butter fats a less than ideal monitoring tool; by the time raised butter fats are detected, the herd is often experiencing periparturient problems and does not need telling they have a problem! For this reason, looking at low milk yields in stale milkers may be preferable.

Low milk protein

Low milk protein can be indicative of low energy status, and this can be linked to poor fertility. Using a threshold of 2.9%, milk protein seems to yield a usable indicator, in that large numbers of cows with milk protein below 2.9% can be taken as indicative that the cow's feeding and energy status may be impacting on fertility performance. Total milk protein production can also be used to take milk yield as well as quality into account, and it has been suggested that good milkers less than 60 DIM should exceed 1 kg milk protein a day, and that amounts below 0.7 kg are a cause for concern (Figure 39.4). However, there is still a yield effect, with high-yielding herds rarely dropping below 0.8 kg and some low yielding, extensively managed herds rarely exceeding 0.7 kg. Probably of greater value is to look at the changes in value – a consistent downward trend would be cause for concern.

The ration

What is being fed?

Investigating the stages and processes between a recommended ration and what the cows actually eat should be central to any audit. Mixer wagons are very commonly used on farm, and can supply valuable information.

- Is the ration the farm decides to feed, the same as the recommendation? Details can get lost in transfer to the loader tractor, ingredients can be omitted or staff members can make changes on their own initiative.
- How does the mixer wagon operator adjust to changes in intake; do they just alter one of the major ingredients, thereby altering the underlying ration formulation? More correctly, they should adjust all ingredients up and down as required. Simple 'loader sheets' can be made up, and modern mixer wagons can make the adjustments within their control boxes.
- How are baled products fed? How is the bale split to adjust for changes in group size? It is not easy!
- How does the 'number of cows' fed relate to the numbers of cows actually in the group?
- How accurately are feeds weighed into the wagon? Free-flowing materials should be reasonably simple to weigh in, but feeds such as silages and straw in blocks or 'sections' can be more difficult. Modern wagons can log exactly what is put into the wagon, and this can be compared to the target ration. The difference between what should have been fed and what was fed can be as great as 20%.
- How was the ration mixed? The function of modern mixer wagons is to reduce the length of long forage (usually straw) short enough that it cannot be sorted out, and to mix all of the ingredients so that the cows cannot pick out the most palatable components while not over-processing the mix and reducing the effective fibre content. The PACE system, on Kennan wagons, and other systems can record the order in which ingredients are added to the mix and the time and speed of mixing between adding successive ingredients. Such information can help with compliance and consistency between different operators.
- How is the finished ration assessed? Producing and feeding TMRs is a key component of modern stockmanship, and the finished mix should be examined at regular intervals. Do the

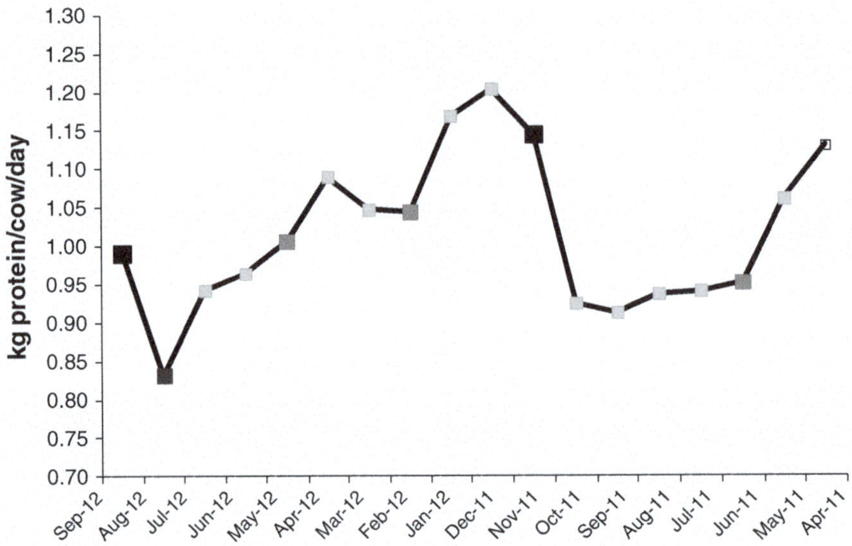

Figure 39.4 Milk protein production (kg/day) in fresh calvers (less than 60 DIM) (derived from NMR records). The size and boldness of the line markers are related to the statistical significance of the differences between successive months.

operators know what the ideal finished ration should look like? Is a Penn State sieve or similar used to assess mixing and processing, is there evidence of excessive sorting with straw and long forage left over?

How much is being eaten?

The key to feeding cows is knowing how much they will eat, and generally maximising their intake. Prediction of intakes is probably the most inaccurate, but most important, part of any rationing software. Any prediction is therefore a first estimate, and in any investigation this should be confirmed. Most units with mixer wagons know the fresh weight fed into the trough, but do not always assume they know how many cows there are in a shed! In-parlour and out-of-parlour feeders can be more difficult to interrogate; they generally work on volume, rather than weight, and are rarely calibrated, although they live in a fairly hostile environment. In addition, all such measurements are on a fresh weight basis and, within reasonable bounds, the moisture content of a ration does not affect intake. It is, therefore, important to assess the dry matter and, hence, the dry matter intake. This can be done simply, cheaply and routinely on farm using a microwave oven or a domestic food dessicator. Measuring and maximising dry matter intake should be a key control point within any on-going nutritional audit.

Lastly, enquire about the level of 'refusals' or 'push-out'. The amounts that farmers will tolerate depends on how difficult it is to remove the refusals from the trough (ideally it should be mechanised) and whether the daily refusals can then be fed back to other lower-ranking groups. Where these issues can be resolved a general target would be 3–5% 'push out' rising to 7–10% for the transition and fresh calver groups.

Forages

Generally, farms will have an NIR-based forage analysis available, but this should be checked for the following:

- When was the sample submitted for analysis? If several months ago, is it still valid to what is being fed now?
- How was the sample collected? Was it a 'face' or a 'core' sample? The former are preferred as the feeding season progresses. Is the sample representative of the forage? How many sub-samples were collected from different bales or across the feed face?
- Does the 'forage type' specified on the analysis relate to the forage being fed? NIR calibrations are forage type specific. If the farm's forage is a bi-crop or a minority crop (such as ensiled lucerne), then a 'wet lab' assessment should be carried out.
- Does the analysis 'fit' the forage you are seeing? The analysis only actually assessed a few grams of forage – how does this relate to the clamp being fed? In addition, the analysis will shift as the clamp is fed out. Carrying out regular oven dry matter assessments is practical and can be very rewarding.
- Feed composition will differ through the clamp, due to differences in plant species and in growing conditions. Routine measurement of dry matters through the season can show considerable variation (see Figure 39.5), and these can be large enough to affect animal performance. Samples should be collected regularly for dry matter assessment.

Forage storage

Carry out a critical appraisal of how the forage is stored and fed out.

- How compacted and anaerobic is the stored forage? It should be difficult to push a hoof-knife into the cut face. Compaction

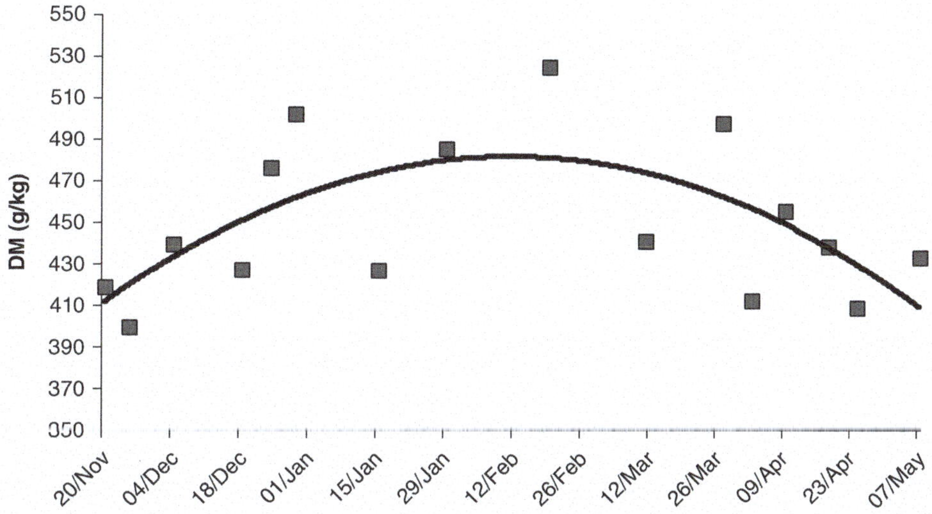

Figure 39.5 Changes in measured dry matter of a large clamp of grass silage through a winter feeding period (each dry matter value is the mean of three samples collected and analysed separately).

is easier with wet feeds, but more difficult as chop length increases.

- How 'tidy' is the face? Maize silage, in particular, will suffer heating and undergo aerobic fermentation if the face is not smooth and tight. There should be minimal lifting and air ingress when feed is removed.
- Top and shoulder waste. How much waste is there, and it is being controlled through the use of salt or vapour-seal barriers? What happens to any mould-contaminated feed? Is it kept out of the cow's ration, or is it thoroughly mixed through the TMR?
- The clamp. Is the drainage away from the clamp face? Is the clamp floor clear of mud, soil and old forage?

Supplementary feeds

Storage: is the feed dry, and are there any signs of contamination or distress during production and transport. Are the stores vermin-proof?

Clinically examine the feeds:

- Visually. Does it look the same colour as other samples, and is it uniform in colour and consistency.
- Smell. Generally, and at a risk of being anthropomorphic, good cattle feeds smell nice. A tobacco or caramel smell may indicate over-heating and damage to the protein. Rancid fat and butyric fermentation smell unpleasant, as do some of the products of mould fermentation.
- Taste. Cows have a sweet tooth. Butyric acid tastes unpleasant; un-palatable feeds such as protected fats, and many of the high DCAB feeds and salts, taste bitter.
- Cost. There are few bargain feeds available to the average dairy farmer – if it sounds too cheap to be true, then it probably is.

The environment

How a ration is presented, how the buildings are laid out, what access the cows have, etc. can have a major impact on herd performance. Bach (2008) looked at 47 milking herds in Spain that were all fed the same TMR made at a central depot. Mean daily yield varied from 20.5 to 33.6 litres, and 56% of this variation was not attributable to the diet. Areas to address are:

Trough design

- How much does the trough hold and how often is it filled? Is there food available at all times?
- If adequate food is available at all times, then there will be some left over when the trough is re-filled. What happens to this feed? Surplus food should be removed, and this is most likely to happen when it can be done mechanically and the surplus feed recovered for feeding to other groups.
- What is the surface of the trough? If it is rough, pitted concrete, it is difficult to clean and cows will have to alter their natural eating pattern of pulling food into their mouths with their tongues.
- How wide is the trough? Troughs that feed from just one side can get a bit narrow and tight against a wall. A bigger issue is where cows access the trough from both sides. They have to be narrow enough to ensure that feed is not left in the centre, but then the nose-to-nose eating can be intimidating for submissive cows.
- How high is the trough floor? Ideally, the trough floor is 100–150 mm above the level the cow stands on, to give her good access and reduce pressure on the front feet.

Space available

Cows are herd animals and, generally, they all do activities such as eating and grazing at the same time; if submissive cows cannot carry out the activity at that time, the social pressure is such that they will often have to move on to the next activity 'un-satisfied'. It is, therefore, important that there is sufficient trough space for all cows to eat at the same time. For lactating animals, the general recommendation is 600–700 mm per cow, with a 10% reduction resulting in a decline in milk yield by 0.75 L/day (Grant, 2011). This rises to 900–1000 mm for transition and freshly calved cows, to avoid restricting intake in submissive animals.

Cow time budgets

The modern daily cow is a busy animal. She needs to spend 12–14 hours a day lying down, five hours a day eating and about three hours a day walking, drinking, grooming and socialising. She also needs to be milked. If the overall milking time each day (time away from the housing/feed areas) exceeds three to four hours a day, she will be compromised. She will maintain her lying time at the expense of feeding time, such that milk yield can fall by 2–3 litres (Grant, 2011). Common on-farm scenarios are.

- 'One man' units, where the cows are pushed out from the cubicle/feed shed before milking, so the cubicles and passageways can be serviced.
- Large units milking three times a day, where large groups spend so long going through the milking process that they are away from their feed for too long.

The cow

Assessment of the cow and of the rumen is a central part of any nutritional audit, and has been reviewed in detail by Atkinson (2009). Key components to assess are:

Clinical disease incidence

Most of the clinical diseases that have a nutritional component are seen around calving, and so will be considered in other chapters. Typical target levels would be:

- Milk fever. Target under 5% of cows calved per year.
- Displaced abomasa. Target:
  - under 8000 L/cow/year target is zero.
  - over 8000 litres target is under 3% of herd.
- Clinical ketosis. Target 2–3% of herd.

Body Condition Score (BCS)

Excessive change in BCS over the production cycle is to be avoided. Ideally, a cohort of cows would be scored regularly through the year, but such data are rarely available. BCS assessment can be rapid, but the results are subjective and can vary widely between different assessors. Such variation would seem to put people off scoring their cows, and data are rarely collected on a routine basis. More commonly, the auditor will have to score cows at the farm visit and, by relating the scores to stage of lactation, build up a picture of how BCS changes over time. When scoring to a five-point scale, targets would be 2.5–3.0 at calving, dropping by a maximum of 0.5 BCS units through to peak milk yield, and regaining this (and no more) through to drying off.

Rumen fill

A five-point scale based on assessment of the left sub-lumbar fossa has been proposed (Atkinson, 2009), with a score of 1 indicating a very empty rumen and poor feed intake, through to a score of 5, as might be seen in a pre-calver where the rumen volume completely obliterates the fossa. Pre-calvers should have very good rumen fill, scoring 4 or more, while milkers will tend to have lower scores (2.5–3.5), as the ration has a higher degradability and faster gut transit time.

Faecal scoring

Faeces can be scored as they lie of the ground, ranging from a watery mass with no structural form (score 1), through to very firm faeces (score 5) that form individual 'balls' similar to horse faeces. Targets would be 2–3 in milkers, with the dung pat being about 2 cm thick and taking the imprint of a boot. Dry cows will have higher scores of around 3–4. Faecal sieving can also be used to assess digestive 'health'. A small 'apple-sized' sample of faeces is placed in a domestic sieve, and washed under running water until the effluent is clear and all rape seed husks have been removed. The ideal is a small volume with a consistent structure, with all fibre particles less than 8 mm long. Increased amounts of residue in the sieve, with longer fibres and undigested feed components, are indicative of poor rumen health.

Cudding activity

Assess cows when they are at rest in the cubicles or loose yards. The target is that more than 60% of cows that are 'idling' will be chewing the cud. If this drops below 50%, with considerable numbers of animals 'doing nothing', this suggests that the ration is short in structural fibre and not stimulating sufficient cudding and rumen buffering. Each cud-ball should be chewed 60–70 times before re-swallowing.

Ruminocentesis

Rumen fluid samples (not collected *per os*) can be used to assess rumen health. The pH of freshly drawn samples can be assessed with a calibrated pH meter, with readings below 5.5 highly indicative of ruminal acidosis. However, feeding patterns and sampling times will affect such readings with a dip in pH seen about two hours after a concentrate feed. The rumen fluid should also be examined microscopically on a warmed microscope slide (blood temperature). Protozoa can readily be seen at low magnifications. These organisms are sensitive to rumen pH and rumen health, with diminished numbers and reduced mobility being indicative of poor rumen conditions.

Time motion studies

Cows are crepuscular by nature, and should eat mainly at dawn and dusk. Modern dairy cows try to maintain this pattern, despite the milking regime we impose on them. If the audit is carried out in the middle of the day, the milkers should have finished eating; if they are still at the trough, do they have enough access, both space and hours in the day? By contrast, it may be desirable that stale cows and 'far off' dry cows are eating most of the day, as this suggests we have constrained energy intake to match their requirements.

Blood sampling

A range of detailed and comprehensive 'metabolic profiles', based on blood sampling selected animals, have been defined. However, the cost of such wide-ranging assessments are considerable, and limit their application. The predominant nutrient of interest is energy, and much can be gained by concentrating solely on β-hydroxybuterate (BHB) in the milkers and non-esterified fatty acids (NEFAs) in the dry cows. BHB levels can be measured cowside, using equipment developed for human diabetes patients. The method is quick and cheap, and can be carried out by trained farm staff. The ease and low cost allow all cows to be sampled, and at the optimal time. At routine intervals, all cows from 4–10 days post-calving should be sampled, and an on-going picture of energy status built up over several sampling sessions. Energy status in transition cows is better assessed using NEFAs, trying to take samples 10–4 days before calving, and then correcting the exact timing once the cow has calved.

References

Atkinson, O. (2009). Guide to the rumen health visit. *In Practice* **31**, 314–325.

Bach, A., Valls, N., Sloans, A. and Torrent, T. (2008). Associations between non-dietary factors and dairy herd performance. *Journal of Dairy Science* **91**, 3259–3267.

Dyk, P.B., Emery, R.S. and Liesman, J.L. (1995). Pre-partum nonesterified fatty acids in plasma are higher in cows developing periparturient health problems. *Journal of Dairy Science* **78**(Suppl. 1), 264.

Grant, R. (2011). *Cow comfort economics.* Procedures of Dairy Day at Miner Institute, NY, USA, Dec 2011.

CHAPTER 40

The Farm Audit: Udder Health, Mastitis Milk Quality and Production

Andrew Biggs

Learning objectives

- Appreciate the scope of the farm audit.
- Appreciate the direct costs and indirect costs.
- Appreciate the application of the measure, manage and monitor construct.
- Appreciate why data analysis, risk assessment and infection profiles are important 'measures'.
- Understand the important key performance indicators and target values.
- Understand the importance of identifying herd transmission patterns.

Introduction

Mastitis is one of the most common and costly diseases of dairy cattle and, while disease prevalence and incidence varies generic aims to minimise its impact on health, welfare productivity and profit remain. Trends within the dairy industry the world over are of increasing herd size. This simple trend is complicated by variations in production systems, such that nutrition, cow environment (housing, pasture-based or a mix) and milk harvesting have tended to become polarised into those systems using a high degree of technological innovation and input, and those that are simple low-input low-output systems. As a consequence, dairy industries vary around the world according to the local culture, environment, business models and opportunities and market opportunities. Differences in available foodstuffs, local breed characteristics, and market requirements and opportunities, influence the choices and aspirations of dairy farmers. It is very important that these business and health aspirations are fully understood, such that any goals and targets set as part of a herd health plan or trouble shooting visit are appropriate.

Herd health planning is an active process and can be summarised as 'Measure, Manage, Monitor'. The cyclical process continually evaluates health status by measuring health and performance parameters, applying appropriate and achievable management control measures, and then monitoring changes by measuring health and performance parameters, adjusting and continually refining the management control measures. This allows for realistic short, medium and long term goals and targets to be set. Targets should be farm-specific and set to encourage improvement without being unattainable in the time frame set.

A Mastitis Farm Audit should be modelled on the 'measure, manage, monitor' approach of herd health planning.

The 'measure' component encompasses three broad areas of:

- Data analysis.
- Risk assessment.
- Infection profile (Schukken *et al.*, 2012).

As a consequence, the herd-level diagnosis of contagious or environmental is more appropriate than the simplified classical contagious or environmental characteristics of the predominant bacteria isolated. The significance of the isolation of any potential mastitis-causing bacteria will be influenced by the prevalence and transmission patterns.

Holistic farm audit: characterising the farm

- Geographic, topographical and climatic characteristics, for example: climate (temperature, seasonal variation, altitude, rainfall), land type, drainage and available food sources.
- Infrastructure, labour availability and market opportunities, for example: transport links, access to trained or trainable work force, availability of first time buyer or ability for producer retailer approach, liquid milk or processed milk market.

Bovine Medicine, Third Edition. Edited by Peter D. Cockcroft.

- Production system. For example:
  - Housing.
    - Permanently housed.
    - Permanently at pasture.
    - Seasonal mixture of housed and pasture-based at a herd or production group level.
  - Housing type.
    - Cubicles – (see Table 40.1).
    - Straw yard – loose housed (Table 40.2).
    - Cow byre – tie stall.
  - Cow type
    - High yielding.
      - Pure bred, often pedigree (e.g. Holstein Friesian)
    - Low-yielding.
      - Possible cross bred (e.g. Channel Island cross)
  - Production profile
    - High, medium or low yield..
    - Once, twice, three or four times a day milking.
  - Milk harvesting.
    - High tech – with sensor technology, ACRs and possibly automated PMTD.
      - AMS/VMS/robot milking.
      - High capacity semi-automated milking parlour.
    - Low tech.
      - Hand milking.
      - Less automated milking parlour.

Milk quality audit

Bulk tank milk

Bulk milk sold from dairy farms has to comply with quality targets, which vary around the world. Bulk Milk Somatic Cell Count (BMSCC) is an indirect measure of mastitis prevalence and represents a weighted average individual cow SCC, influenced by each cow's yield but, importantly, only for those cows contributing milk to the bulk tank. Total Bacterial Count (TBC) or Total Viable Count (TVC) is a hygiene measure of bacterial contamination of bulk milk, which has largely been superseded by Bactoscan for regular routine hygienic monitoring of ex-farm milk sales.

Table 40.1 Advantages and disadvantages of cubicle housing (FAWC, 1997).

Advantages	Disadvantages
Low quantity of bedding required.	Passageways and cubicle bases contaminated with slurry.
Opportunity to use alternative bedding materials and mats which can further reduce usage of straw.	Higher risk of lameness and leg damage.
Lower risk of environmental mastitis.	
Higher stocking rate.	

Table 40.2 Advantages and disadvantages of straw yards (adapted from FAWC, 1997).

Advantages	Disadvantages
Relatively low incidence of lameness.	Large quantity of bedding required.
Less risk of damage to knees, hips and hocks.	Relatively high level of management.
	Higher risk of environmental mastitis.
	Feeding and loafing passageways contaminated with slurry.
	Lower stocking rate.

Milk quality is required to be within certain thresholds for example according to European law (EU directive 92/46 EEC 9):

- The SCC must not exceed a geometric average over three months of 400 000 cells/ml, with at least one test per month.
- The bacterial count (TBC/TVC) must not exceed 100 000 cells/ml, based on a rolling geometric average over a two month period, with at least two samples per month.

Bactoscan has no legal standing, but is used throughout the world. Additional information regarding the relationship between TBC, TVC and Bactoscan can be found at: http://www.food.gov.uk/multimedia/pdfs/mb_009_feb2001.pdf.

Box 40.1 Target values for BMSCC and Bactoscan count

> Target BMSCC 100–150 000 cells per ml
> Target Bactoscan < 20 000 cells per ml

BMSCC is influenced by the individual cows contributing to the bulk milk tank, in proportion to their cell count and the volume of milk they are producing. The percentage contribution of each cow can be calculated as the proportion each cow's total cell count production (cow milk yield multiplied by its cell count), as a proportion of the total cell count in the bulk milk tank (total volume of milk in the bulk tank multiplied by the BMSCC).

The economic impact of increased BMSCC can be divided into:

- Financial penalties applied by the first time buyer. Penalties vary according to milk contract.
- Reduced milk production (Figure 40.1).
- An increased risk of clinical mastitis.

Bactoscan is influenced by the various sources of bacteria that can be found in bulk milk and include the following:

- Bacteria entering the milk supply from:
  - Dirty teat surface.
  - Milk from missed clinical cases allowed to enter the bulk tank.
  - Unit drop-offs onto dirty milking parlour floor.
- Poor milking machine wash up.
- Poor milk refrigeration.
- Unsanitary bulk milk tank.

Bacteria associated with increased Bactoscan include:

- Coliforms – environmental/faecal contamination/poor teat preparation
- Thermodurics (laboratory pasteurisation count) – poor wash up routine
- Pseudomonads/Psycotrophs – poor milk cooling
- Mastitis causing bacteria (e.g. *Staph aureus, Mycoplasma or Strep uberis*) – missed clinical cases (see tables below)

The economic impact of an increased Bactoscan is predominantly from the financial penalties applied by first time buyers and will vary according to the milk contract.

Individual cow milk

Herds that perform regular individual cow dairy herd improvement (DHI) milk recording have access to a large dataset of milk quality information, including individual cow somatic cell count (ISCC), which can be used to evaluate the dynamic aspects of intramammary infections over time. Computerisation of such

Parameter	Interpretation
TBC (total bacterial count) or TVC (total viable count).	The TBC/TVC is the total number of colony forming units from 1 ml of milk, measured using a standard microbiological laboratory technique.
Thermoduric count or laboratory pasteurisation count (LPC).	Thermoduric bacteria can withstand relatively high temperatures, and high counts are associated with a problem with the milk machine washing routines.
Psychrotrophs count.	Psychrotrophs are environmental bacteria. They grow even at bulk tank refrigeration temperatures and will reach high levels if held at cold temperatures for prolonged periods. They also increase when either there is a poor milk cooling or a dirty environment.
Pseudomonads count.	Pseudomonads come from the environment but are not of non-enteric origin. Now often used instead of psychotroph counts.
Coliform count.	The coliform count indicates the amount of faecal contamination of the teat and udder. and therefore of parlour hygiene. High levels will be seen when the environment is poorly maintained and pre-milking teat preparation is inadequate.
Mastitis pathogens.	Presence of potential mastitis pathogenic bacteria in bulk milk indicates presence in herd. Absence does not mean the pathogen is not in the herd.

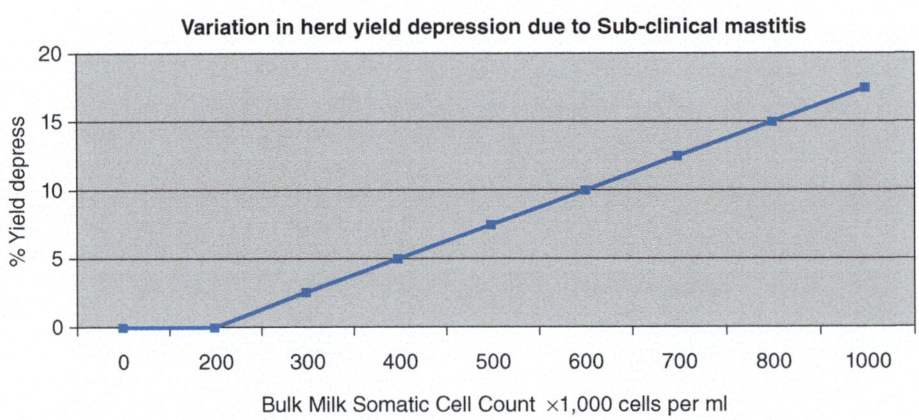

Figure 40.1 The decrease in herd milk yield with increasing bulk milk somatic cell count due to sub-clinical mastitis prevalence.

large datasets allows the changes to the implied infection status of cows to be monitored as they move above or below a given SCC threshold over time. Varying the SCC threshold will vary the sensitivity (Sn) and specificity (Sp) of indicating a cow as infected or uninfected. A threshold of 200 000 cells per ml at a composite cow level, as with DHI SCC data, gives a reasonably balanced Sn and Sp. However, to increase the Sp of a cow being uninfected a lower threshold is more appropriate See Box 40.3.

Problem	TBC/ TVC	Thermo-duric	Psychrotrophs/ Pseudomonas	Coliform
Mastitis	H			
Contaminated teat surfaces	H		H	H
Wash up problem	H	H		
Refrigeration problem	H	H	H	H

H = High

Box 40.2 Target values for differential TBC/TVC

Total Bacterial count	<5,000 cfu/mL
Coliform	<20 cfu/mL
Thermodurics (LPC)	<175 cfu/mL
Psycotrophs	<500 cfu/mL
Staph aureus	<50 cfu/mL
Strep uberis	<200 cfu/mL

Strep agalactiae and *Strep dysgalactiae* should not be present.

Box 40.3 Target values individual cow SCC (high specificity)

ISCC – < 150 000 cells/ml for multiparous cows
<100 000 cells/ml for heifers

Mastitis costs audit

Mastitis costs will vary around the world and will depend on milk value and the costs of drugs, dairy chemical and labour. Although it is useful to be aware of the detail of direct, indirect and preventative costs on a particular farm most often the direct costs are the ones recognised by the farmer as having the most impact on farm profitability.

- Direct costs attributable to mastitis – easily identified and quantified.
  - Treatment costs – drugs.
  - Reduced milk sales from discarded milk during treatment and withhold period.
  - Labour costs.
  - Veterinary surgeon time (if required).
  - Loss of the value of cow and potential production from fatal cases.
  - Milk price – financial penalties or loss of bonus on pence per litre (ppl).
- Indirect costs attributable to mastitis – less easily quantified.
  - Reduced yield subsequent to a case of mastitis.
  - Increased risk of repeated cases later in lactation.
  - Increased risk of culling.
  - Spread to other cows resulting in increased intramammary infections.
  - Loss of genetic potential from herd from forced culling.
  - Potential financial penalties once milk returned to tank via:
    - effects on BMSCC and TBC/Bactoscan;
    - antibiotic violation.
- Preventative management costs.
  - Labour:
    - maintaining hygienic cow accommodation/environment;
    - appropriate hygienic effective milking routine;
    - regular DHI individual cow milk recording;
    - maintaining accurate clinical and drying off records;
    - regular analysis and appraisal of SCC and clinical records;
    - potential segregation of cows based on udder health status.
  - Consumables:
    - pre-milking teat preparation – (paper towels gloves etc);
    - teat disinfectant – (pre and post milking);
    - dairy chemicals – (parlour cleaning and cluster disinfection);
    - antibiotic milking cow, dry cow and internal teat seal tubes;
    - diagnostic sampling.

Analysis of data audit

Herd diagnosis of transmission patterns

Analysis of clinical mastitis data from farm records and sub-clinical data from DHI data can yield useful information for new, repeat, chronic and cure rates. However, 'diagnosing' the herd transmission patterns as predominantly contagious or predominantly environmental goes beyond this, and gives a better indication of where management efforts should be concentrated. Increasingly, it is being recognised that, although the predominant bacteria isolated from mastitis and high SCC cases can give an indication of potential contagious or environmental behaviour, some strains can behave in a non-typical way.

While diagnosing the behaviour or transmission patterns of mastitis causing pathogens within a herd is important to reach a herd-level diagnosis of contagious or environmental, it is also important to identify their likely origin in terms of dry period origin or lactation origin.

This results in four potential categories of mastitis characterisation:

- Dry period environmental.
- Dry period contagious.
- Lactation environmental.
- Lactation contagious.

It is possible for a herd to have more than one transmission and origin pattern simultaneously, or for the herd characteristics to change over time. This makes the 'Monitor' part of 'Measure, Manage, Monitor' essential in keeping up with the potential changing epidemiology of mastitis on a particular farm.

Herd-level diagnosis from pattern analysis

Analysis of herd data, including DHI SCC data, clinical data and calving dates, allows transmission patterns and likely origin of intramammary infections to be inferred:

1. Important characteristics of contagious transmission patterns:
   - Long duration of intramammary infections (IMIs)
   - Relatively high BMSCC
   - Multiple clinical episodes from a single quarter – (recurrent cases)
   - High cow SCC in DHI data in months before clinical episodes
   - Strong link between the prevalent existing infections and likelihood of new infections with the same pathogen.
   - Positive correlation between the prevalence of existing infections (% chronic high-SCC cows) and risk of new infections (% new high-SCC cows).
2. Important characteristics of environmental transmission patterns:
   - Relatively short duration of intramammary infections (IMIs)
   - Potentially low BMSCC
   - High incidence of clinical cases without presence of contemporaneous long duration IMI's
   - Low cow SCC in DHI data in months before clinical episodes
   - High incidence of periparturent IMIs and clinical cases
   - No link between the prevalent existing infections and likelihood of new infections with the same pathogen.
   - Negative correlation between the prevalence of existing infections (% chronic high-SCC cows) and risk of new infections (% new high-SCC cows)
3. Important characteristics of new infections of dry period origin:
   - Most commonly environmental pathogen and transmission patterns: cows are not being milked to facilitate contagious spread.
   - High incidence of new IMIs in early lactation:
     - >8% index clinical cases within 30 days of calving (1 in 12 cows calving in analysis period) (Bradley and Green, 2008).
     - >5% cows with failure of dry period protection. Failure of dry period protection is defined by cows switching from a low SCC prior to drying to a high SCC at the first milk recording within 30 days post-partum.
4. Important characteristics of infections of lactation origin:
   - Can be either environmental or contagious pathogens and transmission patterns:
     - >17% index clinical cases in cows more than 30 days calved (2 in 12 cows calving in analysis period) (Bradley *et al.*, 2008).
     - >5% new IMI's based on increase from below 200 000 cells per ml threshold to above threshold at DHI recording other than first DHI recording within 30 days of calving.

Clinical data analysis

- Incidence: number of cases per 100 cows per year.
- Severity: sick cows or even fatalities.
- Response to treatment: recurrence rates.
- Stage of lactation: fresh calved or later in lactation (Figure 40.2).
- Predominantly environmental or contagious behaviour (see characteristics list above).
- Predominantly dry period origin or lactation origin (see characteristics list above).
- Seasonality: time of year.
- Age of cows affected: heifers or older cows.

Clinical mastitis targets

Parameter	Target	Interference
Mastitis rate (cases per 100 cows)	30	40
% herd affected	20%	30%
% recurrence rate	<10%	15%
Tubes per cow in herd per year	1.5	2.5
Tubes per case	4	6
Cull rate for mastitis	<2%	5%
Dry cow mastitis (summer mastitis)	<1%	5%

Sub-clinical data analysis

- BMSCC.
- Individual SCC records.

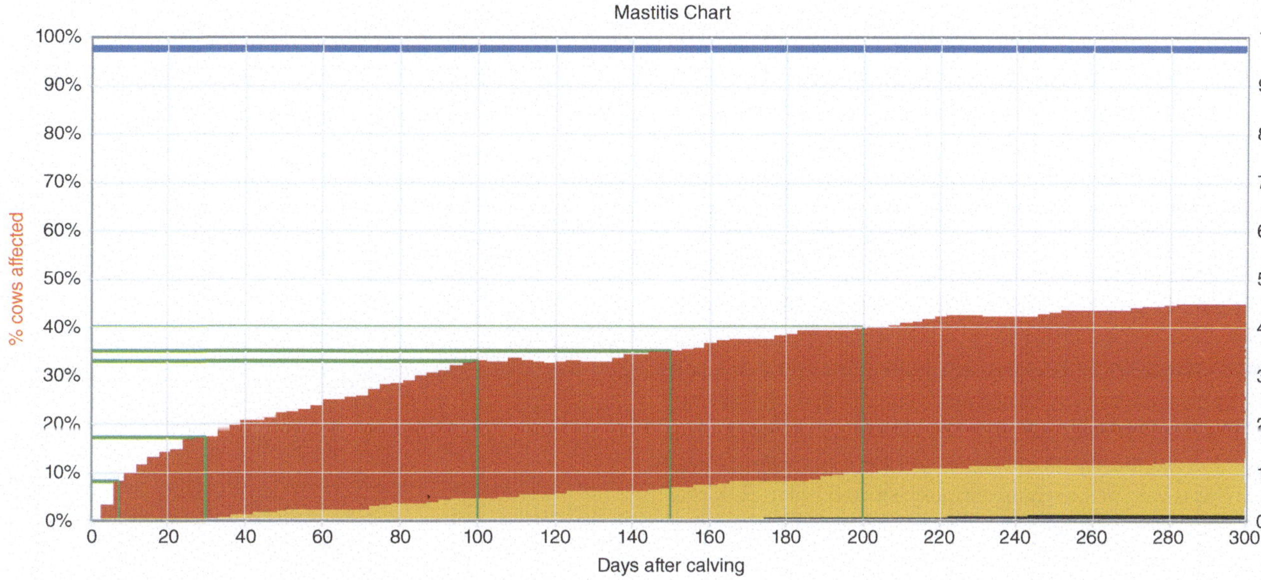

Figure 40.2 Survival curve for index and repeat cases of clinical mastitis cases (red = index cases and orange = repeat cases) (Interherd+ PAN Livestock Services). Target for index mastitis cases in cows calved 30 days or less is 8.5%, or 1 in 12. This herd has 18% cases in cows calved 30 days or less, and is likely to have a dry period origin mastitis problem.

- new infection rates.
- non-recovered new infection rates.
  - proportion of new infection that fail to cure by the next monthly DHI recording.
- prevalence of chronic infections.
- prevalence of cows with SCC > 200 000 cells per ml.
- dry-period performance.
- net transmission ratios over a time period or over the dry period.
  - gives an approximation of the change in prevalence of infection calculated as the ratio of apparent new infections to apparent cured infections and is calculated as follows:
  - number of cows moving upwards through the 200 000 cells per ml threshold (apparent new infections) divided cows moving downwards through the 200 000 cells per ml threshold (apparent cured infections).

Net transmission ratios over a time period or over the dry period

- Ratios < 1 indicate an improving situation with a decreasing prevalence as the number of apparent new infections is less than the number of apparent cures.
- Ratios of > 1 indicates a worsening situation with an increasing prevalence as the number apparent new infections is greater than the number of apparent cures.

Sub-clinical mastitis target values for SCC dynamics during lactation

Proportion of lactating herd (cows)	Target
acquiring new intramammary infections per month	<5%
that is chronically infected (last two SCC > 200 000 cells per ml)	<5 %
above 200 0000 cells per ml in any one month	<10%

Target values for SCC dynamics across the dry period and interpretation of SCC changes before drying off and after calving

DHI cow SCC Before dryoff	After calving	Reason	Target
LOW	LOW	New infection prevented	>80%
LOW	HIGH	New infection acquired	<5%
HIGH	LOW	Existing infection cured	<5%
HIGH	HIGH	Existing infection not cured or cured and new infection acquired	<10%

SCC dynamics during dry period:
SCC status

LOW ≤ 200,000 cells per ml
HIGH ≥ 200,000 cells per ml

Risk assessment audit

Herd diagnosis of transmission patterns

A structured approach to assess the management influences on mastitis disease patterns is required to ensure all areas are considered. A risk assessment tool has been developed, following a literature review (Dufour *et al.*, 2011), and includes six categories, culminating in an overall risk score for the herd. The categories include Biosecurity, Milking Procedures, the Milking System, Treatments, Hygiene/Housing and Susceptibility Management.

Data is collected and standardised from a questionnaire, and actual observations and measurements compiled, so that a score can be obtained for each category. For each of the six categories, a general score, based on the opinion of the assessor, is also added. This is valuable, as many farmers are aware of the key risk factors for udder health, and are practicing the identified best management practices for udder health. However, the actual quality of implementation of the best management practices differs dramatically between farms. It is not acceptable to ask a question and score on the basis of the answer, so an 'on farm' assessment is required to give a score that reflects the reality of what is being applied.

For example, post-milking teat disinfection may be being practised but, if the spray is being directed horizontally as the cows leave the parlour, the general score by the assessor will be low, to reflect the poor execution of what is known to be a known best management practice which might otherwise have scored highly. The scoring system is illustrated in Table 40.3.

Milking parlour audit

Mechanical functional audit

- Static test
  - Vacuum reserve – ISO standard
  - Liner change frequency – black rubber liners every 2500 milkings
- Dynamic test
  - Pulsation rate and ratio
    - Rate 55 to 65 per minute
    - Ratio = (a + b)/(c + d)
      - range 55 : 45 and 70 : 30 – often 60 : 40
      - a (opening phase)
      - b (milk flow or milk out phase) > 30%
      - c (closing phase)
      - d (closed phase) > 15%
      - Time > 200 ms for good teat massage
  - Automatic Cluster remover (ACR) take off switch point and delay – 400 ml per minute switch point with five second delay
  - Three times a day milking requires a higher switch point e.g. 500 ml per minute

Milking routine audit

- General cleanliness of parlour.
- Wash down walls before start and between 'rows'.
- Wash outside of clusters when soiled.
- Quiet and stress free – little shouting, no dog.
- Wear appropriate clothes – waterproof/apron, disposable gloves.
- Teat prep and cleanliness.
- Pre-milking teat dip (Pre-MTD) – full coverage all teats – 10 ml dipping, 15 ml spraying per cow per milking.
- Foremilking.
- Lag time – 60 to 90 seconds – bimodal flow – dry milking.
- Dip-strip wipe-apply.
- Time and motion – batch, sequential, territorial and group.
- Unit alignment – long milk tube (LMT) clips – pull excess on ACR string.
- Under-milking – poor prep and premature ACR removal (bimodal flow).
- Over-milking – slow milkers weights used to machine strip.
- Observe unit removal – clamping off LMT if no ACR – no pulling of udder sideways – manual or ACR.
- Post-milk teat dip (PMTD) – soon after unit removal – full coverage all teats.
- Cow audit.
- Mastitis detection – how effective – often under-diagnosed.
- Treatment protocols.
- Teat condition score (Figure 40.3).
- Hygiene score (Figure 40.4).
- Body condition score (Table 40.4).
- Faecal consistency score (Schreiner & Ruegg, 2003).

Housing/environment audit

Pasture management

- Avoid cows remaining on same pasture for more than two weeks. Graze two weeks and rest four weeks (Green *et al.*, 2007).
- Ensure sufficient drainage to avoid flooding or significant poaching.
- Track and gateway management.
- Fly control.

Housing – ventilation

- Ensure that there is adequate ventilation throughout the building – if insufficient, forced (mechanical) ventilation can be used to ensure adequate control of temperature and humidity.
- Check that cows do not show a preference for certain areas of the building.
- The air inlet area should be 2–4 times the outlet area, with an outlet area of ≈ 0.10–0.15 m^2 per adult cow.

Table 40.3 Risk assessment summary of a dairy farm with a high risk for contagious transmission. A score of 80 is high, between 60 and 80 is medium, and less than 60 is low (after Dufour *et al.*, 2011).

Category	Score	Indicative of transmission pattern	Key issues
Biosecurity	31%	Contagious	Purchase animals without testing.
Milking procedures	82%	Contagious	Excellent teat dip procedure.
Milking system	55%	Contagious	Short d-phase, no equipment maintenance plan.
Treatments	70%	Both	Good sops, no subclinical treatment protocol defined.
Hygiene/housing	69%	Environmental	Hygiene score moderate.
Susceptibility management	82%	Environmental	Good nutrition, breeding plan.
Overall risk for the farm	71%		

Data Capture Form: Teat End Scoring (Hyperkeratosis)

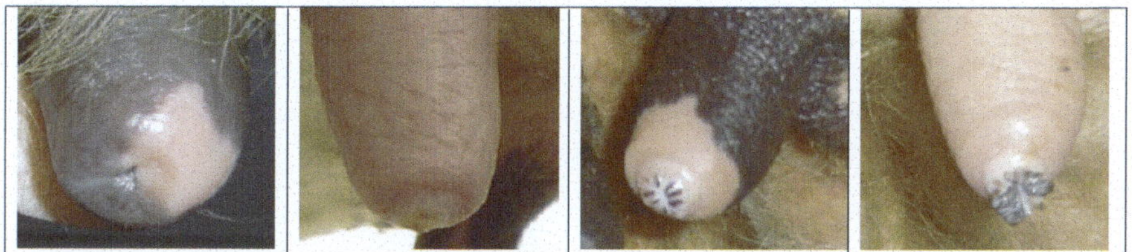

Score N	Score S	Score R	Score VR
No ring.	Smooth ring.	Rough ring.	Very rough ring.
No callosity ring present at the teat end.	A smooth or slightly rough callosity ring. Parakeratosis.	Hyperkeratosis of the teat epidermis and eversion of the teat end.	Hyperkeratosis of the teat epidermis and keratin fronding of the teat orifice. Severe teat end eversion.

Figure 40.3 Teat end scoring system DairyCo Mastitis Control Plan.

Table 40.4 Target body condition scores.

Stage of lactation	Target body condition score (scale 1–5)
At calving	2.5–3.0
60 days in milk	2.0–2.5
200 days in milk	2.5–3.0
Drying off	2.5–3.0

- Make use of the 'stack' effect where possible – an open ridge > 200 mm wide is usually required along the length of the building.
- Manage moisture sources and ensure that water is directed away from the building (avoid leakage from drinking systems, rain goods such as gutters and downpipes and roof leaks).

Slurry management and scraping routine

- All passageways, loafing areas and feed areas should be scraped out at least twice daily.
- Automatic scraping systems, if present, should be run sufficiently often such that passageways are kept clean, and slurry does not overflow the sides of the scrapers.
- There should be sufficient slopes to facilitate effective drainage, such that pooling of liquid in passageways and feed areas is minimised.

Housing cubicles

- Bedding: sand, straw, sawdust, recycled paper, power station ash.
- Bedding material application frequency.
- Base: mattress or mat.
- Size: length, width – breed-dependent.
- Head rail/brisket board: position – breed-dependent.

Data Capture Form: Hygiene Scoring

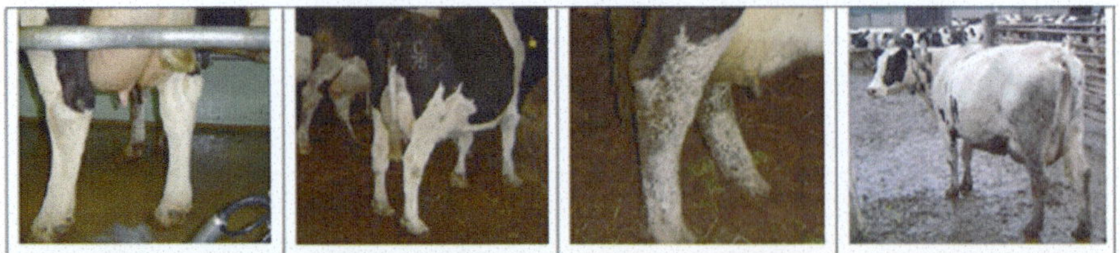

Score 1	Score 2	Score 3	Score 4
<5% of the foot to hock distance is contaminated. Dry hooves	6 to 20% of the foot to hock distance is contaminated. Dry hooves	20 to 40% of the foot to hock distance is contaminated, OR Hooves are very dirty	>40% of the foot to hock distance is contaminated and/or the hooves are soaked in mud
Udder is free of dirt	Udder is slightly dirty (2 to 10% dirty)	Udder is dirty (10 to 20% of the surface)	>30% of the udder is coated with caked on dirt

Figure 40.4 Hygiene scoring system DairyCo Mastitis Control Plan.

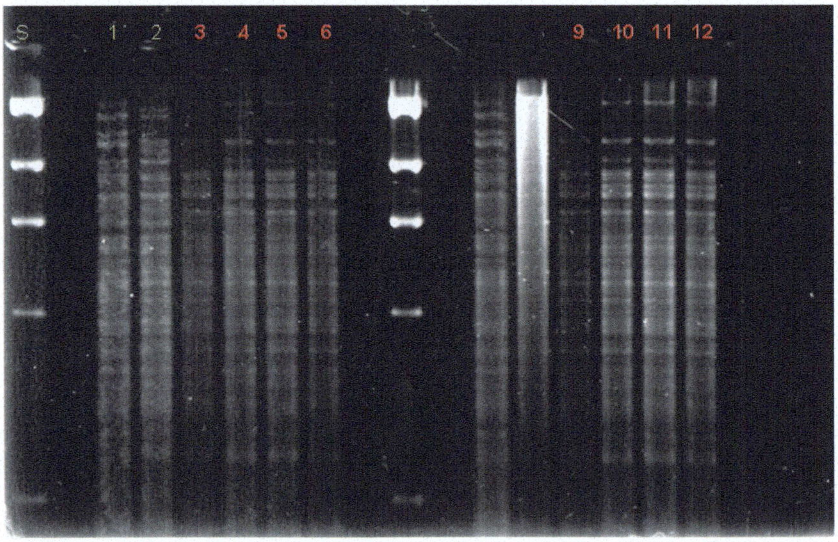

Figure 40.5 Molecular strain typing techniques such as Pulse Field Gel Electrophoresis (PGFE).

- Dung channel: number of times a day scraped out.
- Overcrowding: stocking rate.
- General hygiene: overall cleanliness.
- Humidity/ventilation.

Housing yards

- Bedding: sand, straw, sawdust, recycled paper.
- Bedding material application frequency and frequency of complete cleaning out.
- Water trough position: wet bedding.
- Access points in and out of bedded area.
- Overcrowding: stocking rate.
- General hygiene: overall cleanliness.
- Humidity/ventilation.

Infection profile

Data analysis and risk analysis gives a good insight into actual and likely transmission patterns leading to a herd-level diagnosis. However, recent advances in molecular strain typing has the potential to give further insights into the epidemiology of the bacteria involved.

The infection profile in a herd is made up from the various bacteria identified from IMIs in the herd and, just as importantly, the specific characteristics of the identified bacteria. The distribution of the bacterial species involved in IMIs gives an indication of the likely predominant transmission patterns on the farm. Many species involved might suggest an environmental problem. However, the presence of any one individual bacterial species is not sufficient information to make a herd diagnosis on the infection transmission pattern.

The isolation of one species with persistent infections and contagious abilities, such as *S. agalactiae*, would imply contagious problems for the herd, while the isolation of many species might imply environmental problems. However, the identification of *S. agalactiae* in a herd does not necessarily imply a contagious mastitis problem until the prevalence and transmission patterns have been evaluated. If the prevalence of IMIs with *S. agalactiae* in the herd is very low, or molecular strain typing identifies it as *S. agalactiae* of human origin, with little 'cow adaptation' or contagious spread, then the isolation of *S. agalactiae* may be of minor significance at a herd level.

Equally, if *Kebsiella* spp. is identified as the predominant cause in a clinical mastitis outbreak, and molecular strain typing shows a clonal (few strains) rather than non-clonal (multiple strains, typical of infections of environmental origin) infection transmission pattern with persistent infections, it is highly likely that contagious spread is occurring with a pathogen which is classically described to behave in an environmental manner.

Molecular strain typing techniques, such as Pulse Field Gel Electrophoresis (PGFE) (Figure 40.5), Matrix Assisted Laser Desorption/IonizationTime of Flight Mass Spectrometry (MALDI-TOF MS), and micro-arrays, have the potential to identify persistent infections within a quarter of the time, and shed light on transmission patterns.

References

Bradley, A.J., Breen, J.E. and Green, M.J. (2008). Mastitis pattern analysis – a fresh look at the analysis of bovine mastitis: Part 2 – clinical mastitis data. *UK Vet* **13**, 1–5.

Dufour, S., Frechette, A., Barkema, H.W., Mussell, A. and Scholl D.T. (2011). Effect of udder health management practices on herd somatic cell count. *Journal of Dairy Science.* **94**, 563–579.

FAWC (1997). *Report on the Welfare of Dairy Cattle.*

Green, M.J., Bradley, A.J., Medley, G.F., and Browne, W.J. (2007). Cow, Farm and Management Factors during the Dry Period that Determine the Rate of Clinical Mastitis after Calving. *Journal of Dairy Science* **90**, 3764–3776.

Schreiner, A. and Ruegg, P.L. (2003). Relationship between udder and leg hygiene scores and subclinical mastitis. *Journal of Dairy Science* **86**, 3460–3465.

Schukken, Y.H., Schmitt-van de Leemput, E., Moroni, P., Welcome, F., Gurjar, A., Zurakowski, M., Gutierrez, C., Ceballos, A. and Zadoks, R. (2012). *Keynote address 27th Proceeding World Buiatrics*, Lisbon, pp. 145–148.

Further reading

Biggs, A. (2009). *Mastitis in Cattle*. The Crowood Press.

Blowey, R.W. and Edmondson, P. (2010). *Mastitis Control in Dairy Herds*, 2nd edition. Farming Press.

Useful websites

BMC: proceedings of conferences, 1998: www.iah.bbsrc.ac.uk/bmc/index.html

BCVA: proceedings, 1993– with membership: www.bcva.org.uk/

NMC: proceedings, factsheets, resources, some without membership: www.nmconline.org/

AABP: proceedings, factsheets, resources, some without membership: www.aabp.org/

IDF: www.fil-idf.org/Content/Default.asp

IAH: www.iah.ac.uk/

UKVet: www.ukvet.co.uk/

NOAH: www.noah.co.uk/

Dutch Udder Health Centre: www.ugcn.nl/

Canadian Bovine Mastitis Research Network: http://www.mastitisnetwork.org/

CHAPTER 41

The Farm Audit: Foot Health, Lameness and Footcare

Nick Bell

Learning objectives

- Appreciate the prevalence and incidence of lameness in dairy herds.
- Appreciate the impact of lameness on welfare, dry matter intake, milk production and fertility.
- Appreciate the direct and indirect economics costs of lameness.
- Understand the importance of mobility scoring as part of a herd lameness management programme.
- Appreciate the importance of early detection and early, effective treatment.
- Appreciate the need and value of preventative and corrective foot-trimming.
- Appreciate the importance of foot hygiene and dry conditions under foot.
- Understand the relationships between lameness and cow time budgets.
- Understand the relationship between lameness and movement methods, distances, surface type and turning movements.
- Understand the importance of transitional cow and heifer management in reducing the risk of lameness.
- Appreciate the importance of conformation and breeding in reducing the risk of lameness.
- Be able to perform an on farm audit of foot health, lameness and footcare.

Introduction

Lameness in dairy cattle is often a complex, multifactorial and dynamic disease, complicated by a variable lag period between cause and the lameness event. Often, lameness is a culmination of several events over the lifetime of the animal, making it a difficult disease for producers to establish the true aetiology and risk factors, and hence correctly identify appropriate control measures. The lameness audit must involve robust assessment of current performance, a review of past events and past performance, and an evaluation of future risks relating to the environment, the type of cow and management. The role of the advisor involves understanding and explaining how the risks are likely to interact to identify cost-effective control points.

Past and current performance

Lameness in dairy herds affects productivity, animal welfare and hence is a quality assurance issue. Various studies have highlighted a high prevalence of lameness, with an apparent rising trend from 16.3% in a US springtime assessment in 1993 (Wells *et al.*, 1993) to 37% more recently in the UK (Barker *et al.*, 2010). Meanwhile, lameness incidence reports are more variable, according to how much formal screening for lameness was used (Archer *et al.*, 2010). Prevalence studies probably quantify lameness more accurately and are more consistent with lameness risk factors, which have intensified on the majority of farms in the last 30 years although, in the absence of epidemiological surveys, the true direction of the trend line remains speculation.

Ultimately, lesion incidence (Table 41.1), gathered with a minimum of monthly screening, remains the most robust way of identifying current trends at farm, nati\nbonal and international levels. This approach will more clearly identify emerging challenges such as the severe, necrotic claw lesions associated with digital dermatitis (Evans *et al.*, 2011). This data allows lesions to be analysed by season and parity, with first lactation animals representing useful cohorts for evaluating current risk factors.

Bovine Medicine, Third Edition. Edited by Peter D. Cockcroft.

Table 41.1 Foot lesion incidence rates (new and repeat limb cases per 100 cows per year) for the three most common lesions affecting dairy cows in the UK.

Lesion causing lameness	Reported and calculated[a] incidence rates cases/100 cows/year (and range‡)	Authors
Sole ulcer	12.2	Rowlands *et al.*, 1983
	15	Clarkson *et al.*, 1996[a]
	13.8	Hedges *et al.*, 2001
	6.2 (0-28.5‡)	Barker, 2007
White line disease	3.8	Rowlands *et al.*, 1983
	12.2	Clarkson *et al.*, 1996[a]
	12.7	Hedges *et al.*, 2001
	5.5 (0-30.7‡)	Barker, 2007
Digital dermatitis	n/a	Rowlands *et al.*, 1983
	4.5	Clarkson *et al.*, 1996[a]
	12.0	Hedges *et al.*, 2001
	2.8 (0-69.5‡)	Barker, 2007

[a]Incidence rate was not reported, but limbs affected and numbers of cows could be used to calculate incidence rate.

Mobility scoring (locomotion or lameness scoring)

Without formal training and regular herd scoring for lameness, the dairy producer's estimate of lameness in their herd can be very inaccurate (Wells *et al.*, 1993; Whay *et al.*, 2003). Whay *et al.* (2003) reported a farmer assessment mean prevalence of 5.7% in their dairy herds; the actual mean prevalence recoded following an assessment in these herds was 22.1%.

Without formal screening, the manager can remain focused on dealing with the severely lame cows visible at the back of the herd at milking, rather than being aware of the cows that are mildly or moderately lame in the middle of the mob. Emerging evidence suggests that most cows transition through mild and moderate stages of lameness before becoming severely lame (Stoye *et al.*, 2014) and, for most lesions, the long term cure rate following correct treatment is vastly improved if treated early (Groenevelt *et al.*, 2014).

The process of mobility scoring involves an assessor observing cows from the side and rear while they walk past. This is often done when the cows are entering or exiting the milking parlour. The assessor uses a standard assessment framework to categorise the cows according to the severity of the signs observed. The spectrum of severity of lameness can make its quantification challenging. Assessing the incidence of specific disorders causing lameness may be inherently flawed if there are no internationally agreed thresholds for lameness and no standardised screening approaches.

Nonetheless, establishing baseline prevalence is a fundamentally important starting point when working with a producer and numerous scoring methods are in use (Whay, 2002). Each scoring system comes with a varying degree of complexity, with scores based on a small number of behavioural signs being easiest for producers to learn, but composite scores based on the full range of behaviours associated with lameness, showing the highest levels of sensitivity and specificity (Flower & Weary, 2002; O'Callaghan *et al.*, 2002). In general, scoring methods use the signs of pain, which include walking at a slower speed, a shortened stride length, an arched back and diminished weight-bearing of affected limbs.

As mobility scoring does not rely on the accuracy of farm records it is a useful starting point for any foot health audit or investigation. For ongoing evaluation, mobility scoring should occur at least four times a year to capture seasonal variation. For enhanced screening of lame cows, scoring at least fortnightly is recommended, although some herds with observant stockmen spotting cows between scoring sessions can manage with monthly intervals or without formal screening at all.

Mobility scoring generates valuable information about which cows to prioritise for treatment by the farm staff (mild lameness and first aid treatment), foot trimmer (routine trims generally) or the veterinary surgeon (lesions requiring extensive debridement or surgery under local anaesthesia). Target values can be set for this parameter and comparative benchmarking can be performed against other similar farms. Some dairy herd health assurance schemes have mobility scoring as a requirement.

A five-category mobility scoring system adapted from Sprecher *et al.* (1997) is presented in Table 41.2 and Figure 41.1. Some of the production losses associated with scores and target values are indicated in Table 41.3. A four-category mobility scoring system adopted in the UK is presented in Table 41.4.

If mobility scores are performed on a regular basis it is possible to categorise the cows in the herd into four categories: not lame; new cases; recovered cases; and chronic cases, according to their relative mobility score on the current (CR) and previous (PR) mobility recording session (Archer *et al.*, 2010). Whichever mobility scoring system is used, the cows are classified as lame or not lame. In the case of the Sprecher system, cows > score 2 (3, 4, 5) would be classified as lame (1), while cows with a score less than or = score 2 (1, 2) would be classified as not lame (0). Each cow is then placed in one of the four categories as follows: PR 0 CR 0 – Not Lame; PR 0 CR 1, New Case; PR 1 CR 0; Recovered. PR 1 CR 1; Chronic. When plotted over time, the dynamics of these four categories can be monitored and trends identified.

Where there is a good consistency between lameness prevalence and recorded incidence, then herd foot trimming and lameness records may be of some value for evaluating lesion incidence. There is international agreement on the terms used for the 15 most common primary foot lesions that producers and foot trimmers should be able to visually recognise (Archer *et al.*, 2010). The commonest lesions show reasonable levels of repeatability (Manske *et al.*, 2002). Laminitis does not feature

Table 41.2 The modified Sprecher five-point mobility scoring system (adapted from Sprecher, 1997; Robinson & Juarez 2011).

Score	Clinical stage	Back standing	Backmoving	Favouring a leg	Gait
1	Normal	Flat	Flat	No	Normal
2	Mildly lame	Flat	Arch	No	Normal
3	Moderately lame	Arch	Arch	No	Shortened stride
4	Lame	Arch	Arch	Yes Bears weight	Abnormal
5	Severely lame	Arch	Arch	Yes Reluctant to bear weight	Abnormal

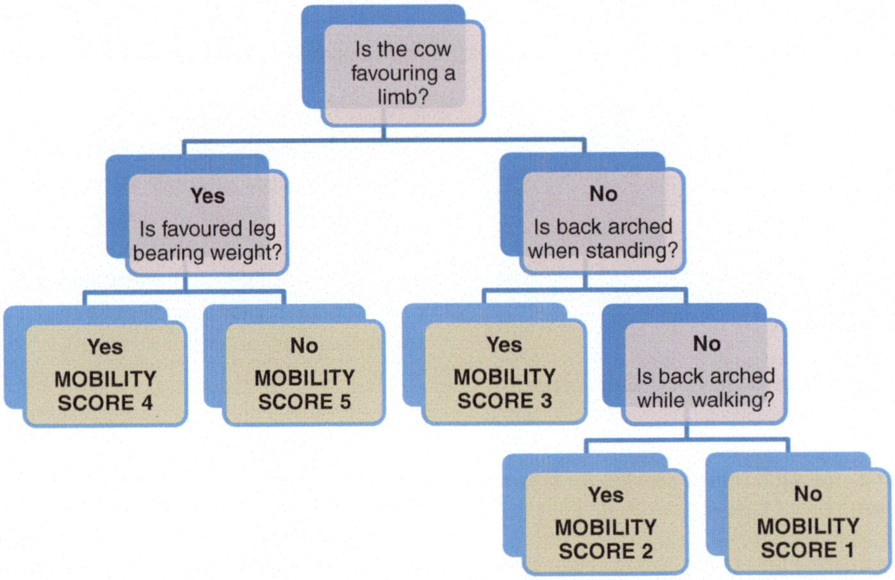

Figure 41.1 How to score cows using the modified Sprecher five-point system (adapted from Sprecher, 1997; Robinson & Juarez 2011)

Table 41.3 The modified Sprecher five-point mobility scoring system – impacts on production and target values (adapted from Robinson & Juarez, 2011).

Score	Clinical stage	Reduction in dry matter intake %	Reduction in milk yield %	Fertility relative risk increase	Target % of herd	Intervention thresholds
1	Normal	0	0		75.0	
2	Mildly lame	1	0	>2	15.0	
3	Moderately lame	3	5	Days to first service	9.0	3 + 4 + 5
4	Lame	7	17	2.8	0.5	>10%
5	Severely lame	16	36	Days open	0.5	4 + 5 > 5%)
				15.6		
				Services/conception 9.0		

on the list, as it is not a term associated with a single visible lesion causing lameness; it represents a disease pathogenesis rather than a lesion causing lameness, and there is still great uncertainty as to whether this disease process occurs commonly in cattle, despite it being frequently discussed.

While it is important to understand the cost of lameness through use of published literature on productivity losses and treatment costs (Esslemont, 2005; Willshire & Bell, 2009), a sense of pride in seeing improvement in herd health may well be sufficient for motivating most producers, who are aware that lameness is costly for their businesses (Leach *et al.*, 2010).

Relating lameness risk factors to past and future events

In the last ten years, there has been a significant shift in understanding of the aetiology and pathogenesis of claw horn lesions,

Table 41.4 The four-point mobility scoring system (adapted from DairyCo).

Score	Mobility	Gait	Suggested action
0	Good	Walks with even weight bearing and rhythm on all four feet with a flat back.	• No action. • Routine (preventative) foot trimming when/if required.
1	Imperfect	Steps uneven (rhythm or weight-bearing) or strides shortened; affected limb or limbs not immediately identifiable.	• May benefit from routine (preventative) foot trimming when/if required. • Further observation recommended.
2	Impaired	Uneven weight-bearing on a limb and is immediately identifiable and/or obviously shortened strides (usually with an arch to the centre of the back).	• Lame and likely to benefit from treatment. • Foot should be lifted to establish the cause. • Should be attended to as soon as practically possible.
3	Severely impaired	Unable to walk as fast as a brisk human pace (cannot keep up with a healthy herd) and signs of score 2.	• Very lame. • Cow will benefit from treatment. • Requires urgent attention, care and further professional advice. • Cow should not be made to walk far and kept on a straw yard or grass. • In the most severe cases culling may be the only possible solution.

from a predominantly nutritional and laminitis associated disease process to a primary biomechanical aetiology. The robustness of the claw is influenced by digital cushion thickness (itself affected by changes in body condition score), as demonstrated by Bicalho *et al.* (2009a), underfoot moisture and slurry consistency (Logue, 1999), and horn quality, in part affected by the ingestion of certain vitamins such a biotin (Hedges *et al.*, 2001), as well as trauma. Claw horn growth rates are influenced by dietary carbohydrate and crude protein levels, among other factors (Vermunt & Greenough, 1995), but claw shape can be managed by appropriate claw trimming regimes. This shift in understanding has had profound implications for the priorities to be reviewed within the lameness audit, which should have an appropriate balance of environmental, managemental (including a broad consideration of feeding and cow behaviour at the feed barrier) and animal assessments. Whenever possible, performance should be assessed using suitable animal-based outcome measures, with an evaluation of future risk and more detailed troubleshooting when performance needs improving. The usual topics to be reviewed at lameness audit could include those outlined in Table 41.5, which are usually best assessed at milking *and* between milkings.

Early detection and early, effective treatment

Lameness is invariably caused by a variety of diseases and, in most instances, cows will not recover without treatment. In a 60 herd study assessing risks for lameness in first lactation, delays to treatment and factors resulting in ineffective treatment was the largest risk factor for severe lameness (Bell *et al.*, 2009). Delays to treatment will allow lesions causing lameness to progress to more chronic and, in some instances, irreversible states involving bony exostoses (Blowey & Inman, 2012), often affecting more than one limb. The ability of the farm team to promptly detect and skilfully treat lameness will have a marked affect on controlling levels of severe lameness where there has been a problem.

Early detection and early, effective treatment risk assessment:

- Is lame cow spotting performed as a dedicated task on a routine basis (at least fortnightly, if not daily) by someone who is capable of recognising lameness (but independent of foot trimming)?
- Are cows easily and clearly identifiable from a distance?
- Are lesions caught at an early stage prior to deep, well-established infections within the foot?
- Are the persons performing routine foot trimming and lame cow treatments competent, if not proficient, and are these people available on any day of the year?
- Is skilled labour provision sufficient to cope with numbers of lame cow and routine foot trims?
- Are facilities sufficient for throughput of animals in a manner safe for operator and animal, with time necessary for treating more challenging cases?

Routine preventative and corrective foot trimming

The high-yielding dairy cow managed predominantly indoors will typically experience excessive net claw horn growth (growth exceeds wear). Increased toe length in relation to the heel depth,

Table 41.5 Topics to review at a lameness audit. To conduct the audit, the assessor must evaluated lameness prevalence, lesion incidence, foot and leg lesions in a sample of animals, cow flow, standing times and various farm staff activities. This is usually best done by making observations at around milking, and assessing foot health at trimming.

Area of husbandry	Measure of performance (ideally outcome measures)
Early detection and early, effective treatment	Severe lameness prevalence Chronic lameness prevalence Overall lameness prevalence
Routine foot trimming	Toe length and other aspects of foot shape Proportion of cows receiving a scheduled trim Proportion of cows lame within one month following a scheduled trim
Foot hygiene and dry conditions underfoot	Foot cleanliness score
Routine foot disinfection (foot bathing)	Digital dermatitis size score and grade (in infected herds)
Lying behaviour (lying comfort)	Actual lying times and number/duration of bouts Hock swelling and ulceration *At different sites around shed*: Behaviour of cows as they interact with cubicles (rising restrictions) Standing index/cow comfort index Cubicle use index Cubicle occupancy
Penning times	Turnaround time at milking for each group at each milking, measured from moment of first disturbance to when cows returned to beds (and feed/water)
Cow flow at milking and other times	Cow behaviour and time to move between areas (watching for raised head behaviour and concrete slips) Mean/median group stocking rates and maximum group stocking rates
Walking surfaces	Slip rates on walking surface Patterns of foot lesion found at foot trimming (routine and lame cow trims) Slow cow flow in spite cows having room to pass each other comfortably
Youngstock management	Lameness prevalence and sole ulcer incidence in first lactation
Feed barrier design and management	Behavioural observations and feed position of cows at feed barrier High prevalence of front foot lameness relative to hind feet (>10%)
Feeding	Body condition score and body condition score loss in early lactation
Breeding	Review of family predispositions
Transition cow management	All risks coinciding during the transition period

reducing foot angle, often starts prior to first calving. Sole overgrowth and medio-lateral claw imbalance will be most common in early lactation. Exceptions are the extensively managed cow walking long distances on tracks. Vermunt & Greenough (1995) reviewed factors contributing to claw wear and growth.

When there is little or no claw overgrowth and a low incidence of lameness, then foot trimming is unnecessary and may even be harmful. However, lame cows with claw horn lesions will require some therapeutic foot trimming, and housed herds will invariably experience toe overgrowth, sole overgrowth or an imbalance of medial and lateral claws. If left uncorrected, then claw overgrowth has a tendency to worsen and foot angle becomes flat, raising the risk of lameness. In situations when wear exceeds growth, then cows develop lesions causing lameness, such as thin soles, sole bruising, sole penetrations, white line lesions and toe ulcers. When wear and growth are both very high, such as cows housed on coarse sand, soles may be worn flat. On units with high wear and sole trauma, abaxial wall wear, with a characteristic overgrowth of the central sole area, is observed (Telezhenko *et al*., 2009).

Toe length, foot angle, medio-lateral claw imbalance, sole overgrowth and heel erosion can all be assessed at milking in most parlours. Toe length is undoubtedly the easiest feature to score, with the aid of a simple measuring guide. It is important to allow some degree of interpretation, as optimal toe lengths vary with age and breed (first lactation heifers have short toes relative to cows). Cull cows may be left out of recent trim events, and some lame cows will have pathologically larger claws, which cannot be corrected.

An alternative, and perhaps better, means of assessing the need for trimming and the effectiveness of current on farm practices is to examine some feet lifted in the foot-trimming facilities. This allows an assessment of the entire trimming process, from shedding cows, loading into the crush, the ease

Table 41.6 Possible timings of routine foot trimming.

Timing	Rationale
4–8 weeks before first calving	Correct foot angle and overgrowth prior to highest risk period in the animal's productive life. Most benefit for animals on high plains of nutrition, especially if loose on straw yards or similar without scraped concrete feed barriers.
60–80 days after first calving 80–180 days after calving (multiparous cows)	To correct sole overgrowth and foot angle after the period when horn overgrowth has occurred in response to sole bruising and trauma in the fresh period.
Drying off (up to 2 weeks before to 4 weeks after)	Correct foot angle and overgrowth prior to highest risk period.
Before turn-out	Spring calving herds.
Midwinter	Autumn calving herds.

with which a cow is restrained and the foot lift, the skills of the personnel performing the foot trimming and finally the validity of the lameness data captured.

Optimal timing of foot trimming will vary according to individual animal factors and some seasonal variation. Foot checks (feet lifted and claws trimmed if necessary) are typically performed at certain points through a cow's life, but the evidence for optimal generic timings is lacking. Over-trimming is a real hazard that needs careful monitoring. Table 41.6 outlines some common timings of foot checks.

The most widely adopted foot trimming technique is the Dutch five-step method, as summarised in Table 41.7, with various proposed modifications. For cows that are never housed, then steps 1–3 become obsolete. Assessing the skills of the personnel conducting routine trims and lame cow treatments will require a detailed understanding of optimal foot trimming methods. The evidence base for treatment protocols is still weak (Potterton *et al.*, 2011).

Routine preventative and corrective foot trimming risk assessment:

- Mismatch of foot trimmer availability and scheduled routine trim.
- Poor facilities and maintenance of equipment.
- Not following principles of Dutch five-step foot trimming: common faults include over-trimming of soles, axial wall, abaxial wall and/or heels.
- Extended calving intervals.
- Extended intervals between trims.
- High levels of carbohydrate and protein in diet.
- Old, smooth concrete.
- Extensive use of rubber matting on walkways or loose housing without exposure to some abrasive floor surfaces.
- Very abrasive walking surfaces, including asphalt, acid-eroded concrete, abrasive cow tracks or coarse sand bedding.

Foot hygiene and dry conditions underfoot

Moisture and slurry underfoot are substantial risk factors for infectious disorders such as digital dermatitis, as well as reducing the robustness of the claw by eroding heel horn and softening the sole or the white line horn. However, cost-effective interventions after buildings have been erected can be difficult to determine.

Foot hygiene and dry conditions underfoot risk assessment:

- Narrow, overstocked alleys preventing cow flow, creating congested areas and being prone to slurry build-up.
- Automatic scrapers.
- Alleys in housing without a 2–3% fall.
- Pools of slurry or water present in the house or walkways.
- Incomplete scraping in general or in specific areas.
- Poorly drained tracks, gates or troughs in fields.

Routine foot disinfection (foot bathing)

Inevitably cows feet come into contact with slurry and pooled water or urine contaminated with faecal matter. For any cow this presents a risk, particularly if digital dermatitis is endemic within the herd. Animals may be susceptible by virtue of genetic predisposition (Scholey *et al.*, 2010, 2012), age (naivety), periparturient immunosuppression, bovine viral diarrhoea or other immunosuppressive states.

Numerous biocidal agents appear efficacious for use within foot bath (Laven & Logue, 2006; Bell *et al.*, 2014). Local legislative restrictions may mean that only certain biocides are licensed for use on-farm.

When evaluating foot bathing protocols, it is important to check that an appropriate disinfectant or treatment is being used, that the concentration is correct, that the baths are being renewed at the correct intervals and that there is a correct frequency of use. This will inevitably mean checking the dimensions of the foot bath, watching cows walk through the solution to ensure that feet are being exposed to solution, and reviewing levels of disease on feet.

As the frequency of use appears to be important for many herds, finding ways of making foot bathing part of the milking routine is important for compliance. Including dry cows and, when relevant, youngstock as part of a foot bathing regime, may also be extremely important for gaining overall control of infection.

Routine foot disinfection (foot bathing) risk assessment:

- Infection uncontrolled in youngstock.
- No foot bathing of dry cows.
- No proactive treatment of active lesions other than foot bathing.
- Use of a biocide that does not tolerate faecal contamination.

Table 41.7 Dutch five-step method, adapted from Toussaint Raven (1985).

Steps	Instruction	Illustration
1a	Trim toe length to the correct length, starting with the medial claw of hind feet and lateral claw of front feet. Healthy claws should be measured from where the claw horn is firm at the coronary band and, as a guide, will measure for Holstein Friesians: • 7 cm at 22–24 months old; • 7.5–8 cm for mature animals.	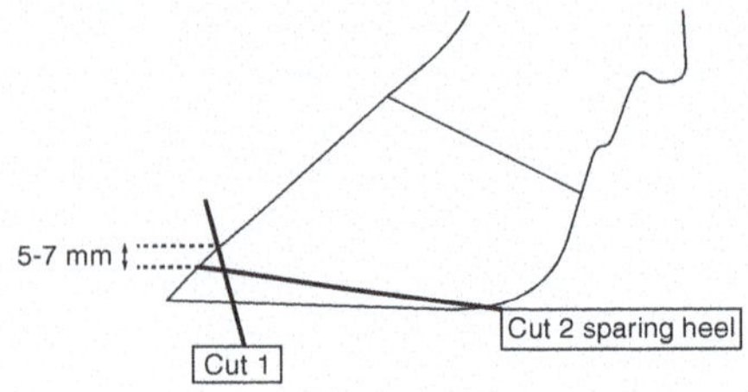
1b	Reduce thickness of sole at toe to 5–7 mm, sparing the heel, while creating a stable weight-bearing surface from and across the toe. Extra toe thickness should be allowed if there is dorsal wall curvature which is not straightened.	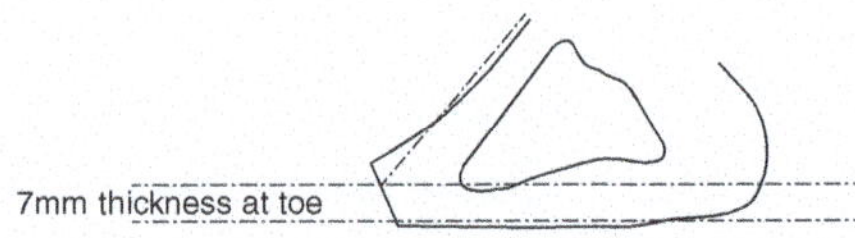
2	Restore balanced weight bearing between medial and lateral claws, but not at all costs.	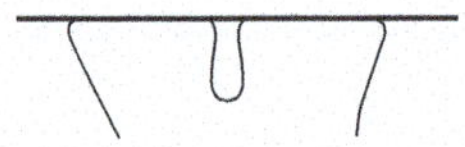
3	Hollow out the central sole region sufficiently to allow materials to drain from the inter-digital space and for weight-bearing surface to be transferred from the lateral hind claw to the wall.	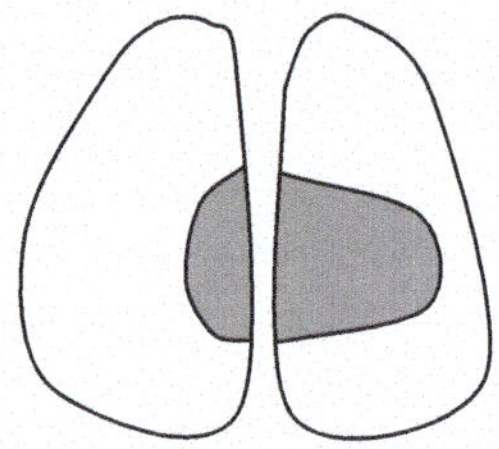
4	If a painful lesion present, create a difference in heel height through use of an orthopaedic block on a sound claw or by trimming down the plantar two-thirds of the lateral hind claw or palmar two-thirds or the medial foreclaw.	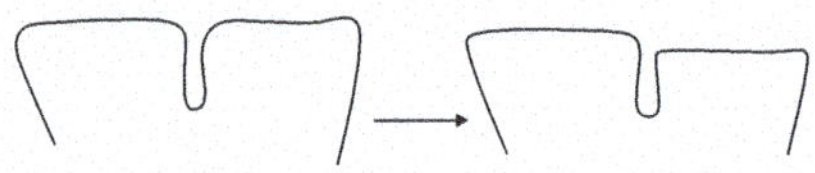
5	Remove loose horn, ridges of horn and fissures of heel erosion. Trimming should be conservative, restricted to the heel of the medial hind claw and not within the toe triangle of the lateral hind claw.	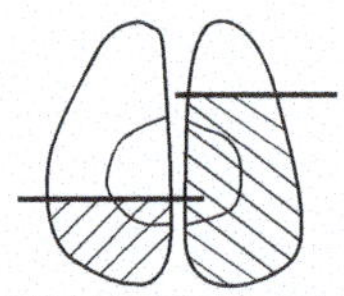

- More than one cow per litre of foot baths solution remaining prior to replenishment.
- Low concentration of biocides used (in relation to standard recommendations).

Assessing lying behaviour (lying times)

Total lying time and normal distribution of lying bouts through the day can be important for the prevention of some claw horn lesions, such as sole ulcers and white line lesions, and possibly for productivity. Lying times can be measured directly, and new technology allows potentially sophisticated analysis. Without tools for individual or herd measurement, then other spot measures, such as standing index, need to be used (Cook *et al.*, 2005).

Bed surface appears to be highly important, and hock swelling may give indications of bed cushioning (although slipping in yards, mycotoxicosis and *Mycoplasma bovis/weyonii* may occasionally be implicated) while hock ulceration may indicate a problem with surface abrasiveness. Stocking rates over

100% will result in reduced lying times (Fregonesi *et al.*, 2007). However, there may be many other important limiting factors affecting lying behaviour which could be more significant, such as bed comfort or cubicle dimensions. Aspects of cubicle divider design include neck rail position, obstruction in the forward lunge or bob space, and bed width. Heat stress and windy conditions will influence lying behaviour. In addition to lying comfort, any factors resulting in differential preference for beds may cause problems of competition, displacement and disturbance and, hence, reduced lying times.

Lying behaviour (lying times) risk assessment:

- Anything other than deep, dry bedding systems (deep sand, straw, wood chip, recycled manure are generally best).
- Evidence of hock injury or Beds hard to knee test.
- Infrequent bedding, exposing hard lying surfaces.
- Cubicle or building fixtures that interferes with lying down or rising (lunge and bob behaviour).
- Differential preferences – differences in bed cushioning, differences in bed dimensions, exposure to varying climatic conditions (winds or intense sun).
- Poor ventilation or heat abatement.
- Variations in stocking rate (beds, feed, water or yard space).

Penning times and time budgets

Estimating standing times at milking and for other events can be useful in estimating if time budgets for milking cows are being compromised. Time budgets published by Cook *et al.* (2004) can be used to estimate a maximum penning time. However, prolonged penning represents a risk, and some cows can tolerate prolonged standing times if pressures on other elements of the time budget are low. For example, a low-yielding cross-breed, managed with low stocking rates and excellent lying comfort, can tolerate more standing at milking than a high-yielding Holstein, zero-grazed and given a hard rubber mat with sawdust bedding system.

Penning times and time budgets risk assessment:

- Large milking groups (particularly if groups merged, say, during a summer grazing period).
- Slow milking staff/milking routines.
- Feeding and bedding up not done during milking.
- Systems involving one man moving cows, cleaning beds, milking cows, bedding and feeding.
- Shutting all cows off beds to allow teat end closure for 30 minutes after the last cow is milked.
- Overstocked feed barrier.
- Narrow feed passage, cubicle passages, or cross-passages.
- Blind-ending passages.
- Infrequent cross-passages especially if passageways are deemed narrow.
- Long pens times for AI, PD, foot trimming or other routine health events.
- Long pen times during mucking-out.
- Unnecessarily long lock-up times with locking yokes.
- Waiting to cross roads or other groups of cows.

Cow flow at milking and other times

When cows are forced to move, as invariably happens at milking, some cows demonstrate flight behaviour, not only from the personnel fetching cows, or dogs if they are used, but also from more dominant cows, when they are forced into closed proximity. Chesterton (2004) found patterns of lameness due to white line disease differed in first lactation heifers, compared with multiparous cows. Heifers had more lesions in front medial claws, typical of injuries incurred through escape manoeuvres, while multiparous cows had lesions of the hind feet, more likely to occur as cows drove their way through other cows. Fixed period observations of cow behaviour at herding can identify the frequency with which flight behaviours and slip events are occurring in relation to human, dog or cow pressures.

The speed with which cows move from housing or fields to the collecting area reveals deficiencies in walking comfort (see later) and other obstacles causing bottlenecks. A short delay due to a bottleneck in cow flow on a single day is of little significance but, multiplied up two or three times daily for months or years, it can represent a substantial labour expense, as well as a source of lameness. Examples might include a poorly placed water trough on a track bend, a 90-degree turn in a walkway, or a physical narrowing.

In the collecting yard, cows may move voluntarily into the milking parlour or may require force, through use of a physical or electric backing gate. Clearly, the backing gate is undesirable for foot health, as forced movements cause foot trauma. Methods of enticing cows into the parlour requires cows to be receiving compound in the parlour, or cows must be hungry and seeking food after milking. Unpleasant experiences, like poorly adjusted milking equipment, stray voltage or an aggressive milker, can quickly undo any enticement.

Re-training herds can be troublesome, but observations of cows in the collecting yard, and as they enter the parlour, can reveal personnel behaviours impeding cow flow, slowing up milking and causing foot lesions. It can appear counterintuitive that providing generous space for cows to stand in the collecting yard allows cows to enter more quickly, but the space provides room for re-ordering from herding order to milking order, and prevents congestion at the entrance to the parlour. Repeated fetching of cows inevitably results in cows turning and foot trauma. Personnel should be made aware of the risk of claw trauma when cows are raising heads above the rumps of other cows. Rubber matting may mitigate the trauma to some degree, but any source of cow flight behaviour should be strongly discouraged.

As cows exit the parlour, then the same principles of flow apply, with 90 or 180 degree turns and physical or behavioural bottlenecks being common findings. Foot baths and sorting gates may be sited too close to the parlour, preventing dispersal and overtaking as necessary. Again, rubber matting may reduce the impact of trauma. Rubber yard mats appear most beneficial for increasing the speed with which cows move away from the parlour after milking.

The importance of cow flow also applies to cow sheds. Cows will spend most of their time lying down and feeding. Most cow traffic will be between these areas. The balance between alley widths and cross-passage frequency and width remains a best guess in the absence of any data on cow movements. Most old sheds have alley widths that easily block as cows turn behind feeding or perching cows. A common source of obstruction is bulling cows. When cows are provided with $3\,m^2$ of separate loafing area, then many of the bulling cows prefer to spend time in these areas. Overall, Holsteins should have at least $4\,m^2$ per cow of concrete alleys, but typically $7\,m^2$ per cow allows cow flow and slurry depths to be better managed in twice daily milking routines.

Other aspects of housing design that can have a major effect on cow flow have already been covered in lying comfort. Recommendations for water trough space are stated as enough for 10% of the herd to drink at once (6–10 cm per cow in group). Perhaps the siting of water, and ensuring sufficient flow of clean, palatable water is more important, with regular cleaning, as well as encouraging cows away from bottlenecks in the cow flow around buildings. Commonly, they are sited on narrow cross-passages. Water troughs sited in high-demand areas, such as on the parlour exit, need to have a large dispersal area and high water pressure, to prevent congestion associated with waiting cows.

Cow flow at milking and other time budgets risk assessment:

- Hurried herding by personnel or, worse still, dog or person in vehicle.
- Backing gates, particularly electric.
- No bell or buzzer on backing gate.
- No CCTV or automatic cut-off on backing gate.
- Herd expansion ahead of facility provision.
- Batch calving, resulting in overstocked transition pens.
- Mismatch between stocking rates, particularly feed barrier and bed space.
- Long penning times, which adds pressure to densely stocked sheds.
- High stocking rates for groups containing freshly calved cows and first lactation heifers.
- Reliance on outdoor space at times when weather may be unsuitable.
- Sub-optimal Transition cow management.

Walking surfaces

Slats are a significant risk to foot health, despite the advantages of being able to manage slurry and minimise the pooling of moisture and slurry. The disadvantages of slats may be mitigated to a large degree with rubber matting. The findings from concrete-slatted systems allow some degree of extrapolation of risk to various patterns of concrete groove, which remain largely uninvestigated. Old, grooved concrete has been found to be a risk factor for lesions such as white line.

New concrete can represent a significant hazard. The concern about the caustic nature of lime in new concrete remains unproven. The common usage of high pH desiccants in beds should cast serious doubt over the validity of this theory. However, the physical roughness, abrasiveness and pointedness of some textures set into new concrete represents a significant hazard to claws, and requires careful evaluation.

Cow track surfaces and management of cows on them is a significant risk factor for white line lesions, sole penetrations and thin soles.

Walking surfaces risks assessment:

- Slatted concrete without rubber.
- Grooved or harshly patterned concrete.
- Abrasive concrete, particularly combined with a sharp (non-marine) ballast.
- Sharp or large stone on tracks.
- Long distances walked.
- Poor drainage, resulting in mud and pools of water or slurry.

Youngstock management

First lactation heifers are particularly vulnerable to new cases of lameness. The size and severity of claw lesions at lesion scoring increases at each and every lactation, but overall deterioration is largest in first lactation (Offer *et al.*, 2000). This may be due to an under-developed digital cushion (Raber *et al.*, 2006), due to heifers being unaccustomed to using facilities such as cubicles, or due to low social ranking, resulting in displacement from feed or lying space.

Youngstock management risk assessment:

- No or insufficient cubicle training prior to the transition period.
- Heifers calving under- or over-conditioned.
- Heifers coming in straight from pasture onto concrete immediately after calving.
- Heifers grouped with lactating cows.

Feed barrier design and management

Relatively little research has been done on the impact of feed barrier design and management on foot health. De Vries *et al.* (2004) demonstrated that stocking rates influence the number of negative interactions, and Endres *et al.* (2005) showed that barrier designs with divisions between feed positions also help reduced bullying behaviours. Other aspects of feed barrier design, including height of feed base, the position of neck rail and frequency of pushing up feed have not been well investigated. Blackie *et al.* (2011) showed that lame cows delay feeding behaviour until after sound cows had fed, presumably to reduce chances of negative interactions.

Feed barrier design and management risk assessment:

- Insufficient feed space (stocking rates under 0.7 m feeding width space per Holstein Friesian).
- Overstocked fresh pen.
- Narrow feed passage (cows unable to pass in both directions and feed simultaneously).
- If not using feed troughs, then not pushing up 4–8 times per day.

Feeding

With the recent shift in understanding of the aetiology of claw horn lesions, it is easy to overlook some significant feeding-related risk factors. Sub-acute ruminal acidosis is still considered by many to be the explanation for why foot health improves with biotin supplementation at 20 mg/head/day (Hedges *et al.*, 2001). Any practices that result in significant body condition score loss, particularly in the period between calving and peak yield, will significantly increase the risk of claw lesions (Bicalho *et al.*, 2009b). This could include the feeding of high crude protein and carbohydrate levels to drive milk production, rather than achieve yield through high dry matter intakes. The consistency of the slurry will also affect foot cleanliness, thereby influencing infection pressure for conditions such as digital dermatitis and interdigital necrobacilosis.

Feeding risk assessment:

- Adverse behaviour of cows at the feed barrier (displacement, competing or stretching for feed).
- Any feeding practices resulting in extreme BCS loss, thin cows, sub-acute ruminal acidosis and loose faeces.
- Diets unbalanced, deficient or outside recommended safe limits, particularly for starch/carbohydrate, crude protein, minerals and biotin.

Breeding

Many producers have been selecting for leg set and foot angles for many generations, and the evidence would suggest, with current indices, that this looks unlikely to keep pace with the increasing risk to foot health (Stott *et al.*, 2005). Locomotion, as a selection index, may have improved the situation slightly, but the evidence is lacking. The provision of alternative indices with positive health traits may provide a solution to this problem in future, but is not easy to evaluate on farm. In the meantime, there is little that can be done to evaluate risk, other than to be aware of sires to avoid.

Some breeds and cross-breeding may provide a more immediate solution for some producers, but the impact of these approaches remains unquantified. Genomics may offer a technological solution, particularly for conditions like digital dermatitis, predisposition to which appears to be coded for on a number of defined single nucleotide polymorphisms (Scholey *et al.*, 2010).

The main area which the veterinarian can evaluate with respect to breeding is the effectiveness of the culling policies. Dams with lameness or poor conformation of a genetic nature should not be re-bred or, at the very least, should be served using beef semen. Ultimately, the facilities and management can often be improved to account for the changing genotype of the modern dairy cow, and decisions about breeding are often more related to productivity to maintain production for the business. Nonetheless, there is an important role for the vet to make clients aware of the need to successfully match standards of management and resources to the increasing needs of the modern dairy cow, in order to be profitable from this approach.

Breeding risk assessment:

- Inbreeding and line breeding.
- Use of known, high risk bulls.
- Insufficient replacement heifers to operate a culling policy for foot health.

Transition cow management

The transition period is the period when changes occur to the suspensory apparatus within the foot; when cows enter negative energy balance; when cows are less likely to lie down; when they have to adjust to sudden social changes, resulting in alterations in rank; and when immunosuppression is most likely. It should come as no surprise that minimising the risks during transitions can reduce the devastating interactions that lead to lameness in later lactation and then subsequent lactations thereafter. The lameness advisor should use this understanding to emphasise the importance of management during this period.

Final comment

Many lesions causing lameness become chronic and irreversible. Improving lameness without extensive culling requires several years of consistently improved management and effective preventative measures. Measuring performance, especially in first lactation heifers, will demonstrate improvements, but expectations need managing from an early stage to avoid disappointment, as lameness control programmes take several years to develop fully and achieve tangible results.

References

Archer, S., Bell, N.J. and Huxley, J.N. (2010). Lameness in UK dairy Cattle: A review of the current situation. *In Practice* **32**, 492–504.

Barker, Z.E. (2007). *Epidemiology of Lameness in Dairy Cows.* PhD thesis, Warwick.

Barker, Z.E., Leach, K.A., Whay, H.R., Bell, N.J. and Main, D.C.J. (2010). Assessment of lameness prevalence and associated risk factors in dairy herds in England and Wales. *Journal of Dairy Science* **93**, 932–941.

Bell, N.J., Bell, M.J., Knowles, T.G., Whay, H.R., Main, D.C.J. and Webster, A.J.F. (2009). The development, implementation and testing of a lameness control programme based on HACCP principles and designed for heifers on dairy farms. *Veterinary Journal* **180**, 178–188.

Bicalho, R.C., Machado, V S. and Caixeta, L.S. (2009a). Lameness in dairy cattle: A debilitating disease or a disease of debilitated cattle? A cross-sectional study of lameness prevalence and thickness of the digital cushion. *Journal of Dairy Science* **92**, 3175–3184.

Bicalho, R.C., Machado, V.S. and Caixeta, L.S. (2009b). Lameness in dairy cattle: A debilitating disease or a disease of debilitated cattle? A cross-sectional study of lameness prevalence and thickness of the digital cushion. *Journal of Dairy Science* **92**, 3175–84.

Blackie, N., Amory, J.R., Bleach, E. and Scaife, J. (2011). The effect of lameness on lying behaviour of zero grazed Holstein dairy cattle. *Applied Animal Behaviour Science* **134**, 85–91.

Blowey, R.W. and Inman, R. (2012). Is there a case for reassessing hoof-trimming protocols? *Veterinary Record* **171**, 592–593.

Chesterton, R.N. (2004). *Linking farm physical conditions, herd management and cow behaviour to the distribution of foot lesions causing lameness in pasture-fed dairy cattle in New Zealand*, pp.200–202. Maribor, Slovenia.

Clarkson, M.J., Downham, D.Y., Faull, W.B., Hughes, J.W., Manson, F.J., Merritt, J.B., Murray, R.D., Russell, W.B., Sutherst, J.E. and Ward, W.R. (1996). Incidence and prevalence of lameness in dairy cattle. *Veterinary Record* **138**, 563–567.

Cook, N.B., Bennett, T.B. and Nordlund, K.V. (2004). Effect of free stall surface on daily activity patterns in dairy cows with relevance to lameness prevalence. *Journal of Dairy Science* **87**, 2912–22.

Cook, N.B., Bennett, T.B. and Nordlund, K.V. (2005). Monitoring indices of cow comfort in free-stall-housed dairy herds. *Journal of Dairy Science* **88**, 3876–3885.

DeVries, T.J., von Keyserlingk, M.A.G. and Weary, D.M. (2004). Effect of Feeding Space on the Inter-Cow Distance, Aggression, and Feeding Behaviour of Free-Stall Housed Lactating Dairy Cows. *Journal of Dairy Science* **87**, 1432–1438.

Endres, M.I., DeVries, T.J., von Keyserlingk, M.A.G. and Weary, D.M. (2005). Short Communication: Effect of Feed Barrier Design on the Behaviour of Loose-Housed Lactating Dairy Cows. *Journal of Dairy Science* **88**, 2377–2380.

Esslemont, R. (2005). The costs of lameness in dairy herds. *UK Vet* **10**, 41–49.

Evans, N.J., Blowey, R.W., Timofte, D., Isherwood, D.R., Brown, J.M., Murray, R., Paton, R.J. and Carter, S.D. (2011). Association between bovine digital dermatitis treponemes and a range of 'non-healing' bovine hoof disorders. *Veterinary Record* **168**, 214.

Flower, F. and Weary, D. (2002). Testing measures of lameness: Using behaviour to predict presence and severity of hoof lesions in dairy cattle. *Journal of Dairy Science* **85**, 247.

Fregonesi, J.A., Tucker, C.B. and Weary, D.M. (2007). Overstocking reduces lying time in dairy cows. *Journal of Dairy Science* **90**, 3349–3354.

Hedges, J., Blowey, R.W., Packington, A.J., O'Callaghan, C.J. and Green, L.E. (2001). A longitudinal field trial of the effect of biotin on lameness in dairy cows. *Journal of Dairy Science* **84**, 1969–1975.

Laven, R.A. and Logue, D.N. (2006). Treatment strategies for digital dermatitis for the UK. *The Veterinary Journal* **171**(1), 79–88.

Leach, K.A., Whay, H.R., Maggs, C.M., Barker, Z.E., Paul, E.S., Bell, A.K. and Main, D.C.J. (2010). Working towards a reduction in cattle lameness: 1. Understanding barriers to lameness control on dairy farms. *Research in Veterinary Science* **89**, 311–317.

Logue, D.N. (1999). Report on the workshop on the biology of lameness (Funded by MDC & Scottish Office). *Cattle Practice* **7**, 321.

Manske, T., Hultgren, J. and Bergsten, C. (2002). Prevalence and interrelationships of hoof lesions and lameness in Swedish dairy cows. *Preventive Veterinary Medicine* **54**, 247–263.

O'Callaghan, K.A., Cripps, P.J. and Murray, R.D. (2002). Behavioural indicators of pain associated with lameness in dairy cattle. *Research in Veterinary Science* **72**, 10.

Offer, J.E., McNulty, D. and Logue, D.N. (2000). Observations of lameness, hoof conformation and development of lesions in dairy cattle over four lactations. *Veterinary Record* **147**, 105–109.

Potterton, S., Bell, N.J., Whay, H.R., Main, D.C.J. and Huxley, J.N. (2011). *A Review of the Peer Reviewed Literature on the Treatment and Prevention of Foot Lameness in Cattle Published Between 2000 and 2011* [Online]. DairyCo. Available at: http://www.google.co.uk/url?sa=t&rct=j&q=&esrc=s&frm=1&source=web&cd=1&ved=0CDMQFjAA&url=http%3A%2F%2Fwww.dairyco.org.uk%2Fnon_umbraco%2Fdownload.aspx%3Fmedia%3D10391&ei=riCeUZTvGqTl4QTiiID4Bg&usg=AFQjCNF3lmTzwo6xqJxuXg3X648aDEOB-w&sig2=ecIkAKiZ5b8AoiMMAvXsKA&bvm=bv.46865395,d.bGE (Accessed 23/5/13).

Raber, M., Scheeder, M.R.L., Ossent, P., Lischer, C.J. and Geyer, H. (2006). The content and composition of lipids in the digital cushion of the bovine claw with respect to age and location – a preliminary report. *Veterinary Journal* **172**, 173–7.

Robinson, P.H. and Juarez, S.T. (2011). *Locomotion Scoring Your Cows: Use and Interpretation.* Department of Animal Science University of California, Davis, CA.

Rowlands, G.J., Russel, A.M. and Williams, L.A. (1983). Effects of season, herd size, management system and veterinary practice on the lameness incidence in dairy cattle. *Veterinary Record* **113**, 441–445.

Scholey, R.A., Ollier, W.E.R., Blowey, R.W., Murray, R.D. and Carter, S.D. (2010). Determining host genetic susceptibility or resistance to bovine digital dermatitis in cattle. *Advances in Animal Biosciences* **1**, 2–2.

Scholey, R.A., Blowey, R.W., Murray, R.D., Smith, R.F., Cameron, J., Massey, J.P., Ollier, W.E. and Carter, S.D. (2012). Investigating host genetic factors in bovine digital dermatitis. *Veterinary Record* **171**, 624.

Sprecher, D.J., Hostetler, D.E. and Kaneene, J.B. (1997). A lameness scoring system that uses posture and gait to predict dairy cattle reproductive performance. *Theriogenology* **47**, 1179–1187.

Stott, A.W., Coffey, M.P. and Brotherstone, S. (2005). Including lameness and mastitis in a profit index for dairy cattle. *Animal Science* **80**, 41–52.

Telezhenko, E., Bergsten, C., Magnusson, M. and Nilsson, C. (2009). Effect of different flooring systems on claw conformation of dairy cows. *Journal of Dairy Science* **92**, 2625–2633.

Toussaint Raven, E. (1985). *Cattle footcare and claw trimming*. Farming press Ltd, Suffolk, UK.

Vermunt, J.J. and Greenough, P.R. (1995). Structural characteristics of the bovine claw: horn growth and wear, horn hardness and claw conformation. *British Veterinary Journal* **151**, 157.

Wells, S.J., Trent, A.M., Marsh, W.E. and Robinson, R.A. (1993). Prevalence and Severity of Lameness in Lactating Dairy-Cows in a Sample of Minnesota and Wisconsin Herds. *Journal of the American Veterinary Medical Association* **202**, 78–82.

Whay, H. (2002). Locomotion scoring and lameness detection in dairy cattle. *In Practice* **24**, 444–449.

Whay, H.R., Main, D.C.J., Green, L.E. and Webster, A.J.F. (2003). Assessment of the welfare of dairy cattle using animal-based measurements: direct observations and investigation of farm records. *Veterinary Record* **153**, 197–202.

Willshire, J.A. and Bell, N.J. (2009). An Economic Review of Cattle Lameness. *Cattle Practice* **17**, 136–141.

CHAPTER 42

Reproductive Technologies: On-Farm Applications

Tim Parkinson

Learning objectives

- Appreciate how oestrus detection can be improved.
- Understand how the oestrous cycle can be synchronised and manipulated.
- Appreciate the advantages and limitations of oestrus synchronisation and fixed-time AI programmes.
- Understand how ovarian superstimulation can be achieved, and the expected outcomes.
- Appreciate the factors which influence the outcomes of artificial insemination, including the use of sexed semen.
- Be familiar with embryo collection and transfer techniques and the expected outcomes.
- Be familiar with *in vitro* embryo production and the expected outcomes.

The aim of this chapter is to provide veterinarians with the learning outcomes to be able to give appropriate advice with regards to the on-farm applications of reproductive technologies.

Oestrus detection and its improvement

Detection of behavioural oestrus

Prediction of the fertile period of the bovine oestrous cycle has traditionally relied upon detection of behavioural changes that occur around the time of ovulation, particularly sexual receptivity ('oestrus behaviour'), which can be observed as willingness to allow the male to approach and mount and, uniquely amongst domestic animals, female-to-female mounting. Cows also show other behavioural changes, such as social association with cows that are in a similar reproductive status (formation of 'sexually active groups'), a decline in time spent feeding, and increased locomotion and vocalisation.

There are also physiological changes associated with the follicular phase, such as changes in the characteristics of reproductive-tract mucous secretions and a nadir of circulating progesterone concentrations, which also have the potential to allow detection of oestrus. In addition, the timing of oestrus can be controlled pharmacologically, which can be used to allow insemination at a time that is based upon the predicted state of the ovarian cycle rather than upon any direct observation of the cow. Observation of oestrus behaviour forms the mainstay of oestrus detection programmes and, in turn, depends upon:

- The observational skills of the stock manager;
- The timing, place and frequency of observations;
- Accurate recording of cows' identities;
- The ability and willingness of the cow to display oestrus;
- The size and calving pattern of the herd.

Oestrus detection rate is closely related to the herd's reproductive outcomes (notably its submission, conception and final pregnancy rates). Likewise, poor oestrus detection accuracy (i.e. in terms of false positive rate) can markedly impair first service conception rates (Morton, 2000). Oestrus detection rates are relatively low for herds that calve all year round, and the figures reported by Kinsel & Etherington (1998) of a mean detection rate of 48% and a range of 23–64% for Canadian dairy herds would be typical. These low rates are due, at least in part, to smaller sexually active groups (van Vliet & van Eerdenburg, 1996), the difficulty that many herd managers experience in maintaining concentration upon oestrus detection over a long period of time, and the pressure of other farm tasks that have to be done every day (O'Connor, 2007). Conversely, oestrus detection rates in seasonally calving herds can often be in excess of 90% (Morton, 2000), primarily because of the large sexually active groups and the short period of time over which oestrus detection has to be undertaken.

The effectiveness of oestrus detection is generally increased by observing cows in situations in which they are likely to display oestrus (Plate 42.1) which, in turn requires that they are likely to be undisturbed, such as while in cubicle yards, 'loafing'

Bovine Medicine, Third Edition. Edited by Peter D. Cockcroft.

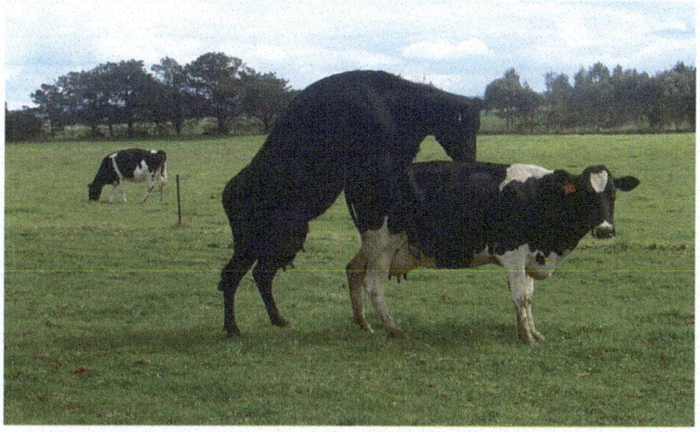

Plate 42.1 Oestrus is best detected when cows are undisturbed. At pasture, once cows have finished grazing, is one of the best situations for oestrus detection. Reproduced with kind permission from J Malmo.

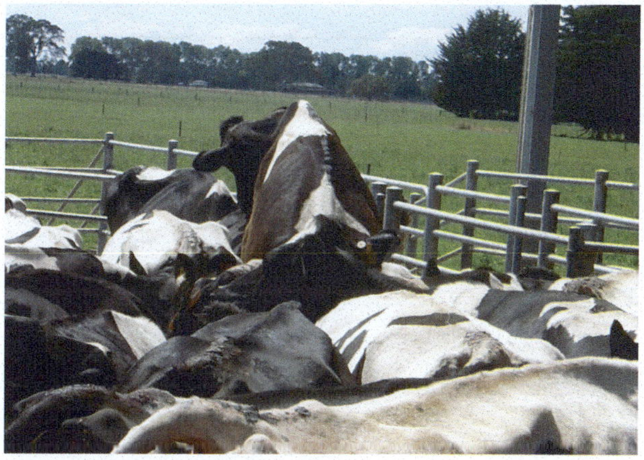

Plate 42.2 Accurate oestrus detection in collecting yards is difficult to achieve. Cows are less likely to display oestrous behaviour, it is difficult to record identities, and it is often unclear whether the cow that is being mounted is standing voluntarily. Reproduced with kind permission from J Malmo.

areas, or at pasture (Esslemont & Bryant, 1976). Conversely, cows are less likely to display oestrus behaviour when held in collecting yards, during milking, when feeding or when moving along farm tracks (Pennington *et al.*, 1986), and it is more difficult to accurately identify cows that are in oestrus under such circumstances (Plate 42.2). Slippery conditions underfoot and poor quality cubicle housing, with low ceiling heights, are also associated with poorer display of oestrus behaviour. It is commonly held that cows more commonly display oestrus by night than by day; while this may be true, it is more likely due to being undisturbed by other farm activities by night, rather than to an intrinsic diurnal pattern of behaviour (Albright & Arave, 1997). Thus, the absolute time of observation is not critical, but it is essential to avoid periods during which the cows are disturbed. Two to four observation sessions, each of 15–30 minutes duration, critically, of undisturbed cows, can achieve oestrus detection rates of 75–85%, even in year-round calving herds.

Recent years have seen a progressive decline in the intensity of oestrus behaviour. The duration of oestrus has decreased, the number of mounts has declined and the duration of each mount has reduced, to the extent that a significant proportion of cows fail to display classic oestrus behaviour during the follicular phase of the cycle. One of the methods that has been suggested for combating this decline is formalising the observation secondary behaviours associated with oestrus (van Vliet & van Eerdenburg, 1996), to provide an overall 'score' (Table 42.1).

Table 42.1 Scoring scale for observed signs of oestrus behaviour (van Vliet & van Eerdenburg, 1996). Reproduced with permission of Elsevier.

Oestrus signs	Scoring scale
Non-mounting signs	
Mucous vaginal discharge	3
Cajoling	3
Restlessness	5
Sniffing of the vagina of other cow	10
Resting with chin on other cow	15
Mounting signs	
Mounted by other cow but not standing	10
Mounting (or attempting) other cows	35
Mounting headside of other cow	45
Standing heat	100

With 2–3 × 30 minute observation periods per day, oestrus is deemed to occur when a minimum total of 50 points is accumulated over a 24 hour period.

Improving oestrus detection

The negative consequences of poor oestrus detection upon herd reproductive performance and, consequently, upon farm profitability, has been repeatedly presented over a great many years. Even so, failure to understand (or perhaps to act upon) this relationship is often the core issue affecting herds with poor reproductive performance. Thus, Sprecher *et al.* (1995) noted that herds with reproductive problems characteristically either: failed to maintain adequate breeding records; failed to observe for oestrus on a daily basis; failed to separate oestrus detection from working on other farm tasks; or had underfoot conditions that were so poor that cows would not display oestrus behaviour. Other problems, unrelated to oestrus detection, included poor control of body weight and poor management of post-partum uterine infections.

Thus, the first means by which oestrus detection can be improved is to ensure that herd managers detect oestrus properly and keep proper records. O'Connor (2007) re-emphasised the importance of ensuring the responsibility for oestrus detection is assigned to an (named) individual, who has been adequately trained. Nothing changes, however; as long ago as the 1970s, Esslemont was showing the greater effectiveness of oestrus detection by trained versus untrained staff (Esslemont, 1974).

Table 42.2 Aids to the detection of oestrus in cows. Based on Parkinson *et al*. (2010).

Method	Use	Advantages	Disadvantages
Based upon mounting behaviour			
Tail paint (Plate 42.3)	Paint applied over the tail head is removed when cows are mounted by each other.	Improves results from visual detection alone.	Needs considerable experience to decide if cows with partially removed paint are actually in oestrus.
Heat-mount detectors (e.g. KaMar, Bulling Beacon)	Capsule applied over the tail head is broken when the cow is mounted, turning the capsule red.	Gives a more clear-cut result than tail paint in cows that are only mounted a few times.	Capsule can burst by rubbing, or if a cow is unable to avoid a single mount when she in not in oestrus.
Oestrus detection patches (e.g. Estrotect) (Bonato *et al*., 2012)	Patch applied over tail head; removal of surface layer reveals a bright undercolour when the cow is mounted.	Gives a more clear-cut result than tail paint, but fewer false positives than capsules.	Missed oestrus events can occur when devices are not checked or are rubbed in cubicles.
Electronic heat mount detectors (e.g. Heatwatch) (Palmer *et al*., 2010)	Applied over tail head; records mounts electronically.	Accurate provided cows stand to be mounted.	Relatively expensive as it requires specialized equipment.
Teaser bulls	Chin-bull marker shows which cows have been mounted.	Positive indication of oestrus.	Presence of intact bulls in the herd, bulls become disinterested with time, small risk of spreading venereal disease.
Based upon increased activity			
Pedometers	Increased walking activity is measured as an indicator of oestrus.	Improves results above what is commonly achieved by visual detection.	Relatively expensive as it requires specialized equipment; moderate sensitivity and specificity.
Neck-mounted activity monitors (e.g. Heatime) (Aungier *et al*., 2012)	Increased movement activity is measured as an indicator of oestrus.	Improves results above what is commonly achieved by visual detection.	Relatively expensive as it requires specialized equipment; moderate sensitivity and specificity.
Based on physiological changes			
Method	**Use**	**Advantages**	**Disadvantages**
Milk progesterone	Monitor cycle and do fixed time AI when concentration falls.	Very accurate if done carefully.	Expensive. Inaccurate if not done carefully.
Vaginal mucous resistance	Daily monitoring of vaginal resistance.	Independent of behavioural signs.	Invasive.
Milk composition and temperature	In-line measurement during milking.	Fully automated, so minimizes requirement for human observation.	High capital input. Validation of results is not complete.

Aids to oestrus detection

Once basic aspects of stockmanship have been addressed, there are a variety of aids that can be used to help improve oestrus detection (Table 42.2, Plate 42.3).

Methods based on the detection of mounting activity (e.g. tail paint, heat mount detectors) are, of course, predicated upon the assumption that mounting actually does occur. This is by no means a given in the light of the overall reduction in duration and intensity of oestrus expression, and the further reduction in the intensity of mounting behaviour in housed versus pastured cows (Palmer *et al*., 2010). Likewise, the effectiveness of activity-based monitors can be limited by circumstances such as tie-stall housing (Felton *et al*., 2012), or even the duration of grazing, and the distance from between paddocks and the milking shed (Sakaguchi, 2011).

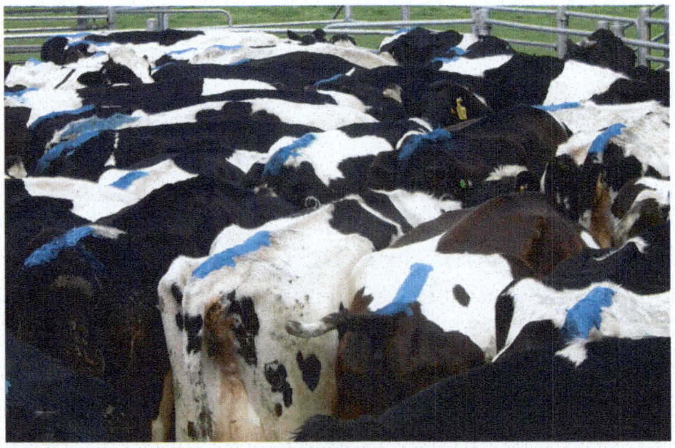

Plate 42.3 A herd of cows with tail paint freshly applied. Reproduced with kind permission from J Malmo.

Thus, while technological aids can augment behavioural observations, their accuracy, in terms of both false positive and false negative detections of oestrus, suggest that they are not yet in themselves better than well-managed behavioural detection. Importantly, though, the results that are achieved by most technological aids to oestrus detection are much better than national average oestrus detection rates based on observation alone. In this context, Holman *et al.* (2011) showed that combining data from observation and activity monitors gives detection efficiency improved from than either method alone, while Morton (2000) similarly showed that combining the use of tail paint with behavioural observation gives better result than either method in isolation (Table 42.3).

Manipulation and synchronisation of the oestrous cycle

Oestrus synchronisation and fixed-time AI programmes

In year-round calving intensive systems, the twin problems of low conception rates and low oestrus detection rates result in simply not getting enough cows pregnant: oestrus detection rates of ≈50%, combined with conception rates of ≈30%, mean that pregnancy rates per cycle of around 15% are by no means uncommon. In these circumstances, there are substantial benefits to using protocols that synchronise ovulation and allow for fixed timed AI (FTAI) without oestrus detection (Bo & Mapletoft, 2012). In seasonally calving, pasture-based systems, in which post-partum feed supply is usually the limiting factor in reproductive performance, treatment of cows in anovulatory anoestrus is often the main concern, since achieving 365-day calving intervals remains imperative in these systems to synchronise feed demand with pasture supply. Regardless of this, it is preferable that treatment regimens can both induce oestrus in anoestrous cows and synchronise it in cycling cows.

The basis of the mode of action of prostaglandin $F_{2\alpha}$ for oestrus synchronisation is that it causes luteal regression. Removal of the negative feedback effect of progesterone upon luteinising hormone (LH) allows ovulation of the next dominant follicle. Because such systems rely upon the removal of an active *corpus luteum*, they require that cattle are cycling. The most common variant is double administration of $PGF_{2\alpha}$ (typically 11 days apart; Figure 42.1a), which ensures that there is a responsive *corpus luteum* at the time of the second treatment.

While there are many slightly different permutations of time intervals between treatments, all $PGF_{2\alpha}$–based protocols suffer from the common limitation that the interval between $PGF_{2\alpha}$ administration and oestrus/ovulation is quite variable. This is largely because such regimes mostly fail to control the development of the follicular wave. Hence, FTAI at a single time is generally too imprecise for good conception rates so, more than one FTAI is needed, often in addition to observation to detect the 10–15% of animals that come into oestrus later than expected. Despite these shortcomings, where $PGF_{2\alpha}$-based protocols are used in animals that are known to be cycling (e.g. well-grown maiden heifers), or in combination with limited oestrus detection, they can significantly advance mean conception date in seasonal (Figure 42.1b) and non-seasonal (Figure 42.1c) herds.

Control of the follicular wave appears to be critical to the success of oestrus synchronisation and induction programmes, primarily in order to ensure that the time of ovulation is regulated, with enough precision to give acceptable conception rates after breeding by a single FTAI. In principle, the follicular wave is controlled by:

1 Ablating the dominant follicle that is present at the start of the programme;
2 Inhibiting ovulation until the new dominant follicle has developed;
3 Precisely controlling the time of ovulation of that follicle (Wiltbank *et al.*, 2011; Figure 42.2).

A pre-existing dominant follicle can be removed either by causing it to regress or to ovulate. Older oestrus synchronisation regimes used oestradiol to cause follicular regression, but withdrawal of the use of oestradiol esters in cattle means that these protocols are no longer used in the EU. Alternatively, gonadotropin-releasing hormone (GnRH) is given to induce an LH surge, which causes ovulation and, thereby, removes the dominant follicles. The GnRH also induces follicle stimulating hormone (FSH) surges, which recruits a new cohort of follicles to start a new follicular wave. Luteinisation of the ovulated follicle causes a rise in progesterone concentrations (Pursley & Martins, 2012), which, by maintaining LH concentrations at basal values, precludes ovulation during the follicular growth phase.

In some programmes, especially those used in deeply anoestrous cows (in which the presence of an LH-responsive follicle at the start of the programme is by no means certain), progesterone concentrations are maintained or augmented by the use of an intravaginal progesterone-releasing insert (Stevenson *et al.*, 2006; McDougall, 2010). Progesterone concentrations are

Table 42.3 Oestrus detection practices and detection rates in seasonal-calving herds. Reproduced with permission of Dairy Research and Development Corporation.

Heat detection practices used	% of herds having high (>94%) estimated heat detection rates
Neither paddock checks nor HMD used	32%
Paddock checks but not HMD used	50%
HMD but not paddock checks used	59%
Both paddock checks and HMD used	89%

HMD: heat mount detector.
From Morton (2000).

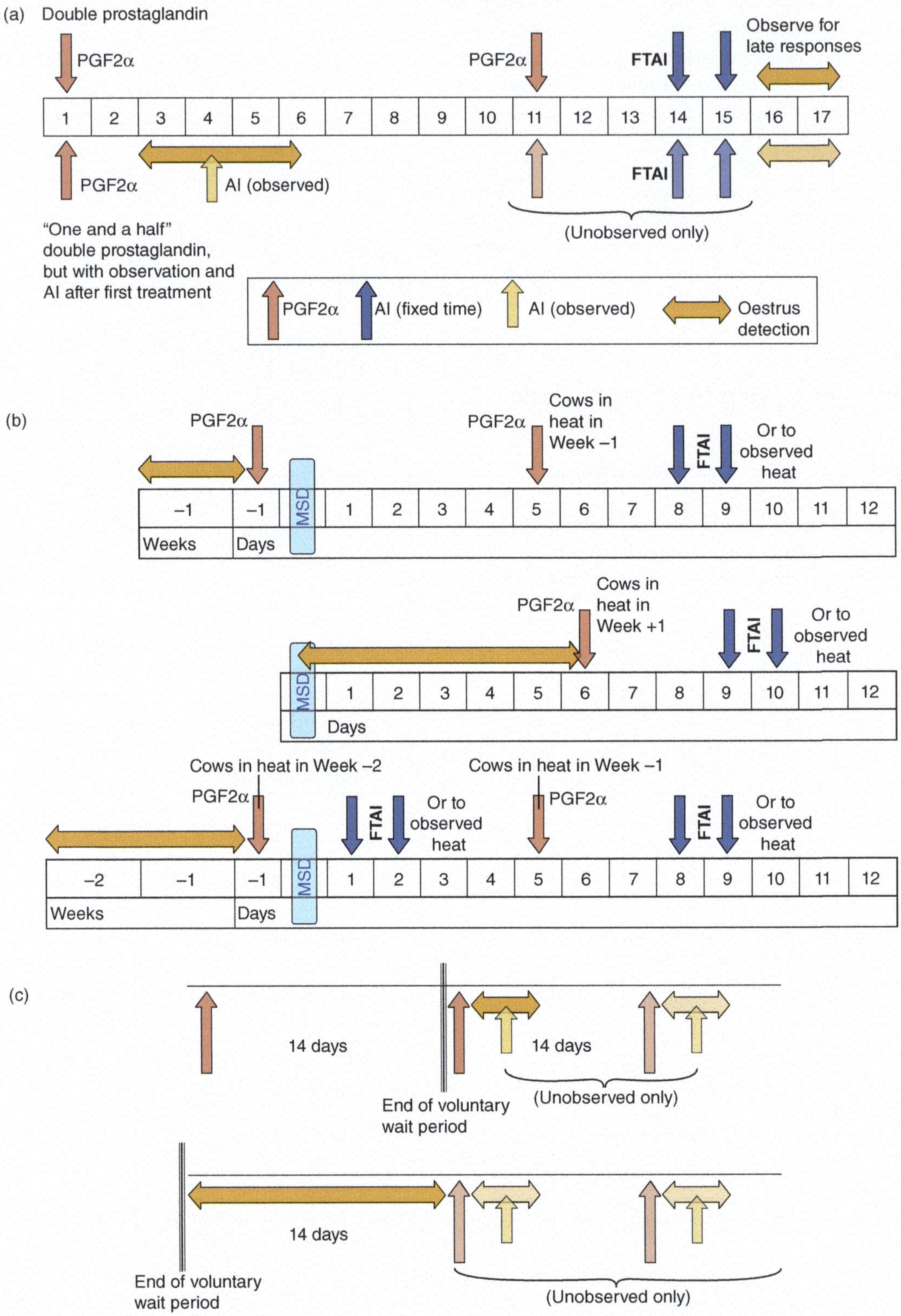

Figure 42.1 a) Standard 11-day double $PGF_{2\alpha}$ oestrus synchronisation programme, using fixed time AI (above) or oestrus detection and insemination after the first PG administrations (below). b) $PGF_{2\alpha}$-based oestrus synchronisation programmes for use in seasonal-calving herds: single 'why wait' (upper), modified 'why wait' (middle) and double 'why wait' (lower). Insemination to detected oestrus usually results in better conception rates than does fixed time insemination. MSD = mating start date. Adapted from Morton *et al*. 2003. c) $PGF_{2\alpha}$-based oestrus synchronisation programmes for use in non-seasonal calving herds. 'Aggresive prostaglandin' (upper). Cows not detected in oestrus after the $PGF_{2\alpha}$ given at the end of the voluntary wait period are re-treated 14 days later. 'Regular prostaglandin' (below): cows not inseminated within 14 days of the end of the voluntary wait period are treated with PG (and every 14 days thereafter until they conceive). Adapted from Morton *et al*. 2003.

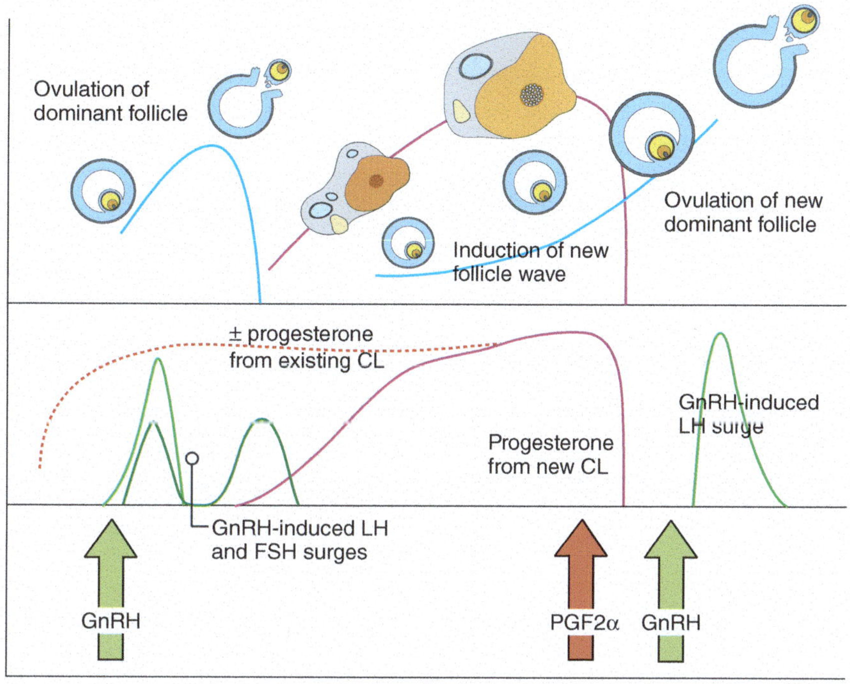

Figure 42.2 Mechanism of action of GnRH-PGF2α-GnRH (GPG, Ovsynch) protocols for synchronising oestrus in cattle.

thereafter abruptly reduced by administration of $PGF_{2\alpha}$ and/or removal of the intravaginal insert. Finally, ovulation is caused by a second dose of GnRH, given 48–56 hours after the $PGF_{2\alpha}$. Such protocols ('GPG' or 'Ovsynch'), form the basis for most current oestrus synchronisation and induction programmes. There are many variants on this basic theme, some of which are summarised in Figure 42.3.

Ovsynch programmes can improve herd fertility by:

- Removing the need for oestrus detection
- Increasing the number of cows that are inseminated per cycle
- Probably, but not conclusively, increasing per-service conception rate.
- Reducing the calving to conception interval

Per-service conception rates to FTAI after a GPG programme vary according to breed, dairying system and time post-partum. For example, in intensively managed North American Holstein cattle, figures of between 30–5% are common (e.g. DeJarnette & Marshall, 2003; Colazo *et al.*, 2009), whereas McDougall (2010) achieved rates of >60% in Jersey/Holstein-Friesian cattle managed at pasture. Body condition score has a substantial effect: conception rate in cows with BCS ≤ 2.75 (1–5 scale) was 23% versus 53% in cows with BCS >2.75 (Galvao & Santos, 2010).

The response to GPG is highly dependent upon the stage of the follicular wave at the start of the programme, largely as it determines whether or not ovulation of the dominant follicle occurs in response to the first GnRH. If the follicle does not ovulate, it may persist through the treatment regimen and eventually ovulate in response to the second GnRH – or, it may regress at an unpredicted time, resulting in unregulated emergence of the next follicular wave and ovulation of an immature oocyte. Fertility in both of these circumstances is poor.

Secondly, it depends upon the progesterone concentrations after ovulation, such that fertility appears to be highest when the progesterone secreted by an existing *corpus luteum* is augmented by the GnRH-induced *corpus luteum*. All of these factors seem to be ideal when the GPG programme is started on days 5–9 (and are optimal when started on days 6 or 7) of the cycle; ≈90% of cows ovulate when GnRH is given within this time window, versus <50% during the remainder of the cycle (Wiltbank *et al.*, 2011). In order to improve the chances of a cow being on days 5 or 6 of the cycle at the start of a GPG programme, various methods of 'pre-synchronisation' have been developed (Figure 42.4). These add materially to the cost and, because of their complexity, can result in non-compliance with treatment regimes. However, they are advocated for the improvements in synchronisation and fertility that they provide.

The only comprehensive meta-analysis of the responses to oestrus synchronisation programmes is that undertaken by Raibee *et al.* in 2005, using trials completed up to 2003. Outcomes were very variable between trials, but there were small improvements in the relative risk (RR) of pregnancy (final

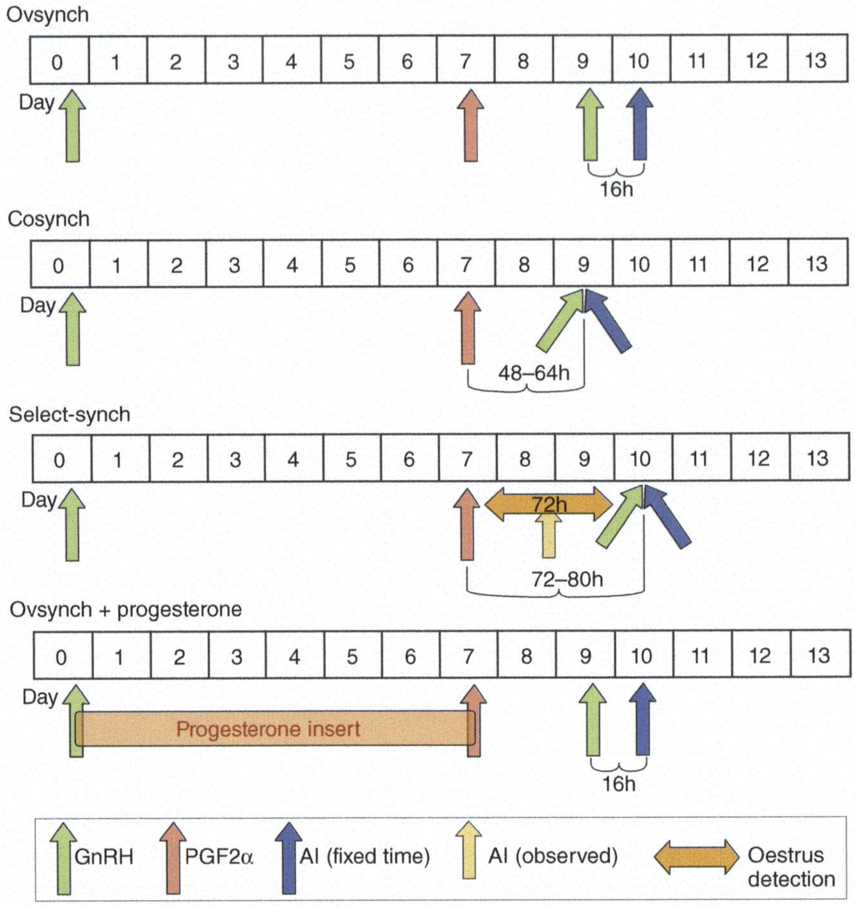

Figure 42.3 Variations of the Ovsynch theme: cosynch, in which the final GnRH is given at the same time as FTAI; select-synch, in which there is a period of oestrus detection before a (delayed) GnRH and FTAI to cows not observed in oestrus, and the addition of progesterone to better induce oestrus in anoestrous cows and to control LH secretion during the period of follicular growth. Adapted from DeJarnette 2010 and MacDougall 2010.

pregnancy rate) in Ovsynch compared to natural breeding (RR: 1.04; 95% CI: 0.36–3.23), $PGF_{2\alpha}$-based synchronisation (RR: 1.11; 95% CI: 0.31–2.64), or Select-synch (RR: 1.08; 95% CI: 0.38–3.10). Its effectiveness was improved by pre-synchronisation (RR (Ovsynch): 0.89; 95% CI: 0.71–1.22).

More recent trials have given similar results. Stevenson (2011) showed better synchronisation, but only a non-significant increase in pregnancy rate after pre-synch (double $PGF_{2\alpha}$ pre-synchronization) programmes, compared to Ovsynch. Double Ovsynch programmes may give better results; Giordano *et al.* (2012) reported 39% per-service conception rate for a double Ovsynch versus 30% for simple Ovsynch programmes. This recently developed protocol has not yet, however, been subjected to meta-analysis. Miller *et al.* (2007) compared fertility outcomes of herds bred to synchronised versus detected oestrus in US herds between 1995 and 2004, showing a reduction of 17 days between calving and first service, and of nine days open in favour of synchronised oestrus.

Ovarian superstimulation

Superstimulation of the ovary (formerly known as 'superovulation') is a critical component of the embryo technologies (recovery and transfer of embryos, ovum pick-up and *in vitro* fertilisation) that are now widely used as means of accelerating genetic selection and facilitating international traffic in genetics in the cattle-breeding industries (Greve & Callesen, 2005). Recent improvements in understanding of the regulation of follicular development and, in particular, of the dynamics of the follicular wave, have allowed for better control and simpler protocols for ovarian superstimulation.

In principle, superstimulation relies upon circumventing the physiological limitations of one ovulation per bovine oestrous cycle by administration of exogenous FSH at around the time of emergence of a follicular wave (Aerts & Bols, 2010). Before details of the bovine follicular wave had been properly elucidated, early superovulation regimens were based on empirical evidence that the best responses were obtained if stimulation

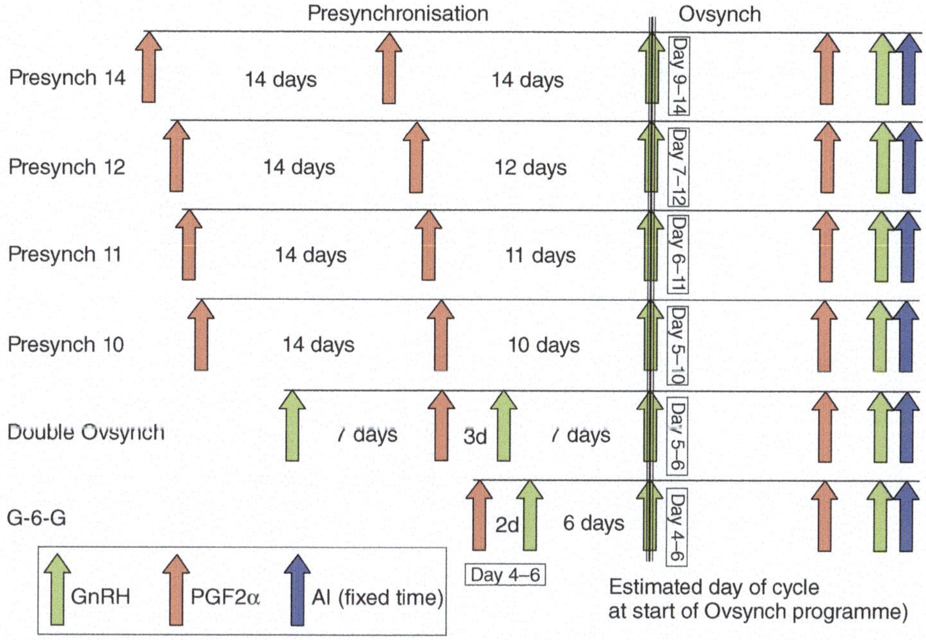

Figure 42.4 Methods of pre-synchronisation before a GPG programme, to control the stage of the follicular wave at the start of synchronisation. Presynch programmes rely upon double PGF2*α* programmes to control the wave; double Ovsynch and G-6-G programmes employ various components of the GPG programme to control the wave. Adapted from Stevenson 2011, 2012.

began at around days 8–12 after oestrus. This is a time which, subsequently, has been recognised as encompassing the emergence of the second follicular wave in cows with either two- or three-wave oestrous cycles (Mapletoft & Bo, 2012).

In most currently used protocols, stimulation is achieved by using either a single injection of equine chorionic gonadotrophin (eCG) or multiple injections of pituitary-extracted porcine or equine FSH. Thereafter, the luteal phase is terminated with $PGF_{2\alpha}$ to induce ovulation. Multiple insemination is usually recommended, typically 12 and 24 hours after the onset of oestrus (as detected or at a fixed time), and commonly with two straws of semen per insemination (Figure 42.5a). Some protocols, particularly those based upon eCG, also add GnRH (or hCG) at around the onset of oestrus to control the timing of ovulation.

The major problems with superstimulation are that:

- The response is highly variable in terms of numbers of follicles, numbers of ovulations and numbers of transferrable embryos.
- Insemination needs to be a fixed time to obviate the need for oestrus detection.
- Many regimes are complicated, resulting in a risk of poor treatment compliance.

The response to superstimulation varies greatly, and has been the biggest single problem with developing standardised regimes for embryo transfer. Numbers of recovered embryos vary wildly (a range of 0–60 has been reported), 20% of donors produce no embryos, and the response is affected by breed, age, nutrition, farm and handling (Hesser *et al.*, 2011). Some of the variation is due to the intrinsic characteristics of the individual cow's ovary; individual animals consistently produce similar numbers of embryos at repeated superstimulations, probably as a result of effects upon the follicular hierarchy that were sustained *in utero* (see Evans *et al.*, 2012). How nutrition affects superstimulation is not well understood: on the one hand, it is clear that animals that are in an unbalanced nutritional state have poor responses (Sartori *et al.*, 2007); yet evidence for an improved response after nutritional supplementation is equivocal at best (Velazquez, 2011).

Both eCG and abattoir-recovered FSH have variable amounts of LH-like activity. The presence of LH during the stimulation phase is detrimental to the response, either through premature activation of the oocyte, premature luteinisation or premature ovulation (Aerts & Bols, 2010), all of which lead to decreased fertilisation rates and embryo production. Some protocols therefore now incorporate progesterone, either as a norgestoment implant or as an intravaginal insert (e.g. Rivera *et al.*, 2011; Martins *et al.*, 2012). Such protocols also have the advantage that endogenous LH secretion is suppressed (which can be a problem when endogenous progesterone concentrations are too low to fully inhibit LH), and that the timing of the fall of progesterone concentrations can be more precisely controlled (i.e. by withdrawal of the exogenous source) by relying upon $PGF_{2\alpha}$-induced luteolysis.

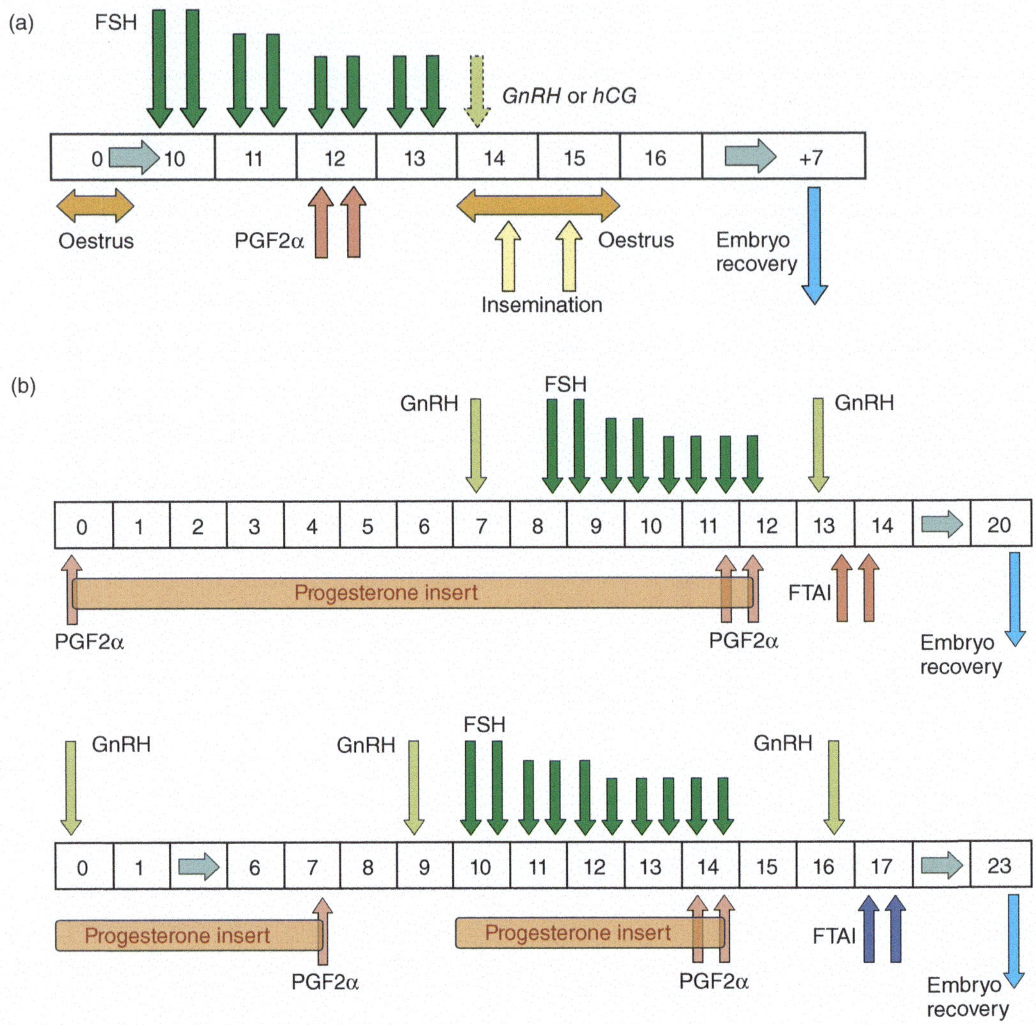

Figure 42.5 a) A commonly used method of inducing ovarian superstimulation for embryo collection in cattle. The timing of the start of FSH treatment represents a compromise for the timing of the start of the follicular wave in 2- and 3-wave cows. b) Different regimens for the incorporation of progesterone into ovarian superstimulation and embryo collection programmes. Adapted from Rivera *et al.* 2012.

The half-life of eCG is long, so only a single administration is needed, but that of FSH is short, so it has to be given frequently (12 hourly). Consequently, it is not rare for mistakes to be made in giving the multiple injections that are required in FSH-based regimens. Moreover, as biological products, both have a non-negligible risk of transmitting disease (Mapletoft & Hasler, 2005). Perhaps, in the long term, recombinant production of FSH isoforms whose half-life is extended by hyperglycosylation may solve these problems (Hesser *et al.*, 2011). In the meantime, combinations of FSH and eCG have been developed as a way of reducing the total number of treatments that are needed.

For example, the final two or four injections of FSH have been replaced by a single dose of eCG, which has resulted in comparable (or, in some cases, better) results than the standard 8-dose FSH protocol (Mapletoft & Bo, 2012). Additionally, slow-release formulations of FSH have been assessed experimentally but, at the time of writing, are probably not sufficiently advanced for commercialisation (Bo *et al.*, 2010).

Variability can also be reduced by controlling the follicular wave before the start of the superstimulation protocol. While oestradiol is a very effective way of doing this, its use is not permitted within the EU. As an alternative, regimes similar to those used for controlling the follicular wave in oestrus synchronisation programmes can be used (Baruselli *et al.*, 2011). Examples of regimes that both control the follicular wave and which can be used for fixed-time AI are shown in Figure 42.5b.

Despite these improvements in superstimulation programmes and, hence, embryo recovery rates, all remain dependent upon natural processes of ovulation and fertilisation. Some of the disadvantages posed by these processes can be circumvented by collection of oocytes directly from the ovary for use in *in vitro* fertilisation. The numbers of oocytes that can be collected is generally much greater than the number of fertilised embryos, but the ultimate success of such technology depends upon the success of *in vitro* fertilisation and culture of the embryo to a transferrable (blastocyst) stage (Baruselli *et al.*, 2012; see below).

Artificial insemination

Artificial insemination (AI) is the most widely used reproductive technology in cattle breeding. Many dairy cows are bred exclusively by AI, and almost all are inseminated at least once. It is less widely used in extensive beef suckler herds, because of difficulties of oestrus detection and yarding of cattle for insemination, but is relatively common in more intensive beef production systems.

The primary reason that AI is used is to provide relatively cheap access to high-quality genetics. Typically, AI sires have breeding values (BV) for dairy or beef production that are within the top 1% of the national herd. Hence, in dairy herds, AI is generally used for genetic improvement of the next generation of milking cows. It is used for genetic improvement in beef herds, too, but is primarily used as a source of high BV terminal sires. Artificial insemination provides a cheap and rapid means of disseminating new strains, such as occurred in the UK in the 1970s and 1980s, when the Holstein breed was introduced. Historically, an important reason for the development of AI was the control of venereal diseases (campylobacteriosis and trichomonosis), which were endemic in national cattle herds in the 1940s and 1950s. Although it is now less commonly used as a means of controlling these diseases, it remains an extremely effective means of doing so.

Because of the necessity for accurate oestrus detection and for drafting and yarding of cattle for insemination, some herd managers choose to use either a short period of AI or to use entirely natural service sires. Using appropriate bull management regimens (e.g. optimising the bull-to-cow ratio, rotation of groups of bulls, pre-season breeding soundness examinations), good fertility outcomes can be achieved, albeit at the cost of genetic progress. Lima *et al.* (2009) showed higher pregnancy rates on day 223 postpartum in cows that were exposed to continuous natural service (84%) than those that underwent Ovsynch synchronisation followed by a series of progesterone-based resynchronisations (75%).

Conversely, systems that use a short period of AI, followed by natural service, give variable results. Lima *et al.* (2012) showed higher 84-day pregnancy rates after three rounds of fixed-time AI, followed by natural service, than after a single round (65% versus 54%), although no difference in 231-day rates (both 81%). However, de Vries *et al.*, (2005) little difference between all-AI, all natural service and mixed AI/natural service regimens in the winter, whereas pregnancy rates were higher to natural service in the summer. Evidence from uncontrolled studies (Parkinson *et al.*, 2004) suggest that final (day 90) pregnancy rates to a short period of AI (0.5–1.5 cycles), followed by natural service, can be as high as 95%.

Voluntary wait period

Cows are first bred to AI after a postpartum 'voluntary waiting period' (VWP). The VWP is allowed so that cows can complete uterine involution and resume regular oestrous cycles, so it should not be less than 42 days. On the other hand, a VWP of >63 days inevitably result in calving intervals of >365 days (which is still important in seasonal-calving systems). Dairy herds in Australia with the highest 100-day in-calf rates all had VWP of ≤ 55 days (Morton, 2000), a figure which corresponds closely to the 53 and 56 days reported for US herds (Caraviello *et al.*, 2006; Miller *et al.*, 2007). Inchaisri *et al.* (2011) showed that the optimal VWP differs between cows, but for most it is <56 days, 37% have an optimal VWP of six weeks, 63% <8 weeks and only 10% of >10 weeks.

Generally, it is better to inseminate most cows at the first oestrus after the completion of the VWP (regardless of its duration) than to delay for a further cycle (Steeneveld & Hogeveen, 2012). However, for very high-yielding cows or cows with a persistent lactation, a longer VWP (extended by up to 60 days) may be economically preferable (Arbel *et al.*, 2001) or difficult to avoid, despite negative economic consequences (Inchaisri *et al.*, 2010).

Timing of insemination

The optimal timing of insemination after detected oestrus was established in the early days of the AI industry. The original recommendation (the 'am-pm rule') was that cows first detected in oestrus in the morning should be inseminated that same afternoon, while those detected in oestrus in the afternoon should be inseminated the next morning. Alternatively, if there is only a single insemination period each day, cows first detected in the morning should be inseminated that morning, while cows detected in the afternoon should be inseminated the following morning.

Large-scale studies show that conception rates do not differ between the once-a-day inseminations and the 'am-pm' protocol (summarised by Dransfield *et al.*, 1998), nor is there any difference when liquid, rather than cryopreserved, semen is used (Viswanath *et al.*, 2004). Morton (2000) confirmed that there is no advantage to twice- versus once-daily inseminations, although there can be an interaction between insemination frequency and oestrus detection practices, such that changing from twice- to once-daily insemination may be associated with poorer reproductive performance.

Peak conception rates occur at around 4–16 hours after the onset of oestrus, whether insemination occurs after detected oestrus (Dransfield *et al.*, 1998) or at a fixed time (Dorsey *et al*, 2011). Conception rate falls dramatically once insemination is delayed beyond 24 hours (Figure 42.6). The optimum timing of AI is a compromise between numbers and ageing of the sperm and ageing of the oocyte (Saacke *et al.* 2000). Early insemination achieves inadequate pregnancy rates due to high levels of unfertilised ova (i.e. because there are insufficient capacitated sperm at the site of fertilisation), although the survival of the fertilised embryos is high. Late insemination achieves inadequate pregnancy rates, due to poor embryo quality (i.e. due to loss of developmental capacity of an aged oocyte), despite a high fertilisation rate, and is accompanied by an increased level of early embryonic death.

Bull and inseminator efficacy

Conception rates achieved by the semen produced from commercial AI organisations is monitored by 'non-return rate' (i.e. the proportion of cows that are not re-presented for insemination within a fixed period of time). This figure, which is higher than conception rate, is nonetheless very highly correlated with it and can be used to give a rapid indication of any problems that an individual sire may develop. Outliers whose conception rate is below the acceptable range are generally withdrawn from semen production for AI, either temporarily or permanently, depending upon whether the defect is likely to improve. Some low fertility can be explained with reference to gross changes in semen quality, or by the ability of individual sires' semen to withstand cryopreservation. Recent work, however, suggests that DNA fragmentation may be an accurate predictor of the fertility of AI sperm (Karoui *et al.*, 2012), which may obviate the need for field monitoring through non-return rates.

It is, therefore, far more common for infertility due to poor semen quality to have arisen due to mishandling of the cryopreserved semen during its distribution (rare), its on-farm storage (common), or its thawing and subsequent handling (very common). Semen does not generally survive thawing and re-freezing so, when an on-farm storage container 'runs out' of liquid nitrogen, disastrous conception rates will

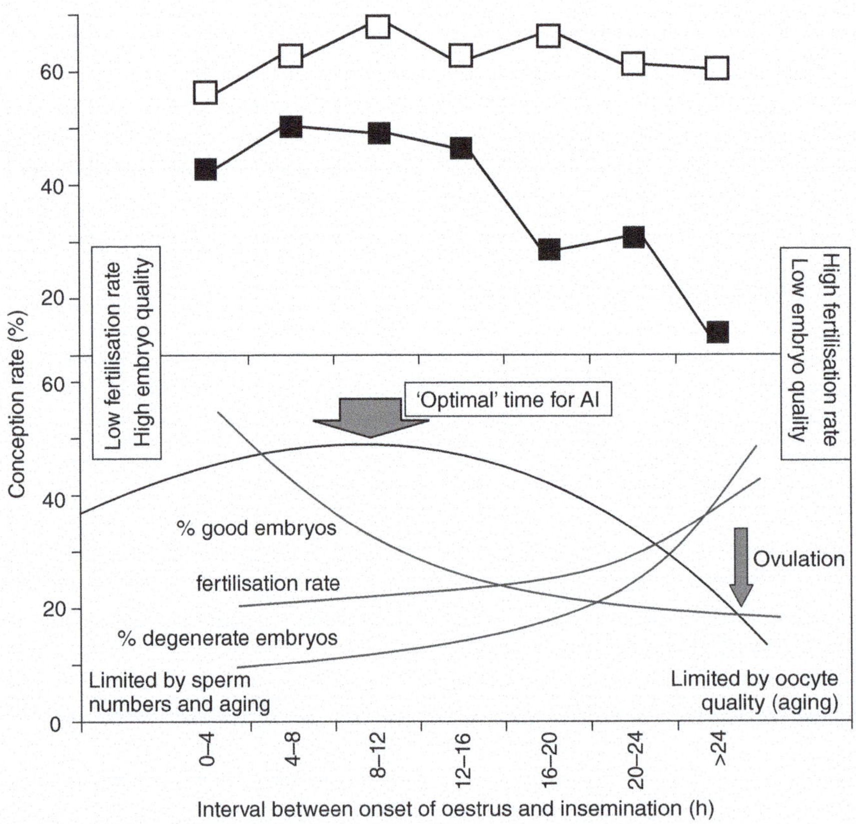

Figure 42.6 Timing of artificial insemination of cows, based on optimising the fertilisation rate and the quality of the ensuing embryo. Data from Dransfield *et al.* (1998: filled squares), Dorsey *et al.* (2011: open squares) and Saacke *et al.* (2000: lower panel).

generally ensure. Poor handling of straws during removal from the storage tank can result in partial thawing of those which are returned to storage, again resulting in sperm damage. Poor temperature control (water that is too hot or too cold) during and after thawing can also result in impaired fertility.

Inseminator proficiency is probably the main factor affecting the success of insemination. Non-return rates achieved by AI centre technicians are closely monitored, and individuals whose rates fail to meet an acceptable standard are either retrained or dismissed. Farmer-inseminators ('DIY inseminators') are not subject to any such scrutiny and, hence, while average results do not differ from centre technicians, their results are much more variable (Morton, 2000; Buckley *et al.*, 2003). Buckley *et al.* (2003) showed that DIY inseminators achieve a range of conception rates from 28% to 68%. Morton (2000) showed that 13% of DIY inseminators achieved conceptions rates that were >5% above AI centre technician average. However, 45% were >5% below, and 12% were >15% below, centre technicians. The worst DIY inseminators' conception rates were >30% below centre technicians.

It appears that those who achieve high rates do so by optimising the timing of insemination to the onset of oestrus, and by meticulous attention to optimal insemination practice, whereas those who achieve poor rates pay less attention to detail, often as a result of not having (or taking) enough time for the task. Neither the conception rates, nor the return on capital, are optimal until the third season after changing from natural service to DIY AI (Shaw & Dobson, 1996), probably due mainly to the development of inseminator proficiency with time.

Sexed semen

The ability to control the sex of offspring by sorting X- and Y-bearing sperm has been a longstanding goal of cattle breeding. Of the many methods that have been tried, separating on the basis of the greater mass of DNA in an X- than in a Y-bearing sperm is the only one that has so far proved reliable. Sperm are stained with a non-damaging DNA-binding dye, and then are separated by flow cytometry on the basis of the increased fluorescence of X- compared to Y- bearing cells (Seidel, 2007).

The technology of sperm sorting has now progressed to a point at which 90–95% accuracy of separation can be achieved (Dejarnette *et al.*, 2009; Trigal *et al.*, 2012). However, the problems remain that the process remains quite slow, with the consequence that relatively low numbers of sperm have to be used per insemination. Also, the sorting process damages sperm, and that damage is additive to the damage caused by cryopreservation (Frijters *et al.*, 2009). Consequently, the conception rates to insemination by sexed semen are generally lower that those for conventional AI.

The benefits from using sexed semen in the dairy industry are primarily related to increasing the number of heifer calves available as herd replacements. Currently, virtually all heifer calves have to be used and the rate of production of heifers is barely sufficient to keep up with demands for replacements. Although it is attractive to envisage that the use of sexed semen might allow for greater female-side selection, de Vries *et al.* (2007) calculated that ≈60% of female calves would still have to be used as replacements, meaning that only ≈10% of the selection intensity that can be achieved through male-side selection could be attained. However, there is little merit to using sexed semen to try to augment male-side selection, as the benefits are almost entirely confined to selection upon milking cows (Khalajzadeh *et al.*, 2012).

Conception rates to sexed semen are typically ten percentage points lower than those to conventional semen. In Holstein heifers, first service conception rates were 56% for conventional AI, versus 45% for sexed semen (DeJarnette *et al.*, 2009). Sexed semen can be used for fixed time AI, although the success is much more dependent upon the stage of follicular development at the time of insemination than for conventional semen. In *Bos indicus* beef cows, Sa Filho *et al.* (2012) found that the conception rates to fixed time AI were 59% versus 57% for conventional and sexed-semen insemination, when the dominant follicle was ≥ 9 mm at the time of insemination, compared with 50% versus 32%, when the follicle was <9 mm. Similarly, the optimal timing of fixed time insemination is a little later for sexed semen than conventional AI; Sales *et al.* (2011) showed that insemination with sexed semen 60 hours after progesterone removal gave a conception rate of 32%, compared with 16% at 54 hours.

Such studies indicate that conception rate to sexed semen is at least partly dependent upon the synchronisation of insemination to the time of ovulation. Attempts to improve conception rates by increasing the number of sperm in the insemination dose have not been rewarding, as the response seems to depend more upon the characteristics of the individual bull than upon sperm numbers *per se* (Frijters *et al.*, 2009; DeJarnette *et al.*, 2011). As the correlation for individual bulls' conception rates when used for conventional or sexed-semen AI is only modest, it appears that, for the time being, either bulls will have to be selected for the ability of their sperm to survive sorting, or lower conception rates will have to be accepted.

Embryo transfer and *in vitro* embryo production

Embryo transfer (ET) has become widely used since practical methods of collection and implantation were developed in the 1970s/80s. Its initial stimulus was for the rapid dissemination of 'new' genetics, including the introduction of European beef breeds into North America and of the US/Canadian Holstein breeds into Europe. Subsequently, it has become the preferred means of exporting germ plasm around the world, since transporting embryos obviates the costs and welfare issues associated with live animal transport; the disease risks associated with importing embryos are much less than those associated with live animals; and implantation into 'local' recipients means that a degree of acclimatisation and immunity to local diseases can be acquired before birth.

Recent years have therefore seen ET developing as a major exporting industry for 'improved' cattle genetics. Also, with increased repeatability and reliability of multiple-ovulation embryo transfer (MOET) procedures, genetic testing of dairy sires is increasingly based on the lactational performance of sisters, rather than that of daughters (as in traditional progeny testing), thereby reducing the time (and, hence, costs) of sire-proving schemes (Mapletoft & Hasler, 2005). The main on-farm uses of ET are, therefore:

- Production of embryos for export, often to developing nations.
- Rapid multiplication of a new breed or bloodline.
- For breeding bulls for use in AI, and for breeding their sisters for assessment of lactation performance.

The methods of ET that were developed in the 1980s have recently been supplemented by *in vitro* methods of embryo production. Use of *in vitro* embryo production (IVP) technologies in commercial cattle breeding was hampered for a long time by an inability to maintain embryos *in vitro* to a point at which they can be implanted into a recipient. Methods of embryo culture have now been developed to an extent which, while not devoid of shortcomings, has allowed IVP to become a commercially viable component of cattle breeding.

Depending upon the purpose of the ET programme, the sex ratio of offspring can potentially be manipulated by the use of sexed semen, either *in vivo* or for IVP (Hayakawa *et al.*, 2009; Barcelo-Fimbres *et al.*, 2011).

Collection and transfer of embryos

Embryo transfer consists of three processes:

- Collection of fertilised embryos from a donor.
- Evaluation and/or storage of the embryos.
- Implantation into a donor.

Donor cows can be prepared by ovarian superstimulation (see above), or single embryos can be collected after natural oestrus and mating. Embryos are collected non-surgically, using a transcervical catheter that is manipulated into position *per rectum*. A two-way catheter (e.g. the Foley catheter) is preferred by most operators, but three-way catheters are also used, and specialised embryo collection catheters are available. Cows are usually given epidural anaesthesia to reduce straining, and the perineum is carefully cleaned to avoid faecal contamination of the reproductive tract. The catheter is advanced through the cervix, using either a stylet within the catheter or a cervical dilator to aid its passage – the cervical canal of the heifer in particular can be exceedingly difficult to navigate.

Most operators advance the catheter deep into each uterine horn separately, and flush the horn and the utero-tubal junction with a series of small aliquots (25–50 mL) of flushing medium (commonly Dulbecco's phosphate buffered saline, supplemented with either 1% foetal calf serum or 1–2% bovine serum albumin (BSA), plus antibiotics (Bruck Bøgh & Greve, 2009)). Current research is attempting to replace animal-derived products such as BSA in embryo handling media (Hasler, 2010), primarily as a means of reducing the risk of disease spread.

Flushings are passed through a 70 μm filter to remove somatic cellular debris, and then embryos are eluted from the filter and evaluated for quality. By day 6 or 7, embryos should have reached compacted morula, compacted blastocyst, blastocyst or expanded blastocyst stages; less developed embryos are unlikely to develop. They are also graded according to well-established criteria (Linder & Wright, 1983; Farin *et al.*, 1995):

- Grade 1 (excellent): Spherical, symmetrical, uniform cells
- Grade 2 (good): Minor imperfections (e.g. a few extruded blastomeres, irregular shape)
- Grade 3 (poor): Numerous imperfections, (e.g. extruded blastomeres, degenerated cells, cells of varying sizes, many large vesicles)
- Grade 4 (degenerate)

Grade 1 and 2 embryos are much more likely to result in pregnancies than are Grade 3 (Linder & Wright, 1983). Moreover, quite subtle morphological features, such as blastomere colour, the extent of compaction, timing of blastocyst formation and expansion and diameter of the embryo, are linked with embryo quality, ultrastructure, gene expression and ability to survive cryopreservation (Van Soom *et al.*, 2003).

The development of effective methods of cryopreserving embryos has greatly increased the efficiency of the technology, liberating it from the requirement of immediately available recipients (Mapletoft & Hasler, 2005). Current methods of freezing and thawing embryos are typically slow, multistage processes, but much research is being devoted to simplification of these methods, especially for one-step, on-farm, thawing of embryos (Youngs *et al.*, 2010). Nonetheless, pregnancy rates achieved with cryopreserved high-grade embryos are very similar to those achieved by direct transfer (Leibo & Mapletoft, 1998).

Where embryos are to be directly implanted, the recipients should be prepared by a parallel oestrus synchronisation protocol, which aims to ensure that ovulation is closely synchronised with that of the donor as possible (Figure 42.7). Synchrony between donor and recipient is a major determinant of success, with more than 24 hours asynchrony being associated with a marked reduction in pregnancy rate (Linder & Wright, 1983). It is preferable that morulae should be transferred to day 6

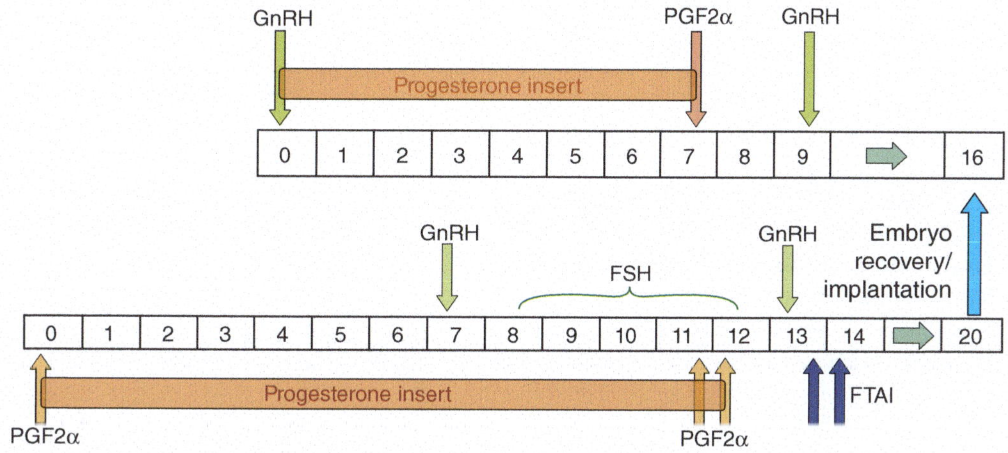

Figure 42.7 Synchronisation of recipients (above) with the donor (below) for direct transfer of embryos into the recipient. Control of the follicular wave with a GPG programme gives better results than a simple double-$PGF_{2\alpha}$ regimen, although the latter can also be used. Adapted from Baruselli *et al*. 2011.

recipients and blastocysts to day 7 recipients (Bruck Bøgh & Greve, 2009). Embryos are implanted through the cervix into the mid-uterine horn ispilateral to a *corpus luteum*. Pregnancy rates are highly dependent upon the operator, particularly as any trauma to the uterus that results in bleeding markedly impairs success.

The OIE *Terrestrial Animal Health Code* requires that embryos are washed by changing media ten times before transfer or cryopreservation. Additionally, embryos for export are treated with trypsin to remove BVD and bovine herpes viruses from the surface of the zona pellucida. Van Soom & Nauwynck (2008) noted that it is more difficult to remove viruses from the zona of *in vitro* than *in vivo* derived embryos.

In vitro embryo production

In vitro embryo production has been developed as both a means of increasing the usage of oocytes from an individual female, and of circumventing some of the inefficiencies of the ovarian supersimtulation process that underpins ET. Currently, around one-third of the embryos produced worldwide are derived from IVP (Baruselli *et al.*, 2012). There are four steps in the process:

- Collection of oocytes, either *in vivo* or after slaughter.
- Oocyte maturation and sperm capacitation *in vitro*.
- Fertilisation.
- *In vitro* culture of the embryo to a point at which it can be implanted into a recipient.

For IVP in cattle, it is preferable that the final stages of oocyte maturation have taken place before *in vitro* fertilisation, although there is a reasonably high level of correlation between the developmental competence of the oocyte during *in vitro* maturation and the diameter of the follicle from which is was collected. It is also preferable that follicles are collected at around the time of wave emergence, rather than when dominance has occurred (Blondin *et al.*, 2012). Collection twice per week appears to be the optimal frequency to maximise numbers of follicles while avoiding the presence of dominant follicles (Boni, 2012).

Follicles can be collected with or without ovarian stimulation, although more oocytes, with better capacity for embryo development, can be collected after synchronisation of the follicular wave or after a modest level of ovarian stimulation with FSH over 2–3 days (Rodriguez *et al.*, 2010), followed by a period of FSH deprivation ('coasting': Blondin *et al.*, 2012). Responses are better in cows that are neither in negative energy balance nor overfed, are better in *B. indicus* than *B. taurus* cattle (Baruselli *et al.*, 2012), and may be better in beef (Angus) than dairy (Holstein) animals (Ratto *et al.*, 2011).

Oocytes are collected as cumulus-oocyte complexes (COC) by transvaginal ultrasound-guided follicle aspiration, usually from follicles of a minimum diameter of ≈5 mm. COC are classified according to the number of layers of cumulus cells and the appearance of the oocyte: those with at least two layers of cumulus cells and homogenous oocyte cytoplasm are used for embryo production. Interestingly, COCs that are just beginning to undergo apoptosis give better responses than do those that are highly compacted (Blondin & Sirard, 1995). It is relatively easy to induce oocyte nuclear maturation *in vitro*, but cytoplasmic maturations is more difficult to induce. Consequently, the developmental competence of the embryo is highly dependent upon the conditions under which the COC is matured (Blanco *et al.*, 2011). Fertilisation can either be with unsorted or sexed semen.

Difficulty in culturing the fertilised oocyte through to a transferrable (blastocyst) stage has been a major limitation to IVP. Initially, this was achieved by *in vivo* culture in the oviduct of sheep and, later, by co-culture with oviduct cells *in vitro*. Most embryos are now cultured in defined media, although details of the ideal composition of such media remains under investigation (Block *et al.*, 2011).

In vitro-produced embryos can be cryopreserved, but they are rather more fragile than *in vivo*-produced embryos; or they can be directly implanted into recipients after culture to the blastocyst stage. The best recipients are virgin heifers, preferably those that have undergone an oestrus synchronisation programme that tightly controls the time of ovulation (see above). Because the early uterine environment affects the epigenetic programming of the foetal genome, it is important that the nutritional management of recipients is optimised (Marinho *et al.*, 2012). Typical results are that around 6–15 oocytes can be recovered at each collection, of which most (>80%) are suitable for processing. Cleavage (fertilisation) rates are ≈80%, but development to blastocyst stage is only ≈40%. Thus, 1–2 transferrable embryos result per collection. Transferred embryos typically result in a 30–40% pregnancy rate (Hasler *et al.*, 1995; Ratto *et al.*, 2011).

Setting aside the technical issues of IVP, the main problems of the method have been that a proportion of calves exhibit various developmental abnormalities. Specifically, IVP embryos are more likely to result in abnormalities (Greve & Callesen, 2005; Farin *et al.*, 2006) which, together, are known as the 'abnormal offspring syndrome':

- Failure to establish the pregnancy.
- Failure of growth and development of the foetus and placenta (including hydrallantois), resulting in abortion.
- Defects of growth and development of the foetus and placenta that allow the pregnancy to go to term. but do not allow survival of the foetus in the neonatal period.
- Less severe abnormalities of development that allow the pregnancy to go to term and the neonate to survive.

These abnormalities are believed to arise as a result of epigenetic changes occurring during the various *in vitro* maturation and culture stages, which persist through foetal development and, thereafter, into adult life. One particularly interesting group of genes which may be affected are those for insulin-like growth factor receptor 2, which appears to have significant roles in the elongation of the trophoblast and in the development of key organs during the period of organogenesis (Farin *et al.*, 2010).

References

Aerts, J.M.J. and Bols, P.E.J. (2010). Ovarian follicular dynamics. A review with emphasis on the bovine species. Part II: Antral development, exogenous influence and future prospects. *Reproduction in Domestic Animals* **45**, 180–187.

Albright, J.L. and Arave, C.W. (1997). *The Behaviour of Cattle*. CAB International, Wallingford, UK.

Arbel, R., Bigun ,Y., Ezra, E., Sturman, H. and Hojman, D. (2001). The effect of extended calving intervals in high-yielding lactating cows on milk production and profitability. *Journal of Dairy Science* **84**, 600–608.

Aungier, S.P.M., Roche, J.F., Sheehy, M. and Crowe, M.A. (2012). Effects of management and health on the use of activity monitoring for estrus detection in dairy cows. *Journal of Dairy Science* **95**, 2452–2466.

Barcelo-Fimbres, M., Campos-Chillon, LF. and Seidel GE. (2011). *In vitro* fertilization using non-sexed and sexed bovine sperm: sperm concentration, sorter pressure, and bull effects. *Reproduction in Domestic Animals* **46**, 495–502.

Baruselli, P.S., Ferreira, R.M., Sales, J.N.S., Gimenes, L.U., Sa Filho, M.F., Martins, C.M., Rodrigues, C.A. and Bo, G.A. (2011). Timed embryo transfer programs for management of donor and recipient cattle. *Theriogenology* **76**, 1583–1593.

Baruselli, P.S., Sa Filho, M.F., Ferreira, R.M., Sales, J.N.S., Gimenes, L.U., Viera, L.M., Mendanha, M.F. and Bo, G.A. (2012). Manipulation of follicle development to ensure optimal oocyte quality and conception rates in cattle. *Reproduction in Domestic Animals* **47**(Suppl. 4), 134–141.

Blanco, M.R., Demyda, S., Moreno Millán, M. and Genero, E. (2011). Developmental competence of *in vivo and in vitro* matured oocytes: A review. *Biotechnology and Molecular Biology Review* **6**, 155–165.

Block, J., Hansen, P.J., Loureiro, B. and Bonilla, L. (2011). Improving post-transfer survival of bovine embryos produced *in vitro*: Actions of insulin-like growth factor-1, colony stimulating factor-2 and hyaluronan. *Theriogenology* **76**, 1602–1609.

Blondin, P. and Sirard, M.A. (1995). Oocyte and follicular morphology as determining characteristics for developmental competence in bovine oocytes. *Molecular Reproduction and Development* **41**, 54–62.

Blondin, P., Vigneault, C., Nivet, A.L. and Sirard, A.M. (2012). Improving oocyte quality in cows and heifers – what have we learned so far? *Animal Reproduction* **9**, 281–289.

Bo, G.A. and Mapletoft, R.J. (2012) New approaches to superovulation and fixed-time AI in dairy cattle. *Cattle Practice* **20**, 19–28.

Bo, G.A., Carballo Guerrero, D., Tribulo, A., Tribulo, H., Tribulo, R., Rogan, D. and Mapletoft, R.J. (2010). New approaches to superovulation in the cow. *Reproduction, Fertility and Development* **22**, 106–112.

Bonato, G.L., Cunha, M.O., Santos, R.M. dos and Carneiro, L.C. (2012). Estrotect efficiency in identifying estrus in crossbred dairy cows. *Brazilian Journal of Veterinary Research and Animal Science* **49**, 19–23. [Portugese]

Boni, R. (2012). Ovum pick-up in cattle: a 25 year retrospective analysis. *Animal Reproduction* **9**, 362–369.

Bruck Bøgh, I. and Greve, T. *Assisted Reproductive Technologies* (2009). In: Noakes, D.E., Parkinson, T.J. and England, G.C.W. (eds). *Veterinary Reproduction and Obstetrics*, 9th Edition, pp.855–894. Elsevier, Edinburgh.

Buckley, F., Mee, J., O'Sullivan, K., Evans, B., Berry, D. and Dillon, P. (2003). Insemination factors affecting the conception rate in seasonal calving Holstein-Friesian cows. *Reproduction, Nutrition, Development* **43**, 543–555.

Caraviello, D.Z., Weigel, K.A., Fricke, P.M., Wiltbank, M.C., Florent, M.J., Cook, N.B., Nordlund, K.V., Zwald, N.R. and Rawson, C.L. (2006). Survey of management practices on reproductive performance of dairy cattle on large us commercial farms. *Journal of Dairy Science* **89**, 4723–4735.

Colazo, M.G., Gordon, M.B., Rajamahendran, R., Mapletoft, R.J. and Ambrose, D.J. (2009). Pregnancy rates to timed artificial insemination in dairy cows treated with gonadotropin-releasing hormone or porcine luteinizing hormone. *Theriogenology* **72**, 262–270.

de Vries, A., Steenholdt, C. and Risco, C.A. (2005). Pregnancy rates and milk production in natural service and artificially inseminated dairy herds in Florida and Georgia. *Journal of Dairy Science* **88**, 948–956.

de Vries, A., Overton, M., Fetrow, J., Leslie, K., Eicker, S. and Rogers, G. (2007). Exploring the impact of sexed semen on the structure of the dairy industry. *Journal of Dairy Science* **91**, 847–856.

DeJarnette, J.M. (no date) *Ovsynch, co-synch, presynch and kitchensynch: how did breeding cows get so complicated*? At: http://www.selectsires.com/programs/docs/ovsynch_cosynch_presynch.pdf. Accessed 30/9/12

DeJarnette, J.M. and Marshall, C.E. (2003). Effects of pre-synchronisation using combinations PGF2α and (or) GnRH on pregnancy rates of Ovsynch- and Cosynch-treated lactating Holstein cows. *Animal Reproduction Science* **77**, 51–60.

DeJarnette, J.M., Nebel, R.L. and Marshall, C.E. (2009). Evaluating the success of sex-sorted semen in US dairy herds from on farm records. *Theriogenology* **71**, 49–58.

DeJarnette, J.M., Leach, M.A., Nebel, R.L., Marshall, C.E., McCleary, C.R. and Moreno, J.F. (2011). Effects of sex-sorting and sperm dosage on conception rates of Holstein heifers: Is comparable fertility of sex-sorted and conventional semen plausible? *Journal of Dairy Science* **94**, 3477–3483.

Dorsey, B.R., Kasimanickamb, R., Whittier, W.D., Nebel, R.L., Wahlberg, M.L. and Hall, J.B. (2011). Effect of time from estrus to AI on pregnancy rates in estrous synchronised beef heifers. *Animal Reproduction Science* **127**, 1–6.

Dransfield, M.B.G., Nebel, R.L., Pearson, R.E. and Warnick, L.D. (1998). Timing of insemination for dairy cows identified in estrus by a radiotelemetric estrus detection system. *Journal of Dairy Science* **81**, 1874–1882.

Esslemont, R.J. (1974). Economic and husbandry aspects of the manifestation and detection of oestrus in cows. I. Economic aspects. *ADAS Quarterly Review* **12**, 175–184.

Esselmont, R.J. and Bryant, M.J. (1976). Oestrous behaviour in a herd of dairy cows. *Veterinary Record* **99**, 472–475.

Evans, A.C.O., Mossa, F., Walsh, S.W., Scheetz, D., Jimenez-Krassel, F., Ireland, J.L.H., Smith, G.W. and Ireland, J.J. (2012). Effects of maternal environment during gestation on ovarian folliculogenesis and consequences for fertility in bovine offspring. *Reproduction in Domestic Animals* **47**(Suppl. 4), 31–37.

Farin, P.W., Britt, J.H., Shaw, D.W. and Slenning, B.D. (1995). Agreement among evaluators of bovine embryos produced *in vivo* or *in vitro*. *Theriogenology* **44**, 339–349.

Farin, P.W., Piedrahita, J.A. and Farin, C.E. (2006). Errors in development of fetuses and placentas from *in vitro*-produced bovine embryos. *Theriogenology* **65**, 178–191.

Farin, C.E., Farmer, W.T. and Farin, P.W. (2010). Pregnancy recognition and abnormal offspring syndrome in cattle. *Reproduction, Fertility and Development* **22**, 75–87.

Felton, C.A., Colazo, M.G., Ponce-Barajas, P., Bench, C.J. and Ambrose, D.J. (2012). Dairy cows continuously-housed in tie-stalls failed to manifest activity changes during estrus. *Canadian Journal of Animal Science* **92**, 189–196.

Frijters, A.C.J., Mullaart, E., Roelofs, E.M.G., van Hoorne, R.P., Moreno, J.F., Moreno, O. and Merton, J.S. (2009). What affects fertility of sexed bull semen more, low sperm dosage or the sorting process? *Theriogenology* **71**, 64–67.

Galvao, K.N. and Santos, J.E.P. (2010). Factors affecting synchronisation and conception rate after the Ovsynch protocol in lactating Holstein cows. *Reproduction in Domestic Animals* **45**, 439–446.

Giordano, J.O., Wiltbank, M.C., Guenther, J.N., Pawlisch, R., Bas, S., Cunha, A.P. and Fricke, P.M. (2012). Increased fertility in lactating dairy cows resynchronised with Double-Ovsynch compared with Ovsynch initiated 32 d after timed artificial insemination: resynchronisation with double-ovsynch. *Journal of Dairy Science* **95**, 639–653.

Greve, T. and Callesen, H. (2005). Embryo technology: implications for fertility in cattle. *Scientific and Technical Review (OIE)* **24**, 405–412.

Hasler, J.F. (2010). Synthetic media for culture, freezing and vitrification of bovine embryos. *Reproduction, Fertility and Development* **22**, 119–125.

Hasler, J.F., Henderson, W.B., Hurtgen, P.J., Jin, Z.Q., McCauley, A.D., Mower, S.A., Neely, B., Shuey, L.S., Stokes, J.E. and Trimmer, S.A. (1995). Production, freezing and transfer of bovine IVF embryos and subsequent calving results. *Theriogenology* **43**, 141–152.

Hayakawa, H., Hirai, T., Takimoto, A., Ideta, A. and Aoyagi, Y. (2009). Superovulation and embryo transfer in Holstein cattle using sexed sperm. *Theriogenology* **71**, 68–73.

Hesser, M.W., Morris, J.C. and Gibbons, J.R. (2011). Advances in recombinant gonadotropin production for use in bovine superovulation. *Reproduction in Domestic Animals* **46**, 933–942.

Holman, A., Thompson, J., Routly, J.E., Cameron, J., Jones, D.N., Grove-White, D., Smith, R.F. and Dobson, H. (2011). Comparison of oestrus detection methods in dairy cattle. *Veterinary Record* **169**, 47–52.

Inchaisri, C., Jorritsma, R., Vos, P.L.A.M., van der Weijden, G.C. and Hogeveen, H. (2010). Economic consequences of reproductive performance in dairy cattle. *Theriogenology* **74**, 835–846.

Inchaisri, C., Jorritsma, R., Vos, P.L.A.M., van der Weijden, G.C. and Hogeveen, H. (2011). Analysis of the economically optimal voluntary waiting period for first insemination. *Journal of Dairy Science* **94**, 3811–3823.

Karoui, S., Diaz, C., Gonzalez-Marin, C., Amenabar, M.E., Serrano, M., Ugarte, E., Gosalvez, J., Roy, R., Lopez-Fernandez, C. and Carabano, M.J. (2012). Is sperm DNA fragmentation a good marker for field AI bull fertility? *Journal of Animal Science* **90**, 2437–2449.

Kerbrat, S. and Disenhaus, C. (2004). A proposition for an updated behavioural characterisation of the oestrus period in dairy cows. *Applied Animal Behaviour Science* **87**, 223–238.

Khalajzadeh, S., Nejati-Javaremi, A. and Mehrbani Yeganeh, H. (2012). Effect of widespread and limited use of sexed semen on genetic progress and reproductive performance of dairy cows. *Animal* **6**, 1398–1406.

Kinsel, M.L. and Etherington, W.G. (1998). Factors affecting reproductive performance in Ontario dairy herds. *Theriogenology* **50**, 1221–1238.

Leibo, S.P. and Mapletoft, R.J. (1998). Direct transfer of cryopreserved cattle embryos in North America. *Proceedings of the 17th Annual Convention of the American Embryo Transfer Association*, pp. 91–98.

Lima, F.S., Risco, C.A., Thatcher, M.J., Benzaquen, M.E., Archbald, L.F., Santos, J.E.P. and Thatcher, W.W. (2009). Comparison of reproductive performance in lactating dairy cows bred by natural service or timed artificial insemination. *Journal of Dairy Science* **92**, 5456–5466.

Lima, F.S., Bisinotto, B.S., Ribeiro, E.S., Ayres, H., Greco, L.F., Galva, K.N., Risco, C.A., Thatcher, W.W. and Santos, J.E.P. (2012). Effect of one or three timed artificial inseminations before natural service on reproductive performance of lactating dairy cows not observed for detection of estrus. *Theriogenology* **77**, 1918–1927.

Linder, G.M. and Wright, R.W. (1983). Bovine embryo morphology and evaluation. *Theriogenology* **20**, 407–416.

Mapletoft, R.J. and Bo, G.A. (2012). The evolution of improved and simplified superovulation protocols in cattle. *Reproduction, Fertility and Development* **24**, 278–283.

Mapletoft, R.J. and Hasler, J.F. (2005). Assisted reproductive technologies in cattle: a review. *Scientific and Technical Review (OIE)* **24**, 393–403.

Marinho, L.S.R., Untura, R.M., Morotti, F., Moino, L.L., Rigo, A.G., Sanches, B.V., Pontes, J.H.F. and Seneda, M.M. (2012). Large-scale programs for recipients of *in vitro*-produced embryos. *Animal Reproduction* **9**, 323–328.

McDougall, S. (2010). Effects of treatment of anestrous dairy cows with gonadotropin-releasing hormone, prostaglandin, and progesterone. *Journal of Dairy Science* **93**, 1944–1959.

Miller, R.H., Norman, H.D., Kuhn, M.T., Clay, J.S. and Hutchison, J.L. (2007). Voluntary waiting period and adoption of synchronised breeding in dairy herd improvement herds. *Journal of Dairy Science* **90**, 1594–1606.

Morton, J. (2000). *The InCalf Project. Progress report No. 2.* Dairy Research and Development Corporation, Melbourne, Vic, Australia.

Morton, J., Larcombe, M. and Little, S. (2003). *The InCalf Book for Dairy Farmers.* Dairy Australia, Werribee, Victoria.

O'Connor, M.L. (2007). Estrus detection. In: Youngquist, R.S. and Threlfall, W.R. (eds) *Current Therapy in Large Animal Theriogenology*, 2nd Edition, pp. 270–278. Saunders-Elsevier, St Louis, Missouri.

Palmer, M.A., Olmos, G., Boyle, L.A. and Mee, J.F. (2010). Estrus detection and estrus characteristics in housed and pastured Holstein–Friesian cows. *Theriogenology* **74**, 255–264.

Parkinson, T.J., Frear, M. and O'Leary, D. (2004). *Use of bulls in larger dairy herds.* Proceedings of the Dairy3 Conference, Rotorua. **2**, 41–48.

Parkinson, T.J., Vermunt, J.J., Malmo, J. and Weston, J.F. (2010). Reproduction and disorder of the reproductive system. In: Parkinson, T.J., Vermunt, J.J. and Malmo, J. (eds). *Diseases of Cattle in Australasia*, pp. 414–502. New Zealand Veterinary Association, Wellington, New Zealand.

Pennington, J.A., Albright, J.L. and Callahan, C.J. (1986). Relationships of sexual activities in estrous cows to different frequencies of observation and pedometer measurements. *Journal of Dairy Science* **69**, 2925–2934.

Pursley, J.R. and Martins, J.P.N. (2012). Impact of circulating concentrations of progesteroneand antral age of the ovulatory follicle on fertility of high-producing lactating dairy cows. *Reproduction, Fertility and Development* **24**, 267–271.

Rabiee, A.R., Lean, I.J. and Stevenson, M.A. (2005). Efficacy of ovsynch program on reproductive performance in dairy cattle: a meta-analysis. *Journal of Dairy Science* **88**, 2754–2770.

Ratto, M.H., Peralta, O.O.A., Mogollon, G., Strobel, P. and Correa, J. (2011). Transvaginal ultrasound-guided cumulus oocyte complexes aspiration and in vitro embryo production in suckled beef and lactating dairy cattle on pasture-based management conditions. *Animal Reproduction Science* **129**, 1–6.

Rivera, F.A., Mendonc, L.G.D., Lopes, G., Santos, J.E.P., Perez, R.V., Amstalden, M., Correa-Caldero, A. and Chebel, R.C. (2011). Reduced progesterone concentration during growth of the first follicular wave affects embryo quality but has no effect on embryo survival post transfer in lactating dairy cows. *Reproduction* **141**, 333–342.

Rodriguez Villamil, P., Tribulo, A., Ramos, M., Ongaratto, F. and Bo, G. (2010). Comparision of oocyte recovery rates and morphology obtained by OPU after different hormonal treatments in cattle. *Proceedings of the 26th World Buiatrics Congress*, Santiago, Chile.

Sa Filho, M.F., Girotto, R., Abe, E.K., Penteado, L., Campos Filho, E.P., Moreno, J.P., Sala, R.V., Nichi, M. and Baruselli, P.S. (2012). Optimizing the use of sex-sorted sperm in timed artificial insemination programs for suckled beef cows. *Journal of Animal Science* **90** 1816–1823.

Saacke, R.G., Dalton, J.C., Nadir, S., Neble, R.L. and Bame, J.H. (2000). Relationship of seminal traits and insemination time to fertilization rate and embryo quality. *Animal Reproduction Science* **60–61**, 663–677.

Sakaguchi, M. (2011). Practical aspects of the fertility of dairy cattle. *Journal of Reproduction and Development* **57**, 17–33.

Sales, J.N.S., Neves, A.H., Souza, A.H., Crepaldi, G.A., Sala, R.V., Fosado, M., Campos Filho, E.P., de Faria, C., Sa Filho, M.F. and Baruselli, P.S. (2011). Timing of insemination and fertility in dairy and beef cattle receiving timed artificial insemination using sex-sorted sperm. *Theriogenology* **76**, 427–435.

Sartori, R., Bastos, M.R., Mollo, M.R. and Martins, A.C. (2007). Influence of feed intake on embryo production in cattle. *Acta Scientifica Veterinaria* **35**, Suppl. 3, s874–s878.

Seidel, G.E. Overview of sexing sperm. (2007). *Theriogenology* **68**, 443–446.

Shaw, C. and Dobson, H. (1996). Reproductive and financial impact of a do-it-yourself artificial insemination programme compared with keeping a bull. *Veterinary Record* **139**, 594–597.

Sprecher, D.J., Farmer, J.A., Nebel, R.L. and Mather, E.C. (1995). The educational implications of reproductive problems identified during investigations at Michigan dairy farms. *Theriogenology* **43**, 373–380.

Steeneveld, W. and Hogeveen, H. (2012). Economic consequences of immediate or delayed insemination of a cow in oestrus. *Veterinary Record* **171**, 17–22.

Stevenson, J.S. (2011). Alternative programs to presynchronise estrous cycles in dairy cattle before a timed artificial insemination program. *Journal of Dairy Science* **94**, 205–217.

Stevenson, J.S. (2012). *To presynch or not to presynch?* At: http://www.hoards.com/E_reproduction/REP33. Accessed 30-9-12.

Stevenson, J.S., Pursley, J.R., Garverick, H.A., Fricke, P.M., Kesler, D.J., Ottobre, J.S. and Wiltbank, M.C. (2006). Treatment of cycling and noncycling lactating dairy cows with progesterone during Ovsynch. *Journal of Dairy Science* **89**, 2567–2578.

Trigal, B., Gómez, E., Caamano, J.N., Muñoz, M.J., Moreno, J., Carrocera, S., Martin, D. and Diez, C. (2012). *In vitro* and *in vivo* quality of bovine embryos in vitro produced with sex-sorted sperm. *Theriogenology* **78**, 1465–1475.

Van Soom, A. and Nauwynck, H.J. (2008). Risks associated with bovine embryo transfer and their containment. *CAB Reviews: Perspectives in Agriculture, Veterinary Science, Nutrition and Natural Resources* **3**(060), 7 pp.

Van Soom, A., Mateusen, B., Leroy, J. and de Kruif, A. (2003). Assessment of mammalian embryo quality: what can we learn from embryo morphology? *Reproductive BioMedicine Online* 7, 664–670.

Van Vliet, J.H. and Van Eerdenburg, F.J.C.M. (1996). Sexual activities and oestrus detection in lactating Holstein cows. *Applied Animal Behaviour Science* **50**, 57–69.

Velazquez, M.A. (2011). The role of nutritional supplementation on the outcome of superovulation in cattle. *Animal Reproduction Science* **126**, 1–10.

Vishwanath, R., Mells, J., Johnson, D.L. and Xu, Z.Z. (2004). Effect of timing of insemination of dairy cows with liquid semen relative to the observation of oestrus. *Proceedings of the New Zealand Society of Animal Production* **64**, 140–142.

Wiltbank, M.C., Sartori, R., Herlihy, M.M., Vasconcelos, J.L.M., Nascimento, A.B., Souza, A.H., Ayres, H., Cunha, A.P., Keskin, A., Guenther, J.N. and Gumen, A. (2011). Managing the dominant follicle in lactating dairy cows. *Theriogenology* **76**, 1568–1582.

Youngs, C.R., Leibo, S.P. and Godke, R.A. (2010). Embryo cryopreservation in domestic mammalian livestock species. *CAB Reviews: Perspectives in Agriculture, Veterinary Science, Nutrition and Natural Resources* 5(060), 1–11.

CHAPTER 43

Optimising Herd Fertility: the Farm Audit

Rob Smith

Learning objectives

- Understand the key performance indicators and target values used to measure performance.
- Understand the factors to consider when setting targets.
- Understand the factors which impact on fertility and the information that needs to be gathered during the farm audit.

The aim of this chapter is to provide the veterinarian with a structured explanation of key elements that affect fertility and outline KPIs and target values that can be used measure performance. Investigative approaches to sub-optimal performance will be presented.

Introduction

Reproduction in dairy cows has two main outcomes: production of a calf that has economic value (which may be a replacement heifer); and the stimulation of a new lactation. The targets for reproductive performance for a herd are dependent on the farming system adopted which, in turn, should be focused on efficient delivery of the milk supply contract the farm is aiming to fulfil. The two extremes to consider are; seasonal (spring) calving, to synchronise peak lactation with peak grazed grass availability producing milk for manufacturing; and all year round calving, to fulfil a 'level dairy' supply contract (often $\pm$ 10% of a set volume per month) to meet all year round demand for liquid milk. Autumn calving to supply peak demand from conserved feed and purchased concentrate, and then utilise grazed grass at turn-out in the spring to meet the lower demands of late lactation, can also be a viable system. Mixtures of these systems on one unit can be adopted but, when auditing performance, it needs to be clear if this is a result of planned breeding and rational financial justification, or if it is a result of poor herd performance and an inability to reach fertility targets.

After calving, a cow must overcome a series of physiological hurdles for conception to take place (Table 43.1).

Failing to overcome a hurdle reduces the likelihood of an animal conceiving at the required time. Thus, the time from calving to overcoming these hurdles, and the proportion of animals that have done so by a set time, can be used as performance indicators and, also, as an early warning system that herd management is not going to achieve the required pattern of conceptions. Thus the time from calving to overcoming these physiological hurdles can be used as key performance indicators. Once the breeding period starts for the group or an individual, the percentage of animals served and also identified pregnant per three weeks (the length of an oestrous cycle), and by set periods after calving or into the breeding period, also generates KPIs (Table 43.2).

Types of KPI

KPIs can be divided into those that determine the proportion of a cohort that have a particular outcome to an event (e.g. the proportion pregnant to a service), and the time to that event (e.g. calving to conception interval). These two types can be combined in KPIs determining the proportion that have had a particular outcome by a determined time (e.g. the percentage of animals which have conceived by 100 days after calving, the '100 day in calf rate'). These can be taken from 'failure' plots of calving to conception for a cohort (Figure 43.1).

The exact number of days after calving to be used has been hotly debated. One hundred days seems appropriate for seasonal calving herds, but 120 days may better differentiate adequately performing, high-yielding, all year round calving herds. If the performance of a cohort is monitored, then time to event data will get worse as the average time from calving of the cohort get longer and further animals conceive.

Culling or continuing to serve management decisions also impact on the KPI and its interpretation. The number of animals

Bovine Medicine, Third Edition. Edited by Peter D. Cockcroft.

Table 43.1 Post-calving period: key performance indicators and target values.

Time relative to calving	Event	KPI	Notes
-72hours	Induction of parturition	% induced target 0%	NZ target < 4%.
0	Intervention at calving	% assisted calving Target < 4%	Analyse by bull. Use of easy calving bulls.
1–12 hours	Delivery of foetal membranes	% retention of foetal membranes (over 12 hrs) Target < 2%	Related to dry cow nutrition and milk fever.
1–21 days	Involution of uterus and expulsion of contents	Score involution at post natal/ pre-breeding check	Related to dry cow nutrition and milk fever.
7–28 days	Resolution of uterine bacterial contamination	% endometritis at 28+ days Target < 10%	28+ days post-calving.
14–28 days	Resumption of ovarian cyclicity	% with CL and single or twin dominant follicles under 20 mm diameter, or signs of oestrus at post natal/pre-breeding check 28 days+ after calving. Target 100% (See Peake *et al.*, 2011)	No CL = not ovulated. Small ovaries with no metoestrus bleeding = anoestrous. Single versus multiple dominant follicles at pre-breeding and ONO examinations – suggest oestradiol production is not sufficient so FSH not suppressed. Fate of first dominant follicle depends on LH pulse frequency – main determinate is energy balance or stressors.
14–35 days	First display oestrus	Days to 1st recorded oestrus Target <42 days	80% of 1st ovulation show no oestrus expression due to lack of progesterone priming.
Until start of service	Oestrus	% observed in oestrus prior to service period Target dependent on VWP but ideally 100%. Seasonal herds under 65+% investigate	Write in 21-day diary to predict time of next oestrus to focus oestrus observation.

that are culled for failure to conceive should be monitored. The 100 days in calf and 200 days not in calf rates, using the number of animals calved and ever eligible to be served as the denominator (rather than the number who survive to these times), are relatively immune to the effects of involuntary culling.

The size of the cohorts, and time over which cohorts are selected to produce a KPI, are important for their validity and timeliness. Large cohort size avoids observed changes being influenced by natural variation but, in small herds, this means that the cohort covers a long period of time, so problems are not detected early. Conversely, natural variation is not identified as 'a problem', either. The cohort is traditionally all the animals that have had a particular event occur in that calendar year or rolling 12-month period. For example, the interval from one calving to next calving of all animals that calve in a calendar year is the calving index for a herd.

The main problem with this approach is that it is very historical. Conceptions that make up the current calving index occurred 9–21 months earlier. The management factors that may have led to failure to conceive may have occurred 12–24 months ago or more. Changing current practices in response to historical, rather than contemporary, data runs the risk of making erroneous decisions.

This has been addressed in some computer programmes by production of three-month as well as 12-month rolling averages and use of control charts, such as cumulative sums (cu-sum), which show changes in the trends. It is still a matter of judgement as to how long a trend needs to occur before remedial action is indicated. The delay in confirming the outcome of pregnancy, possible from four weeks after service, but delayed until the end of the breeding period on some farms, also adds a delay. Using non-return to oestrus as a proxy for pregnancy carries the danger of interpreting anoestrus as pregnancy (Box 43.1). Statistical analysis has not yet encroached into this area, but determining the appropriate critical probability before a trend can be said to not be due to natural variation needs careful consideration. The classical scientific $p = 0.05$, or 1 in 20 times it will be due to natural variation, will be too stringent, and 1 in 5–10 may be more appropriate, given the time lag in production of the underlying data.

Table 43.2 Service period: key performance indicators and target values.

KPIs for the service period End of voluntary waiting period (VWP) in all year round herds (42–60 days after calving) Earliest service date (ESD) in seasonally calving herds calculated back from the planned start of calving – 282 days			
Time relative to calving	Event	KPI	Notes
First 21-day period	Oestrus detection and Service	• % served in first three weeks of breeding season (first service submission rate). Target 100%. • Calving to first service interval. • VWP/ESD to first service interval. Target 11 days. • % conceived in first three weeks of breeding season. Target 65%. • % served by 80 days post-calving. Target 70–100%, depending on system.	
First and subsequent 21-day periods	Oestrus detection and Service	• Calving to conception. • VWP/ESD to conception. • All services submission rate. • Pregnancy rate by service number. • 6th and 9th week (from start of breeding season) in calf rates. For seasonal herds. Targets 80 and 96 % respectively. • 100 or 120 day (after individual cows calving) in-calf rates for all year round herds. Target 60%. • 200 day not in-calf rate <10%.	120 day in calf rate suggested as better differentiator of good verses poor performance in higher yielding all year calving herds.
14 days after service	Maternal recognition of pregnancy	• Failure leads to return to oestrus at normal 18–24 day interval	All inter-service interval information assumes the original service is to a correctly identified oestrus.
	Late embryonic death	• Irregular inter-oestrus intervals over 24 days	See Figure 43.6.
	Diagnosis of pregnancy	• % positive of those undergoing pregnancy diagnosis (PD) • Cow presented for service are those not re-served so depends on pregnancy rate and submission rate.	Target 100%, but realistic target dependent on timing of PD after service. After one possible oestrus, i.e. before 36 days – 88% After two possible oestrus, i.e. after 48 days – 96%
	Abortion	• Target 2%	Abortion more likely in twin pregnancies, which are more common in higher-yielding cows. Investigate all abortions.

High numbers of returns (low non-return rate) is a definitive sign of low pregnancy rate. Return within 18 days suggests incorrectly timed original service. This can be used as an indicator that there is a fertility problem and other animals may also not be pregnant. However, high non-return rates can be due to a return to anoestrus, reduced oestrus expression and low submission rate. Confirmation of pregnancy by a specific method such as palpation or ultrasonography per rectum, pregnancy associated glycoprotein assay is strongly advised to ensure these assumptions are not misplaced.

Averages must be used with caution. Data may be extremely skewed, and medians may give a better representation of the herd performance than means. However, the distribution of the data is also important. This is readily appreciated if we consider calving to conception interval (Figure 43.2). If an animal conceives early, it will dry off early, have a short lactation and produce less milk. If an animal conceives at 40 days post-calving, for example, and is given a dry period of 60 days and a gestation length of 285 days, it will only lactate for 265 days. Classically, the rate the yield reduces after peak is 3% per week (Wood's

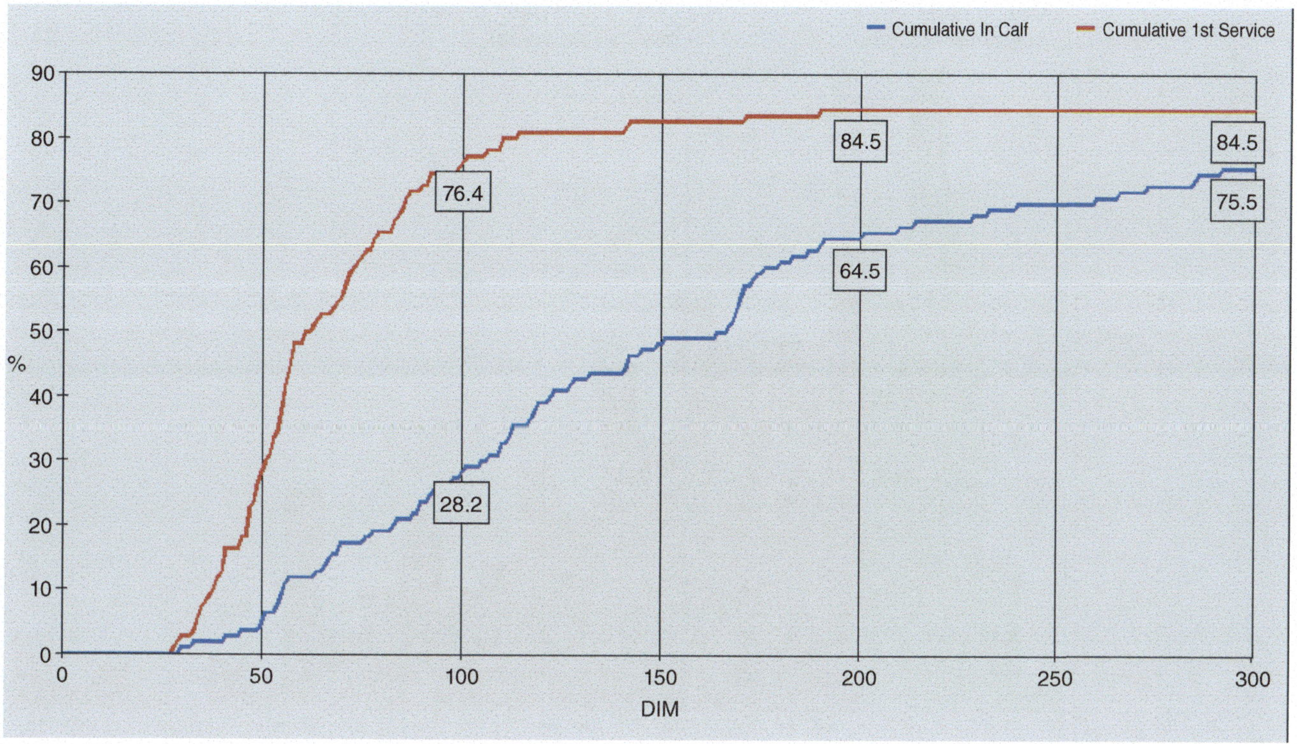

Figure 43.1 Failure curve showing the % of animals having a first service and conceived with time after calving. Value at 100 days is the 100 day in calf rate. Value at 200 days is the 200 day not in calf rate. (Program: *TotalVet QMMS/SUMIT* Software).

Box 43.1 Non-return rate (NRR)

If animals are not re-served they may be pregnant. The non-return rate, the number of animals that have not returned to oestrus by a specified time after service, may be used to indicate pregnancy. This may be non-return by:

- 35 days (NRR35) for dairy cows who would then get a pregnancy diagnosis on veterinary fertility visits every two weeks,
- 49 days (NRR49) used for grazing animals in New Zealand-type system;
- 56 days (NRR56) used by AI companies as a proxy for bull semen pregnancy rate as, at least in the UK, they do not have access to actual farm data so they assume not being asked to return to re-serve an animal correlates with actual number of animals becoming pregnant.

curve), but being pregnant will suppress lactation further. The animal will be dried off and calve again within the year and the ratio of days lactating to days dry will be lower, and the overall yield per year will be lower than if the animal had conceived later. Also, in many herds, the pregnancy rate is lower when animals are served earlier, so overall the cost of a pregnancy is higher, as more services are required. Cows that conceive later have more days milking, but also have more days milking at a lower yield, and the next peak lactation is delayed. There are also health, energetic and economic consequences of being fed more than they require for production. Putting fat on and then losing it is, overall, less efficient than eating food directly for production, and increased body condition score increases the likely amount of BCS loss after calving and also the risk of fatty liver and other post-partum diseases. Cows that do not conceive until after target will produce less milk per year, as they have more days of lower yield in their lifetime. A herd with a mixture of cows at these two extremes may have the same mean and median calving to conception interval as a herd where all cows were on target, but would have less milk produced per cow per year. In seasonally calving herds, these animals will also calve either earlier than the feed supply, or too late to make full and efficient use of it. A tight pattern is also important to reduce both pathogen build-up in the environment and the need to prolong calving supervision.

It should be recognised that, even in poorly managed herds, many cows show good reproductive performance. Any changes aimed to improve the average must not reduce the fertility of these cows. The animals within the herd with the problem should be identified. By determining what risk factors they have, compared to their well-performing herdmates, it is possible to gain an insight into the underlying causes, and to formulate possible

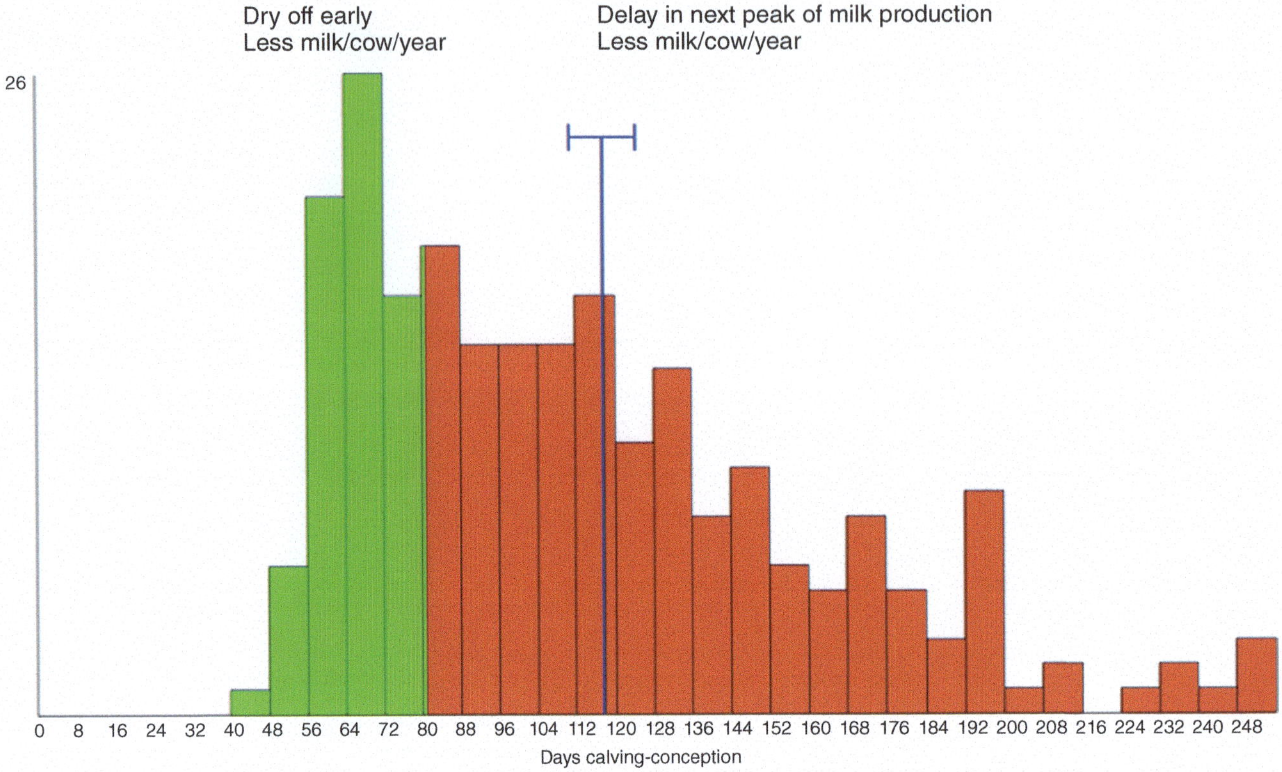

Figure 43.2 Calving to conception spread. Green animals below 80 days, red above. Mean (blue line) 118 days, median 105 days. (Program: *Interherd*, Pan Livestock Services).

Box 43.2 Pregnancy rate verses conception rate

The percentage of ova that are fertilised by a correctly timed service may be as high as 80%. A variable proportion of these 'conceptions' are lost prior to the diagnosis of 'pregnancy'. The physiologically purist view is that the percentage of animals served that are subsequently detected as pregnant should be termed 'pregnancy rate', to ensure it is understood that the percentage of services resulting in an initial conception (conception rate) is higher and not measurable on farm, but that good management and disease control may reduce the number of conceptions lost prior to pregnancy diagnosis. This appears to be an uphill battle, as recently pregnancy rate (shortened to 'Preg rate') has been used to describe the percentage of animals eligible for service (i.e. after the ESD[1] or VWP[2] and not pregnant) that are served within a rolling three-week period and are subsequently detected as pregnant. Thus, it is a combination of submission rate and pregnancy rate (using the above ideal terminology). It has also been termed 'fertility factor' or 'fertility efficiency'.

Disagreements regarding terminology should not detract from increasing use of the percentage of animals eligible for service that are served within a rolling three-week period and are subsequently detected as pregnant as the single most timely indicator of overall fertility.

[1]Earliest service date (ESD) in seasonally calving herds, calculated back from the planned start of calving – 282 days.
[2]Voluntary waiting period (VWP) in all year round herds (usually 42–60 days after calving)

strategies to focus intervention on those animals that would benefit from it without risking reducing the performance of others. See Table 43.3 for examples of such subgroup analysis.

Rather than analysis of data from defined cohorts, data can be used as it is produced by adding it to cumulative sum (cu-sum) charts, giving a more rapid indication of performance. They have been traditionally used for service outcome, but can be used to relate occurrence of periparturient disease and subsequent service and conception by target time after calving (Figure 43.3). Looking at the date when the gradient of the graph changes allows the exact time the trend in fertility changes to be pinpointed. If management changes, such as alterations in feeding (silage clamp (bunker) or grazing paddocks), are recorded in the farm diary and marked on the graph (Figure 43.4), then their influence on fertility can be determined. This can be done for different groups or cohorts (e.g. higher- and lower-yielding cohort, heifer and cows), to detect patterns.

There is also a cost to an animal becoming pregnant. Under circumstances where cost of pregnancy are high (high staff and semen costs, low pregnancy rate, a small difference in cost

Table 43.3 Examples of measuring subgroup performance using subgroup KPI outcomes.

Subgroup	Comments
All fertility KPIs by milk production cohort (ideally in relation to genetic potential: high, intermediate, low)	Poorer fertility in higher-producing animals suggests they have poorer energy balance. Conversely, poorer fertility in lower yielding animals suggest poor health/disease, affecting both yield and fertility.
Service outcome by AI technician	Used to monitor technician performance. Farm staff may be compared by pregnancy rate to their services and cu-sums may be drawn for each to see how they vary over time. AI companies may use non-return rate at 56 days to monitor staff performance. Random variation depends on number served, but a ≥ 5 percentage point difference is worthy of discussion. May be due to types of animals served.
Service outcome by time of service after calving	As negative energy balance may last for 60+ days post-partum, and the developing ovum may be influenced by its environment, earlier services at 40–50 days after calving may be more successful than those 80–100 days after, when the ovum has developed during negative energy balance.
Calving to first service and conception and service outcome by parity	If first calved heifers have a poor performance and are in the same group as cows, this suggests increased stress. Competition for resources including water, feed and cubicles may be responsible. If older higher-yielding cows have a poor performance, this suggests negative energy balance and inadequate diet energy density and/or lameness.

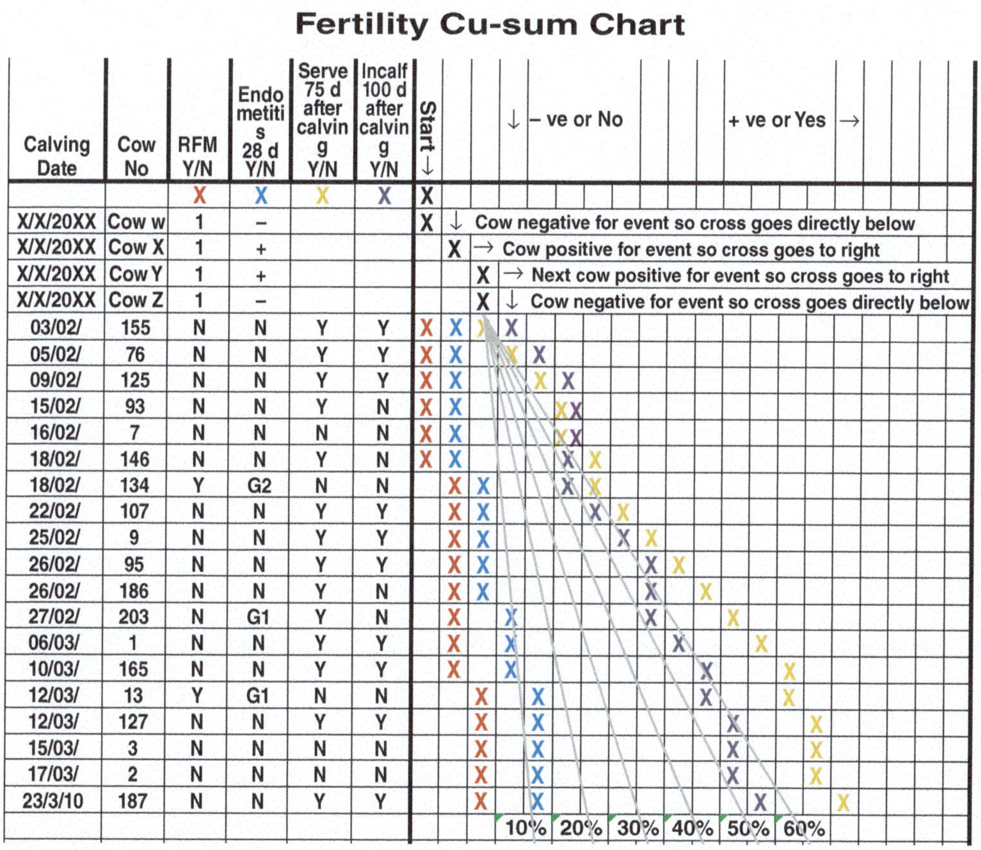

Figure 43.3 Cumulative sum control chart for periparturient disease and service and conception by target time after calving. Explanation of how a cu-sum is constructed are on the first four lines, and blank chart can be printed off and used in the farm office. Milk fever and other metabolic conditions can be added (program: Microsoft *Excel*).

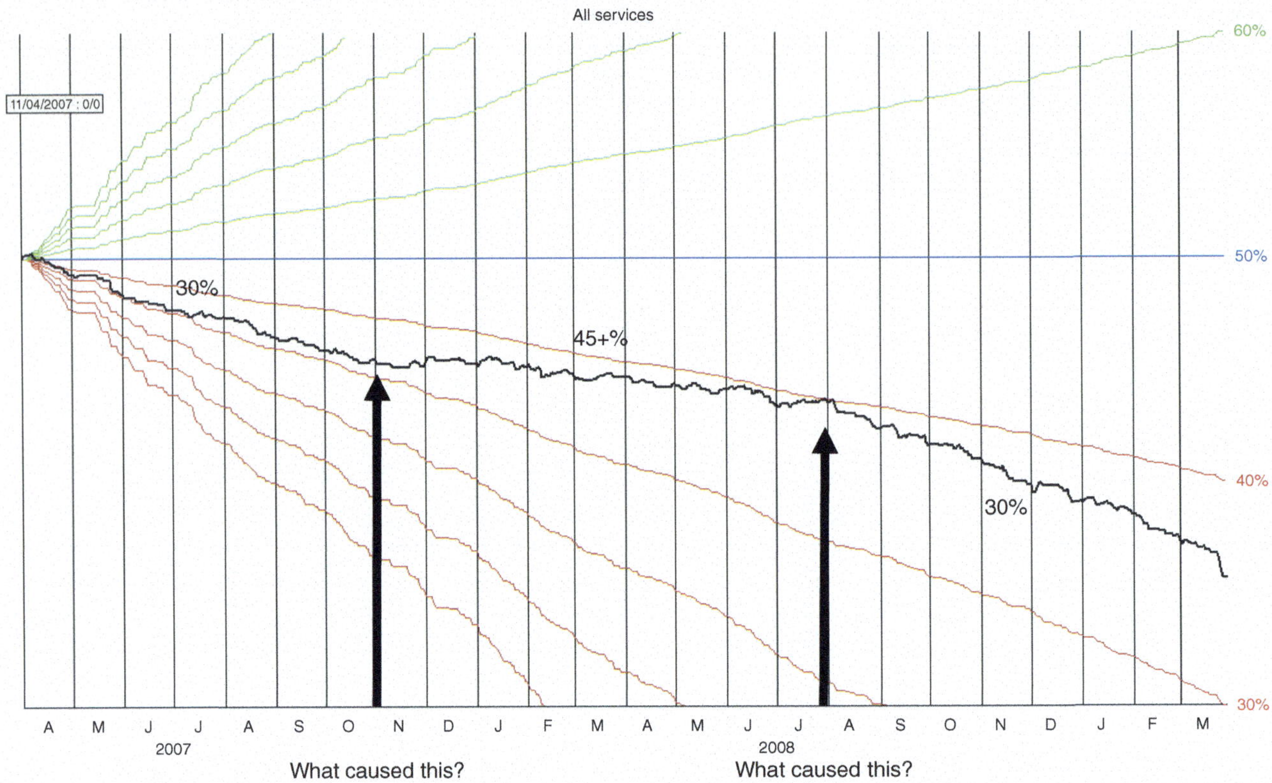

Figure 43.4 Cumulative sum control chart for service outcome over time (black line). Positive outcome = line goes up. Negative outcome = line goes down. Services are in time order but even time per month. Green, blue and red lines are calculated indicating different pregnancy rates. Arrows point to where the gradient of the black line changes, indicating change in herd pregnancy rate (program: *Interherd*, Pan Livestock Services).

between an in-calf or freshly calved cow and the income from a cull cow) and benefit is low (cows have a flat lactation curve, so the difference between peak and late lactation is small and purchase costs of replacement animals are low), re-serving animals may not be economically beneficial (De Vries, 2006). Some farmers will state that pregnancy rates are too low if animals are served too soon after calving, so they employ a long, voluntary waiting period. This can exacerbate post-calving problems in subsequent lactations, as the cows that have extended lactations may put on body condition as they are fed for a higher yield than they are producing. They then have reduced dry matter intake and lose body condition score after calving, thus reducing the likelihood of conception in the next lactation. Good management may overcome these problems, but their potential needs to be recognised when voluntary waiting period is decided.

Fertility KPIs, specifically the 120 day in calf rate and the percentage of heifers not mated by 17 months of age, have been suggested as indicators of poor animal welfare in a herd (Nyman *et al.*, 2011). Many welfarists are not comfortable with production being an indicator of welfare, but good management underpins both good fertility and good welfare. Induction of parturition to maintain tight calving patterns became very common in New Zealand, and concerns regarding consumer perception resulted in national targets of under 4% of any herd being induced having been set by the industry (Anon, 2010). There are welfare concerns regarding other fertility practices. Some organic farming standards do not allow management use of exogenous reproductive hormones. The percentage of animals receiving induction of oestrus, or fixed time insemination protocols, may become KPIs to monitor these practices in the food supply chain.

The capabilities of the farm staff also need to be audited. Recording service outcome by the person who identified the oestrus (both staff and any automated system and the signs observed) and who inseminated the animal is useful. This can also instil healthy competition, but success, rather than just submission for service, needs to be used, otherwise erroneous services can result. The timing between services, the inter-service interval, can indicate the quality of oestrus detection. The interpretation of inter-service intervals histograms, available in several programs, are shown in Figure 43.5. Embryonic loss can also affect these patterns, so submission rate data (see Box 43.3) should also be used to assess oestrus detection. Studies from diverse populations indicate that around 10%

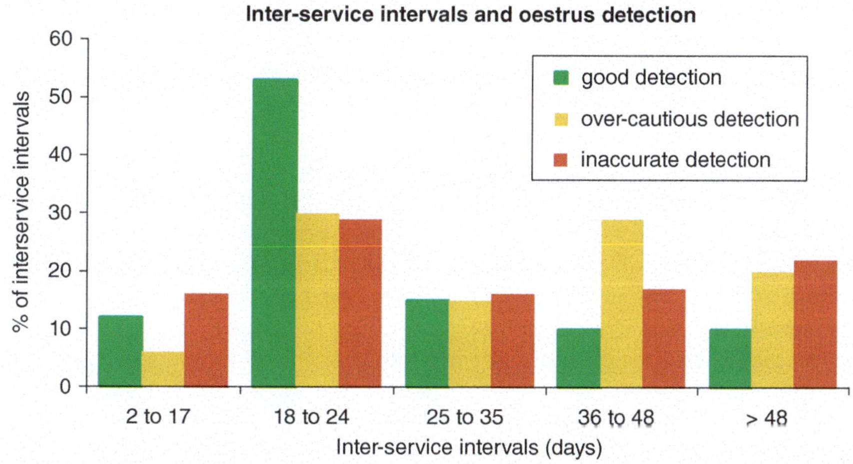

Figure 43.5 Interpretation of inter-service interval histogram. Ideally, repeat services would occur in the 18–24 day period; target over 55%.Target ratios between number of animals with inter-service intervals in different periods have also been suggested such as 5 : 1 between number of animals with inter-service intervals of 18–24 days and number with 36–48 days intervals. (Adapted from Anon, 1984).

Box 43.3 Submission Rate

Submission rate is the percentage of animals past the ESD or VWP, and thus eligible for service, which are served in a three week period. Two variations can be produced:

1 *First Service Submission rate*. This is either the percentage of animals served in the first three weeks of the breeding period, for seasonal herds, or the percentage of animals served in the first three weeks after the voluntary waiting period, in all year round herds. This is related to return to cyclicity after calving and oestrus detection efficiency. A variation is to identify animals which have not received a first service after the ESD/VWP, and determine the percentage which are serviced in a rolling three-week period. This is the timeliest piece of data available on farm, as it can be calculated for the last three weeks at any time, although numbers of animals may be low, so interpret with caution.

2 *All services submission rate*. The percentage of animals eligible to be served that are served in a rolling three-week period. It is a reflection of oestrus detection and cyclicity. Animals are eligible if they have passed the ESD/VWP and are not pregnant. *This parameter can only be calculated once pregnancy diagnosis has been confirmed.*

The later after service pregnancy diagnosis is performed, the higher the percentage pregnant should be.

For example: 40% pregnant to the service and 80% submission/oestrus detection rate of non-pregnant animals at subsequent services, 18–24 days and 36–48 days later.

If 100 cows are served 40 cows would be pregnant. 60 cows *should* be seen at the return to oestrus 21 days later but, because the oestrus detection rate is only 80%, 12 cows are not re-served and are also presented for PD, so a total of 52 cows are presented for PD and 40/52 are pregnant. 40/52 = 77% .

If the animals are presented for PD after two possible cycles, then there are 12 animals not detected in oestrus at the first service. 12 × 0.2 = 2 animals are not detected at the second possible oestrus, so only 42 animals will be presented; 40 out of 42 = 95% are in calf.

This makes the all-services submission rate more historical than the first service submission rate – how historical depends on when the pregnancy diagnosis takes place. It is less sensitive to delays in return to cyclicity after calving than is first service submission rate.

of animals are submitted for AI when milk progesterone is high, suggesting they are in luteal phase. Strategic use of milk progesterone samples to indicate to staff that cows are not in oestrus can be an aid to re-training.

Planning the farm visit

If the veterinarian is not familiar with the farm, it is best to obtain baseline information via a standard questionnaire, and review any fertility data available, prior to visiting the farm. This allows the veterinarian to be aware of major problems, so that questions can be more focused, and any anomalies between answers provided and evidence from data can be tactfully discussed. Many herd managers are aware of the ideal, and will discuss this with a good degree of understanding. All staff involved in fertility management need to be involved, so that what actually happens on the farm can be determined. The drivers causing the farm to operate differently from this ideal, and the factors that may prevent improvement, need to be identified. This may range from financial or infrastructural, to lay belief in a different way of working or cause of disease.

Looking at the cows

The veterinarian should walk the farm, accompanied by farm staff. The general environment and cow comfort should be assessed. Locomotion, cleanliness and hock lesion scores can be recorded systematically, or as part of the overall impression of cow welfare. Specific issues, such as quality of floor surface, passageway width, size and access time to loafing area, cow group size and composition (for example, heifers or all non-pregnant cows in the same group), determine the likelihood that cows can express oestrus. The number of groups, the arrangement of buildings, training and experience of staff, staff time allocated will determine how easily any oestrus could be observed.

The signs that are used to determine oestrus should also be discussed. In some studies, only 50% of cows displayed standing oestrus. Secondary signs, such as chin resting and sniffing of the vulva, may be used to help improve submission rate. Suggestions on how to improve these parameters, based on realistic options for the farm, should be suggested in the report.

If a specific problem has been detected during pre-visit data analysis, fertility examination of cows in an identified risk group can be performed. These are contemporary data, but only a snapshot, so findings should not detract from overall conclusions gained from analysis of longitudinal data.

If no records of body condition score are available body condition scores can be determine for a selection of animals from each key management group to assess the potential amount of body condition score change occurring but be aware that they may not reflect relative differences throughout the year when food availability may vary. It may stimulate the vet and farm staff to commence longitudinal monitoring.

Individual risk factors for poor fertility are outlined in the HACCP (Chapter 44). Recent research suggests that stressors interact, and a mild stressor that would not have reproductive consequences on its own can interact with another, resulting in reproductive failure (Figure 43.6; Peake *et al.*, 2011). For example, increased somatic cell count on its own did not affect the proportion of animals ovulating, but potentiated the effect of lameness, significantly reducing the number of lame, high cell count cows that ovulated (Morris *et al.*, 2009).

Setting targets

The ultimate targets for the farm will depend on the farming system, and possible targets are outlined in Tables 43.1 and 43.2. Interim targets should be agreed with the farm staff for the next breeding period, and reviewed before further, progressively tougher targets are set approaching the ultimate target. This aids morale and incentivises staff to focus on the task of submitting cows for service. If farm staff expect to fail, because the targets are initially set too high, they will not be well motivated and nothing will be achieved. Computer programs such as the *Interherd+* program in the UK, and the *InCalf* project in Australia, set a target of the top 25% percentile, or the average of the top 25% of farms for a KPI. This means that 25% of farms are already meeting that standard. They can then be given the top 10% performance as a goal. Those in the top 10% are usually driving themselves, so will be aware of their performance and already actively monitoring it.

Infectious disease monitoring using bulk tank milk samples is inexpensive. The monitoring scope and schedule will depend on the disease status and vaccinations used on farm. Bulk tank samples can be tested for leptospirosis, BVD and IBR (Johne's and liver fluke are additional options which may be of interest on some farms). A testing frequency of every three months may be appropriate, with the outcomes being closely scrutinised for changes in status. Vaccination strategies and the number of

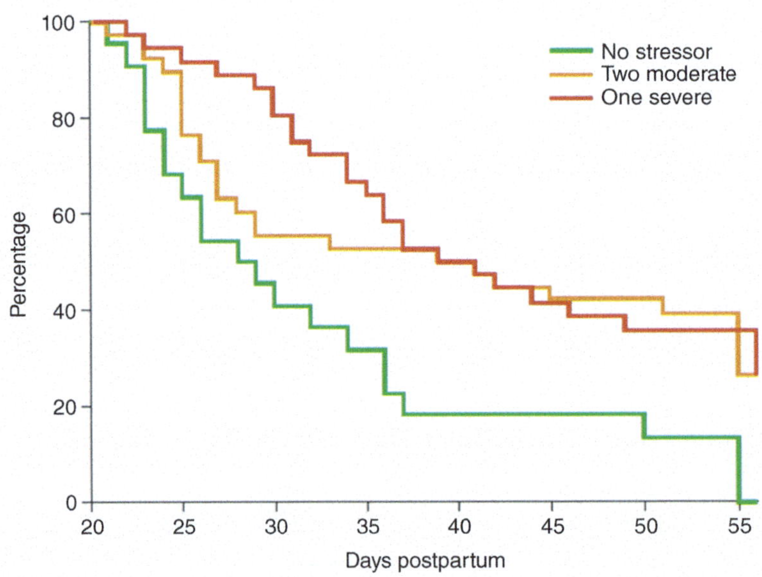

Figure 43.6 Failure plot of time to first luteal phase after calving for animal with one, mild, two mild or one severe stressor (lameness, sub-clinical mastitis and body condition score loss). From Peake *et al.* (2011).

animals not vaccinated should be reviewed, as many animals are not vaccinated at the correct schedule, to maximise immunity at the appropriate time relative to service. Ideally, all abortions should be investigated and any requirements of national animal health legislation, such as notification of suspicion of disease, must be followed.

Conclusion

Fertility is intrinsically linked with milk production. Fertility performance is a bellwether for quality of the animal environment, overall management and nutrition. To have a positive influence on fertility, the veterinary surgeon needs to be an active part of the herd management team, meeting with the herd manager, agricultural advisor and nutritionalist, and should be actively monitoring up-to-date fertility information. Selecting the correct KPIs for the farming system employed and the data available are key to auditing herd fertility. A dairy herd health questionnaire to assist in the process can be found in Annex 43.1 at the end of this chapter.

References and other sources of information

Anon (1984). *Dairy Herd Fertility*. Her Majesty's Stationary Office, London. ISBN: 0 11 242715 4.

De Vries, A. (2006). Economic value of pregnancy in dairy cattle. *Journal of Dairy Science* **89**, 3876–85.

Dobson, H., Smith, R.F., Royal, M.D., Knight, C.H. and Sheldon I.M. (2007). The High-producing Dairy Cow and its Reproductive Performance. *Reproduction in Domestic Animals* **42**(Suppl. 2), 17–23.

DairyAustralia Incalf project: http://www.dairyaustralia.com.au/Animals-feed-and-environment/Fertility.aspx

DairyCo Pd+ fertility improvement programme: http://www.dairyco.org.uk/technical-information/fertility/pdplus/

Holmes, C.W., Brookes, I.M., Garrick, D.J., Mackenzie, D.D.S., Parkinson, T.J. and Wilson, G.F. (2002) *Milk Production from Pasture, Principles and Practices*. ISBN 0 473 08308 6. Massey University Press.

Morris, M.J., Walker, S.L., Jones, D.N., Routly, J.E., Smith, R.F and Dobson, H. (2009) Influence of somatic cell count, body condition and lameness on follicular growth and ovulation in dairy cows. *Theriogenology* **71**, 801.

New Zealand Veterinary Council Induction of Calves (2010). (http://www.vetcouncil.org.nz/documentation/Other/Operational Guidelines_InductionOfCalving.pdf, accessed 24/2/2013.

Nyman, A.K., Lindberg, A. and Sandgren, C. H. (2011) Can pre-collected register data be used to identify dairy herds with good cattle welfare? *Acta Veterinaria Scandinavica* **53**(Suppl. 1), S8.

Peake, K.A., Biggs, A.M., Argo, C.M., Smith, R.F., Christley, R.M., Routly, J.E. and Dobson, H. (2011) Effects of lameness, subclinical mastitis and loss of body condition on the reproductive performance of dairy cows. *Veterinary Record* **168**, 301.

Refsdal, A.O. (2000) To treat or not to treat: a proper use of hormones and antibiotics. *Animal Reproduction Science* **60**, 109.

DAIRY HERD HEALTH QUESTIONNAIRE

GENERAL:

Name:.. Telephone No:..

Address:.. Best time to telephone:.........................

....

Staff

Name	Experience	Training	Duties	Specific responsibilities	Financial interest in business?

What farm records are available? Milk Recording Y/N..........................Organisation.......................Feed Analysis................................

Agricultural adviser...

On-farm computer system..

Herd Size:

Unweaned calves ....
Heifers under 1 year........................
Heifers over 1 year..........................

Cows lst lact...............................
Cows over 5 lact........................
Cows total ....

Quota (owned).. (leased in/out)...

Milk contract:... **Profile required: seasonal/level/other** ....
(other contracts/profiles that may be available...)

Other farm enterprises...

Last 12 months herd changes:

Cows bought...........................
Heifers bought......................
Calves bought........................

Cows sold...................
Heifers sold...............
Calves sold.................

Farmer perception:

What are your main aims?...
....

What are the main farm problems that concern you?..
....
....

1 FERTILITY AND CALVING

Intended calving pattern – All year/Autumn/Spring

Actual calvings each month (most recent 12 months)

Jan.	Feb	March	April	May	June	July	Aug	Sept.	Oct.	Nov.	Dec.

Earliest service date/s ....End of service period/s..

Voluntary Waiting period (VWP)

Policy for any variation of VWP

Cow numbering: All/Some/None   Freeze brand/Jumbo tag/Neck band/None

Oestrus detection:

Who is involved?   Timing and duration of observations

Area for oestrus expression (e.g. outside loafing area), ...passageway width.............................

All non-pregnant cows grouped together? Y/N Group sizes

Heat detection aids - Kamar/Paint/Bull/RMS/automated system (.....................)/other

When checked/ who responsible?   Any automated alerts (email/text) Y/N to whom?

% within 30 days of VWP without an active device on?

% of heats detected after VWP actually served....................

Bulling cow records kept – Y/N

18–24 day returns diary kept – Y/N   Any automated alerts (email/text) Y/N to whom?

Metoestrous bleeding checked Y/N   added to returns diary for 16–22 days? Y/N

Service methods used

% Service Natural ....AI............ET recipient planned...........ET repeat breeder

Number of bulls
System used (running with cows – single or team/supervised mating)
Rest/work cycle for bull
Bedding access, feeding arrangements (cow TMR = increased BCS) body condition score
Mobility scores
Semen tested before use /annually?   Y/N copy of latest report

AI Procedures

DIY A.I./Technician AI/mix – specify

Who?   Training history of AI staff (Compare pregnancy rates)

Policy for use of sexed semen

Policy for use of mixed semen (Fertility+)

Review AI flask management and refill arrangements.
(Consider post thaw motility test semen if poor pregnancy rates)

Location of AI...............restraint (crush/yoke/gate/stall/other..................
Duration of isolation from cows..................from food................

AI Sire selection criteria:

Bull breeds used – heifers.............................. Cows....................
(Review PTA/EBVs of bulls)

Service Management

% serves after full synchronisation protocols 1st service........ 2–4th service .... 4th+service ....
% serves after Prostaglandin for Oestrus not observed 1st......... 2–4th........... 4th+...........
Policy for post natal checks (7–21 days PP?)..% of animals seen
Policy for pre-breeding checks (28–42 days PP?)...% of animals seen
Policy for oestrus not observed/not seen Bulling cows ....% of animals seen
Policy for cows 4th service+/over 80–100 days into breeding period
(e.g. mixed semen straw/double service/day 10–12 GnRH/Progesterone supplementation/ other......................).

Pregnancy diagnosis Some/All/None Timing of PD

Method – Who? Manual/Ultrasound/Milk progesterone/Milk PAG/other

% Abortions......................
% investigated? Diagnosis?

Bulk milk Antibody classification for BVDv, IBR, Lepto.

Fertility Records:

Calving index..
Calving – 1st Service...
Pregnancy rate...
Number of culls for poor fertility...

Reproductive Disease Events
% Dystocia (any intervention at calving)
Assisted (Farmer). ....
Assisted (Vet).................
No. calves born dead
% Retained foetal membranes (over 12 hours after calving)
% Metritis
% Endometritis grade 1...........grade 2...........grade 3.............
Seasonal trends?
Trend of disease with dry/transition cow nutrition (grazing) Y/N
Trend of disease with dry/transition cow stocking density Y/N

Have you had any cow deaths around calving? ....

Type of freshly calved cow housing........
Average time in freshly calved cow group after calving: heifer..............cow................

Mobility
Does herd mobility score? Review score distribution and history
Routine foot trimming?
Recording of lame cows and lesion type

% lesion detected by type heifers...........cows............

Is there a heifer group after calving?

Feed barrier space per cow (feed face competition)

Body Condition Score (Score min 20 or if less all of management group)

Review records and plot individual cow BCs changes if possible or assess each group now and calculate assumed changes.

Low yielders 2–3 months prior to drying off
Far off dry cow group
Close to calving dry cow group
Freshly calved cows
Cows 2–3 months after calving

CHAPTER 44

A Hazards Analysis Critical Control Point Approach to Improving Reproductive Performance in Lactating Dairy Cows

I.J. Lean, A.R. Rabiee and N. Moss

Learning objectives

- Appreciate how the HACCP approach can improve reproductive performance.
- Appreciate the need for risk assessment in reproductive management.
- Appreciate the critical control points in reproductive performance.
- Appreciate the critical management control points to maintain and improve fertility.
- Appreciate the need to monitor and review the corrective measures and risk management procedures associated with reproductive performance.

Introduction

Hazards analysis critical control point (HACCP) methods are used in many industries to provide quality outcomes. A HACCP includes design of a production process, decomposition diagram, identification of hazards, risk assessment, definition of critical control points and critical management points, active monitoring of the process, planning corrective measures and risk management procedures. These have been used to manage reproduction in dairy herds for some time (Lean *et al.*, 2000). The HACCP provides a logical framework to understand reproduction as a series of time-related events and actions needed to improve reproductive performance. Factors under the direct control of farm managers are the focus.

A critical part of quality assurance is to ensure that outcomes are measured accurately, and effective systems for recording and analysing data are a prerequisite for optimal reproductive performance.

Defining optimal reproductive outcomes

Reproductive efficiency targets are better based on measures indicating the proportion of cows becoming pregnant over a given period of time, or before a target time – for example, 21 day pregnancy rates, percentage pregnant by 100 days after calving (all year round herds, AYR) or percentage of cows pregnant by six weeks after the start of mating (seasonally calved herds (SCH) and split-calving herds). Other goals include a low percentage of cows not pregnant by the time after calving, so that it becomes necessary to cull for reproductive failure, a satisfactory conception rate and low rates of abortion.

The interval from calving to conception for a herd (or mating to conception) can be expressed mathematically as a cumulative survival curve that is determined by more than 100 different factors. However, the equation can be simplified to:

$$fn(t) = t_1 \pm \frac{C}{F \times M \times ODR} \tag{44.1}$$

Where:

t_1 = time to first breeding after calving or mating
F = female fertility (0–1)
M = male fertility (0–1)
ODR = ovulation detection efficiency (0–1)
C = cycle length of the cow.

All other factors are nested within these major factors. For example, factors relating to the quality of semen and delivery of

Bovine Medicine, Third Edition. Edited by Peter D. Cockcroft.

fertile sperm into the female tract are described within the factor 'male fertility'. A single management change may impinge on two or three of the measures in the equation. While absolute failure in male or female fertility or heat detection will result in no pregnancies, minor failures in several areas will lower pregnancy conception rates or delay conception unacceptably. This conceptual framework has been used to develop the HACCP outline (Table 44.1, Figure 44.1).

Calf and heifer rearing

Farmers exercise control over heifer rearing in two main areas; the nutritional plane of growth and insemination age. The following goals reflect successful heifer rearing management.

Targets

1 Heifers able to enter the herd at a maximum of 24 months of age and compete with older cows for feed and other resources. Body weights at breeding for dairy heifers are; 350kg for Holstein, 225kg for Jersey, 350kg for Brown- Swiss, 275kg for Ayrshire breeds.
2 Heifers achieve return to oestrus after calving at the same time as adult cows.
3 Heifers become pregnant at the same rate as adult cows.
4 Optimal body condition score at calving is 3.5 (1–5 scale).

Risk factors influencing heifer performance

- High rates of mortality can limit the number of herd replacements that are available. Actions: Use vaccination programs to control risks of loss.

Table 44.1 A HACCP approach to achieving 80% of cows pregnant by 100 days after calving or within six weeks of mating start date.

Key factors	Implications	Secondaryfactors	Comments and time-related hierarchy
Time to first breeding	Failure to breed early minimises the number of matings before milk production declines, making cows less profitable		***First area of time-related failure.*** Previous lactation and heifer rearing influence results 6–12 months later.
	An area that is very amenable to change for little cost	Farmer policy	Delay results from inattention or desire to increase conception rates.
	Can be modified by hormonal therapy with progesterone and $PGF_{2\alpha}$	Anoestrus	Small heifers not well grown, poor body condition at calving, disease.
		Therapeutic agents	Prostaglandin or progesterone programmes can shorten the period to first breeding.
Detection of ovulation	A precondition to mating, unless hormonal therapy with fixed-time inseminations is used		***Second area of time-related failure.***
		Farmer factors	Requires time, a few committed people; heat detection aids can help; prostaglandin or progesterone use can increase sensitivity.
	Using hormonal programs to increase the number of cows in heat at one time increases oestral display or fixed time insemination	Cow factors	Display time can be very short and display is influenced by prevalence of oestrus, nutrition, environment and temperature.
	Detecting returns to oestrus	Farmer factors	Reapply heat detection aids after oestrus.
Male fertility	Semen quality is affected by many issues outside the control of the farm	Semen factors	***Third area of time-related failure.***
		Semen storage	Tank maintenance and semen handling should be regularly assessed.
		Inseminator factors	Do-it-yourself inseminators at more risk of failure than professionals.
		Bull fertility	Potential problems may be reduced by vaccination for campylobacteriosis and physical examination.
Female fertility	The most complex of the factors		***Fourth area of time-related failure.***
		Disease	Metritis, cystic ovarian disease, lameness and mastitis are associated with delay in conception.
		Nutrition	Influences time to oestrus, oestrus display and conception.
		Genetics	Increased potential for body tissue mobilisation may be reducing fertility.
Cycle length	Can be changed by hormonal manipulation		

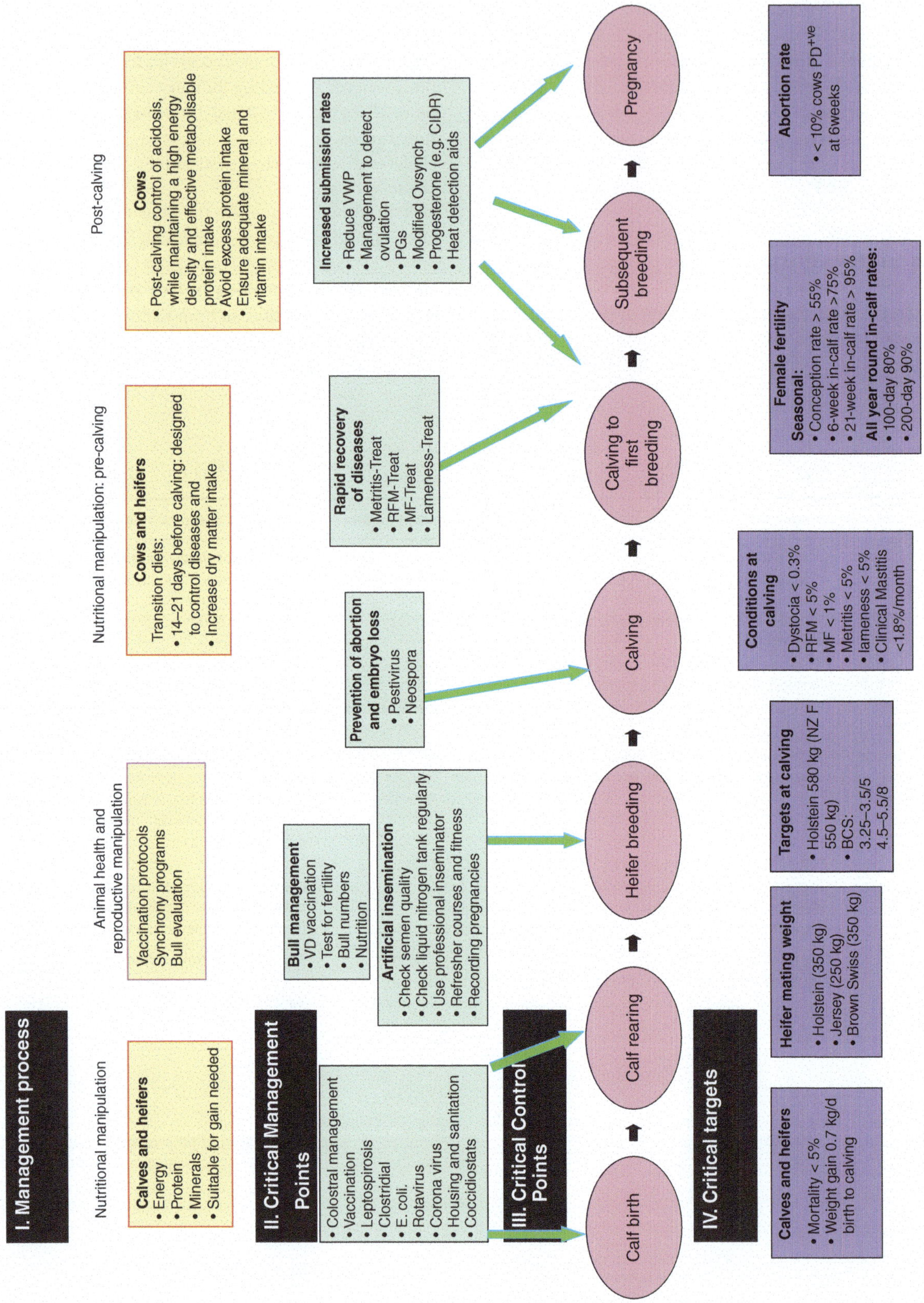

Figure 44.1 Reproductive performance process.

- Nutritional factors causing poor growth delay herd entry or result in low body condition and weight. Many forages are deficient in energy, protein, vitamins and minerals. Action: Risk of deficiencies (or excesses) should be assessed and corrected.
- Parasites control programs are a critical part of achieving satisfactory heifer performance.
- Disease conditions that result in poor heifer growth are well outlined in Chapter 37. These should not be ignored for their potential to limit performance.

Critical management points

- Care of the pregnant cows to provide healthy calves: Two-thirds of the growth of the unborn calf occurs during the last 6–8 weeks before birth. The cow should be provided an adequate balanced diet to provide the calf with sufficient nutrients to ensure a strong, healthy calf at birth. See 'Transition feeding' in Chapter 38 for recommendations.
- Colostrum: Calves should receive four litres of high quality colostrum within the first four to six hours after birth.
- Rearing: Critical target – Holsteins gain approximately 0.7 kg per day to 24 months old. Higher rates of gain and earlier herd entry ages have been recommended (van Amburg *et al.*, 1998).
- Underfeeding energy and protein results in heifers weighing much less, but smaller differences in skeletal size. Undersized heifers will not exhibit first oestrus until they are many months older than normal sized heifers (Canfield & Butler, 1990; Rhodes *et al.*, 1995, 1996). Achieving body weight targets at first calving due to feeding and management increases milk yield (Dobos *et al.*, 1994; Dobos, 1999) and reproductive performance.
- Feeding more energy than is required may result in over fat heifers and possibly permanent udder damage with reduced lactation yield.
- Hoffman *et al.* (1996) emphasised the use of skeletal measurements to define replacement heifer size. Optimal body condition score at calving was determined to be 3.5 (1–5 scale). Body condition scores more than 3.5 have been demonstrated to increase the probability of metabolic problems (Grummer *et al.*, 1995) and dystocia (Hoffman *et al.*, 1996) and to reduce milk yield (Waltner *et al.*, 1993).

Time to first breeding after calving

This factor is a major determinant of time to conception. Long voluntary waiting periods before cows are submitted for breeding can be a problem in year round mating systems. In seasonal breeding herds, long calving intervals are associated with increased intervals from calving to first breeding, and can also be associated with very short intervals between calving and first insemination, because late-calving cows have a short interval after calving to mating start. Shorter calving intervals are associated with reducing intervals to first breeding, increasing efficiency of oestrus detection, and increasing the number of cows submitted for AI between 55 and 85 days post-partum (Macmillan & Watson, 1973; Pelissier, 1978; Schneider *et al.*, 1981).

From a HACCP perspective, the critical goals in optimising the time to first breeding are:

1 Cows should resume normal oestrous cycles within 30–45 days after calving.
2 Cows that are cycling should be submitted for breeding, to ensure that more than 80% are mated within 80 days of calving (non-seasonal calving) or six weeks of mating start date (seasonal calving).
3 Cows in seasonal herds should calve sufficiently early to allow a minimum of 20 days from calving to mating start date.

Critical control points

These include appropriate hormonal treatments to induce oestrus and nutritional management. The cause of post-partum anoestrus may be abnormal follicular maturation without ovulation, presence of an ovarian cyst, true anoestrus or normal cyclic ovarian activity with no observable signs of oestrus.

- Body condition score: time to first breeding is influenced by body tissue reserves. Cows in body condition score <3.0 (scale 1–5) or <4 (scale 1–8) have increased intervals to first mating and more risk of conception failure (Pryce *et al.*, 2001; Garnsworthy & Topps, 1982; Curtis & Lean, 1998; McDougall *et al.*, 2001; Morton, 1999; Stagg *et al.*, 1995; Bossis *et al.*, 1999). Cows in higher body condition scores have shorter intervals to re-establishing cyclicity after calving, but over-conditioned cows (body condition score >3.5 (scale 1–5)) have a longer interval to first breeding and reduced fertility (Butler & Smith, 1989; Rukkwamsuk *et al.*, 1999). These may be partially mediated through metabolic disorder associated with excessive weight loss (Moss, 2001) or increased risk of post-partum disease (Curtis & Lean, 1998).
- Incidence of anoestrus cows: post-partum anoestrus, defined as cows not detected in oestrus and that do not have a CL on either ovary, is a major factor lowering submission rates in SCH (Jubb *et al.*, 1989; McDougall *et al.*, 1995; Xu & Burton, 1998). Anoestrus can cause significant economic loss, primarily because of the management requirements to maintain a seasonally concentrated calving pattern. McDougall *et al.* (1998) reported that post-partum anoestrus is the most common form of infertility for dairy cows in New Zealand, and affects up to 20% of cows >45 days postpartum. Cows with poor body condition score and negative nutrient balance are more likely to be anoestrus (Burke *et al.*, 1998). Therefore, feeding strategy can influence the incidence of anoestrus cows.

- Policy to breed: Webster *et al.* (1997a) found that the manager's target for time to first mating was a significant factor determining differences in reproductive performance between best performing AYR herds and those worst performing. Better performing herds planned to mate cows earlier. The SCH were more effective in submitting cows for mating than AYR (Morton, 1999).
- Hormonal manipulations can be used to increase the density and detection of ovulation. Many programs have been developed that will allow a shorter interval from calving to mating.
- Periparturient disease: Diseases such as retained placenta, metritis, milk fever, ketosis and lameness all increase the period to mating.
- Dietary energy intake can influence the luteal function in heifers and resumption of cyclicity (Villa-Godoy *et al.*, 1990).

Critical management points

Actions

- Optimise body condition, either during heifer rearing or in the previous lactation. *From a HACCP perspective, this is the first point at which an assessment needs to be made.* The target is a body condition score of 3.25–3.5 (scale 1–5) or 4.5–5.5 (scale 1–8) by the completion of lactation; for Holstein heifers, 580 kg of body weight before calving should be achieved.
- Submit cows for breeding. This is, in part, a policy decision and mating should start from 45 to 55 days after calving in AYR.
- Therapeutic agents can be used to meet targets. Ovsynch (and variations on this), prostaglandin, prostaglandin/gonadotropin releasing hormone and progesterone programs can increase submission rates and the prevalence of oestrus and ovulation, thereby increasing ovulation detection efficiency. See Chapters 42.

Detection of ovulation

Lactating dairy cows have poor reproductive performance due to low fertility and a low rate of estrus detection. Oestrus detection efficiency is ≤ 50% in most dairy herds (Barr, 1975, Bosworth *et al.*, 1972, Esslemont, 1974, King *et al.*, 1976, Hazen and Laurent, 1991, Stevenson and Britt, 1994, Westwood *et al.*, 2002).

Targets

1 Accurate (highly specific) and sensitive detection of cows in oestrus that ovulate
2 Minimal labour requirements to achieve these goals.

Critical control points

Sub-oestrus is responsible for 80–90% of cases of post-partum anoestrus in dairy cows during the breeding period (Mialot & Badinand, 1985; Tefera *et al.*, 1991; Humblot & Grimard, 1996). About half of all oestrus-related behaviour is not detected in post-partum cattle (Stevenson & Britt, 1977; Hanzen & Laurent, 1991; Westwood *et al.*, 2002). Factors that influence the ability to achieve the HACCP target are:

- Environmental factors: those that negatively impact on the effectiveness of a heat detection program (O'Connor, 2000) include: housing vs. pasture conditions, poor footing surfaces such as slippery concrete, foot and leg lameness, a lower prevalence of other cows in oestrus, summer, and very high or low environmental temperatures. Cows show oestrus more in the morning and afternoon than in the middle of the day.
- Size of dairy herd: as dairy herds increase in size, the problem of poor detection of oestrus is amplified, because the labour input per cow decreases.
- Nutritional and production management of the herd: cows that had less reliance on mobilised body tissue, lower milk production, and lower genetic merit, were more likely to display oestrus. Importantly, cows that ate 6 kg of dry matter per day more than herd-mates in the week of ovulation were 26 times more likely to express signs of oestrus at ovulation. A cow was twice as likely to show heat at ovulation when another cow was simultaneously on heat (Westwood *et al.*, 2002).

Critical management points

From a HACCP monitoring standpoint, it is generally too late to identify heat detection failure from records. It is better to use indices that identify the number of cows anticipated in oestrus over a 21-day period, and assess whether the expected proportion of cows is being detected. A failure to detect 80% of anticipated oestrus events in a period should trigger an investigation into reproductive or management failure.

Solutions to the problem of inadequate detection of oestrus include: an increase in the frequency of daily checks of cows for oestrus activity; use of aids for oestrous detection, including tail paint, heat mount detectors, pedometers, pressure transducers on the tail head of the cow; and judicious use of hormones to synchronise oestrus in groups of cows.

Actions

Heat detection can be improved by:

- Establish standard operating procedures (SOP) for oestrus detection: cows should be observed at times and locations where they are likely to express oestrus (i.e. where cows have a good footing surface and few obstacles to hinder interaction). Cows should be observed at least three times a day. The average oestrus period lasts less than eight hours, and twice-daily observation will miss many cows. For some cows, there is relatively little opportunity even for vigilant herdsmen to observe heat.

- Use heat detection aids: these should augment, but not necessarily replace, visual detection. A strategy of increasing the sensitivity of heat detection with more sensitive heat mount detectors can increase the number of false positives, unless these aids to heat detection are interpreted with caution. All heat detection aids require management decisions for suspect cows, information interpretation and regular maintenance.
- Having fewer people dedicated to the task of heat detection may improve reproductive performance (Webster *et al.*, 1997a), suggesting that knowledge of the cows and individual behaviour is an aid in heat detection.
- Record all heats and use these data to predict oestrus.
- Synchrony methods increase the density of cows in heat and group interaction. Cows in heat and cows that will be in heat in the next 48 hours form sexually active groups. Inducing heat and/or ovulation with hormonal treatments increases the probability of detecting oestrus, and some methods allow timed insemination.
- Minimise lameness: balanced diets which prevent ruminal acidosis will reduce the risk of lameness. Track preparation is critical for pastured herds and cows should not be left on concrete or in moist conditions for too long. Lame cows should be examined and treated.

Male fertility

Bull

Artificial insemination is widely used in dairy herds; however, bulls are commonly used to mate cows that fail to conceive, or as strategy to obviate the need for heat detection and insemination. In order to adequately exploit the use of natural service in the dairy herd, appropriate selection and management of bulls should be included in the HACCP. It is also vital to prevent the disastrous economic consequences of sub-fertile bulls; regular evaluation of their reproductive performance is required.

The critical goals in using bulls are:

1 To improve the sensitivity and specificity of heat detection.
2 To improve pregnancy rates, because more cows are detected in true oestrus and serviced.
3 To reduce the labour involved in heat detection.
4 To reduce the cost of semen, equipment and personnel, and to eliminate inefficient semen handling in artificial insemination.

Critical control points

The perception is that pregnancy rates improve when natural service is used, because more cows are detected in true oestrus and serviced, and greater doses of semen are present in the female reproductive tract. However, management of dairy bulls is very important, as poorly managed natural service programs will decrease fertility compared to AI. Factors that influence bull performance are detailed below.

- Breeding soundness: Approximately 11% of yearling bulls are either sterile or sub-fertile at 12–14 months of age. Breeding soundness examinations show that 4% of proven sires develop fertility problems between breeding seasons.
- The risks of venereal diseases, such as vibriosis and trichmonasis, are an important consideration when using natural service.
- Lameness in bulls can impair the bull's ability to serve and can result in testicular degeneration and reduced fertility. Bulls can suffer from excess hoof wear if they have prolonged contact with concrete.
- Adult bulls that carry excessive weight relative to their body frame may be more reluctant to mount and have reduced libido (Jorgensen, 1998; Monke, 1988; Monke, 2002).
- Heat stress can reduce male fertility by decreasing sperm concentration and motility, and increasing morphologically abnormal sperm. A negative effect of heat stress on libido is less well documented.
- Gossypol toxicity: Gossypol, from diets containing cottonseed products, may reduce bull fertility, due to an increase in the number of abnormal sperm. This effect should not be overstated, but the risk should be recognised.
- Bulls should be of adequate stature to mate cows.
- Bull power needs to be enough bulls to cover number of cows in heat at mating, especially when using synchrony programs.
- Inflammatory conditions that result in pyrexia can depress sperm count for 6–8 weeks.

Critical management points

The management of bulls in dairy farms using natural service is critical to success.

- Adult bulls need to be fed to maintain body condition and not gain excessive weight. An average of daily gain of about 1.0 kg between 6–18 months of age is a reasonable goal. Thereafter, the average daily gain should slowly decline. An optimum adult weight for adult, large breed, dairy bulls is 1000 kg, but bulls should culled before achieving this weight. Bulls should be culled once they weigh more than 150% of adult cow weight.
- Bulls should be selected at least 60–90 days before the breeding season, to allow for vaccinations to prevent clostridial and major viral disorders; anthelmintic treatment and breeding soundness should be conducted before using the bull in a herd.
- Basic reproductive examination of bulls includes: measurement of scrotal circumference, clinical examination of the genitalia; assessment of the conformation of the bull (with particular emphasis on legs and feet); and observation of coitus. Semen evaluation may also help to detect bulls that are producing abnormal semen but are normal on clinical examination (Hueston, 1988, Chenoweth, 1992; Chenoweth, 2000; Kastelic *et al.*, 2000). The ultimate test of breeding soundness is the density and number of conceptions for each bull.

- The effect of heat stress on bulls can be minimised by providing water, access to shade, and ensuring that bulls are not overused during hot weather.
- Yearling and two-year-old bulls have a lesser semen capacity, and should be used in greater numbers when oestrus synchronisation programs are used, and as follow-up bulls for AI programs where a large number of females are expected to return to oestrus.
- Use bulls when they are aged between 18 months and three years of age. Bulls should be culled on age (four years old), weight and function. Sexual activity of the bulls is greater when several sires are used with a group of cows. However, dominant bulls will tend to serve more cows than others. Implementation of a rotational roster will contribute to maintaining sexual interest (Furman & Hughes, 1989; Chenoweth, 2000).
- A general recommendation is to use one bull per 30 non-pregnant cows or heifers. If synchrony programs have been employed in large herds, large numbers of cows can return to oestrus over a few days. We recommend that up to one bull per eight females be used in very tight synchrony programs. One or two reserve bulls should be used on a rotational basis (Hueston, 1986; Furman & Hughes, 1989).
- Venereal disease, vaccination and surveillance: dependent upon the region, vaccination may be recommended to reduce the risk of venereal disease. Vaccines are available for vibriosis (Chenoweth & Larsen, 1992), and trichomonosis (for use in females in the USA (Risco, 2000)). Clinical surveillance and diagnostic testing to detect the presence or incursion of venereal disease is advisable (Monke, 1986; Howard *et al.*, 1990; Chenoweth & Larsen, 1992).
- Draft bulls from the herd during the milking to reduce hoof damage (Parkinson and Vermunt, 2000).

Artificial insemination

The critical goals in using AI are;

1. To increase the utilisation of sires that can disseminate desirable genetics.
2. To reduce the risk of introducing venereal diseases to the herd.
3. To eliminate the danger to humans and cows.
4. To eliminate or reduce the work and expense of keeping and handling bulls.
5. To ensure that pregnancy rates using AI meet or exceed those using bulls.

Critical control points

The following factors determine the percent of resulting pregnancies from AI;

- Errors in sensitivity and specificity of oestrus detection increase semen costs and the interval from calving to conception (Risco, 2000).
- Female fertility level of the herd.
- Fertility of semen used. Some determinants of semen fertility are not under the direct control of the farm manager – principally, the handling and processing of semen from the bull to the point of sale of semen. Fertility of semen varies and monitoring is needed.
- Inseminator efficiency. Poor handling and thawing of semen, and incorrect site of deposition of semen, may be contributing factors to the poorer performance of do-it-yourself (DIY) inseminators than professional inseminators (Morton, 1999).

The percentage of pregnancies resulting from AI is the product of these four factors, and not their average. When these factors are multiplied, their product or percentage of pregnancies is less than the lowest factor (see equation 44.1).

Critical management points

- Bulls that are selected for AI should be monitored andrologically for soundness, and semen periodically examined for normality. These processes are outside the scope of farm management, but the performance of the bulls used for AI should be monitored across farms to identify those with poor fertility.
- Once semen is on farm, procedures should be in place to ensure that the viability of the semen is maintained. Control measures include: regular monitoring of the semen tank to ensure that nitrogen levels are adequate to keep temperatures optimal; use of a narrow mouth tank to avoid temperature fluctuations; and adequate storage conditions for the vacuum tank to prevent damage to the tank.
- Insemination procedures: semen should be thawed in warm water. No more than three straws should be routinely thawed at a time.
- Further training: regular refresher courses in artificial insemination are recommended for DIY inseminators in order to evaluate semen handling and placement.
- Conception rate comparisons are a useful method of detecting possible emerging problems. Comparisons should be made between inseminators, parities, and between natural and artificial breeding.
- Awareness of fatigue and lack of practice are factors influencing AI performance. In SCH, there can be a hiatus of several months in AI, and inseminators may be in poor physical condition to inseminate a large number of cattle. Even with practice, large numbers of cattle submitted for AI following heat synchrony programmes can pose physical challenges. Specific recommendations on the number of inseminations attempted in a day will depend on the degree of fitness and experience of the operator.

Female fertility

Assessment of the female herd fertility is difficult. Confounding factors such as male fertility, heat detection specificity, and timing of breeding ensure that it is difficult to isolate variance associated with female fertility. The critical goals in female fertility are;

1 To reduce the incidence of metabolic diseases by implementing appropriate nutritional management.
2 To reduce the risk of reproductive disorders after calving (such as retained placenta and metritis).
3 To achieve a high submission rate; 85–90% by 100 days after calving in AYR or over six weeks after mating start in SCH, with > 75% submitted within three weeks.
4 To maintain conception rates per service above 50% and pregnancy rates above 95% by the end of breeding season.
5 To achieve a high milk production without compromising fertility
6 To reduce the incidence of anoestrus.
7 To implement hormonal treatments that increase submission and conception.

Critical control points

The most important questions regarding female fertility raised in recent years are those relating to the effects of long-term genetic selection for increased milk and milk solids production. Increased milk production is associated with lower fertility, but it is not clear that this association is causal. The association may result from nutritional management to increase milk production, or changes in the physiology of the cows, resulting from genetic selection for increased milk production. While there is a negative association between high production and reproduction, this not mean that higher production necessarily results in lower reproductive performance. For example, Morton (1999) found that higher producing herds had higher fertility.

If we consider the reduction in fertility to represent a metabolic disorder, this predicts that diets can be developed to achieve high production but maintain reproduction. Key risk factors that contribute to female fertility are detailed below.

- Genetic selection for high milk production: the estimated heritability of fertility is low: 0–0.03 (Hansen *et al.*, 1983). Consequently, negative associations between milk yield and fertility may be of limited long-term impact. Importantly, for an individual dairy farm, these changes in genetic merit have very little immediate impact.
- Negative nutrient balance (NNB): excessive mobilisation of body tissue appears to a major cause of lowered fertility. Following parturition, dry matter intake needs to increase 2–3 fold in order to meet the nutrient demands of milk production. However, the increase dry matter intake after calving is not as rapid as the increase in nutrient output in milk, resulting in a nutrient deficit. While the term Net Energy Balance (NEB) has been used to describe the deficit between energy intake and energy output in cows, the term should be strictly applied to energy, as other nutrient deficits occur during this period. In particular, protein is mobilised from body tissue in early lactation; mineral and vitamin fluxes are more difficult to determine, but are also negative. A preferable term to NEB is net nutrient balance (NNB). Westwood *et al.* (2002) found that by breaking NNB into its determinants, which are milk solids production and feed intake, and including body weight change as a separate variable, provided greater understanding of the factors influencing time to conception. Cows in the upper quartile of dry matter intake were 26 times more likely to show oestrus at first ovulation than those in the lower quartile, while those in the higher quartile of milk production were 11 times less likely to show oestrus at first ovulation than herd mates in the lower quartile of milk production. Conception rates are adversely influenced by NNB at, or preceding, the time of first insemination.
- BCS and bodyweight loss: loss of body condition (BCS) after calving is greater for cows in higher body condition (Garnsworthy & Topps, 1982), and loss of BCS or weight is negatively associated with reproductive performance (Westwood *et al.*, 2002) and may be greater in high genetic merit animals (Pryce *et al.*, 2001). After calving, loss of body weight leads to an increase in concentrations BHB and NEFA in blood (Lean, 1994). Concentrations of blood cholesterol, the substrate for progesterone synthesis, also reflect BCS and nutrient balance (Lean, 1994; Moreira *et al.*, 2000). Pregnancy rates to a timed insemination program were lower for low-BCS cows (Moreira *et al.*, 2000). Many workers have found an optimal BCS in which cows should calve of 3.25–3.5 (scale 1–5), 4.5–5.5 (scale 1–8) or 4.5–5.5 (scale 1–10). Loss of body weight may also influence concentrations of progesterone. Progesterone has an important role in normal fertilisation, embryo transport and embryo survival (Garcia-Winder *et al.*, 1986; Mee *et al.*, 1991). Peripheral progesterone concentrations during the post-partum ovulatory cycle are reduced by NEB (Villa-Godoy *et al.*, 1988; Spicer *et al.*, 1990; Staples *et al.*, 1990). Cows with the lowest energy status after calving had lower progesterone levels during their third oestrous cycles (Villa-Godoy *et al.*, 1988). Level of feeding has a key role in controlling progesterone concentrations in blood and also progesterone metabolism in dairy cattle (Rabiee *et al.*, 2001a).
- Protein concentration in the diet: there has been a long term awareness of the problems of feeding excessive protein (Butler & Smith, 1989). Westwood *et al.*, (2002) found that feeding more rumen-degradable protein and greater loss of bodyweight was associated with significantly lower probability of conception at first service. A meta-analysis of available studies strongly supported findings from individual studies and meta-regression showed, that the negative effects of protein on conception were explained by increased soluble protein intake (Lean *et al.*, 2012).
- Reproductive disorders: retained placenta, metritis and ovarian cysts are major factors reducing the risk of conception

(Curtis & Lean, 1998; McDougall, 2001; Moss, 2001). Morton (1999) also found that these factors and lameness markedly reduced fertility. Gröhn & Rajala-Schultz (2000) reported that cows with retained placentae, metritis and ovarian cysts had 14%, 15% and 21% lower conception rates, respectively, when compared to cows without these conditions.

These findings, and others on female fertility, can be expressed as follows: increased genetic merit for milk production places cows at greater risk of body tissue mobilisation; cows with less herd dominance and excessive body condition are placed at greater risk of increased body tissue mobilisation; cows that mobilise more body tissue, cows on diets high in rumen-degradable protein and cows that have peri-parturient diseases are at more risk of reproductive failure.

Critical management points

Optimal reproductive efficiency will be achieved when each cow conceives at the most desirable interval from calving, whether in a seasonal or non-seasonal herd. This will only be achieved if the factors influencing female fertility are controlled. Previously critical management points include factors that influence female fertility, such as optimal body condition score before calving.

- From a HACCP perspective, excessive body condition > 3.5 (scale 1–5) or 6 (scale 1–8) should be avoided, because dry matter intake is lower in these cows, and cows are more likely to have a negative nutrient balance. These cows will deposit fat in the liver, resulting in hepatic lipidosis and ketosis.
- Provision of diets that reduce the risk of metabolic disease after calving is critical to both prevention of disease and maximising dry matter intake after calving.
- Ensuring energy intake to minimise body weight loss. Feeding management should be designed to maintain a high energy density (11.5–12 MJ, 36% NSC) and sufficient fibre to maintain rumen stability (NDF > 30% of DM). Acidosis should be avoided, as this depresses feed intake and may be associated with lowered fertility. The inclusion of some fat source(s), in diets where fat is < 5%, into the ration within the first 30 days post-partum may result in an improvement in energy status and, consequently, conception/pregnancy rates of cows. Fat supplements can improve energy balance and reduce the risk of metabolic diseases such as ketosis. Inclusion of fat, especially fats that can provide conjugated linoleic acids, often derived from oil seeds, can positively influence fertility (Thatcher *et al.*, 2002). Part of this effect may be mediated through reduced body tissue loss (Rabiee *et al.*, 2012). However, linoleic (C18:2) and linolenic fatty acids (C18:3) are classified as essential fatty acids and must be supplied in the diet, because the double bonds between the Δ-9-carbon and terminal methyl group of fatty acids cannot be inserted by mammalian biological processes. This has important implications for pasture-fed cows that can receive substantial amounts of C18:2 and C18:3 in the diet, and may explain some of the very good reproductive performance achieved in well-fed and -managed pastured herds. Consequently, the diet should contain 5% of dietary DM, as fats high in C18:2 and C 18:3 that can reach the small intestine, or contain commercial supplements of these fats.
- Early detection of cows that fail to get pregnant and are not in oestrus may aid nutritional and reproductive management of the herd.
- Treatment of reproductive disease: timely treatment of reproductive disorders will improve fertility of cows affected by these disorders. Effective treatments for metritis include antibiotic infusions (Roberts, 1986) and prostaglandins treatments 14–28 days after calving (Burton & Lean, 1995).
- Exogenous hormonal manipulation of reproductive cycle: manipulations that are effective in increasing conception rates in cows, include prostaglandins (Macmillan *et al.*, 1987; Burton & Lean, 1995) and gonadotrophin-releasing hormone at the time of mating (Morgan & Lean, 1993), particularly in repeat breeders.

In brief, from the HACCP management approach, female fertility can be best managed by ensuring that pre-calving nutrition maintains appetite and reduces periparturient disease (Chalupa *et al.*, 1997; Lean *et al.*, 1998), and that appetite and feed intake are maintained after calving. Feeding systems should minimise the effects of competition for feed and diets should be balanced, in respect to the protein and energy contents and structure.

Conclusions

The process of examining the management tasks required to achieve good fertility identified a series of time-related critical

Table 44.2 Ten steps to getting cows in calf: a HACCP approach.

Cattle Production Consultants: Ten steps to getting cows in calf – a HACCP approach.		
1	Calf management and heifer growth	Record all events
2	Adequate body weight in two-year-olds (580kg)/BCS at calving 3.25 (1–5 scale)	
3	Smooth transition periods: minimise disease	
4	Minimise BCS loss	Monitor
5	Short VWP 45–60days	
6	Heat synchrony programs early treatment of anoestrus	
7	Use heat detection aids	
8	Optimise male fertility	Review regularly
9	Re-detection of heats/early detection of non-pregnant cows	
10	Prevent abortion	

Table 44.3 Ten steps to getting cows in calf: a checklist.

Step	Critical control points	Critical management
1	Calf management and heifer growth	• Colostrum management (4L high quality within 6-12 hours) • Early introduction to concentrates and high quality forages • Adequate nutrition between weaning and joining (Aim 0.6–0.7 kg/day) • Parasite control and vaccination • Select easy calving sires/breeds (beware of beef if no data!)
2	Adequate body weight in two-year-olds (580kg)/BCS at calving (3.25/5)	• Monitor growth rates • Supplementary feed when pasture quality poor • Feed transition rations to heifers
3	Smooth transition periods-minimise disease and maintain appetite	• Prevent milk fever • Maintain nutrient balance/prevent ketosis • Stimulate appetite • Adapt rumen • Stimulate udder development
4	Minimise BCS loss after calving (<1/5 BCS)	• Flows from points 2 and 3 • Adequate access to supplements (concentrates and forages) – trough/bunk/feeder space (70 cm/head) balanced rations
5	Short VWP 45–60days	• Facilitated mentally if you make the decision • Facilitated physiologically by points 2–4 conception rates down a little but compensated for by increased pregnancies by 100 days
6	Heat synchrony programs and prevention or early treatment of anoestrus	• 14-day PG programs • CIDRs useful but not a panacea – is it worth treating anoestrous cows in non-seasonal herds? • More cows on increases sensitivity of heat detection, helps with labour organisation
7	Use heat detection aids	• Augments visual heat detection • No farmer sees every heat • Many cows on at night only or for only 2–6 hours
8	Optimise male fertility	• Check semen, inseminator technique, tank • Inseminator fitness (NB if batch mating) • Bulls must be fit and fertile • Adequate bull power (NB if batch mating – 3–6 per 100 cows) • Vibrio vaccinated (if appropriate)
9	Re-detection of heats/early detection of non-pregnant cows	Paint/KaMaR all cows until tested pregnant (50% of cows back in 21 days if CR = 50%)
10	Prevent abortion	• Lepto- vaccinate • Vibrio- vaccinate • BVD vaccinate • Neospora – dogs? • Salmonella – nutrition/freedom from lactic acidosis – vaccinate if major problem • Biosecurity protocols

management points that can be used both to reduce the risk of management failure and as a tool to focus diagnostic efforts. Good fertility is only achieved by careful attention to all aspects of reproductive management. Table 44.2 indicates the ten steps to getting cows in calf using a HACCP approach. Table 44.3 provides a detailed checklist of the ten steps.

References and further reading

Bailey, L.F. and McLennan, M.W., McLean, D.M. Hartford, P.R. and Munro, G.L. (1973). The use of dexamethasone trimethylacetate to advance parturition in dairy cows. *Australian Veterinary Journal* **49**, 567–573.

Barr, H.L. (1975). Influence of oestrus detection on days open in dairy herds. *Journal of Dairy Science* **58**, 246–247.

Beam, S.W. and Butler, W.R. (1997). Energy balance and ovarian follicle development prior to the first ovulation postpartum in dairy cows receiving three levels of dietary fat. *Biology of Reproduction* **56**, 133–142.

Beam, S.W. and Butler, W.R. (1999). Effects of energy balance on follicular development and first ovulation in postpartum dairy cows. Review. *Journal of Reproduction and Fertility* (Suppl.) **54**, 411–24.

Beam, S.W. and Butler, W.R. (1998). Energy balance, metabolic hormones, and early postpartum development in dairy cows fed prilled lipid. *Journal of Dairy Science* **81**,121–131.

Beardsley, G.L., Muller, L.D., Garverick, H.A., Ludens, F.C. and Tucker, W.L. (1976). Initiation of parturition in dairy cows with dexamethasone. II. Response to dexamethasone in combination with estradiol benzoate. *Journal of Dairy Science* **59**, 241–247.

Beckett, S.D. and Lean, I.J. (1997). Gonadotrophin-releasing hormone in postpartum dairy cattle, a meta-analysis of effects on reproductive efficiency. *Animal Reproduction Science* **48**, 93–112.

Bell, A.W. (1995). Regulation of organic nutrient metabolism during transition from late pregnancy to early lactation. *Journal of Animal Science* **73**, 2804–19. Review.

Bell, A.W., Slepetis, R. and Ehrhardt, R.A. (1995). Growth and accretion of energy and protein in the gravid uterus during late pregnancy in Holstein cows. *Journal of Dairy Science* **78**, 1954–61.

Bossis, I., Wettemann, R.P., Welty, S.D., Vizcarra, J.A., Spicer, L.J. and Diskin, M.G. (1999). Nutritionally induced anovulation in beef heifers, ovarian and endocrine function preceding cessation of ovulation. *Journal of Animal Science* **77**, 1536–1546.

Bostedt, H., Peche, E. and Stroble, K. (1980). Effect of GnRH applied immediately postpartum on the course of the puerperium and the fertility of cows after placental retention. Berliner and Muchener. *Tierarztliche Wochenschrift* **93**, 184–188.

Bosworth, R.W., Ward, G., Call, E.P. and Bonewitz, E.R. (1972). Analysis of factors affecting calving intervals of dairy cows. *Journal of Dairy Science* **55**, 334–338.

Britt, J.H., Kittock, R.J. and Harrison, D.S. (1977). Frequency of ovarian follicular cysts, reasons for culling and fertility in Holstein Friesian cows given gondaotrophin releasing hormone at two weeks after parturition. *American Journal of Veterinary Research* **38**, 749–751.

Burke, J.M., Hampton, J.H., Staples, C.R. and Thatcher, W.W. (1998). Body condition influences maintenance of resistant first wave dominant follicle dairy cattle. *Theriogenology* **49**, 751–760.

Burke, J. M., Staples, C. R., Risco, C. A., De La Sota, R. L. and Thatcher, W. W. (1996). Effect of feeding a ruminant grade Menhaden fish meal on reproductive and productive performance of lactating dairy cows. *Journal of Animal Science* **74**(Suppl. 1),263.

Burton, N.R. and Lean, I.J. (1995). Investigation by meta-analysis of the effect of prostaglandin F2α administered post partum on the reproductive performance of dairy cattle. *Australian Veterinary Journal* **136**, 90–94.

Butler, W.R. (2000). Nutritional interactions with reproductive performance in dairy cattle. *Animal Reproduction Science* **60–61**, 449–457.

Butler, W.R. and Smith, R.D. (1989). Interrelationships between energy balance on postpartum reproductive function in dairy cattle. *Journal of Dairy Science* **7**, 676–783.

Canfield, R.W. and Butler, W.R. (1990) Energy balance and pulsatile LH secretion in early postpartum dairy cattle. *Domestic Animal Endocrinology* **7**, 323–330.

Carroll, D. J., Hossain, F. R. and Keller, M. R. (1994). Effect of supplemental fish meal on the lactation and reproductive performance of dairy cows. *Journal of Dairy Science* **77**, 3058–3072.

Cavalieri, J., Flinker, L.R., Anderson, G.A. and Macmillan, K.L. (2003a). Characteristic of oestrus measured using visual observation and radiotelemetry. *Animal Reproduction Science* **76**, 1–12.

Cavalieri, J., Eagles, V.E., Ryan, M. and Macmillan, K.L. (2003b). Comparison of four methods for detection of oestrus in dairy cows with resynchronized oestrous cycles. *Australian Veterinary Journal* (under review).

Cavalieri, J., Eagles, V.E., Ryan, M. and Macmillan, K.L. (2003c). Role of the sensitivity of detection of oestrus in the submission rate of cows treated to resynchronize oestrus. *Australian Veterinary Journal* (under review).

Cavalieri, J. and Macmillan, K.L. (2002). Synchronization of oestrus and reproductive performance of dairy cows following administration of oestradiol benzoate or GnRH during a synchronized pro-oestrus. *Australian Veterinary Journal* **80**, 486–493.

Cavalieri, J., Eagles, V.E., Ryan, M. and Macmillan, K.L. (2000). Patterns of onset of oestrus and reproductive performance of dairy cows enrolled in controlled breeding programs. In: *Proceedings of the Australian and New Zealand Combined Dairy Veterinarians Conference* 15–19 May 2000. Le Lagon Resort, Port Vila, Vanuatu. Massy University, Palmerston North. 161–182.

Chalupa, W. Sniffen, C., Hoover, W. (1997). Adoption of technology, The way to the future? *Current Topics in Dairy Production* **2**, 1.

Chenoweth, P.J. (1992). A new bull breeding soundness evaluation form. *Proceedings of the Annual Meeting of the Society for Theriogenology* **63**.

Chenoweth, P.J. (2000). Rationale for using breeding soundness evaluations. *Compendium of Continuing Education for the Practising Veterinarian* **22**, S48–S54.

Chenoweth, P.J. and Larsen, R.E. (1992). Selection, use and management of natural service bulls. In: Van Horn, H.H. and Wilcox, C.J. (eds). *Large dairy herd management*, pp. 209–218. Champaign, Am. Dairy Sci. Soc.

Chew, B.P., Erb, R.E., Randel, R.D. and Rouquette, F.M.,Jr. (1978). Effect of corticoid induced parturition on lactation and on prepartum profiles of serum progesterone and the estrogens among cows retaining and not retaining fetal membranes. *Theriogenology* **10**, 13–25.

Clayton, R.K. (1984). Induction of parturient in cattle during the later stages of pregnancy, A comparison of three treatment methods. *Veterinary Record* **114**, 113–114.

Curtis, M.A., Lean, I.J. (1998). Path analysis of metabolic and antioxidant risk factors for periparturient and postparturient conditions and reproductive performance in dairy cows. XX World Buiatrics Congress, Sydney **2**, 809–818.

Cusack, P.M.V. and Perry, V. (1995). The effect of feeding whole cottonseed on the fertility of bulls. *Australian Veterinary Journal* **72**, 463–466

Davis, K.L. and Macmillan, K.L. (2001). Controlled calving with induction of parturition on day 274 of gestation in dairy cows. *Proceedings of the New Zealand Society of Animal Production* **61**, 184–186.

Dobos, R.C., McPhee, M.J., Spence, S.A. and Hegarty, R.S. (1994). Comparison of non-linear functions for describing the growth of dairy heifers in northern New South Wales. In, *Proceedings of the Australian Society of Animal Production* **20**, 374.

Dobos, R.C. (1999). *Growth and development of Friesain heifers*. PhD thesis, University of Sydney.

Dohoo, I.R., Martin, S.W., McMillan, I. and Kennedy, B.W. (1984). Disease, production and culling in Holstein-Friesian cows. II. Age, season and sire effects. *Preventive Veterinary Medicine* **2**, 655–670.

DRDC report (1997). *Heifer liveweight and reproductive performance.*

Drackley, J.K. (1999). ADSA Foundation Scholar Award. Biology of dairy cows during the transition period, the final frontier? *Journal of Dairy Science* **82**, 2259–2273.

Erb, H.N., Smith, R.D., Oltenacu, P.A., Guard, C.L., Hillman, R.B., Powers, P.A., Smith, M.C. and White, M.E. (1985). Path model of reproductive disorders and performance, milk fever, mastitis, milk yield, and culling in Holstein cows. *Journal of Dairy Science* **68**, 3337–3349.

Esslemont, R.J. (1974). Economic and husbandry aspects of manifestation and detection of oestrus in cows. III. The detection of estrus. *Agricultural Development Advisory Service Quarterly Review* **15**, 83–95.

Etherington, W.G., Martin, S.W., Bonnett, B.N., Johnson, W.H., Miller, R.B., Savage, N.C., Walton, J.S. and Montgomery, M.E. (1988). Reproductive performance in dairy cows following treatment with cloprostenol 26 and/or 40 days postpartum. A field trial. *Theriogenology* **29**, 565–575.

Etherington, W.G., Kelton, D.F. and Adams, J.E. (1994). Reproductive performance of dairy cows following treatment with fenprostalene, dinoprost or cloprostenol between 24 and 31 days postpartum, a field study. *Theriogenology* **42**, 739–752.

Ferguson, J.D. (1991). Nutrition and reproduction in dairy cows. *Veterinary Clinics of North America* **7**, 483–507.

Ferguson, J.D., Sklan, D., Chalupa, W.V. and Kronfeld, D.S. (1990). Effects of hard fats on in vitro and in vivo rumen fermentation, milk production, and reproduction in dairy cows. *Journal of Dairy Science* **73**, 2864–2879.

Furman, J.E. and Hughes, M.A. (1989). Breeding bull management. *Compendium of Continuing Education for the Practising Veterinarian* **11**, 95–98.

Garcia-Winder, M., Lewis, P.E., Deaver, D.R., Smith, V.G., Lewis, G.S. and Inskeep, E.K. (1986). Endocrine profiles associated with lifespan of induced corpora lutea in postpartum beef cows. *Journal of Animal Science* **62**, 1353–1362.

Garnsworthy, P.C. and Topps, J.H. (1982). The effect of body condition of dairy cows at calving on their food intake and performance when given complete diets. *Animal Production* **35**, 113–119.

Garverick, H.A. (1976). Induction of parturition in dairy cattle. In: Wilcox, C.J.; Van Horn, H.H., Harris, Jr., B., Head, H. H., Marshall, S.P., Thatcher, W.W., Webb, D.W. and Wing, J.M. (eds). *Large Dairy Herd Management*, pp. 231–246. University Presses of Florida.

Gröhn, Y.T. and Rajala-Schultz, P.J. (2000). Epidemiology of reproductive performance in dairy cows. *Animal Reproduction Science* **60–61**, 605–14. Review

Grummer, R.R., Hoffman, P.C., Luck, M.L. and Bertics, S.J. (1995). Effect of prepartum and postpartum dietary energy on growth and lactation of primiparous cows. *Journal of Dairy Science* **78**, 172–180.

Hansen, L.B., Freeman, A.E., and Berger, P.J. (1983). Association of heifer fertility with cow fertility and yield in dairy cattle. *Journal of Dairy Science* **66**, 306–314.

Harrison, J. H., McNamara, J. P. and Kincaid, R. L. (1995). Effect of whole cottonseeds and calcium salts of long-chain fatty acids on performance of lactating dairy cows. *Journal of Dairy Science* **78**, 181–193.

Hanzen, C.H. and Laurent, Y. (1991). Applications des progestagénes an traitment de l'anoestrus fonctionnel dans l'espéce bovine. *Annales de Médecine Vétérinaire* **135**, 547–557.

Hayes, D.P., Pfeiffer, D.U. and Morris, R.S. (1998). Effects of calving induction on subsequent milk yield and reproductive performance of cows from seasonally mated New Zealand dairy herds. *New Zealand Veterinary Journal* **46**, 97–101.

Heinrichs, A.J., Kierman, N.E., Graves, R.E. and Hutchinson, L.J. (1987). Survey of calf and heifer management practices in Pennsylvania. *Journal of Dairy Science* **70**, 896–902.

Heinrichs, A.J. (1996). *The importance of heifer raising to a profitable dairy farm*. In: Proceedings of the National Conference on Calves, Heifers, and Dairy Profitability, Harrisburg, PA. Northeast Reg. Agric. Eng. Serv., Ithaca, NY.

Hoffman, P.C. and Funk, A. (1992). Applied dynamics of dairy replacement growth and management. *Journal of Dairy Science* **75**, 2504–2516.

Hoffman, P.C., Brehhm, S.G., price, S.G. and Prill-Adams, A. (1996). Effect of accelerated postpuberty growth and early calving on lactation performance of primiparous Holstein cows. *Journal of Dairy Science* **79**, 2024–2031.

Howard, T.H. Bean, B and Hillman, R. and Monke DR. (1990). Surveillance for persistent bovine viral diarrhea virus infection in four artificial insemination centres. *Journal of the American Veterinary Medical Association* **196**, 1951–1955.

Hueston, W.D. (1986). Reproductive management programs for dairy bulls. In: Morrow, D.A. (ed). *Current therapy in Theriogenology*, vol. 2, Diagnosis, treatment and prevention of reproductive diseases in small and large animals, pp. 395–400. Pheladelphia, WB Sunders.

Hueston, W.D., Monke, D.R. and Milburn, R.J. (1988). Scrotal circumference measurements on young Holstein bulls. *Journal of the American Veterinary Medical Association* **192**, 766–768.

Humblot, P. and Grimard, B. (1996). *Le Point Vétérinaire* **28**, 917–925.

Jochle, W. (1993). Forty years of control of the oestrous cycle in ruminants, progress made, unsolved problems and potential impact of sperm encapsulation technology. *Reproduction, Fertility and Development* **5**, 587–594.

Jorgensen, N.A. (1998). *Bull nutrition*. Proceedings of 12th Technical Conference on Artificial insemination and Reproduction. pp. 88–93. Colombia, National Association of Animal Breeders.

Jubb TF, Brightling P, malmo J, Larcombe, Anderson GA and hides SJ. (1989). Evaluation of a regimen using a progesterone releasing intravaginal device (CIDR) and PMSG as a treatment for post partum anoestrus in dairy cattle. *Australian Veterinary Journal* **66**, 334–336.

Kastelic, J., Cook, R.B. and Coulter, G.H. (2000). Scrotal/testicular thermoregulation in bulls. In: Chenoweth, P.J. (ed). *Topics in bull fertility*. http//www.ivis.org.

King, G.J., Hurnik, J.F. and Robertson, H.A. (1976). Ovarian function and estrus in dairy cows during early lactation. *Journal of Animal Science* **42**, 688–692.

Langford, S.H. (1979). Induction of parturient in cows. *New Zealand Veterinary Journal* **27**, 107–108.

Larson, L.L. and Ball, P.J.H. (1992). Regulation of estrous cycles in dairy cattle, a review. *Theriogenology* **38**, 255–267.

Lean, I.J. (1994). *Calf to cow, care and profit*. University of Sydney.

Lean, I.J., Galland, J.C. and Scott, J. (1989). Relationships between peak milk yield, lactational persistency and fertility in dairy cows. *Theriogenology* **31**,1093–1103.

Lean, I.J., Wade, L.K. and Rajczyk, Z.K. (1998). *Managing dynamic change, Disease prevention and increased production in the periparturient cow*. XX World Buiatrics Congress, Sydney **2**, 799.

Lean I.J., Rabiee A.R., Moss N. (2000) A Hazards Analysis Critical Control Point Approach to Improving Reproductive Performance in Lactating Dairy Cows. *Asian-Australasian Journal of Animal Sciences* **13**(Suppl), 266–269.

Lean, I.J., Celi, P., Raadsma, H., McNamara, J. and Rabiee A.R. (2012). Effects of dietary crude protein on fertility, Meta-analysis and meta-regression. *Animal Feed Science and Technology* **171**, 31- 42.

Lee, A.J. (1997). The interplay of feeding and genetics of heifer rearing and first lactation milk yield, A review. *Journal of Animal Science* **75**, 846–851.

Leslie, K.E. (1981). *Effect of gonadotrophin releasing hormone on reproductive performance in dairy cows with retained placenta*. MS thesis, University of Guelph.

Lucy, M.C., Staples, C.R., Thatcher, W.W., Erickson, P.S., Cleale, R.M., Firkins, J.L., Clark, J.H., Murphy, M.R. and Brodie, B.O. (1992). Influence of diet composition, dry-matter intake, milk production and energy balance on time of postpartum ovulation and fertility in dairy cows. *Animal Production* **54**, 323–331.

Malmo, J. (2002). Bull management; Dairy Farm. In: *Encyclopedia of Dairy Sciences*, pp. 205–209. Academic Press. Elsevier Science.

Malmo, J. and Beggs, D. (2000). Reproductive management programs for seasonal calving dairy herds. In: *Proceedings of the Australian and New Zealand Combined Dairy Veterinarians Conference, Vanuatu*, pp, 229–240.

Malmo, J. (1991). In: *Dairy Med. Prod.* University of Sydney Post Graduate Committee in Veterinary Science, Proceedings. 161, 477.

Macmillan, K.L. (1979). Calving patterns and herd production in seasonal dairy herds. Proc. NZ Soc. *Animal Production* **39**, 168–174.

Macmillan, K.L. and Clayton, D.G. (1980). Factors influencing the interval to postpartum oestrus, conception date and empty date in an intensively managed dairy herd. *Proceedings of the New Zealand Society of Animal Production* **40**, 236–239.

Macmillan, K.L. and Watson, J.D. (1973). A.B. in New Zealand dairy herds. II. Interactions between conception rate and submission rate on the proportion of the herd reported in calf to A.B. *New Zealand Journal of Experimental Agriculture* **1**, 309–314.

Macmillan, K.L. Day, A.M., Henderson, H.V. and Allison, P.A. (1987). Some effects of injecting a PGF2α (Lutalyse) during the post-partum period on the subsequent fertility of dairy cows. *Proceedings of the New Zealand Society of Animal Production* **47**, 65–68.

Macmillan, K.L., Lean, I.J. and Westwood, C.T. (1996). The effects of lactation on the fertility of dairy cows. *Australian Veterinary Journal* **73**,141–147.

Macmillan, K.L., Pearce, M.G., MacDonald, K.A., Copeman, P.J.A. and Kilgour, R. (1985). Effects of varying feeding time on diurnal calving patterns in dairy cows. *Proceedings of the New Zealand Society of Animal Production* **45**, 35–37.

McDougall, S. (2001). Effects of periparturient diseases and conditions on the reproductive performance of New Zealand dairy cows. *New Zealand Veterinary Journal* **49**, 60–67.

McDougall, S. and Rhodes F. (1998). Diagnosis and treatment of non-cycling cows. In: 75th NZVA Conference, Rotorua, NZ, pp. 219–228.

McDougall, S., Burke, C. R., Macmillan, K. L. and Williamson, N. B. (1995). Patterns of follicular development during periods of anovulation in pasture-fed dairy cows after calving. *Research in Veterinary Science* **58**, 212–216.

McDougall, S., Cullum, A.A., Anniss, F.M. and Rhodes, F.M. (2001). Treatment of anovulatory anoestrous postpartum dairy cows with a gonadotropin-releasing hormone (GnRH), prostaglandin F2α, GnRH regimen or with progesterone and oestradiol benzoate. *New Zealand Veterinary Journal* **49**, 168–172.

Mee, M.O., Stevenson, J.S. and Minton, J.E. (1991). First postpartum luteal function in dairy cows after ovulation induced by progesterone and gonadotropin-releasing hormone. *Journal of Dairy Science* **74**, 1573–1581.

Mellado, M. and Reyes, C. (1994). Association between preparturient disorders and reproductive efficiency in Holstein cows in Northern Mexico. *Preventive Veterinary Medicine* **19**, 203–212.

Mialot, J.P. and Badinand, F. (1985). L'Anoestrus chez les bovines. In: Française de Buiatrie (ed). *Miex Connaître, Comprendre et amîtriser la fécondité bovine*. Maisons_Alfort, France. Tome II, pp. 217–233.

Moller, K. and MacDiarmid, S.C. (1981a). The reproductive performance of New Zealand dairy cows after induction of calving. *New Zealand Veterinary Journal* **29**, 172–172.

Moller, K. and MacDiarmid, S. (1981b). The economy of induced early parturition in New Zealand dairy herd. *New Zealand Veterinary Journal* **29**, 165–167.

Monke, D.R. (1988). *On-farm management of bull intended for AI service*. Proceedings of the 12th technical Conference on Artificial Insemination and Reproduction, pp. 68–79). Columbia, National Association of Animal Breeders.

Monke, D.R. (1986). Noninfectivity of semen from bulls infected with bovine leucosis virus. *Journal of the American Veterinary Medical Association* **188**, 823–826.

Monke, D.R. (2002). Bull management; Artificial insemination centers. In: *Encyclopedia of Dairy Sciences*. Academic Press. Elsevier Science, pp. 198–204.

Moran, J.B. (1993). *Calf rearing – a guide to rearing valves in Australia*. Victorian Department of Agriculture, Melbourne.

Moran, J.B. (1996). Improved management systems for dairy replacement heifer. In, *Proceedings of the Australian Society of Animal Production* **21**, 71–72.

Moreira, F., Risco, C., Pires, M.F.A., Ambrose, J.D., Drost, M., DeLorenzo, M. and Thatcher, W.W. (2000). Effect of body condition on reproductive efficiency of lactating dairy cows receiving a timed insemination. *Theriogenology* **53**, 1305–1319.

Morgan, W.F. and Lean, I.J. (1993). Gondadotrophin-releasing hormone treatment in cattle, a meta-anlysis of the effects on conception at the time of insemination. *Australian Veterinary Journal* **70**, 205–209.

Morton, J. (1999). *The InCalf Project: A progress report*. Dairy Research and Development Corporation, Melbourne, Australia.

Morton, J.M. (2000). The InCalf Project–some risk factors reproductive performance in Australian dairy herds. *Proceedings of the Australian and New Zealand Combined Dairy Veterinarians Conference, Vanuatu*, pp, 229–240.

Morton, J.M. and Butler, K.L. (1995a). Direct effects of induced parturition on subsequent reproductive performance of dairy cows from commercial herds in south-western Victoria. *Australian Veterinary Journal* **72**, 293–295.

Morton, J.M. and Butler, K.L. (1995b). Reductions in milk production after induced parturition in dairy cows from commercial herds in south-western Victoria. *Australian Veterinary Journal* **72**, 241–245.

Morton, J.M. and Butler, K.L. (1995c). The effects of induced parturition on the incidence of clinical disease and mortality in dairy cows from commercial herds in south-western Victoria. *Australian Veterinary Journal* **72**, 1–4.

Moss, N. (2001). *The epidemiology of subfertility in Australian dairy cows.* PhD Thesis, University of Sydney.

Nash, J.G., Ball, L. and Olson, J.D. (1980). Effect on reproductive performance of administration GnRH to early postpartum dairy cows. *Journal of Animal Science* **50**, 1017–1021.

Nation, D. P. Morton, J. Cavalieri, J. Macmillan, K.L. (2001). Factors associated with the incidence of 'Phantom cows' in Australian dairy herds. *Proceedings of the New Zealand Society of Animal Production* **61**, 180–183.

Nebel, R.L., and McGilliard M.L. (1993). Interactions of high milk yield and reproductive performance in dairy cows. *Journal of Dairy Science* **76**, 3257–3268.

Obese, F.Y. (2003). *Characterisation of variation in selected insulin-like growth factors and insulin-like growth factor binding proteins in pasture-fed lactating dairy cows.* PhD thesis, University of Melbourne, Victoria. Australia.

O'Connor, M. (2000). Eight factors contribute to highly effective heat detection. In: *Herd Management System.* Zinpro Animal Nutrition Publication.

Palmquist, D. L. and Jenkins, T. C. (1980). Fat in lactation rations, Review. *Journal of Dairy Science* **63**, 1–14.

Parkinson, T.J. and Vermunt, J.J. (2000). Management of bulls in dairy herds. In: *Proceedings of the Australian and New Zealand Combined Dairy Veterinarians Conference,* 191–206.

Peeler, E.J. and Otte, M.J. (1994). Inter-relationship of periparturient disease in dairy cows. *Veterinary Record* **134**, 129–132.

Pelissier, C.L. (1978). Fertility problems under large herd management. In: Wilcox, C.J. (ed). *Large herd dairy management*, p. 201. University Presses Florida, Gainesville.

Pryce, J.E., Coffey, M.P. and Simm, G. (2001). The relationship between body condition score and reproductive performance. *Journal of Dairy Science* **84**, 1508–1515.

Rabiee, A.R., Macmillan, K.L. and Schwarzenberger, F. (2001a). Progesterone metabolism in ovariectomised non-lactating Holstein-Friesian cows treated with progesterone with two levels of feed intake. *Animal Reproduction Science* **66**, 35–46.

Rabiee, A.R., Macmillan, K.L. and Schwarzenberger, F. (2001b). The effect of level of feed intake on progesterone clearance rate by measuring faecal progesterone metabolites in grazing dairy cows. *Animal Reproduction Science* **67**, 205–214.

Rabiee, A.R., Macmillan, K.L. and Schwarezenberger, F. (2001c). Progesterone clearance rate in lactating dairy cows treated with a CIDR device with two different levels of milk yield. *Reproduction Nutrition Development* **41**, 309–319.

Rabiee, A.R., Macmillan, K.L. and Schwarezenberger, F. (2002a). Plasma, milk and faecal progesterone concentrations during the oestrous cycle of lactating dairy cows with different milk yields. *Animal Reproduction Science* **4**, 121–131.

Rabiee, A.R., Macmillan, K.L., Schwarzenberger, F. and Wright, P.J. (2002b). Effects of level of feeding and progesterone dose on plasma and faecal progesterone in ovariectomised cows. *Animal Reproduction Science* **73**, 185–95.

Rabiee, A.R., Breinhild. K., Scott, W., Golder, H.M., Block, E. and Lean, I.J. (2012). Effect of fat additions to diets of dairy cattle on milk production and components, A meta-analysis and meta-regression. *Journal of Dairy Science* **95**,1–23.

Radostits, O.N. (1974). Symposium, Recent advances in calf rearing. *Journal of Dairy Science* **58**, 436–470.

Rhodes, F.M., Fitzpatrick, L.A., Entwistle, K.W. and Déath, G. (1995). Sequential changes in ovarian follicular dynamics in *bos indicus* heifers before and after nutritional anoestrus. *Journal of Reproduction and Fertility* **104**, 41–49.

Rhodes, F.M., Entwistle, K.W. and Kinder, J.E. (1996). Changes in ovarian function and gonadotropin secretion preceding the onset of nutritionally induced anestrus in *bos indicus* heifers. *Biology of Reproduction* **55**, 1437–1443.

Rhodes, F.M., McDougall, S. and Ververk, G.A. (2001). Reproductive performance of dairy cows not detected in oestrus but with a detectable corpus luteum, in response to treatment with progesterone, oestradiol benzoate and prostaglandin F2α. *New Zealand Veterinary Journal* **49**, 13–17.

Risco, C.A., Chenoweth, P.J. Larsen, R.E., Velez, J., Shaw, N., Tran, T. and Chase, C.C. (1993). The effect of gossypol in cottonseed meal on performance, hematological and semen traits in post pubertal Brahman bulls. *Theriogenology* **40**, 629–633.

Risco, C.A. (2000). Management and economics of natural service sires on dairy herds. In: Chenoweth, P.J. (ed). *Topics in bull fertility.* IVIS: www.ivis.org.

Roberts, S.J. (1986). *Veterinary Obstetrics and Genital Diseases*, 3rd edition. Woodstock, S.J. Roberts.

Roche, J.F., and Diskin, M (2001). Resumption of reproductive activity in the early postpartum period cows. *BSAS* (Diskin, M.G. ed.) Occasional Publication **26**, 31–42.

Rukkwamsuk, T., Wensing, T. and Kruip, T.A.M. (1999). Relationship between triacylglycerol concentration in the liver and first ovulation in postpartum dairy cows. *Theriogenology* **51**, 1133–1142.

Ryan, D.P., Snijders, S., Yaakub, H. and O'Farrell, K.J. (1995). An evaluation of estrous synchronization programs in reproductive management of dairy herd. *Journal of Animal Science* **73**, 3687–3695.

Schneider, FJ, Shelford, J.A., Peterson, R.G. and Fisher, L.J. (1981). Effects of early and late breeding of dairy cows on reproduction and production in current and subsequent lactation. *Journal of Dairy Science* **64**, 1996–2002.

Seykora, A.I., and MacDaniel, B.T. (1983). Heritabilities and correlations of lactation yields and fertility for holsteins. *Journal of Dairy Science* **66**, 1486–1493.

Sklan, D., Bogin, E., Avidar, Y. and Gur-arie. S. (1989). Feeding calcium soaps of fatty acids to lactating cows, effect on production, body condition, and blood lipids. *Journal of Dairy Research* **56**, 675–681.

Sklan, D., Kaim, M., Moallem, U. and Folman, Y. (1994). Effect of dietary calcium soaps on milk yield, body weight, reproductive hormones, and fertility in first parity and older cows. *Journal of Dairy Science* **77**, 1652–1660.

Son, J., Grant, R.J. and Larson, L.L. (1996). Effects of tallow and escape protein on lactational and reproductive performance of dairy cows. *Journal of Dairy Science* **79**, 822–830.

Spalding, R.W., Everett, R.W., and Foote, R.H. (1975). Fertility in New York artificially inseminated Holstein herds in dairy herd improvement, *Journal of Dairy Science* **58**, 718–723.

Spanski, N.A., Drackley, J.K., Davis, C.L. and Jaster, E.H. (1997). Utilization of supplemental triglycerides or free fatty acids by calves from 4 to 10 weeks of age. *Journal of Dairy Science* **80**, 573–85.

Spicer, L.J., Tucker, W.B. and Adams, G.D. (1990). Insulin-like growth factor-I in dairy cows, relationship among energy balance, body condition, ovarian activity, and estrous behaviour. *Journal of Dairy Science* **73**, 929–937.

Stagg, K., Diskin, M.G., Roche, J.F., Sreenen, J.M. (1995). Association between FSH concentrations and follicle growth during normal oestrous cycle and nutritional anoestrus in heifers. *Journal of Reproduction and Fertility* **15**, 66 (Abstract).

Staples, C.R., Thatcher, W.W. and Clark, J.H. (1990). Relationship between ovarian activity and energy status during the early postpartum period of high producing dairy cows. *Journal of Dairy Science* **73**, 938–947.

Stevenson, J.S. and Britt, J.H. (1977). Detection of oestrus by three methods. *Journal of Dairy Science* **60**, 1994–1998.

Stevenson, J.S. and Britt, J.H. (1994). Detection of estrus by three methods. *Journal of Dairy Science* **60**, 1994–1998.

Taylor, V.J., Beever, D.E. and Wathes, D.C. (2000). Plasma IGF-I, energy balance status and ovarian function in dairy cows producing average and high milk yields in the early postpartum period. *Journal of Reproduction and Fertility Abstract series* **26**, 34–35.

Taylor, C., Rajamahendran, R. (1994). Effect of mid-luteal phase progesterone levels on the first wave dominant follicle in cattle. *Can. Journal of Animal Science* **74**, 281–285.

Tefera, M., Humblot, P., Chaffaux, S. and Thibier, M. (1991). Epidémiologi et thérapeutique de l'infertilité fonctionnelle de la vache laitiére. *Recueil de Médecine Vétérinaire* **167**, 335–345.

Thatcher, W.W., Santos. J., Staples, C.R. and Mattos, R. (2002). *The science of Omega-3 fatty acids on dairy cows reproduction. Journal of Dairy Science* ADSA series. Québec, Canada.

Van Amburg, M.E., Galton, D.M., Bauman, D.E., Everett, R.W., Fox, D.G., Chase, L.E. and Erb, H.N. (1998). Effects of three prepubertal body growth rates on performance of Holstein heifers during first lactation. *Journal of Dairy Science* **81**, 527–538.

Villa-Godoy, A., Hughes, T.L., Emery, R.S., Chapin, L.T. and Fogwell, R.L. (1988). association between energy balance and luteal function in lactating dairy cows. *Journal of Dairy Science* **71**, 1063–1072.

Villa-Godoy, A., Hughes, T.L., Emery, R.S., Enright, W.J., Ealy, A.D., Zinn, S.A. and Fogwell, R.L. (1990). Energy balance and body condition influence luteal function in Holstein heifers. *Domestic Animal Endocrinology* **7**, 135–148.

Voges, H., Horner, G.W., Rowe, S. and Wellenberg GJ. (1998). Persistent bovine pestivirus infection in the testes of an immunocompetent, non-viraemic bull. *Veterinary Microbiology* **61**, 165–175.

Waltner, S.S. McNamara, J.P. and Hillers, J.K. (1993). Relationship of body condition score to production variables in high producing dairy cattle. *Journal of Dairy Science* **76**, 3410–3419.

Webster, F.B., Lean, I.J., Kennedy, D., Phillips, K. (1997a). A case-control study to identify farm factors affecting fertility of dairy herds, univariate description of factors. *Australian Veterinary Journal* **75**, 266–273.

Webster, F.B., Lean, I.J., Curtis, M.A. (1997b). A case-control study to identify farm factors affecting fertility of dairy herds, multivariate description of factors. *Australian Veterinary Journal* **75**, 262–265.

Westwood, C.T., Lean, I.J., Garvin, J.K., Della Vedova, J.J. (1997). Heat detection in the dairy cow. *Current Topics in Dairy Production* **1**, 58.

Westwood, C.T., Lean, I.J. and Garvin, J.K. (1998). A study to identify factors affecting resumption of ovarian activity, successful conception and pregnancy in lactating dairy cows, Multivariate description of factors. XX World Buiatrics Congress, Sydney **2**, 635.

Westwood, C.T., Lean, I.J. and Garvin, J.K. (2002). Factors influcing fertility of Holstein dairy cows, A multivariate description. *Journal of Dairy Science* **85**, 3225–3237.

Williamson, N.B. (1996). The economics of reproductive management programs in large and medium dairy herds. *Bovine Practitioner* **30**, 15–20.

Wiltbank, M.C., Gumen, A. and Sartori, R. (2002). Physiological classification of anovulatory conditions in cattle. *Theriogenology* **57**, 21–52.

Xu, Z.Z., Burton, L.J. and Macmillan, K.L. (1996). Reproductive management of lactating dairy cows following oestrus synchronization with progesterone, oestradiol and prostaglandin. *New Zealand Veterinary Journal* **44**, 99–104.

Xu, Z.Z. and Burton, L.J. (1998). Synchronization of estrus with PGF2α administration 18 days after a progesterone treatment in lactating dairy cows. *Theriogenology* **50**, 905–915.

Xu, Z.Z. and Burton, L.J. (1999). Reproductive performance of dairy heifers after estrus synchronization and fixed-time artificial insemination. *Journal of Dairy Science* **82**, 910–917.

Xu, Z.Z. and Burton, L.J. (2000). Estrus synchronization of lactating dairy cows with GnRH, progesterone, and prostaglandin F2α. *Journal of Dairy Science* **83**, 471–476.

Young, I.M. and Anderson, D.B. (1986). First service conception rate in dairy cows treated with dinoprost tromethamine early post partum. *Veterinary Record* **118**, 212–213

Zulu, V.C., Sawamukai, Y., Nakada, K., Kida, K. and Moriyoshi, M. (2002). Relationship among insulin-like growth factor-I, blood metabolites and post-partum ovarian function in dairy cows. *Journal of Veterinary Medical Science* **64**, 879–885.

CHAPTER 45

Practice-Based Dairy Health Planning and Plans

Jonathan M.E. Statham

Learning objectives

- Appreciate the purpose of herd health plans and herd health planning.
- Appreciate the application of the measure, manage and monitor construct in herd health management.
- Be aware of the relationship between herd health assurance schemes and herd health planning.
- Be aware of the relationship between cattle health schemes and herd health planning.
- Appreciate the historical development of herd health planning and management.
- Understand the challenges in implementing herd health planning and production management plans.

Introduction

A Herd Health Plan (HHP) is a document which describes health planning (HP) on a particular farm – a process of measuring (using good record keeping), managing (through treatment and prevention strategies) and further monitoring of health and reproductive performance, to ensure the welfare of animals and support the profitability of the farm business. The process should be evidence-based. This 'cycle' of events is shown in Figure 45.1.

The purpose of health planning (HP) is primarily to prevent disease and improve animal health and production by introducing long-term strategies focusing on the whole herd. Planning should be designed to reduce the losses from disease and reproductive failure. This can be achieved for diseases caused by a single pathogen by preventing the entry of the infection into the herd, and by controlling and eradicating the disease where present. Reducing the risk of multifactorial diseases may require changes to the management and the environment and the use of vaccines, where appropriate.

Although the component parts are often familiar clinical procedures, genuine HP is differentiated by this long-term, whole-herd approach, and by taking ownership of the process through an effective vet-farmer partnership. Dairy health planning offers an opportunity for veterinary practitioners to engage with their farm clients in a proactive fashion and to deliver genuinely preventative medicine at the hub of the farm team. Although this is not a new concept, it is still significantly under-exploited in general veterinary practice, and this chapter seeks to outline a framework which may be utilised to explore these opportunities.

Dairy health planning

A starting point for the development of a herd health plan is to define the scope of data that is required. This decision is dependent on discussion of the herd needs by veterinarian and farmer. A basic list might include:

- Infectious disease status: BVD, IBR, Leptospira, Johne's disease and *Neospora caninum*.
- Reproductive performance: calving to conception interval, conception rate, submission rate.
- Mastitis: clinical mastitis rate, subclinical mastitis rates (new infections; chronic infections; first infections).
- Lameness: herd mobility scores and lesion records.
- Youngstock health: mortality rates, calf pneumonia and calf scour incidence.
- Nutrition and metabolic disease (incidence of ketosis, LDA, milk fever, milk protein and fat).
- Culling rate (reasons): voluntary and involuntary.

Financial measurement should not be overlooked; the business performance of the farm unit should be included in the farm

Bovine Medicine, Third Edition. Edited by Peter D. Cockcroft.

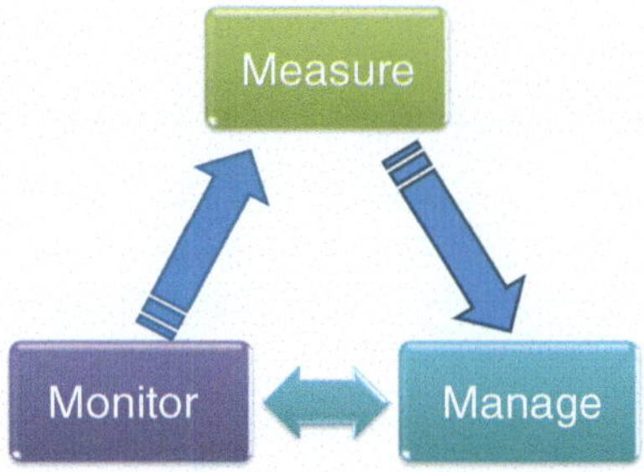

Figure 45.1 The Measure, Manage and Monitor cycle.

audit. Analysis of variable and fixed costs is essential in achieving a thorough understanding of the constraints or motivators acting on a herd.

Motivation to record herd health data is supported by positive feedback in the form of herd health reports, in the style of the farm audit. Shaping the appropriate level of data recording is an important role for the veterinary practice. Inadequate data recording clearly undermines the ability of the farmer-veterinarian partnership to implement change on the basis of robust evidence. However, excessive and unstructured data recording is also demotivating, by demanding inappropriate levels of time and resource with limited opportunity to deliver real improvement in herd performance as a result.

Disease monitoring

Single-agent infectious disease: testing

The range of diagnostic tests available to measure single-agent infectious disease continues to increase. Decision-making requires a balanced understanding of the sensitivity and specificity of the tests alongside economic cost benefit. Although serology remains the herd-level surveillance tool of choice for many agents, increasing use is made of other methods, such as PCR. Consideration should be made of appropriate sample sizes and age groups to be measured. For example, cost effective herd level screening for BVD may be achieved through blood sampling a strategic cohort of 6–10 homebred youngstock from each management group, using the BVD antibody ELISA. However, consideration must be made regarding colostral antibody status, so sampled animals should be at least eight months old and unvaccinated, if interpretation is to be possible.

The Cattle Health Certification Scheme (CHeCS) standards ensure that herd health status in one single-agent disease health scheme is comparable to that in all other schemes in the UK. Close collaboration by CHeCS with other countries ensures that licensed schemes in the UK are compatible with those in other countries, in terms of what must be measured to determine a defined herd health status. Table 45.1 summarises some examples of the processes that may be required for achieving health accreditation. These may change with time, and may vary dependent upon the scheme.

Multifactorial and management diseases: what data are required and how will they be measured?

In the same way that laboratories have developed CHeCS accredited health schemes for single-agent disease control, milk recording organisations (MROs) have developed a series of tools and services to measure multifactorial/managemental disease. Although these services are predominantly based on software tools for milk recording purposes, they have the ability to record health and fertility events, medicine usage, birth dates and cattle movement information. Veterinary access to

Table 45.1 Examples of herd accreditation scheme requirements.

Disease	How to become accredited
BVD	• A serological check test is carried out on five calves from each management group (9–18 months). • A second check test is carried out 12 months later. • Accredited status is obtained if all results are negative.
Johne's	• Subject to herd history, two or three herd tests are carried out on all animals two years of age and older, at intervals of 12 months. • Accredited status is obtained if all results are seronegative.
IBR	• Two herd tests are carried out at an interval of between four weeks and 12 months. • All animals 12 months of age and older, plus non-homebred younger animals, must be sampled. • Accredited status is obtained if all results are seronegative.
LEPTO	• Two herd tests are carried out at an interval of between five and 12 months. • All animals over 24 months, plus any stock of 12–24 months that are intended for breeding, must be tested. • Accredited status is obtained if all results are seronegative.

data through online tools allows analysis of farm trends and benchmarking comparisons to be made. Co-ordinated health schemes are beginning to emerge from these services (Statham, 2011).

A variety of tools are available to facilitate the recording of management dairy data globally. Simple paper-based systems are still appropriate for some herds but, in general, software packages are a prerequisite of modern dairy data recording. *Interherd* and *Interherd +* (NMR, UK), *Total Vet* (QMMS, UK) and *DairyComp 305* (USA) are three such systems which support recording of dairy data, the generation of action lists and the analysis of herd problems.

What to measure and how to achieve reliable and interpretable data collection are real challenges in the commercial farm situation. How motivated are the farm team to collect accurate data? How consistent are diagnostic definitions across the farm team or the wider practice or national benchmark group?

For example, in measuring mastitis performance, how confident can the herd veterinary surgeon be that clinical mastitis is being recorded in a reliable and repeatable fashion? How is mastitis being detected? There are several options: foremilking, inspection of in-line filters, milk conductivity, udder change, CMT tests or the somatic cell counts from the routine milk recording visit. When are subclinical cases really missed clinical cases of mastitis? How robustly, therefore, can inter-herd comparisons be interpreted in benchmarking systems?

Standardisation can significantly improve the quality of data recording, and may form part of farm team knowledge exchange programmes. These issues should not be overlooked when interpreting the increasingly sophisticated software tools available to record and present data for analysis.

Interpretation of the data

Veterinary input is then vital to utilise the recorded data. There are two main stages: risk assessment and risk management.

Risk assessment

Risk assessment involves the comparison of recorded data for the key performance indicators with target values, in order to judge whether performance is satisfactory or unsatisfactory. The analysis may be carried out either by comparing the herd performance to other, similar herds (benchmarking), or monitoring the changes in performance of the herd over time (longitudinal assessment). Benchmarking offers an opportunity for motivating herd improvement through competitive interaction with a regional peer group. Delivered on a regular basis, benchmarking offers a route to regular comparison of performance. However, benchmarking is potentially controversial, as poorly performing herds may be demotivated by this process. Longitudinal comparison of improvement, or deterioration in performance, will indicate the outcomes in response to implemented changes. A range of data analysis tools are viable to facilitate this process.

Risk management

Risk management represents the key opportunity for bespoke veterinary input. If risk assessment reveals a deficit in herd performance, the opportunity then exists for veterinary advice to promote improvement. This is appropriate on many levels, from reproductive deficits to high clinical mastitis rates and poor mobility performance. It is essential that advice is delivered on the basis of evidence-based analysis. Computer-based tools allow the analysis of large amounts of data generated by larger herds, but simple paper-based analysis may be perfectly adequate – for example, a Cu-Sum chart of pregnancy diagnoses, or pattern of mastitis cases in the first month of lactation out of every 12 cows calved (Green *et al.*, 2007).

Further evidence gathering may be required from the initial benchmarking exercise to identify the component risk factor(s). For example:

- **Reproductive performance:**
  A declining conception rate (CR) may prompt further investigations. These may include nutritional metabolic profiling, forage analysis, ration analysis, body condition score analysis and rumen fill scoring. In addition, infectious disease monitoring may be justified, and a review of artificial insemination technique and semen quality. Seasonal trends in CR may indicate changes in grazing strategy, or the need for supplementary feeding. Poor CR for a specific batch of semen may indicate poor handling or a problem with liquid nitrogen storage.
- **Mastitis:**
  A high clinical mastitis rate may prompt both a milking time visit to review milking routine and parlour performance, as well as an environmental assessment to review housing space, hygiene and ventilation factors.
- **Lameness:**
  A deterioration in the herd mobility score may prompt a review of hoof care protocols, as well as further assessment of environmental factors, such as cubicle design and cow flow dynamics.

A clear and concise strategic direction of outcomes and targets available to all the farm and veterinary team should be provided.

Knowledge exchange, training and standard operating procedures

The opportunity to deliver knowledge exchange (KE) and training on-farm is an integral aspect of this process. Regular training, to drive good performance in milking routine or heat detection, is an opportunity to achieve improvement and to avoid the negative effects of producing a HHP which nobody on the farm implements or complies with. Genuinely listening to the concerns of the farm team, and including feedback into the HP process, improves compliance with suggested change.

Similarly, standard operating protocols (SOPs) and bespoke tools, such as vaccination calendars, are essential vehicles for delivery of the HHP.

Monitor

The outcomes of any management change should inform future veterinary herd health input, and so the monitoring step in this health planning process is critical. Only by constantly iterating management advice can the performance in relation to change be assessed, and further change and improvement be achieved. A static template plan begins to be redundant the day it is written. Monitoring includes ongoing recording and benchmarking of key endemic disease and reproductive parameters, such as clinical mastitis rates, herd mobility and submission rate, in addition to surveillance of infectious disease.

This dynamic monitoring exercise offers a further opportunity for veterinary presence on-farm. The role of paraprofessionals in the veterinary team may include both the gathering of data, such as mobility scoring or teat scoring at milking time, and also collecting samples such as milk or faeces for surveillance. New graduates can also play a fuller part in this process, which provides high intellectual challenges and enables earlier participation at a higher level than traditional reactive work.

History of health panning in the UK

GB 'Cattle Health Initiative' (2006–2008)

In the aftermath of the foot and mouth disease (FMD) outbreak of 2001 in the UK, a review of livestock farming by the Department of Food, Environment and Rural Affairs (DEFRA) led to the publication of the GB Animal Health and Welfare Strategy (AHWS). The overall objective of the AHWS was to achieve higher standards of animal health and welfare, and to develop a more sustainable livestock industry.

The FHP 'Cattle Health Initiative' (CHI) project (2006–2008) was pivotal to the delivery of the AHWS in England, and was based on three of its principles:

1. Working in partnership.
2. Understanding roles and responsibilities.
3. Prevention is better than cure.

Health planning (HP), or 'Farm Health Planning' (FHP), as it was referred to, was central to DEFRA's strategies for animal health/welfare, veterinary surveillance and provision of future veterinary services in the UK (Woods, 2007). Through the promotion of 'positive animal health', FHP aimed to enhance animal well-being, farming profitability and veterinary practice viability, and to gather data for input into improved veterinary surveillance systems. The purpose was to facilitate the development and uptake of HP, which practising veterinarians would then offer as a private service to their farming clients.

This initiative was driven partly by the desire to avoid a repetition of the recent FMD and BSE outbreaks in the UK. Other significant factors were the decline in agricultural incomes (which had reduced the uptake of traditional veterinary services), changes to meat hygiene regulations and European Community (EC) subsidies, and the UK Competition Commission's enquiry into veterinary medicines. It was, however, not a new concept, and it had been promoted in major drives by the veterinary profession both in the 1930s and the 1960s (Woods, 2007, 2008), with similar aims.

Farm assurance schemes

Additionally, the drive for farm assurance in the UK in the late 1990s marked an important opportunity for veterinary engagement with the industry and it was important that this opportunity was taken energetically (Sibley, 2000). Farm assurance sought to promote consumer confidence in the delivery of appropriately managed food production from British farms. The provision of a (veterinary) 'Health Plan' became an early requirement of Great Britain Farm Assurance schemes. The British Cattle Veterinary Association (BCVA) engaged positively with the production of health plans, and developed health planning software, together with education and training to support its use. A Herd Health Plan (HHP) has been described as 'a document which describes a method intended to monitor, treat and prevent health problems, ensure welfare of animals and aims to be cost-effective for the farm business' (Sibley, 2000, 2006).

A HHP for the purpose of farm assurance would include:

- Legislation and welfare.
- Medicines and residues.
- Youngstock health.
- Reproduction.
- Mastitis.
- Lameness.
- Nutrition.
- Infectious disease control.

The table in Annex 45.1 at the end of this chapter shows all areas included in the Health and Performance Monitoring Plan, and all areas needed to be complied with for a signed Certificate of Conformity to be issued. If incomplete, a Health Plan would be issued but would not be signed.

Health plans and herd health planning

Unfortunately, requirements of early assurance schemes could often be met without any real engagement with the veterinarian-farmer partnership, and some 'plans' represented little more than a tick-box exercise. The drive to promote active health planning was undermined by the production of such generic 'plans', imposed to satisfy retailer requirements for farm assurance rather than reflecting a true working summary of herd health in action. Dairy farmers could opt out of working with their veterinary surgeons on the production of a health plan, avoiding a professional veterinary fee, but also potentially missing the opportunity to address more fundamental herd health issues.

There consequently developed a misconception of the contrast between the production of a static herd health plan versus the delivery of genuinely dynamic herd health planning.

Bell *et al.* (2006) evaluated HP on 61 dairy farms. 48% of farmers stated that their plan was no longer an active document, and did not consider that the plan was of any benefit; 18% considered that the plan did not have to reflect what was happening on the farm; and 50% of the farmers' comments about HP included negative opinions about additional bureaucracy, the lack of perceived benefit and the feeling that planning was a poor use of their time.

If HP was to be adopted, it needed to be accepted by farmers as effective. 43 of the farmers did make positive comments about having a HHP; plans were considered useful for managing herd problems, improving liaison with vets, and as a training aid for new employees. However, the focus of these comments was largely centred on the production of a document, not on the process of dynamic herd improvement described by proactive veterinary involvement in the farm team.

Wapenaar & Hall (2011) investigated the differences in opinions of farm veterinary surgeons and dairy farmers regarding Herd Health Plans (HHP) and Herd Health & Production Management (HH&PM). Two comparable questionnaires, one for vets and one for farmers, were distributed throughout the UK. For the purpose of this study HHPs were defined as 'the current paper document issued by the British Cattle Veterinary Association or other organisations'. The HH&PM was defined as 'regular scheduled farm visits that go beyond the "one-off" tasks such as pregnancy diagnosis, castrations and dehorning; the purpose being to prevent disease and/or improve animal health and production by introducing long-term strategies focusing on the herd as a whole.'

Veterinarians and farmers respondents differed when listing the 'major roles' of the veterinarian on the farm. Although vets saw 'optimising milk production' and 'being an independent advisor' as important roles, this did not seem to be perceived as such by the farmer. Furthermore, when presenting themselves to clients, veterinarians seemed to favour the 'friend of the farmer' style approach; a much smaller proportion of farmers seemed to prefer this approach. The majority of farm respondents (81%, $n = 98/121$) valued the discussions with their veterinarian, and it was apparent from the relatively small proportion of vets instigating a discussion on farm (26%, $n = 33/125$), that there is an opportunity for a more proactive approach from veterinarians.

When asked 'What is your opinion on the current HHP?' (options: 'No opinion', 'Useful document', 'Useless document' and 'Other, please specify'), 44% of vets and 44% of farmers considered it a 'Useful document'. A minority of respondents, (27% of vets and 16% of farmers) regarded the HHP as a 'Useless document'. 40% of veterinarians described their opinion with detailed comments in the 'Other' category; 'Usefulness varies from farm to farm depending on attitude, but mainly useless'; 'Potentially useful but often over-complicated and flawed'; 'Potentially useful, but ignored by farmer; initial discussion is useful'. Most of the specific comments could be summarised as 'potentially useful', 'usefulness varies per client', and 'useful if improved and updated'.

However, dynamic *measurement* of performance did become a requirement of the Great Britain Farm Assurance, and any plan produced after 1 April, 2010 required evidence of a health review having taken place. The Red Tractor marketing logo appeared on over £10bn of UK food products by 2010. Great Britain dairy farm assurance scheme standards were therefore re-branded the 'Red Tractor Farm Assurance – Dairy Standards' to reinforce the link between assured status and the eligibility for product to carry the logo. Rather than just simply putting a new signature and date on the front of the health plan document, there was a need to show evidence of a regular collation of the incidence of health conditions and performance, together with an indication that these results were satisfactory or otherwise.

As a minimum, this requirement for dynamic performance monitoring included lameness, mastitis, and culling rates and reasons, with results then available to evaluate disease levels, assess the effectiveness of current preventative measures and allow performance benchmarking. This could then indicate the need for any modifications of the prevention and treatment protocols.

To quote the assurance document, '*It is strongly recommended that the health planning process, including the development of the Health Plan and the annual review, is conducted in conjunction with the farm veterinary surgeon. Apart from providing an objective overview of the situation, the breadth of experience and technical knowledge of the veterinarian can be extremely valuable in proposing practical, cost-effective solutions to improving the health and welfare status of the herd.*' This represented a very strong steer towards veterinary involvement (but fell short of making a veterinary health plan compulsory), and a recognition by the industry that active health planning is essential to farm performance and the image of the dairy industry.

Farmers, and their veterinarians, could produce a health plan in a variety of formats, so long as they incorporated the same aspects of planned preventative and treatment measures and other procedures. The scheme provided a template for the health plan and review, found as an appendix to the standards manual, or could be downloaded from the scheme website (www.assureddairyfarms.org.uk). Similarly, for the review, if the health records data were maintained in other formats, such as charts or farm/web-based computer systems, then this need not be duplicated.

UK cattle health schemes

In addition to state-sponsored schemes such as those concerned with eradication and control of bovine tuberculosis and brucellosis, a wide range of commercial cattle health schemes have emerged to facilitate these processes (Statham, 2011):

- accredited laboratory-based schemes aimed principally at controlling single-agent infectious disease;
- schemes based on milk recording data, aimed principally at control of management disease.

Single-agent schemes

Cattle Health Certification Standards (UK)

Cattle Health Certification Standards (UK), abbreviated to CHeCS, www.checs.co.uk, is a self-regulatory body for Cattle Health Schemes in the UK. It is a non-trading organisation established by the British cattle industry for the control and eradication of non-statutory diseases by a set of standards to which all licensed Cattle Health Schemes must adhere (Duncan, 2000). It addresses control of BVD, IBR, Leptospirosis, Johne's disease and, recently, *Neospora caninum*.

Biosecurity Risk-Assessments Tools

Prior to embarking on a CHeCS cattle health scheme programme, it is advised that a biosecurity risk assessment is carried out for the premises to facilitate better understanding of the aims of the scheme. This can be done independently or through the Biosecurity module in web-based 'MyHealthyHerd.com'. General biosecurity should be assessed covering, cattle, people and animals. In addition to this, a disease specific risk assessment should be carried out covering disease risk status, vaccine status, surveillance status and control/current status.

SAC also support health planning software which facilitates the production of health plans.

HerdWise (NML)

The Johne's Screening Programme is run as 'HerdWise' by National Milk Laboratories (NML) and administrated by the NMR Group. The scheme requires regular structured measurement of individual animal Johne's status. The herd veterinary surgeon produces a flexible package for the specific farm to provide testing and consultancy. The programme then uses the same milk samples taken by NMR at the monthly recording, and charges are based on the number of cows in the herd. Some introductory understanding of the level of prevalence of Johne's in the herd can be obtained by using a 30-cow targeted screen (i.e. selecting 30 high-risk cows – old/sick/reduced production-or screening cull cows as they exit the herd (Statham, 2011)).

Control of management or multifactorial disease

No single body assumes responsibility for certification of management or multifactorial disease controls, but farm assurance schemes evolved to drive the recording of food production from herds with a known health status and, recently, a number of industry initiatives, such as the DairyCo Mastitis Control Plan (www.dairyco.org.uk), have emerged in the UK. These are discussed below.

DairyCo Mastitis Control Plan

Expert systems are emerging with a genuine evidence base to support decision making in health planning. They still require clinical veterinary judgement to complement epidemiological modelling, but have a significant role to play:

The national mastitis control initiative, led by DairyCo (www.dairyco.org.uk) in partnership with the University of Nottingham and QMMS Ltd, was a good example of an industry-led partnership scheme set up to control endemic disease (in this case, mastitis) in the UK (dairy) cattle population. The scheme was the first of its kind and reached more than 750 dairy herds and 150 veterinary surgeons and advisors by the beginning of 2012.

Practitioners were registered with the scheme (www.mastitiscontrolplan.co.uk) and underwent two days of intensive CPD training, led by RCVS-recognised specialists and concentrating on the use and interpretation of data patterns within herds, herd-level diagnosis and implementation of the DairyCo Mastitis Control Plan. The original research (Bradley *et al.*, 2007; Green *et al.*, 2007) showed, on average, a 20% reduction in the incidence rate of cows affected with clinical mastitis after 12 months in herds that put the Plan in place. This example of health planning provides an opportunity to control one of the most costly and debilitating diseases in cattle, both in the UK and worldwide, and could also be used as a blueprint for other endemic disease.

Lameness Control Schemes

The 'Healthy Feet Project', with the Bristol Cattle Lameness Programme, stated:

'The aim of the Healthy Feet Project is simple; we want to help reduce lameness in dairy cattle on UK farms and encourage farmers, vets and advisors to work together.'

Support from DEFRA and the Tubney charitable trust facilitated a website which provided key information and tools for lameness control (www.cattle-lameness.org.uk). The GB levy body DairyCo adopted the findings of the Bristol project, and rolled out the DairyCo Healthy Feet Programme. This offers a multi-level resource aimed at producers, including a mobility mentor scheme delivered by veterinarians and other mobility professionals.

Working with the dairy industry in 2008, DairyCo launched a new ground-breaking cattle mobility score, which became the industry standard for measuring mobility and lameness in UK dairy herds. The score was developed as a result of research carried out by the industry and DairyCo over the previous 18 months, and it aimed to free industry from the confusion between different locomotion scoring methods.

A number of major UK milk buyers and supermarkets have promoted uptake of the scheme over the last two years, with the aim of improved UK dairy cow welfare through reduced lameness.

DairyCo produced a mobility DVD that contained information about the best possible location to mobility score, and advice on scoring frequency. It also had information on, and examples of, the points to look for when scoring cattle into each category (www.dairyco.org.uk).

Planning versus management – where are we now?

Confusion exists between the production of a static herd health plan (HHP) and the active process of health planning (HP) that a preferred term may become herd health and production management (HH&PM). 'Health planning' implies something which may be rigid or dictated, and so 'management' may be a better term to describe the interactive and dynamic nature of the process which requires daily attention.

The veterinary profession is ideally positioned as 'custodians' to manage this balance. However, other advisors will take on this role if veterinarians do not choose to be involved, or fail to genuinely listen to the needs of their farming clients. Veterinarians need to engage farmers in active HH&PM, and will need to find different strategies and motivators to achieve success with different individuals.

Kristensen & Enovoldsen (2008) compared perceptions of 16 Danish dairy farmers and 18 veterinary surgeons. The veterinary surgeons surveyed believed that farmers' primary focus was on production and profit. However, the farmers valued teamwork and animal welfare more. The rankings are presented in Table 45.2.

Table 45.2 Perceptions of veterinarians and farmers (Kristensen & Enovoldsen (2008). Reproduced with permission of Kristensen and Enevoldsen.

Priority rank	Veterinarians	Farmers
1	Production	Teamwork
2	Animal welfare	Animal welfare
3	Knowledge dissemination	Knowledge dissemination
4	Teamwork	Production

In addition, Bigras-Poulin (1985) found that Ontario farmers' socio-psychological characteristics were more important to farm performance than the herd level variables describing production, health and fertility. People take actions for a variety of reasons, including relative income standing, risk aversion, a feeling of uncertainty, employee satisfaction, and subjective well-being.

It is important to appreciate that HH&PM goes beyond simple economics to achieve improvement, and requires a genuine working vet-farmer partnership with an emphasis on teamwork.

References

Amory, J.R., Barker, Z.E., Wright, J.L., Mason, S.A., Blowey, R.W. and Green, L.E. (2006). LAMECOW at the University of Warwick: A study of lameness in dairy cattle. *Cattle Practice* **14**, 123–125.

Bell, N.J., Main, C.J., Whay, H.R., Knowles, T.G., Bell, M.J. and Webster, A.J.F. (2006). Herd health planning: farmers' perceptions in relation to lameness and mastitis. *Veterinary Record* **159**, 699–705.

Bennett, R.M., Christiansen, K., Clifton-Hadley, R.S. (1999). Direct costs of endemic diseases of farm animals in Great Britain. *Veterinary Record* **145**, 376–377.

Bigras-Poulin, M., Meek, A.H., Martin, S.W. (1985). Attitudes, management practices, and herd performance – a study of Ontario dairy farm managers. II Associations. *Preventive Veterinary Medicine* **3**, 241–250.

Bradley, A.J., Leach, K. A., Breen, J.E., Green L.E., and Green M.J. (2007). Survey of the incidence and aetiology of mastitis on dairy farms in England and Wales. *Veterinary Record* **160**, 253–258.

Burr, P. (2004). Health Schemes: Are they only for the minority? *Cattle Practice* **12**(4), 255–257.

Caldow, G.L. (2001). Herd Health Security: The role of laboratory tests. *Cattle Practice* **9**(2), 105–110.

Duncan, A. (2000). Cattle Health Certification Standards (UK) (CHeCS). *Cattle Practice* **8**(3), 319–320.

Esselmont, R.J. and Kossaibati, M.A. (2002). The costs of disease and poor fertility in dairy herds. *Daisy Report* **5**, 5–21; 117–125.

Gibbens, N. (2009). *Animal Health 2008: The Report of the Chief Veterinary Officer*. DEFRA publication.

Green, M.J., Leach, K. A., Breen, J.E., Green, L. E., Bradley, A.J. (2007). National intervention study of mastitis control in dairy herds in England and Wales. *Veterinary Record* **16**, 287–293.

Kristensen, E.L. and Enovoldsen, C. (2008). A mixed methods inquiry: How dairy farmers perceive the value(s) of their involvement in an intensive dairy herd health management program. *Acta Veterinavia Scandinavica* **50**, 50.

Lowe, P. (2009). *Unlocking Potential: A report on veterinary expertise in food animal production*. DEFRA.

Sibley, R. (2000). Planning Health care on dairy farms. *In Practice* **22**, 405–406.

Sibley, R. (2006). Developing health plans for the dairy herd. *In Practice* **28**, 114–121.

Statham, J.M.E. (2006). Benchmarking or Business Opportunity? Using milk recording data to expose your clients weaknesses. *Cattle Practice* **14**, 49–56.

Statham, J.M.E. (2008). A review of the BCVA Health Planning Initiative and Future Direction. *Cattle Practice* **16**(2), 107–115.

Statham, J.M.E. (2011). Cattle Health schemes; 2.Multifactorial or management diseases. *In Practice* **287**, 33; 282–285.

Wapenaar, W. and Hall, J. (2011). Opinions and practices of vets and dairy farmers towards herd health 1 management in the UK. *Veterinary Record* **170**(17), 441.

Whitaker, D.A., Kelly, J.M., Smith, S. (2000). Disposal and disease rates in 340 British dairy herds. *Veterinary Record* **146**, 363–367.

Woods, A. (2007). The farm as clinic: veterinary expertise and the transformation of dairy farming, 1930–1950. *Studies in History and Philosophy of Biological and Biomedical Sciences* **38**, 462–487.

ANNEX 45.1: HEALTH & PERFORMANCE MONITORING PLAN

The table below will be completed annually. The incidence will be monitored and reviewed on a bimonthly basis as part of the herd health scheme benchmarking service.

*Health and performance information that **must** be collated for monitoring:*

	No. of cases		Farm target(s) (total or per-100 cows – delete as appropriate)	Comments, observations (e.g. pattern in timing, common causes)
	Total	Per 100 cows*		
Lameness				DD and sole ulcers
Mastitis				
Culling rate				
Main reasons for culling	1 Cell counts 2 Lameness 3 Fertility			
Involuntary culls, i.e. number of animals that died/emergency slaughtered (on-farm)				
Calf Mortality – 0–24 hours (incl. stillborn)				
Calf Mortality – 24 hours–42 days				
Abortions				

*To determine number of cases per 100 cows, calculate: $\frac{\textit{Total number of cases}}{\text{Total number of cows}} \times 100$

PART B COMPLETED BY:

Name: Role on farm: (e.g. farmer, herdsman, vet)

Declaration:

The information recorded within Part B, to the best of my knowledge, is accurate and a true reflection of incidences on the farm. Where required, relevant records will be provided to the vet to undertake the annual herd health review.

Signed: (farmer/ herdsman) Signed: (and vet if applicable)

Date:

*Health and performance information it is **recommended** is collated for monitoring:*

	Number of cases		Farm target (s)	Comments, observations
	Total	per 100 cows		
Health and welfare				
Mobility scoring – Score 2 and 3 cows (impaired and severely impaired mobility)				Number of cows scored = Date of most recent scoring = / /
Milk fever				
Hypomagnesaemia ('staggers')				
Retained foetal membranes				
No. of assisted calvings				
Survivability and productivity				
Fertility parameters Days to 1st service Conception rate (%) Calving interval (days) Females reaching second calving				
Average number of Lactations				
Average milk yield (state whether yield is related to days, lactation etc). Cows Heifers				
Average milk quality (12 months) Butterfat % Protein % Bactoscan Somatic Cell Count Urea				

FARM NAME Farm

PART C – HEALTH AND PERFORMANCE REVIEW

VET REVIEW OF DATA AND RECOMMENDATION OF ACTIONS/ PRIORITY AREAS

This section must be completed by a veterinary surgeon, at least annually. As part of the vet review, the vet may need access to the records that have been used to collate data (e.g. medicine records). NB: The vet is *not* expected to validate or verify data collated by the farmer – they are required to review it and make recommendations based on what they have seen. Farmers are not bound by the scheme to act upon vet recommendations.

I have reviewed data and health and performance records (where available) related to:

- Lameness [ ] Tick if seen
- Mastitis [ ]
- Culling and mortalities [ ]
- Fertility, reproductive disorders and calving problems [ ]
- Metabolic disorders [ ]
- Calf diseases [ ]
- Other diseases and conditions [ ]
  (list any others seen)

And as part of the review I have also inspected:

- Cows in milk [ ] Tick if seen
- Calves [ ]
- Dry cows [ ]
- Other youngstock [ ]
- Stock bulls [ ]

other (list)

And recommend that the following priorities are acted upon within the specified timeframe:

	Priority	Actions to address	Complete by
1.			
2.			
3.			

The relevant sections (to these priorities) of the Herd Health Plan should also be updated.

The priorities and actions I recommend above are based upon the data and facts provided to me and the cows inspected on the day. As such, the effectiveness of my recommendations could be limited by the accuracy of the information provided and whether the cows seen are a true reflection of the herd.

Veterinary surgeon name: Veterinary practice:

Veterinary surgeon's signature Date of review

CHAPTER 46

Organic Dairy Farms

Kathryn Ellis

Learning objectives

- To be aware of the structure of the legislation pertaining to organic farming in the EU and UK.
- To understand of the major differences in the management of organic dairy farms.
- To understand the regulations pertaining to the treatment of organic dairy cattle with veterinary medicines.
- To understand the challenges associated with organic dairy farming with respect to udder health, nutrition and parasite control.

Introduction to organic farming

In the United Kingdom (UK), the number of registered organic holdings has increased dramatically in the last 15 years, with numbers of organic cattle continuing to increase (DEFRA, 2011). Although organic farming is still supplying a 'niche' market, representing around 4% of the UK farmed land area and < 5% of cattle (fewer than 1% of prime cattle slaughtered are organic), there is a widespread distribution of holdings. Having an understanding of the organic farming system, including the associated regulations, is important in order to provide appropriate veterinary services to organic clients and their livestock.

Organic farming has its origins in early 20th Century Europe, with the Soil Association, formed in the UK in 1946. It is defined by the principles outlined in Figure 46.1, and can be viewed as an holistic approach to farming. In practice, this means that farmers utilise some or all of the following techniques: Use of legumes (such as clover) to fix nitrogen; Recycling of manures and crop wastes; mechanical control of weeds; operation of a 'closed farm system' with respect to nutrients; crop rotations to minimise disease build-up; mixed and rotational grazing to reduce parasite burdens; growing resistant crop varieties; minimising chemical and/or veterinary therapeutic drug usage.

Organic farming regulations

In the European Union (EU), organic food production is regulated by Council Regulation (EC) 834/2007; this is the most recent update of the EU regulations, which came into effect in January, 2009. This legislation outlines the baseline EU standards, farming practices and inspection of organic producers and processors. Despite organic production having a recognised following for many decades, there has been a Livestock Annex in the EU regulations only since August 2000. Each member state of the EU must abide by the baseline EU regulations but, in addition, each is also at liberty to add to the regulations (i.e. to make them more stringent).

In the UK, the EU legislation is interpreted via The Compendium of UK Organic Standards (Anon, 2006) and overseen by the relevant agricultural departments of each devolved region: In England by Department of Environment, Food and Rural Affairs; in Scotland by the Scottish Government; in Wales by the Welsh Government. The basic UK standards for organic production and processing are legally enforced by the Organic Products Regulation 2004.

Organic farming certification

In the UK there are nine DEFRA-approved organic certification bodies (Table 46.1). Each of these certification bodies has its own set of rules for organic production, based on the underlying EU and UK legislation, although in some cases additional requirements are set, over and above the baseline regulations.

Bovine Medicine, Third Edition. Edited by Peter D. Cockcroft.

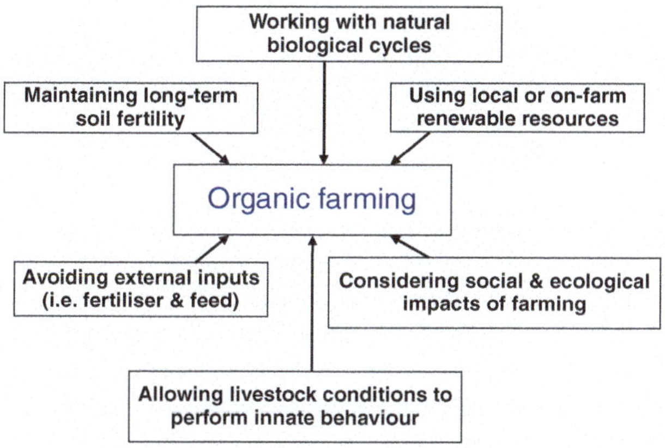

Figure 46.1 Principles defining organic farming systems.

For a producer to be a registered organic farm, the following steps should have been completed:

1 The producer has registered with one of the certification bodies.
2 The producer is following that certification body's production standards.
3 The farm has a farm conversion plan, if it is converting from non-organic production, and/or a subsequent organic farming management plan for maintenance following conversion.
4 The farm is subject to annual inspection from the certification body's own inspectorate, whereby the holding is audited with respect to inputs, crop treatments, livestock feeds, livestock movements, livestock treatments and health records, to ensure the producer is abiding by the rules of production.

If all of the above procedures are completed to the satisfaction of the certifier, the producer may then call his/her produce organic.

Conversion to organic production

Conversion to organic production generally entails a minimum of a two-year soil conversion period for the farm. The livestock on the holding have a variable conversion period, dependent on animal species: for example, a dairy cow should be managed organically for a minimum of nine months before her milk can be sold as organic; a suckler cow must be managed for 12 weeks before her offspring (not the cow herself) can be sold as organic. Animals raised for organic meat production have to be born and raised organically to be sold as organic. Usually, the conversion period is associated with a reduction in farm yields due to reduced stocking densities and different feeding practices. There is a great deal of advice available for producers wishing to convert to organic production systems, including information on the funding available to support producers in the conversion period when they have reduced yields, but are not able to sell organic produce (see 'Useful Sources of Information' at the end of this chapter).

Organic management regulations

A stipulation of the UK regulations (Anon, 2006) is that a herd health plan is required, '*ensuring the proper control of disease and the encouragement of positive animal welfare … This must be provided for by a plan drawn up by the farmer, preferably working in partnership with a veterinary surgeon and agreed between them during and after conversion, to develop and operate an organic livestock system which conforms to these Standards. The plan must ensure the development of a pattern of health building and disease control measures appropriate to the particular circumstances of the individual farm and allow for the evolution of a farming system progressively less dependent on allopathic veterinary medicinal products*'.

This is a great opportunity for veterinarians to become involved in herd health work with organic dairy clients, as prevention of disease (and evidence-based medicine) is central to the organic approach.

Other general issues that relate to organic dairy herd health management include:

Table 46.1 Approved organic certification bodies in the UK.

Name of certification body	Comments	Website address
Soil Association Certification Ltd		www.soilassociation.org/certification
Scottish Organic Producers Association (SOPA)		www.sopa.org.uk
Organic Farmers and Growers (OFG)		www.organicfarmers.org.uk
Biodynamic Agricultural Association		www.biodynamic.org.uk
Irish Organic Farmersand Growers Association		http://iofga.org/
Organic Trust Limited	Republic of Ireland-based body	http://www.organic-trust.org/
Quality Welsh Food Certification Ltd	Lamb and beef only	http://www.wlbp.co.uk/organic_overview
Ascisco Ltd	Minor section of Soil Association	www.soilassociation.org/certification
Organic Food Federation		www.orgfoodfed.com

1 Farms should operate generally under a closed herd policy where possible, although up to 10% bought-in replacements are allowed per annum.
2 Livestock must be fed on a 100% organic ration, which is preferably home grown (up to 50% can be bought in if needed).
3 Weaned animals should be fed a minimum of 60% dry matter intake of forage.
4 Calves must have access to whole milk for three months and be group housed after seven days old; if done, disbudding and or castration must be done before three months old.

Veterinary medicines use and withdrawal periods

Although one of the aims of organic production systems is to minimise the use of veterinary medicines, if there is a clinical justification for treatment of an animal then it is permissible to do so under the organic regulations. Under EU and UK regulations, recommendations are that phytotherapeutic (e.g. plant extracts), homoeopathic products and trace elements, should be used in preference to chemically synthesised allopathic veterinary medicinal products or antibiotics, *provided that their therapeutic action is effective for the species of animal, and the condition for which the treatment is intended.* If no such alternative product is available or deemed to be effective then, under veterinary guidance, the use of veterinary medicine is permitted.

Veterinary medicinal products must be authorised in accordance with current European and UK legislation, and appropriate records must be kept detailing the animal treated, the indication for treatment, the product used, the batch number and the withdrawal period. The baseline EU and UK requirement is that the withdrawal period on treatments is twice that stated on the product's datasheet, with the Soil Association requiring three times the duration of withdrawal. A product with a zero withdrawal period (for example a prostaglandin analogue) has an automatic 48 hour withdrawal period under organic rules. Any off-datasheet use requires application of the standard withdrawal periods (28 days meat). In addition, the Soil Association requirements restrict the use of certain other drug classes, such as third and fourth generation cephalosporins and fluoroquinolones, to very specific instances of individual animals under treatment.

An animal in an organic production system may receive no more than three *courses* of veterinary allopathic treatment per year, or one course if the animal is to be killed before it is one year old. A course of treatment is defined as: '*a course of treatment shall mean all necessary measures taken to restore the animal to health following a particular disease episode*'. It is important to be aware that multiple administrations of a product, or simultaneous administrations of two products – for example, administration of a non-steroidal anti-inflammatory drug concurrently with an antimicrobial to treat a foot lameness for more than one day – would be considered to be one course of treatment. Vaccines and parasite treatments are not included as courses of treatment, although some certification bodies prefer use of reduced valency vaccines, where possible.

Preventive veterinary treatments are prohibited which, in dairy systems, means that blanket antimicrobial dry cow therapy is not permitted. Nor are herd-based reproductive treatments permitted (for example, heifers would not be allowed to be treated to synchronise oestrous). No growth promoters are permitted; however, under current EU regulations, hormonal growth promoters are not permitted anyway in non-organic production.

It is important to realise that strategic therapy use is allowed, when supported with evidence of a requirement; therefore, the strategic administration of an anthelmintic to a part, or the whole, of a group of animals would be permissible, if supported with evidence of need to do so, such as poor liveweight gains or a high faecal egg count in a group of grazing animals. It is equally important to emphasise that animals are *not required to show clinical disease or, in the worst case, die, before treatments can be administered.* National or international disease control measures are allowed; a recent example of this is the blanket use of Bluetongue (BTV 8) vaccination to control disease in Europe.

Overall, preventive herd health is key in reducing the requirement for veterinary therapy; an aim of all producers, organic or otherwise. However, it is vital for veterinary surgeons working with organic producers to communicate with their clients and the client's organic certification body when discussing preventive health measures, and when considering the requirements for treatment of organic livestock, to ensure that there is no compromise in animal welfare or the producer's livelihood.

Herd health planning

When considering herd health planning for organic dairy farms, it is important to remember the essential differences in production compared to non-organic systems. However, it is also important to emphasise the similarities to non-organic systems; many of the same production diseases, such as mastitis, infertility and lameness, are as much of a problem as they are on non-organic herds (Marley *et al.*, 2010; Ahlman *et al.*, 2011), and the endemic infectious diseases, such as Bovine Virus Diarrhoea (BVD) and Infectious Bovine Rhinotracheitis (IBR) are equally important.

Veterinary surgeons advising organic clients must be aware of the production principles of organic farming and the specific requirements of both the individual farm circumstances and the certification body with which the producer is registered (Vaarst *et al.*, 2011). A useful UK-based source of advice and information is the Organic Compendium, an on-line resource available at http://www.organicvet.co.uk/. In certain situations, organic regulations may lead to different risks of disease prevalence (e.g. with regards to nutrition, udder health and parasite control), and these are discussed further in the sections below.

Health challenges in organic dairy systems

Nutrition

The milk price paid to producers has fluctuated in recent years and, although organic producers receive a higher price per litre of milk than non-organic producers, the differential does not easily cover the increased costs of production. Therefore, successful organic dairy farming requires high standards of stockmanship and a suitable farm geographical environment. Some producers have chosen to have a spring calving pattern and thus seek to maximise milk production from grazed grass. Whatever system is used, the key is to maximise the efficient use of quality forage, whether grazed or conserved. Organic concentrates are expensive to grow and/or buy and, economically and environmentally, it makes most sense to be an efficient user of forage.

Since the requirement is to have a daily 60% minimum DMI as forage, forages must be highly palatable. In the summer, this means careful use of grazed pasture (Figures 46.2 and 46.3); grass sward quality should be optimal, and the clover component of the pasture is not excessive so as to avoid pasture bloat. In winter, it is essential to have good quality silage(s) available. Herds that tend to perform best are those with the ability to grow multiple forage sources on-farm, such as whole-crop wheat, or mixed crops such as cereals undersown with clovers for ensiling. Although some organic producers feed only forage to their cows, the lower milk yields tend to make these systems more marginal, and can be associated with significant fluctuations in body condition score of the cows. Despite the costs associated with feeding concentrate or grain feeds, the returns overall, in terms of milk production potential from cows and improved herd health, tend to justify the expense of moderate concentrate feeding (Blair, 2001).

In herds feeding poor quality forages, the main effects are reduced milk yield overall, or reduction in milk protein percentage. Poor body condition score – or body condition score loss – in the cows can also indicate inadequate energy supply. It is advisable to include regular body condition scoring at key points of the dairy cow's cycle (drying off, calving, breeding), to allow a herd-level picture of energy balance to be developed (Mulligan, 2012).

The transition period is critical in terms of individual (and herd) dairy cow and herd health, irrespective of production system, with increased likelihood of the subsequent development of several important diseases associated with poor transition management. This applies just as much in organic herds, even those with lower milk yields, and benchmarking farms with respect to the incidence of diseases such as milk fever, ketosis, left displaced abomasum, retained placenta and lameness is very important (Mulligan, 2012).

There is some debate as to whether Holstein cows are suitable for organic dairy production, given their genetic predisposition to partition energy towards milk. This does, to an extent, depend upon stockmanship, as there are numerous very successful Holstein organic dairy herds in the UK, on which cows graze excellent quality pastures in the summer that are well managed, and are fed high-quality mixed forages in the housed period. Therefore, when appraising an organic farm, consideration should be given to what that farm is capable of in terms of home-grown feed production and feeding systems, as to whether cows with a genetic potential to produce large volumes of milk are suitable.

Udder health

In the UK, there is no milk payment structure based on bulk milk somatic cell count (BMSCC) for organic producers; therefore, there is less incentive for producers to keep such a tight control on BMSCC, compared to non-organic producers. So long as the rolling three-month geometric mean BMSCC is below the EU limit of 400 000 cells per ml, milk can be sold. In effect, this, and the fact that blanket antimicrobial dry cow therapy is not permitted, means that organic dairy herds tend to have higher BMSCCs than non-organic herds (Ellis, 2005; Prins *et al.*, 2012).

Nevertheless, addressing udder health is important on organic farms, as a high BMSCC is associated with reduced milk yield, increased clinical mastitis cases and, therefore, discard of mastitic milk, as well as increased culling rates. The traditional approaches to mastitis control serve well to help improve udder health: milking machine maintenance, rapid detection and treatment of clinical mastitis cases, high standards of hygiene during milking, identification and separation of high cell count/chronic mastitis cows and appropriate treatment or culling, high standards of hygiene in the cows' environment, whether housed or at pasture (Ellis *et al.*, 2007), and good background herd health and nutrition to optimise the cows' immune function. The key differences with organic systems are in the treatment of mastitis cases and approach to the dry cow.

Ideally, to reduce spread of infection and improve animal welfare, cows with clinical mastitis should be indentified and treated as soon as possible. In practice, this depends on skilled milking personnel who can identify clinical cases accurately and quickly. In addition, the use of individual cow somatic cell count information is very useful in keeping track of cows with chronic consistent or intermittent high cell counts. Treatment of mild to moderate new cases of clinical mastitis can involve intra-mammary antimicrobial administration and use of non-steroidal anti-inflammatory drugs.

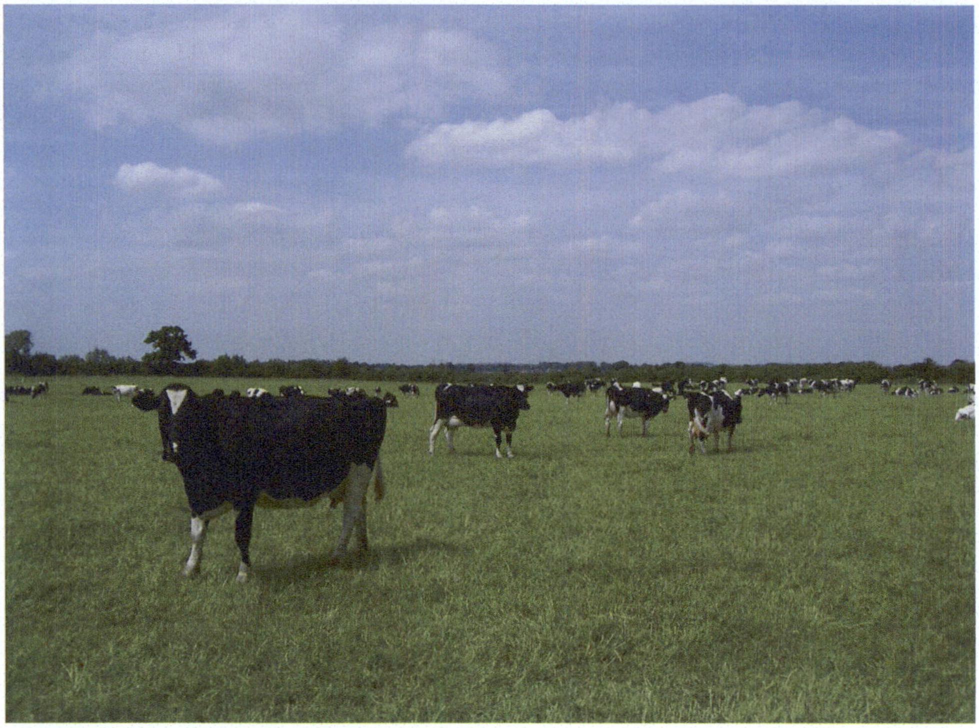

Figure 46.2 Organic Holstein cattle grazing mixed grass and clover swards in the summer.

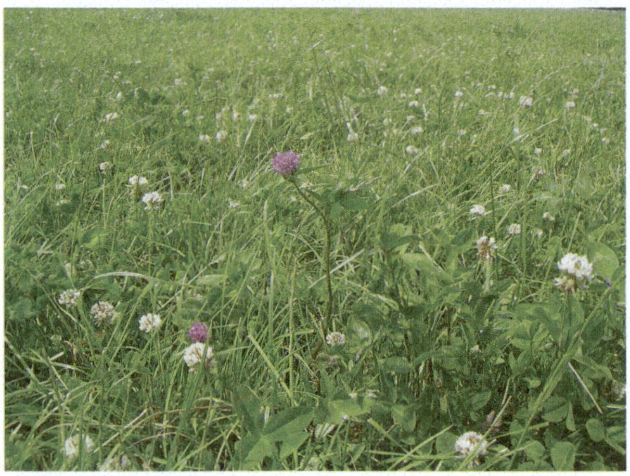

Figure 46.3 An example of a mixed grass and clover sward for grazing, containing ryegrass and both red and white clover.

The use of homoeopathic remedies is often practised (Ellis, 2005), but it is not proven that these are effective and it can be argued that the rapid, judicious use of antimicrobial therapy at an early stage of infection may lead to a net reduction in use overall. Other supportive therapies, such as udder massage and stripping out of affected quarters, can be very helpful in alleviating signs in affected cows. Treatment of severe cases of mastitis, in which affected cows are recumbent and likely to have some degree of endotoxic shock, should be undertaken by the veterinarian.

The use of internal teat sealants in cows at drying-off has enabled organic herds to have an effective control measure to reduce mastitis acquired during the dry period, and these products are highly recommended. On an individual basis, antimicrobial dry cow therapy can be administered to cows with known increasing somatic cell counts or a history of clinical mastitis prior to drying-off. In cases of chronic mastitis/high somatic cell counts, affected quarters can be dried-off early (without the use of antimicrobials).

Controlling mastitis with minimal antimicrobial use is a challenge. The key components are to optimise the hygiene practices in the herd at milking and in the environment, and to identify infected cows accurately and rapidly. An approach to Udder health management of clinical mastitis is shown in Box 46.1 and dry cow management in Figure 46.2 and Box 46.1.

Parasite control

Control of parasitic infections in non-organic livestock is typically based on appropriate grazing management and the use of parasiticides and vaccines, where available. Because all animals in a group at any one time are assumed likely to be exposed to similar degrees of parasite challenge, it is common practice to treat all members, in order to reduce the impact of the challenge

Box 46.1 Udder health management: clinical mastitis

Clinical mastitis recording and treatment guide

Clinical signs

Grade 1	New case of mastitis in previously normal quarter. Few (<5) clots/flakes in fore milk. Rest of milk looks normal. No heat, pain or firmness in udder. Cow bright, with no other signs of illness.
Grade 2	New case of mastitis in previously normal quarter OR a grade 1 case that still has signs at next milking. Many (>5) clots/flakes in foremilk +/− also in main milk. No heat, pain or firmness in udder. Cow bright, with no other signs of illness.
Grade 3	Clots throughout milk. Heat, firmness or pain in udder. Cow bright, with no other signs of illness.
Grade 4	Changes in milk (may be watery, bloody or clotty). Heat, firmness or pain in udder. Cow is dull, depressed and may be down. May have a high (>38.5°C/101°F) or low (<38.5°C/101°F) temperature.

Suggested treatment protocol for clinical mastitis cases

Grade 1	Strip out quarter fully at *first* milking with signs. Apply udder salve and massage quarter, apply teat dip. ***Check for signs at next milking***. If clear of signs at next milking, leave. If still has signs, treat as Grade 2. Record case and treatment in medicines record and on mastitis record.
Grade 2 and Grade 3:	Strip out quarter fully at *first* milking with signs. Use lactating cow intra-mammary tube in affected quarter according to datasheet. After quarter is stripped/milked out wear gloves, clean and disinfect teat end with spirit wipe. Insert syringe nozzle *just inside* the teat opening and empty contents into teat. Massage the teat to disperse antibiotic up into udder. Apply teat dip. Mark cow with tail/foot tape or spray. Record treatment in medicines record and on mastitis record.

Milk is to be withheld for 2 × datasheet recommendation from last treatment

Check for change in signs at next milking.

If signs worsen or do not respond after a standard course of treatment, seek veterinary advice.

Grade 4 — Get veterinary attention immediately.

The cow is very sick and will need injectable antibiotics, anti-inflammatory and other supportive treatments.

Record treatment in medicines record and on mastitis record.

Box 46.2 Udder health management: dry cow therapy administration and monitoring

Administering dry cow therapy

- Dry-off all cows abruptly.
- Do not administer dry cow therapy during milking – keep the cows back and treat them at the end.
- Wear clean disposable gloves.
- Clean teats if dirty.
- Wipe dry with paper towel.
- Use iodine pre-dip/spray.
- Wipe dry with paper towel.
- **Thoroughly** clean and disinfect the teats (do far side first) using spirit wipes/spirit soaked cotton wool, and allow to dry.
- Strip out (in reverse order – near side first) any remaining milk by hand.
- A re-clean teat ends with spirit and allow to dry.
- Administer product – (either internal teat sealant or antibiotic dry cow tube) do near side teats first and only *partially* insert tube cannula.
- Dip teats in post milking teat dip or use external teat sealant in the summer.
- Mark cows as having been treated.
- Separate cows into a dry cow group and allow to stand for at least 30 minutes to allow teat to close.
- Record details of cows treated in the medicines book.
- **Antimicrobial dry cow tubes** - ORGANIC MILK WITHDRAWAL PERIOD IS 2X DATASHEET RECOMMENDATION AFTER TREATMENT.
- **Internal teat sealant dry cow tubes**
  - Do not massage product up into gland after application.
  - Remember to check product has been stripped out by calf at first milking after calving.
  - Organic withdrawal period is 48 hours.

Other points to remember:

- Fly control in the summer.
- Clean housing/environment in summer and winter.
- Correct nutrition and body condition scores for dry cows.

MONITORING THE USE OF DRY COW THERAPY

- **Cows that abort or calve early**
  Isolate aborting cows and check whether you need a brucellosis test. (Consider veterinary investigation for infectious agents other than *Brucella* spp. of all aborting cows.)
  Once health status is assured, and if cow had an antibiotic dry cow product remember to observe organic milk withdrawal period before milk goes in the tank. If in doubt about residues after withdrawal period, get a milk sample checked – you can use an on-farm kit, DelvoSP, or send to a lab.
  If you have any questions seek veterinary advice.
- **Monitoring efficacy of dry cow therapy**
  Use CMT in first week of lactation on cows known to have had high SCCs prior to drying off. This can identify problem quarters/cows and management decisions can then be made (i.e. milking order or possible culling).
  Monitoring the individual cow SCCs in last three milk recordings of previous lactation and first three milk recordings of new lactation will help assess the effectiveness of their dry-cow management.
  Obtain milk samples from clinical mastitis cases (all grades) occurring in the first month of lactation and submit a proportion for bacteriology. (Check first before sending).
  Keep recording all mastitis cases (in dry period or in lactation).
- **Chronically infected cows**
  Chronically infected cows are less likely to respond to dry cow therapy. *Therefore,* remember that older cows, with higher SCCs, with more infected quarters, (particularly with *Staph. aureus* infections), will not respond well.
  Cows with >3 cases of mastitis in the same quarter in one lactation or > 5 cases of mastitis in all quarters in one lactation, should be considered *carefully* as priority cull cows.

and subsequent transmission. The option of mass treatment is actively discouraged by organic farming systems; hence, the emphasis is on early detection of clinical or subclinical cases against a background of lower stocking densities, good nutrition and favourable management (Anon., 2006). Data on parasite burdens in organic dairy cattle are limited, but do suggest there may be a greater challenge in organic dairy cattle and youngstock (Svensson *et al.*, 2000; Sato *et al.*, 2005; Ellis *et al.*, 2011) leading to significant reductions in growth rates at grass (Figure 46.5).

Assessment of challenge is not always easy. Faecal egg counts (FEC) are the most widely used parameter to evaluate gastrointestinal nematode infections of ruminants. Although they are commonly used because of their relative convenience, FEC (particularly single time point FEC) are not necessarily reliable measures of the magnitude or species composition of worm burdens, nor effects on performance (Brunsdon, 1971; Gasbarre *et al.*, 1996; Nogareda *et al.*, 2006), and phenotypic variation in faecal egg output is well recognised (Gasbarre *et al.*, 1996). Faecal egg counts are more reliable indicators of gastrointestinal parasite infection in younger cattle than in cows (Gross *et al.*, 1999) and, even in these, the window of useful time is limited. It has been shown that FEC reflect parasite exposure approximately five to ten weeks after turnout in first grazing season calves (Shaw *et al.*, 1997; Eysker & Ploeger, 2000). After housing, no correlation between faecal egg counts and exposure exists, and only plasma pepsinogen concentrations and ELISA measurement of parasite antibodies are viable candidates for monitoring (Dorny *et al.*, 1999; Eysker and Ploeger, 2000).

Blood pepsinogen concentrations have been used since 1965 as a diagnostic tool for ostertagiosis in cattle (Anderson *et al.*, 1965). It has been demonstrated that blood pepsinogen concentrations can correlate with abomasal pathology and infection burdens of abomasal nematodes (Ploeger *et al.*, 1990a, 1990b, 1990c; Berghen *et al.*, 1993; Ploeger *et al.*, 1994; Dorny *et al.*, 1999), although the relationship is not always straightforward, because the amount and duration of parasite larval challenge, and the age of the animal, can have effects on pepsinogen concentrations measured.

Recent advances in herd-health monitoring have involved the use of an ELISA-based milk *O. ostertagi* (MOO) test to

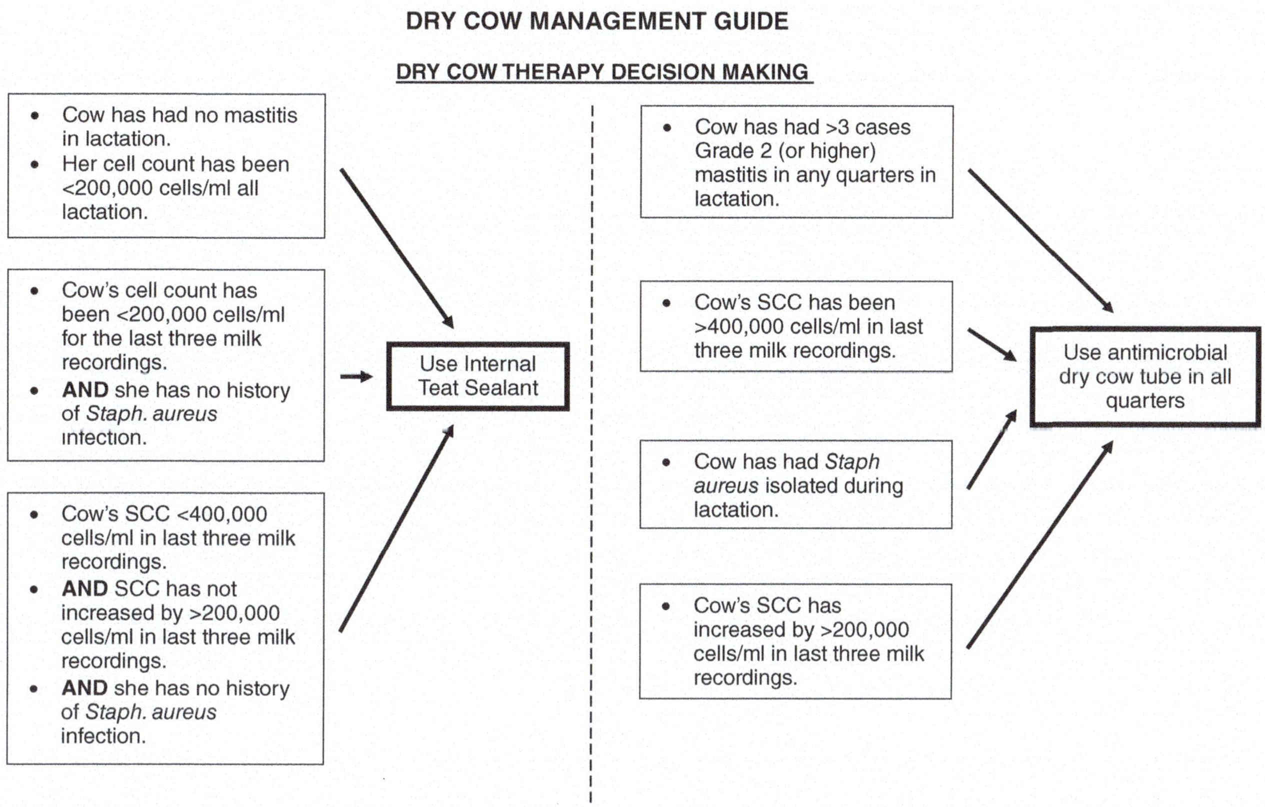

Figure 46.4 First grazing season organic dairy youngstock, showing marked variation in size following significant gastrointestinal parasite challenge.

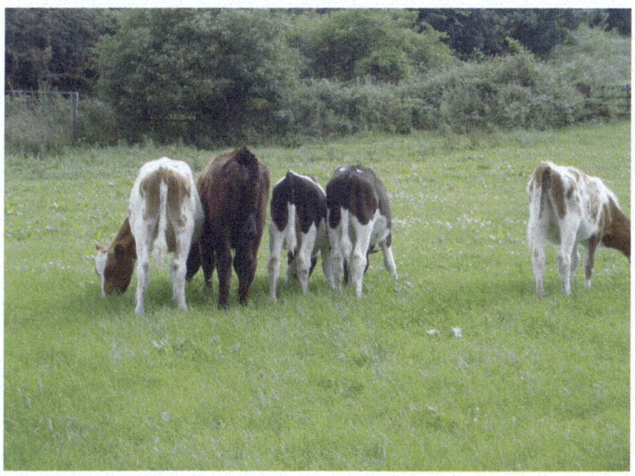

Figure 46.5 Udder health management: dry cow therapy decision making guide.

determine the concentration of antibody against *O. ostertagi* in individual animal or bulk-milk samples (Höglund *et al.*, 2010). It is generally recognised that a wide between-host variation exists in the ability to develop an antibody response against gastrointestinal nematode antigens, implying that an ELISA may not be very appropriate for diagnosis in individual animals (Eysker & Ploeger, 2000). On a practical scale, bulk milk ELISAs can be very useful in herd monitoring (Forbes *et al.*, 2008). The major disadvantage of using milk as a substrate is that it can only be used to monitor adult, lactating cattle.

In recent years, fluke infection of cattle has become more prevalent in the UK (Pritchard *et al.*, 2005), which has been attributed to a generally warmer and wetter climate (Mas-Coma *et al.*, 2000). Control of fluke infection in grazing cattle, particularly organic cattle, is difficult to achieve without the support of flukicide therapy; many of the pasture management techniques, such as fencing off wet areas, are costly and are impractical in wet regions, such as the western areas of the UK. Fluke infection can have effects on the productivity of dairy cattle of all ages (reduced growth rates and poorer milk yield) and can predispose to other infections (e.g. Salmonellosis), as well as acting in synergy with gastrointestinal nematodes to produce clinical disease (Schweizer *et al*, 2005).

The simplest way of dealing with parasitic infections is to use anthelmintics and/or flukicides when clinical disease appears, but this approach can be accompanied by heavy production losses in the group, and it is highly questionable from a welfare point of view (Vercruysse & Claerebout, 2001). Acceptance of a certain degree of production loss without compromising welfare may be an option in organic production systems, in which a central ethos is not necessarily to maximise production (Thamsborg *et al.*, 1999). However, it is important to consider that calving replacement dairy heifers at 24 months old is the most economically and environmentally effective aim (Garnsworthy, 2004), so any reduction in heifer growth rate at grass will compromise this ideal.

Securing sufficient exposure to induce immunity, but without compromising health, in youngstock through an integrated approach based primarily on grazing management, supported by herd monitoring, seems more likely to be successful in addressing the organic aims. Although grazing rotation alone does not prevent parasite infection (Kristensen *et al.*, 2006), careful pasture rotations have been used to control parasitic gastroenteritis (PGE) in first season grazing animals (Eysker *et al.*,1998; Dimander *et al.*, 2003). However, critical to this approach is the importance of recognising seasonal and yearly variation in PGE challenge from the same pastures (Dimander *et al.*, 2003; Nogareda *et al.*, 2006) and substantial larval overwintering on rotationally grazed pastures (Dimander *et al.*, 2003). Assessing risk factors for disease, and its impact on health and production, must be given high priority in organic farming, as this is a system which emphasises the importance of animal welfare (Thamsborg *et al.*, 1999).

Thus, in summary, monitoring parasitism should include a combination of liveweight gain, FEC, plasma pepsinogen assessment and ELISA milk testing. The precise combination should be formulated following discussion between the producer and the veterinary surgeon, as to the most pragmatic approach on an individual farm basis.

Ideally, dairy youngstock in their first grazing year should not be turned out onto paddocks that have had first grazing season animals on them in the second half of the previous year, as such paddocks may have significant, residual larval nematode populations. However, in reality, especially in a situation where there is marginal grazing habitat and permanent pasture, such as that found on some organic farms, there is limited flexibility that can be achieved in grazing rotations, leading to repeated use of certain fields for youngstock as they are unsuitable for lactating cattle. Although organic stocking rates are lower than those in conventional farming systems, where grazing is marginal (as may be the case in some more extensive systems), selective behavioural grazing patterns may mean that animals are, in reality, grazing smaller 'useful' areas and, hence, being exposed to high concentrations of infective larvae (Thamsborg *et al.*, 1998).

Practical measures to surmount this problem are not easy. In theory, these may include increasing the period of time spent between grazing periods, or to ensure that adult cattle are grazing after youngstock whenever possible, to 'mop up' larvae that will have been cycled through first grazing season animals. In reality, logistical issues of accessibility of pastures to lactating cattle that need to walk to a milking parlour twice daily, and pasture quality to support the nutritional needs of lactation, mean that rotation with adult cattle in less-favoured pastures is difficult. Given these logistical constraints, appropriate use of anthelmintics is justified in organic systems to ensure good health and welfare standards.

Recent work investigating the potential for targeted selective treatments (TST) in sheep (Kenyon *et al.*, 2009) and cattle (Höglund *et al.*, 2009) would be seen to be highly relevant to organic systems to reduce parasitic disease and minimise anthelmintic use. This also applies to evidence-based strategies to minimise the development of anthelmintic resistance, as described by Taylor (2010). This endoparasite control programme, entitled 'Control of Worms Sustainably' (COWS) is designed to minimise the development of anthelmintic resistance, and is now being recommended for adoption in the UK. This approach includes, amongst other recommendations, using anthelmintic only when necessary following monitoring of faecal egg counts, and preserving susceptible worms on the pasture by not treating adults cows or a small percentage of the healthy youngstock.

Summary

Organic dairy farming can be challenging, but many principles of the epidemiology of disease and of appropriate animal husbandry are similar to non-organic systems. Veterinarians should be aware of the organic regulations, so they can advise their clients appropriately to ensure healthy, productive livestock.

References

Ahlman, T., Berglund, B., Rydhmer, L. and Strandberg, E. (2011). Culling reasons in organic and conventional dairy herds and genotype by environment interaction for longevity. *Journal of Dairy Science* **94**, 1568–1575.

Anderson, N., Armour, J., Jarrett, W.F., Jennings, F.W., Ritchie, J.S. and Urquhart, G.M. (1965). A field study of parasitic gastritis in cattle. *Veterinary Record* **77**, 1196–1204.

Anon. (2006). Compendium of UK Organic Standards. Published by DEFRA. Available at: http://archive.defra.gov.uk/foodfarm/growing/organic/standards/pdf/compendium.pdf

Berghen, P., Hilderson, H., Vercruysse, J. and Dorny, P. (1993). Evaluation of pepsinogen, gastrin and antibody response in diagnosing ostertagiasis. *Veterinary Parasitology* **46**, 175–195.

Blair, R. (2001). Feeding Organic Cattle. In: *Nutrition and Feeding of Organic Cattle*, pp232–243. CABI, Wallingford, Oxfordshire.

Brunsdon, R.V. (1971). Trichostrongyle worm infection in Cattle. *New Zealand Veterinary Journal* **19**, 203–212.

DEFRA (2011) United Kingdom Organic Statistics. Available at: http://www.defra.gov.uk/statistics/files/defra-stats-foodfarm-environ-organics-statsnotice-110811.pdf

Dimander, S.O., Höglund, J., Uggla, A., Sprondly, E.,Waller, P.J. (2003). Evaluation of gastro-intestinal nematode parasite control strategies for first-season grazing cattle in Sweden. *Veterinary Parasitology* **111**. 193–209

Dorny, P., Shaw, D.J. and Vercruysse, J. (1999). The determination at housing of exposure to gastrointestinal nematode infections in first-grazing season calves. *Veterinary Parasitology* **80**, 325–340.

Ellis, K.A. (2005). *Studies of the Composition of Milk Produced on Organic and Conventional Dairy Farms in the UK*. PhD Thesis, University of Liverpool.

Ellis, K.A., Innocent, G.T., Mihm, M., Cripps, P., McLean, W.G., Howard, C.V. and Grove-White, D. (2007). Dairy cow cleanliness and milk quality on organic and conventional farms in the UK. *Journal of Dairy Research* **74**, 302–310.

Ellis, K.A., Jackson, A., Bexiga, R., Matthews, J., McGoldrick, J., Gilleard, J. and Forbes, A.B. (2011). Use of diagnostic markers to monitor fasciolosis and gastrointestinal nematodes on an organic dairy farm. *Veterinary Record* **169**(20), 524.

Eysker, M. and Ploeger, H.W. (2000). Value of present diagnostic methods for gastrointestinal nematode infections in ruminants. *Parasitology* **120**, S109–S119.

Eysker, M., van der Aar, W.M., Boersema, J.H., Githiori, J.B. and Kooyman, F.N.J. (1998). The effect of repeated moves to clean pasture on the build up of gastrointestinal nematode infections in calves. *Veterinary Parasitology* **76**, 81–94.

Forbes, A.B., Vercruysse, J. and Charlier, J. (2008). A survey of the exposure to *Ostertagia ostertagia* in dairy cow herds in Europe through the measurement of antibodies in milk samples from the bulk tank. *Veterinary Parasitology* **157**, 100–107.

Garnsworthy, P. C. (2004). The environmental impact of fertility in dairy cows: a modelling approach to predict methane and ammonia emissions. *Animal Feed Science and Technology* **112**, 211–223.

Gasbarre, L.C., Leighton, E.A., Bryant, D. (1996). Reliability of a single fecal egg per gram determination as a measure of individual and herd values for trichostrongyle nematodes of cattle. *American Journal of Veterinary Research*. **57**, 168–171.

Gross, S.J., Ryan, W.G., Ploeger, H.W. (1999). Anthelmintic treatment of dairy cows and its effect on milk production. *Veterinary Record* **144**, 581–587.

Höglund, J., Morrison, D.A., Charlier, J., Dimander, S.O. Larsson, A. (2009). Assessing the feasibility of targeted selective treatments for gastrointestinal nematodes in first-season grazing cattle based on mid-season daily weight gains. *Veterinary Parasitology* **164**, 80–88.

Höglund, J., Dahlström, F., Engström, A., Hessle, A., Jakubek, E., Schnieder, T., Strube, C. and Sollenberg, S. (2010). Antibodies to major pasture borne helminth infections in bulk tank milk samples from organic and nearby conventional dairy herds in south-central Sweden. *Veterinary Parasitology* **171**, 293–299.

Kenyon, F., Greer, A.W., Coles, G.C., Cringoli, G., Papadopoulos, E., Cabaret, J., Berrag, B., Varady, M., Van Wyk, J.A., Thomas, E., Vercruysse, J. and Jackson, F. (2009). The role of targeted selective treatments in the development of refugia-based approaches to the control of gastrointestinal nematodes of small ruminants. *Veterinary Parasitology* **164**, 3–11.

Kristensen, T., Thamsborg, S.M., Andersen, H.R., Soegaard, K. and Nielsen, A.L. (2006). Effects of grazing system on production and parasitism of dairy breed heifers and steers grazing wet marginal grasslands. *Animal Science* **82**, 201–211.

Marley, C. L., Weller, R. F., Neale, M., Main, D. C. J., Roderick, S. and Keatinge, R. (2010). Aligning health and welfare principles and practice in organic dairy systems: a review. *Animal* **4**, 259–271.

Mas-Coma, S., Valero, M.A. and Bargues, M.D. (2000). Climate change effects on trematodiases, with emphasis on zoonotic fascioliasis and schistosomiasis. *Veterinary Parasitology* **163**, 264–280.

Mulligan, F. J. (2012). A herd Health Approach to Dairy Cow Nutrition and Production Diseases of the Transition and Early Lactating Dairy Cow. *Key Note Lectures and Round Table Proceedings of the 27th World Buiatrics Congress, Lisbon, Portugal*, pp. 89–96.

Nogareda, C., Mezo, M., Uriarte, J., Lloveras, J. and del Campillo, M.C. (2006). Dynamics of infestation of cattle and pasture by gastrointestinal nematodes in an Atlantic temperate environment. *Journal of Veterinary Medicine Series. B – Infectious Disease and Veterinary Public Health* **53**, 439–444.

Ploeger, H.W., Kloosterman, A., Eysker, M., Borgsteede, F.H.M., Vanstraalen, W. and Verhoeff, J. (1990a). Effect of Naturally-Occurring Nematode Infections on Growth-Performance of 1st-Season Grazing Calves. *Veterinary Parasitology* **35**, 307–322.

Ploeger, H.W., Kloosterman, A., Borgsteede, F.H.M. and Eysker, M. (1990b). Effect of Naturally-Occurring Nematode Infections in the 1st and 2nd Grazing Season on the Growth-Performance of 2nd-Year Cattle. *Veterinary Parasitology* **36**, 57–70.

Ploeger, H.W., Kloosterman, A., Bargeman, G., Vonwuijckhuise, L. and Vandenbrink, R. (1990c). Milk-Yield Increase After Anthelmintic Treatment of Dairy-Cattle Related to Some Parameters Estimating Helminth Infection. *Veterinary Parasitology* **35**, 103–116.

Ploeger, H.W., Kloosterman, A., Rietveld, F.W., Berghen, P., Hilderson, H. and Hollanders, W. (1994). Quantitative estimation of the level of exposure to gastrointestinal nematode infection in first-year calves. *Veterinary Parasitology* **55**(4), 287–315.

Prins, D.G.J., Barrett, D.C. and Ellils, K.A. (2012). *Production performance of organic dairy farms in the United Kingdon between 2001 and 2010*. Abstract Proceedings of the 27th World Buiatrics Congress, Lisbon, Portugal, 253.

Pritchard, G.C., Forbes, A.B., Williams, D.J.L., Salimi-Bejestani, M.R. and Daniel, R.G. (2005). Emergence of fasciolosis in cattle in East Anglia. *Veterinary Record* **157**, 578–582.

Sato, K., Bartlett, P.C., Erskine, R.J. and Kaneene, J.B. (2005). A comparison of production and management between Wisconsin organic and conventional dairy herds. *Livestock Production Science* **93**, 105–115.

Schweizer, G., Braun, U., Deplazes, P. and Torgerson, P.R. (2005). Estimating the financial losses due to bovine fasciolosis in Switzerland. *Veterinary Record* **157**, 188–193.

Shaw, D.J., Vercruysse, J., Claerebout, E., Agneessens, J. and Dorny, P. (1997). Gastrointestinal nematode infections of first-season grazing calves in Belgium: General patterns and the effect of chemoprophylaxis. *Veterinary Parasitology* **69**, 103–116.

Svensson, C., Hessle, A. and Höglund, J. (2000). Parasite control methods in organic and conventional dairy herds in Sweden. *Livestock Production Science* **66**, 57–69.

Taylor, M.A. (2010). *Sustainable worm control strategies for Cattle. A Technical Manual for Veterinary Surgeons and Advisors.* COWS, EBLEX and Dairy Co. www.eblex.org.uk and www.dairyco.org.uk.

Thamsborg, S.M., Jorgensen, R.J. and Nansen, P. (1998). Internal parasitism of steers grazing extensively at different stocking rates. *Acta Veterinaria Scandinavia* **39**, 311–323.

Thamsborg, S. M., Roepstorff, A. and Larsen, M. (1999). Integrated and biological control of parasites in organic and conventional production systems. *Veterinary Parasitology* **84**, 169–186.

Vaarst, M., Winckler, C., Roderick, S., Smolders, G., Ivemeyer, S., Brinkmann, J., Mejdell, C.M., Whistance, L.K., Nicholas, P., Walkenhorst, M., Leeb, C., March, S., Henriksen, B.I.F., Stöger, E., Gratzer, E., Hansen, B. and Huber, J. (2011) Animal Health and Welfare Planning in Organic Dairy Cattle Farms. *The Open Veterinary Science Journal* **5**(Suppl 1: M5), 19–25.

Vercruysse, J. and Claerebout, E. (2001). Treatment vs non-treatment of helminth infections in cattle: defining the threshold. *Veterinary Parasitology* **98**, 195–214.

Useful sources of information

The **DEFRA** website (http://www.defra.gov.uk) has links to the following:

- Compendium of UK Organic Standards (September 2006)
- Guidance Document on European Union Organic Standards (December 2008)
- Council Regulation (EC) 834/2007, implemented by Commission Regulation (EC) 889/2008 and Commission Regulation (EC) 1235/2008
- **SAC Organic** website: http://www.sac.ac.uk/consulting/services/i-r/organic/
- **Organic Centre Wales** has information on business management and producers: http://www.organiccentrewales.org.uk/
- **Elm Farm Research Centre** has information on all aspects of organic farming: http://www.organicresearchcentre.com/
- **Organic Compendium**. Gives advice on disease-specific issues as well as general herd-health and welfare advice. Available at: http://www.organicvet.co.uk/
- **Business Link** website. Government website giving information on business set-up and management. See: http://www.businesslink.gov.uk/bdotg/action/layer?topicId=1083732127&furlname=organic&furlparam=organic&ref=http%3A//archive.defra.gov.uk/foodfarm/growing/organic/index.htm&domain=www.businesslink.gov.uk

SECTION VI

Beef Cattle Herd Health

CHAPTER 47

Beef Suckler Cow Diseases: Monitoring and Surveillance

Phil Scott

Learning objectives

- Appreciate the important diseases in suckler cows.
- Understand the different sources of information and the evidence they provide to support risk analysis and decision-making.
- Appreciate the role of biosecurity and herd health planning is disease prevention.

Introduction

Establishing the absolute and relative importance of disease prevalence and economics is important in setting priorities and shaping the control and prevention strategies at a national, regional and farm level. The aim of this chapter is to present some of the current information and sources of information that are available to help the veterinarian in their evidenced-based decision making. The information can also be used to provide convincing justifications for appropriate intervention strategies.

The relative importance of diseases depends largely on the beef cattle production system, whether a breeding herd which sells weaned calves or a finishing unit/feedlot. While it is possible to extract basic production figures from most of the veterinary practice's beef herds, accurate benchmarking proves very difficult, because there are no reliable national statistics. Recently, the Cattle Health and Welfare Group (CHAWG) of Great Britain has published its first report of disease incidence data to help primary producers and the industry, including veterinarians and government, set a framework so that progress can be gauged and reported on an ongoing basis. The report includes the most recent statistics on the cattle sector and on disease incidences. While the data are not complete, they represent the most accurate information available to veterinarians upon which to base decisions.

National biosecurity

The CHAWG report makes interesting reading, and veterinary practitioners in Great Britain will be surprised by figures that show, despite the report describing Great Britain as a discrete biosecurity unit, that more than 31 000 cattle were imported into Great Britain in 2010. These cattle represent a serious biosecurity risk, as evidenced by importation of pregnant cattle in 2008 that gave birth to calves congenitally infected by bluetongue virus (BTV-8).

The total GB cattle population in 2011 was 8.34 million on just under 66 000 holdings. In 2011, there were just over 12 000 dairy producers, with an average herd size of 127 cows, and around 45 000 beef suckler farms. Seventy percent of cattle were on premises that kept over 150 head, and these accounted for a quarter of all holdings.

Ten most important cattle health and welfare issues

A number of GB cattle sector organisations were contacted to come up with their lists of the top ten cattle health and welfare issues, to obtain an understanding of what the industry itself feels are its main problems (lists not ranked in order of importance). The lists showed close agreement between the dairy and beef sectors (Table 47.1). It should, however, be noted that many of these issues are multi-factorial and have genetic, nutritional and on-farm management components.

Bovine Medicine, Third Edition. Edited by Peter D. Cockcroft.

Table 47.1 Ten most important diseases of beef and dairy cattle in Great Britain (not ranked in order of importance).

Beef	Dairy
Fertility	Fertility
Mastitis	Mastitis
infectious bovine rhinotracheitis	Lameness
Bovine Viral diarrhoea	Bovine viral diarrhoea
Johne's disease	Johne's disease
Liver fluke	Bovine tuberculosis
Nutrition	Nutrition
Calf pneumonia	Calf pneumonia and scour
Calf scour	Parasitic gastroenteritis/lungworm
Parasitic gastroenteritis/lungworm	Genetics

The limitations of such lists are immediately apparent, as evidenced by including 'fertility' rather than dytocia in the beef cattle list; bovine tuberculosis (b-TB) is not considered a problem in beef cattle, because many beef herds are located in Scotland, which is officially b-TB free.

Farm animal health planning

According to DEFRA, around 60% of livestock farmers had a written farm animal health plan in 2012 (up from 58% in 2009), and 41% of farmers use their health plan on a routine basis to impose disease management decisions. Sixty four percent of farmers claimed always to source livestock from farms where the health status is known, and 34% do so sometimes.

Sources of information used in the CHAWG report

Food chain information

Food chain information is often limited, but is very useful for monitoring diseases/infestations where there are pathognomonic changes such as liver fluke. In 2011, up to 30% of cattle livers were condemned at slaughter, due to *Fasciola hepatica* (liver fluke) infestation.

Scanning surveillance

Scanning surveillance in GB is regarded as a valuable method of detecting new and emerging diseases. However, scanning surveillance depends upon the following sequence of events:

1 Observation by livestock keeper.
2 Notification to a veterinary practice.
3 Notification to Animal Health Veterinary Laboratory Agency or Scottish Agricultural College laboratory.

Disease surveillance findings are published for all species monthly in the *Veterinary Record* and in species-specific, quarterly 'Emerging Threats Reports'. In addition to this, Disease Trend Reports are routinely produced to help monitor changes in numbers of diagnoses and affected holdings across years. Quoted examples of the success of scanning surveillance in GB include sarcoptic mange and bovine neonatal pancytopaenia (BNP).

However, there are reports of diseases such as congenital pseudomyotonia, which was detected and reported by veterinary clinicians but which would not have been detected at necropsy, even with detailed histopathological investigation. There was a gap of 18 months between the first suspected cow with bovine spongiform encephalopathy and official description of the disease. The importance of an accurate clinical examination is critical to the investigation of unusual cases. Recent technologies, such as mobile telephones which capture video clips, allow veterinary clinicians in farm animal practice to communicate with specialists in veterinary schools and other centres, both nationally and internationally. Transmission of ultrasound recordings and radiographs, and even auscultated sounds, allows more objective and informed dialogue between parties.

Mortality

By recording deaths by the return of individual cattle passports, cattle movement records (British Cattle Movement Records; BCMS) provide some information on cattle mortality rates. In 2008, approximately one in 13 beef suckler calves (7%) died in their first six months of life. About 240 000 adult cattle die each year of unknown causes on farms. This latter statistic requires urgent investigation, and is a major source of essential information presently lost to farmers and their veterinary advisors. The traditional facility for gross necropsy at knackeries and other collection centres has been lost in many countries. While such data presented many limitations, gross lesions could be readily observed. Lungworm infestation, blackleg and chronic suppurative foci would be good examples of diseases that would be readily and reliably detected at necropsy of fresh cadavers.

Fertility data

Age at first calving

According to English Beef and Lamb Executive (EBLEX), a target of calving beef heifers at two years old or 24 months of age is achievable, yet the national average for both Wales and England is approximately 34 months.

Calving period

Data on the calving period in suckler herds are limited. English data from enterprise costing surveys showed calving periods in the range of 20–22 weeks for average lowland and less favoured area (LFA) suckler herds, respectively, for 2010/11. Calving periods for hill, upland LFA and lowland suckler herds in Scotland were 16, 15 and 14 weeks, respectively for 2010. Ideally, producers should be aiming for a compact calving period of between 9–12 weeks.

The average calving interval for suckler cows calving in England and Wales in 2010 was relatively similar ranging between 440 and 446 days. This suggests that 21% more calves are possible from the same number of cows by improving herd fertility and by reducing the calving interval to an average of 365 days for all cows in the herd. These data are supported by reports of high levels of bull infertility. However, such investigations are more often undertaken after detection of a high barren rate during a pregnancy diagnosis test, or following an extended calving period. These fertility parameters are invaluable to those veterinary practitioners with a proactive approach. It provides evidence with which to convince their farming clients of the financial value of bull breeding soundness assessments ahead of the service period, rather than after a problem has arisen.

Barren rate

Information on barren suckler cow rates is scarce. English data from enterprise costing surveys show barren cow rates in the range of 6.3–8.1 barren cows per 100 cows exposed to the bull across all the lowland and LFA suckler herds surveyed in 2010. The industry benchmark for barren rate is less than 5% of females exposed to the bull.

Calf diseases

Neonatal diarrhoea

Scouring was the most common disease in young calves and the greatest single cause of death. Between 2003 and 2012, AHVLA tested around 10 000 submissions from neonatal calves with diarrhoea. A diagnosis was reached in approximately 75% of submissions, with isolation rates of rotavirus (42%), cryptosporidiosis (40%), bovine coronavirus (9%) and colibacillosis (8%). Over 32% of 1300 samples in another UK survey from scouring calves were positive for cryptosporidia, with 29% positive for rotavirus, 17.7% for bovine coronavirus, and 3.8% for *E. coli*. While these data describe relative isolation rates of likely enteropathogens, it is important to remember that rotavirus and cryptosporidia are also commonly isolated from clinically healthy calves.

While highly effective vaccines are available to control rotavirus, coronavirus and enterotoxigenic *E. coli*, only 10–15% of beef cows are vaccinated nationally to control calf scour. These data are very valuable to practitioners, and highlight opportunities to promote real preventive medicine programmes.

Calf pneumonia

Data on respiratory disease in the CHAWG report were less extensive, and largely relied on estimates from textbooks more than a decade old. While respiratory disease pneumonia was the most common reason for death or poor performance from weaning to 10 months old, estimated average costs were £82 per suckler calf. Of this, 40% was accounted for in veterinary fees and drugs and 60% resulted from lost production. These figures are no longer accurate, as beef price have doubled in the past ten years.

Paratuberculosis

Johne's disease was estimated to cost the UK cattle industry up to £13m annually. The herd prevalence was over 34% in UK in 2009, but is now estimated to be over 50% where farmers have engaged in awareness activities such as bulk milk testing in dairy herds.

BVD

There are various estimates of the costs of BVD to the cattle industry in GB. It has been estimated that eradicating BVD could be worth £50–80 million to the Scottish cattle industry over ten years. Furthermore, BVD is estimated to cost the UK cattle industry up to £61 million annually.

A market report in 2008 indicated that 50% of beef suckler herds had been recently exposed to BVD and figures from 1648 herds tested in 2011 found that the prevalence of exposed herds had increased to 62%. In Scotland, 27.8% of 3424 beef herds sampled between September 2010 and April 2011 showed evidence of exposure to BVD.

These data and costings are more useful in regional and national campaigns for control and/or elimination. Adoption of effective vaccination programmes in herds within the veterinary practice's clients can often be more effective when costs from a local herd are presented while maintaining anonymity.

Surprisingly, animal welfare has been highlighted as a reason for the control of BVD in Scotland. While persistently-infected BVD youngstock may suffer chronic pneumonia, many infected animals achieve market weight without an increased disease incidence. There are few data that would support the argument that BVD presents a greater animal welfare concern that any other infectious disease.

Leptospirosis

A market report in 2008 indicated that 35% of suckler herds had confirmed or suspected leptospirosis. Figures from 1648 herds tested in 2011 found that 43% of herds had been exposed to leptospirosis. In these surveys, the distinction between seroconversion and disease with production losses is not clearly stated. However, many farms with employees vaccinate cattle against leptospirosis to limit zoonotic risk and to comply with health and safety policy.

IBR

A market report in 2008 indicated that 28% of beef herds had confirmed or suspected IBR. Once again, there is no clear distinction made between vaccination and exposure to virus, and convalescence from clinical disease. These data should be regarded on a national basis, and highlight the importance of biosecurity measures.

Vaccination

A recent study on 71 farms using a BVD vaccine found that 21% of farmers vaccinated using the incorrect dose of vaccine or by the wrong route, nearly 50% had the wrong time interval between doses, only 24% managed to complete the primary course of a vaccination four weeks before service, and 34% kept a vaccine bottle open for more than a month in contrast to the guidelines of only ten hours.

Cattle health schemes

Cattle Health Certification Standards (CHeCS) is the regulatory body for the ten cattle health schemes operating in the British Isles for monitoring, control and eradication of disease for IBR, Leptospirosis, Johne's Disease and BVD. Currently, 14 000 UK herds (14% of national herd – dairy : beef ratio around 40 : 60) are in some form of disease monitoring, control and/or eradication under a CHeCS accredited scheme.

Key intervention points for important diseases in beef suckler herds are provided in Chapter 48.

CHAPTER 48

Beef Suckler Herd Health: Key Intervention Points

Phil Scott

Learning objectives

- Understand the key interventions in the following categories:
  - Introduced stock.
  - Calf scours.
  - Respiratory disease.
  - Welfare.
  - Productivity and fertility.
- Appreciate the importance of herd health planning.

The ten most important diseases and problems of beef cattle as determined by producers are listed in Table 48.1 alongside proposed key interventions. It is clear that key interventions can be planned well in advance of many of these diseases, but biosecurity measures are becoming much more important as producers seek to establish herds free of specific diseases. According to DEFRA, around 60% of Great Britain's livestock farmers had a written farm animal health plan in 2012, and 41% of farmers used their veterinary herd health plan on a routine basis to impose disease management decisions. Industry surveys have also consistently shown that farmers value independent veterinary advice above all others sources for their herd management. This chapter aims to highlight key intervention points where veterinary practitioners can have a significant effect on the health of the beef herd and, thereby, improve welfare, productivity and profitability.

Key intervention areas – health

Selection of replacement breeding stock

The selection of replacement breeding stock is critical to the health status of the beef herd, and risk assessment takes into account several factors, including:

- Health status of herd of origin
- Quarantine facilities
- Biosecurity of the herd, and biocontainment of diseases already present
- Vaccination policy outlined in the veterinary herd health plan.

Health status of herd of origin; pre-purchase disease screening

The main source of disease on a farm is the purchase of infected animals. Contact with diseased animals at the farm perimeter is a lower risk, but can be significant in certain situations such as infectious bovine rhinotracheitis (IBR) and bovine viral diarrhoea virus (BVDv). Vector-borne diseases, such as Bluetongue and Schmallenberg virus, have caused problems in northern Europe. However, there is no potential control barrier at farm level.

Paratuberculosis (Johne's disease), BVDv, salmonellosis, bovine tuberculosis, Leptospirosis, IBR and Bluetongue are some examples of common infectious diseases that can be introduced onto a beef farm following purchase of infected stock. Parasitic infestations, including liver fluke and lungworm, can also be introduced with purchased stock. Purchased calves can also introduce enteropathogens and respiratory disease viruses. Introduced stock can, therefore, potentially introduce seven of the ten most important diseases onto a beef farm.

Pre-movement testing for bovine tuberculosis is routinely undertaken in some countries, and the necessary cattle handling affords the opportunity to test for other diseases, such as paratuberculosis, BVDv, IBR, and leptospirosis, although seronegative test results have to be interpreted with caution for some diseases. However, this profile of the vendor's herd allows the veterinary practitioner to give the client more informed advice. The present disease status of the purchaser's own herd is another important determinant in disease control, because it is not uncommon for purchased cattle from high health status herds to succumb to disease, such as IBR, already endemic in the purchaser's herd.

Bovine Medicine, Third Edition. Edited by Peter D. Cockcroft.

Assessing risk template

A simple risk analysis for beef farmers to highlight the importance of farm biosecurity. This example uses BVDv, but the same format applies to other diseases.

Assessing the risk of introducing BVDv onto your farm from neighbouring farms.

Do you share common grazing? What is your perimeter fencing?

	Risk
Double perimeter fence	Low
Shared common grazing	High
Single perimeter fence	High

Explanation of risk assessment:

BVDv can be readily spread from an infected animal to your cattle by direct contact over a fence.

The important biosecurity objective in all diseases is to prevent (or minimize) cross-contamination of an animal's infected body fluids (faeces, urine, saliva, respiratory secretions, discharges from abortion/calving etc.) to other animals, feed and equipment.

Selection of purchased animals (if not closed herd)

Risk of introducing BVDv onto your farm from purchased livestock

Do you buy clean cattle (bulling heifers) or pregnant cattle?

	Risk
Purchase clean cattle	Nil
Purchase pregnant cattle	High

Explanation of risk assessment:

Infection of the foetus less than 110–120 days of gestation may lead to the birth of a live calf persistently infected (PI) with BVD virus. The dam would test antibody positive and therefore this source of infection could be missed on a routine screen.

Do you screen purchased livestock?

	Risk
Purchase BVDv accredited stock	Nil
Purchase vaccinated stock from vaccinated herd	Low
Purchase stock from unknown source	High

Explanation of risk assessment:

Select all necessary purchased animals from known BVDv health status herds to reduce the risk of infection.

Vaccination will not control BVD if the animal is already infected with the virus.

Purchasing stock from unknown sources greatly increases the possibility of BVDv infection.

Blood sample all purchased non-pregnant cattle from unknown source for BVD antibody; a positive antibody result indicates prior exposure or vaccination. If seronegative (no antibody) the laboratory will test for the presence of antigen (virus). All antigen positive cattle (persistently infected, PIs) must be rejected. Any pregnant cattle in the same batch must also be rejected because of the risk of infection of the developing foetus (see above).

Are cattle isolated following purchase (until blood test results are available)?

	Risk
Isolate purchased stock	Nil
Mix with other cattle	High

Strict isolation prevents contact between animals after arrival on farm and reduces the risk of spread BVDv as well as other infectious agents. Purchased cattle can be mixed with other cattle once their BVDv status has been determined.

Do you restrict entry of people/vehicles onto your farm?

	Risk
Restrict entry	Nil
Free movement of all visitors/vehicles etc	Low

BVD virus could be transmitted by vehicles, equipment, clothing and shoes of people (veterinarians, contractors, other farmers, salesmen, service personnel) who move between herds but the risk is considerably less than movement of infected stock.

Figure 48.1 Risk assessment template using BVDv as an example.

Vaccination

BVD can be controlled by initial vaccination which comprises two doses 3–4 weeks apart before first service followed by booster vaccination at 12 months' intervals. If all breeding females are vaccinated then this will control disease by preventing BVD infection of the developing foetus during pregnancy and production of PI calves.

BVD eradication is possible following whole herd blood testing and elimination of all PI carrier animals. If farmers go for eradication then strict herd biosecurity measures must be maintained to prevent re-introduction of virus infection as the herd will soon become naïve and fully susceptible to infection.

Risk of introducing BVDv onto your farm from purchased livestock

	Risk
Purchase BVDv accredited stock	Nil
Purchase vaccinated stock from vaccinated herd	Low
Purchase stock from unknown source	High

Explanation of risk assessment:

Vaccination of a PI calf will not provide protection against BVD and this animal will remain a potent source of infection.

Risk of BVDv spreading on your farm from purchased livestock

	Risk
Blood test all cattle before purchase – all cattle antigen negative.	Nil
Vaccinate purchased cattle, no blood testing	High

Vaccination of a PI calf will not provide protection against BVD and this animal will remain a potent source of infection however the impact will be limited when all cattle on the farm have been vaccinated.

Figure 48.1 (*continued*)

Table 48.1 Beef producers' ten most important diseases in Great Britain (not ranked in order of importance), and proposed key interventions.

Diseases/problems	Key intervention
Fertility - dystocia	Genetics, management
Mastitis - chronic	Management, dry cow therapy
Infectious Bovine Rhinotracheitis	Biosecurity, vaccination
Bovine Viral Diarrhoea	Biosecurity, vaccination
Johne's Disease	Biosecurity, biocontainment
Liver Fluke	Biosecurity, strategic treatments
Nutrition	Management
Calf Pneumonia	Housing, management, vaccination
Calf Scour	Housing, management, dam vaccination
Parasitic Gastroenteritis /Lungworm	Management, strategic treatments

Quarantine facilities

Strict quarantine of all purchased cattle, and those animals returning to the herd from shows and other events, is inadequate on most farms. Many farmers mistakenly consider a calving box to be a 'quarantine' facility. The recommended minimum quarantine period is four weeks, to allow signs of disease to become apparent; all disease screening tests should have been undertaken before purchase and movement onto the farm. All necessary vaccinations should be undertaken during this quarantine period.

Biosecurity of the herd, and biocontainment of diseases already present

Biosecurity aims to reduce/prevent the introduction of new diseases onto a beef operation from outside sources. The important biosecurity objective in all diseases is to prevent (or minimise) cross-contamination of an animal's infected body fluids (e.g. faeces, urine, saliva, respiratory secretions, discharges from abortion/calving) to other animals, feed and equipment.

BVDv is often used as an example of risk analysis in the veterinary herd health plan to alert farmers to the potential dangers from diseases not present in the herd. A simple risk analysis template for beef farmers to highlight the importance of farm biosecurity is presented in Figure 48.1.

BVD can be introduced onto the farm by the introduction of:

- Cattle incubating disease.
- Apparently healthy cattle that are persistently-infected with the virus (PIs).
- Cow infected during pregnancy now carrying a persistently-infected foetus.
- Direct contact with neighbouring infected cattle.
- Purchase of a seronegative non-pregnant animal that has acquired a transient infection during trade, and then transmits this to a newly pregnant susceptible animal in the destination herd.

BVD virus can be transmitted by vehicles, equipment, clothing and shoes of people (veterinarians, contractors, other farmers, salesmen, service personnel) who move between herds, but the disease risk is considerably less than the movement of infected stock.

Biocontainment refers to reducing/preventing the movement of infectious diseases on the farm. Biocontainment measures are especially important for diseases such as paratuberculosis and salmonellosis, and include:

- Maintain good hygiene in buildings/yards, and calving boxes in particular.
- Minimise faecal contamination of food, water and pasture (e.g. by raising feed and water troughs, strip grazing, use of mains/piped water rather than surface/pond water).
- Avoid spreading yard manure onto pasture.

Quarantine and vaccination of introduced cattle

All purchased cattle must complete the vaccination policy outlined in the veterinary herd health plan before entering the herd. The primary vaccination course, for diseases such as leptospirosis and BVD, requires two injections, 3–4 weeks apart, which corresponds to a recommended quarantine period of four weeks. Anthelmintic and flukicide treatments may also be necessary during the quarantine period.

Summary of key interventions for introduced stock:

- Pre-purchase testing of all cattle for specific diseases.
- Quarantine of all introduced cattle.
- Effective biosecurity and biocontainment.
- Vaccination, anthelmintic and flukicide treatments, where appropriate.

Management of disease

The health of an individual animal depends on a balance between the genotype of the host, the pathogen and the environment – the so-called 'epidemiological triad'. In 2008, approximately one in 13 beef suckler calves (7%) that were born alive died within the first six months of life.

This section will focus upon the key interventions for calf scour and calf pneumonia, which were listed as two of the top ten diseases of beef cattle.

Neonatal diarrhoea

Between 2003 and 2012, 75% of samples submitted from over 10 000 neonatal calves with diarrhoea in GB yielded a potential enteropathogen; rotavirus (42%), cryptosporidiosis (40%), bovine coronavirus (9%) and colibacillosis (8%). These data are invaluable to veterinary practitioners, because there are highly effective vaccines available to control rotavirus, coronavirus, and enterotoxigenic *E. coli*. However, only 10–15% of beef cows are vaccinated nationally to control calf scour. Veterinary practitioners can use these results to promote real preventive medicine programmes.

Timely vaccination is only one component of disease prevention; adequate dam nutrition is essential to ensure adequate accumulation of immunoglobulins in the udder, then ingestion of colostrum within the first six to 12 hours of birth (passive antibody transfer – PTA). Field studies have consistently shown failure of PTA on many beef farms, with a consequently high incidence of septicaemia/bacteraemia, neonatal diarrhoea and respiratory disease. Total plasma protein, readily measured on a refractometer, is a cheap method to assess PTA in calves. Plasma protein concentration in newborn calves is around 40–45 g/L, increasing to around 60–65g/L 12–24 hours after ingesting good quality colostrum. While colostrum evaluation using a colostrometer, which measures specific gravity, is useful in dairy herds, poor quality colostrum is not a problem in beef cattle unless the cows are poorly fed during late gestation (when they would present in poor body condition at calving), or they have chronic mastitis is several quarters.

Summary of key interventions for calf scour

- Dam vaccination.
- Adequate passive antibody transfer.
- Environmental hygiene.
- Dam nutrition.
- Mastitis prevention.

Respiratory disease

There are a large number of respiratory vaccines available worldwide, often combining several attenuated strains of respiratory viruses, including bovine respiratory syncytial virus (BRSV), parainfluenza-3 (PI-3), and inactivated infectious bovine rhinotracheitis (IBR). There are several vaccines containing inactivated bacteria, mainly *Mannheimia haemolytica*. Recent advances have included the development of live IBR marker vaccines (gE negative), which permit vaccination while undertaking an elimination programme, whether on a local, regional or national basis. Attenuated live BRSV vaccine can be administered by the intranasal route from three weeks old.

Recent surveys have estimated that approximately 60% of farm buildings used to house cattle over the winter months in the UK have inadequate ventilation.

The challenge for veterinary practitioners is to identify and attempt to minimise all risk factors, which may include:

- Respiratory viruses and bacteria.
- Overcrowding.
- Poor ventilation.
- Concurrent parasitic infestations; lungworm, parasitic gastroenteritis and lice.
- Poor nutrition.
- Procedures such as dehorning and castration.
- Trace element deficiencies.

While it may be possible to isolate recognised bacterial pathogens from various sites in the respiratory tract, interpreting the results can be problematic, as many of these bacteria exist as commensals.

In many herd disease situations, addressing housing deficiencies listed above and completing the respiratory virus vaccination programmes ahead of the major risk period, whether housing or crowding, should significantly reduce the incidence of respiratory disease. Such a programme necessitates the collection of appropriate samples from an earlier outbreak of respiratory disease; the types of samples collected will be dictated by the veterinary practitioner's knowledge of the likely causal organisms.

Antibiotic metaphylaxis

Whole group antibiotic injection/medication when 10–33% of the group show signs of respiratory disease, referred to as antibiotic metaphylaxis, is practised in many situations to control disease. The introduction of single injection long-acting macrolide antibiotics has resulted in whole-group antibiotic therapy with no subsequent disease monitoring, despite the recurrence of disease in 15–25% of cases, referred to as treatment failures in the promotional materials produced by pharmaceutical companies.

An increasing number of peer-reviewed field studies have shown that, in an outbreak of respiratory disease, antibiotic treatment of only febrile cattle (>39.7°C) reduces antibiotic usage and associated costs. Indiscriminate antibiotic usage in farm animals has been highlighted by the OIE and EU authorities as a major concern. Antibiotic metaphylaxis to treat respiratory disease in cattle will come under increasing scrutiny, especially when there is a large body of peer-reviewed evidence that treatment of only febrile cattle is necessary. Veterinary practitioners should now act to promote vaccination to prevent respiratory disease and treat only those cattle that are febrile, but also monitor their response to antibiotic therapy, otherwise certain antibiotics, namely fluoroquinolones and fourth generation cephalosporins, may be restricted to human medicine. Few veterinarians could reasonably argue against increasingly prudent and transparent use of antibiotics.

Herd management

Housing and handling facilities require improvement on many farms. Parasite control is important throughout the grazing season, and effective strategies should be detailed in the veterinary herd health plan. Treatment of cattle before the winter confinement/housing period is essential to control parasitic gastroenteritis, particularly ostertagiosis, lungworm, liver fluke and pediculosis. While anthelmintic and flukicide combination products are available (e.g. ivermectin and chlorsulon), the convenience of single treatment should not outweigh the most beneficial treatment times.

Key interventions

- Calf vaccination.
- Prompt antibiotic treatment of sick animals.
- Environment/housing improvements.
- Parasite control, especially lungworm and liver fluke.

Welfare

Major improvements in beef cattle welfare could be achieved by:

- Reducing disease prevalence figures.
- Reducing mutilations.
- Reducing dystocia prevalence.

There have been many attempts to define animal welfare. In the view of the Farm Animal Welfare Committee (FAWC), welfare encompasses both physical and mental health and, for farm animals, it is largely determined by the skills of the stock workers, the system of husbandry and the suitability of the genotype for the environment. Veterinary surgeons are experts in animal health, but it is the consideration of the mental well-being of our patients that differentiates animal welfare from animal health; calves confined in slatted veal crates may be healthy, but do not have a good life, and many would reason that they may not have a life worth living.

Animal sentience (the capacity to experience or feel in a way that is analogous to human experience) has been one of the most controversial aspects of the application of science to animal welfare. However, it is difficult to argue with the current position that all vertebrate animals (and some others) are sentient. Farm animals are recognised as sentient beings within the EU Treaty of Amsterdam, 1999.

Some pain and distress is considered unavoidable in livestock husbandry with current knowledge and farming practice, but the goal should be to minimise its occurrence. Difficult ethical and agricultural decisions have to be made when dealing with suffering, sometimes by imposing a lesser act that may still cause short-term pain or distress but provide long-term relief for the individual or group. The long-term goal should be to eliminate the source of the problem through improved disease control, husbandry and breeding to avoid this lesser act.

There has been a rapid growth of animal welfare assessment on farms. This was originally done by focusing on the resources available to the animal, but is now increasingly looking at the animal itself, based upon both health and behaviour. Veterinary practitioners can have a positive impact on animal welfare in beef herds by encouraging good management reflected in appropriate cow body condition scores, achievement of target weight gains, absence of infestations such as pediculosis, and very low prevalence of lameness and mastitis.

When assessing any welfare problem, it is necessary to consider the intensity and duration of suffering, the number of animals involved, and the alternatives to promote well-being. Equally important is the ability to improve welfare through existing sound husbandry, with good stockmanship assisted by an effective veterinary herd health plan.

Inflammatory diseases are a major source of pain in animals. From a veterinary standpoint, inflammation can readily be identified as localised heat and swelling, sensitivity to palpation, and loss of function. Inflammation induces alterations in pain processing, which may have serious long-term consequences for the animal. Long-term pain causes a hyperalgesic state, in which animals become more sensitive to painful stimuli and are adversely affected by stimuli that would be innocuous to normal individuals (allodynia).

The Five Freedoms are the cornerstone of UK government and industry policy and for the basis for the Codes of Recommendations for the Welfare of Livestock:

- Freedom from hunger and thirst, by ready access to fresh water and a diet to maintain full health and vigour.
- Freedom from discomfort, by providing an appropriate environment, including shelter and a comfortable resting area.
- Freedom from pain, injury and disease, by prevention or rapid diagnosis and treatment.
- Freedom to express normal behaviour, by providing sufficient space, proper facilities and company of the animal's own kind.
- Freedom from fear and distress, by ensuring conditions and treatment which avoid mental suffering.

The Farm Animal Welfare Council has made many recommendations on health and disease in many of its previous reports, reinforcing the benefits of active animal health planning managed with veterinary input, the importance of preventive measures and good husbandry. A key document that provides an overview and strategic goals for farm animal welfare for the next 20 years is the *Report on Farm Animal Welfare in Great Britain: Past, Present and Future* (2009). The FAWC report on stockmanship highlights the important role and responsibility of stockpeople in managing disease and avoiding suffering. There is increasing awareness of the benefits of training, accreditation and continuous professional development, and considerable progress has been made on industry strategies for training and skills development such as the National Animal Disease Information Service (nadis.org.uk).

Mutilations

'The lesser of two evils' is the argument used for mutilations. This is covered by Banner's second principle: 'the harm requires justification and must be outweighed by the good'. One simple utilitarian answer is that a brief period of pain, lasting a few minutes or hours, is acceptable when weighed against the positive experiences gained over months or years of a life that was otherwise worth living. The principle is: 'any harm which is justified by the second principle ought, however, to be minimised as far as is reasonably possible'.

There are legal requirements for local anaesthesia for disbudding/dehorning, and castration beyond certain age limits, which vary between regions of the world. Many published studies have recorded less pain after Burdizzo castration than either surgical castration or elastrator ring, yet Burdizzo castration is rarely undertaken, either by farmers or by veterinarians. Injection of a NSAID prior to castration further reduces observed indicators of pain, but is rarely undertaken, presumably for perceived cost reasons. Individual veterinary surgeons can impact upon calf welfare by adopting scientifically proven and more welfare-friendly procedures with NSAID administration before, rather than after, the procedure.

Dystocia

The negative productivity impact of dystocia has been discussed elsewhere in this chapter, alongside management changes to reduce its prevalence. The welfare consequences of a difficult calving must not be ignored, because trauma leads to inflammation and infection and, inevitably, to pain. The most serious consequences of dystocia include: fatal haemorrhage from ruptured middle uterine artery; ruptured uterus and death from septic peritonitis; and septic metritis associated with retained foetal membranes. Antibiotics and non-steroidal anti-inflammatory drugs should be administered daily for three to five days to counter endotoxaemia.

Key interventions

- Improve/select herd genetics to reduce dystocia prevalence.
- Reduce disease prevalence.
- Reduce/avoid mutilations, change technique (e.g. Burdizzo method) or procedure if mutilation is considered essential.
- Greater use of NSAID drugs by veterinarians and farmers.
- Better farm planning for emergency situations, such as prolonged drought and other extreme weather conditions.

Productivity

The major factors increasing beef herd productivity include a compact calving period and a low barren rate. Dystocia has a major negative effect on subsequent breeding performance. Bull fertility is critical in natural service beef herds.

A target of calving beef heifers at two years old or 24 months of age is achievable, yet the national average for both Wales and England in a recent survey is approximately 34 months. English data from enterprise costing surveys showed calving periods in the range from 20–22 weeks, when producers should be aiming for a compact calving period of 9–12 weeks. The average calving interval for suckler cows calving in England and Wales in 2010 was similar, ranging between 440 and 446 days. These figures indicate that 21% more calves could be produced from the same number of cows by improving herd fertility and reducing the calving interval to an average of 365 days for all cows in the herd. English data from enterprise costing surveys show barren cow rates in the range of 6.3–8.1 barren cows per 100 cows exposed to the bull, when the industry benchmark is less than 5%.

Affects of dystocia upon subsequent breeding performance

Researchers have noted that the number of cows detected in oestrus during a 45-day artificial insemination period was 14% lower in those requiring assistance than in those calving with no difficulty. Conception to artificial insemination was six per cent lower in cows experiencing dystocia than in those without dystocia. Pregnancy rate after the entire breeding season (70 days) was 16% lower in cows that had been assisted (85% versus 69%). The pregnancy rate among cows that had caesarean deliveries was 26.6% lower (52.4% versus 79.0%) than the herd average.

In two studies at the United States Meat Animal Research Center (MARC), Clay Center, Nebraska, calf losses within 24 hours of birth averaged four percent for those born with little or no assistance, compared to 16% for those requiring assistance. In a Hereford herd at the United States Livestock and Range Research Station, Miles City, Montana, 57% of all calf losses were caused by dystocia. Dystocia in two-year-olds was 3–4 times higher than three-year-olds, and three-year-olds had about twice as much difficulty as four-year-olds. The predominant type of dystocia affecting two-year-old heifers was absolute foetal oversize.

Birth weight and length of gestation are determined by genotype of the calf, maternal genetic effects and environmental effects. Bulls with low estimated breeding values for birth weight have been selected for mating heifers, but the positive genetic correlation between birth weight and mature weight mean that the progeny of these bulls tend to have lower weaning weights. However, these data must be viewed on a herd basis, whereby much lower dystocia rates using high EBV bulls will result in greater herd profitability, despite lower weaning weights. Unfortunately, there are few comparisons of the likely profitability of high and low EBV beef bulls from commercial beef herds; such data would be very helpful, both to beef producers and their veterinary advisors.

No differences in the birth weight of calves have been observed in response to variation in feeding in mid-pregnancy, and variable responses in birth weight, and the incidence of dystocia to feeding in the third trimester of pregnancy, have been reported. Variability in the incidence of dystocia in response to feeding level in the third trimester of pregnancy makes it difficult to make recommendations for the feeding of heifers at this stage of gestation. More research is needed into the effects of nutrition in early gestation on foetal and placental development in cattle.

Pre-breeding fertility checks of heifers include trans-rectal palpation for freemartins and pregnancy, and must be undertaken for all purchased replacement breeding females.

Bull breeding soundness examinations are considered to be an integral component of the beef herd health plan, and must be undertaken before the start of the breeding season.

Key interventions

- Compact calving period – body condition scores/nutrition.
- Low barren rate – fertile bulls, cows well-fed.
- Reduce/eliminate dystocia – bull genetics.
- Ensure bulls are fertile; pre-breeding soundness checks.

Profitability

There are many factors that influence the profitability of a beef enterprise. Veterinary advisors tend to focus upon disease prevalence rates, and their direct and indirect costs, without looking at the economics of the whole enterprise. The lack of business expertise within the veterinary profession was highlighted in a recent UK government report, referred to as the Lowe Report, 'Unlocking Potential – a report on veterinary expertise in food animal production'.

It is all too easy to abstract estimates of the costs of individual disease events from various publications, and two examples are detailed below:

Dystocia

The total cost of a slightly difficult calving was estimated to be approximately £110, and of a seriously difficult calving between £350 and £400. The economic costs of dystocia have been estimated to be four times greater than treatment costs alone.

Respiratory disease

Pneumonia was the most common reason for death or poor performance from weaning to ten months old, with estimated average costs of £82 per beef calf.

However, these data alone may not act a stimulus for change; for example, costs of lameness in dairy cows have been published for the past 40 years, but lameness prevalence remains at unacceptably high rates around 20% in the UK. From a veterinary input, improved farm profitability will result from increased productivity and reduced disease prevalence. Such improvements are most likely achieved by implementing, and regularly updating, the veterinary herd health and management plan. Few veterinary practitioners have the necessary skills to interpret and advise farmers on the financial management of their enterprises; specialisation in cattle medicine is more likely to provide rewards for both farmer and veterinarian.

Key interventions

- Constantly update veterinary herd health and management plan

References and further reading

Farm Animal Welfare Council (2009). *Report on Farm Animal Welfare in Great Britain: Past, Present and Future.*

Farm Animal Welfare Council (2007). *Report on Stockmanship and Farm Animal Welfare.*

Ritchie, H.D. and Anderson, P.T. (1994). Calving Difficulty in Beef Cattle. In: *The Beef Cattle Handbook*. Beef Improvement Federation.

Hickson, R.E., Morris, S.T., Kenyon, P.R. and Lopez-Villalobos, N. (2006). Dystocia in beef heifers: a review of genetic and nutritional influences. *New Zealand Veterinary Journal* **54**, 256–264. http://archive.defra.gov.uk/foodfarm/policy/animalhealth/vservices/pdf/lowe-vets090806.pdf

CHAPTER 49

Auditing Beef Cow Herd Reproduction

George Caldow and Iain Riddell

Learning objectives

- Understand the importance of standardisation of reproduction data in beef herds
- Be able to perform the following audits:
  - General herd audit.
  - Barren cow audit.
  - Calf mortality audit.
  - Bull audit.
  - Assessing the body condition of the cows.
- Be able to analyse the data and further investigate unresolved problems.

Background and introduction

The production of beef from the beef cow herd has been an important part of cattle production throughout the world. In the European Union (EU), 40% of the beef produced comes from 12 million beef cows out of a total cow population of 36 million. Traditionally, beef cow herds have been low input systems, and are often associated with low profitability and, therefore, a lack of investment. However, beef cows have the ability to graze marginal land that will not support intensive crop production, and to convert poorer pasture into high-quality protein and energy in systems that satisfy the welfare needs of the animals, giving beef cow herds an important role in the agricultural output of hill and upland or range areas throughout the world (Figure 49.1). Their grazing activity is also considered to be more compatible with the conservation needs of these areas, compared to that of small ruminants.

Despite the low input, the basic goal remains to produce one live calf per cow per year from an animal calving for the first time at two years of age, and producing seven to nine calves in its lifetime (Figure 49.2). This is in recognition of the feed cost of the cow being the highest variable cost in the system.

The assessment of output can be refined by measuring the total weight of calf produced at weaning (standardised to 200 days) to the total weight of the cows mated. This can be expressed as a ratio, and the aim is to exceed 0.5. Therefore, a system that utilises relatively small- to medium-sized maternal breeds (less than 600 kg), mated to terminal sires to produce calves with a rapid growth rate, will be most efficient, but only if the fertility of the herd is high and there is low calf mortality. The herd physical performance targets required to achieve this efficiency have been defined as at least 94% cows successfully weaning a calf from a nine week breeding season where 65% of the cows conceive in the first three weeks.

Matching the nutritional requirements of the cows to the natural growing cycle of the pasture is the single most important consideration for the system. This is made easier by the ability of the animal to undergo an annual cycle of storing body condition that is used for maintenance and pregnancy during the months when pasture is not growing. To harness this efficiently, the body condition of the animals must be monitored and fine-tuned by intervention to prevent excessive body condition increasing the risk of dystocia or poor body condition, resulting in prolonged post-partum anoestrus.

It is therefore clear that, in most situations, seasonal calving should be timed to ensure that, after calving, cows have a good supply of grass to allow them to satisfy their nutritional priorities (Table 49.1), and to build up nutritional reserves to support them during the period of the year when pasture is not productive. Cows that achieve body condition score 2.5 (on a range of 1–5, where 1 is emaciated and 5 is obese) by mating will be able to satisfy the first eight of the nine priorities, and satisfactory fertility will follow.

However, as the gestation length for terminal sire breeds is often closer to 295 days than the 285 days of many of the maternal breeds, there is a further constraint to the system. Cows may have as little as 65 days to return to ovarian cyclicity and to conceive, if they are to achieve the target of one calf every

Bovine Medicine, Third Edition. Edited by Peter D. Cockcroft.

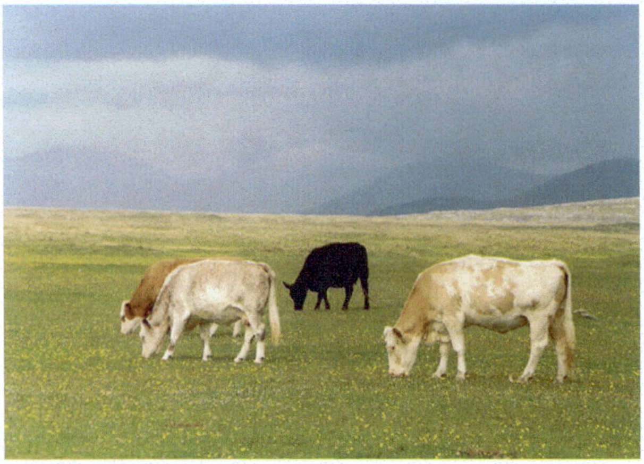

Figure 49.1 Beef cows have the ability to graze marginal land that will not support intensive crop production, and to convert poorer pasture into high-quality protein and energy in systems.

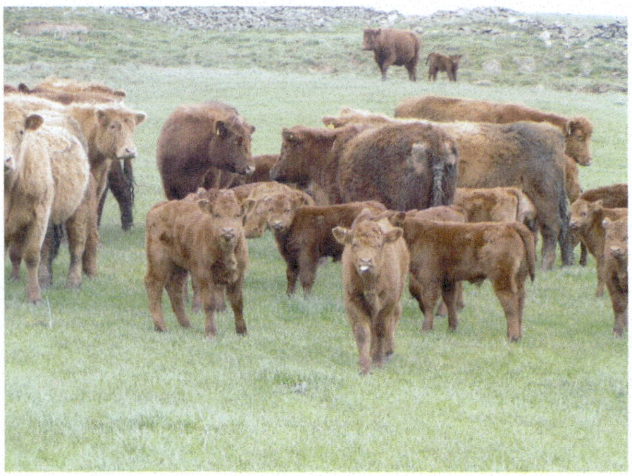

Figure 49.2 The basic goal remains to produce one live calf per cow per year from an animal calving for the first time at two years old, and producing seven to nine calves in its lifetime.

year. Therefore, it can be very difficult to achieve the targets of biological efficiency recognised above for herds where the cow breed is a large cow, based on a dairy cross animal, and terminal sires with a long gestation length are used. In recognition of this, in Scotland, a management blue print has been defined covering the five key areas for beef cow herd managers to address with the support of their advisers or vets (Table 49.2).

The five-point plan is the starting point for the 'Plan, Do, Check, Adjust' management cycle for beef cow producers, and the cattle practitioner should seek to have an integral part in this management process. Where the veterinary practitioner carries out pregnancy diagnosis for the herd, there is an opportunity to enter the cycle at the 'Check' stage and, for herds with poor results, this is an easy opportunity. The practitioner must therefore be able to carry out the relevant audit to analyse and identify the root causes of any production failure, and be able to offer the appropriate advice to help get fertility back on track.

Table 49.1 Nutritional priorities of the beef cow (adapted from Short & Adams, 1988). Reproduced with permission of Agricultural Institute of Canada.

1	Basal metabolism
2	Activity
3	Growth
4	Energy reserves
5	Maintenance of pregnancy
6	Lactation
7	Additional energy reserves
8	Oestrus cycles and initiation of pregnancy
9	Excess energy reserves

Table 49.2 Five-point plan for beef cow herd fertility (adapted from Caldow *et al.*, 2007). Reproduced with permission of British Cattle Veterinary Association.

1	Heifer management	Early breeding and target growth rates to be mated at 15 months after reaching 65% of mature body weight. Recognise that animals continue to have growth requirements until after their third pregnancy (85% of mature body weight at second mating and 95% at third), and must be given preferential treatment if the growth targets are to be met and prolonged anoestrus avoided. Select and manage heifers to calve as early in the breeding season as possible, and always in the first three weeks.
2	Bulls: soundness and fertility	Breeding soundness examinations carried out on all bulls prior to breeding season. Bulls should meet the breeding standards in use in each country (e.g. physically sound, scrotal circumference > 34 cm, ≥ 50% progressive motility of spermatozoa).
3	Manage cow condition and nutrition	To achieve condition score 2.5 at mating. Know the target condition scores for calving, mating and weaning for the system, and avoid excessive weight loss, particularly after calving. To know what intervention is necessary to achieve targets.
4	Avoid difficult calvings	Select bulls on EBVs; prevent over-fat cows. Bulls should be selected on neutral or short gestation length and positive direct calving ease. Where herds are rearing their own replacements, then selecting for maternal calving ease is also important. Cows should not exceed body condition score three at calving.
5	Maintain herd health	The major diseases that impact on fertility and cow longevity should be managed through herd health planning and biosecurity. In many countries, this will address BVDV, venereal campylobacter infection and paratuberculosis control and prevention.

Standardisation of reproduction data in beef herds

In contrast to the situation in the dairy herd, it can often seem that there is little data available to analyse in the beef cow

Table 49.3 Standardisation of data.

Denominator	Comment	Numerators	Target/interference
Number of females mated.		Number of calves weaned. Number of abortions. Number of still births. Number of live calves.	94% <2% 0 95%
The number of females that calve at full term.	Excludes abortions, defined as under-sized calves born outside of the calving season. Includes cows producing a stillborn calf.	Number of females that calve in each three week period of breeding season.	Target of 65% in first three weeks; 97% in nine weeks.

herd. However, the information required is straightforward and recorded in some way in most herds. The most useful source of data is often the herdsman's diary. Here, information on calving dates, calving assistance, treatments, etc. is stored. Where that source of data is unavailable, a more basic analysis can be derived from the age distribution of the herd, drawn from existing databases. For example, in many EU countries, the animal identities and date of birth can be downloaded from the national animal movement database, and used to infer a calving distribution.

To facilitate the analysis of fertility in the beef herd, it is necessary to use a standardised approach to collecting and presenting the data (Table 49.3). The primary denominator in auditing beef herd reproduction is the number of breeding females that are mated. The number of cows calving and the number of calves weaned are expressed against this. In addition, the same denominator can be used for the proportion of cows that are barren, abort, produce a stillborn calf or a live calf.

The number of cows mated is less useful for examining calving spread, and the alternative is the number of cows that calve at full term. Where natural mating is used, the service date is unknown, and differentiating between late abortions and stillbirths is difficult. However, this can be resolved by recording a calf that is born dead, but of normal size, as a stillbirth, and including it in this denominator. A female that produces undersized and dead calf or calves born before the calving season has started should be recorded as an abortion and excluded from this denominator. The total number of females that produce a full-term calf can then be used as the denominator for the proportion of cows calving in each three-week period of the breeding season.

Assessing calf viability is less straightforward (Figure 49.3). Using the number of cows that calve as the denominator is simple, but it does not accommodate twin births, which can be expected to occur at the rate of 2% or more, depending on the breeds that make up the herd. Excluding stillborn calves has some logic, but stillbirths can be a significant component of the losses in this area. The favoured denominator is the number of calves born, and this is calculated by adding the number of twin births to the total number of cows that calve (Table 49.4). The number of stillbirths, deaths within 48 hours of age and deaths from 48 hours to weaning, can all be expressed against this denominator (Table 49.4).

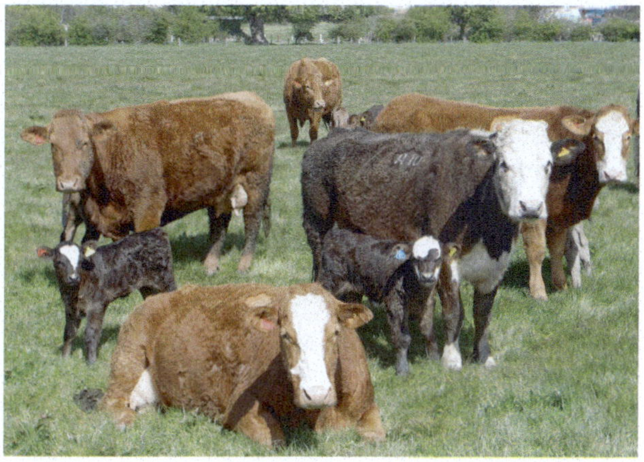

Figure 49.3 Assessing calf viability should form part of the audit.

Table 49.4 Assessing calf viability.

		Parameter	Target/ interference
The number of calves born.	Includes twins and stillbirths.	Number of stillbirths.	0
		Number of deaths within 48 hours of birth.	<2%
		Number of calves that die from 48 hours after birth.	0

The final element is the standardisation of the start of the calving season to allow assessment of calving spread. As gestation lengths to the same bull can vary up to ten days, it is important to introduce a fix for this by adding 285 days to the day the previous breeding season started, and nominate this as the start of the calving season. Cows that calve prior to this can be pushed into the first three weeks (Caldow *et al.*, 2007). This creates a discrete calving period that can be split into three-week intervals and gives a better illustration of fertility, although it must be recognised that there is an artificial inflation of the numbers calving in the first period.

Auditing fertility in the beef cow herd

As already stated the most obvious point of contact for the veterinary practitioner is the visit to carry out pregnancy diagnosis for the herd and this opportunity should be used to collect and analyse the available production data for the herd. To get the most from this opportunity the herd manager should be asked to provide information on the calving season just passed and to have this available before the visit scheduled for the pregnancy diagnosis. This should include information on the following areas:

1 General herd audit: this will include all the data detailed in Table 49.3, and provide the three key performance indicators (KPI): the percentage of cows producing a live calf; length of the calving season; the percentage of cows that calve in the first three weeks of the calving season. This will allow an immediate assessment of the reproductive efficiency of the herd.
2 Barren cow audit: once all the non-pregnant animals have been identified, the next step of the process begins. A table should be created for all the cows identified as non-pregnant (Table 49.5). Even where the number of barren cows falls below the interference level (5%), it is important to complete this exercise, as it can still identify problems that can be overcome to increase output in future. For example, animals calving for the first time represent only around 15% of the cows in most herds, and most losses from this age group can be prevented by modifying their management. It should also be recognised that an extended breeding season can be used to hide a barren cow problem. In these cases, a similar audit can be carried out for all cows calving beyond the first nine weeks of the calving season.
3 Calf mortality audit: this should include stillbirths. The most important information in this analysis is age of the dam, identity of the sire (which may not be known) and calving date. Ultimately, the cause of death provides the most useful information but, without a systematic necropsy being carried out on every calf, this information is often of low value.
4 Bull audit: all bulls that have been used in the herd at the current and previous breeding season should be listed, and the key EBVs that relate to fertility should be listed – gestation length, calving ease direct, and calving ease maternal. The breed society websites provide access to the databases that include all EBVs for registered bulls, and all that is needed is the bull's official ear number to locate the animal's details within the database.
5 Assessing the body condition of the cows: at the time of pregnancy diagnosis, this is likely to be unrewarding as, in most herds, pregnancy diagnosis will be carried out at the end of the grazing season, when body condition should be optimal. Nevertheless, focus particularly on the body condition of the younger animals, and oldest animals may show whether under-nutrition is likely to have been a problem.

Analysing the data

The general audit allows an overall assessment of where the herd is without identifying the root cause of any shortfalls in productivity. In general, most deficits can be related back to the five-point plan, but the challenge is then to use the information collected in audits 2, 3 and 4 to pinpoint what the issues are. Thus, first and second calvers being over-represented in the barren cow analysis indicates that the heifer management programme needs to be re-assessed, and it can also be an indicator that the nutritional management of the entire herd is suboptimal. Other common findings are that cows that were assisted at calving, or older cows, or those that last calved at the end of the calving season, are over-represented.

Where there is any indication of a problem with stillborn calves and mortality in the first 48 hours, an underlying dystocia problem is likely to be the root cause, with either nutritional management (calving cows in excessive body condition) or one or more bulls having poor calving traits. This can usually be resolved by examining the bull audit data.

Further investigation

Not every audit will result in the identification of a root cause. A recent incursion of infectious disease, for example, will tend to affect all categories of breeding females in the herd equally.

Table 49.5 Barren cow audit.

Cow identity	Age at last calving	Date of last calving	Degree of calving assistance	Sex of calf	Birth weight of calf	Twins Yes/no	Bulling group

Chronic poor reproductive performance can be seen due to copper deficiency in association with molybdenum excess, and will result in high barren rates and long, flat calving distributions. In these situations, further investigation will be required. A sample of the cows should be bled and tested appropriately. Where serological screening is carried out, a negative result is often the most valuable, producing an unequivocal answer that a particular infectious agent was not involved. Otherwise, a cautious interpretation of the significance of the presence of specific antibody is required.

In regions where *Campylobacter fetus venerealis* and *Tritrichomanas foetus* are present, then appropriate investigative techniques should be considered to identify these agents.

Where a root cause is not identified, the entire bull stud should be subjected to a breeding soundness investigation.

Plan, do, check, adjust

The pregnancy diagnosis visit provides the most common contact point for the cattle practitioner to integrate their expertise into the reproductive management of the herd, but some herds may use lay contractors to carry this out. Other opportunities should be sought, and health planning in the UK and Eire has offered an obvious opportunity. The challenge is to use an approach based on the collection and analysis of data, and to put the practitioner to the fore at each of the checkpoints in the 'plan, do, check, adjust' management cycle. The methodology outlined here can form the foundations of a data-based approach to health planning, and to the fertility audit of the beef cow herd.

References

Caldow, G., Riddell, I., Stuart, H. and Lowman, B. (2007). Improving efficiency of the beef cow herd. *Cattle Practice* **15**(2),138–144.

Short, R.E. and Adams, D.C. (1988). Nutritional and hormonal interrelationships in beef-cattle reproduction. *Canadian Journal of Animal Science* **68**, 29–39.

CHAPTER 50

Farm Audit – Replacement Beef Heifers

Robert L. Larson

Learning objectives

- Understand the important husbandry practices that impact heifer development.
- Understand how heifer development practices impact the productivity, welfare, health and hence profitability of beef cows.
- Be able to compile and perform a farm audit questionnaire focused on replacement beef heifer development.
- Be able to indicate appropriate values for key performance indicators.
- Be able to communicate the important outcomes of the farm audit.

Audit: measurable outcomes

- Adequate weight per day of age at weaning.
- Confirmed structural soundness (sound feet and legs, absence of genetic defects).
- Implementation of planned vaccination protocol to enhance herd immunity to pregnancy-wasting diseases.
- Breeding soundness evaluations of yearling heifers (reproductive tract scoring (RTS), estimating pelvic area, and determining yearling weight) conducted.
- Breeding soundness examination of bulls conducted prior to breeding season.
- Bulls selected based on appropriate predictions of sires' genetic influence on progeny performance (EPD/EBV for milk production, growth, and calving ease/birth weight).
- High percentage of heifers respond to synchronisation system (if utilised).
- Length of first breeding season is limited and timed to start before the mature herd breeding season.
- Pregnancy percentage to artificial insemination (AI) breeding and percentage of each cohort becoming pregnant by 21-day intervals, determined by palpation or ultrasound assessment of the uterus.
- Adequate body condition/body weight at time of palpation for pregnancy determination for first pregnancy.
- Adequate body condition/body weight at start of first calving season.
- Calving distribution by one-week, two-week or three-week intervals, calving difficulty scores, pregnancy loss between pregnancy determination via palpation and calving determined for each cohort.
- Adequate body condition score prior to start of second breeding season.
- Adequate body condition score at time of weaning first calf.

Introduction

Productivity for beef cattle herds has been shown to be increased when a high percentage of heifers become pregnant early in the first breeding season, and economic return is enhanced when primiparous heifers conceive for a second pregnancy as two-year-olds (Lesmeister *et al.*, Patterson *et al.*, 2003). Proper development of beef replacement heifers starts with selection of heifers at, or prior to weaning, and continues through a period of moderate growth from weaning to the start of a short, controlled breeding season at about one year old. Heifers should be mated to bulls at low risk of contributing to a high percentage of the heifer cohort experiencing dystocia.

Once pregnant, the replacement heifers need to continue to grow throughout pregnancy and to give birth to a live, healthy calf at slightly less than a cohort-median of two years old. Management of primiparous replacement females continues through a period of post-partum anoestrous. While longer than for multiparous cows, this anoestrous period is short enough to allow resumption of fertile cycles prior to the start of the next breeding season. Because beef heifers typically reach puberty

Bovine Medicine, Third Edition. Edited by Peter D. Cockcroft.

around one year of age, gestation lasts over nine months, and beef cattle herds are typically managed to calve in a single two- to three-month time period each year; at any time of year, at least two, and usually three, cohorts of replacement heifers one year apart in age (between birth and being confirmed pregnant for their second gestation) are present within a herd. Therefore, when auditing the performance of one replacement heifer cohort, information gleaned may be utilised, not only to adjust the management of the cohort that provided the data, but also to improve the management of other cohorts of nulliparous or primiparous heifers currently in the herd.

I have made several assumptions based on North American production constraints that probably have wide, but not necessarily universal application. These assumptions influence subsequent management recommendations and include:

1 The greatest expenses in a beef cattle production system are the fixed cost of land and depreciation on cattle, facilities, and equipment (Lawrence, 1997).
2 Feed costs, distinct from grazing costs, are the most significant variable cost and are large expenses in the overall production system (Lawrence, 1997).
3 Other significant costs for beef cow herds include interest payments for capital and wages for family and hired labour (Lawrence, 1997).
4 Forage resources vary in quantity and quality throughout the year, with some months having relatively poor forage production.
5 Nutrient requirements for beef cows vary, based on the stage of gestation and level of lactation.
6 Cohorts of mature cows (multiparous; three years and older) in moderate body condition receiving adequate nutrition have a period of postpartum anoestrous lasting an average of 50–60 days (Lents *et al.*, 2008; Cushman *et al.*, 2007).
7 Cohorts of primiparous two-year-old cows in moderate body condition receiving adequate nutrition have a postpartum anoestrus that averages 80–100 days (Ciccioli *et al.*, 2003; Berardinelle & Joshi, 2005).
8 About 60–70% of matings between a cycling cow and fertile bull will result in pregnancy that can be detected 50 days later (BonDurant, 2007).

These constraints lead to a number of goals to minimise land and depreciation costs per dollar-value of calf production, while

Table 50.1 Reproduction goals to minimise fixed and variable costs per dollar-value of calf production in beef cattle herds.

Goal	Target
Limit breeding season length for mature (primiparous and multiparous) cows.	65 days (maximum 90 days)
A high percentage of cows exposed to bulls become pregnant and maintain that pregnancy at least 50 days. (i.e. pregnancy percentage determined 50+ days after the end of the breeding season).	95% (minimum 90%)
A high percentage of cows exposed for breeding become pregnant to matings that occurred in the first 21 days of the breeding season.	65% (minimum 60%)
A high percentage of cows exposed for breeding become pregnant to matings that occurred in the first 42 days of the breeding season.	85% (minimum 80%)
Start the breeding season for heifers earlier than the start of the mature cow breeding season.	45 days (minimum 30 days)
Limit breeding season length for heifers.	65 days (minimum 45 days) (maximum 65 days)
The average body weight by 400 days old (immediately pre-breeding) for a cohort of replacement heifers should ensure high likelihood that nearly all of the cohort has reached puberty.	65% of mature weight (minimum 60%)
By the start of the mature cow calving season (i.e. six to eight weeks prior to the onset of heifer breeding), a high percentage of heifers in a replacement cohort should have palpable uterine and ovarian characteristics consistent with having attained puberty.	65% (minimum 60%)
A high percentage of replacement heifers exposed to bulls become pregnant and maintain that pregnancy at least 50 days (i.e. pregnancy percentage determined 50+ days after the end of the breeding season).	>90% (minimum 90%)
A high percentage of replacement heifers exposed for breeding become pregnant to matings that occurred in the first 21 days of the breeding season.	65% (minimum 60%)
The average body weight by the onset of the calving season for a cohort of replacement heifers should ensure a high likelihood that nearly all of the cohort is in adequate body condition to minimise risk of dystocia due to nutrition and that the postpartum anoestrous period will not be extended.	85% of mature weight (minimum 80%)

controlling non-grazing feed costs as well as capital and labour costs (Table 50.1).

An important goal is to have a controlled breeding (and, subsequently, calving) season that results in calves being born at the same time each year (365-day herd calving interval). Cows should be limited to a 65- to 90-day calving season to manage cow herds so that periods of the cow production cycle that have the highest nutrient requirements are matched with the months of the year with the highest forage production. In order to ensure adequate production of calves to offset land, depreciation, feed, interest, labour and other costs, a high percentage of the cows exposed to bulls for breeding each year should become pregnant and carry that pregnancy to birth of a healthy calf. Another goal is to have a high percentage of cows conceiving early in the breeding season, with all or most of the herd appropriately matching the high nutritional requirement periods of high lactation and late gestation foetal growth with the best forage production, as well as to have the herd's calves as old (and therefore heavy) as possible at the time of weaning.

Cows that conceive in the first 21 days of the breeding season have 61–81 days from calving until the start of the next controlled breeding season, and cows that conceive in the second 21 days of the breeding season have 40–60 days between calving and the start of the next breeding season. Cows that conceive more than 42 days after the start of the breeding season are not likely to have completed the period of post-partum anoestrus and to be cycling at the start of the following breeding season. Because two-year-old primiparous cows have a longer period of post-partum anoestrus than older cows, they need to calve no less than 1–20 days prior the start of the expected first calving date for the mature herd for this age cohort to be cycling at the start of their second breeding season. This can be accomplished with a 45-day heifer breeding season that begins 45 days prior to the start of the mature cow breeding season or a 30-day heifer breeding season that begins 30 days prior to the start of the mature cow breeding season.

Onset of puberty in beef heifers

Age at onset of puberty

In order for heifers born in a 65-day calving season to reach puberty by the start of a breeding season that starts 45 days prior to the start of the mature cow breeding season, the heifers must reach puberty by 335–400 days old. Puberty is reached when the beef heifer is able to express oestrous behaviour, ovulate a fertile oocyte and obtain normal luteal function (Moran, 1989). Mean age at puberty for cohorts of North American beef heifers is typically 350–425 days, with some variation around this estimate (Gasser *et al.*, 2006; Yilmaz *et al.*, 2006; Beck, 2005; Basarab *et al.*, 2011; Shaffer *et al.*, 2011). Therefore, to ensure that a high percentage of heifers are pubertal by the start of a breeding season that proceeds the mature herd breeding season, the heifers must be born early in the calving season, and the heifer breeding season cannot precede the mature cow breeding season by more than 45 days. In addition to selecting replacements from heifers born early in the calving season, age at puberty can be decreased by selecting for breeds with a younger age at puberty, selecting within a breed for younger age at puberty, or crossbreeding with another breed that has a similar or younger age at puberty (Short *et al.*, 1990).

Weight at onset of puberty

Age is not the only determining factor influencing the onset of puberty in beef heifers, body weight is also considered an important variable (Nelsen *et al.*, 1982). Mean body weight at puberty for *Bos taurus* breed heifers such as Angus, Hereford, Charolais, or Limousin is about 60% of mature weight (Dziuk & Bellows, 1983; Wiltbank *et al.*, 1985). Dual purpose breed heifers such as Braunvieh, Gelbvieh, or Red Poll tend to reach puberty at an average of about 55 percent of mature weight, and *Bos indicus* heifers, most commonly Brahma or Brahma-cross, are older and heavier at puberty than the other beef breeds – about 65% of mature weight (Laster *et al.*, 1972, 1976, 1979; Stewart *et al.*, 1980; Sacco *et al.*, 1987).

Other factors can also have some influence on the onset of puberty, and include: exposure to bulls (Pennel *et al.*, 1986; Roberson *et al.*, 1991); time of year (heifers born in the fall reach puberty at a younger age than heifers born in the spring; Schillo *et al.*, 1983); and exposure to progestrogens (Short *et al.*, 1976; Gonzalez-Padilla *et al.*, 1975; Spitzer, 1982). Using the conservative value of 65% of mature body weight as a target weight for the start of the breeding season results in a needed average daily body weight gain of 0.5–1.0 kg per day (1.1–2.2 lbs. per day) from weaning to breeding for typical beef herds.

Diet effects on onset of puberty

High starch diets appear to influence the age and/or weight at puberty. Ciccioli *et al.* (2003) reported that heifers with a higher starch intake had lower weight at puberty, compared to a isonitrogenous-isocaloric diet with higher fibre, even though the two diets resulted in the same body weight and fat reserves (Ciccioli *et al.*, 2003). Similarly, Gasser *et al.* (2006) found that heifers fed a higher starch diet were younger and lighter at puberty than heifers fed a lower NE control diet when the treatments were started at 99 days of age (Gasser *et al.*, 2006). In contrast, other studies have shown that while high grain diets decrease the age at puberty, weight at puberty was increased (Short & Bellows, 1971; Hall *et al.*, 1995,).

Meeting, but not grossly exceeding, the target weight is important for heifer fertility and production. Developing heifers on a high plane of nutrition (both energy and protein) from weaning to breeding results in earlier puberty (Wiltbank *et al.*, 1969; Oeydipe *et al.*, 1982) improved udder development (Bond & Wiltbank, 1970), and increased pregnancy percentage compared with a low plane of nutrition (Short & Bellows, 1971; Patterson *et al.*, 1989). This difference in pregnancy percentage is probably at least partially due to differences in pituitary function of heifers fed a low-energy versus a high-energy diet. Day *et al.* (1986) found that heifers developed on a low-energy diet failed to exhibit an increase in luteinising hormone (LH) pulse frequency, at a time when heifers developed on an adequate diet exhibited increased LH pulse frequency and attained puberty.

Assessment of reproductive soundness of replacement beef heifer cohorts

Reproductive tract scoring

The reproductive tract scoring (RTS) system was developed to subjectively classify pubertal status, using size of the uterus and ovaries estimated by palpation per rectum. The system assigns a score to each heifer using a five-point scale, where a score of 1 is considered an immature tract, and scores of 4 and 5 are considered a cycling tract (Anderson *et al.*, 1991).

An RTS of 1 is used to describe heifers with infantile reproductive tracts that are not near the time of puberty when palpated. These heifers have small, flaccid tracts and small ovaries with no significant structures. Heifers may be assigned a RTS of 1 because:

1 they are simply too young to fit into the breeding season being planned;
2 they are too light to reach their target weight and are not able to express their genetic potential for reaching puberty; or
3 they were implanted with a steroid hormone growth-promoter near the time of birth.

Heifers assigned a RTS of 2 have slightly larger uterine diameter, but tone is still lacking and the ovaries have very small follicles. Heifers described as having a RTS of 3 have some uterine tone, and larger uterine diameter than heifers with more immature scores. Heifers assigned either a score of 4 or 5 are considered cycling, as indicated by good uterine tone and size and easily palpable ovarian structures. RTS 4 is assigned to heifers that have large follicles but do not have a palpable corpus luteum (CL). Heifers with a RTS of 5 are similar in uterine and ovarian size, tone, and structure when palpated per rectum, as compared to RTS 4 heifers, except that a CL is palpable.

The scores assigned with the RTS system are able to predict the reproductive performance of yearling heifers, especially for pregnancy percentage to synchronised breeding and to pregnancy percentage at the end of the breeding season. Heifers with more mature reproductive tracts had higher pregnancy percentage and calved earlier (Patterson & Bullock, 1995).

Heifers should be evaluated and assigned an RTS about six to eight weeks prior to the breeding season. If deficiencies are found this far ahead of planned breeding, management changes can result in an increased number of heifers reaching puberty by the start of the breeding season. If the heifers are evaluated too far ahead of the breeding season (>8 weeks), the heifers are likely to be young and to have lower tract scores that do not truly reflect their potential to reach puberty before the breeding season.

A reasonable goal is to have at least 80%, and up to 90% or more, of replacement heifers cycling at the start of the breeding season. A group is likely to reach this goal if 65% of the heifers are classified as cycling (scored as RTS 4 or 5), and most of the remainder of the heifers are RTS 3 when evaluated 6–8 weeks before breeding. In order to reach the goal of at least 80% of heifers in a replacement pool cycling at the start of the breeding season, nutrition must remain adequate for continued growth from the time of RTS evaluation until breeding.

If a low percentage of heifers are cycling at the time of RTS evaluation and many of the heifers are scored as 3, management changes must be instituted immediately. These changes may include:

1 increasing the plane of nutrition so that increased weight gain will allow the heifers to reach target weight by the start of the breeding season;
2 holding the heifers over to breed six months later, to calve in an alternate calving season;
3 marketing the heifers for feeder cattle and finding another source of replacements.

If a large percentage of the heifers evaluated are RTS 1 or 2, the cohort will not have good reproductive success in a breeding season that starts in 6–8 weeks, and the heifers should be managed as feeder heifers and another source of replacements found.

Pelvic area assessment

The use of pelvic measurement at one year old as a tool to decrease the risk of dystocia has been described extensively since the late 1970s (Neville *et al.*, 1978; Holtzer & Schlote, 1984; Deutscher, 1985). Veterinarians have used pelvic area measurements of yearlings because the major cause of dystocia is a disproportionately large calf, compared to the heifer's pelvic area. The correlation between yearling and two-year-old pelvic areas is 0.70 (Neville *et al.*, 1978); therefore, measuring pelvic area as a yearling is beneficial for predicting pelvic size at the time of parturition. Pelvic area is moderately to highly heritable (0.44–0.61) so, after a few years of measuring heifers used to produce replacements, producers can increase the average pelvic size of the herd (Benyshek & Little, 1982; Morrison *et al.*, 1984).

Critics of using pelvic area measurements to decrease dystocia point out that pelvic area is also positively correlated to mature cow size and calf birth weigh (Laster, 1974; Price & Wiltbank, 1978). If producers place selection pressure on heifers by selecting for increasingly larger pelvic area, calf birth weight will also increase, and the risk of dystocia is not likely to decrease (Basarab *et al.*, 1993). A number of researchers have shown that selection based on pelvic area alone did not significantly reduce the risk of dystocia in groups of heifers (Naazie *et al.*, 1989, Van Donkersgoed *et al.*, 1990; Whittier *et al.*, 1994).

Rather than using pelvic area measurement to select for maximum pelvic size, this tool should be used to set a minimum pelvic size as a culling criterion (such as 150 cm^2 at a year of age), without assigning preference for heifers that exceed the minimum. In addition, by including mature weight as a selection criterion, heifers with a genetic predisposition for small pelvic area are culled without increasing mature size.

Comprehensive breeding soundness examination of beef heifer cohorts

An effective way to evaluate the reproductive soundness of yearling heifers in a ranch setting is by using yearling weights, RTS and pelvic area measurements together to describe the maturity and reproductive soundness of the heifer cohort. These three criteria are closely correlated in that, within a set of heifers with similar genetic makeup, one should expect higher tract scores in heifers that have heavier yearling weights, and these heifers should also have greater pelvic area than lighter-weight heifers.

Because we expect yearling weight, RTS and pelvic area all to be related, one should make note of heifers, or groups of heifers, where that relationship is not strong. Heifers that have reached their target weight and have a high RTS, but which have a small pelvic area, may have a genetic predisposition for a small pelvis. Another example where heifers do not perform as expected is the case where heifers are implanted with a growth promoter near the time of birth. Often, these heifers have very adequate yearling weights and pelvic areas, but RTS indicate tract immaturity.

Pelvic area tends to increase more rapidly near the time of puberty than during the pre-pubertal period (Bullock & Patterson, 1995). This knowledge is useful when examining pelvic area data, in that a heifer that has a RTS of 5 and is of adequate yearling weight, but has a small pelvis, has a high probability of having a small pelvis at the time of calving as a two-year-old. In contrast, a heifer with the same pelvic area, that has a RTS of 2 and has not reached her target weight, may very well have an adequate pelvis at calving, if management changes are made so that she reaches puberty and becomes pregnant.

Nutrition during first gestation

The target weight concept can be continued for planning nutritional requirements through pregnancy. A heifer should weigh 80–85% of her mature weight at the time of calving as a two-year-old. The nutritional demands of pregnancy increase as gestation progresses. These demands occur not only due to foetal growth, but also due to uterine/placental growth and metabolism involved with the foetal/maternal interaction and exchange of nutrients and waste.

Heifers calving in subjectively determined body condition scores (BCS) of 4, 5, or 6 (on a 9-point scale) respectively, had calves with progressively heavier birth weights, but dystocia score was not influenced by BCS at calving (Spitzer *et al.*, 1995). Heifers with greater weight gains pre-partum had calves with heavier weaning weights than did heifers with moderate weight gains (Spitzer *et al.*, 1995). Greater BCS at calving resulted in more heifers in oestrus and more heifers pregnant by 40 and 60 days of the subsequent breeding season (Spitzer *et al.*, 1995). When body weight or condition loss occurred during the middle third of pregnancy, increased nutrient intake one to three months before calving substantially improved pregnancy percentage, compared to cows that continued to lose weight (Selk *et al.*, 1988). However, cows that maintained weight throughout the last half of pregnancy had higher pregnancy percentage than those that lost weight and had to gain it back later, even though pre-calving BCS were similar between the two groups (Selk *et al.*, 1988).

Nutrition following first parturition

During the first 80–100 days following parturition, a heifer must continue to grow at about 0.23 kg per day (0.5 lbs/day), support lactation for a suckling calf, resume fertile oestrous cycles and conceive for a second pregnancy. The maintenance nutritional requirements for lactating heifers average about 20% higher than that for non-lactating heifers (but requirements are greatly affected by milk production potential). In beef cattle, peak lactation occurs at approximately 60 days post-partum and maximum yield has been reported to range from 4.1 kg/day to 13.6 kg/day (9–30 lbs/day) (National Research Council, 1996).

Energy and protein requirements post-calving greatly exceed that of mid-gestation heifers, and even late gestation heifers. These higher demands make it difficult to add body condition to heifers once lactation begins. Because post-calving condition score and energy balance control ovulation, and condition scores of 6 or greater are required for high conception percentage in primiparous heifers, both body condition at calving and level of nutrition post-partum are critical control points affecting pregnancy percentages (Wright *et al.*, 1992; DeRouen *et al.*, 1994). Ciccioli *et al.* (2003) showed that primiparous cows fed to gain more weight for the first 71 days postpartum had a shorter interval to first post-partum oestrus and ovulation, a larger dominant follicle at first oestrus, and higher pregnancy percentage at the first oestrus, compared to cows fed to gain less weight.

Bull fertility

To ensure that bulls can deliver fertile semen to the reproductive tract of heifers, a thorough breeding soundness examination to evaluate semen quality, structural soundness and health of all breeding bulls should be done a few weeks prior to the start of the breeding season. Once the breeding season begins, producers should spend time observing activity in the breeding pasture, to make sure that bulls are searching out heifers that are in heat and that they are able to mount and complete the act of breeding. It is particularly important during the first 20 days of the breeding season to visually evaluate bulls frequently, to ensure normal ambulation and lack of injuries to the penis, prepuce, or testicles. Mounting indicators glued to heifers' tail heads, or chin ball markers on bulls, can be valuable tools to evaluate the number of heifers or cows of mated per day or per week in a breeding pasture (depending on frequency of observation). If 80–100% of non-oestrus synchronised heifers are cycling at the start of the breeding season, 4–5% on average should be bred each day. If the number is below this level, either the females are not cycling, or the bulls are not detecting heifers in heat.

It is also important to monitor the breeding pasture from about day 20 to day 30 or 40, as females that fail to conceive to the first mating return to heat. If 65% of the herd became pregnant during the first 20 days of the breeding season then, on average, less than 2% of the herd should be bred each day of the second 20 days of the breeding season. If, on average, 4–5% of the cows were bred each day of the first 20 days of the breeding season, but 2% or more are being bred during the second 20 days, it is likely that the bulls are not successfully causing conception, and the cause needs to be investigated immediately.

Determining success of beef cattle breeding season

Determining the percentage of heifers that become pregnant by the end of the breeding season allows one to identify heifers that are not pregnant, and to determine the best marketing plan for those animals. In addition, if more pregnant heifers are available than are needed as herd replacements, the excess can be marketed to herds needing pregnant animals. A goal of 90% or more of heifers in the replacement pool being pregnant at the end of the breeding season is achievable in good heifer management systems.

If heifers are synchronised and bred by artificial insemination (AI), bulls should be held out of the breeding pasture for two weeks following the last day of AI breeding, so that the percentage becoming pregnant to the AI mating can be accurately determined early in gestation via foetal aging by uterine palpation or ultrasound examination. 65–70% or more of the heifers identified in oestrus and bred artificially should become pregnant to AI. If heifers are treated with a protocol designed to synchronise ovulation for timed mating, information about the number of heifers displaying oestrous behaviour is lost and cannot be evaluated; but if 90% of heifers are cycling and 90% of the cycling heifers respond to the synchronisation protocol, the same 65–70% success to AI mating will result in 53–57% of timed-inseminated heifers becoming pregnant to AI. Failure to meet this goal could indicate inaccurate determination of oestrus (or poor percentage cycling, or poor synchronisation success, if using a timed-insemination protocol), poor semen delivery by the AI technician, poor semen quality or poor condition of the females (stress, high environmental temperature, losing weight).

Auditing beef replacement heifer management

Proper management of replacement heifer cohorts from weaning, until they are confirmed pregnant with their second calf approximately two years later, requires careful attention to meeting growth and reproductive goals at specific auditing time points. Because of the two-year time frame encompassed by beef heifer replacement management, between one and three heifer cohorts, each a year apart in age, may be evaluated at each of four auditing events (Figure 50.1).

In a spring-calving herd, the first auditing event in the calendar year takes place 60–90 days prior to the expected start of the calving season (Table 50.2).

At this time, pregnant mature females are evaluated to ensure that they are approaching the onset of calving in good body condition (BCS 5–6 on a 9-point scale), and the body weight of heifers in their first gestation is such that they are meeting weight gain goals, so that they will reach 80–85% of their mature weight by the onset of calving. As the two-year-old replacement heifers begin to calve, this cohort should be audited to determine if 15% or fewer (or a herd-specific goal) have difficulty during parturition, and that less than 2% of heifers confirmed as pregnant in early- to mid-gestation fail to calve due to gestational loss (Table 50.3).

The onset of the mature cowherd calving season overlaps with several important auditing events (Table 50.4). The mature cowherd should be audited to determine the percent of parturitions that are classified as dystocia, and this risk should not exceed 5%. In addition, fewer than 2% of cows confirmed pregnant earlier in gestation should fail to carry their calves to term. This time period (onset of mature cowherd calving) occurs approximately six weeks prior to the start of the replacement heifer breeding season, which precedes the cow breeding season by 30–45 days – which is an ideal time to assess the reproductive soundness of the yearling heifer cohort.

Yearling replacement heifer cohorts should be evaluated to ensure that nearly all heifers have reached a body weight that is 60–65% of their predicted mature weight, and that 65% of

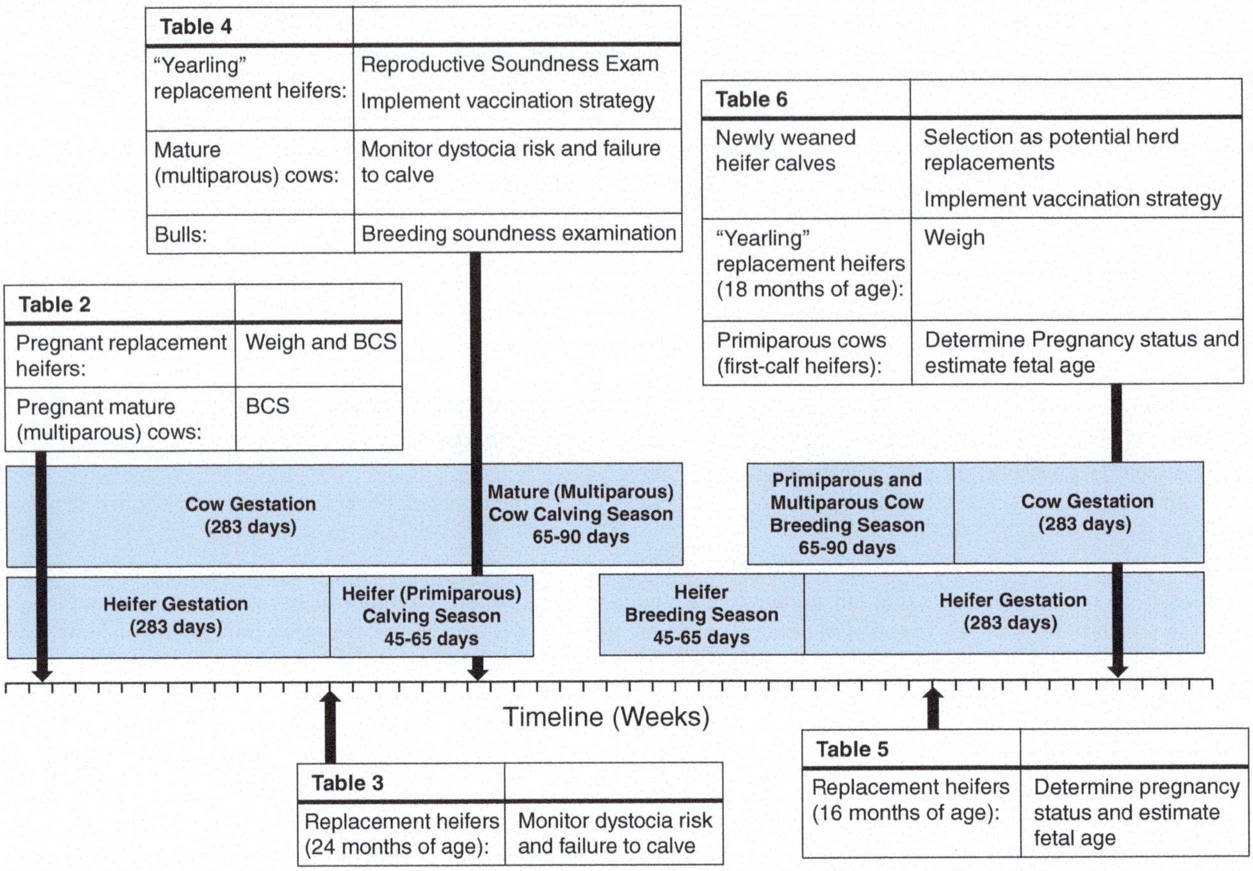

Figure 50.1 Time line of heifer development audits from weaning until a confirmed second pregnancy.

Table 50.2 Audit of key indices 60–90 days prior to the expected start of calving to ensure high replacement beef heifer reproductive efficiency.

Cohort	Audit: measurable outcomes	Intervention if goals not attained
Pregnant replacement heifers (approximately 21 months old).	Average daily weight gain since breeding that is meeting target gains from breeding to first calving (80% of mature weight).	If weight gain is not sufficient to ensure reaching 80–85% of mature weight by the time of calving, increase nutrient density of diet and re-evaluate in 45–60 days.
	Good body condition (BSC 6 on a 9-point scale).	Minimum median cohort body condition score of 6 on a 9-point scale (maximum median cohort body condition score of 7 on a 9-point scale).
Multiparous cows.	Moderate body condition (BSC 5 on a 9-point scale).	Minimum median cohort body condition score of 5 on a 9-point scale (maximum median cohort body condition score of 6 on a 9-point scale).

the heifers are cycling and have palpable evidence of having reached puberty. In addition, pelvic area can be measured, and heifers evaluated to ensure that they meet minimum standards. Because a successful breeding season depends on both fertile females and males, bulls should be selected and evaluated 4–6 weeks prior to the start of the breeding season, with a thorough breeding soundness examination to ensure that sufficient fertile bulls are available for the desired bull to heifer ratio.

If the yearling replacement heifer cohort met all of the auditing criteria leading up to the breeding season, and they were exposed to fertile bulls, the result should be excellent reproductive efficiency. To audit the success of the breeding season, the yearling

Table 50.3 Audit of key indices at the time the heifer cohort is expected to begin calving to ensure high replacement beef heifer reproductive efficiency.

Cohort	Audit: measurable outcomes	Intervention if goals not attained
Two-year-old replacement heifers	<15% (or herd-specific goal) of replacement heifers have dystocia	Re-evaluate selection criteria for bulls used for mating heifers. Select bulls with calculations of parental expected phenotype estimations (e.g. Expected Progeny Difference – EPD, or Expected Breeding Value – EBV) that ensure low risk of dystocia. Investigate energy, protein, or mineral deficiencies that could contribute to dystocia.
	<2% of replacement heifers classified as pregnant fail to calve.	Initiate an investigation of possible infectious, toxic, or endocrine causes of abortion.

Table 50.4 Audit of key indices at the time the mature-cow herd is expected to begin calving to ensure high replacement beef heifer reproductive efficiency.

Cohort	Audit: measurable outcomes	Intervention if goals not attained
'Yearling' Replacement heifers (six weeks prior to onset of heifer breeding season).	65% of heifers should have palpable uterine and ovarian characteristics consistent with having attained puberty. Mean body weight of cohort should be nearly 65% of average mature cow body weight.	The heifer breeding season starts in about six weeks. If the heifers are under-weight and immature, and can reach target weight within six weeks, increase energy level of diet. If a small percentage of the heifers are likely to have initiated fertile cycles (puberty) by the start of breeding, consider selling the heifers as feeders and purchasing replacements.
	Exceed 130–150 cm^2 pelvic area.	Cull heifers that have palpable evidence of reaching puberty that are below pelvic area cut-off.
	100% of yearling replacement heifers receive appropriate vaccinations for pregnancy-wasting diseases.	Institute appropriate vaccination protocol for pregnancy-wasting diseases.
Mature cows (primiparous and multiparous).	<5% (or herd-specific goal) of cows have dystocia.	Re-evaluate selection criteria for bulls used for mating heifers. Select bulls with calculations of parental expected phenotype estimations (e.g. EPD, EBV) that ensure low risk of dystocia. Investigate energy, protein, or mineral deficiencies that could contribute to dystocia.
	<2% of cows classified as pregnant fail to calve.	Initiate an investigation of possible infectious, toxic, or endocrine causes of abortion.
Bulls selected to mate with 'yearling' heifers.	Sufficient bulls will pass a complete breeding soundness examination to ensure an appropriate bull : heifer ratio.	Obtain sufficient number of bulls to ensure an appropriate bull : heifer ratio.

Table 50.5 Audit of key indices 100 days after start of heifer breeding season to ensure high replacement beef heifer reproductive efficiency

Cohort	Audit: measurable outcomes	Intervention if goals not attained
'Yearling' replacement heifers (approximately 16 months old)	90% of heifers are pregnant following a 45–65 day breeding season. 60–65% of heifers exposed to bulls are pregnant from a mating during the first 21 days of the breeding season.	Evaluate replacement heifer target age and weight at start of breeding season, and adjust for next cohort to ensure that nearly all are pubertal prior to breeding. Evaluate breeding soundness of bulls.

Table 50.6 Audit of key indices at the time calves are weaned (e.g. 150–250 days old) to ensure high replacement beef heifer reproductive efficiency.

Cohort	Audit: measurable outcomes	Intervention if goals not attained
Newly weaned heifer calves.	Age: heifers selected for potential replacements must be born in the first 42 days of the calving season. Genetics: calculations of parental expected phenotype estimations (e.g. EPD, EBV) exceed herd-specific cut-offs. Parental and heifer phenotype: feet, leg, and udder confirmation exceed herd-specific cut-offs.	If insufficient numbers of suitable replacements are identified, consider purchasing appropriate replacements from another herd with health status at least as high.
	100% of replacement heifers receive appropriate vaccinations for pregnancy-wasting diseases.	Institute appropriate vaccination protocol for pregnancy-wasting diseases.
'Yearling' heifers pregnant with first calf (approximately 18 months old).	Average daily weight gain since breeding that is meeting target gains from breeding to first calving (80–85% of mature weight).	If weight gain is not sufficient to ensure reaching 80% of mature weight by the time of calving, increase nutrient density of diet and re-evaluate in 45–60 days.
Primiparous cows (a.k.a. first-calf heifers) (approx. 30 months old).	Pregnancy percentage: 95% of cows exposed to bulls should be pregnant in a 65–90 day breeding season (90% minimum). Pregnancy distribution: 60–65% of first-calf heifers exposed to bulls are pregnant from a mating during the first 21 days of the breeding season.	Evaluate body weight and body condition at calving, and adjust for next cohort to ensure that nearly all are cycling prior to breeding. Evaluate breeding soundness of bulls.

heifers should be evaluated for pregnancy status when foetal age can be accurately estimated, usually not later than 100 days after the onset of the breeding season (Table 50.5).

If the heifer breeding season lasts 65 days, examining heifers for pregnancy status 100 days after the start of breeding results in gestational ages between 35–100 days. By determining gestational age of the foetuses at this time, the veterinarian can determine the percentage of the cohort that became pregnant to the AI mating (if used), as well as determine if 65% of the cohort became pregnant in the first 21 days of the breeding season. The overall reproductive success for a 45- to 65-day breeding season should result in at least 90% of the replacement heifer cohort becoming pregnant. If uncertainty exists for the pregnancy status of some heifers, those that are not confirmed pregnant can be re-examined later in gestation.

The final replacement heifer auditing event in the calendar year for spring-calving beef herds occurs at the time of calf weaning and determination of the pregnancy status for the mature herd (Table 50.6). At this time, there are three cohorts of replacement heifers to be evaluated. The youngest is the heifers that are being weaned. The newly weaned heifers selected for inclusion in the replacement cohort should have been born no later than 42 days after the start of the mature herd calving season, and they should meet genetic and phenotype selection criteria for the herd. The heifers that were weaned a year earlier should be in mid-gestation of their first pregnancy, and should be evaluated to ensure that they are gaining weight at the rate necessary to reach 80–85% of their mature weight by the end of gestation. The pregnancy status of the replacement cohort that is nursing their first calves should meet the auditing goal of 95% pregnant following a 65–90 day breeding season, with 60–65% of the cohort having become pregnant in the first 21 days of the breeding season.

Summary

Implementing an auditing system that evaluates replacement beef heifers at critical time points, from weaning until their second pregnancy is confirmed, allows veterinarians and beef producers to remove nearly all the risk associated with developing herd replacements. Heifer cohorts that meet or exceed all the audited growth and reproduction goals are likely to have high reproductive efficiency, and to have a positive impact on herd production and profitability. Management of cohorts that fail to meet audit goals can be altered to correct the problem, or to minimise the negative effect by the next auditing event. This auditing approach to replacement heifer development capitalises on veterinary skills and services, and implements a systematic veterinary-client relationship that benefits beef producers, veterinarians, and the cattle herd.

References

Anderson, K.J., Lefever, D.G., Brinks, J.S. and Odde, K.G. (1991). The use of reproductive tract scoring in beef heifers. *Agri-Practice* **12**(4), 19.

Basarab, J.A., Rutter, L.M. and Day, P.A. (1993). The efficacy of predicting dystocia in yearling beef heifers: I. Using ratios of pelvic area to birth weight or pelvic area to heifer weight. *Journal of Animal Science* **71**, 1359–1371.

Basarab, J.A., Colazo, M.G., Ambrose, D.J., Novak, S., McCartney, D. and Baron, V.S. (2011). Residual feed intake adjusted for back fat thickness and feeding frequency is independent of fertility in beef heifers. *Canadian Journal of Animal Science* **91**, 573–584.

Beck, P.A., Gunter, S.A., Phillips, J.M. and Kreider, D.L. (2005). Development of replacement heifers using programmed feeding. *Professional Animal Scientist* **21**, 365–370.

Benyshek, L.L. and Little, D.E. (1982). Estimate of genetic and phenotypic parameters associated with pelvic area in Simmental cattle. *Journal of Animal Science* **54**, 258–263.

Berardinelle, J.G. and Joshi, P.S. (2005). Introduction of bulls at different days. *Journal of Animal Science* **83**, 2106–2110.

Bond, J. and Wiltbank, J.N. (1970). Effect of energy and protein on oestrus, conception rate, growth and milk production of beef females. *Journal of Animal Science* **30**, 438–444.

BonDurant RH. (2007). Selected diseases and conditions associated with bovine conceptus loss in the first trimester. *Theriogenology* **68**, 461–473.

Bullock, K.D. and Patterson, D.J. (1995). *Pelvic growth in beef heifers and the effects of puberty*. Proceedings: Beef Improvement Federation 27th Research Symposium and Annual Meeting. Sheridan, Wyoming, 1995, pp.171–173.

Ciccioli, N.H., Wettemann, R.P., Spicer, L.J., Lents, C.A., White, F.J. and Keisler, D.H. (2003). Influence of body condition at calving and postpartum nutrition on endocrine function and reproductive performance of primiparous beef cows. *Journal of Animal Science* **81**, 3107–3120.

Cushman, R.A., Allan, M.F., Thallman, R.M. and Cundiff, L.V. (2007). Characterization of biological types of cattle (Cycle VII): Influence of postpartum interval and oestrous cycle length on fertility. *Journal of Animal Science* **85**, 2156–2162.

Day, M.L., Imakawa, E., Zalesky, D.D., Kittok, R.J. and Kinder, J.E. (1986). Effects of restriction of dietary energy intake during the prepubertal period on secretion of luteinizing hormone and responsiveness of the pituitary to luteinizing hormone-releasing hormone in heifers. *Journal of Animal Science* **62**, 1641–1648.

DeRouen, S.M., Franke, D.E., Morrison, D.G., Wyatt, W.E., Coombs, D.F., White, T.W. *et al.* (1994). Prepartum body condition and weight influences on reproductive performance of first-calf beef cows. *Journal of Animal Science* **72**, 1119–1125.

Deutscher, G.H. (1985). Using pelvic measurements to reduce dystocia in heifers. *Modern Veterinary Practice* **66**, 751–755.

Dziuk, P.J. and Bellows, R.A. (1983). Management of reproduction of beef cattle, sheep and pigs. *Journal of Animal Science* **57**(Suppl. 2), 355.

Gasser, C.L., Grum, D.E., Mussard, M.L., Fluharty, F.L., Kinder, J.E. and Day, M.L. (2006 Induction of precocious puberty in heifers I: Enhanced secretion of luteinizing hormone. *Journal of Animal Science* **84**, 2035–2041.

Gonzalez-Padilla, E., Ruiz, R., LeFever, D., Denham, A. and Wiltbank, J.N. (1975). Puberty in beef heifers. III. Induction of fertile oestrus. *Journal of Animal Science* **40**, 1110–1118.

Growth patterns for pelvic dimensions and other body measurements of beef females. *Journal of Animal Science* **47**, 1080–1088.

Hall, J.B., Staigmiller, R.B., Bellows, R.A., Short, R.E., Moseley, W.M. and Bellows, S.E. Body (1995). composition and metabolic profiles associated with puberty in beef heifers. *Journal of Animal Science* **73**, 3409–3420.

Holtzer, A.L.J. and Schlote, W. (1984). Investigations on interior pelvic size of Simmental heifers. *Journal of Animal Science* **59**(Suppl. 1), 174.

Laster, D.B. (1974). Factors affecting pelvic size and dystocia in beef cattle. *Journal of Animal Science* **38**, 496–503.

Laster, D.B., Glimp, H.A. and Gregory, K.E. (1972). Age and weight at puberty and conception in different breeds and breed crosses of beef heifers. *Journal of Animal Science* **34**, 1031–1036.

Laster, D.B., Smith, G.M. and Gregory, K.E. (1976). Characterization of biological types of cattle. IV. Postweaning growth and puberty of heifers. *Journal of Animal Science* **43**, 63–70.

Laster, D.B., Smith, G.M., Cundiff, L.V. and Gregory, K.E. (1979). Characterization of biological types of cattle (Cycle II). II. Postweaning growth and puberty of heifer. *Journal of Animal Science* **48**, 500–508.

Lawrence, J. (1997). *Determinants of Cow-Herd Cost of Production*. A.S. Leaflet R1446, Beef Research Report, Iowa State University.

Lents, C.A., White, F.J., Ciccioli, N.H., Wettemann, R.P., Spicer, L.J. and Lalman, D.L. (2008). Effects of body condition score at parturition and postpartum protein supplementation on oestrous behaviour and size of the dominant follicle in beef cows. *Journal of Animal Science* **86**, 2549–2556.

Lesmeister, J.L., Burfening, P.J. and Blackwell, R.L. (1973). Date of first calving in beef cows and subsequent calf production. *Journal of Animal Science* **36**, 1–6.

Lucy, M.C., Billings, H.J., Butler, W.R., Ehnis, L.R., Fields, M.J., Kesler, D.J. *et al.* (2001). Efficacy of an intravaginal progesterone insert and an injection of PGF2a for synchronization of oestrus and shortening the interval to pregnancy in postpartum beef cows, peripubertal beef heifers, and diary heifers. *Journal of Animal Science* **79**, 982–995.

Moran, C., Quirke, J.F. and Roche, J.F. (1989). Puberty in heifers: A review. *Animal Reproduction Science* **18**, 167–182. Gasser.

Morrison, D.G., Williamson, W.D. and Humes, P.E. (1984). Heritabilities and correlations of traits associated with pelvic area in beef cattle. *Journal of Animal Science* **59**(Suppl 1), 160 (Abstract).

Naazie, A., Makarechian, M.M. and Berg, R.T. (1989). Factors influencing calving difficulty in beef heifers. *Journal of Animal Science* **67**, 3243–3249.

National Research Council (1996). *Nutrient Requirements of Beef Cattle*, 7th edition. National Academy of Sciences, Washington DC.

Nelsen, T.C., Long, C.R. and Cartwright, T.C. (1982). Postinflection growth in straightbred and crossbred cattle. II. Relationships among weight, height and pubertal characters. *Journal of Animal Science* **55**, 293–304.

Neville, W.E., Mullinix, B.G., Smith, J.B. and McCormick, W.C. (1978). Growth patterns for pelvic dimensions and other body measurements of beef females. *Journal of Animal Science* **47**, 1080–1088.

Oeydipe, E.O., Osori, D.I.K., Aderejola, O. and Saror, D. (1982). Effect of level of nutrition on onset of puberty and conception rates of Zebu heifers. *Theriogenology* **18**, 525–539.

Patterson, D.J. and Bullock, K.D. (1995). *Using prebreeding weight, reproductive tract score and pelvic area to evaluate prebreeding development of replacement heifers*. Proceedings: Beef Improvement Federation 27th Research Symposium and Annual Meeting. Sheridan, Wyoming, pp. 174–177.

Patterson, D.J., Corah, L.R., Kiracofe, G.H., Stevenson, J.S. and Brethour, J.R. (1989). Conception rate in Bos taurus and Bos indicus crossbred heifers after postweaning energy manipulation and synchronization of oestrus with melengestrol acetate and fenprostalene. *Journal of Animal Science* **67**, 1138–1147.

Patterson, H.H., Adams, D.C., Klopfenstein, T.J., Clark, R.T. and Reichert, B. (2003). Supplementation to meet metabolizable protein requirements of primiparous beef heifers: II. Pregnancy and economics. *Journal of Animal Science* **81**, 563–570.

Pennel, P.L., Zalesky, D.D., Day, M.L., Wolfe, M.W., Stumpf, T.T., Azzam, S.M. *et al.* (1986). Influence of bull exposure on initiation of oestrous cycles in prepubertal beef heifers. *Journal of Animal Science* **63**(Suppl. 1), 129 (Abstract).

Price, T.D. and Wiltbank, J.N. (1978). Predicting dystocia in heifers. *Theriogenology* **9**, 221–249.

Roberson, M.S., Wolf, M.W., Stumpf, T.T., Werth, L.A., Cupp, A.S., Kojima, N. *et al.* (1991). Influence of growth rate and exposure to bulls on age at puberty in beef heifers. *Journal of Animal Science* **69**, 2092–2098.

Sacco, R.E., Baker, J.F. and Cartwright, T.C. (1987). Production characteristics of primiparous females of a five-breed diallel. *Journal of Animal Science* **64**, 1612–1618.

Schillo, K.K., Hansen, P.J., Kamwanja, L.A., Dierschke, D.J. and Hauser, E.R. (1983). Influence of season on sexual development in heifers: age at puberty as related to growth and serum concentrations of gonadotropins, prolactin, thyroxine and progesterone. *Biology of Reproduction* **28**, 329–341.

Selk, G.E., Wettemann, R.P., Lusby, K.S., Oltjen, J.W., Mobley, S.L., Rasby, R.J. and Garmendia, J.C. (1988). Relationships among weight change, body condition and reproductive performance of range beef cows. *Journal of Animal Science* **66**, 3153–3159.

Shaffer, K.S., Turk, P., Wagner, W.R. and Felton, E.E.D. (2011). Residual feed intake, body composition, and fertility in yearling beef heifers. *Journal of Animal Science* **89**, 1028–1034.

Short, R.E. and Bellows, R.A. (1971). Relationships among weight gains, age at puberty and reproductive performance in heifers. *Journal of Animal Science* **32**, 127–131.

Short, R.E., Bellows, R.A., Carr, J.B., Staigmiller, R.B. and Randel, R.D. (1976). Induced or synchronized puberty in beef heifers. *Journal of Animal Science* **43**, 1254–1258.

Short, R.E., Staigmiller, R.B., Bellows, R.A. and Greer, R.C. (1990). Breeding heifers at one year of age: Biological and economic considerations. In: *Proceedings 39th Annual Beef Cattle Short Course*. pp 93–106. Univ. of Florida, Gainesville.

Spitzer, J.C. (1982). Pregnancy rate in peripubertal beef heifers following treatment with Syncro-Mate B and GnRH. *Theriogenology* **17**, 373–381.

Spitzer, J.C., Morrison, D.G., Wettemann, R.P. and Faulkner, L.C. (1995). Reproductive responses and calf birth and weaning weights as affected by body condition at parturition and postpartum weight gain in primiparous beef cows. *Journal of Animal Science* **73**, 1251–1257.

Stewart, T.S., Long, C.R. and Cartwright, T.C. (1980). Characterization of cattle of a five-breed diallel. III. Puberty in bulls and heifers. *Journal of Animal Science* **50**, 808–820.

Van Donkersgoed, J., Ribble, C.S., Townsend, H.G.G. and Janzen, E.D. (1990). The usefulness of pelvic measurements as an on-farm test for predicting calving difficulty in beef heifers. *The Canadian Veterinary Journal* **31**, 190–193.

Whittier, W.D., Eller, A.L. and Beal, W.E. (1994). Management changes to reduce dystocia in virgin beef heifers. *Agri-Practice* **15**(1), 26–32.

Wiltbank, J.N., Kasson, C.W. and Ingalls, J.E. (1969). Puberty in crossbred and straightbred beef heifers on two levels of feed. *Journal of Animal Science* **29**, 602–605.

Wiltbank J,N., Roberts, S., Nix, J. and Rowden, L. (1985). Reproductive performance and profitability of heifers fed to weigh 272 or 318 kg at the start of the first breeding season. *Journal of Animal Science* **60**, 25–34.

Wright, I.A., Rhind, S.M., Whyte, T.K. and Smith, A.J. (1992). Effects of body condition at calving and feeding level after calving on LH profiles and the duration of the post-partum anoestrous period in beef cows. *Animal Production* **55**, 41–46.

Yilmaz, A., Davis, M.E. and Simmen, R.C.M. (2006). Analysis of female reproductive traits in Angus beef cattle divergently selected for blood serum insulin-like growth factor I concentration. *Theriogenology* **65**, 1180–1190.

CHAPTER 51
Cattle Housing: Design and Management

Jamie Robertson

Learning objectives

- Understand the relative importance of environmental factors on animal physiology.
- Understand the relative importance of environmental factors on pathogen survival.
- Be able to discern which of the key environmental factors may be impacting on health in individual case and group situations; moisture, air quality, air speed, temperature or mechanical impact.
- Be able to decide which design aspect of a building or system is contributing to failure to manage the key environmental variables.
- Be able to source information on design parameters including ventilation competence.
- Be able to compile a farm audit questionnaire and perform an audit.
- Be able to communicate the important outcomes of the farm audit.

Environmental impact

The weather is the constant, changeable bundle of environmental factors that influence so much of what the producer and the practitioner have to consider with regard to animal health. The basic appreciation of the pressures placed by climate on cattle production is a major reason for attempting to modify that climate and placing animals in a shelter or a building. The impact of sun, wind and rain are all modified by housing livestock, but not always to the benefit of animal health and welfare.

Respiratory infections in cattle are a classic example of a health risk that can be strongly influenced by the weather. Consideration of risk periods in the UK would indicate that periods of high humidity coinciding with lower wind speeds can be associated with an increased prevalence of respiratory symptoms in cattle of all ages. Similarly, there can be a relationship between periods of extreme diurnal air temperature variation and increased risk of respiratory infection. Alban *et al.* (1999) describe an analysis of the trigger factors for outbreaks of enzootic pneumonia in ten Danish dairy herds, with outdoor climate playing a key role. Periods of increased respiratory symptoms were associated with seven day averages of cold (0°C) and higher-humidity weather, compared with colder temperatures (−5°C) and marginally lower humidity. Many authors have similar results, which should direct the practitioner towards an understanding of the reasons why and, thereby, to formulating management strategies to deal with the problems.

It has been suggested that any assessment of the contribution of the environment, and particularly the built environment, to any animal health problem should be carried out not by initial examination of the building 'design', but by diagnosis of which particular environmental variable is influencing the problem. Buildings are complex, many designs are inappropriate, and tomorrow they may function in a different manner. The assessment process of a health problem that may have a significant environmental component needs only to consider the role of moisture, air speed, air quality and temperature. If there is a problem, there will either be too much or too little of one or more of these vital ingredients. If the relevant environmental variable can be identified, there is a much greater probability that the practical limitations of a specific building or system can be identified.

Air speed

The effect of shelter on the physiology of cattle is substantial, whether from wind speed, rainfall or solar gain. The main

Bovine Medicine, Third Edition. Edited by Peter D. Cockcroft.

impact on cattle in the UK and northern Europe is from the energy losses and potential physiological stress caused by wind chill, whereby the negative effect of air speed across an animal is compounded by low air temperatures. There are problems for health and welfare at higher temperatures, too, and the combination of higher metabolic rates from high genetic potential animals and increased duration of housing means that air speed needs to be managed to support health at both ends of the thermal comfort range.

Adult cattle are not typically considered to be under physiological pressure from UK weather conditions. A small degree of shelter is beneficial, and the benefits are greater for animals on lower energy intakes. It is instructive, however, to consider the impact of air speed on the lower critical temperatures of growing and adult stock, and to make a judgement as to whether air speed at any particular location may be contributing to physiological stress.

The situation presented by young cattle under UK winter weather conditions is actually quite clear. It is entirely predictable that youngstock less than four weeks old will be subjected to cold stress, and that the duration of stress will be massively and significantly influenced by the air speed at animal level. Table 51.1 refers to the lower critical temperatures of youngstock, and reference to weather data indicates that, with air temperature as a single environmental factor, young cattle in the UK are predictably at risk of physiological stress in the winter months. Table 51.2 shows the confounding effect of temperature, air speed and damp on the LCT of youngstock.

The impact of the environmental variables of air temperature, air speed, rainfall and solar radiation have been successfully modelled to estimate the thermal losses from cattle. In a series of experiments with scale models and full scale trials, Jones & Bruce (1985) and others demonstrated the thermal dynamics of different cattle systems provided with different levels of shelter. Growing cattle are not exempt from the risk of thermal stress under typical housing conditions, particularly when feed intake drops for any reason and the built environment is less than competent. Table 51.3 demonstrates that, even at 200–300 kg live weight (LW), animals with reduced intake of a high metabolisability diet will be below their lower critical temperature (LCT) during ambient winter conditions, even before the impact of damp bedding or elevated air speeds are taken into consideration.

The idea that housing is protecting cattle from thermal stress needs to be checked on site. Damp bedding and wet floors are too common to be ignored, and the air speed between buildings and pens and along walkways and feeding areas is often higher than the ambient conditions.

Table 51.1 Lower critical temperature of calves. Reproduced with permission of University of Exeter.

Effect of air speed, calf weight and feed level on lower critical temperature (Webster, 1981)

Type of calf	Lower critical temperature °C at air speeds of:	
	0.2 m/sec	2.0 m/sec
New born (35 kg)	+9	+17
One month old (50 kg)	0	+9
Veal calf (100 kg)	−14	−1

Table 51.2 Lower critical temperature of youngstock. Reproduced with permission of Aberdeen, Scottish Farm Buildings, Investigation Unit.

Metabolisability	Live weight gain kg/day	LTC °C 100 kg heifers of large breed		
		Air speed		Damp bed
		0.5 m/sec	2.0 m/sec	
0.5	0	11.9	20.9	17.9
	0.25	8.2	17.2	14.2
	0.5	3.1	12.1	9.1
	0.75	−4.2	4.8	1.8
	1	−15.5	−6.5	−9.5
0.7	0	14.7	23.7	20.7
	0.25	12.6	21.6	18.6
	0.5	10	19	16
	0.75	6.6	15.6	12.6
	1	2.2	11.2	8.2

Air quality

The role of air quality can be critical in the survival rates of many pathogens. The impact on respiratory pathogens has been demonstrated clearly in the work of C.S Cox and others (Cox, 1987), and needs to be considered for other cattle environmental pathogens such as *E. coli* and *S. uberis*. Improving the air quality substantially reduced the survival rate of aerosolised *E. coli* compared with less fresh air. The physical factors relevant to this association are relative humidity (RH), temperature and open air factor (OAF), and all determine survival and decay rates of a number of bacteria and viruses involved in animal health problems. The aerial environment can produce surface inactivation of bacteriophages during aerosolisation of particles and, while the damage may be temporary, the effect will be to reduce infectivity rates. In addition, the ability of a bacteriophage to survive and return to original infectivity depends on the surrounding nutrients in the environment and the broader picture of air quality. Exposure to fresh air circulation is vital to respiratory health and also for environmental mastitis when either *E. coli* or *S. uberis* are present within a straw-bedded structure or on the surface of cubicles (Robertson, 2010).

Table 51.3 The impact of diet, intake, live weight and breed on LCT at air speed 0.5 m/sec. Reproduced with permission of Aberdeen, Scottish Farm Buildings, Investigation Unit.

Metabolisability	Live weight gain	Lower critical temperature (°C) for cattle of live weight:				Lower critical temperature (°C) for cattle of live weight:			
		100 kg	200 kg	300 kg	500 kg	100 kg	200 kg	300 kg	500 kg
		Bulls of large mature size				Bulls of small mature size			
0.5	0	7.5	2.8	−0.5	−5.4	7.5	2.8	−0.5	−5.4
	0.25	5.1	0.4	−3	−8.2	3.9	−0.8	−4.2	−9.5
	0.5	2	−2.6	−6.2	−11.6	−0.9	−5.4	−9.1	−14.7
	0.75	−1.9	−6.4	−10.1	−15.8	−7.6	−11.7	−15.6	−21
	1	−7	−11.2	−15.1	−21.2	−17.4	−20.5	−24.6	−31.5
0.7	0	10.7	6.5	3.5	−2.7	10.7	6.5	3.5	−0.9
	0.25	9.3	5.1	2	−4.4	8.7	4.4	1.3	−3.3
	0.5	7.7	3.4	0.3	−6.3	6.2	1.9	−1.3	−6.1
	0.75	5.7	1.4	−1.8	−8.6	3	−1.2	−4.5	−9.6
	1	3.2	−0.9	−4.2	−11.4	−1.1	−5	−8.5	−14

Moisture

Competent flooring, drainage, roofing and management all impact on moisture levels within a building, and the design, use and management of materials can all effect the competence of hygiene practices. However, a prime factor that mediates the interaction of the built environment, moisture and animal health is ventilation.

Ventilation is the mechanism by which the accumulated airborne waste products from cattle systems are removed from a building and replaced by clean, fresh air. Two of the main constituents of animal house air that are non-pathogenic, but have a significant role in animal health and productivity, are heat (energy) and moisture. The target of good building design is to manage the expected dynamics of heat and moisture to the extent that they are not allowed to accumulate. It is the accumulation and excess of heat and moisture within animal systems that increases the probability of physiological stress, increases non-productive animal behaviours, and frequently provides an improved environment for bacterial and viral survival. Competent ventilation is an absolute requirement to manage heat and moisture in cattle buildings.

There has been much conflicting information concerning the design of ventilation for naturally ventilated buildings. This is unfortunate, because the original model that became internationally accepted was published in 1975 (Bruce, 1975), and has been republished by DairyCo (2012). The requirements are for an appropriately sized area in the roof structure to let the expected thermal and moisture load to be exhausted by the warmed air rising. The effect of the exhaust air leaving the building is to bring an equal volume of clean, fresh air into the building. and for a reasonable distribution of that air amongst the cattle.

Naturally ventilated buildings are ventilated most of the time (>80%) by the power of the wind. This can be well managed, but the negative aspects of air speed need to be kept under control. Apart from high-yielding cattle housed under warmer conditions, there is a design requirement to control air speed to below 2 m/sec at animal height, with a target of 0.5 m/sec.

Approximately 50% of all cattle buildings assessed for ventilation capacity alone are not competent. The most common failings are:

- inadequate outlet area in the roof;
- inadequate air inlet area in the walls;
- poor distribution of air inlets, leaving areas of poor air movement.

Conversely, some buildings are designed and/or managed so that there is too much air speed over the cattle.

Building competence

Moderation of climate by building structures is obvious, but there are two major areas where housed animal systems are not fulfilling requirements. The first is in the competence of the building designs, whereby one or more features that are intended to protect animals from extremes of climate either accentuate an environmental pressure or create a new one. The second area of default is in the materials, construction and maintenance of animal buildings.

To take the aspects of building construction, materials and maintenance first, there are a number of areas where the practitioner can check to see if any of these factors may contribute to an environmental influence on health. The most common failure is that buildings and surfaces are not constructed as they are detailed at the design stage. For example, floor slopes and floor surfaces that are not competent can lead to pooling of wastes, increase moisture levels in a building, increase numbers of dirty cattle and contribute to mastitis and foot problems. Any subsequent losses are a result of increased pressure on the cattle or increased environmental support of commensals and pathogens. Losses will not be diminished until the source of the original problem is corrected. Attention to detail in the construction of ventilation systems is also variable, and failure to apply planned design detail is a common observation.

Clear design parameters have been available since 1990, and current details relevant to dairy cow housing are available in Dairy Housing: a best practice guide (DairyCo, 2012) and, for beef cattle, in Better Cattle Housing Design (EBLEX, 2013).

Materials used in cattle buildings have been subject to very little design attention over the past 20 years, leaving a range of threats and opportunities with respect to cattle health. The main focus should be on how the physical and chemical properties of a material contribute to a building system that is productive and sustainable. In animal husbandry terms, the system needs to support health and provide a return of investment. However, in the UK at least, there appears to be a devotion to concrete and steel, with some timber used for cladding. While the durability of concrete and steel is hard to question (even if the investment appraisal is often lacking), their thermal properties mean that they cannot be supportive of a positive environment for young cattle under UK winter conditions. They are, in effect, cold materials.

Steel cladding and, especially, steel roofing can contribute to a predictable environmental risk for young stock. Steel is a good conductor of energy and will transfer heat in and out of a building rapidly. Thus, a steel-clad space for youngstock will nearly always be as cold as the ambient air temperature, apart from when the sun is shining, when there can be significant solar gain. The result is a building that will be cold through the winter, apart from days of bright sun, followed by cold, clear nights, when the diurnal air temperatures inside the structure will be at a maximum range, providing ideal conditions for respiratory stress.

The final physical aspect of buildings and their contribution to environmental competence is maintenance. Generally, cattle buildings in the UK are of simple design and construction, and need little maintenance. Relevant areas of weakness are the competence of concrete surfaces and maintenance of gutters and downpipes. A building for 200 cows might have 1500 m^2 of concrete cubicles and floors and, in a location with 1000 mm of rainfall per annum, will manage 1500 tonnes of rainwater from just one roof. The potential for supporting the survival and spread of pathogens is substantial if the building structure is not well maintained.

Floors

The physical impact of animal hooves, tractors and scrapers on concrete floors will produce a smoother surface over time. This will significantly impact on animal health and welfare, as well as human health and safety. Grooving of concrete floors has appreciable cost benefits, with benefits accruing from:

- Improved cow confidence and movement.
- Safer environment for bulling.
- Reduction in foot problems and associated costs.
- Reduced risks of animal slips/injury/culling.
- Improved drainage of surface water.

There are field-based reports that grooving previously unsatisfactory concrete flooring has improved fertility in herds, with the assumption being that cattle were showing a standing heat better and were standing for longer, making it easier to be recognised. Cow comfort is of significant benefit to cattle health and productivity, and the floor plays a major part. Rubber matting is being used increasingly as a cost-effective investment in cattle housing, not only for cubicle mats but also for feeding stances and slats:

- Increased lying comfort.
- Improved heat insulation.
- Improved slip resistance.
- Reduced risks of slips/injury/culling.
- Enhanced weight gain (on slats).

Hygiene

In a study designed to investigate those management factors that may have an influence on shedding rates of *Eschericia coli* 0157 by beef cows, the state of being housed was considered the most important of the influencing factors (Synge *et al.*, 2003). While the potential interactions between factors in and around housing are complex, the authors site further work that found that feed mangers and water bowls had the highest possible rates of positivity for VTEC 0157.

Pen hygiene has a major role to play on animal health. A restricted spatial environment will always increase infection pressures on stock, and excretion of viable pathogens into the pen environment can be better managed. For example, the average duration of shedding of *Salmonella Dublin* from groups of calves on four endemically infected herds was found to be 17 days (Neilsen *et al.*, 2006), and is indicative of the need to provide a 'sick pen' in order to manage animal health at a herd level.

There is major benefit to be gained from improving the standards of hygiene in calf housing. Too many systems are not competent in cleanability, drainage, moisture levels, and air quality and air speed, and the practitioner is too often asked to solve health problems without an honest appraisal of the calf house environment.

Light

There should be an appropriate amount and duration of lighting to ensure that welfare needs are met.

Table 51.4 Appraisal of housed cow behaviour: a checklist.

Cow behaviour			Yes/No check
Variable	**Detail**	**Cause/effect**	
Macro	Cow location within shed – preferred locations?	Significant environmental differences within shed	
	Stance – alert/submissive	Environmental stress?	
	Productivity?	Appropriate for feed/ genetics/system.	
	• Appropriate access to water	Feed area too exposed?	
	• Appropriate access to feed	Must suit demand.	
	• Appropriate space per animal		
	Nervousness? • Bullying • Poor building layout • Stray voltage • Restricted visibility	• poor access feed/water • poor access lying areas • dark, single entry/ exit?	
	Coat/hair condition – stark, or heavy hair growth	Indicative of cold and/or exposure	
Micro	Leg/hock lesions	Cubicle length, bedding	
	Foot/claw condition	Floor surface/condition/ pooling. Poor slats.	
	Dirty lower legs	Excess dirty water, pooling, poor drainage in walkways, short/long cubicles	
	Dirty udder/teats		
	Damaged teats/tails	Cubicle width/poor separation between beds	
	Neck lesions	Poor feed barrier design	
	Sweating	Poor ventilation	
		Too much solar gain	

Artificially increasing day length, combined with bolstering natural levels of light within a building, has been shown to be of benefit to dairy cows. Work undertaken at Bangor University demonstrated a 6% yield increase when cows were subjected to longer light periods with more intense light (Farm Energy Centre, 2001). Similar work in the USA has shown yield increases between 5–16% (Dahl, 1997). Cows should be exposed to between 16–18 hours of light each day to achieve the benefits of long-day photoperiod. The level of light required to trigger the response is around 200 lux.

As with any stimulation of milk production, long-day photoperiod treatment will pull an increase in dry matter intake (DMI), but in response to higher milk production rather than the opposite. In other words, cows do not eat more and then produce more milk. Rather, they produce more milk and consume more feed to meet the increased demand for energy to make that milk. Given a typical 2.5 kg/day response to long day photoperiod, a 1 kg/day increase in DMI should be planned for to support a higher milk yield.

It is widely accepted that photoperiod modulates the establishment of post-partum oestrous cycles and conception rates, with significant reduction in calving to oestrus periods and improved conception rates, compared with cows without 18L : 6D light supplementation.

Light for dry cows

Research from the USA suggested there are benefits to be obtained from manipulating daylight length for dry cows (Wall, 2005). The study agreed with work presented in 2000 (Miller, 2000), which demonstrated that dry animals which were subjected to a photoperiod which included eight hours daylight (>200 lux) and 16 hours of darkness (20 lux), produced 3.2 kg/day more milk than dry cows subjected to a more typical eight hours darkness and 16 hours daylight. This practice is significantly easier to achieve during the winter months, although dry animals housed in early spring and autumn may also benefit.

The observations above means that dry cows should not remain under the same lighting as lactating cows. Light intensity above 50 lux has been shown to decrease melatonin concentrations, which is the normal feedback of a period of adequate 'dark'.

Mechanistically, it appears that prolactin has a causal relationship with the observed dairy performance effects during the dry period, and also on immune function, via altered sensitivity to prolactin (Dahl & Petitclerc, 2003). There is a clear improvement in cellular immune function in cattle on short-day photoperiod (SDPP) relative to long-day photoperiod. The relationship with immune function is a further reason for management

Table 51.5 Visual appraisal of the building: a checklist.

Building visual appraisal			Yes/No check
Variable	**Detail**	**Cause/effect**	
Orientation	Prevailing wind direction?	Influences wind chill, air quality within unit, water ingress, ventilation efficiency, solar gain.	
	Low frequency but harsh weather direction?	Probability of wind chill, low temperatures.	
Protection	Walls and surrounding structures • Total: lack of fresh air. • Competent under most weathers? • Partial – draughts? • Exposed – wind chill, rain?	 • Common on exposed sites. • Target requirement. Increases outside air speed. Underestimated in UK.	
	Gaps below doors and gates.	High wind chill at animal height.	
	Solar gain – negative effects: • Roof lights excessive? • Roof materials. • Insulation?	Good light, too much heat? Thermal properties – tin is poor; heats and cools rapidly. Not yet common in UK.	
	Solar gain – positive effects: • Roof lights. • Access to direct sunlight.	Value of natural light.	
Moisture	Areas of standing damp, high straw usage, lowered stocking density, poor air quality, etc.	Increased moisture levels often beneficial to bacterial and viral survival, will decrease LCT, and will reduce ambient temperatures.	
Floors	**Drainage:** • Competent. • Partial. • Poor.	If a floor is not competent, it will never be competent until it is changed.	
	Too rough, too smooth.	Risks of mechanical foot/leg damage.	
Lighting	Light ≥ 200 lux; dark ≤ 20 lux.	Major impact on reproductive efficiencies and milk yields.	
Materials	Concrete and steel extensive. Tin roofing. Straw quality? Sawdust quality? Recycled materials? • Shredded timber. • Shredded plasterboard. • Gypsum.	Significant heat sink. Poor insulation properties. Moulds, mycotoxins, dust. Moulds, mycotoxins, dust. • timber/screws, nails. • teat lesions/H_2S risk • H_2S risk in slurry	
Surrounding buildings	Major impact on fresh air delivery, ventilation effectiveness, disease transmission.	Contributory factor to problems?	

to pay attention to the detail of lighting, with the prospect of minimising negative environmental impact on health by astute control of the housing conditions. The DairyCo housing guide (DairyCo, 2012) contains practical guidance on lighting requirements and installation of lighting systems.

Biosecurity

The idea of using space as a health management tool is well established. Physical isolation of animals will inherently reduce the opportunities for either importing or exporting pathogens,

Table 51.6 Ventilation appraisal: a checklist.

Ventilation Appraisal Variable	Detail	Effect	Yes/No check
Ventilation – natural	Is ventilation competent? Animal location indicating clean/stale areas? Signs of condensation? • Stained purlins • Dark staining of roof sheets • Cobwebs	Stale air? Areas of building not ventilated? Dominant cows in preferred locations. Ventilation is principal mechanism for removing airborne moisture from building.	
	Excess accumulation of moisture in bedding?	Excessive straw use; dirty cows, mitigation by reduced stocking density.	
	Smell • Damp. • Traces of ammonia.	Poor air quality.	
	Adequate outlet in roof (ridge)?	Ball park 0.04 m^2 per calf, rising to 0.1 m^2 per adult.	
	Adequate inlet area in side walls?	Minimum twice the outlet area; optimum four times outlet area.	
	Inlets very open – no restriction of air speed.	Air speeds↑↑ = lower LCT; reduce productivity, increase risk of immune suppression.	
	Inlet area shared with older animals?	Sharing pathogens?	
	Inlets pulling dirty air from area with older animals?	Sharing pathogens (e.g. from adjacent buildings)?	
	Dirty air spilling in from adjacent poorly ventilated spaces with older cows?	For example, collecting yards.	
Ventilation – mechanical	Clean fans and components? Positive pressure fans (blowing): • Blowing clean air or dirty air? • Is air intake inside or outside building? • Is air distributed through a duct?	Clean blades worth 10% efficiency. Air is only as clean as the source air. As air travels through a building it will accumulate moisture, gases, heat, dusts and microbes.	
	Is there adequate outlet in roof?	Inadequate outlets increase the risk of airborne disease transmission within a space.	
	Negative pressure fans (sucking): • Is fan located where stale air will accumulate naturally? • Is fan effective?	Impact of negative pressure fan is extremely local. Fan needs to be located where stale air accumulates naturally.	
Cooling fans	Is the air driven by cooling fans leaving the building?	Check for accumulations of stale air within buildings	
	Is air driven by cooling fans directed across the backs of cows?	Cooling effect of 1–2°C requires elevated air speed across cows' backs.	
	Addition of fine water spray.	Creates additional cooling.	

and the scale of any space between a source of pathogen and a potential host is usually significantly associated with the degree of risk. However, a number of false assumptions or misconceptions may be observed in practice, and the difficulty with these is that the participants may well be expecting a degree of protection or risk management for their business which is actually not present:

- Effective separation distance for respiratory pathogens is >3 km.
- Spatial correlation for *Salmonella Dublin* outbreaks estimated at between 2–17 km, depending on regional prevalence and other factors (Erksbøll & Nielson, 2007).
- The 'footprint' of downwind impact of one building on another is 10–15 times a building height, such that it is predictable that aerosols will be drawn downwards in vigorous eddies within that range.
- Biosecure separation is seldom achieved in practice within commercial cattle farms.

Physical and biological security is seldom achieved at herd/farm level in the cattle sector. In many ways, this provides an opportunity for improving cattle health; improving conditions around farms will limit the casual spread of pathogens. The attention to detail in infrastructure, resources and training required for effective biosecurity can be observed in many parts of the commercial poultry sector. The key issues practiced are:

- Effective security of boundaries; front gate for personnel and vehicles, building physical security against vermin, foot dips for inter-building hygiene.
- Structures that are designed to be cleanable.
- Standard operating procedures for cleaning and disinfection.
- Management practice that monitors effectiveness.
- Effective isolation facilities.

With reference to the impact of environmental factors on health management, there is opportunity to improve both individual animal and herd biosecurity by application of simple observations:

- Physical barriers, if competent, can be very effective.
- Upwind is always 'cleaner' than downwind.
- Distance will reduce effective dose rates in many circumstances, but will seldom eliminate risk at within farm level.
- Surfaces, materials, slopes and drainage that are suitable for cleaning, are easier to clean.
- The ability to provide a dry environment, or a period of dryness and cleanliness, decreases survival rates of many pathogens.

Appraisal of buildings

Checklists for the appraisal of buildings are provided above in Tables 51.4 (Cows), 51.5 (buildings) and 51.6 (ventilation).

References

Alban, L., Larsen, L.E., Chriel, M., Tegtmeier, C. and Nielsen, T.K. (1999). *The occurrence of clinical outbreaks of enzootic pneumonia in calves in ten Danish Dairy herds during the winter 1996–1997: Descriptive results.* Proceedings, Bristol 24th–26th March, Society for Veterinary Epidemiology and Preventative Medicine, pp. 118–130.

Bruce, J.M. (1975). Natural ventilation of cattle buildings by thermal buoyancy. *Farm Building Progress* **42**, 17–20.

Bruce, J.M. (1986). Lower critical temperatures for housed beef cattle. *Farm Building Progress* **84**, 23–28.

Cox, C.S. (1987). *The aerobiological pathway of microorganisms.* John Wiley & Sons, Chichester. ISBN 0 471 91170 4

Dahl, G.E. (1997). Effects of Long Daily Photoperiod on Milk Yield and Circulating Concentrations of Insulin Growth Factor – 1. *Journal of Dairy Science* **80**, 2784–2789.

Dahl, G.E. and Petitclerc, D. (2003). Management of photoperiod in the dairy herd for improved production and health *Journal of Animal Science* **81**, 11–17.

DairyCo (2012). *Dairy Housing: a best practice guide.* www.dairyco.org.uk/resources-library/technical-information/dairy-housing-a-best-practice-guide/

EBLEX (2013). *Better Cattle Housing Design.* http://www.eblex.org.uk/returns/brp/

Erksbøll, K. and Nielson, L.R (2007). *Distances between neighbouring herds of relevance for local spread of Salmonella Dublin between cattle herds on Denmark.* Proceedings, Helsinki , 28th – 30th March, Society for Veterinary Epidemiology and Preventative Medicine, pp. 51–62.

Farm Energy Centre (2001). *Supplemental Light for Dairy Cows.* TN67.pm65/11.01

Jones, C.G. and Bruce, J.M (1985). Shelter studies using thermal models of cattle. *Progress in Biometeorology* **2**, 83–98.

Miller, A.R.E. (2000). Effects of Photoperiodic Manipulation During the Dry Period of Dairy Cows. *Journal of Dairy Science* **83**, 962–967.

Nielsen L.R., Van Den Borne B.H.P. and Van Schaik G. (2006) *Estimation of infection transmission parameters for* Salmonella Dublin *in young dairy calves.* Proceedings, Exeter 29th–31st March, Society for Veterinary Epidemiology and Preventative Medicine, pp. 179–190.

Robertson, J. (2010). *Ventilation and its impact on mastitis control.* Proceedings of the British Mastitis Conference, Sixways, Worcester, 63–73.

Synge, B.A., Chase-Topping, M.E., Hopkins, G.F., McKendrick, I.J., Thomson-Carter, F., Gray, D., Rusbridge, S.M., Munro, F.I., Foster, G. and Gunn, G.J. (2003). Factors influencing the shedding of verocytotoxin-producing *Escherichia coli* 0157 by beef suckler cows. *Epidemiologial Infections* **130**, 301–312.

Wall, E.H. (2005). Effect of Short-day Photoperiod During the Dry Period on the mammary Gland of the Dairy Cow. *Journal of Dairy Science* **88**, 3145–3148.

Webster, A.J.F. (1981). *Weather and infectious diseases in cattle.* Proceedings, BVA Congress, 17–20 September 1981, University of Exeter.

Further reading

CIGR Handbook of Agricultural Engineering Volume II, Animal Production & Aquacultural Engineering (1999). The American Society of Agricultural Engineers, ISBN 0-929355-98-9. www.cigr.org/documents/CIGRhandbookVol2.pdf

CHAPTER 52

Bovine Respiratory Disease (BRD): Diagnosis, Prevention and Control

Peter D. Cockcroft

Learning objectives

- Understand the role of the veterinarian in the control and prevention of bovine respiratory disease.
- Appreciate the important risk factors in the epidemiology of the disease.
- Understand the further investigative techniques, samples and diagnostic tests that can be employed to characterise an outbreak or high incidence of BRD.
- Appreciate how the risk of BRD can be reduced.

Introduction

This chapter will review the diagnosis, prevention and control of respiratory disease in dairy calves, weaned suckler calves and growing beef animals entering the feedlot or being finished in semi-intensive finishing systems. Respiratory disease caused by lungworm (*Dictyolcaulus viviparous*), chronic lung infections (*Trueperella pyogenes*), fog fever (L-tryptophan), 'metastatic' pneumonia (e.g. caudal vena-cava syndrome) and upper airway conditions (e.g. necrotic laryngitis) will not be covered in this chapter.

Bovine Respiratory Disease (BRD) is a common and important condition in feedlots and growing, housed cattle. These respiratory syndromes are often known collectively as bovine respiratory disease (BRD), and may include 'shipping fever', 'enzootic calf pneumonia' and the bovine respiratory disease complex (BRDC). The veterinarian has an important role in the identification and assessment of risk factors – the diagnosis and characterisation of the causal pathogens, the selection of appropriate vaccines and protocols for the recognition, isolation and treatment of affected animals.

In beef feedlots there is an increased risk of BRD, with high morbidity and mortality rates. Bovine respiratory disease causes decreased weight gains, decreased feed utilisation, decreased carcass quality and increased prophylaxis and therapy costs, leading to enormous economic losses. A national survey of the US beef industry (NAHMS, 2000) found that 14.4% of cattle placed in US feedlots acquired the disease. This disease accounts for 75% of all disease outbreaks in feedlots, and is responsible for 50–70% of all feedlot mortalities (Loneragan *et al.*, 2001; Edwards, 2010). The direct and indirect costs of each treated case have been estimated at US$ 92 (Schneider *et al.*, 2009).The cost to the industry is several billion dollars in treatment, prevention and control (Griffin, 2006; Snowder *et al.*, 2007).

Urban-Chmiel & Groom (2012) have reviewed the control and prevention of BRD, with a focus on feedlots, which summarises much of the recent literature. Reviews on BRD can also be found in Cooper & Brodersen (2010a). Cusack *et al.* (2004) provide a review of the epidemiology and medicine of bovine respiratory disease in feedlots. Taylor *et al.* (2010a, 2010b) reviewed the risk factors and preventative measures used in bovine respiratory disease. Lorenz *et al.* (2011) reviewed the literature on calf housing and pneumonia. Other chapters in this book also provide additional information.

The pathogens

Recognised pathogenic viruses are: bovine pestivirus (bovine viral diarrhoea virus (BVDV), infectious bovine rhinotracheitis (BHV-1, IBR) bovine parainfluenza-3 (PI-3), corona virus and bovine respiratory syncytial virus (BRSV). The bacteria commonly isolated from clinical BRD have been identified as *Mannheimia haemolytica* (formerly *Pasteurella haemolytica*),

Bovine Medicine, Third Edition. Edited by Peter D. Cockcroft.

Pasteurella multocida, *Histophilus somni* (formally *Haemophilus somnus*) and *Mycoplasma bovis*. These bacteria can all be found as commensal in the upper airways. Bovine viral diarrhoea virus (BVDV) appears to play an important role, both in terms of immune suppression and synergistic effects with other pathogens.

Epidemiology

Bovine respiratory disease complex is associated with risk factors which lower the immune system and increase the susceptibility to viral and bacterial pathogens. The risk factors include stressors such as transport, and environmental conditions such as high dust levels and humidity levels. Viral, bacterial or mycoplasmal pathogens can cause primary disease, but may also compromise the defence mechanisms of the respiratory system, allowing other pathogens to become established in the lower airways. Mixed infections in BRD are common. Most cases of BRD in feedlots occur in the first three weeks following arrival and decline up to week 12.

Housed dairy calves and weaned suckler calves

The risk of pneumonia is related to the pathogenic challenge and the competency of the calf's natural defence mechanisms. The pathogenic load is dependent upon the ventilation rate of the house, the humidity, the stocking density and the prevalence of pathogens in the group. The calf's natural defences consist of the immune system and the upper airway defence mechanisms that reduce the risk of infection reaching the lower airways. The immune system is supplemented by the successful passive transfer maternal immunoglobulins in the neonate by the timely ingestion of sufficient quantities of colostrum. Stress will reduce the capability of the immune system to combat infections, due to the release of cortisol, causing immunosuppression. Castration, dehorning/disbudding, handling and weaning are examples of stressors. Cold may also be a stress in cooler northern winters, unless sufficient dry bedding is supplied.

The accumulation of noxious gases such as ammonia can reduce the efficiency of the natural physical defences such as the mucco-ciliary escalator in the trachea, with an increased risk of pneumonia. Urine and faeces release ammonia into the atmosphere. The provision of dry straw and regular removal will reduce the concentration of ammonia in the air, and increased ventilation rates will also reduce ammonia concentrations. Ammonia levels of less than 10 ppm are recommended. Higher humidity is associated with higher and more viable pathogen loads in the air. In housed cattle in winter, humidity often exceeds 85%, and it can be difficult to reduce this.

The pathogenic load is usually increased by mixing animals from different sources and by mixing different age groups. The older calves pose a higher risk to the younger calves. This co-mingling increases the range of pathogens that the younger calves are exposed to.

Calves which are kept in stable groups have a lower risk of pneumonia compared to constantly changing dynamic groups. This may be due to increased social stress or an increase in the pathogenic challenge. Age-matched groups also have a reduced risk. The use of appropriately designed, managed and sited outdoor hutches reduces the risk of pneumonia, compared to groups of calves housed indoors. Individual pens indoors also reduce the risk, compared to grouped housed calves. Legislation in the EU requires calves to have sight of other calves, and to be able to touch other calves if kept in individual pens. Calves must only be kept in individual pens up to the age of eight weeks.

Lorenz *et al.* (2011) have reviewed the literature and have referenced the following parameters for calf housing: at least four air changes per hour are needed in winter and up to 40 in summer. Natural ventilation is achieved through wind and the stack effect in monopitch or pitched houses, given that adequate air outlets (ridge opening: 5 cm width for every 3 m width of the building) and inlets (eave openings: at least half the space of ridge openings), as well as sufficient difference in height between the openings is provided (not less than 1.5 m, but preferably 2.5 m).

Recommended air space per calf is not less than 6 m^3 up to six weeks, and 10 m^3 up to 12 weeks old. Problems can arise in naturally ventilated calf barns in cold and damp wintry conditions, when it can be impossible to keep relative humidity below an acceptable level of 85%. Additionally, ventilation is often compromised by the closing of air inlets in an attempt to prevent cold stress for the calves. If calves are housed in individual pens indoors, the barn climate often does not reflect the microclimate in the pens. Ventilation is impaired, with an increasing numbers of solid panels surrounding the calf (solid walls in the back or front of the pen, top covers), leading to an increase in airborne microbes. Poly tents are now being used for dairy calf rearing, which have fan-driven ventilation systems that need to be regulated according to ambient temperatures and humidity levels.

Weaned suckler calves and the risk of pneumonia

Suckler calves are often spring-born in the northern hemisphere, and are normally weaned at 5–9 months of age. The calves which are not being retained as replacements will either enter an intensive feedlot system, or be raised in a semi-intensive system. Semi-intensive systems alternate housing in the cooler months with grazing in the warmer months. The best method to reduce the stress of weaning in cow and calf systems has not been clearly defined, with methods including sudden separation, line contact and the use of nose clips. Spring-born calves are housed in autumn and fed silage and concentrates. Dehorning, castration, vaccination and anthelmintic treatment are procedures which may also be timed to occur at weaning followed, in many cases, by immediate housing. Ideally, these events should occur 4–6 weeks before housing, and spaced to reduce the level of stress. Introducing concentrates in the form of creep feed before housing is beneficial. If the animals are destined for the feedlot or calf sales, this pre-conditioning will reduce the morbidity and mortality from BRD.

Pre-disposing factors for BRD in feedlot cattle

Animals destined for the feedlots or fattening yards experience a number of potential stressful changes. These may include: transport with variable journey times, routes and types of transport; handling (loading, unloading, induction); dehydration due to restricted availability or unfamiliarity with the water supply; hunger due to restricted availability or familiarity; co-mingling and regrouping; extremes in temperature; high humidity; and excessive dust.

Taylor *et al.* (2010a) have reviewed the scientific evidence for predisposing BRD factors. They reported that many factors are confounded in published studies and that appropriate studies are lacking for many of the factors currently thought to be important. Transport, sale barn calves, comingling and BVDV PI calves were risk factors which were supported by the research literature.

Host factors, environmental and management factors have been reviewed by Urban-Chmiel & Groom (2012). The risk of BRD is often increased with management practices that increase stress. These practices include weaning, transportation, diet changes, high stocking density, handling, and surgical procedures (dehorning, castration). Mixing of cattle, leading to changes in social structures, has been shown to be detrimental. Animals associated with a greater risk of BRD include: young cattle; cattle which have had long journey times; cattle purchased from sale yards; cattle purchased from vendors or regions whose cattle have a history of BRD; pens of cattle sourced from multiple vendors; and cattle in poor condition.

The disease

Some pathogens produce a specific clinical profile of signs. For example, RSV may cause lung emphysema with a characteristic crackling sound on lung field auscultation, whereas IBR may produce a severe tracheitis with paroxysmal coughing when the trachea is palpated. There may also be a severe conjunctivitis. Other outbreaks include multiple pathogens. Secondary bacterial infections are considered to be important in pneumonic disease pathology.

Death from BRD can occur within 24–36 hours of the onset of clinical signs, depending upon the causal pathogen(s). The infection can become chronic, with widespread, permanent lung fibrosis, adhesions and abscesses, with a decrease in performance. Early recognition and treatment of BRD is important to minimise these adverse changes. Signs of respiratory disease include: discharge from the eyes, nose and mouth; coughing; rapid, shallow breathing; extended head; red nose and dry muzzle; staring coat depression; lethargy; isolation; reduced appetite; pyrexia; dyspnoea; and increased respiratory rate and dehydration. Animals with rectal temperatures over 40°C and clinical signs should be treated. Sub-clinical or unrecognised BRD is apparent from abattoir surveys, where lung lesions are often present in animals which have no treatment record.

Pyrexia may be present 24–36 hours before other clinical signs are recognised. Once an outbreak has been recognised, measuring the temperatures of the remaining animals in the group will identify the pyrexic animals, which can then be treated early in the course of disease.

In housed, grouped calves, moving among the group and forcing them to stand and move allows the identification of affected animals due to the increase in dyspnoea and breathing rate. These animals are often reluctant to rise, and do not come up to feed when food is replenished in the food trough. If affected, dairy calves are individually penned, then anorexia is more easily noted and the temperature can be taken, as little restraint is required.

Further investigations

Once a provisional clinical diagnosis of BRD has been made, further characterisation of the problem may be required. Although diagnostic testing can provide valuable information when investigating the causes of respiratory disease within a group, veterinarians and producers should agree on the diagnostic question, testing goals and use of results, before submitting samples (Cooper & Brodersen, 2010b). The animals to be tested or sampled should be representative, untreated and in the early stages of the disease.

A clinical history and the following information should be obtained, so that the results can be interpreted in context (Cooper and Brodersen, (2010b):

1. Age range of affected animals and ages of animals sampled.
2. Age of onset or number of days since arrival (stocker or feedlot operation) and progression in herd.
3. Environment or housing or bedding.
4. Mortality and morbidity in comparison to past averages for groups. Changes in mortality and morbidity over the course of the problem.
5. Duration of illness of affected animals and individuals selected for sampling.
6. Duration of problem in the herd.
7. Clinical signs and sequence of onset. Changes in signs or severity since onset.
8. Treatments and their response. Any treatment given to animals sampled.

9 Common factors among affected animals.
10 Changes in management, preceding the onset of problem (new feed, new source, feed quality, component quantity).
11 Vaccination history.
12 Quarantine and isolation, if any.
13 Biosecurity efforts, if any.
14 Veterinarian's suspicion of problem's cause.
15 Owner's suspicion of problem's cause.

Although nasal and nasal pharyngeal swabs have been used to isolate IBR associated with disease, the significance of bacterial isolates is more difficult to interpret, as the pathogenic bacteria, such as *Mannhaemia haemolytica* and *Mycoplama bovis*, can be present as commensals. The preferred sampling technique is bronchio-alveolar lavage. This technique is described in Chapter 15. These samples can be used for cytology, viral indirect immuno-fluorescence tests (IFATs), bacterial and mycoplasmal culture, lungworm larval and PCR analysis. Ideally, samples from three or more affected animals should be samples, so that pathogen profiles can be compared. Faecal samples can be taken to screen for L3 *Dictyocaulus viviparous*. Serology can be used to indicate exposure to viral pathogens, but rising titres are necessary to confirm an active infection. The latter requires two blood samples, three weeks apart. A sample size of 6 is often recommended.

Post-mortem examinations can be usefully performed on sick, untreated, euthanised animals, or animals found dead within the last few hours. Confirmation that the cause of death was pneumonia is useful, and samples from untreated fresh cadavers may yield useful isolations and antimicrobial sensitivities. The following samples are suggested: lung section with affected/unaffected area (fresh and fixed in formalin), bronchial and tracheal lymph nodes (fresh and fixed in formalin), and serum. Histopathology, PCR, serology and bacterial culture may be able to characterise the pathology and causative agents responsible (Cooper & Brodersen, 2010b).

Treatment

Chapter 23, on the selection and use of antimicrobials, provides some useful guidelines for the treatment of pneumonia. Early recognition, isolation and treatment will minimise current and future production losses. The affected animal should be removed to the hospital pens. Isolated hospital pens with low stocking densities for sick animals are recommended. This will reduce the stress on the affected animal, allow closer observation and treatment, and increase the access to water and food. It will also reduce the pathogen challenge within the pen.

Records should include the identification of the animal, the admission date, weight, treatment dates, treatment regime, dosage rates, withholding period, date moved into the recovery pens and the outcome of treatment. Treated cattle should be identified by using distinct ear tags (Cooper & Brodersen, 2010b).

Selection of an antimicrobial is dependent upon several factors which may include: route of administration (subcutaneous administration may be preferable to intra-muscular injections), the length of action, the withdrawal times, and the sensitivity of the pathogen and the anticipated time of slaughter at finishing. Resistance to *Mannheimia haemolytica* and *Pasteurella multocida* is common, but variable between regions (Cusack *et al.*, 2004).

Non-steroidal anti-inflammatory drugs (NSAIDs) have been shown to reduce pyrexia, diminish the severity of clinical signs, and lung pathology, and improve average daily weight gains in calves with respiratory disease when compared to untreated calves or calves only treated with antimicrobials.

Other therapeutic agents such as bronchodilators (e.g. clenbuterol) and mucolytics (e.g. bromohexine) may have a beneficial effects, but are rarely used. Bromhexine can increase pulmonary concentrations of oxytetracycline, sulfonamides and erythromycin. Millophylline causes broncho-dilatation by relaxation of smooth muscle, increased contractility of the diaphragm, increased mucco-ciliary clearance and increased performance of the right and left ventricular contraction with a diuretic effect. Although historically used in individual severe cases, this class of drug is not licensed for food-producing animals. Diuretics may be beneficial in reducing lung oedema, but they can increase the severity of any pre-existing dehydration and increase the viscosity of the mucous. Hypertonic saline has also been used in cases of calf pneumonia to reduce lung congestion.

BRD control programmes

Taylor *et al.* (2010b) reviewed the evidence for currently promoted preventive measures. They found studies were lacking which provided strong evidence for many of the commonly held beliefs for a range of preventative measures used in pre-conditioning. However, the experimental designs may not have provided sufficient power to identify important factors. They found that weaning and vaccination prior to sale had some benefits, and that metaphylaxis reduced mortality, morbidity and improved growth rates although the cost benefit was more variable.

Prevention and control objectives should be targeted to reduce the stressors, minimise the pathogen challenge, increase immunity and control environmental factors which reduce natural upper airway defences.

In beef feedlots, some of these objectives can be achieved by purchasing calves directly from breeders rather than through sale yards, preferably from breeders who yard-weaned calves. Ideally, the supplier should have a high health status and would be IBR- and BVD-free.

Conditioning or backgrounding for a period of 30–45 days of the weaned calves destined for the feedlot is considered to be beneficial. This involves penning the calves in confined spaces to condition them to the feedlot pens. In addition, similar feeding troughs and watering tanks to those in the feedlot, with hay and limited quantities of concentrate, are provided. This transition period avoids otherwise abrupt changes, when they are introduced into the feedlot. It also ensures that calves have been weaned, castrated and dehorned for 30–45 days before entry into the feedlot. During this time, they should be processed (vaccinated, de-wormed, vitamin injections). Vaccination 4–6 weeks prior to entry to the feedlot is ideal to ensure immunity has developed. Vaccination at the point of entry will provide little protection during the high-risk first two weeks in the feedlot. Monitoring for persistently infected BVD animals, and removing them before entering the feedlot, may have merit in some situations.

Using low-stress stock-handling techniques, minimising journey times and avoiding extreme temperatures during the journey to the feedlot are advisable.

On arrival, sick animals should be identified and removed to the hospital pens. Dust should be kept to a minimum. Industry standards for stocking densities should be based upon finishing weight, and group sizes should be carefully controlled. Once the group is established in the feedlot, movements and additions to the group should be minimised. There should be regular monitoring of cattle for signs of BRD, and removal of affected animals to hospital pens. Metaphylactic antibiotics may be used following an adverse BRD risk assessment. The use of metaphylaxis and vaccinations are discussed in more detail below.

Metaphylaxis

Metaphylaxis is the mass medication of animals to prevent the development of disease in animals at risk, or in those animals incubating the disease. It is associated with a reduction in mortality and morbidity rates, and an increase in weight gain due to respiratory disease in beef feedlots. The use of mass medication, in the form of metaphylaxis, is controversial, although cost-effective outcomes have been demonstrated in large feedlots in North America. Up to a 50% reduction of in morbidity, and up to a 25% reductions in mortality have been reported (Urban-Chmiel & Groom, 2012).

A recent meta-analysis of North American studies estimated a decrease in mortality and morbidity of 2% and 26%, respectively, for animals that received antimicrobial treatment on arrival in the feedlot. The average daily weight gain was 0.11 kg higher in these animals, compared with calves not receiving metaphylactic treatment. Reductions in the prevalence of lung lesions at the abattoir have been reported.

Metaphylaxis may be administered parenterally, in the water and in the feed, depending on the product. Administration is usually upon entry, or within a few days following arrival to the feedlot, although it is sometimes administered before transport to the feedlot. The timing and length of action of the metaphylaxis should coincide with the highest risk of BRD, which is usually during the first three weeks. The goal is to strategically implement metaphylactic therapy where it will provide optimum benefits. It has been suggested that metaphylaxis may also be useful to cover the period of risk if vaccination only occurs at the point of entry into the feedlot or housing. Because of the cost of metaphylaxis, and the growing concern regarding antibiotic use in production animals, it is usually reserved for calves assessed to be at high risk. High-risk calves may include recently abruptly weaned, unvaccinated, comingled, transported, non-conditioned calves. The use of metaphylaxis should be reserved for high-risk situations where no other strategies can mitigate the risk to an acceptable level.

Products that have been used for metaphylaxis include oxytetracyclines, ceftiofur, florfenicol, tilmicosin and tulathromycin. In the United States, those approved for metaphylaxis have included: tilmicosin, florfenicol, tulathromycin and ceftiofour (Urban-Chmiel & Groom, 2012). A large number of papers have compared the impact of different regimens and antimicrobials on morbidity, mortality, growth rates and the cost. Readers are referred to these papers, so that the evidence and context is detailed.

The decision to metaphylactically administer any class of pharmaceutical products is based on clinical signs, expected illness rates in the group, and prior evidence of product efficacy (Nickell & White, 2010). General guidelines that have an impact on the decision to administer metaphylactic treatment for BRD include:

1 the clinical appearance of the cattle on arrival;
2 current (and expected) morbidity/mortality patterns;
3 feed consumption;
4 elevated body temperature; and
5 efficacy of products labelled for the control of BRD (Pollreisz, 1991).

The decision for metaphylactic intervention should be based on a risk assessment, although it is often administered on the basis of the precautionary principle.

Vaccination

There are a number of vaccines available against the common respiratory pathogens. These vaccines are marketed in a variety of different combinations. The literature is still unclear about the quantitative efficacy and economics of vaccination in the feedlot, due to the multifactorial nature of the condition.

The vaccines available vary between countries but include: *Mannhaemia haemolytica*, *Pasteurella multocida*, *Histomonus sommnii*, IBR, RSV. PI3 BVD. IBR modified live, gene-deleted (gE) modified live virus and inactivated marker vaccines, to distinguish vaccination from field virus infection, have been developed and are commercially available. Protective immunity takes take 1–3 weeks to develop in an immune-competent animal. Vaccination is therefore best delivered as part of a pre-conditioning programme, rather than at point of entry into the feedlot.

References and further reading

Cooper, V.L. and Brodersen, B.W. (2010a). Bovine Respiratory Disease. *Veterinary Clinics of North America: Food Animal Practice* **26**(2), 191–417.

Cooper, V.L. and Brodersen, B.W. (2010b). Respiratory Disease Diagnostics of Cattle. *Veterinary Clinics of North America: Food Animal Practice* **26**(2), 409–416.

Cusack, P.M.V., McMeniman, N. and Lean, I.J. (2004). The medicine and epidemiology of bovine respiratory disease in feedlots. *Australian Veterinary Journal* **82**(3), 154–156.

Edwards, T.A. (2010). Control methods for bovine respiratory disease for feedlot cattle. *Veterinary Clinics of North America: Food Animal Practice* **26**, 273–284.

Griffin, D. (2006). Antibiotic metaphylaxis to control respiratory disease. *Cattle Production Library* **CL-606**, 1–6.

Loneragan, G.H., Dargatz, D.A., Morley, P.S. and Smith, M.A. (2001). Trends in mortality ratios among cattle in us feedlots. *Journal of the American Veterinary Medical Association* **219**, 1122–1127.

Lorenz, I., Earley, B., Gilmore, J., Hogan, I., Kennedy, E. and More, S.J. (2011). Calf health from birth to weaning. III. housing and management of calf pneumonia. *Irish Veterinary Journal* **64**, 14.

NAHMS (2000). *Feedlot '99 Part II: Baseline Reference of Feedlot Health and Health Management.* USDA, APHIS, National Animal Health Monitoring System.

Nickell, J.S. and White, B. (2010). Metaphylactic Antimicrobial Therapy for Bovine Respiratory Disease in Stocker and Feedlot Cattle. *Food Animal Practice* **26**(2), 287–300.

Pollreisz, J.H., Bechtol, D.T. and Upson, D.W. (1991). Problems and practice in mass medication of beef cattle. *Veterinary Clinics of North America: Food Animal Practice* **7**(3), 659–68.

Schneider, M.J., Tait, R.G. Jr., Busby, W.D. and Reecy, J.M. (2009). An evaluation of bovine respiratory disease complex in feedlot cattle: Impact on performance and carcass traits using treatment records and lung lesion scores. *Journal of Animal Science* **87**, 1821–1827.

Snowder, G.D., Van Vleck, L.D., Cundiff, L.V., Bennett, G.L., Koohmaraie, M. and Dikeman, M.E. (2007). Bovine respiratory disease in feedlot cattle: Phenotypic, environmental, and genetic correlations with growth, carcass, and longissimus muscle palatability traits. *Journal of Animal Science* **85**, 1885–1892.

Taylor, J.D., Fulton, R.W., Lehenbauer, T.W., Step, D.L. and Confer, A.W. (2010a). The epidemiology of bovine respiratory disease: What is the evidence for predisposing factors? *Canadian Veterinary Journal* **51**, 1095–1102.

Taylor, J.D., Fulton, R.W., Lehenbauer, T.W., Step, D.L. and Confer, A.W. (2010b). The epidemiology of bovine respiratory disease: What is the evidence for preventive measures? *Canadian Veterinary Journal* **51**, 1351–1359.

Urban-Chmiel, R. and Groom, R.D.L. (2012). Prevention and Control of Bovine Respiratory Disease. *Journal of Livestock Science* **3**, 27–36.

CHAPTER 53

Farm Audit of Beef Cattle Nutrition

Colin Morgan

Learning objectives

- Understand the basic principles of ruminant digestion.
- Appreciate the requirements for energy, protein, minerals and vitamins.
- Be able to audit the adequacy of diets for suckler cows and growing and finishing animals.

Introduction

An audit of the nutrition of beef cattle requires assessment of the animal's status and production targets (nutrient requirements) and the status of the feeds it is offered (nutrient composition and amount). To do this it is necessary to consider the animal requirements in terms of energy, protein, major minerals, trace elements and vitamins and at the same time ensure efficient rumen function. To provide a rationale for inclusion of these factors in the audit, it is useful to review briefly digestion and the derivation of requirements. A more detailed description is given by McDonald *et al.* (2011).

Ruminant digestion

The anatomy of the ruminant digestive tract dictates that rumen fermentation by microbes is anterior to normal mammalian digestion. Thus, the rumen microbes act directly on feeds before the enzymes produced in the abomasum and small intestine. Efficient ruminant production systems depend on optimum rumen function, and the needs of the rumen microbes must be considered first. The microbes ferment carbohydrates (sugars, starch and fibre) to volatile fatty acids (VFA – principally acetic, propionic and butyric acids), yielding energy for their growth. Since the reticlulo-rumen is anaerobic, fermentation is not complete to carbon dioxide and water, and the host animal absorbs the VFA from the rumen and can extract the remaining energy by cellular oxidation.

Over 70% of the animal's energy requirements are met by the VFA. Fats are not fermented in the rumen, but unsaturated fats are hydrogenated. The fibre-fermenting microbes are sensitive to high levels of fat in the diet. The fatty acids, especially unsaturated fatty acids, coat the fibre and impede fermentation, and some fatty acids are toxic to the microbes. Digestion and absorption of fats occurs in the small intestine.

Microbes also break down nitrogen-containing compounds in feeds (such as protein and amino acids) to ammonia, which is incorporated into microbial protein. These microbes can also use non-protein nitrogen compounds and thus can 'upgrade' these materials to microbial protein. The microbes and undegraded feed proteins pass out of the reticulo-rumen, are subjected to the digestive enzymes in the abomasum and small intestine, and are absorbed as amino acids. Thus, the host animal receives a mixture of amino acids derived from microbial and feed protein, the majority being from the microbes.

The importance of fibre and managing starchy feeds

Optimum microbial fermentation occurs when the pH is maintained at around 6.5 to 7 by absorption of the VFA produced and their neutralisation by bicarbonate in saliva. Thus, chewing activity is important, and sufficient long fibre must be given to maximise chewing time. In practice, rations should have a minimum of 30% forage with sufficiently long fibre particles. Large meals of starchy concentrates are fermented rapidly with minimum chewing, and the acids produced can reduce the rumen pH below the optimum for fibre digestion. At the extreme, the acids kill the fibre-digesting microbes and attack the rumen wall, leading to acidosis. The acid conditions and lack of rumen motility also increase the incidence of bloat. Therefore, supplements of

Bovine Medicine, Third Edition. Edited by Peter D. Cockcroft.

concentrate feeds should be fed in small quantities and, if large amounts are required, they should be split into more than one daily meal. Special feeding practices are required for intensive ('barley beef') rations.

Energy requirements

The energy in feeds available for use by the ruminant is the metabolisable energy (ME), which is the gross energy (GE) of the feed, less the energy in the faeces, urine and methane produced by microbial fermentation in the gut. The ME is used with differing efficiencies according to its use (maintenance, growth, lactation, etc.), the ME content of the feed, and the level of feeding. Low-ME foods are fibrous, require more work for digestion and have lower efficiency of use.

At high levels of feeding, feeds pass through the gut more rapidly, with less time for digestion and, thus, they have lower energy values. The animal's requirement for energy is expressed as net energy (NE), and for maintenance depends on the metabolic body weight of the animal. The NE requirement for growth is a function of the weight of the animal and the rate of weight gain, being higher for heavier (more mature and more fat) animals and for higher rates of gain (more fat). Breed type (early, medium and late maturing) and sex (bull, steer or heifer) are also taken into account in the calculation of the net energy value of gain.

The NE requirement for lactation depends on the milk yield and composition and the requirement for pregnancy increases with time. The NE supplied by a diet is calculated as its ME × efficiency of use (km for maintenance and kp for production). Since the ME of the diet is not known until it is formulated, working with feed ME values would involve an iterative process of formulation. However, this can be avoided if the NE values of the individual feeds, combined for maintenance and production (NEmpMJ/kgDM), are used.

$$
\begin{aligned}
\text{Em} &= \text{NE for maintenance (MJ/d)} \\
\text{Ep} &= \text{NE for production (MJ/d)} \\
\text{km} &= 0.019\text{ME(MJ/kgDM)} + 0.503 \\
\text{kp} &= 0.0424\text{ME(MJ/kgDM)} + 0.006 \\
\text{kmp} &= \text{NE required/ME required} \\
&= (\text{Em} + \text{Ep})/(\text{Em/km} + \text{Ep/kp}) \\
\text{NEmp} &= \text{ME (MJ/kgDM)} \times \text{kmp}
\end{aligned}
$$

For a more accurate calculation, an adjustment for the level of feeding should also be included. The full list of equations for the calculation of net energy requirements is given by AFRC (1993). Combining these net energy requirements with the efficiencies of use of ME, and including the calculation of the level of feed correction for each feed, is a lengthy calculation and is best done using a spreadsheet. When the need to consider the potential food intake of the animal is also included, a ration formulation program is essential for the audit of a ration.

Protein requirements

The ruminant, like all animals, requires protein (amino acids) for maintenance, growth, lactation, etc. However, as noted above, the requirement is met mainly from microbial protein produced in the rumen. Therefore, the requirements of the rumen microbes need to be considered first, in order to ensure efficient rumen fermentation. The microbes require energy and nitrogen. The feed energy available to the microbes is in the form of fermentable metabolisable energy (FME), which is the ME of the feed less the energy in fats and fermentation acids in feeds such as silage.

Nitrogen compounds in feeds provide degradable nitrogen, and the efficiency of its capture into microbial protein depends on the rate of release of the nitrogen. If the nitrogen is released too quickly, the ammonia produced may not be matched with the FME, and wastage will result. Excess ammonia is absorbed from the rumen and converted to urea in the liver, then excreted in the urine. The nitrogen captured by the microbes is the effective rumen degraded nitrogen or protein (ERDP). The extent of degradation of the food protein depends on the feed type and on the time spent in the rumen, and is shorter at higher levels of feeding. The ERDP required by the microbes for growth is related to the FME in the diet and the level of feeding. At high levels of feeding, microbial growth is more efficient, and more ERDP is required per MJ FME. Feed protein that is not degraded by the rumen microbes passes to the small intestine, where it provides digestible undegraded dietary protein (DUP).

The animal's requirement to meet its needs for maintenance and production is in terms of metabolisable protein (MP). For maintenance, this depends on the weight of the animal. For growth, it depends on weight, weight gain, breed type and sex. For lactation, it depends on yield and milk protein content. For pregnancy, it increases with time.

The amino acids absorbed from digested microbial protein and DUP are used with differing efficiencies, according to the use to which they are put: maintenance, growth, lactation, pregnancy. The full list of equations for the calculation of MP requirements is given by AFRC (1993), although it has been recognised that the requirement for maintenance is too low, and a calculation similar to that of INRA (1989) or NRC (2000) is more appropriate. Again, the calculations of supply of FME and ERDP, and the subsequent supply of DUP and microbial protein to the small intestine and of MP requirements, although straightforward, are lengthy, and the use of a spreadsheet or ration formulation program is recommended.

Table 53.1 The metabolic role, effects of deficiency and dietary requirements of minerals and vitamins (adapted from McDonald *et al.*, 2011).

Element or vitamin	Role	Effects of deficiency	Requirement/ kg diet DM
Calcium	Bone and teeth, transmission of nerve impulses	Rickets, osteomalacia, milk fever	4–7 g*
Phosphorus	Bone and teeth, energy metabolism	Rickets, osteomalacia, depraved appetite, poor fertility	3–4 g*
Potassium	Osmoregulation, acid-base balance, nerve and muscle excitation	Retarded growth, weakness	7 g
Sodium	Acid-base balance, osmoregulation	Dehydration, poor growth	1 g*
Chloride	Acid-base balance, osmoregulation, gastric secretion	Alkalosis	2 g
Sulphur	Structure of amino acids, vitamins and hormones, chondroitin	Equivalent to protein deficiency (urea-supplemented diets)	2 g
Magnesium	Bone, activator of enzymes for carbohydrate and lipid metabolism	Nervous irritability and convulsions, hypomagnesaemia	1–3 g*
Iron	Haemoglobin, enzymes of electron transport chain	Anaemia	40 mg
Copper	Haemoglobin synthesis, enzyme systems, pigments	Anaemia, poor growth, depigmentation of hair and wool, swayback	12 mg
Cobalt	Component of vitamin B_{12}	Pining (emaciation, anaemia, listlessness)	0.3 mg
Iodine	Thyroid hormones	Goitre; hairless, weak or dead young	0.5 mg, or 2 mg if diet contains brassicae
Manganese	Enzyme activation	Retarded growth, skeletal abnormality, ataxia	40 mg
Zinc	Enzyme component and activator	Parakeratosis, poor growth, depressed appetite	40 mg
Selenium	Component of glutathione peroxidase, iodine metabolism, immune function	Myopathy, secondary thyroid deficiency	0.12 mg
Vitamin A	Sight, epithelial tissues	Blindness, epithelial infection	2000–4000 iu*
Vitamin D	Calcium absorption	Rickets	300–750 iu*
Vitamin E	Antioxidant	Muscle degeneration, liver damage	25 iu

*Requirements for the major minerals and vitamins A and D should be calculated for individual cases.

Major mineral, trace element and vitamin requirements

The role of these nutrients and the effects of deficiency are summarised in Table 53.1. The requirements for the major minerals are calculated according to the needs for maintenance and production and should be estimated for each specific case. The requirements for trace elements are usually expressed as concentration in the diet dry matter. For further information of mineral and vitamin nutrition, see McDonald *et al.* (2011) and, for a detailed description of mineral nutrition, see Suttle (2010).

Auditing feed composition

For concentrate feeds published tables of nutrient composition (e.g. AFRC, 1993; McDonald *et al.*, 2011) are usually adequate for ration formulation purposes, unless the material is uncommon or is suspected to vary in composition. The case is different for forages. Whereas the composition of straws do not vary greatly (ME around 6.5 MJ/kgDM and CP 40 g/kgDM), there is variation in the composition of hays (ME 7.5–9.5 MJ/kgDM, CP 70–100 g/kgDM), and an analysis of the material being fed will assist the formulation of accurate rations. For silages, it is essential the analysis is carried out, since silages vary considerably in composition (DM 150–600 g/kg, ME 8–12 MJ/kgDM, CP 80–190 g/kgDM), and assuming an 'average' composition could lead to large errors in ration formulation, with inappropriate quantities and types of supplement being fed and target performance being missed.

Auditing beef cattle nutrition

Suckler cows

The aim of beef cow nutrition is to produce a healthy, viable calf, adequate milk for its growth, for the cow to re-breed annually

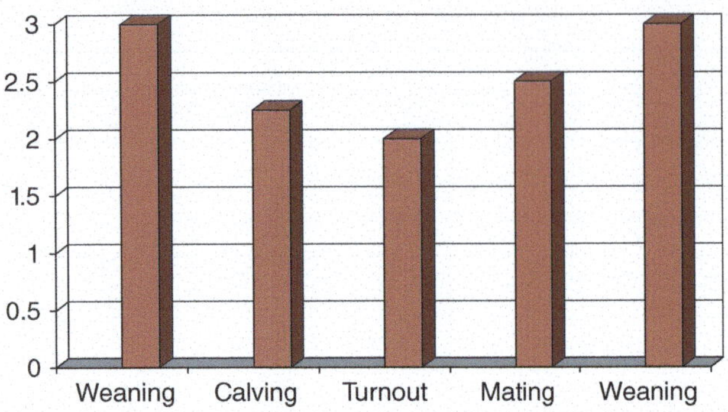

Figure 53.1 Target condition scores for spring calving cows.

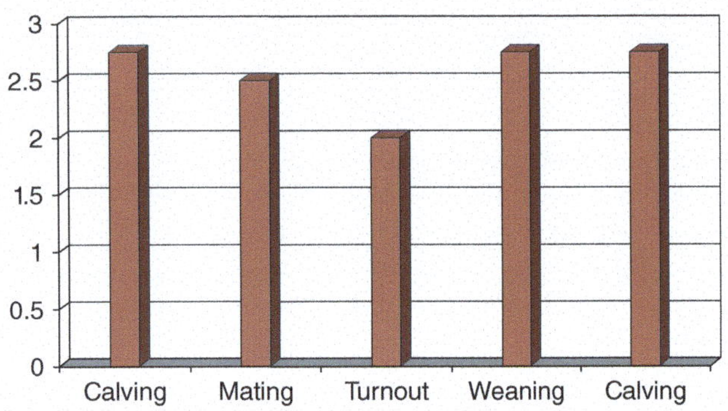

Figure 53.2 Target condition scores for autumn calving cows.

and to maintain the cow in a fit, but not fat, condition. In addition, feed costs during the winter need to be kept under control to ensure profitability. Research has shown that increasing energy intake to lactating cows has only small effects on milk yield and calf growth rate, but a large effect on cow weight and body condition score. For pregnant cows, high body condition scores are associated with difficult calvings. Conversely, excessive mobilisation of fat and the resulting low body condition score will cause difficulty in re-breeding. Thus condition score can be used as a guide to feeding levels, and targets can be set for each stage of the production cycle – see Figure 53.1 for spring calving and Figure 53.2 for autumn calving cows: scale 0 (very thin) to 5 (over fat).

For spring calving cows, the requirements are for maintenance and for the growing calf and associated membranes. Although the nutrient requirements increase exponentially through pregnancy, it has been shown that cows can be fed at a flat rate through the winter. This avoids high levels of feeding near to term, which may encourage high calf birth weights with the associated calving difficulties. Thus, the calculation of requirements can be set at around eight weeks before birth. The target condition scores are shown in Figure 53.1 and, assuming one unit of condition score is equivalent to 13% of live weight, an appropriate weight change for the winter feeding period can be calculated.

For a 650 kg cow at the appropriate CS of 3 (on a 1–5 scale) at the start of the winter, a loss in weight of 0.3 kg/day will result in a CS of around the target 2.25 at calving. Taking into account the pregnancy requirement at eight weeks before calving, the daily ME requirement for the winter is then around 75 MJ.

In order to meet protein requirements, diets must be formulated to provide the rumen microbes' requirement for ERDP, which for silage/straw-based rations is 500 g/day, and for straw/concentrate-based rations is 560 g/day. Once the ERDP requirement has been met, the digestible amino acids supplied by microbial protein in the small intestine will be sufficient to satisfy the animal's requirement for MP (332 g/day). This is usually achieved with diets containing around 90 g CP/kgDM.

Autumn calving cows housed at CS 2.75 can lose around 0.25 CS units to the end of mating (a live weight loss of 0.2 kg/day in a 650 kg cow) and, if she is giving 10 kg milk, the ME requirement is around 120 MJ/day and the ERDP requirement on a silage-based diet is 800 g/day. The MP requirements of the cow (745 g/day) will be met by microbial protein, and diets with around 110 gCP/kgDM are usually sufficient. Once the cow is in calf, a saving on feed costs can be made by reducing the ME allowance to 95 MJ/day.

All diets should contain an appropriate suckler cow mineral and vitamin supplement.

Growing and finishing cattle

For rapid rumen development, it is essential that dairy-bred early weaned calves receive fibrous and concentrate (starchy) feeds. Fibrous feeds (ideally straw or hay) will ensure growth in size of the rumen/reticulum. Starchy feeds are required, since the VFA produced from them encourages the development of absorptive papillae on the surface of the rumen wall. Suckled calves from the beef herd should be offered concentrates as a creep feed before weaning, to encourage rumen development and ease the transition from milk to solid feeds at weaning.

Table 53.2 Net energy (NE MJ/d) and metabolisable protein (MP g/d) requirements of growing cattle.

Weight gain kg/d		**0.6**	**0.8**	**1.0**	**1.2**
Live weight kg					
200	NE	25	27		
	MP	336	381		
300	NE	32	36	39	
	MP	393	435	476	
400	NE		43	48	52
	MP		489	527	564
500	NE			55	61
	MP			581	617
600	NE			63	68
	MP			637	673

Table 53.3 Metabolisable energy (ME MJ/d), effective rumen degradable protein (ERDP g/d) and digestible undegradable dietary protein (DUP g/d) requirements of growing medium maturity steers on a silage-based diet (silage ME 10.6 MJ/kgDM, CP 130 g/kgDM) or straw-based diet.

Weight gain kg/day		**0.6**		**0.8**		**1.0**		**1.2**	
Live weight kg		Silage	Straw	Silage	Straw	Silage	Straw	Silage	Straw
200	ME	45	45	49	50				
	ERDP	310	358	361	413				
	DUP	138	108	151	118				
300	ME	61	59	67	67	73	75		
	ERDP	408	472	474	545	551	626		
	DUP	133	92	133	88	125	77		
400	ME			83	81	91	91	99	102
	ERDP			577	662	671	762	757	854
	DUP			121	66	100	42	81	20
500	ME					106	106	116	118
	ERDP					778	884	881	993
	DUP					85	17	55	0
600	ME					118	119	130	133
	ERDP					878	992	993	1117
	DUP					77	4	40	0

Newly weaned calves respond to a source of DUP, as their rumen function is still developing.

Once weaned, the ration should contain a balance of roughage and concentrate appropriate to the performance required to meet the target slaughter weight. Straw or hay-based diets will require a supplementary energy feed and a protein source to satisfy the ERDP requirements. Usually, the rumen microbial protein will supply the MP required by the host animal. In rapidly growing young animals, the microbial protein may not be sufficient, and a protein supplement that is a good source of DUP (e.g. soya bean meal) will be required.

On silage-based diets, cereal supplements are usually sufficient unless the silage is low in CP (<110 gCP/kgDM) or the ration is for rapidly growing bulls, where a supplement with around 180 gCP/kgDM may be beneficial. Nutrient requirements should be calculated for each group of animals, with knowledge of the nutrient content of the feeds being used. Clearly, it is not possible to give nutrient requirements for all situations for growing and finishing animals here, but examples of NE and MP requirements are given in Table 53.2 and ME, ERDP and DUP requirements for cattle on a silage and straw-based diets are given in Table 53.3. A mineral and vitamin supplement should always be included in the ration.

Practical steps in the farm audit of nutrition

In order to carry out an audit of the nutrition of beef cattle, it is necessary to ensure that the calculated ration is appropriate for the stock (weighing stock and checking target performance), that the ration on paper is actually being fed (check for wastage and cleaning out of troughs), and that this is actually being eaten by the cattle (adequate trough space and time for all to consume their allowance). This involves:

- Checking of scales used to weigh feeds and their regular calibration; calibration of buckets, etc. which are used to provide feeds by volume (very important for material given in small quantities, e.g. mineral and vitamin supplements).
- Analysis of feeds given (ME, crude protein, oil, fibre, and an estimate of FME, degradability of protein and, where required, measurement of mineral, trace element and vitamin content).
- Checking and regular calibration of scales used to weigh animals.
- Condition scoring of cows at appropriate times during the year, but especially at housing in the autumn for spring calving cows, to set weight changes to meet targets at calving.
- Regular weighing of growing/finishing cattle, to check if on target.
- Formulation of rations and calculation of feed requirements for the winter period.
- Assessment of feed supplies (amount in silage pit or bales, hay and straw bales, bulk grain stores) and the necessity to buy in supplements to meet protein and mineral and vitamin requirements.

If there are problems that are suspected to be associated with nutrition and feeding, the following checks should be carried out in addition:

- Adequacy of nutrient supply.
- Adequacy of fibre content and length of fibre particles in the ration (minimum 30% long fibre with a minimum particle length of 25 mm).

- Amount of starchy concentrates given and size of concentrate meals (maximum of 0.5 kg/100 kg live weight in each meal).
- Amount and type of fat in the ration, being careful of the incorporation of high levels of co-products from the human food industry, such as biscuit meal (which are high in fat) and draff (a by-product of the brewing and distilling industry) at more than 50% of the dry matter.

References

AFRC (1993). Energy and Protein Requirements of Ruminants. An advisory manual prepared by the AFRC Technical Committee on Responses to Nutrients. CAB International, Wallingford, UK.

INRA (1989). Ruminant Nutrition: Recommended Allowances and Feed Tables. Editor: Jarrige, R. INRA, Paris, France.

McDonald, P., Edwards, R.A., Greenhalgh, J.F.D., Morgan, C.A., Sinclair, L.A., and Wilkinson, R.G. (2011). *Animal Nutrition*, 7th Edition. Pearson Education Limited, Harlow, UK.

NRC (2000). *Nutrient Requirements of Beef Cattle.* Seventh Revised Edition, 1996 (Update 2000). National Academy Press, Washington, DC.

Suttle, N.F. (2010). *Mineral Nutrition of Livestock*, 4th Edition. CABI, Wallingford, UK.

Further reading

Crawshaw, R. (2001). *Co-Product Feeds.* Nottingham University Press, Nottingham, UK.

Ewing, W.N. (1997) *The Feeds Directory, Vol. 1: Commodity Products.* Context, Leicestershire, UK.

Ewing, W.N. (2002). *The Feeds Directory Branded Products Guide.* Context, Leicestershire, UK.

MAFF (1990). *UK Tables of Nutritive Value and Chemical Composition of Feedingstuffs.* Rowett Research Institute, Aberdeen.

Roy, J.H.B. (1980). *The Calf*, 4th Edition. Butterworths, London, UK.

CHAPTER 54

Audit of Semi-Intensive Beef Finishing Systems

Peter D. Cockcroft

Learning objectives

- To understand the production system.
- To appreciate the target growth rates and carcase quality targets.
- To understand the common health problems and associated risk factors at grass and housing.
- To understand prevention and control of the common diseases.
- To be able to audit a semi-intensive beef finishing system and formulate a health management plan.

The aim of this chapter is to provide useful information to enable veterinarians to construct and perform an audit of a semi-intensive beef finishing systems from weaning to slaughter. The rearing of bull beef in more intensive systems and feedlot cattle will not be described here. An overview of the suckler calf and dairy beef calf production systems is included. The major health problems encountered are briefly described. The risks associated with housing design and management are highlighted. A checklist to assist the audit process is provided.

Introduction

Semi-intensive beef rearing and finishing systems are production enterprises in which the growing cattle spend one or two summers out at grass before slaughter. The animals are either weaned calves from the suckler (cow and calf) herd, or from the dairy herd which use, either continental or traditional beef breeds.

The veterinarian and the audit process

In order to ensure that veterinary advice is appropriate, it is important that an audit is performed to obtain a clear understanding of the current practices, performance and the aims of the enterprise. The audit should identify the current resources, the processes and the values of the key performance indicators. It should include the current biosecurity protocols, housing and environment, breeding management, nutrition and feeding, preventative health care, husbandry protocols and standard operating procedure, and records kept.

The outcomes of the audit should be compared to the best current practices, and the values of key performance indicators compared to appropriate target values. One measure which takes into account all elements of production is the margin achieved from each 1 kg of finished beef per year. This parameter includes the start and finish weights, growth rates, losses, feeding costs, and can even include the effect of subsidies. Herd health programmes that use the 'measure, manage and monitor' approach can then be devised, prioritised, costed, discussed and selectively implemented.

The total feed costs increase as the feed conversion ratios (FCRs) becomes poorer and the cattle are kept for longer, but the use of cheaper home-grown forage may compensate. When investigating different types of finishing systems, the relationships between feed costs, FCR and fixed cost structure on the farm need to be understood.

Carcase grading and differential tissue growth

It is important for the veterinarian to be aware of the factors that influence the carcase classification for which differential payments will be made, and to appreciate the farmer's target carcase objectives. Over-fat carcases at slaughter will cost the producer money in unnecessary feeding costs and downgrading.

There are significant breed differences in the age at which the rate of fattening occurs. Fattening occurs sooner in early-maturing traditional breeds (e.g. Hereford and Aberdeen

Bovine Medicine, Third Edition. Edited by Peter D. Cockcroft.

Angus) when compared to late-maturing continental breeds (e.g. Charolais and Simmental). There are also gender differences. Heifers lay down fat earlier than steers. Steers lay down fat earlier than bulls. Breeds and individuals with good conformation will yield a higher proportion of high value hindquarter lean meat, compared with animals with a poor conformation. Double-muscled breeds have this advantage. Carcases in the EU are classified using the EUROP Europe, using E for excellent, U, R, O and P for poor. Conformation classes U, O and P are subdivided into better (+) and poorer (-) classes. Fatness is scored from 1 (leanest) to 5 (fattest), with 4 and 5 subdivided into fatter H and Leaner L classes.

Suckled calf production and associated health problems

The weaned calf is the primary output from the beef suckler herd, and it is important to maximise the number of calves produced and raised. The highest mortality rates are recorded for dystocia, stillbirth and weak calves and neonatal diseases. An achievable target up to four weeks of age would be a mortality rate of 4% or less.

Dystocia due to feto-pelvic disproportion is most commonly recognised in beef heifers, and may be due to foetal oversize or a narrow pelvic, due to immaturity or over-conditioning. Mal-presentations and twins are also a cause of dystocia. Hypocalcaemia, under-nutrition and vitamin E and selenium deficiencies may also contribute to uterine inertia, leading to an apparent dystocia. The risk of dystocia can be reduced by using bulls with an easy calving estimated breeding value, calving down at a condition score of 2.5 (scale 1–5) at a minimum of 85% of the mature body weight. The selection of replacement heifers, using appropriate pelvic measurements, can be used to reduce the risk. If the mating date is accurately known, parturition can be induced if the gestation becomes prolonged beyond 278 days and foetal oversize is predicted. Increased supervision may enable the early recognition of dystocia and reduce losses by appropriate intervention.

Abortions can result in significant losses, and may be a consequence of a number of infectious agents, including IBR, BVD, Leptospirosis, *Campylobacter foetus venerealis, Brucella abortus* (not in the UK), Salmonella, *Listeria moncytogenes, Bacillus licheniformis, Neospora caninum* and mycotic abortion.

Loss of foetuses following pregnancy diagnosis at 60 days should not exceed 2%, and higher figures should be investigated. Nutritional deficiencies such as iodine and vitamin E/selenium can result in stillborn and weak calves. Manganese deficiency, when pregnant cows are fed silage without supplementation, can result in calf joint laxity and dwarfism. Bovine neonatal pancytopaenia (BNP), following the ingestion of colostrum, is now rare and is likely to decline following the withdrawal the BVD vaccine (PregSure®), which is considered to be a risk factor.

Hypothermia, mis-mothering and the failure of passive transfer of maternal immunoglobulins are well recognised. Coli-septicaemia, joint ill, navel ill, enteritis (rota, corona-virus, cryptosporidia, salmonella) and pneumonia are important neonatal diseases. These can be mitigated by reducing or eliminating the risk factors. This includes using clean calving paddocks, navel dipping, and by ensuring the timely intake of colostrum, vaccinating the dams (Rota/Corona/*E. coli*) and treating the affected calves promptly. Necrotic enteritis is usually encountered at 2–4 months old. The condition has a poor prognosis and is of unknown aetiology.

The growth of the calf up to the point of weaning is dependent upon the cow's milk supply, the pasture, and creep feeding of a cereal based mix in a dry, sheltered location which only the calves can access. The timing and amount of creep feeding will depend on whether the calf is autumn- or spring-born. For autumn-born calves, creep feed should be available during the winter housed period and is usually fed *ad lib* up to a maximum of 2.5 kg daily, but it is discontinued when they are turned out onto pasture in springtime. For spring-born calves, supplementation is usually only provided in the late summer before housing and weaning.

When to wean should be a decision based on feed supply and cow condition. Once the calf is 6.5 months (200 days) old, 75% of its nutrient requirement should be from feeds other than milk. Feeding the cow on expensive silage and concentrates to produce milk is very wasteful once the calf is itself able to eat silage and concentrates. If suckling calves are causing excess loss of body condition from the cow, they should be weaned immediately.

Weaning is stressful for the calf and, in spring-born calves, this may coincide with housing. Autumn-born calves are often weaned during mid-summer. Transport, mixing and housing of calves increases the risk of pneumonia from shipping fever (*Mannheimia haemolytica, Pasteurella multocida*), IBR, RSV, PI3, BVD and mycoplasma infections. There is a temptation also to include vaccination, castration, worming and dehorning at the point of weaning and housing, but this should be resisted due to the increased stress, despite the saving in labour costs.

Weaning is a good time to weigh the calves and record their weights. Endoparasitic gastroenteritis may be a risk, depending on the pasture contamination once the calves are consuming larger quantities of grass. Spring-born calves may be at increasing risk towards late summer and autumn, before weaning. Autumn-born calves will be at a similar risk which coincides with mid-summer weaning. Control and monitoring strategies need to be implemented. Lungworm and liver fluke infections should also be considered in the late summer and autumn grazing period. Trace element supplementation with copper, selenium, cobalt and iodine may be required.

Vaccinating several weeks before housing will ensure that immunity is developed before the risk increases upon housing. Lice infestation is common, and treatment of the entire group for lice is a wise precaution at housing. An evaluation of the proposed stocking densities, bedding arrangements and airspace is recommended. An analysis of the proposed feeding budget diet composition and the target growth rates is a worthwhile exercise. Winter feed cost is a high variable cost in all of these semi-intensive systems, and should be used strategically. Creep feed will often be made available to weaned spring born calves to support the growth rates up to the autumn calf sales.

Autumn-born calves are often housed and fattened for slaughter at 15–18 months, during the second housing period. They may receive treatment for larval fluke and potential hypo-biotic endoparasites, such as *Ostertagia ostertagia* at housing. Once weaned and housed, the spring-born calves are fed on a store ration which supports a growth rate of 0.7 kg/day, to minimise the winter feed costs. A mineral vitamin supplement is required. Compensatory growth is strategically achieved during the following grazing season.

Spring-born calves will be finished off during their second grazing season, which will require a strategic endoparasite control programme and monitoring plan, unless clean grazing is available. Mineral and trace element supplements may be required.

Performance target values for winter-finishing suckler calves are presented in Table 54.1, and grass-finishing suckler store cattle in Table 54.2.

Table 54.2 Targets for grass finishing suckler-bred store cattle.

	Charolais/Limousin/Simmental crosses	
	Steers	Heifers
Overwintering		
Feeding period (months	6	6
Start weight (kg)	250	230
Daily gain (kg	0.8	0.6
Cereal (kg)	200	–
Silage (tonnes, 25% DM)	4.0	4.0
Turnout weigh t(kg)	400	350
Grass-finishing		
Feeding period (months)	5	4
Daily gain (kg)	1.0	0.9
Cereal (kg)	75	35
Overall stocking rate (cattle/ha)	4.0	4.3
Slaughter weight (kg)	550	460
Carcase weight (kg)	310	255
Main carcase class (EUROP)	U4l	U4l

Semi-intensive dairy beef production systems and associated health problems

A significant quantity of beef produced in the UK comes from bull calves born into the dairy herds. These may be pure-bred dairy calves, or may be the product from the strategic use of a beef bull. The latter may increase with the availability of sexed semen. Theses calves may be castrated to become steers, or kept entire to be finished as bull beef. Rearing bull beef are best suited to intensive indoor rearing due to safety considerations.

The calves from the dairy herd destined for beef production may be removed to a specialised calf rearing unit at seven days old. These calves are usually weaned at 7–10 weeks old and sold at 12–15 weeks old. Calves should be obtained in age-matched batches from a rearer with a high health status (BVD and IBR free) at 12–15 weeks old from the same source, and should be consuming 1 kg of concentrate per day and hay. They may be either spring-born or autumn-born (or in between) and will follow the same rearing programme as beef suckled calves once they reach 6–9 months old.

The difference between the two systems is the requirement for earlier creep feed to compensate for the absence of milk once weaned. The comparative target weight gains for dairy-bred calves and suckler calves are shown in Table 54.3. Calves from

Table 54.1 Targets for winter-finishing suckled calves.

	Angus/Hereford crosses	Charolais/Limousin/Simmental crosses	
	Steers	Steers	Heifers
Feeding period (months)	5	6	5
Start weight (kg)	320	350	310
Daily gain (kg)	0.9	1.0	0.8
Cereal (kg)	300	550	225
Silage (tonnes 25% DM)	3.2	3.4	3.5
Stocking (cattle/ha)	11	10	10
Slaughter weight (kg)	445	525	425
Carcase weight (kg)	250	295	235
Main carcase class (EUROP)	R/–U4L	–U/U + 4L	–U4L

Table 54.3 Target weight gains at grass for dairy bred and suckler calves.

Type	First grazing season (kg/day)	Second grazing season (kg/day)
Continental × dairy steers	0.85	0.90
Continental × dairy heifers	0.75	0.85
Suckler calves (steers)	1.10 (plus creep feeding)	0.90
Suckler calves (heifers)	0.95 (plus creep feeding)	0.85

the dairy herd will have a higher intake of grass and an earlier exposure to worm eggs on the pasture from mid-June onwards, which may increase the risk of higher endoparasite burdens, depending on the grazing management and the timing of turnout onto grass.

The aim of the 18–20 month beef system using autumn-born steer and heifer calves is to achieve target growth rates of 0.9 kg/day during the first winter, 1.0 kg/day during the summer grazing season and 1.0 kg/day from housing to slaughter, to 550 kg at 18–20 months old. The target values for the age weight and growth rate are shown in Table 54.4.

The aim of the spring-born beef system for spring born steers and heifer calves is to finish the cattle at the end of their second grazing season with a carcase weight of 290 kg, to maximise performance from grazed grass and to reach market specification weight by 18–20 months old. Animals spend two-thirds of their lifetime at grass in this system, and the proportion of time spent in the house is minimised. Target values for age, weight and growth rate are given in Table 54.5.

Housing

In cooler northern hemisphere climates, winter housing is common. The construction and design is important to facilitate ventilation, feeding management and cleaning-out. Welfare codes and industry standards should be checked for compliance with floor space and air allowances. The allowance should be based upon the final weight expected. Alternatively, there should be a plan to extend the pen size. Absolute and relative inlet and outlet sizes are important in a building with a central ridge, so that the 'stack' effect removes moisture and harmful gases. Space boarding in the walls and sides can facilitate the movement of air, provided the ingress of rain is minimal. Solid floor and slats may be used. The most common is a solid floor, with a lying area covered with straw and a feeding area which may be solid or slatted. Straw should be replaced every six weeks with dry straw.

Animals from eight weeks to six months of age should be kept in groups of no more than 20, and no more than 40 animals should share the same air space. If concentrate is fed periodically, there is a need to ensure access through the provision of appropriate trough space. A previous history of recurrent problems with pneumonia may reflect poor ventilation or poor management practices. Signs of condensation may be suggestive of poor airflow with discoloured timbers. The presence of nearby elevated structures can severely affect the airflow.

Health management: turnout and the grazing period

There are a range of common diseases in the semi intensive system. The risk factors for some of these diseases occur either during the housing period (e.g. pneumonia) or the grazing period (e.g. endoparasities). Clostridial vaccinations are important to protect against the following diseases: Blackleg (*C. chauvoei*) Malignant oedema, *C. septicum*, *C. novyi*, *C. chauvoei*, *C. sordelli*), Tetanus (*C. tetani*),

Table 54.4 Target live weights for autumn-born Holstein heifers finishing at 20 months.

Month	Age	Stage	Weight	Weight gain during preceding period
January (Year 1)	15 weeks	Bought in	120 kg	–
April (Year 1)	7 months	Turnout	200 kg	0.9 kg/day
November (Year 1)	14 months	Housing	410 kg	1.0 kg/day
May (Year 2)	20 months	Slaughter	580 kg 290 kg (carcase)	1.0 kg/day

Table 54.5 Target live weights for spring-born Angus and Hereford × heifers and steers finishing at 20 months.

Month	Age	Stage	Weight	Weight gain during preceding period
July (Y1)	16 weeks	Bought in	120 kg	–
October (Y1)	7 months	Housing	210 kg	1.0 kg/day
April (Y2)	14 months	Turnout	410 kg	0.7 kg/day
November (Y2)	20 months	Slaughter	550 kg 290 kg (carcase)	1.0 kg/day

Black disease (*C. novyi* type B), Botulism (*C. botulinum*), Enterotoxaemia, *C. perfringens* (particularly Type D), Bacilliary haemoglobinuria, *C. novyi* type D (formerly *C. haemolyticum*) and Abomasitis in calves (*C. sordelli*). A primary course should be given during calfhood, and an annual booster is advisable. A supplementary Vitamin ADE injection during the housing period may avoid marginal deficiencies on poor quality diets.

After weaning, at grass, it is important that there is an endoparasite monitoring and control programme in place for parasitic gastroenteritis (PGE), lungworm and liver fluke. For PGE, this may include turnout onto clean pastures, delay of turnout onto clean pastures and/or strategic monitoring and treatment. Occasionally, white muscle disease (Vitamin E/Selenium deficiency) is seen at turnout, due to increased exercise and physiological demand. Copper, cobalt, selenium and phosphorous deficiencies may become apparent during the first or second season at grass. Frothy bloat may be induced at grass, depending upon the pasture composition and grass growth patterns. Gradual introduction to fast-growing grass/legume pastures, using time-limited exposure or strip grazing, will reduce the risk.

Clinical signs of PGE may include scouring, poor growth rates or weight loss and sub-mandibular oedema. Post-mortem examinations will reveal high total worm counts. Faecal egg counts are useful. Serum pepsinogen has been used to indicate abomasal infections of *O. ostertagia*. Field trials to assess growth response from drenching can be used, but other diagnostic methods are preferred.

In liver fluke infections, there is often a history of previous infections on the property or part of the farm, with summer infection usually the most common in the UK. Abattoir feedback may confirm the presence of adult fluke. Clinical signs include submandibular oedema, scouring and weight loss. Post-mortem examinations may reveal adult fluke in the liver. Blood biochemistry can be used to identify the liver damage associated with high liver fluke infestation. Liver fluke eggs will be present in the faeces if there are mature fluke in the liver bile ducts. There is an ELISA test which will indicate group exposure to the parasite.

In areas known to be deficient in either copper, cobalt, selenium or phosphorous, monitoring is a wise precaution. With copper deficiency, liver samples are the most reliable sample (deficient <0.1 mmol/kg DM). Samples can be obtained by liver biopsy or from the abattoir. Blood biochemistry measuring plasma copper (deficient <5 μmol/L) and ceruloplasmin (deficient <5 U/L) are diagnostically useful. Pasture analysis to assay copper, molybdenum and sulphate, to determine if other factors are interacting to cause deficiency, or copper alone, can be helpful. The clinical signs include colour coat changes, apparent joint enlargement and poor growth rates. In selenium deficiency, the following parameters values indicate deficiency: blood glutathione peroxidase <10 units, blood selenium <0.25 μmol/L, liver selenium <2.5 nmol/kg DM and pasture selenium deficient <0.02 mg/kg DM.

The clinical signs of white muscle disease are sudden death, stiff gait and collapse and apparent dyspnoea when the intercostal muscles are affected. The following parameter values indicate cobalt deficiency: plasma vitamin B12 <0.1 mmol/L, liver vitamin B12 <75 nmol/kg wet weight, liver cobalt deficient <1.0 μmol/kg dry matter, and pasture cobalt deficient <0.1 mg/kg DM. The clinical signs include poor weight gain and anaemia. Phosphorus deficiency is characterised by pica (eating bones and rubbish), poor growth, soft bones and bone fractures. In phosphorous deficiency, blood and bone ash calcium and phosphorus parameter values are abnormal.

Coccidiosis can occur at pasture (usually *E. alabamenisis*), and this should be considered when scouring and poor weight gains are observed on heavily stocked or previously (and recently) stocked pasture. Exposure to culicoides infected with bluetongue virus and Schmallenburg virus may occur at pasture, and vaccines are available for both conditions. Towards the end of the summer, the risk of lungworm rises, and the strategic use of anthelminitics can be used to avoid clinical disease. There is a live oral vaccine that can be given before turnout, which is very effective, but this is more commonly used in dairy heifers.

At grass, when the population of flies increases, outbreaks of infectious kerato-conjunctivitis (New Forest eye) may occur, which can be severe, with a high mobidity. There is bepharospasm, epiphora and corneal ulceration in one or both eyes. Mustering or collecting the cattle in yards for processing may increase the risk. Close monitoring and the strategic use of pour-on preparations or ear tags will be helpful in high risk areas. Withdrawal times must be carefully considered if the animals are near finishing. This condition is sometimes seen at housing, due to the close contact. In tick areas, louping ill, basesiosis and tick-borne fever (*Cytoectes phagocytophilia*) may need to be considered, in addition to the tick infestation *per se*.

Health management: housing

Pneumonia is an important and common condition of housed growing cattle. Ideally, castration, weaning, vaccination should not occur together or at the time of housing, as the stress will increase the risk of pneumonia. Vaccinations six weeks prior to housing is the best practice, so that protection is more fully developed by the time of the cattle are housed and at greatest risk. Vaccines against IBR. RSV,BVD, PI3 and *Mannheimia haemolytica* are available. Serology may be useful in identifying potential pathogens in a sub-sample of the group, and may be used to select appropriate viral vaccines. An all in/all out policy, no mixing of different groups or ages, animals at housing, adequate ventilation by using the correct stocking density, and adequate feeding space, with humidity and dust kept to minimum, will reduce the risk of pneumonia.

Treatment of all the animals in the group which are to be housed together for lice (*Linognathus vituli* (sucking), *Bovicola*

Table 54.6 Semi-intensive beef audit checklist.

Farm profile
- Size and purpose
- Production system
  - Suckler cow and calf
  - Steers and heifers (Dairy × beef crosses)
- Objectives of enterprise
- Stock numbers and turnover

Housing
- Type of housing
- Space allowance
  - Floor space
  - Air space
- Group size
- Shared air space
- Housing inlets and outlets
- Management
- Bedding
- Trough space
- Lighting
- Water
- Management

Bioscurity protocols

Records KPIs and target values
- Mortality
- Growth rates
- Age and weight at slaughter
- Classification of carcase
- Number of animals slaughtered

Weaning programme

Feeding
- Creep feed
- Transition to housing diet
- Winter feeding budget
- Composition and adequacy of diet
- Pasture assessment
- Weight for age
- Growth rates

Health programmes
- Vaccines programmes
  - Clostridial
  - Pneumonia
  - IBR
  - RSV
  - PI_3
  - BVD
  - *Mannheimia haemolytica*
  - Bluetongue
  - Schmallenberg
- Endoparasite control
  - Clean grazing
  - Delayed turnout
  - Antihelmintics program
    - At grass
    - At housing
  - Faecal egg counts
    - Faecal egg reduction tests
  - COWS strategy
- Ectoparasite control
  - Evidence of lice
  - Lice control at housing
  - Liver fluke control
    - At grass
    - At housing
  - Lungworm
    - Vaccination
    - Strategic antihelmintic
    - Monitoring program
  - Supplements (Se, Co, Cu)
- Major health problems (checklist)

Health monitoring programmes
- Health records
  - PGE
  - Feacal egg counts
  - Pepsinogen
  - Post-mortem examination
- Liver fluke
  - ELISA
  - Fluke
  - Lungworm
  - Post-mortem examination
  - Abattoir returns
- Antihelmintic resistance
  - Feacal egg reduction test
- BVD PI testing
- Pneumonia
  - Serology
  - Bronchio-alveolar wash – IFAT
- Mineral deficiencies
  - Cu
  - Co
  - Se

bovis (biting) louse, *Haematopinus eurysternus* (sucking) and *Selenoptes capillatus* (sucking) is common at housing. Lice populations often increase rapidly, due to close contact. Lice infestations cause pruritus, anaemia, and reduce the FCE. Treatment may also be necessary for larval fluke and hypobiotic *O.ostertagia* to avoid type II ostertagiasis. A transitional diet to allow the rumen to adapt to the higher energy diets fed in the winter housing period is recommended. During this transitional period, B1 deficiency, with the attendant nervous signs may be seen, due to the rapid production of thiamainases by bacteria in the rumen. Sub-acute or acute acidosis may also occur if access to higher energy diets is too rapid and uncontrolled. Free gas bloat may be observed as a consequence of the ruminal stasis.

The checklist in Table 54.6 may be used as a starting-point to develop a more targeted audit questionnaire.

CHAPTER 55

Beef Cattle Feedlots – How to Measure, Manage and Monitor

Mandi Carr

Learning objectives

- Appreciate the role of the beef feedlot in quality beef production.
- Understand how the veterinarian can contribute to the success of the feedlot enterprise.
- Be aware of the important and common conditions in beef feedlots.
- Understand how to measure, manage and monitor performance in the beef feedlot.
- Appreciate the key performance indicators and target values to measure performance.

Introduction

This chapter will provide a framework to enable beef cattle veterinarians to measure, manage and monitor risk in a beef feedlot. It will briefly scope across the common and important conditions that have a high impact on health, welfare, productivity and profitability.

Understanding the beef cattle feedlot

Feedlotting involves the provision of an artificial environment in which animals are placed in a confined area and required to consume a pre-determined diet for the purpose of production. Beef cattle are placed in a feedlot because poor quality pasture feed limits the cattle's ability to reach marketable weight. Also, consumers in both the domestic and export markets demand a consistent supply of beef, resulting in pressure to supply quality and quantity every day of the year.

Cattle sourced from farms or saleyards are transported to the feedlot by road, rail or sea. Legislation, codes of practice and quality assurance programs govern the transport requirements. Cattle arriving at the feedlot are generally tired and uncomfortable, so it is important that they are given time to settle, offered good quality hay and have access to fresh water.

Within a week of arrival, cattle will undergo a process called 'induction'. This involves gathering key details such as breed, age, sex and weight, so that cattle with similar attributes can be housed together. Cattle are given an individual identification tag (usually electronic) to enable their progress to be followed, and a colour-coded lot number management tag that is easily visible from a distance. Vaccinations, vitamin injections and treatment for internal/external parasites are also given, along with hormone growth promotants (HGPs), depending on the customer's requirements. Cattle are then yarded together, based on attributes that best suit the market destination (domestic or export).

It is important that cattle have enough space to exhibit normal behaviour and access to fresh clean water, and that feed is available *ad lib*. Diets are formulated by nutritionists to be palatable and nutritionally balanced, providing sufficient protein, energy, fibre, minerals and vitamins for production, maintenance and health, ensuring that digestive upsets are minimised. Final weights depend on the market destination, the number of days on feed and the diet provided. Typically, cattle stay at the feedlot for 50–120 days.

Cattle are observed daily by staff trained in animal welfare, husbandry and handling. Cattle appearing sick, shy feeders and poor doers are identified, removed from the pen and treated. Water troughs, feed bunks and the pen environment are checked and cleaned as required. Effective environmental management is essential for sustainable production. Manure

Bovine Medicine, Third Edition. Edited by Peter D. Cockcroft.

is regularly removed from the pens, composted and generally sold to farms, nurseries and market gardeners. Any run-off from the pens is collected in ponds and used to irrigate crops. Strict environmental legislation ensures that soil, water and air pollution is prevented. Consultants provide advice on nutrition and the environment, with veterinarians generally overseeing the animal health program.

Once cattle reach marketable weight, they are transported for processing. Reducing stress by minimising transport time, time in lairage, and preventing mixing of cattle at the processing facility, maximises cattle health and welfare, leading to better beef eating quality.

Common conditions impacting on cattle performance in the feedlot

There are four important factors that affect the profitability of a beef feedlot: the buying price of store cattle; the selling price of finished cattle; the cost of the diet; and the performance of the cattle. Buying price, selling price and feed costs have many external influences, and are often out of the control of the feedlot. Cattle performance, however, is largely influenced by management of the feedlot. Purchasing healthy animals, minimising stress, providing a comfortable feedlot pen environment, establishing a good surveillance system and the use of vaccines and antimicrobial agents, when necessary, is essential to the control and prevention of disease within the feedlot and ultimately, cattle performance.

The major objective on arrival at the feedlot is to get cattle onto a diet (which results in rapid growth) as quickly as possible, while minimising the morbidity and mortality associated with a change in diet and environment. However, the constant movement of cattle into and out of the feedlot makes the control of infectious diseases challenging. Constant exposure to pathogens, the stress of co-mingling, nutritional background, feeding management, and animal husbandry practices, all affect the prevalence of disease in the feedlot. Infectious diseases of the respiratory tract are a major cause of morbidity and mortality in the first 30–45 days after arrival in the feedlot, while digestive diseases are a potential threat within the first 30 days of arrival. The top three conditions that impact on cattle performance in beef feedlots are respiratory disease, digestive disorders and heat stress (Table 55.1).

Table 55.1 Common conditions impacting cattle performance in the feedlot.

Condition	Causes	Susceptibility	Signs	Treatment
Respiratory disease	*Pasteurella multocida* *Mannheimia haemolytica*. *Histophilus somni* *Trueperella pyogenes* *Mycoplasma* species. IBR virus. BVDV. BRSV. PI3 virus.	High: first 30–45 days. Medium: any time	Cattle off feed. Nasal discharge. Fever. Depression. Coughing. Laboured breathing. Extended head and neck. Open mouth breathing. Increased respiratory rate.	Remove from pen. Less competitive environment. Antimicrobials. Anti-inflammatories. Easily digestible diet (e.g. lucerne).
Digestive disorders (grain poisoning)	Transition period too fast. Grain milled too fine	High: first 30 days Low: >50 days on feed	Kicking at abdomen. Grinding of teeth. Diarrhoea. Cattle off feed. Depression. Bloat Staggering. Death.	Remove from pen. Magnesium oxide (or sodium bicarbonate). Good quality hay. Antimicrobials. Rumenotomy. Rumen transfaunation.
Heat stress	High daytime temperatures with high humidity and no wind. High overnight temperatures. Cattle on >100 days on feed. Cattle with large amounts of subcutaneous fat. Dark-coloured cattle.	High: >100 days on feed. High: Cattle with large amounts subcutaneous fat. High: Dark-coloured cattle.	Seeking shade. Refusal to lie down. Reduced food intake. Crowding near water trough. Agitation. Reduced rumination. Open mouth breathing. Excess salivation. Ataxia. Collapse. Convulsions. Death.	Provide shade and sprinklers. Increase salt content of diet. Highly digestible, high energy diet. Decrease handling. Decrease stocking rate.

Respiratory disease

Most deaths within a feedlot result from respiratory disease (Loneragan *et al.*, 2001). Varying degrees of lung consolidation, necrosis, fibrin deposition, abscess formation and pleural effusion are found at necropsy. Common bacterial causes are *Pasteurella multocida*, *Mannheimia haemolytica*, *Histophilus somni*, *Trueperella pyogenes*, and the *Mycoplasma* species. Common viral causes are infectious bovine rhinotracheitis (IBR) virus (bovine herpes virus type 1), bovine viral diarrhoea virus (BVDV), bovine respiratory syncytial virus (BRSV) and parainfluenza 3 (PI3) virus.

Identifying cattle at risk of developing respiratory disease is of paramount importance. Treating high risk cattle at 'induction' with metaphylactic antimicrobials can reduce morbidity and mortality by about 50% and improve weigh gain by approximately 10% (Smith *et al.*, 1994; Young, 1995; Guthrie *et al.*, 2000). Daily observation of high-risk cattle, monitoring the pen environment and aggressive treatment programmes are essential to minimising the effect of respiratory disease. Necropsy examinations on all deaths is necessary to establish a diagnosis and ensure accurate management of associated sick cattle.

Digestive disorders

Digestive disorders are the second leading cause of mortality and morbidity in a feedlot. The most common cause is grain overload, also called grain poisoning or acidosis. Ingestion of too much grain, too quickly, results in an excessive build-up of lactic acid in the rumen, creating ruminal acidosis. Absorption of this lactic acid results in metabolic acidosis. Milling grain too fine is a common factor in grain overload, as is attempting to transition cattle onto the finisher diet too fast.

Identifying cattle that are not coping with the change in diet is essential in managing the effects of digestive disorders. Monitoring rumen pH is a useful tool in identifying cattle with acidosis (pH 5–5.5). These cattle can then be treated to restore the balance of the rumen. If a large proportion of the pen is suffering from acidosis, the transition period can be lengthened, or the milling process altered.

Once cattle are over the transition period and are consuming the required amount of finisher ration, digestive disorders become less common.

Heat stress

Hot weather can have a significant impact on cattle performance within the feedlot. High temperatures, with high humidity and no wind, especially if the overnight temperature remains high for several nights in a row, can predispose cattle to heat stress. Cattle with large amounts of subcutaneous fat (usually cattle on >100 days of feed) and dark-coloured cattle are highly susceptible.

Management is of paramount importance in the control and prevention of heat stress in feedlots. Cattle must have the ability to obtain shade. Good airflow is important, as is access to fresh, cool, clean drinking water. Decreasing stocking density, decreasing handling, and ensuring correct manure management, are all important strategies in controlling heat stress. Changing the diet to include salt, and providing a highly digestible, high-energy diet that produces less metabolic heat, are also important tools.

Heat stress results in decrease feed consumption, decreased weight gains and increased susceptibility to disease. Early identification of factors that can lead to heat stress is critical in preventing a cascading set of events.

Measuring, managing and monitoring risk

Feedlot management affects cattle performance through its effect on feed intake, weight gain and herd health. Any factor that causes stress can result in increased incidence of disease in the feedlot. Selection of healthy cattle to enter the feedlot, a transport system that minimises distance travelled and minimises stress (adequate rest and feeding periods if travelling long distances), a good induction process, transition period, feedlot pen environment, feeding system, and surveillance system, are essential in successfully limiting the economic impact of disease on the feedlot. Recording information at all these stages helps to establish trends, identify new problems and document progress (Table 55.2).

The decision of what type of cattle to purchase and where to purchase them from requires a risk analysis. Purchasing a uniform group of feeder calves or yearling cattle from one source will limit the incidence of disease, but the cattle may cost more, resulting in a smaller gross margin. Disease is generally always higher in weaned calves and cattle purchased from several sources. Developing a reporting system that regularly informs the buyer of the condition of the cattle received and their subsequent performance will assist the buyer in the type of cattle required to be purchased. Developing a standard operating procedure (SOP) for suppliers, involving age, weight, minimum weaning time, minimum castration/dehorning times, pre-vaccination schedule and pre-parasite treatment schedule, is useful to ensure that cattle entering the feedlot are pre-condition to the feedlot environment.

Transporting cattle the shortest time possible to the feedlot is economically most feasible. Transportation equipment and facilities should meet legislative standards, and be able to comfortably transport cattle regardless of the season. Feedback to transport companies on the condition of the cattle at arrival, and the subsequent performance of the cattle, including the incidence of disease, is critical. Measuring distance travelled against performance of the cattle is a key factor in advising where cattle can be sourced from.

Assessing the cattle at induction is of paramount importance. Determining their ability to cope with a change in diet and environment, and identifying those cattle not adjusting well, is

Table 55.2 Checklist for managing, measuring and monitoring risk in the feedlot.

Category	Hazard/risk assessment	Manage	Measure	Monitor
Purchasing cattle	Source 1 One source 2 Several sources	Pre-conditioning cattle 1 Vaccination (Clostridial diseases, *Mannheimia haemolytica*, IBR, PI3, BVDV) at least 3 weeks prior to entry. 2 Castration/De-horning at least 3 weeks prior to entry. 3 Weaned for a minimum of 45 days prior to entry. 4 Treated for internal and external parasites at least 3 weeks prior to entry. 5 Source – farm vs. saleyard.	Performance of cattle 1 Average daily gain (ADG) >1.8 kg/day. 2 Transition period <4 days 3 Health /sickness <10%. 4 Source performance farm vs. saleyard.	Performance of cattle from each individual source 1 Average daily gain (ADG) <1 kg/day poor. 2 Transition period >10 days poor. 3 Health/sickness >10% poor. 4 Feedback to buyers/source.
Transportation	Distance. Equipment and facilities. Arrival procedure – unloading.	Local vs. state vs. interstate. Regulatory and legislative controls.	Distance travelled hours vs. days. Performance of cattle vs. distance travelled. Health of cattle vs. distance travelled. Condition of cattle at arrival.	Performance of cattle vs. distance travelled. Transport regulations and legislation. Performance of cattle vs. transport company. Health of cattle
Induction Process	Timing. Pre-conditioning of cattle. Health of cattle at arrival.	<7 days post-arrival. SOP pre-conditioned cattle. SOP non-conditioned cattle. Lot number. Align attributes to market.	Breed, age, sex, weight. Vaccination, internal/external parasites, vitamin, HGPs. Individual and lot identification.	Health of cattle 1 Individual. 2 Lot. Performance of cattle 1 ADG. 2 Transition onto feed. 3 Transition into environment. 4 Market specifications. Job record sheet.
Cattle not performing	1 Sick cattle. 2 Poor doers. 3 Shy feeders. 4 'Bullers' (cattle being ridden all the time).	Observation – pen riders 1 Trained in cattle behaviour and handling. 2 Early recognition of poor performing cattle	Number of sick animals <5%. Number of poor doers < 1.5%. Number of shy feeders. Number of bullers. Number requiring treatment < 10%. Type of treatment. Number returning to pen. Performance of cattle (ADG). Necropsy findings.	<3% cull rate for poor performance. <1.5% mortality rate. <10% morbidity rate. <15% treatment rate. Disease outbreaks. Necropsy reports.
Nutrition	Transition diet. 1 Milling of grain. 2 Type of grain. 3 Use of molasses Finisher diet. Market specifications. 1 Domestic. 2 Export.	Pre-condition cattle. Transition onto feed over 16 days. Feed available at all times. Use of maize in diet. Feed at same time each day. Finisher diet of 80% concentrate and 20% roughage. Market specifications 1 Domestic. 2 Export. Water intake.	Consumption 2.5–3% of body weight. Incidence of acidosis. Wheat > barley > oats > maize. Number not adapting to diet. Amount molasses in diet. Time of feeding. Feed in trough at all times. Number making market specifications. Water intake 30–80 kg per day, depending on weather.	Consumption <1.5% body weight poor. Transition period <21 days. Number not adapting 1 Pre-conditioned <2%. 2 Not pre-conditioned <20%. Molasses <10%. Incidence of acidosis < Number making market specifications. Water intake <30 kg per day critical. Job record sheets.

Table 55.3 (*continued*)

Category	Hazard/risk assessment	Manage	Measure	Monitor
Facilities	Drainage. Space per head . Protection from wind, rain, snow, excessive heat, sunshine. Feed bunk. 1 Space. 2 Protection from weather damage. Water availability.	Slope 3–6%. 9–15 m^2 per head. 2.76 m^2 per head. 250–460 mm per head. 1–1.5 m cover. Quality of water. Water trough space 250–300 mm per head.	Manure management. 1 Depth of manure 25–50 mm after cleaning Stocking density. SOP pen maintenance.	ADG decreases with increase in depth of manure. Health of cattle. Performance of cattle. Job record sheets.
Record keeping	Poor record-keeping procedures.	Staff training. Development SOPs	Staff performance. Records being kept – others required?	Identify trends. Identify new problems. Document progress.

critical to minimising future disease problems. Early recognition and aggressive treatment will minimise losses due to poor performance.

It is desirable that cattle are fed at the same time each day, to reduce the incidence of digestive upsets, and that cattle have feed in the troughs at all times. It is important that excessive amounts of feed are not put out, as feed can become stale. To minimise wastage of feed, it is critical to estimate the amount of feed required by the pen, so there is little left over each day. A 200 kg animal requires 6–7 kg of feed to gain 1 kg of live weight; a 600 kg animal requires 12–14 kg of feed to gain 1 kg of live weight. Covered feed bunks will provide added comfort to cattle when eating, and protect the feed from weather damage. Feed bunk space ranges from 25–30 cm per head for yearling cattle to 38–46 cm per head for bullocks.

Stocking rates are influenced by the size of the cattle and the environment. Cattle require between 9–15 square metres per standard cattle unit (600 kg live weight animal), and even as high as 25 m^2 with some accreditation schemes. Dusty and boggy conditions need to be avoided, and protection from wind, rain, snow, excessive heat and sunshine is essential.

Manure management is a critical factor in the success of the feedlot. It is an integral part of the operation, with approximately 1–2 tonnes of manure per head needing to be removed each year. Manure has a high nutrient value and is very suitable as a fertilizer, so the financial returns need to be optimised. Typically, a 450 kg animal produces about 5–6% of live weight as manure each day, with 85–90% of this being water and 10–15% being solid material. Stocking rate and animal live weight have a significant impact on the moisture added to the pen environment, and to the rate of manure accumulation. The frequency of pen cleaning must be adjusted to match the accumulation of manure. The result of pen cleaning should be a smooth, uniform surface that promotes good drainage and improves cattle performance.

A key factor in minimising disease problems within a feedlot is to have a good surveillance system in place. Daily observation by people trained in cattle handling and behaviour is essential in early recognition of poor-performing or sick cattle. Aggressive treatment or procedures can then be undertaken to avoid significant weight loss.

Records are essential in understanding the incidence of disease in the feedlot, the response to treatment and production performance. Daily morbidity and mortality statistics and treatment records should be kept and analysed monthly. Cull rates due to poor performance should be less than 3%; morbidity rates less than 5%; mortality rates less than 1%; and treatment rates less than 10%. A disease summary, based on post-mortem results and treatment records, should be produced and analysed. The diseases treated, treatments used, the outcome of treatments, average length of treatment and fatality rates should all be recorded. They should be correlated to necropsy results, and matched to the epidemiology of mortality rates, including the number of days the animal was in the feedlot, when signs were observed and if treatment was initiated. Mortalities should be classified into preventable and non-preventable mortalities, where preventable mortalities are those that are considered to be due to inadequacies in management or feedlot personnel.

A performance summary should be completed when each lot is marketed. Average daily gain, total feed consumption, feed conversion efficiency ratios, mortality, morbidity, treatment costs per head and culling rates should all be analysed.

Something that cannot be overemphasised is the importance of records in identifying individuals and pens not performing to their potential, identifying new problems and documenting progress.

Conclusion

Feedlots have an important influence on regional, state and national economies. They provide a finishing mechanism for the beef industry, as well as a significant value-adding mechanism for the local community. Managing risk in the feedlot ensures the feedlot's financial viability and sustainability.

References

Clark, T. (2006). *Guidelines for the Establishment and Operation of Cattle Feedlots in South Australia*, 2nd Edition.

CSIRO (1992). *Australian Model Code of Practice for the Welfare of Animals - Cattle*. Standing Committee on Agriculture, CSIRO Publications, Victoria, Australia.

Guthrie, C.A., Laudert S.B. and Zimmerman, A.G. (2000). Metaphylaxis for undifferentiated bovine respiratory disease. *Compendium on Continuing Education for the Practising Veterinarian* **22**(3), S62.

Irsik, M., Langemeier, M., Schroeder, T., Spire, M. and Roder, J.D. (2006) Estimating the Effects of Animal Health on the Performance of Feedlot Cattle. *Bovine Practitioner* **40**(2), 65–74.

Loneragan, G.H., Dargatz, D.A., Morley, P.S. and Smith, M.A. (2001). Trends in mortality ratios among cattle in US feedlots. *Journal of the American Veterinary Medical Association* **219**(8), 1122–1127.

Radostits, O.M. (2000). *Alberta Feedlot Management Guide*. Dept of Internal Medicine, Western College of Veterinary Medicine, University of Saskatchewan.

Radostits, O.M. and Blood, D.C. (1985). *Health and Production Management in Beef Feedlots in Herd Health: A Textbook of Health and Production Management of Agricultural Animals*. WB Saunders Company.

Smith, R.A. (2004). *Feedlot Diseases and Their Control*. Proceedings 23rd World Buiatrics Congress, Quebec, Canada.

Smith, R.A., Gill, D.R. and Van Koevering, M.T. (1994). A comparison of tilmicosin and ceftiofur for treatment of bovine respiratory disease. *Bovine Practitioner* **28**, 35–37.

Young, C.A. (1995). Antimicrobial metaphylaxis for undifferentiated bovine respiratory disease. *Compendium on Continuing Education for the Practising Veterinarian* **17**, 133–142.

CHAPTER 56

Organic Beef Farms

Kathryn Ellis

Learning objectives

- To be aware of the structure of the legislation pertaining to organic farming in the EU and the UK.
- To understand the major differences in management of organic beef farms.
- To understand the regulations pertaining to treatment of organic beef cattle with veterinary medicines.
- To understand the challenges associated with organic beef farming with respect to optimising forage use, breeding and parasite control.

Introduction to organic farming

In the United Kingdom (UK), the number of registered organic holdings has increased dramatically in the last 15 years, with numbers of organic cattle continuing to increase (DEFRA, 2011). Although organic farming is still supplying a 'niche' market, representing around 4% of the UK farmed land area and < 5% of cattle (fewer than 1% of prime cattle slaughtered are organic), there is a widespread distribution of holdings. Having an understanding of the organic farming system, including the associated regulations, is important in order to provide appropriate veterinary services to organic clients and their livestock.

Organic farming has its origins in early 20th Century Europe, with the Soil Association, formed in the UK in 1946. It is defined by the principles outlined in Figure 56.1 and can be viewed as a holistic approach to farming. In practice, this means that farmers utilise some or all of the following techniques: Use of legumes (such as clover) to fix nitrogen; recycling of manures and crop wastes; mechanical control of weeds; operation of a 'closed farm system' with respect to nutrients; crop rotations to minimise disease build-up; mixed and rotational grazing to reduce parasite burdens; growing resistant crop varieties; minimising chemical and/or veterinary therapeutic drug usage.

Organic farming regulations

In the European Union (EU), organic food production is regulated by Council Regulation (EC) 834/2007. This is the most recent update of the EU regulations, which came into effect in January 2009. This legislation outlines the baseline EU standards, farming practices and inspection of organic producers and processors. Despite organic production having a recognised following for many decades, there has been a Livestock Annex in the EU regulations only since August 2000. Each member state of the EU must abide by the baseline EU regulations but, in addition, each is also at liberty to add to the regulations (i.e. to make them more stringent).

In the UK, the EU legislation is interpreted via The Compendium of UK Organic Standards (Anon, 2006) and overseen by the relevant agricultural departments of each devolved region: in England by the Department of Environment, Food and Rural Affairs (DEFRA); in Scotland by the Scottish Government; in Wales by the Welsh Government. The basic UK standards for organic production and processing are legally enforced by the Organic Products Regulation, 2004.

Organic farming certification

In the UK, there are nine DEFRA-approved organic certification bodies (Table 56.1). Each of these certification bodies has its own set of rules for organic production, based on the underlying EU and UK legislation, although in some cases additional requirements are set, over and above the baseline regulations.

Bovine Medicine, Third Edition. Edited by Peter D. Cockcroft.

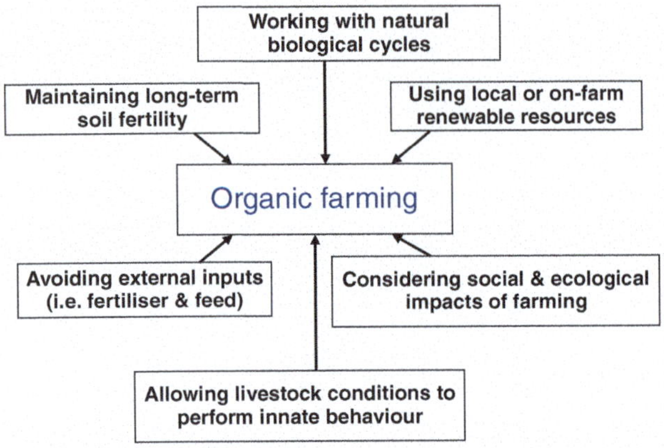

Figure 56.1 Principles defining organic farming systems.

For a producer to be a registered organic farm, the following steps should have been completed:

1 The producer has registered with one of the certification bodies.
2 The producer is following that certification body's production standards.
3 The farm has a farm conversion plan if it is converting from non-organic production, and/or a subsequent organic farming management plan for maintenance following conversion.
4 The farm is subject to annual inspection from the certification body's own inspectorate, whereby the holding is audited with respect to inputs, crop treatments, livestock feeds, livestock movements, livestock treatments and health records to ensure that the producer is abiding by the rules of production.

If all of the above procedures are completed to the satisfaction of the certifier, the producer may then call his/her produce 'organic'.

Conversion to organic production

Conversion to organic production generally entails a minimum of a two-year soil conversion period for the farm. The livestock on the holding have a variable conversion period, dependent on animal species. For example, a dairy cow should be managed organically for a minimum of nine months before her milk can be sold as organic; a suckler cow must be managed for 12 weeks before her offspring (not the cow herself) can be sold as organic. Animals raised for organic meat production have to be born and raised organically to be sold as organic. Usually, the conversion period is associated with a reduction in farm yields, due to reduced stocking densities and different feeding practices. There is a great deal of advice available for producers wishing to convert to organic production systems, including information on the funding available to support producers in the conversion period when they have reduced yields but are not able to sell organic produce (see the section on useful information at the end of the chapter).

Organic management regulations

A stipulation of the UK regulations (Anon, 2006) is that a herd health plan is required, '*ensuring the proper control of disease and the encouragement of positive animal welfare … This must be provided for by a plan drawn up by the farmer, preferably working in partnership with a veterinary surgeon and agreed between them during and after conversion, to develop and operate an organic livestock system which conforms to these Standards. The plan must ensure the development of a pattern of health building and disease control measures appropriate to the particular circumstances of the individual farm and allow for the evolution of a farming system progressively less dependent on allopathic veterinary medicinal products.*'

This is a great opportunity for veterinarians to become involved in herd-health work with organic dairy clients as prevention of disease (and evidence based medicine) is central to the organic approach.

Sources of stock

When a farm is converted to organic production, the existing livestock can be retained but can never be sold as organic.

Table 56.1 Approved organic certification bodies in the UK.

Name of certification body	Comments	Website address
Soil Association Certification Ltd		www.soilassociation.org/certification
Scottish Organic Producers Association (SOPA)		www.sopa.org.uk
Organic Farmers and Growers (OFG)		www.organicfarmers.org.uk
Biodynamic Agricultural Association		www.biodynamic.org.uk
Irish Organic Farmers and Growers Association		http://iofga.org/
Organic Trust Limited	Republic of Ireland-based body	http://www.organic-trust.org/
Quality Welsh Food Certification Ltd	Lamb and beef only	http://www.wlbp.co.uk/organic_overview
Ascisco Ltd	Minor section of Soil Association	www.soilassociation.org/certification
Organic Food Federation		www.orgfoodfed.com

However, the progeny of cows can be sold as organic, following the required conversion period for both land and stock. Cows must be managed organically for at least 12 weeks before calving, to enable the calves to be sold as organic. Breeds must be suitable for local conditions.

Replacements

Producers are encouraged to breed their own replacements or to buy from other organic farms. However, up to 10% of the breeding herd can be replaced each year, from conventional herds, by heifers which have not produced a calf.

Calves

Calves from organic dairy herds can be reared for organic beef production, provided the production system complies with organic standards throughout.

If a calf dies, a replacement calf may be purchased and fostered on. If the calf comes from a conventional (non-organic) herd, it may not be sold for organic meat. Non-organic heifer calves may be used as replacements.

Stores

Conventional store cattle may not be finished as organic. Organic store cattle purchased from other organic farms may be finished organically, but are often in short supply. As some parts of the country are suited for suckled calf production, and other areas more suited for finishing cattle production, weaned suckled calves can be sold from organic rearing to finishing units.

Bulls

Stock bulls can be purchased from conventional farms provided they are subsequently managed to organic standards. Hired bulls can be used, provided they are managed organically while they are on the farm. The use of AI is permitted.

Veterinary medicines use and withdrawal periods

Although one of the aims of organic production systems is to minimise use of veterinary medicines, if there is a clinical justification for treatment of an animal then it is permissible to do so under the organic regulations. Under EU and UK regulations, recommendations are that phytotherapeutic (e.g. plant extracts), homoeopathic products and trace elements, should be used in preference to chemically-synthesised allopathic veterinary medicinal products or antibiotics, *provided that their therapeutic action is effective for the species of animal, and the condition for which the treatment is intended.* If no such alternative product is available or deemed to be effective then, under veterinary guidance, the use of veterinary medicine is permitted.

Veterinary medicinal products must be authorised in accordance with current European and UK legislation, and appropriate records must be kept detailing the animal treated, the indication for treatment, the product used, the batch number and the withdrawal period. The baseline EU and UK requirement is that the withdrawal period on treatments is twice that stated on the product's datasheet, with the Soil Association requiring three times the duration of withdrawal. A product with a zero withdrawal period (for example a prostaglandin analogue) has an automatic 48 hour withdrawal period under organic rules. Any off-datasheet use requires application of the standard withdrawal periods (28 days meat). In addition, the Soil Association requirements restrict the use of certain other drug classes, such as third and fourth generation cephalosporins and fluoroquinolones, to very specific instances of individual animals under treatment.

An animal in an organic production system may receive no more than three *courses* of veterinary allopathic treatment per year, or one course if the animal is to be killed before it is one year old. A course of treatment is defined as: '*a course of treatment shall mean all necessary measures taken to restore the animal to health following a particular disease episode*'. It is important to be aware that multiple administrations of a product, or simultaneous administrations of two products – for example, administration of a non-steroidal anti-inflammatory drug concurrently with an antimicrobial to treat a foot lameness for more than one day – would be considered to be one course of treatment. Vaccines and parasite treatments are not included as courses of treatment, although some certification bodies prefer use of reduced valency vaccines, where possible.

Preventive veterinary treatments are prohibited which, in most cases in beef systems, does not have a significant impact. The major effects of this are that herd- based reproductive treatments are not permitted (for example, animals would not be allowed to be treated to synchronise oestrous in a group for a fixed time service). No growth promoters are permitted; however, under current EU regulations, hormonal growth promoters are not permitted in any non-organic production.

It is important to realise that strategic therapy use *is* allowed, when supported with evidence of a requirement; therefore, the strategic administration of an anthelmintic to a part of, or the whole of, a group of animals would be permissible, if supported with evidence of need to do so, such as poor live weight gains or a high faecal egg count in a group of grazing animals. It is equally important to emphasise that *animals are not required to show clinical disease or, in the worst case, die, before treatments can be administered.* National or international disease control measures are allowed, a recent example of this is the blanket use of Bluetongue (BTV 8) vaccination to control disease in Europe.

Overall, preventive herd health is key in reducing the requirement for veterinary therapy; an aim of all producers, organic or otherwise. However, it is vital for veterinary surgeons working with organic producers to communicate with their clients and with the client's organic certification body, when discussing preventive health measures and when considering the requirements for treatment of organic livestock, to ensure there is no compromise in animal welfare or the producer's livelihood.

Herd health planning

When considering herd health planning for organic beef farms, it is important to remember the essential differences in production compared to non-organic systems. However, it is also important to emphasise the similarities to non-organic systems. Many of the endemic infectious diseases, such as Bovine Virus Diarrhoea (BVD) and Infectious Bovine Rhinotracheitis (IBR) are equally important. Veterinary surgeons advising organic clients must be aware of the production principles of organic farming and the specific requirements of both the individual farm circumstances and the certification body with which the producer is registered.

A useful UK-based source of advice and information is the Organic Compendium, an online resource available at: http://www.organicvet.co.uk/. Herd health work on organic beef units should be aimed at producing high quality beef animals for slaughter as efficiently as possible, with minimal use of concentrate feed for finishing. To obtain the optimum organic beef price, the finished animal must have a good conformation; it is not enough just to be organic. In addition, those producers selling store animals must have high health status calves that will go on to perform well on the finishing unit. Specific issues relating to nutrition, parasite control and breeding are discussed below.

Organic beef management and performance

As organic regulations require a minimum of 60% DMI as forage, this effectively eliminates the use of high quantities of cereal to finish organic beef cattle (i.e. no barley beef systems). In Europe, organic beef production is based around suckled beef production (Figure 56.2), with subsequent finishing, either on farm of origin or by specialist finishers, of cattle on forage-based rations. Spring-calving herds suit the organic system better, as they are able to utilise spring grass growth better at the time of peak energy requirement (see sections on nutrition and reproduction below).

Choice of breed is important; this is largely dependent on farm location, with traditional 'hardy', easier calving beef breeds such as Highland, Welsh Black and Shorthorn type cattle faring well, particularly on marginal or upland organic units. Calf weights at birth, 200 days old and 300 days old are useful indicators of performance (the latter figures reflecting forage availability), but are not always easy to obtain on commercial farms. Average daily calf live weight gains should be comparable with non-organic systems, and in the order of 0.8–1.0 kg live weight per day (Frost *et al.*, 2009; Peers, 2009). Forage-finished organic beef can be achieved at 17–22 months of age (Younie, 2001).

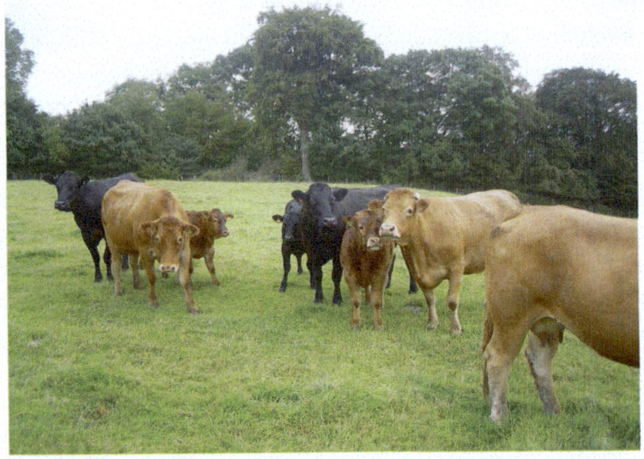

Figure 56.2 In Europe, organic beef production is based around suckled beef production.

The management system of an individual farm is dependent on the farm's location and any other enterprises on the unit. Some herds are successfully outwintered, and others are part, or entirely, housed over winter. Organic regulations stipulate that wholly slatted housing is not acceptable for beef units; therefore, producers must either have bedded accommodation or partly covered slats.

Spring calving has many advantages, as it minimises the conserved forage requirements and can avoid some of the health problems associated with housing young calves in winter. Weaning is a stressful procedure for both cows and calves, and provision of creep feed (either concentrates or high quality forage) to calves, in addition to nose-to-nose contact, can help reduce stress. It is advisable to avoid weaning, housing, castration and dehorning in a short space of time, due to the associated stress leading to reduced immunity. Ideally, all calves should be castrated and dehorned by three months old if possible (dependent on handling facilities and the likelihood of fly problems).

Overall animal performance should be similar to non-organic units, but financial performance can be very variable. This is affected by the lower stocking densities on organic units, but compensated for by the potential for higher return for finished beef and, in general, lower forage costs due to no fertiliser costs. The economics of the organic beef sector are subject to fluctuation and making long term, wide ranging financial predictions is difficult. In general, those producers able to finish cattle make the better margins rather than those selling stores (Younie, 2001).

Feeding organic beef cattle

Grass and white clover swards are the basis of most organic beef systems. However, as with organic dairy farming, having access to alternative sources of forage can be beneficial. Making the best use of home-grown forage is essential, both grazing and conserving. Often, on beef farms, only one cut of silage is taken in order to maximise yield. The difficulty can be that this results in forage with lower energy content, and requires some degree of supplementation (Peers, 2009). It has been recommended that farmers should aim to take two cuts of silage to maximise both quality and quantity, or to introduce a second forage source, such as whole crop cereals or peas (Younie, 2001).

It is important to analyse conserved forages to enable a balanced ration to be formulated. Forage type, soil type, climate and crop management can all significantly affect forage quality, so forage analysis can enable more accurate assessments of ration suitability. In practice, on beef units, the regular use of body condition scoring of beef cows is the most important tool that can indicate nutritional status (Figure 56.3). Spring-calving cows should have a body condition score of 3.0 at housing, 2.5 at calving and 2.0 at turnout. Control of body condition score can be achieved in the autumn by adjusting weaning date; delayed weaning can reduce body condition score, whereas earlier weaning can allow the cow to increase condition.

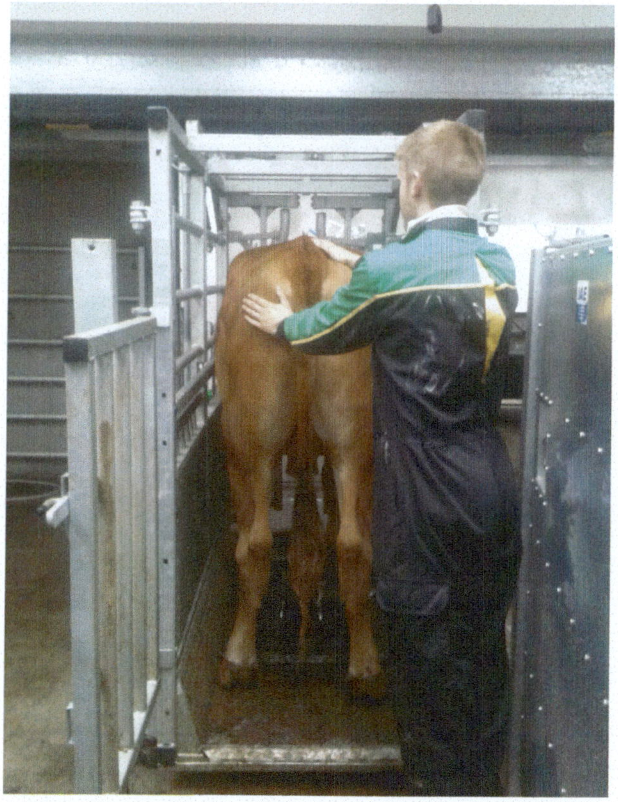

Figure 56.3 The regular use of body condition scoring of beef cows is the most important tool that can indicate nutritional status.

Given the high proportion of forage in organic finishing rations, the limitations of poor quality forage can quickly be apparent, with live weight gains varying between 0.4–1.0 kg/day on different forage energy densities (Peers, 2009). Thus, addition of concentrate may be needed to enable animals to be finished.

Reproductive management

Calving rates of 95% are achievable on organic beef units (Peers, 2009), but maintaining correct body condition score in suckler cows is key in terms of optimising fertility. Cows that are losing excessive amounts of body condition after calving will be difficult to get back in calf. Calving in the spring is intuitively easy in an organic system, as the spring grass can be utilised to increase the plane of nutrition of the cows at the time when energy demands are highest. It is not permitted to synchronise groups of cows to manage fertility; however, on an individual cow basis, the use of progesterone intra-vaginal devices can be a useful adjunct. Nevertheless, it should be emphasised that a successfully managed organic herd should require minimal reproductive drug input. Isolated cases of endometritis can be treated (e.g. with prostaglandin).

Bulls should be subject to the same health and reproductive assessment as on non-organic farms, with careful consideration of biosecurity, in particular with regards to infectious diseases such as bovine virus diarrhoea and Johne's disease (these issues are covered elsewhere).

Parasite control

Spring-born suckled calves grazing with their dams should have been exposed to a moderate gastrointestinal nematode challenge, and thus have started to develop some immunity in their first grazing season. An anthelmintic treatment at housing may or may not be needed; this depends on variation in parasite challenge, both between farms and even within a single farm between different years (see the section on organic dairy cattle parasite control for more information). The decision to treat may be based on overt clinical signs, or based on sub-optimal live weight gains. Plasma pepsinogen concentration can be monitored at housing, where values should be interpreted on a group basis, rather than in individuals. High concentrations of pepsinogen can be used as an indicator to treat the group. Although this approach offers some merit in terms of evidence-based decision-making regarding treatment, the high pepsinogen concentrations are indicative of abomasal damage, so therefore there may already be some compromise to the animals' weight gain.

Fluke control is very difficult in the absence of the use of flukicides, especially in the wetter, marginal pastures found in many parts of the UK where beef cattle graze. An organic beef herd health plan must address fluke, and this may include some or all of the following:

1 Use of abattoir feedback to monitor liver damage from fluke.
2 Routine faecal egg counting for fluke at different times of the year – critically at housing and through the winter if out wintered.
3 Use of appropriate flukicide treatment at key times of the year – at, or just after housing, and again in the late winter/early spring if outwintered. Consideration must be given to the very long withdrawal periods on flukicides, which are a consequence of doubling (or more) the standard datasheet recommendation; animals shortly to be slaughtered should be carefully identified, and not treated unless showing clinical disease.

Summary

Organic beef farming in general is not dissimilar to typical forage-based suckler and finishing beef systems. Many principles of the epidemiology of disease, and of appropriate animal husbandry, are similar to non-organic systems. The key areas are to maximise efficient use of forage in breeding cows to maintain optimal fertility, and in growing stock to optimise growth rates. Veterinarians should be aware of the organic regulations, so they can advise their clients appropriately to ensure healthy, productive livestock.

References

Frost, D., Morgan, M. and Moakes, S. (2009). *A farmer's guide to organic upland beef and sheep production*. Organic Farming Centre, Wales.

Peers, D. (2009) *Organic Beef and Sheep nutrition. Institute of Organic Training and Advice.* Results of Organic Research: Technical Leaflet **3**.

Younie, D. (2001) *Organic and Conventional Beef Production – a European Perspective*. Presented at 22nd Western Nutrition Conference, University of Saskatchewan, Saskatoon, Canada.

Useful sources of information

The DEFRA website (http://www.defra.gov.uk) has links to the following:

- Compendium of UK Organic Standards (September 2006)
- Guidance Document on European Union Organic Standards (December 2008)
- Council Regulation (EC) 834/2007, implemented by Commission Regulation (EC) 889/2008 and Commission Regulation (EC) 1235/2008
- SAC Organic website: http://www.sac.ac.uk/consulting/services/i-r/organic/
- Organic Centre Wales has information on business management and producers: http://www.organiccentrewales.org.uk/
- Elm Farm Research Centre has information on all aspects of organic farming: http://www.organicresearchcentre.com/
- Organic Compendium. Gives advice on disease-specific issues as well as general herd-health and welfare advice. Available at: http://www.organicvet.co.uk/
- Business Link Website. Government website giving information on business set-up and management. See: http://www.businesslink.gov.uk/bdotg/action/layer?topicId=1083732127&furlname=organic&furlparam=organic&ref=http%3A//archive.defra.gov.uk/foodfarm/growing/organic/index.htm&domain=www.businesslink.gov.uk
- Department of Agriculture and Rural Development Northern Ireland: Organic Beef production information available at: http://www.dardni.gov.uk/ruralni/index/bussys/organic_production/organic_beef_and_sheep/beef_and_sheep_beef.htm
- Institute of Organic Training and Advice (IOTA). Various aspects of organic farming advice for producers. http://www.organicadvice.org.uk/

CHAPTER 57

Marketing Beef Cattle Practice

Brad J. White

Learning objectives

- Beef veterinarians add value to client operations, and an appropriate marketing strategy is key to generating synergistic veterinary-client relations.
- Refining the practice brand involves defining the current practice identity and the practice's competitive advantages, in order to improve clarity in client expectations.
- Preferences of target clients influence how the types of services the practice offers are valued.
- Implementing a packaged, convenient service program is a vehicle to capture value from practice strengths and client preferences.
- A communications plan outlines how the practice will share information on the practice brand and service programs with new and existing clients.

Introduction

Beef producers employ an increasingly complex array of tools to generate a high quality product in an efficient manner. Improved management techniques, biological innovation, technological advances and changing consumer expectations influence how beef producers manage their operations. These changes also modify what beef producers expect from their veterinarian, as well as the value that producers place on specific veterinary services. The opportunity for the beef practitioner is not only to provide the high quality services desired by their clientele, but also to receive adequate financial compensation for these efforts.

Not utilising common business practices, such as designing a practice marketing strategy, may limit practitioners from reaching their income potential (Cron *et al.*, 2000). Veterinarians often freely provide information on preventative health programs, management techniques and disease management strategies to their clients. This advice adds value to the client operation by improving herd performance and decreasing health costs, but one challenge for the beef practitioner is providing services in a manner resulting in adequate compensation for the provision of this information. Adding value to a product (or client's herd) is not the same as the veterinarian capturing value from providing the information, and a plan should be created to most effectively capture value from the provision of specific goods or services.

Consider the example of preconditioning programmes in beef calves. Disease in the post-weaning phase causes detrimental performance and economic impacts (Irsik *et al.*, 2006; Babcock *et al.*, 2009; Reinhardt *et al.*, 2009), and several preventative health management techniques have been shown to reduce the risk of post-weaning disease (Step *et al.*, 2008; Roeber *et al.*, 2001; Arthington, 2008); therefore, the natural assumption would be that, if producers properly managed their calves prior to weaning, they should be paid more for these calves at the time of sale. Producers add value to calves by employing a preventative health strategy, but they may not be adequately compensated for these efforts unless the value added program is coupled with a system to capture this added value.

Preconditioned calves can receive a higher price when they are marketed through specific programmes that facilitate effective communications between buyers and sellers, but may not receive a higher price if the calves are marketed without effective seller-buyer interaction (King *et al.*, 2006). This example illustrates the importance of creating a comprehensive system that not only adds value to producer operations (e.g. applying an appropriate preventative health programme), but also facilitates the capturing of this added value by both the producer and the information provider (e.g. ensuring that cattle are marketed in an appropriate manner).

The idea of marketing often has a negative connotation in beef veterinary practice, as frequently it is misconstrued as analo-

Bovine Medicine, Third Edition. Edited by Peter D. Cockcroft.

gous to 'selling' a product and service by convincing clients to purchase something they would not desire if not coerced. A more accurate depiction of marketing is the creation of a value capture mechanism, facilitating the exchange of information to the producer in return for payment for these services. Increasing client loyalty, improving client retention, and developing new clients are three business practices identified as leading predictors of higher personal income for veterinarians (Volk *et al.*, 2005).

An effective marketing programme for the beef veterinary practice achieves these goals by improving client awareness of products and services available through the practice. A marketing strategy is essential for improving practice growth rate (Burge, 2003), and a survey of mixed-animal practices revealed that the gross income per veterinarian grew at a rate of 13.9% (±3.0) in practices with a marketing plan, compared to 4.4% growth in practices that did not have a marketing strategy (Brusk *et al.*, 2010). Creating a marketing plan is time-consuming, but the final result can be valuable to both the practice and the clientele.

The cornerstone of practice marketing is to plan a comprehensive strategy based on aspects of both the practice and the clients. Although a large part of a beef veterinarian's job is client communications, many veterinary practices do not have a formalised marketing plan. A survey of rural mixed animal practices indicated that only 22% of respondents had a marketing plan for the practice (Brusk *et al.*, 2010). The objective of this chapter is to describe a mechanism for creating a beef practice marketing strategy, including refining the practice brand, profiling target clients, creating service programmes, and creating a client communications plan.

Refining the practice brand

A brand can define the embodiment of all information associated with a product or service or, in other words, a brand represents the customer expectations of the quality and types of services that will be provided by the business. All veterinary practices have an existing brand or perceived value, as determined by their clients. The practice brand may have been carefully crafted following a specific marketing strategy, or the practice identity may have been generated passively, based on past interactions with clients. Whether the practice brand was actively or passively created, the types of services requested and the kind of client attracted to the practice is impacted by how the practice is viewed by customers.

The practice brand influences client expectations, and client satisfaction is based on the relationship between client expectations and the level of service provided. A survey of Tennessee livestock producers revealed that producers who perceived problems obtaining veterinary services cited issues (delay in obtaining services, only haul-in available) that could be related to a mismatch between clinic and client expectations (Jensen *et al.*, 2009). Refining the practice brand to match practice goals and competitive advantages is the first step in the creation of an effective marketing strategy.

Prior to refining the brand, an important step is establishing the current practice identity, or how the practice is viewed by clients. What do clients expect from the practice? The practice may be viewed as a technical service provider, a place to procure products at a reasonable price, or as a knowledge resource for the beef operation. If a client walks in the front door of the practice, what type of services can they expect to receive? Are these client expectations aligned with products or services that provide the practice a competitive advantage? The current practice brand is a starting point, but the brand can be refined if the clientele have changed, or the practice identifies a new potentially competitive advantage in the marketplace.

A competitive advantage differentiates the practice by offering a service or product to clients either at a higher quality or a more economical price, compared to other businesses. Competitive advantages come in many different forms, and each practice must identify the areas where they can excel. A true competitive advantage revolves around a product or service that the practice performs better, or more efficiently, than other businesses, and also generates a reasonable economic return for the practice. Veterinary practices can utilise product sales, technical services or knowledge to create an area of excellence in their practice; however, it is challenging to be truly outstanding in all of these areas. The practitioner should critically evaluate practice strengths, weakness and opportunities, in order to select a specific area to focus efforts. This does not ignore the other facets of the practice but, rather, applying disciplined planning to develop the area with the greatest potential to be a competitive advantage.

Not long ago, veterinary practices held a competitive advantage regarding the sale of most animal health products, because they were the most convenient (or only) source in the community. Today, beef operations anywhere in the country can purchase many biological and pharmaceutical products from a variety of locations, including delivery trucks, feed stores, catalogues, and over the internet. Increased competition leads to decreased margins available for the sale of each product. Thus, as in any market where the products are undifferentiated, the lowest price will most often drive the decision on where to purchase products.

Competing in a commodity marketplace dictates that additional revenue is generated if the practice can adequately increase the volume of sales. This is a reasonable business plan for some practices and, to make the most of this opportunity, management efforts should be allocated to areas such as inventory control. The important concept is to identify an area where the practice can have a distinct competitive advantage, and allocate practice resources to make improvements in this target area.

The practice brand is a valuable asset, and aligning the practice identity with future goals and expected opportunities is an important component of the practice marketing strategy. The value of the brand is not in converting existing clients to adopting new services or procedures but, rather, in attracting the ideal clients to the practice to take advantage of practice strengths.

For example, if the practice identifies a competitive advantage in creating a new replacement heifer management programme, this can be incorporated into the practice brand by establishing the practice as a resource for replacement heifer management. The refined practice brand may not convince all current clients to participate in the new programme but it will be a powerful tool, allowing producers who already desire these services to contact the practice. When the client is already motivated to implement management plans that align with the practice brand, a new, synergistic relationship can be created between practice and client. After the practice identity has been clearly defined, the next step is describing the ideal client for the practice.

Understanding target client preferences

The beef operation business structure and client motivation factors influence which veterinary products and services a particular client views as most valuable. Understanding why clients perceive value in specific veterinary services can be used to customise the marketing strategy to reach specific segments of the beef clientele. All clients need to be treated fairly, but this does not imply that all clients are treated exactly the same.

Practices that modify their fees for a specific service among clients in their practice have been shown to have greater gross income, and higher growth rate in gross practice income, compared to clients who charge the same fee for a service to all clients (Brusk *et al.*, 2010). For example, if the practice decides to develop a replacement heifer programme, the same services and procedures may be offered to all clients, but the how the value of the programme is communicated can be customised to specific clients, based on their underlying motivational factors. Existing and future practice clientele can be segmented into one of three main motivational categories, including lifestyle, commodity, or value-driven operations.

Lifestyle or hobby ranches raise livestock for enjoyment or the personal reward of maintaining a cattle operation. Pride of ownership and convenience are major motivating factors for lifestyle operations, and the value proposition to this type of farm is helping to achieve their specific herd improvement goals. Evaluating the economic feasibility of veterinary services may not be a primary concern for lifestyle operations if the services can be offered in a convenient fashion that improves the quality of the operation. Marketing a replacement heifer programme to lifestyle clients would be focused on the convenience aspects (decreased dystocia, calving in a short window), as well as the pride of ownership (raising the best replacement heifers).

Expense-driven or commodity producers are motivated by the cost of the procedure or service, and these individuals are often considered to be price shoppers. The commodity producer makes a living by producing larger volumes of product on a lower cost basis; therefore, they are often motivated by decreasing expenses, as the opportunity to increase production may be limited by operation size. The appealing proposition to the commodity producer is offering a product at a lower cost relative to competition, or a service that will decrease overall farm expenses. Marketing a replacement heifer programme to commodity clients would be focused on decreasing the costs of raising replacement heifers (least cost rations for growing heifers), and increasing the efficiency of the overall programme (fewer heifers leaving the herd after their first calf).

Value-driven producers require a high level of efficiency in recommendations – or, in other words, they desire the value provided by the service to outweigh the cost of the service. These producers make their income based on selling a quality product at a reasonable price; therefore, they may have higher margins and lower volume, compared to the commodity producer. The appealing proposition to the value-based producer is offering a service that has more perceived value than the expense (e.g. creation of a herd record-keeping programme with production data interpretation). Marketing a replacement heifer programme to value-driven clients would be based on potential improvements in product quality (increased genetic value through artificial insemination, higher weaning weights due to early calving).

Most producers share some traits of each of the three main motivational groups, but understanding what drives the producer's animal health decisions influences how specific programmes are most effectively presented to clients. A useful exercise for the practice is to segment their client base into each of the motivational categories, and then generate a specific plan to reach the producers in each category with a specific offered service.

Creating service programmes

After identifying the practice's competitive advantages and what the clients want from the practice, the next step is coming up with a vehicle to couple what the practice offers and what the client needs into a new packaged service offering. Veterinarians have long realised the value of herd health programmes, but the challenge is implementing the programme in a manner that rewards both the client and the veterinarian. Packaging similar services into a comprehensive programme can help the client to achieve their goals, while also providing the practice with a mechanism to charge fairly for the offered services. Traditional veterinary services can also be coupled with additional offerings that facilitate client implementation of the recommended management changes.

Providing farms with not only an idea for improved management, but also a mechanism for implementation of the recommendations, is a valuable service. This creates a synergistic partnership relationship between the practice and client, focused on achieving a specific goal. The partnership benefits the client through improved production, and can help the practice by increased income. Economic growth rates were compared among practitioners, based on commonly offered services, and two services (herd record management and consulting on genetic decisions) were associated with higher five-year growth rates in gross dollars generated per veterinarian in the practice (White *et al.*, 2010). These two services involve the veterinarian in the farm management decision process, and enhance the partner relationship.

A practice may create a new health programme based on sound medical and management recommendations, but clients may not want to participate in the programme. The practice should evaluate why clients may not follow clinic recommendations in order to increase client compliance and, thereby, lead to increased profitability for the client and veterinarian in a mutually beneficial relationship. Three common reasons why clients do not participate in herd health programmes include reluctance to dedicate necessary resources, perceived complexity of suggestions, or limitations due to labour and time.

The reluctance to dedicate necessary resources toward a specific programme is best overcome by proper understanding of client preferences, as above. An accurate understanding of client needs allows customisation of the programme to the specific segment of the client base. The perceived complexity of suggestions is often related to the plan for implementing the health or management recommendations. As a part of a comprehensive programme, recommendations should not only include what to do, but also how to implement the programme efficiently in a specific operation.

Convenience is a motivating factor for many producers, and creating a comprehensive programme with a turnkey design facilitates ease of client participation. For example, if the client decides to participate in a replacement heifer management programme, the clinic does not simply provide a written summary outlining what should be done but, rather, helps with the procuring of necessary resources, scheduling critical events, and making sure that important milestones are achieved. Labour availability is often a rate-limiting step for the implementation of new health programmes in beef operations. Most operations are busy with daily maintenance tasks associated with feeding and managing the herd. Good ideas may fail to be implemented, even if they have longer term positive impacts, because the client impression is that, in the short term, an allocation of additional time and effort must be added to an already overburdened system.

As an example, a programme to intensively manage replacement heifer reproduction can result in more heifers being bred early in the breeding season, resulting in a more uniform, marketable calf crop, generating greater income for the farm. The programme may include several services, such as reproductive tract scoring replacement heifers, utilising oestrus synchronisation, utilising artificial insemination, and defining an appropriate genetic management plan. These services can be offered by the practice and packaged into a single programme, but the labour and technical skills involved in synchronising and breeding the heifers may present a significant obstacle to programme success.

Veterinary practices can improve client satisfaction by aligning programme participants with a person to assist with heifer synchronisation and breeding. The person assisting the breeding programme can be a clinic employee or not, but the important aspect is that the clinic assisted in eliminating obstacles with programme implementation. This can be set up as a mutually beneficial relationship because, if the clinic hires a person to assist with heifer breeding on multiple farms, the clinic benefits from economy of scale (only have to train one or two people), and the ranch gains by having an experienced, trained person to manage heifer breeding. An additional benefit of this type of management scheme is that the practice retains a high degree of influence on several critical control points influencing programme success. This oversight can lead to increased client satisfaction with results and, ideally, should generate long-term client loyalty.

Creating a comprehensive package of services around a single concept offers benefits to both the veterinary clinic and the clientele. The pricing structure can be relatively traditional; producers are used to paying for labour via a fee-for-service arrangement. Clinics can benefit by capturing greater income, related to the increased number of services used by each ranch. Generating efficient production for the farm fosters sustainability, and allows the farm to continue to retain the services of the veterinarian. The relationship also involves the veterinarian in the farm's decision-making process, and encourages client loyalty.

Client communications plans

The final step in the marketing strategy is determining a clear communications plan to convey the value of clinic services to prospective clients. Effective information transfer between the practice and clients is one of the best ways to ensure full utilisation of available services, and to provide clients with a benefit beyond traditional veterinary services. As a result, client relationships are a key determinant of practice financial success (Volk *et al.*, 2005).

Creating a communications plan requires identification of target client, as well as the specific message to be conveyed. The method used to convey the message will be influenced by the goals of the programme, as well as characteristics of client motivations, as described in previous sections. If the goal is to increase client utilisation of services, the message should be concise, focused on a point of importance for the target client, and repeated multiple times. This requires preparation of the message into a simple format that builds interest in the new programme and stimulates further questioning on the topic. Following the replacement heifer programme example, the message to value-based clients may be distilled into three main points: higher pregnancy rates in replacement heifers; decreased dystocia risk, and increased calf weaning weights. The objective is not conveying how these goals will be achieved but, rather, stimulating interest in the programme for potential follow-up conversations.

Communication plans should not focus only on people external to the clinic. Clinic staff and practice associates are important participants when the goal is to communicate a clear, consistent message from the clinic. Maintaining open communication within the practice allows the clients to hear the same message multiple times, as they interact with everyone who works in the clinic.

After designing a specific message to be conveyed, a strategy should be created for implementing the plan, and this strategy may be active or passive. Does the practice wait for producers to call and schedule herd work? Or does the clinic receptionist send reminders and call to arrange times for herd visits? Active communication allows the clinic to control the flow of information, and to send appropriate messages to clients at critical times. Examples of active communication in the veterinary practice include mailing reminder cards, sending letters describing and promoting specific services, and holding informative meetings for clients. Practices that send clients a newsletter (active communication) have been shown to have higher growth rates in gross income generated per veterinarian (Brusk *et al.*, 2010). Active communication allows the practice to maintain a consistent message to targeted clients.

Planned, active communication is an effective way to transfer information on available services to specific target clients. Effective communication requires spending time on creating a clear, consistent message, focused on a point of importance for the target client, and identifying an effective medium to get the message to the client.

Summary

Beef producer expectations are evolving, and veterinarians have several opportunities to offer valuable services to their clients. Improving client utilisation of practice services requires a plan and a systematic approach. Beef veterinary practices can create a marketing strategy by refining the practice brand, profiling target clients, creating service programmes, and creating a client communications plan.

References

Arthington, J.D., Qiu, X., Cooke, R.F. *et al.* (2008). Effects of preshipping management on measures of stress and performance of beef steers during feedlot receiving. *Journal of Animal Science* **86**, 2016–2023.

Babcock, A.H., White, B.J., Dritz, S.S. *et al.* (2009). Feedlot health and performance effects associated with the timing of respiratory disease treatment. *Journal of Animal Science* **87**, 314–327.

Brusk, A.M., White, B.J., Goehl, D.R. *et al.* (2010). Results of a survey to determine demographic and business management factors associated with size and growth rate of rural mixed-animal veterinary practices. *Journal of the American Veterinary Medical Association* **237**, 1385–1392.

Burge, G.D. (2003). Six barriers to veterinary career success. *Journal of Veterinary Medical Education* **30**, 1–4.

Cron, W.L., Slocum, J.V., Jr., Goodnight, D.B. *et al.* (2000). Executive summary of the Brakke management and behavior study. *Journal of the American Veterinary Medical Association* **217**, 332–338.

Irsik, M., Langemeier, M.R., Schroeder, T.C. *et al.* (2006). Estimating the effects of animal health on the performance of feedlot cattle. *Bovine Practitioner* **40**, 65–74.

Jensen, K.L., English, B.C., Menard, R.J. *et al.* (2009). Livestock producers' views on accessing food-animal veterinary services: implications for student recruitment, training, and practice management. *Journal of Veterinary Medical Education* **36**, 30–38.

King, M.E., Salman, M.D., Wittum, T.E. *et al.* (2006). Effect of certified health programs on the sale price of beef calves marketed through a livestock videotape auction service from 1995 through 2005. *Journal of the American Veterinary Medical Association* **229**, 1389–1400.

Reinhardt, C.D., Busby, W.D. and Corah, L.R. (2009). Relationship of various incoming cattle traits with feedlot performance and carcass traits. *Journal of Animal Science* **87**(9), 3030–42

Roeber, D.L., Speer, N.C., Gentry, J.G. *et al.* (2001). Feeder Cattle Health Management: Effects on Morbidity Rates, Feedlot Performance, Carcass Characteristics, and Beef Palatability. *The Professional Animal Scientist* **17**, 39–44.

Step, D.L., Krehbiel, C.R., DePra, H.A. *et al.* (2008). Effects of commingling beef calves from different sources and weaning protocols during a 42-day receiving period on performance and bovine respiratory disease. *Journal of Animal Science* **86**, 3146–3158.

Volk, J.O., Felsted, K.E., Cummings, R.F. *et al.* (2005). Executive summary of the AVMA-Pfizer business practices study. *Journal of the American Veterinary Medical Association* **226**, 212–218.

White, B.J., Brusk, A.M., Goehl, D.R. (2010). Services and procedures offered by rural food animal veterinarians. *Online Journal of Rural Research and Policy* **5**, 1–8.

APPENDIX I

Vade Mecum of Cattle Conditions

Kiro Petrovski

Index

Bovine Medicine, Third Edition. Edited by Peter D. Cockcroft.

Endocarditis (bacterial)
Endometritis
Enzootic pneumonia
Ephemeral fever
Epidydymitis – see orchitis and epididymitis
Facial eczema
Failure of passive transfer
Fatty liver
Femoral nerve paralysis
Fescue poisoning
Fluoride poisoning
Fly-related dermatoses
Fog fever
Follicular cyst – see Ovarian cystic degeneration
Foot and mouth disease
Foul
Fracture of distal phalanx
Fusobacterium necrophorum abortion
Granular vulvo-vaginitis
Haemorrhagic septicaemia
Heat stress
Hepatitis
Hip dislocation/luxation
Histophilus somni complex
Honker syndrome – see tracheal oedema syndrome
Hydrancephaly
Hydrocephalus
Hypocalcaemia
Hypodermosis – see fly related dermatosis
Hypokalaemia
Hypomagnesaemia
Hypophosphataemia
Infectious bovine rhinotracheitis (IBR)
Infectious necrobacillosis of the foot – see foul
Inherited congenital porphyria
Interdigital dermatitis
Interdigital hyperplasia
Ionophores toxicity
Johne's disease
Ketosis
Laminitis
Lead poisoning
Leptospirosis
Lice
Listeriosis
Liver fluke
Lumpy skin disease
Lungworm pneumonia
Lupine-associated poisoning
Luteal cyst – see Ovarian cystic degeneration
Malignant catarrhal fever
Mange
Mastitis
Mastitis: coliform
Mastitis: gangrenous
Megaoesophagus
Meningitis (bacterial)
Metabolic acidosis – neonatal calves
Metritis
Milk fever –see hypocalcaemia
Milking machine-induced teat lesions
Monensin toxicity – see ionophore toxicity
Mycotoxicosis
Nasal granuloma
Necrotic vaginitis, vestibulitis and vulvitis
Necrotising enteritis
Neonatal septicaemia
Neosporosis
Nervous coccidiosis
Nitrate and nitrite poisoning
Nuisance flies – see fly related dermatosis
Oak poisoning
Obturator nerve paralysis
Ocular squamous cell carcinoma
Oesophageal obstruction (intra-luminal)
Orchitis and epididymitis
Organophosphate poisoning
Otitis externa
Otitis interna – see otitis media and interna
Otitis media/interna
Ovarian cystic degeneration
Oxalate toxicity
Papillomatosis
Papular stomatitis – see bovine popular stomatitis
Parainfluenza
Paralysis of the bladder
Paralysis of the tongue
Parasitic gastroenteritis
Parasitic pneumonia – See lungworm
Pediculosis – see lice
Penile deviation
Penile haematoma
Penis: broken – see penile haematoma
Penis: ruptured – see penile haematoma
Penis: fractured – see penile haematoma
Pericarditis
Petroleum distillates poisoning
Pharyngeal trauma
Photosensitisation
Polioencephalomalacia (B1 deficiency)
Post-partum haemorrhage
Postparturient haemoglobinuria
Psorergatic mange – see mange
Psoroptic mange –see mange
Pyelonephritis
Q-fever
Rabies
Repeated breeder cow
Retained foetal membranes – see retained placenta
Retained placenta
Reticulo-pericarditis – see pericarditis
Rift Valley fever

Rumen alkalosis
Ringworm
Rye grass staggers
Salmonellosis
Salt poisoning
Sarcoptic mange – see mange
Schmallenberg virus disease
Sciatic nerve paralysis
Screw worm infestation – see Fly related dermatosis
Seminal vesiculitis
Septic arthritis
Shipping fever
Simple indigestion
Snake bite
Sole ulcer
Spastic paresis
Spinal disorders
Sporadic bovine leukosis
Stomatitis
Summer mastitis
Sweet clover poisoning
Tarsal and carpal hygroma
Teat lesions
Teat lesions: Environment-induced
Teat trauma
Testicular degeneration
Testicular hypoplasia
Tetanus
Theileriosis
Tick paralysis
Tick-borne fever
Ticks
Tracheal oedema syndrome
Traumatic injuries to the sole
Traumatic reticulo-peritonitis
Trichomoniasis
Trypanosomiasis
Udder impetigo
Udder Oedema
Udder: intertrigo and necrotic dermatitis
Udder: skin disorders
Umbilical hernia
Umbilical infections
Urea poisoning
Urea/ammonia poisoning
Urolithiasis
Urticaria
Uterine inertia
Uterine prolapse
Vagus indigestion
Vertebral body abscess
Vesicular stomatitis
Vitamin A deficiency
Warts – see papillomatosis
White line disease
Winter disentery
Yersiniosis
Yew poisoning

Abomasal displacement

Disease Profile
Relatively common disorder occurring usually within the first six weeks of calving. Often concurrent to other post-partum disorders (e.g. mastitis, retained foetal membranes, metritis, hypocalcaemia, abomasal ulceration). Can be left or right. Left displacement of the abomasums is far more common. Right displacement of the abomasum predisposes to abomasal volvulus. Diet high in easily digestible carbohydrates and low on fibre has often been implicated.

Clinical findings
Left displaced abomasum
Decreased appetite to anorexia, no rumination, rumen atony, drop in milk production and decreased faecal output (drier than normal, or scant and watery). Usually mild abdominal pain, ketosis, sprung last few ribs on the left side with sunken paralumbal fossa. Many cases have positive 'pings' on simultaneous percussion and auscultation over the last 2–3 ribs, and produce splashing sounds on succussion. On rectal examination, rumen displaced abomasum cannot usually be palpated but the rumen may be displaced to right.

Right displaced abomasum
Similar to left displaced abomasums. 'Pings' and sprung ribs on the right side.

Abomasal volvulus
Complete anorexia, heavily depressed milk production, rapidly developing with sudden deterioration. Depressed animal, progressive weakness, toxaemia and dehydration. Sometimes melaena. Metabolic alkalosis, paradoxical aciduria, tachycardia, slower capillary refill time. On rectal examination, in advanced cases the abomasum can be felt. Death from circulatory shock and toxaemia occurs if untreated.

Diagnosis
History, signs, blood biochemistry

Principal differential diagnosis
Torsion of the greater mesentery, generalised peritonitis

Treatment
Returning the displaced abomasum to its original position and supportive treatment. Abomasal re-positioning can be conservative (e.g. rolling) or surgical (toggles, closed suturing, various approaches by laparotomy). Treatment of the concurrent disorders.
Abomasal volvulus – surgical correction of the volvulus. Tachycardia over 80 bpm and capillary refill time above four seconds, usually guarded prognosis.

Control
Balanced diet, maintain fibre intake, rapid increase in rumen volume after calving (administration of 20–40 L of electrolytes through a stomach pump), decrease the prevalence of post-partum disorders, keep cows in optimal body condition. Good transition cow management.

Abomasal impaction

Disease Profile and Aetiology
Impaired or blocked passage of ingesta through the pylorus by fibrous feedstuffs, sand, gravel, bezoars or neurological deficits. Can be acute or chronic. Usually individual cases, but can be an outbreak due to low-quality, indigestible feedstuffs. More common in late gestation cows.

Clinical findings
In-appetence to anorexia, atonic rumen, weight loss, scant faeces, dehydration, metabolic alkalosis, distention of right ventral abdomen. Later recumbency. Often associated with vagal indigestion.

Principal differential diagnosis
Abomasal volvulus and torsion, traumatic reticulo-peritonitis.

Treatment
Surgery or oral mineral oils daily for several days. May need to correct metabolic alkalosis. Grave prognosis.

Control
Prevent ingestion of indigestible feedstuffs, sand, gavel and pica.

Abomasal ulcers

Disease Profile
Partial or perforating damage to the abomasal mucosa and wall. Often subclinical.

Aetiology
Probably associated with stress. Highly fibrous feedstuffs may also be involved. In calves, change from milk to solid feedstuffs. Usually affects calves and high-yielding dairy cows, although all classes may be affected, including bulls.

Clinical findings
Type I: non-perforating, no bleeding, no melena, no clinical signs

Type II: bleeding ulcers usually with melaena, anaemia

Type III: perforating ulcer with local peritonitis

Type IV: perforating ulcer with generalised peritonitis, anorexia, abdominal pain, abdominal distention, sick and depressed animal.

Post-mortem findings
Abomasal ulcers, haemorrhagic, greenish to brownish fluid in the peritoneal cavity, localised to generalised peritonitis

Principal differential diagnosis
Abomasal volvulus and torsion, haemorrhagic bowel syndrome.

Treatment
Type II may need blood transfusion, confinement. Type III antibiotics, confinement. Type IV poor prognosis, intensive supportive therapy.

Control
Gradual introduction of solid feedstuffs to calves. Reduction of stress.

Abortion

Disease Profile
Loss of pregnancy from the end of the second month to full term. Abortion can be caused by any factor that compromises the normal function of the corpus luteum, foetal viability or placental integrity. An abortion rate of 2–5% a year without 'clustering' may be considered as 'normal' incidence. Abortion can be caused by many species of bacteria, fungi and protozoa. Ubiquitous bacteria usually cause sporadic abortion, while specific bacterial and protozoal abortions may occur as herd outbreaks.

Aetiology
NOTE: for specific abortions, see appropriate headings.

Various managerial, iatrogenic, infectious (bacteria, protozoa, viruses and fungi), hormonal, nutritional, toxic, and mechanical risk factors may contribute to the increased incidence of abortion. Any debilitating disorder of a heavily pregnant cow may result in abortion. Any stress (alteration in routine, slippery concrete, dog worrying, low-flying aircraft) may result in abortions. Common iatrogenic factors are rough rectal palpation and administration of corticosteroids, prostaglandins, xylazine or other abortifacients.

Infectious causes of abortion include: ubiquitous bacteria (*Trueperella pyogenes, Escherichia coli, Bacillus* spp., *Streptococcus* spp), abortion secondary to a primary bacterial disease (anthrax, bacillary haemoglobunuria, *Chlamydia* spp., *Histophilus somni* complex, pasterurellosis), contagious bacteria (*Brucella abortus, Campylobacter fetus venerealis, Leptospira* sp., *Listeria monocytogenes, Neospora caninum, Trichomonas fetus, Ureaplasma diverticulum*), viruses (e.g. akabane, bluetongue, bovine virus diarrhoea virus, Schmallenberg virus, foot-and-mouth, IBR/IPV, rift valley fever virus) and fungi (e.g. *Mortierella* spp., *Aspergilus* spp., *Absidia* spp., *Mucor, Pseudallescherichia boydii, Rhizopus,* yeasts).

Nutritional factors include undernourishment, deficiencies of macro- and micro-nutrients (Vitamin A, iodine, selenium, phosphorus), excess of some nutrients (e.g. urea, nitrate) and presence of toxic plants (e.g. macrocarpa, other cypress, *Brassica* spp., sweet clover, hemlock, locoweed) or chemicals (e.g. mycotoxins).

Brucellosis, *Chlamydia*, leptospirosis, listeriosis, foot-and-mouth and *Aspergillus* abortions are associated with a zoonotic risk.

Clinical findings
Finding an aborted foetus, haemorrhagic discharge from external genitalia, return to normal oestrus cycle after confirmed pregnancy, premature lactation. When calf aborted near term, it is difficult to confirm whether is normal calving or premature delivery.

Samples
Foetus, serum, milk samples, bulk milk samples, vaginal swab and placenta are important samples when using the diagnostic laboratory. Food samples may also be useful.

Diagnosis
It is important to exclude the common infectious causes of abortion as a first step,. These may include BVD, *N. caninum*, IBR, Leptospirosis, Brucella (where endemic). It can be difficult to establish the final diagnosis in some cases.

Treatment
Potential complications include endometritis, metritis, retained foetal membranes and infertility.

Control
Biosecurity. Vaccination if appropriate. Isolation of aborted animal until the aetiology is established. Management changes according to the aetiology.

Abscess – subcutaneous

Disease Profile
Accumulation of pus in newly formed cavity in the subcutis. It is common in cattle.

Aetiology
Treuperella pyogenes, Fusobacterium necrophorum, other ubiquitous microorganisms. Common complication of penetrating wounds and grass seed lodgement.

Clinical findings
Acute to subacute development of semi-fluctuating, usually painless swelling, clearly demarcated from the surrounding.

Differential diagnosis
Haematoma

Diagnosis
Needle aspirate, ultra-sonography

Principal differential diagnosis
Oedema, Neoplasia.

Treatment
Drainage by 'generously' lancing the abscess and flushing with copious amount of antiseptic solution (dilute iodine) or sterile saline. Antimicrobials are sometimes used, but these should be reserved for ascending infections or signs of systemic involvement.

Acidosis – rumen

Disease Profile
Dairy cows and feedlot beef cattle are at risk from acidosis due to their high-energy dense diets. Two related but clinically distinct conditions are recognised.

Sub-acute ruminal acidosis (SARA):
There is an increase in the volatile fatty acid concentration, with low concentrations of lactate within the rumen. The rumen fluid pH range is 5.0–5.6. The condition causes production losses as a result of poor rumen function. Cud dropping and tail swishing with loose faeces maybe observed. The condition is relatively common in high-producing dairy cows in the early post-partum period and approaching peak lactation and appetite.

'Acute' ruminal acidosis (ARA)
This disorder can be acute to chronic and severe to mild. The rumen pH in acute rumen acidosis is below 5.0, with high lactate concentrations. In severe cases it can be fatal. The lower pH results in sudden change of the microflora (increase in gram-positive bacteria) and death of protozoa.

Aetiology

SARA is associated with poor transition cow management, and high-energy and low-fibre diets with poor buffering capacity.

ARA is associated the rapid access and fermentation of easily digestible carbohydrates and excess production of lactate, causing a rapid reduction in rumen fluid pH. Excess of easily digestible carbohydrates (e.g. cereal grain overload, access to lush pasture) or imbalanced diet.

Clinical findings

SARA is associated with poor production, reduced fertility, loose faeces, excess tail swishing, increased perineal soiling and cud dropping

ARA
Anorexia, diarrhoea, dehydration, depression, rumen atony, weakness, laminitis, recumbency and death are seen in severe cases. In less severe cases, anoexia and depression are noted. Increased incidence of lameness due to laminitis may be seen in affected herd. Cattle are at increased risk of polioencephalomalacia, due to high demand for B1 during lactate metabolism.

Post-mortem findings
Ruminitis, liver abscesses, enteritis.

Diagnosis
SARA: requires careful evaluation using rumen fluid sampling of a representative group of cows (12). Diagnosis is usually made based upon 25% of the group in the SAR pH range and associated clinical profile.

ARA: clinical findings, pH of rumen fluid, metabolic acidosis.

Treatment
SARA: Lower energy density of diet, and increase the fibre content. Add buffers to the ration.

ARA: Severe cases may need to be euthanased or treated intensively if they are to survive. Rumen fluid 'wash out', intravenous fluids with bicarbonate, antibiotics to control bacteraemia, B1, transfaunation and antimycotics may be used. In less severe cases, a hay diet for several days, oral antacids may be curative.

Control
SARA Correct transition cow management and diet formulation.

ARA Gradual adaptation to new feedstuffs. Balanced diet. Ensure water available at all times. Oral supplementation with antacids. Oral supplementation of feed additives (ionophores – monensin, lasalocid).

Actinobacillosis

Common synonyms
Wooden tongue

Disease Profile
Infection of the soft tissues, usually tongue, after exposure to abrasive feedstuffs, particularly thistles and awns. Common, sporadic, rarely herd outbreak.

Aetiology
Actinobacillus ligniersii. Usually requires mucosal lesion caused by traumatic insults for infection.

Clinical findings
Diffuse swelling of the tongue, from firm to hard, impaired prehension, mastication and swallowing, rapid weight loss.

Post-mortem findings
Firm, usually pale abscess of granulomatous type of the tongue or other soft tissues, sometimes with ulceration and/or sinus.

Diagnosis
Clinical signs, detection of pathogen.

Principal differential diagnosis
Dental disorders, foreign body, disorders affecting oral mucosa, pharyngeal trauma or inflammation.

Treatment
Sodium iodide (not in pregnant cattle). Alternatively, streptomycin (not for use in food-producing animals in many countries) or high doses of oxytetracycline. Oral dosing with isoniazid. Use of soft feedstuffs.

Control
Prevent access to abrasive feedstuffs.

Actinomycosis

Common synonyms
Lumpy jaw

Disease Profile
Granulomatous osteomyelitis of the mandible, maxillae, rarely other bones or organs. Mainly younger cattle with erupting molar teeth.

Aetiology
Actinomyces bovis. Trauma to the oral mucosa is predisposing factor allowing infection. Trauma often around erupting teeth.

Clinical findings
Swelling of the mandible, painless and non-mobile. Later, one or multiple sinuses, discharging viscous 'honey-like' yellowish pus with granules.

Post-mortem findings
Osteomyeltis

Diagnosis
Clinical signs (usual), radiography, demonstration of the microcolonies of *Actinomyces bovis* in the pus.

Principal differential diagnosis
Abscess, impacted feed, foreign body, dental problems, actinobacillosis.

Treatment
Difficult to treat. Advanced cases rarely respond to treatment. Antimicrobials, including sodium iodide (not in pregnant cows), penicillin and isoniazid. Surgical opening and debridement of the affected area are possible but not usually attempted.

Control
Prevent ingestion of abrasive feedstuffs.

Akabane

Common synonyms
Arthrogryposis-hydranencephaly syndrome, Acorn calves, Curly calf disease, Dummy calf disease.

Disease Profile
Regional distribution. Rare. Most likely transmitted by blood-sucking insects (mosquitoes and gnats). Infection of pregnant cattle results in clinical disease. Common in tropics and subtropics. More serious outbreaks in naïve herds.
Notifiable.

Aetiology
Arbovirus.

Clinical findings
Abortion, stillbirths, dystocia. Most notably, serious and often fatal congenital abnormalities of calves (e.g. arthrogryposis, hydraencephaly) and weak calves. Mature cattle are usually asymptomatic. Encephalomyelitis may occur.

Post-mortem findings
Arthrogryposis, hydranencephaly.

Diagnosis
Congenital abnormalities of the foetus. Detection of pathogen. Serology.

Principal differential diagnosis
Bluetongue, BVD, nutritional and toxic disorders.

Treatment
No effective treatment.

Control
Vaccination. Vector control.

Alkalosis – metabolic

Disease Profile
Rumen buffering imbalance resulting from reduced activity of the rumen while saliva is still swallowed, or ingestion of some toxic agents (e.g. urea-non-protein nitrogen). Mild (rumen pH of 7.0 to 7.5) and severe form (rumen pH > 7.5). Common complication is putrefying rumenitis.

Aetiology
Mild form – prolonged anorexia, high-fibre diet.
Severe form – overfeeding or accidental ingestion of non-protein nitrogen (e.g. urea, biuret, ammonium phosphate, some fertilisers).

Clinical findings
Mild form – rumen dysfunction and atony, mild bloat, reduced appetite, signs of abdominal pain, mild metabolic alkalosis and dehydration.
Severe form – rumen atony, anorexia, depression, signs of urea poisoning, vomiting, abdominal pain, muscle tremors, incoordination, tachypnoea, weakness, rapid progression of metabolic alkalosis, dehydration and death.

Post-mortem findings
Severe form – rumen content may smell of ammonia. Fresh rumen content pH > 7.5.

Diagnosis
Clinical signs, rumen content pH.

Principal differential diagnosis
Other forms of indigestion, acidosis, other poisonings.

Treatment
Mild form – treat primary disorder or adjust the diet.
Severe form – oral administration of acidifiers (e.g. acetic acid 4–10 L). Treat metabolic alkalosis and dehydration.

Control
Optimise diet. Prevent uncontrolled access to non-protein nitrogen and fertilisers.

Amyloidosis

Disease Profile
Rare sporadic disorder usually a sequelae of long-lasting inflammatory process elsewhere in the body. Most cases diagnosed soon after calving, usually within two weeks.

Renal amyloidosis causes significant chronic proteinuria, hypoproteinaemia, oedematous syndrome and, in later stages, uraemia with recumbency, coma and death.

Aetiology
Common sites for a focal infection are peritoneum, pneumonia, mastitis and metritis. Extensive amyloid deposition is most common in the liver, spleen and kidney.

Clinical findings
Many cases of amyloidosis are subclinical and not detected in live cattle.

Clinical signs include in-appetence, watery diarrhoea, anasarca and rapid emaciation, due to the protein-losing nephropathy ventral oedema and ascites. The condition is terminal.

Post-mortem findings
Affected organs grossly enlarged with pale, shiny and waxy appearance.

Diagnosis
Signs, serum biochemistry, urine analysis – high protein concentration. Rectal palpation – loss of renal segmentation.

Principal differential diagnosis
Other reasons for wasting cow.

Treatment
No effective treatment is available. If diagnosed early enough, emergency slaughter is advised. Later euthanasia.

Anaphylaxis

Common synonyms
Type 1 hypersensitivity.

Disease Profile
Rare. May occur concurrently with urticaria.

Urticaria, pruritus, angioedema, vascular collapse and life-threatening respiratory distress.

Common precipitating causes includes – vaccines, drugs, hypodermal larvae, insect bites, hormones, blood transfusion and milk allergy.

Aetiology
Contact with an allergen in sensitised cattle.

Clinical findings
Sudden onset of severe respiratory distress, muscle tremors, anxiety, pharyngeal and laryngeal oedema, hypersalivation, dacryorrhoea, fever, pruritus, mild bloat, diarrhoea. Nystagmus, collapse, death. Urticaria may or may not be present. Pregnant cows may abort.

Diagnosis
Signs.

Principal differential diagnosis
Acute bloat, clostridial myositis, lightning strike, acute bronchopneumonia, ingestion of cardiotoxic plants.

Treatment
Epinephrine, corticosteroids, supportive treatment as required. In recently dried off cows – emptying of the udder.

Anaplasmosis

Disease Profile
Tick-borne (*Dermatcentor* spp) rickettsial infection of cattle most common in tropical and subtropical areas. Anaplasmosis is characterised by extravascular haemolysis, anaemia, jaundice, emaciation and death. Mature cattle most susceptible. Calves up to 6 months do not show clinical signs. Mortality in mature cattle of naïve herds may reach 50%. Moving naïve cattle into endemic areas may result in high morbidity and mortality.

Aetiology
Anaplasma marginale and *A. centrale*

Clinical findings
Anorexia, lethargy, fever, atonic rumen, constipation, dark-mucous-covered faeces, rapid weight loss. Anaemia develops in later stages. Abortions may occur in cases of severe anaemia. No haemoglobinaemia and haemoglobinuria.

Post-mortem findings
Severe anaemia, later stages jaundice, petechia in the pericardium, sometimes hepatomegaly.

Diagnosis
Examination of stained blood sample and demonstration of the rickettsia. Other tests for detection of the pathogen.

Principal differential diagnosis
Babesiosis, Leptospirosis, Bacillary haemoglobunuria, Severe gastrointestinal parasitism, Copper toxicity

Treatment
Antimicrobials (the best is oxytetracycline), supportive care, handle animals with care (anaemia may result in hypoxia of the brain). Surviving cattle may remain carriers for long periods.

Control
In some countries vaccines with variable efficacy are available. Tick control. Restricted movement of naïve cattle into endemic areas, particularly during high ticks periods.

Anoestrus

Disease Profile
Failure to exhibit oestrus behaviour at appropriate times. Anoestrus is a normal occurrence in pre-pubertal heifers, during pregnancy and in the post-partum period. It can be a common occurrence in high producing dairy cows. Anoestrus may affect individual cows or be a group/herd problem. Suboptimal nutrition (undernourishment or imbalanced diet) is often characterised as herd problem.

Aetiology
Suboptimal nutrition, genital disorders (usually ovaries and/or uterus), concurrent systemic disorders, lameness. Luteal cysts, acyclic.

Clinical findings
Absence of oestrous behaviour.

Diagnosis
Diagnosing the primary disorder. Rectal palpation and ultrasonography of uterus and ovaries.

Principal differential diagnosis
Pregnancy, missed observations of oestrous behaviour

Treatment
Treat primary disorder.

Control
Improve feeding and oestrus observation ,training in oestrus detection,

Anthrax

Disease Profile
Per-acute or acute septicaemia usually characterised by sudden death. Usually sporadic. Most cases associated with some soil disruption (e.g. ploughing, floods) or drought and close to ground razing. Important zoonosis.

Aetiology
Bacillus anthracis. Spores of this bacillus are very resistant and survive long periods in contaminated material.

Clinical findings
Per-acute – often found dead. May observe fever, depression, dyspnoea, muscle fasciculations, congested membranes, short recumbency followed by death in 1–2 hours.

Acute – Death in 1–2 days.

Rare subacute cases – subcutaneous oedema, rumen stasis, haematuria, significant drop in milk yield, milk blood-tinged

Post-mortem findings
Full necropsy is contra-indicated (prevents contamination of environment and sporulation of the pathogen). Rapid decomposition, absence of rigor mortis, dark/tarry non-clotted blood coming out form natural orifices.

Diagnosis
Preparation of blood smears from tail or ear. Stained polychromatic methylene blue. Characteristic capsulated rectangular bacteria. Personal protection equipment should be used.

Principal differential diagnosis
Toxicity, vena cava syndrome, clostridial disorders, many other septicaemic disorders.

Treatment
Poor prognosis. Extended treatment with antimicrobials.

Control
Correct disposal of the carcass (burning or deep burial away from water sources. Vaccination in endemic areas.

Anticoagulant rodenticide poisoning

Common synonyms
Anticoagulant rodenticide toxicity, Warfarin poisoning.

Disease Profile
Rare. The newer anticoagulant rodenticides (bromadiolene and brodifacoum) more toxic due to the long half-life.

Aetiology
Accidental ingestion of rodent bait or contaminated foodstuffs.

Clinical findings
Usually sudden death.

Haematomas, internal and external haemorrhages, ecchymoses, epistaxis, haematuria.

Post-mortem findings
Widespread haemorrhages.

Diagnosis
Signs, history, blood-clothing profile.

Principal differential diagnosis
Sweet clover poisoning.

Treatment
Vitamin K1. Blood transfusion.

Control
Prevent exposure to anticoagulant rodenticide bites and contaminated feedstuffs.

Aspiration pneumonia

Disease Profile
Sporadic, usually fatal disorder due to development of gangrenous pneumonia. More common in calves with necrotic laryngitis, and mature cows with hypocalcaemia, hypomagnesaemia, acetonaemia, oesophageal obstruction, listeriosis, botulism, ephemeral fever, and lead poisoning.

Aetiology
Usually associated with improper administration of oral liquids or aspiration of regurgitated rumen content in recumbency or due to neural dysfunction.

Clinical findings
Fever, sudden depression, dyspnoea, coughing, foul breath. In protracted cases bilateral copious nasal discharge.

Post-mortem findings
Serious gangrenous pneumonia, usually of cranio-ventral right lobe.

Diagnosis
Signs, post mortem findings, history.

Principal differential diagnosis
Other types of pneumonia, septicaemia.

Treatment
Treatment often unpractical, unsuccessful and uneconomical. May try antimicrobials and steroidal or non-steroidal anti-inflammatories.

Control
Ensure cattle have swallowing reflex before oral administration of liquids.

Aujeszky's disease

Common synonyms
Pseudorabies, Mad itch disease, Infectious bulbar paralysis.

Disease Profile
Acute or peracute viral encephalitis. Primary host is pig with asymptomatic infection. Some remote zoonotic risk may be present.

Aetiology
Herpes virus.

Clinical findings
Peracute – sudden death.

Acute – Paresthaesia, pruritus, excoriation, excessive licking, and self-inflicted skin damage. Aggressiveness or dullness. Fever, rumen atony and bloat, grinding of teeth, bellowing, stamping the feet, proprioceptive deficits, head pressing, circling, nystagmus. Progresses into convulsions, recumbency and death in 1–3 days.

Post-mortem findings
Skin trauma, signs of encephalitis and meningeal hyperaemia.

Diagnosis
History (contact with pigs within 4–7 days from clinical signs), detection of virus, serology, intranuclear eosinophilic inclusion bodies in neurons and glial cells.

Principal differential diagnosis
Nervous ketosis, rabies, lead poisoning, hypomagnesaemia, meningitis.

Treatment
No treatment

Control
Avoid contact with pigs.

Babesiosis

Common synonyms
Red water fever, Piroplasmosis, Bovine malaria.

Disease Profile
Caused by protozoan parasite that causes intravascular haemolysis. Ticks (e.g. *Boophilus, Ixodes, Haemophysalis, Rhipicephalus*) are principal vector. Vertical transmission is rare. Common in areas with ticks. Uncommon in cattle younger than 6 months. After an episode of the disorder natural immunity may last 1–2 years up to life-long, provided continuous exposure to the protozoan. Naïve cattle usually presented with a severe form that may result in death. There is a remote zoonotic risk.

Aetiology
Babesia bovis, B. divergens, B. bigemina, B. major, B. ovata, B. jakimowi.

Clinical findings
High fever, anorexia, depression, sudden drop in milk yield, progressive weakness, haemoglobinuria (red urine), anaemia later development of icterus. Tachycardia, tachypnoea, signs of severe haemolysis and hypoxia. In pregnant cows abortion. Cattle infected with *B. bigemina* may present 'pipe stream' diarrhoea. In endemic areas subacute cases with transient fever, slight anaemia, emaciation and carrier stage are common.

Post-mortem findings
Diffuse pallor, jaundice, oedema, enlarged spleen, liver, kidneys, presence of brown urine in the bladder, petechial and ecchymotic haemorrhages on heart and gastrointestinal tract.

Diagnosis
Signs, detection of *Babesia* on stained blood smears or antibodies (often difficult to interpret).

Principal differential diagnosis
Conditions causing heamaglobinuria: Leptospirosis, bacillary haemoglobinuria, brassica toxicity, post-parturient haemoglobinuria, other reasons of suddenly developing fever and reasons for haematuria.

Treatment
Antiprotozal drugs (e.g. imidocarb dipropionate, diminazene diaceturate, amicarbalide diisethionate, phenamidine diisethionate), whole blood transfusion.

Control
Balancing immunity with the degree of infection. Reducing tick population, vaccination.

Bacillary heamoglobinuria

Disease Profile
Peracute clostridial disorder that occurs after a hepatic insult (e.g. fluke) or trauma. Higher incidence in cattle grazing on irrigated, poorly drained or alkaline pastures. Can occur as an outbreak in feedlot fed on feedstuffs from these areas. Usually rare disorder.

Aetiology
Clostridium haemolyticum.

Clinical findings
Sudden death. Sometimes observed high fever, anorexia, severe depression, abdominal pain, cattle reluctant to move, tachypnoea to dyspnoea, haemoglobinuria.

Post-mortem findings
Rapid rigor mortis, subcutaneous gelatinous oedema, subserosal haemorrhages, jaundice, pale hepatic infarct surrounded by hyperaemic zone, red urine in bladder.

Diagnosis
History, signs, necropsy findings, isolation of causative pathogen, identification of toxins.

Principal differential diagnosis
Leptospirosis, postparturient haemoglobinuria, brassica toxicity, black disease, reasons for haematuria.

Treatment
Rarely successful. Antimicrobials, symptomatic.

Control
Vaccination, fluke control.

Bacillus licheniformis infection

Disease Profile
Mainly where silage fed from a clamp and poorly fermented silage. Usually suckler herds. Incidence about 6% but has been up to 25%. Can occur as an outbreak after exposure to heavily contaminated feedstuffs.

Aetiology
Bacillus licheniformis, an aerobic, Gram-positive spore forming bacterium found in the soil.

Clinical findings
Sporadic abortion in the last trimester. Low birth weight calves. Many calves die within 24 hours from calving. No clinical illness in cows. Thickened placenta. Mastitis.

Post-mortem findings
Thickened, dry and wrinkly placenta. Yellow-brown discolouration. Often oedematous, haemorrhagic and necrotic cotyledons.

Diagnosis
Detection of pathogen. Lesions in the placenta.

Principal differential diagnosis
Other causes of abortion and mastitis.

Treatment
None

Control
Ensure good fermentation of silage. Do not feed mouldy silage to pregnant cattle.

Black disease

Common synonyms
Infectious necrotic hepatitis.

Disease Profile
Rare disorder that may occur as a herd outbreak after sudden exposure to liver insult (e.g. fluke).

Aetiology
Exotoxins of *Clostridium novyi.*

Clinical findings

Peracture – Sudden death.

Acute – Fever to subnormal temperature (decline near death due to toxaemia), depressed appetite, rumen atony, hyperpnoea, weakness, deep abdominal pain, depression, reluctance to move, semi-fluid faeces, sometimes liver enlargement. Death occurs in 1–2 days.

Post-mortem findings

Rapid autolysis, enlarged liver with areas of focal necrosis, sero-sanguineous fluid in serous cavities.

Diagnosis

Detection of the pathogen (usually impression smears), post-mortem findings, history of previous cases, signs.

Principal differential diagnosis

Anthrax, other clostridial disorders.

Treatment

Usually unsuccessful. Large doses of antimicrobials. In face of outbreak mass antimicrobial medication and vaccination.

Control

Vaccination. Avoid liver damage (e.g. fluke control, controlled grazing).

Black spot

Common synonyms

Black spock, wrongly called black pox.

Disease Profile

Typical lesions at the teat end caused by bacteria gaining entry as a result of damage caused by faulty operation of the milking machine, particularly defective pulsation and overstretched liners. May predispose to mastitis.

Aetiology

Staphylococus aureus and *Fusobacterium necrophorum* are most common isolates.

Clinical findings

Typically deep ulcers with raised margins and a centrally positioned black spot.

Treatment

Topical application of antimicrobials. Improve post milking teat disinfection, increase concentration of emollient, correct faulty milking machine.

Control

Correct operation of the milking machine. Routine use of post milking teat disinfection.

Bloat

Common synonyms

Rumen tympany, Ruminal tympany, Tympany, Hooven.

Disease Profile

Distention of the rumen with free gas (secondary bloat) or froth (primary bloat). Relatively common. In young calves due to fermentation of milk or milk replacers in underdeveloped rumen.

Aetiology

Primary bloat – excessive intake of immature legumes or lush pasture with high proportion of clover (saponins). Finely ground grains may also result in froth formation. Secondary bloat – physical blockage of the oesophagus or ruminal stasis (FB choke, neoplasia, bilateral pneumonia, vagus indigestion, chilled water)). In calves – cold milk, drinking rather than sucking.

Clinical findings

Obvious distention of the left flank, if sever bilateral distention, dyspnoea, tachycardia, discomfort, sometimes open mouth breathing, staggering, recumbency. On percussion clear tympanic tone.

Post-mortem findings

Characteristic 'bloat' line on the oesophagus (congestion cranially, pallor caudally).

Diagnosis

Clinical signs, stomach tube.

Principal differential diagnosis

Post-mortem bloating. Diaphragmatic hernia, vagus indigestion.

Treatment

Severe bloat is an emergency. **Free gas bloat**: Relief of the gas (stomach tube or ruminal trochar)

Frothy bloat: Mild to moderate cases use of bloat remedies (surfactants such as polaxalene and silicates, cooking oil, bicarbonate po)) may be enough. If severe: ruminal trochar/rumenotomy.

Calf recurrent bloat – probably best treatment is weaning.

Control

Controlled grazing, use of bloat-prevention treatment with bloat remedies, use of iodophores (monensin, lasalocid), mineral or vegetable oils.

Blood in milk

Disease Profile

Frank blood in the milk is usually due to capillary bleeding or rupture of a blood vessel. It is common post calving. Usually ceases within few days without problems. It may also be a result of a trauma in cows of any stage of lactation. Milk with high intensity colour change may need attention (suspicion of developing a black mastitis).

Clinical findings
Pale-pink to chocolate-coloured milk.

Principal differential diagnosis
Black mastitis, dicoumarol poisoning.

Treatment
Antimicrobials (intramammary) can be administered to prevent mastitis but not essential.

Bluetongue

Disease Profile
An arthropod-borne, non-contagious disorder of ruminants. Main vector are *Culicoides*. Occasionally transmitted by insemination and transplacentally when can cause foetal malformations and abortions. Cattle often with inapparent infection.

Aetiology
Orbivurus (with 24 sero-types).

Clinical findings
Tachypnoea, dyspnoea, followed fever, hyperaemia of lips and muzzle, ulcerations of oral mucosa, cyanotic tongue. Sometimes lameness and muscle necrosis. Lameness may progress to knee-walking or recumbency. Foetal malformations and abortions

Diagnosis
Detection of virus or antibodies.

Principal differential diagnosis
Foot-and-mouth, mucosal disease, foot rot, polyarthritis. Other reasons for foetal malformations and abortion.

Treatment
No specific treatment.

Control
Vaccines available in some countries.

Botulism

Disease Profile
Highly fatal neuroparalytic disorder. Usually isolated cases. Outbreaks may occur when contaminated feedstuffs given to a group of cattle. Contamination of feedstuffs or water with rodents, osteophagia (e.g. phosphorus deficiency) and exposure to poultry manure are common sources.

Aetiology
Ingestion of botulinum toxins produced by *Clistridium botulinum* (types B, C and D).

Clinical findings
Developing flaccid paralysis. Constipated, ataxic on hind limbs, loss of tail tone, later the paralysis progresses cranially and affects large groups of muscles, including intercostal. Due to paralysis of respiratory muscles laboured breathing, difficulties in prehension and drinking water. Sternal recumbency.

Post-mortem findings
Non-specific findings.

Diagnosis
Usually difficult. History may be very important. Detection of toxin in serum of affected cattle is confirmatory. Toxin may be difficult to detect. Detection of toxin in feedstuffs may be of value in epidemiologic investigations.

Principal differential diagnosis
Conditions causing flaccid paralysis and weakness. Hypocalcaemia, downer cow, toxic mastitis or metritis.

Treatment
Toxin is long-acting (weeks to recovery). Supportive care, stomach feeding. Antiserum may be available, but usually uneconomical due to the large dose required. Success expected in slower developing cases (less toxin ingested).

Control
In some countries vaccination available.

Prognosis
Poor

Bovine herpes mammillitis

Common synonyms
Bovine ulcerative mammillitis.

Disease Profile
Not common. Usually seen as a herd outbreak. Increased risk of mastitis. Younger cows and heifers are usually more susceptible. Severity of the clinical signs varies dependent on immune status and age.

Aetiology
Herpes Virus – 2

Clinical findings
Initially swollen, painful teats. Papules that soon transform into short-lived vesicles that rupture and ulceration develops. Large areas of the teat skin may slough leaving large painful ulceration that heals slowly in weeks covered in deep dark scabs that are susceptible to bleeding particularly at milking. Sometimes vesicular and ulcerative changes of the udder skin and oral lesions.

Diagnosis
Signs, detection of virus.

Principal differential diagnosis
Pseudocowpox virus infection, photosensitisation, foot-and-mouth, vesicular stomatitis.

Treatment
Supportive care, segregation of infected cows and milking them last. Increased concentration of iodine post-milking disinfectants with added emollients. Moisturising ointments.

Control
In face of outbreak handle affected cattle with care, segregation and milk last, increased use of emollient in post-milking teat disinfectants.

Bovine immunodeficiency-like virus (BIV)

Disease Profile
Widespread in North America and Europe. Spread is usually vertical through infected milk. Probably spread in other ways. Most animals exposed to infection do not show signs of disease. Experimentally can infect sheep, goats and rabbits by blood transfer. No known risk to man.

Aetiology
Lentivirus possibly of variable virulence.

Clinical findings
Most signs appear to be the exacerbation or extended duration of other diseases. Animals may develop fluctuating pyrexia, often with alimentary or respiratory signs, sometimes dyspnoea, lameness, mastitis and nervous signs with mock aggression. Superficial lymph nodes may be palpably enlarged.

Diagnosis
Introduction of new animals, signs, early leukopenia followed by leukocytosis (mainly a lymphocytosis). Antigen culture producing syncytia, antibody presence by indirect immunofluorescence, ELISA or Western blot tests.

Principal differential diagnosis
BVD, BLAD.

Treatment
None.

Control
Possible to test animals prior to entry to herd if resident herd is naïve.

In most cases no attempt at control or prevention.

Bovine iritis

Common synonyms
Silage eye

Disease Profile
Usually adult animals. Most animals being fed silage, especially big bale. Often soil present in it. It is assumed that there is often abrasion of the eye surface by stalks etc. Usually during winter. The condition can occur in the same animal in different years.

Aetiology
Thought to be due to *Listeria monocytogenes.*

Clinical findings
Sudden onset of painful eye condition. Usually unilateral but can be both eyes. Eyelids often partially or completely closed. Sometimes serous ocular discharge which may become mucopurulent. The iris may show white flecks on it, some have hypopyon. Severe signs may last seven to ten days. Can undergo complete resolution.

Diagnosis
Signs, use of silage.

Principal differential diagnosis
Pink eye, local damage, meningitis.

Treatment
Antibacterials systemic and intraconjunctival (penicillin, oxytetracycline).

Corticosteroids – Intraconjuctivally.

Control
Avoid use of high pH silage or where much soil contamination.

Bovine Neonatal Pancytopaenia (BNP)

Common synonyms
Idiopathic haemorrhagic diathesis; Bleeding calf syndrome, Blood sweating.

Disease Profile
Newborn calves under one month of age. Coagulopathy of young beef and dairy calves in Europe

Aetiology
Auto-immune pathogenesis. Alloantibodies to a BVD vaccine (PregSure®) BVD; Pfizer Animal Health) may play a role in pathogenesis. After increasing evidence for the association between the use of the vaccine and the occurrence of disease the vaccine was withdrawn in 2010.

Clinical findings
Sporadic. Fever, anaemia, melena, epistaxis and petechial haemorrhages internal bleeding. Fatal. Some affected calves found dead. Mortality rate may be as high as 5% in some herds

Diagnosis
Signs. History. Elimination of other causes of neonatal bleeding disorders.

Principal differential diagnosis
Exclusion of primary BVD infections

Treatment
Nil

Control
Historical

Bovine papular stomatitis

Common synonyms
Proliferative stomatitis.

Disease Profile
Primarily affects young cattle. Usually mild and benign but rare severe form exist. May predispose to secondary bacterial infection. Zoonotic disorder.

Aetiology
Parapoxvirus.

Clinical findings
Benign form – Usually asymptomatic. Papules (2 to 10 mm) with raised periphery and depressed centre on the muzzle, nose, oral mucosa (particularly hard palate), oesophagus. May cause fever, but appetite is maintained. Spontaneous regression in several days to 3 weeks.

Severe form – Lesions sometimes ulcerate and spread to the rumen. Weight loss, diarrhoea, hypersalivation. Mortality may reach up to 50%.

No lesions at the coronet.

Diagnosis
Detection of the virus, signs.

Principal differential diagnosis
Foot-and-mouth disease, bovine virus diarrhoea virus, vesicular stomatitis, pseudopox virus.

Treatment
Symptomatic and supportive in severe cases.

Control
Normal biosecurity measures, vaccination with autogenous vaccine has been used.

Bovine respiratory disease complex (BRD)

Common synonyms
Shipping fever

Disease Profile
A non-specific syndrome that covers a wide range of disorders of the respiratory tract. Most commonly seen in feedlot beef cattle. Any age, however, younger cattle at higher risk. Often occurs after some stress factor such as transport, re-grouping

Aetiology
Multifactorial – viruses (Bovine herpes virus 1, parainfluenza 3, respiratory syncytial virus, adenovirus, bovine virus diarrhoea virus, respiratory corona virus), bacteria (*Mannheimia haemolytica, Pasteurella multocida, Mycoplasma bovis, Histophilus somni, Trueperella pyogenes*), parasites, nutrition, husbandry (overcrowding), environment (poor ventilation and sanitation), stress (transport, dehorning) and host susceptibility.

Clinical findings
Reduced to absent appetite, dyspnoea, fever, depression, nasal discharge, coughing, pneumonia (abnormal auscultation lung sounds), death. Often there is epiphora.

Post-mortem findings
Tracheitis, pneumonia of various type and degree, pleural adhesions, abscessation of lungs.

Diagnosis
Necropsy, history, signs, trans-tracheal broncho-alveolar lavage to identify the causative pathogens.

Principal differential diagnosis
Specific pneumonia, lungworms, pleuritis, pulmonary oedema, allergic pneumonia and rhinitis, infectious bovine rhino-tracheitis.

Treatment
Early treatment is essential. Antimicrobials. NSAIDs. Supportive treatment. Isolation of sick cattle. Recovery is usually indicated by reduction of fever, return of appetite and gaining weight.

Control
Minimise stressful events, prevent overcrowding, optimal facilities, nutrition, conditions and management. Vaccination.

Bovine spongiform Encephalopathy

Common synonyms
Mad cow disease.

Disease Profile
Zoonotic new variant CJD. Long incubation period following ingestion of bovine tissue contaminated feed. Affects adult cattle.

Aetiology
Abnormal Prion.

Clinical findings
Slowly progressing. Apprehension, incoordination and highly reactive hyper-excitability to startle test. Progression to recumbency. Invariable fatal.

Post-mortem findings
Histopathology: spongiform encephalopathy

Diagnosis
Clinical signs, brain pathology, rapid prion tests.

Principal differential diagnosis
Rabies, pseudorabies listeriosis, polioencephalomalacia, lead poisoning.

Treatment
No treatment.

Control
Prevent ingestion of contaminated feed.

Bovine tuberculosis

Disease Profile
The incidence of the disease is increasing associated with infection in badgers in the UK and possums in NZ. In many countries control programmes are in place. Many other vertebrate species may be affected and act as reservoir. Some zoonotic risk.

Aetiology
Mycobacterium bovis.

Clinical findings
Often asymptomatic or discovered by routine testing before signs appear.

General tuberculosis: Progressive loss of condition, weakness, fluctuating temperature, variable appetite, sometimes dullness. Enlargement of superficial lymph nodes. Some lymph nodes may rupture and drain.
Localised tuberculosis: Signs depend on the location of the process.

Respiratory form – Chronic respiratory disorder; moist cough (worst in the morning, during cold weather and after exercise), later dyspnoea, tachypnoea, and hyperpnoea. On auscultation and percussion area/s of dullness.

Genital form – Uncommon reason of metritis and abortion. In male chronic indurative orchitis.

Mammary form – Chronic indurating mastitis (sometimes with hypertrophy and enlarged supramammary lymph nodes.

Alimentary form – Chronic dysphagia and diarrhoea intermittently replaced by constipation.

Post-mortem findings
Granulomas in lymph nodes of affected areas, usually lung contains abscesses and pleural nodules.

Diagnosis
Signs, region of country, history, intradermal testing, serology, post-mortem carcass inspection.

Principal differential diagnosis
Johne's disease, chronic parasitism, chronic respiratory tract disorders, chronic mastitis of other nature, bovine leukosis, avian tuberculosis, skin tuberculosis.

Treatment
Not attempted. Diagnosed cattle should be slaughtered.

Control
Strict biosecurity. Test and slaughter policy. Prescribed intermittent testing at herd level. Control of wildlife direct or indirect contact.

Bovine virus diarrhoea infection

Disease Profile
One of most important infectious viral disorders in cattle. Can infect cattle of any age. Persistently infected cattle are major source of virus. Type 1 and Type II. Often mild signs but with high impact on fertility (reabsorption/abortion) with congenital abnormalities. Varying virulence depending on strains. Horizontal and vertical transmission. Persistently infected (PI) animals main index source of virus in outbreaks. PI will eventually develop mucosal disease.

Aetiology
Pestivirus

Clinical findings
Persistent infections – May appear normal to ill-thrift and risk of mucosal disease. Usually result of an infection between 40 and 120–140 days of gestation.
Acute form – Fever, anorexia, depression, usually diarrhoea, keratitis and conjunctivitis. Abortion or congenital abnormalities. Sometimes oral lesions (erosions and ulcerations mainly tongue). Thrombocytopaenia and leukopaenia. Some strains may cause pneumonia often complicated with *Mannheimia haemolytica*. In calves severe leukopaenia with immunosuppression, typically diphasic fever, depression, diarrhoea. Usually a result of an infection of immunocompetent naïve cattle and causes transient infection.

Subacute form – Intermittent diarrhoea, lowered appetite and production, illthrift, starring coat, chronic oral lesions.

Haemorrhagic form – Fever, severe thrombocytopaenia (excessively prolonged bleeding, spontaneous haemorrhages of visible mucosal surfaces), hyphema, pneumonia, diarrhoea and high fatality rate.

Mucosal disease – Fever, anorexia, depression, profuse salivation, erosions and ulcerations in the digestive system, sometimes nares, teats and vulva, profuse foul smelling diarrhoea often with blood and fibrin clots or intestinal casts , invariably fatality. Usually a result of persistent infection in immunotolerant cattle. Most cattle will present mucosal disease before 2 years of age. Chronic form of mucosal disease has been described with similar signs of a milder character.

Pregnant cows/heifers – May cause early embryonic loss, abortion, stillbirths, congenital defects and birth of persistently infected calves.

Post-mortem findings
Mucosal disease characteristic lesions.

Diagnosis
Antigen (ear notch, blood) and antibody ELISA (serology).

Principal differential diagnosis
Other causes of diarrhoea, abortions and thrombocytopaenia. Mucosal disease should also include other causes of oral ulcerations.

Treatment
For acute cases supportive treatment. Cattle with mucosal disease have poor prognosis and should be euthanised. Calves with congenital defects have grave prognosis.

Control
Normal biosecurity measures, vaccination available in some countries. Detect and remove persistently infected cattle from the herd.

Bracken fern poisoning

Disease Profile
A common plant poisoning. Can cause bone marrow suppression, enzootic haematuria, bladder and gastrointestinal neoplasia. Clinical disorder usually seen after ingesting a significant portion of the diet (usually >20%) for extended period of time. Plant is toxic fresh and dry.

Aetiology
Ingestion of *Pteridium aquilinum*. Young plants and rhizomes are more toxic. Known toxins are ptaquiloside (primary importance), quercetin and shikimic acid.

Clinical findings
Bone marrow depression –Thrombocytopaenia and neutropaenia seen first, followed by anaemia. Bloody nasal discharge, petechiae and ecchymoses to visible mucosal surfaces, weakness. Prolonged bleeding, immunosuppression (common secondary bacterial infections characterised with signs of the specific disorder), sometimes fever, anorexia, dullness, dyspnoea.

Enzootic haematuria – Red to dark brown urine (haematuria)

Neoplasia – Signs will depend on location and stage of development of the tumours. Usually ill-thrift, starring coat, diarrhoea, haematuria.

Post-mortem findings
Scattered haemorrhages throughout the body, pale bone marrow, ulceration of gastrointestinal tract, neoplastic changes.

Diagnosis
History, thrombocytopaenia, leukopaenia, haematuria.

Principal differential diagnosis
Thrombocytopaenia of other nature, other causes of haematuria and wasting disease.

Treatment
Response to treatment is usually poor. Remove offended feedstuffs. Nursing care. Antimicrobials to prevent bacterial infections. Blood transfusion may be required.

Control
Avoid excess to large quantities of the plant by grazing or hay. Use of herbicides. Provide alternative diet.

Brassica spp poisoning

Disease Profile
Various forms of the disorder including Heinz body anaemia, goitre, enteritis, polioencephalomalacia, photosensitisation, pulmonary oedema and emphysema.

Aetiology
Ingestion of kale, rape, turnips, cabbage, Brussels sprouts and others from this group of plants in high proportion for prolonged periods. Mature plants are more toxic. Known toxins glucosinolates (isothyocyanate, thyocyanate ions and thiones; cause goitrogenic effects and gastro-intestinal irritation), S-methylcistine sulphoxide (SMCO converted in the rumen into dimethyl disulphide – DMSM; causes Heinz body anaemia). Rape and turnips may also be associated with nitrate poisoning (see appropriate heading).

Clinical findings
Heinz body anaemia – *Per acute* – Sudden death. ;
Acute – Haemoglobuniria (coffee-coloured urine), drop in milk yield, lethargy, dyspnoea, pale mucus membranes, sometimes diarrhoea and icterus.; *Chronic* – Light depression, red-tinged urine.;
Subclinical – Mild anaemia.

Goitre – Enlargement of thyroid, weakness, lethargy, recumbency, weight loss. Feeding *Brassica* spp may result in goitrein offspring.

Enteritis – dysentery, abdominal pain. Sometimes anorexia, atonic rumen, scant, sticky faeces.

Polioenchephalomalacia – see appropriate heading.

Photosensitisation – lightly coloured skin oedema, erythema, blistering, pruritus that may lead to self-inflicted wounds.

Post-mortem findings
Pale or jaundiced carcass, thin blood, residual urine shown signs of haemoglobinuria; goitre.

Diagnosis
History, signs, Heinz body anaemia.

Principal differential diagnosis
Other causes of haemoglobinuia (onion poisoning, post-parturient haemoglobinuria, leptospirosis, babesiosis, anaplasmosis, chronic copper poisoning), anaemia (immunomediated, iatrogenic, haemorrhages), goitre (other plants, iodine deficiency), enteritis (plant poisonings (oak, lavender, oleander), parisites, viruses, bacteria, protozoa), polioencephalomalacia (thiamine deficiency), and photosensitisation (primary or secondary).

Treatment
No specific treatment. Reduce or remove *Brassica* spp from the diet. Blood transfusion, protect from sun, iodine supplementation.

Control
Brassica spp should not exceed 40% of the total diet. Introduce gradually. Hay of silage should be provided before turning cattle into *Brassica* spp paddocks.

Brucellosis

Common synonyms
Bang's disease, Contagious abortion

Disease Profile
Often asymptomatic, contagious disorder. Rare in countries that have introduced eradication schemes. Affected systems are reproductive and sometimes musculo-skeletal. An important cause of abortion in cattle in some countries. Aborted foetus and lochia are heavily contaminated with the causative pathogen. Zoonosis.

Aetiology
Brucella abortus.

Clinical findings
In female cattle often only signs are abortion in the second half of gestation followed with retained foetal membranes, and decreased milk yield.

In bulls may cause orchitis, epididymitis and vesicular seminitis.

Some cattle may develop arthritis of the larger joints of the limbs.

Post-mortem findings
Affected animals rarely have detectable changes. Aborted foetuses usually autolysed with evidence of pneumonia.

Diagnosis
Detection of the pathogen, serology, intradermal testing (brucellin).

Principal differential diagnosis
Other causes of abortion.

Treatment
No treatment undertaken. Isolation and cull.

Control
Normal biosecurity measures. Vaccine is available in some countries (may require state approval).

Calf diphtheria

Common synonyms
Oral necrobacillosis, Necrotic stomatitis, Laryngeal necrobacillosis.

Disease Profile
Most commonly disorder of young, rarely adult cattle. Housed grouped calves at higher risk. Affects mouth, pharynx and larynx. Oral form in younger calves (first few months). Laryngeal form in cattle up to 18 months. Usually associated with injuries to the affected areas (e.g. teething, abrasive feedstuffs, oral dosing) allowing anaerobic conditions. Most common multiple suckling grouped dairy calves.

Aetiology
Fusobacterium nechrophorum. Often mixed with other microbial flora (e.g. other anaerobes or facultative anaerobes).

Clinical findings
Oral form – Swelling of the cheeks, foetid odour on breath, painful feeding.

Laryngeal form – Coughing, inspiratory stridor, difficulty swallowing. Often high fever, anorexia, depression, salivation, swelling of the pharynx/larynx.

On oral examination of affected areas inflamed and necrotic mucosa is often easily detected.

Post-mortem findings
Swelling and inflammation of oral, pharyngeal and/or laryngeal mucosa.

Diagnosis
Signs.

Principal differential diagnosis
Oral or pharyngeal trauma, laryngitis, pharyngeal foreign body

Treatment
Antimicrobials (procaine penicillin is a drug of choice in pure culture infections), non-steroidal anti-inflammatory drugs, supportive treatment. May require tracheotomy/laryngoatomy) (in severe cases) but guarded prognosis.

Control
Avoid abrasive feedstuffs and unhygienic conditions, hygiene multiple suckle milk bar. In face of outbreak isolate affected cattle and treat with antimicrobials as early as first signs seen. Long-acting antimicrobials may be administered metaphylactically in significant outbreaks.

Campylobacter infection

Common synonyms
Vibriosis, Vibrio abortion

Disease Profile
Occasional cause of reproductive or digestive problems. Decreased prevalence due to testing and control in bulls and artificial insemination (AI). Digestive form more common in young cattle.

Aetiology
Reproductive – *Campylobacter fetus* subspecies *venerealis* and rarely *fetus*. Digestive – *C. jejuni* and *C. coli*.

Clinical findings
Reproductive form: Female – Infertility, repeated breeders, irregular inter-oestrus intervals and early embryonic death. Sometimes mucoid to mucopurulent vaginal discharge. Sporadic abortion occurs in mid to late pregnancy.

Male – Asymptomatic. Serve as vectors for venereal transmission.

Digestive form – Usually self-limiting diarrhoea with mucus and blood flecks. Mild fever.

Post-mortem findings
Reproductive form – mucopurulent endometritis; aborted foetuses fibrinous serositis; cotyledons oedematous with tan/brown discolouration.

Digestive from – thickened and reddened ileum, and sometimes jejunum.

Diagnosis
Detection of pathogen. Serology. Signs are non-specific.

Isolation from preputial washing in bull.

Principal differential diagnosis
Reproductive form – infection with *Trichomonas foetus*.
Digestive – other causes of diarrhoea.

Treatment
Antimicrobials. Bulls need long service rest after treatment.

Control
Bull – cull and switch to AI. Infected herds – use of AI for minimum two seasons. Vaccination available in some countries.

Cardiac disease

Common synonyms
Congestive heart failure, Cardiac insufficiency

Disease Profile
Congestive heart failure (CHF) is a syndrome, not a specific disorder. Probably common but seldom recognised. Overt signs of CHF do not appear until compensatory mechanisms of the cardiovascular system have been exceeded. May result from primary cardiovascular disorder or be secondary to disorders in other systems. Primary cardiovascular disorder may be congenital or acquired. Common cardiovascular disorders include myocarditis, cardiomyopathy, valvular defects, pericardial pathology, hypertension, thromboembolism and arteritis. CHF may result from ingestion of cardiotoxic plants (e.g. locoweed [*Oxytropis* and *Astragalus*], oleander, avocado, *Phalaris*, and *Cassia occidentalis*), toxic chemicals (ionophores, gossypol, excessive molybdenum and sulphates), altitude sickness, bronchopneumonia, verminous pneumonia, infection (e.g. *Histophilus somni*, *Staphylococcus* spp, *Streptococcus* spp, *Escherichia* spp, *Salmonella* spp), septicaemia, toxaemia, deficiency disorders (Vitamin E, selenium, copper) and neoplasia (e.g. bovine leucosis, lymphosarcoma).

Aetiology
Failure of cardiac function.

Clinical findings
1) Congenital – May be asymptomatic. Lethargy, exercise intolerance, poor growth, abnormal cardiac sounds, cyanosis and sudden death.

2) Congestive heart failure – Loss in condition, poor exercise tolerance, fast pulse, brisket and ventral oedema, jugular vein distention, positive jugular pulse, diarrhoea. Specific signs of pericarditis, endocarditis, myocarditis and myopathy.

Diagnosis
Signs. Blood culture. Auscultation, pericardiocentesis, ultrasonograpgy, radiography, electrocardiography.

Principal differential diagnosis
Other debilitating disorders, respiratory tract disorders, specific cardiovascular disorders.

Treatment
Seldom practical when signs detected as cardiovascular system is overwhelmed. Symptomatic treatment (inotropics, diuretics, vasodilatators, antiarrhythmic, correct electrolyte balance). Treat the underlying cause.

Caudal vena cava syndrome

Common synonyms
Hepatocaval thrombosis. Pulmonary thromboembolism. Metastatic pneumonia. Vena cava syndrome.

Disease Profile
Rare. Usually consequence of rumenitis or liver abscesses. Metastatic spread of septic emboli to lungs. Hypertension with vascular aneurisms that rupture with haemorrhage. Invariably fatal.

Clinical findings
Cardinal clinical sign is bilateral epistaxis or haemoptysis. Usually acute to peracute. Previous history of recovery from respiratory distress (misdiagnosis). Tachycardia, dyspnoea, crackles and wheezes, haemic murmurs, anaemia.

Post-mortem findings
Disseminated multiple abscesses in the lungs associated with blood vessels. Liver abscesses with involvement of caudal vena cava.

Diagnosis
Signs. Difficult before epistaxis develops. Often misdiagnosed as chronic pneumonia. Epistaxis, wheezes and anaemia are assumed as pathognomonic.

Principal differential diagnosis
Chronic supportive pneumonia, endocarditis.

Treatment
Generally not recommended or successful.

Control
Change diet and feeding management to avoid rumen acidosis.

Cerebellar disease

Disease Profile
Neonatal (at calving) or postnatal (weeks to months from calving). Can be infectious, congenital and genetic (e.g. Holstein, Hereford, Aberdeen Angus) in origin.

Aetiology
Intrauterine infection with BVD, bluetongue, Akabane and Wesselsbron viruses. Genetic factors.

Clinical findings
Lack of control of movement, intention head tremors, ataxia, dysmetria, spasticity and sometimes uni-or-bi-lateral absence of menace response. Proprioception is present. No paresis. Sometimes hydraencephaly and arthrogryposis.

Diagnosis
Suckling, pre-suckling serology.

Treatment
None

Control
Vaccination. Biosecurity protocols. Culling of repeated offenders.

Clostridial gastrointestinal disorders

Common synonyms
Enterotoxaemia, Struck.

Disease Profile
Worldwide. Usually causes outbreaks in rapidly growing, vigorous calves few weeks of age. Peracute and acute form. Risk factors: change in diet, copper deficiency, vigorous nursing the dam.

Aetiology
Clostridium perfringens types A to E. Types usually differ dependent on geographic location.

Clinical findings
Peracute – sudden death.

Acute – Abdominal pain and distention, depression, recumbency and death. Haemorrhagic diarrhoea may or may not appear. Prior to death often convulsions, opisthotonus.

Post-mortem findings
Watery blood, haemorrhagic enteritis, petechial haemorrhages. Type D – also paintbrush haemorrhages of the left sub-endocardium.

Diagnosis
Signs and post-mortem findings are only indicative. Detection of pathogen and/or exotoxins.

Principal differential diagnosis
Anthrax, poisoning, clostridial myositis, distended abomasum, salmonellosis, polioencephalomalacia.

Treatment
Rarely successful. Antimicrobials. Supportive care (fluids, electrolytes). Relieve abomasal bloat. Antitoxin treatment may be beneficial.

Control
Vaccination of the dam and calves. In a face of an outbreak metaphylaxis by antimicrobials or antisera.

Clostridial myositis

Common synonyms
Blackleg, Malignant oedema, False blackleg, Gas gangrene.

Disease Profile
A group of per acute to acute disorders characterised by myonecrosis and rapid death. Usually associated with anaerobic conditions in the muscle tissues anywhere in the body (e.g. injury, bruising, intramuscular injections). Most affected young cattle less than 2 years old in a good body condition. May occur as sporadic cases or as an outbreak. Risk factor is tissue bruising. Outbreaks often after some farm protocol (e.g. yarding), low grazing or flooding.

Aetiology
Exotoxins of various species of *Clostridium (chauvoei, septicum, novyi, sordelli)*. Vegetative forms of the causative pathogens develop only in anaerobic conditions.

Clinical findings
Sudden death. In acute cases severe depression, fever, anorexia, tachypnoea, lameness, recumbency, coma, death within 12–24 hours. Sometimes subcutaneous emphysema, cold area over the affected muscle and crepitus.

Post-mortem findings
Rapid autolysis, darkened, dry emphysematous muscle, sometimes with smell on rancid butter.

Diagnosis
History, signs, post-mortem findings, detection of causative pathogens or exotoxins.

Principal differential diagnosis
Acute poisonings, black disease, anthrax, snakebite.

Treatment
Rarely successful due to the rapid course. Antimicrobials (drug of choice procaine penicillin) around affected tissues. Aggressive surgical debridement to allow aeration. Supportive treatment. Poor prognosis

Control
Vaccination. In face of outbreak simultaneous vaccination and administration of procaine penicillin. Carcasses should be destroyed by deep burial or burning to minimise soil contamination.

Cobalt deficiency

Disease Profile
Common in some geographical areas. Often undiagnosed. More serious in growing calves. Associated with decreased growth, poor feed conversion, ill-thrift and anaemia.

Aetiology
Insufficient oral intake of cobalt.

Clinical findings
Decreased appetite, poor growth, loss of body weight, anaemia, thin skin, poor hair coat, pica, diarrhoea, anaemia and decreased fertility. Increased incidence of ketosis.

Post-mortem findings
Anaemia. Poor hair coat and thin skin.

Diagnosis
Signs, geographical area, Vitamin B_{12} or cobalt levels in blood/liver. Response to treatment.

Principal differential diagnosis
Copper deficiency, selenium deficiency, parasitic gastroenteritis and malnutrition

Treatment
Parenteral Vitamin B_{12} or orally cobalt.

Control
Nutritional supplementation.

Coccidiosis

Disease Profile
Infection by intracellular protozoa, usually asymptomatic and self-limiting with formation of host immunity. Clinical disorder is usually seen in young cattle (often older than 3 weeks) after ingestion of large numbers of oocysts or some stressor (e.g. transport, weaning, dietary change, use of corticosteroids). Sporulation is enhanced in warm, wet environment with plenty of organic matter (unsanitary conditions). Often seen in overcrowded conditions with poor hygiene between batches . Chronic damage to the intestinal mucosa can persist. Can cause serious economic losses in young cattle. Three general forms: gastrointestinal, nervous, chronic. Can occur at grass (especially E. alabamensis).

Aetiology
Eimeria bovis. E. zurnii. E. alabamensis

Clinical findings
Intestinal form

Fever, anorexia, tenesumus. Faeces are foul-smelling and may contain sloughed mucosa and blood. Sometimes diarrhoea.

Nervous form (regional occurrence)

Usually after an episode of milder gastrointestinal form. Progression from depression and incoordination, to muscle tremors, hyperesthesia, convulsions, nystagmus and blindness. High mortality rate.

Chronic form

Predominant signs are suppressed appetite, loose faeces, faeces-stained perineum, loss of condition, poor growth, rough hair coat, decreased resistance to other disorders.

Post-mortem findings
Haemorrhagic enteritis with sloughing of ileum, caecum, colon and rectum.

Diagnosis
Signs, post-mortem findings, detection of pathogens.

Principal differential diagnosis
Gastrointestinal form – Cryptosporidiosis, salmonellosis, gastrointestinal parasitism, mucosal disease. *Nervous form – Histophilus somni* infection syndrome, polioencephalomalacia, lead poisoning.

Treatment
Antimicrobials (anticoccidials and sulphonamides), supportive treatment, better nutrition.

Control
Normal biosecurity measures, better hygiene, feeding off-ground, avoid overcrowding, use of coccidiostats.

Conjunctivitis

Disease Profile
Common. Inflammation often extends to the deeper layers particularly to the cornea.

Aetiology
Conjunctivitis can be primary and secondary. Primary irritation from chemicals or more often foreign bodies and infection. Secondary: BVD, MCF, IBR, Rinderpest, viral pneumonia.

Clinical findings
Photophobia. Ocular discharge. Starts as watery, sometimes progressing to mucopurulent and purulent discharge. Opacity of conjunctiva and sometimes of cornea.

Diagnosis
Signs.

Principal differential diagnosis
Other ophthalmic disorders.

Treatment
Treat the primary cause. Antimicrobials locally and/or systemically.

Contagious bovine pleuropneumonia

Common synonyms
Mycoplasma infection.

Disease Profile
Acute, subacute or chronic highly contagious infection that may present as pleuropneumonia and/or arthritis. Clinical disorder often associated with stressor (overcrowding, sudden weather change, regrouping). Naïve herd often suffer outbreak after introduction of infected beasts. Morbidity may reach 100%. Mortality is usually lower but can reach 70%. Endemic in Africa, East Asia and Southern Europe.

Aetiology
Mycoplasma mycoides mycoides. Often complicated with secondary bacterial infection.

Clinical findings
Fever, anorexia, depression, tachypnoea, dyspnoea often with open mouth, coughing, nasal discharge, abducted elbows. Before death sometimes frothy nasal discharge. Lung field auscultation reveals crepitation, rales, pleuritic friction usually unilateral.

Sometimes arthritis to polyarthritis.

Post-mortem findings
Lung oedema, fluid filled alveoli, fibrinous pneumonia, pleuritis. 'Marbling' effect of lungs. Changes are often unilateral.

Diagnosis
Signs, post-mortem findings, detection of the pathogen.

Principal differential diagnosis
Shipping fever, bovine respiratory complex

Treatment
Aggressive antimicrobial treatment (if not aggressive may favour carrier state).

Control
In face of outbreak isolate affected cattle, place herd under quarantine, optimise feeding regimen. Vaccine available in some countries.

Contracted tendons

Disease Profile
Contracted flexor tendons are probably the most prevalent abnormality of the musculoskeletal system of new-born calves. It is usually due to congenital shortening of the flexor tendons or a sequel of feeding lupine plants to cows in pregnancy. Fore-limbs are more commonly affected, usually bilateral. Older animals may acquire contracted tendons as result of disuse following trauma (fracture) or neurologic disorders (radial nerve paralysis).

Clinical findings
Metacarpo-phalangeal and/or metatarso-phalangeal joints are flexed, sometimes the carpus. In new-born calves the disorder may occur with other congenital abnormalities, such as cleft palate, dwarfism and arthrogryphosis.

The real risk to the calf is often underestimated. Affected calves are unable to rise and fail to suckle enough colostrum with failure of passive transfer of immunoglobulins. Therefore, affected calves are at significantly higher risk of development of navel ill, polyarthritis and meningitis.

Diagnosis
Signs

Treatment
Splinting or ring castes to extend the limbs so the sole is plantigrade often effective. They are left in place for 7–10 days. If severe and poor response surgery (transection of superficial/deep flexor tendons followed by casting is usually successful (but expensive). Should be treated soon after recognition, as the calf gets older, the contracted tendons become less responsive. Mildly affected calves may recover spontaneously.

Copper deficiency

Common synonyms
Falling disease, Peat scours.

Disease Profile
Younger cattle are more susceptible, but may occur at any age. Some geographical locations are known to have problems with copper deficiency (Australia, New Zealand, The USA, The Netherlands and the UK).

Aetiology
Diet contains suboptimal levels of copper (primary) or impaired absorption or metabolism due to excess in diet of sulphur, zinc, molybdenum or iron (secondary).

Clinical findings
Ill-thrift, diarrhoea, anaemia, weight loss, osteoporosis, spontaneous fractures, depigmentation and rough hair coat, infertility, reduced milk yield.

Diagnosis
Signs, detection of low copper levels in blood and particularly in liver sample, response to treatment, in young cattle microcytic and hypochromic, whilst in mature cattle hypochromic and macrocytic anaemia.

Principal differential diagnosis
Parasitism, coccidiosis, poisonings, Johne's disease.

Treatment
Copper supplementation (orally or systemically).

Control
In affected areas regular copper supplementation. Regular metabolic profiling and liver biopsies allow timely intervention.

Copper poisoning

Disease Profile
Occasional incidence of acute, highly fatal poisoning. Younger cattle, particularly milk fed cattle, are more commonly affected. Can be primary or secondary.

Aetiology
Primary – *Acute*: ingestion of large quantities of copper over a short period of time or overdosing by systemic route; *Chronic*: small excess in diet over a long period of time. **Secondary** – ingestion of normal quantities of copper associated with phytogenous components in some plants leading to retention of copper in the liver (e.g. subterranean clover) or accumulation of copper and hepatotoxicity (e.g. *Heliotrupium europaeum, Senecio* spp).

Clinical findings
Depression, anorexia, weakness; abdominal pain, hypersalivation, dark, watery faeces, haemolytic crisis (anaemia, methaemoglobinaemia, haemoglobunuria, nephrosis), mucus membranes icteric or muddy-brown, death.

Diagnosis
Signs, copper levels in liver +/− kidney and brain, increased serum-glutamate-oxaloacetate-transaminase activity in final stages.

Treatment
Treatment is usually unsuccessful once haemolytic crisis has occurred. Oral administration of ammonium molybdate and sodium-thiosulphate or -sulphate, chelation treatment (e.g. D-penicillamine. Supportive treatment-blood transfusions.

Control
Avoid grazing pastures with plants associated with copper toxicity, prevent accidental access to excessive quantities of copper, treatment records to avoid overdosing.

Cowpox

Disease Profile
Rare disorder. Heifers usually at higher risk (lack of exposure). In naïve herds all cows at high risk. Reservoir in nature are rats. Cats hunting rats are believed to act as vector between rats and humans. Humans are most likely vector to cows. Zoonotic.

Aetiology
Orthopoxvirus.

Clinical findings
Lesions are usually located on teats and udder. In severe cases lesions may be also detected in the inguinal region and perineum. In male cattle lesions are typically located on the scrotum. Finally, nursing calves may develop oral lesions.

A typical lesions starts as circular erythema, papule, vesicle and pustule. The pustule ruptures centrally forming a circumscribed crater that dries with brown/red scab. On milking cows, after rupture of the vesicle usually there is formation of circumscribed slow-healing ulcer.

Diagnosis
Signs, detection of the pathogen, detection of intracytoplasmic eosinophilic inclusion bodies.

Principal differential diagnosis
Pseudocowpox, chemical injuries, bovine herpes mammillitis, vesicular disease, foot-and-mouth disease, udder impetigo.

Treatment
No specific treatment. Supportive treatment. Keeping the lesions clean. Improved post milking teat disinfection (e.g. quaternary ammonia compounds) with added emollient. Hydrating and antimicrobial ointments.

Control
Separate infected cows, milk last, infected milkers should not be involved in the process of milking for a few weeks.

Cryptosporidiosis

Disease Profile
Important cause of calf diarrhoea. Caused by coccidian protozoa typically spread by faecal-oral route. May also spread through environment. The parasite is capable of infecting many species of animals. Usually seen in calves 4 days to 3 weeks of age. Asymptomatic infections are common in immuno-competent calves. Zoonotic.

Aetiology
Cryptosporidium parvum. Often mixed infections with viruses, bacteria and coccidia.

Clinical findings
Occasional inappetence and depression in calves. Calf diarrhoea often with tenesmus. Pure infections in immunocompetent calves may be self-limiting and lasts for 1–2 weeks. Often complicated with other pathogens and may result in severe diarrhoea (see appropriate heading).

Post-mortem findings
Inflammation and villus atrophy of the intestines.

Diagnosis
Detection of the pathogen.

Principal differential diagnosis
Other causes of calf diarrhoea (see appropriate headings).

Treatment
In uncomplicated cases no specific treatment. In some countries halofuginone is licensed for use in this condition). Supportive treatment (see appropriate headings).

Control
Keep calf housing clean and dry. Ensure good colostrum management and successful passive transfer. More control see heading 'calf diarrhoea'.

Cystitis

Disease Profile
Relatively common. Individual, rarely herd problem. Common prerequisite is trauma to the bladder wall (uroliths, dystocia) and iatrogenic introduction (catheterisation).

Aetiology
Most common bacteria *Escherichia coli.* Other common bacteria are various corynebacteria.

Clinical findings
Tenesmus and frequent (often unproductive) attempts to urinate. Cattle remain in urination posture for some time after the flow ceased or there is a grunt. Red urine.

Post-mortem findings
Oedema, hyperaemia and haemorrhages of the mucosa.

In protracted cases thickened of the wall and rough mucosa.

Diagnosis
Signs. Urinalysis: haematuria, pyuria,

Principal differential diagnosis
Pyelonephritis, urolithis, urethral obstruction.

Treatment
Antimicrobials 2–3 weeks.

Deep digital sepsis

Disease Profile
Common, spread of superficial conditions of hoof, interdigital disorders or laminitis to deeper structures (Joints, tendon sheaths, bone, soft tissue). Three main routes: interdigital route (most common; necrosis, infection or trauma of the dorsal axial skin of the interdigital space), dorsoabaxial route (superficially located dorsal pouch of the digital interphalageal joint makes it vulnerable) and plantar/palmar route (most often *via* the abaxial white line disease).

Clinical findings
Progressive severe lameness (usually none weight bearing). The coronary band or just proximally to it – swelling and erythema. Frequently fistulous track proximal to the coronary band. In earlier stages there is a joint laxity, later might be fused.

Diagnosis
Signs, radiography.

Principal differential diagnosis
Other reasons for lameness

Treatment
In early stages conservative treatment – large doses of systemic and/or regional antimicrobials, and immobilisation. Joint flush may also be helpful.

In later stages radical treatment – claw amputation or ankylosis.

Deficiency of iodine

Disease Profile
Relatively common. Often underdiagnosed. Primary and secondary (e.g. ingestion of plants that prevent iodine absorption – brassicas, soya meal, sorghum, onions, white clover or primary selenium deficiency). More common in some geographical areas.

Aetiology
Deficient intake or goitrogenic feed stuffs.

Clinical findings
Calves – goitre, weak calves, still-born, alopecia, poor growth, ill-thrift, death.

Mature cattle – poor milk production, poor reproduction, increased incidence of retained placenta.

Bulls – reduced libido and semen quality.

Post-mortem findings
Enlarged thyroids.

Diagnosis
Signs, location, blood T4 (±T3) levels, ultrasonography.

Principal differential diagnosis
Selenium deficiency, cobalt, bovine virus diarrhoea infection, neoplasia of thyroid glands.

Treatment
Parenteral or oral dosing.

Control
Oral supplementation. Avoid using goitrogenic feed stuffs.

Deficiency of manganese

Disease Profile
Probably rare. Can be primary and secondary (excess of calcium and phosphorus; interacts with copper, sulphur, zinc and iron).

Aetiology
Insufficient manganese intake; excess of competitor minerals. Congenital calf deformities following winter housed spring calving beef cows fed a restricted diet of silage without manganese supplementation.

Clinical findings
Neonatal calves – congenital chondrodystrophy, swollen joint, twisted limbs and knuckling.

Calves – poor growth, dry and under pigmented coat.

Mature cattle – impaired fertility.

Diagnosis
Signs. Blood manganese levels.

Principal differential diagnosis
Other reasons for deformed calves.

Treatment
Oral supplementation.

Deficiency of selenium and vitamin E

Common synonyms
Nutritional myodegeneration, White muscle disease.

Disease Profile
Common in many regions. Most commonly in young calves as muscular myodegeneration, failure to thrive or reduced reproductive performance in mature cattle. Decreased immunity (increased incidence of pneumonia and mastitis).

Aetiology
Deficient intake of selenium and vitamin E.

Clinical findings
Acute myodegeneration – death due to heart myonecrosis.

Subacute myodegeneration – stiffness, unwilling to walk, difficulty rising and standing, difficulty sucking. Apparent dyspnoea due to intercostal muscle being affected.

Subclinical – failure to thrive, higher incidence of diarrhoea, pneumonia, stillbirths, retained placenta, abortion and poor fertility.

Post-mortem findings
White muscle myodegeneration, cardiac myodegeneration.

Diagnosis
Signs, bloods concentrations, liver selenium. Response to treatment. Blood biochemistry: elevated CPK, AST, hyperkalaemia and myoglobinuria.

Principal differential diagnosis
Copper deficiency, cobalt deficiency, malnutrition, chronic parasitism.

Treatment
Myocardial myodegeneration unsuccessful. Injectable selenium and vitamin E. Supportive care.

Control
Supplementation with selenium and vitamin E (orally and/or paranterally).

Deficiency of zinc

Disease Profile
Probably common. Often underdiagnosed. Primary and secondary (impaired availability due to high copper and iron). More obvious in young, fast growing cattle.

Aetiology
Deficient zinc intake or high copper and iron.

Clinical findings
Skin – parakeratosis (particularly of the lower limbs, muzzle and perineum), hypopigmentation, poliosis.

Calves – inherited parakeratosis (in Shorthorns), bovine hereditary zinc deficiency (in Holsteins), weak, poor suckle reflex.

Reproductive – poor fertility, prolonged post-partum haemorrhage; male-decreased sperm quality and abnormal morphology of sperm.

General – decreased appetite and milk yield, increased incidence of infectious disorders and lameness, mal-absorptive diarrhoea, night blindness, dacryorrhoea, rhinorrhoea, ptyalism, delayed wound, deformed hornes and hooves.

Post-mortem findings
Parakeratosis.

Diagnosis
Signs, skin biopsy, blood and liver zinc levels.

Principal differential diagnosis
Mange, vitamin A deficiency, other causes of ill-thrift.

Treatment
Oral or parenteral administration of zinc. Supportive care. Preventive administration of antimicrobials.

Control
Oral supplementation.

Degenerative joint disease (DJD)

Disease Profile
Progressive, non-infectious and initially non-inflammatory disorder characterised by primary degeneration of the articular cartilage with variable degrees of peri-articular remodelling of the bony tissue. Primary (inherited) or secondary (nutritional, developmental and traumatic causes). Often seen in older animals (>4 years). The exception may be young bulls (often 6–12 months old) fed on high grain diet.

Clinical findings
The larger weight bearing joints are most often affected, particularly the hip. On examination the affected joint shows effusion and pain. Muscles around affected joint are often wasted.

Diagnosis
Signs

Principal differential diagnosis
Hip dysplasia, septic arthritis, rickets, osteoporosis, nutritional osteopathy due to selenium and vitamin E deficiency.

Treatment
Palliative. Affected cattle are eventually culled.

Dental disorders

Disease Profile
Common, but often undiagnosed. Can be primary or often as a sign of a generalised disorder. Includes periodontal disorders (bone surrounding tooth root), dental staining (e.g. porphyria, fluorosis), defective enamel formation (e.g. fluorosis), dental decay (e.g. caries), irregular wear (e.g. older cattle, abrasive feed stuff, calcium deficiency), dental trauma (e.g. broken tooth), polyodontia and periodontal disorders.

Aetiology
Inherited, congenital or acquired conditions.

Clinical findings
Abnormal chewing/prehension behaviour (e.g. head tilt), reluctance to eat, loss of body condition, halitosis, swelling, hypersalivation. On oral examination the affected area is often easily detected.

Diagnosis
Signs, radiography.

Treatment and management
Usually only in valuable cattle. Treat primary disorder. Tooth extraction, supplemental feeding. Soft, palatable feed stuffs.

Dermatophilosis

Common synonyms
Bovine streptothricosis, Rain scald, Mycotic dermatitis.

Disease Profile
Rare. May occur as outbreaks. Cattle exposed to prolonged wet conditions and close contact. Zebu cattle less susceptible. Occurs in hotter months only.

Ectoparasites are probably important in causing micro lesions to the skin.

Potentially zoonotic.

Aetiology
Infection with *Dermatophilus congolensis*.

Clinical findings
Large areas of skin can become infected. Usually dorsum and limbs. Less common udder in cows and scrotum in bulls. Neutrophilic exudation and scab formation. Matting of hairs ('paint brush'). Infected areas susceptible to fly strike.

Diagnosis
Signs. Detection of pathogen. Seasonality.

Principal differential diagnosis
Papillomatosis, skin lymphosarcoma, dermatophytosis, malignant catarrhal fever, mucosal disease.

Treatment
High doses of antimicrobials. Slow recovery. Provide shelter from rain.

Control
Control ectoparasites. Provide shelter. Farm biosecurity.

Diarrhoea in calves

Common synonyms
Calf scours

Disease Profile
Common disorder that may cause significant economic losses on a particular farm. Calves with severe diarrhoea (often have septicaemia or toxaemia) require urgent intervention. Metabolic acidosis, dehydration, hypoglycaemia and electrolyte imbalances occur

Aetiology
Bacteria (*Escherichia coli, Salmonella* and *Clostridium* spp), viruses (rota-virus, corona-virus, BVD virus), protozoa (*Coccidia, Cryptosporidium* and *Giardia* spp), gastro-intestinal parasitism, and diet-related problems.

E. coli diarrhoea usually seen in calves younger than 5 days, rarely up to 2 weeks of age. *Salmonella* diarrhoea is usually seen in calves older than 10–14 days.

Clostridial diarrhoea is usually seen in rapidly growing, vigorous calves. The most common cause is *C. perfringens* types B and C.

Rotavirus diarrhoea is common in calves 5–7 days up to 3 weeks of age. Coronavirus diarrhoea is usually seen in calves 5–20 days of age.

Coccidial diarrhoea is often caused by *Eimeria zurnii, E. bovis,* and *E. alabamensis* . It is usually seen in calves >3 weeks of age. Cryptosporidial diarrhoea is usually seen in calves 1–3 weeks of age.

Gastro-intestinal parasitism is often seen in calves after weaning up to 2 years of age.

Diet-related diarrhoea in calves may be due to problems with the volume (sudden ingestion of large volume), temperature (sudden change to cold liquid in calves accustomed to drink warm liquid or opposite), type of liquid feed (colostrum, whole milk, skimmed milk, milk replacers), method of feeding (change to bucket feeding in calves accustomed to nipple feeding, large-bore opening of nipples), improper storage of feedstuffs (contamination with toxic material).

Important risk factors: colostrum management and intake (e.g. failure of passive transfer), storage and feeding equipment, age at onset, navel management, housing, grouping strategies, population density, hygiene, environmental conditions, personnel working with calves, previous farm history, and care for cows during pregnancy and colostrogenesis.

The main pathophysiologies associated with diarrhoea are dehydration, loss of electrolytes, metabolic acidosis and hypoglycaemia.

Note: For further information, see under specific headings.

Clinical findings
It is impossible to differentiate the aetiologic agent based on the clinical findings. Diarrhoea may be mild to severe. It can be fatal.

Calves have watery diarrhoea of different colour (yellowish, whitish, greenish, meleana), often with faecal coverings (mucin casts, blood flecks). Severe watery and profuse diarrhoea is common finding with bacterial, viral and protozoal diarrhoea of neonatal calves. This is often associated with dehydration of various degrees, inappetence to anorexia, weakness, depression and signs of shock. In case of septicaemia, there are signs of fever (temperature often above 40.5^{0}C). Later there are usually signs of shock.

With coronavirus, *Salmonella* spp, and *Coccidia*, the diarrhoea is often mixed with flecks of blood and mucin. Cryptosporidial and coccidial diarrhoea may be accompanied by tenesmus. Clostridial disease may or may not be associated with diarrhoea. It is more often seen as a sudden death (peracute form) rather than typical diarrhoea. The acute form of the clostridial disease is typically seen in well-nourished calves with signs of diarrhoea, dysentery, abdominal pain, bellowing and sometimes nervous signs. Gastro-intestinal parasitism is often characterised by wasting syndrome with chronic mild to severe diarrhoea.

Post-mortem findings
E. coli diarrhoea has no specific findings, but there is distended thin walled atonic gut. Coccidia is characterised by haemorrhagic enteritis of ileum, caecum and colon.

Clostridial diarrhoea is characterised by congestion of the lower intestinal mucosa and haemorrhagic enteritis.

Principal differential diagnosis
Other calf disorders (see Failure of passive transfer), congenital problems, kidney failure.

Treatment
TREATMENT:

The aim of treatment is to correct fluid and electrolyte loss, metabolic acidosis (see appropriate heading) and hypoglycaemia. Fluids can be given systemically (usually IV) or orally.

Supportive treatments include antimicrobials (when there is evidence of systemic infection), anti-inflammatories and nursing care. Coccidia can be treated with antimicrobials (oral), particularly sulphonamides and anticoccidials)

Control
CONTROL:

Minimise exposure to potential pathogens (all-in all-out system, improved hygiene, less mixing of calves). For *E. coli, Salmonella,* clostridial and rotavirus diarrhoea vaccination of the dam (in late pregnancy), provides protection if there is a good colostrum intake. Control milk intake. Probiotics may be used prophylactically. Clean and rest buildings after calving and rearing. After an out-break all-in-all-out system, proper sanitation of the facility and rest. For coccidial diarrhoea is important to prevent faecal contamination of feeding and watering facilities, ensure good drainage and avoid overcrowding. Preventive treatment with coccidiostats is sometimes recommended dependent upon the risk analysis.

Digital dermatitis

Common synonyms
Mortellaro, Strawberry foot.

Disease Profile
Important and prevalent condition in Europe, North America and in other regions. Contagious multifactorial disease. Enters the property with recent introductions of infected cattle or through contaminated fomites, particularly hoof trimming equipment. Usually occurs as an epizootic onset of lameness. It causes an epidermitis which is very painful when touched.

Aetiology
Various bacteria from the genus *Spirochetae* (common: *Treponema* spp.), wet conditions, trauma and anaerobic conditions are predisposing factors for development of the disease.

Other organisms may facilitate the establishment and severity of the condition. These may include: *Fusobacterium necrophorum, Guggenheimella bovis, Bacteroides* spp., *Peptococcus* spp., *Prevotella* spp., *Campylobacter* spp. Viruses may also be involved.

Clinical findings
Lameness of a various degree, finding typical lesions. Most common site of lesions palmar/plantar interdigital ridge of the rear foot. Lesions typically ulcerative (superficial ulcerations) with white epithelial margins and longer hairs around it. In the early stages of development, lameness is often not detectable. In chronic cases verrucose fronds of keratin develop. Flank skin in contact with the feet in the lying position can have lesions. Digital dermatitis is thought to potentiate the severity of fusiformis infection creating 'super foul'. This infection progresses rapidly causing infection to the deeper structures of the foot and is difficult to treat successfully.

Diagnosis
Signs.

Principal differential diagnosis
Interdigital necrobacillosis, interdigital dermatitis, heel horn erosion, plantar eczema.

Treatment

The number of recurrent cases is high (more than half).

Treatment can be at a cow or herd level. It is imperative to start the treatment as early as possible. Recurrent or new lesions develop within 7–12 weeks of successful treatment in 50% of cows.

At cow level scrubbing and application of local antimicrobial treatment 3–5 days is required.

Some injectable antimicrobials have digital dermatitis on their data sheets.

At herd level the use of antimicrobial containing footbaths is commonly used.

When the disease is first discovered in a herd, all cattle on the property must be examined and treated promptly. Foot disinfectants and foams are now being used by herd on a regular basis to reduce the prevalence by preventing re-infection.

Control

The key control measures include: A herd approach to biosecurity, timely treatment, reducing environment risk factors and routine foot bathing.

Downer cow

Common synonyms

Recumbent cattle. Downer cow. Downer.

Disease Profile

Common. Recumbent (sternal or lateral) for 12–24. Most commonly around calving or at other times. Bright and alert or depressed and non-responsive. Causes may be metabolic, systemic illness, neurological, and musculo-skeletal conditions Common causes around calving are delayed Tx of hypocalcaemia and pressure neuropathies (calving paralysis).

Primary causes include: pelvic fractures, hip dislocation, hypophosphataemia, paralysis (obturator, sciatic, peroneal, tibial, radial nerve, crushed tail syndrome), hypomagnesaemia, ketosis, fatty liver, rumen acidosis, coliform mastitis, metritis, peritonitis, acute haemorrhage, emaciation, exhaustion, terminal disorder, luxation of gastrocnemius tendon, dystocia, femoral fractures, arthritis, hypokalaemia, botulism, tetanus and any other condition causing prolonged recumbency.

Secondary causes: A down cow is at high risk from ischaemic muscle necrosis when immobile. In addition pressure neuropathies of the tibial and peroneal nerves may occur. Traumatic injuries (fractures, muscle, tendon and ligament rupture) can occur when the animal attempts to rise.

Aetiology

Primary and secondary causes of recumbency

Clinical findings

Primary and secondary causes as above:

Evaluation of secondary causes –

Ischaemic muscle necrosis: hindlimbs, swollen muscles, high AST and CPK values

Prognostic evaluation

In general terms if the primary cause is reversible:

animals that are bright and alert, with attempts to rise and frequent positional movements in recumbency are likely to rise.

animals that: are dull and depressed, make no attempt to rise, remain immobile, frequently go into lateral recumbency, extend their hindlimbs backwards and have clinical signs indicating ongoing iscahemic necrosis have a poor prognosis.

Diagnosis

History, signs.

Treatment

Treat the primary cause:

General care and reducing risk of ischaemic muscle necrosis and neuropathies:

NSAIDs, Turn the animals 5 x/day (odd number), lift 2x/day,

(Mobile flotation tanks are available in some areas)

Easy access to food and water. Provision of shade and shelter from adverse weather.

Soft bedding with good footing (move off concrete)

Remove faeces and clean rear end to avoid urine scald.

Avoid flystrike.

Endocarditis (Bacterial)

Disease Profile

Commonly undiagnosed disorder of cattle. Mass-like lesions on or near the heart valves are caused by haematogenous spread of focal infection somewhere else in the body. Most commonly on the tricuspid valve. More common in mature cattle. Risk factors include, but not limited to: rumen acidosis, focal infection (mastitis, metritis, septic arthritis, omphalophlebitis), traumatic reticulo-peritonitis.

Aetiology

Various bacteria. Most commonly isolated *Trueperella pyogenes* and streptococci. Other common isolates: *Escherichia coli, Klebsiella pneumoniae, Staphylococcus aureus, Fusobacterium necrophorum.*

Clinical findings

Variable and vague clinical signs. Tachycardia, lowered appetite, weight loss, heart murmurs (in approximately 50% of affected cattle). In chronic cases signs of right-sided cardiac insufficiency (ventral oedema, jugular vein distention, tachycardia, hepatomegaly); less frequently signs of left-sided cardiac insufficiency (tachycardia, tachypnoea, dyspnoea, coughing). Fever is an irregular sign.

Diagnosis

Probably the best is by ultrasonography. Signs, blood cultures.

Principal differential diagnosis

Other cardiac disorders

Treatment
Usually unrewarding. Poor to grave prognosis. Long-term antimicrobials. Treatment of signs of heart failure.

Endometritis

Common synonyms
Leucorrhoea, Uterine infection.

Disease Profile
Inflammation of the endometrium, without systemic signs. A common cause of infertility. The incidence rate varies between 2% and 40%. More common in older dairy cows. Usually detected in the first month or two after calving. Characterised by delayed involution and uterine discharge. More common in cows with dystocia, induced calving, twins, retained placenta, metritis and clinical ketosis.

Aetiology
Treuperella pyogenes is consistently found. Mixed infections are almost a rule (*Streptococcus* spp, *Escherichia coli, Fusobacterium necrophorum, Prevotalla melaninogenica*). As a rule of thumb infections within the first week from calving are Gram-negative, later Gram-positive.

Clinical findings
Mucopurulent to purulent discharge from the vagina or detected on vaginal examination. On rectal examination sometimes delayed involution.

Diagnosis
Signs, vaginal examination, rectal ultrasonography.

Principal differential diagnosis
Pyometra, metritis.

Treatment
Antimicrobials (systemic or intrauterine) and/or prostaglandins. Self-cure is common.

Control
Optimised management and nutrition to prevent dystocia, retained placenta, metritis and clinical ketosis.

Enzootic bovine leukosis

Common synonyms
Lymphosarcoma, Leukaemia, Malignant lymphoma.

Disease Profile
Except Europe, Australia and New Zealand infection in dairy cattle is relatively common. However, clinical disease rare and occurs in mature cattle. Majority transmission horizontal (iatrogenic and management procedures). Notifiable.

Aetiology
Retro-virus.

Clinical findings
Most common inapparent. Persistent lymphocytosis.

Clinical signs variable dependent on the organ/s affected by developing tumour.

Digestive form – capricious appetite, melaena, diarrhoea.

Nervous form – progressive posterior paraparalysis.

Ocular form – progressive exophthalmos.

Lymphatic form – enlarged lymph nodes.

Respiratory form – dyspnoea, wheezes, stertor.

Cardiac form – muffled heart sounds, enlarged percussion field.

General appearance – progressive but slow developing weight loss, oedema of dependent body regions, hydrothorax, ascites.

Post-mortem findings
Lymphadenopathy.

Diagnosis
Serology, necropsy. Signs only mildly indicative.

Principal differential diagnosis
Dependent on the affected region.

Treatment
No treatment.

Control
Many countries have eradication programmes. Biosecurity. Isolation of infected, test and slaughter, colostrum feeding only from non-infected cows, disinfection of instruments, single-needle use, control of blood-sucking insects, new rectal sleeve for each animal.

Enzootic pneumonia

Common synonyms
Calf pneumonia, Viral pneumonia.

Disease Profile
Very common, particularly in housed young cattle (less than 6 months). Peak incidence at age of one to one and a half month. Usually high morbidity and low mortality. Common risk factors include bought-in calves, failure of passive transfer, overcrowding, larger group size, mixed ages, inadequate housing, poor ventilation, high humidity, stress of weaning, disbudding, castration, and winter months.

Aetiology
Multi-factorial. Usually combination of virus, bacteria and management factors (see risk factors in disease profile).

Common causative agents: *Mycoplasma bovis, M. dispar,* other *Mycoplasma* spp, *Ureaplasma* spp. *Mannheimia haemolytica, Pasteurella multocida, Histophilus somni, Trueperella pyogenes,* viruses (parainfluenza-3, bovine adenovirus, bovine coronavirus, bovine respiratory syncytial virus, bovine virus diarrhoea virus, bovine infectious rhinotracheitis virus).

Clinical findings
Acute onset. Multiple beasts. Fever, depression, anorexia, polypnoea, dyspnoea, muco-purulent nasal discharge, epiphora, harsh dry cough. On auscultation of cranio-ventral lobes abnormal respiratory sounds (loud harsh breath, squeaks, hums, wheezes, crackles). Cough easily elicited by compression of the trachea.

Post-mortem findings
Cranio-ventral lung consolidation, fibrinous pleuritis, emphysema, congestion and oedema of the lung. Often signs of bovine respiratory complex.

Diagnosis
Sings, post-mortem findings, detection of pathogens (nasopharyngeal swabs, transtracheal bronchoalveolar lavage), serology.

Principal differential diagnosis
Bovine respiratory complex, Aspiration pneumonia, Lungworm pneumonia, congenital heart disorders, *Histophilus somni* syndrome.

Treatment
Antimicrobials. Failure to respond to treatment is common in case of virus and *Mycoplasma* spp infections or where the lung pathology is advanced. Non-steroidal anti-inflammatory drugs. Supportive treatment.

Control
Usual measures of biosecurity. Avoid risk factors. Adopt all-in-all-out system. Vaccination. In case of outbreak isolate sick calves and consider metaphylaxis with antimicrobials.

Ephemeral fever

Common synonyms
Three day fever, Three day sickness, Dengue fever

Disease Profile
A seasonal (warmer moths), arthropod-transmitted (*Culicoides, Anopheles, Culcine, Culex*) viral disorder of the tropical areas of Africa, Asia and Australia. Usually occurs as an outbreak in large number of cattle (morbidity up to 80%) in a short period (can be epidemic). Mortality is rare, except in well-conditioned cattle. The spread is dependent on prevailing weather patterns.

Aetiology
Rhabdovirus.

Clinical findings
Short duration bi- or poly-phasic fever, depression, sudden drop in milk yield, muscular fasciculation to stiffness, lameness, lymphadenopathy, recumbency, atony of rumen, drooling (impaired swallowing) and anorexia. Some cattle become paralysed for few hours up to a week or more.

Post-mortem findings
Rare mortality. Polyserositis, oedematous lymph nodes,

Diagnosis
Detection of virus or antibodies.

Principal differential diagnosis
Hypocalcaemia, Acute laminitis.

Treatment
No specific treatment. Supportive care. Fluids may need intravenous administration (swallowing problem). Prevent secondary bacterial infections. Nursing care similar to downer cow. Avoid unnecessary disturbance.

Control
In some countries vaccine is available.

Chlamydial abortion

Common synonyms
Epizootic abortion

Disease Profile
Uncommon but can result in high levels of abortion. A potential zoonosis.

Aetiology
Infection with *Chlamydia psittaci*. May arise following contact with sheep.

Clinical findings
Suppurative placentitis, with thickened placenta and vaginal discharge. May be drop in milk, pyrexia and nasal discharge. Some subsequent infertility.

Post-mortem findings
Placentitis with thickened placenta.

Diagnosis
Impression smears from placenta, culture of placental tissues. Serology of dam and foetus.

Principal differential diagnosis
Other causes of abortion.

Treatment
Antibacterials (injectable) – In in-contact animals use long-acting oxytetracycline or other suitable antibiotics. Isolate all aborting cattle.

Control
Prevent contact between sheep and cattle especially at lambing, and vaccinate sheep. Isolate all aborting cattle until after all discharges cease and dispose of the placentas.

Facial eczema

Disease Profile
Hepatogenous photosensitivity to sunlight due to ingestion of pyrrolydiones (sporidesmins) produced by the fungus *Pithomyces chartarum*. The fungus is a saprophyte of dead plant material under climatic conditions of warmth and moisture. Manifested as cutaneous hypereasthesia. Common in autumn in New Zealand. Occasionally Australia, South Africa and Europe. High morbidity and low mortality. Common risk factors: spore count in pasture, low grazing, previous exposure to sporidesmins and stocking rate.

Aetiology
Sporidesmins A to H toxicosis.

Clinical findings
Usually first sign in drop in milk production. Cutaneous erythema and oedema of lightly pigmented areas, particularly ears, face, udder, dorsum of the trunk and vulva. Restlessness, shade seeking, pruritus. Additionally, cattle with signs of photosensitivity and pigmented animals show anorexia, depression, jaundice. Rarely haemoglobinuria and hepatic encephalopathy.

Post-mortem findings
Acute phase – swollen liver with thickened bile ducts.

Chronic phase – extensive hepatic fibrosis. The left lobe is more affected.

Diagnosis
Signs, elevated gamma glutamyltfansferase (GGT).

Principal differential diagnosis
Other causes of photosensitivity.

Treatment
Remove from sunlight, provide shade and allow grazing at night. Antihistamines early in the course. Provide zinc sulphate in drinking water.

Control
Spore count monitoring, avoid low grazing, manage pasture to minimise dead leaf material, zinc supplementation just before and during risk periods.

Failure of passive transfer

Disease Profile
Very common on some farms. Risk factors include poor colostrum quality and quantity (e.g. care for cows during pregnancy and colostrogenesis, age of cow, volume of colostrum harvested per cow), poor ingestion (e.g. loss of appetite, competition), poor absorption (e.g. enteritis).

Clinical findings
Increased incidence of infection (e.g. diarrhoea, septicaemia, meningitis, infection of the umbilical remnant, septic arthritis, pneumonia and ill thrift) and decreased weight gain.

Diagnosis
Signs. Low GGT. Total Protein levels, Low ZST.

Treatment
In calves < 24h old oral colostrum. In calves >24h old transfusion of full blood from mature cows.

Control
Force-fed colostrum, feed high-quality colostrum, vaccinate dams, feed colostrum of cows producing <9L of colostrum at first milking. Provide antibiotic cover for identified at risk calves?

Fatty liver

Common synonyms
Hepatic lipidosis, Fat cow syndrome.

Disease Profile
Excessive accumulation of fat in the liver of periparturient cows. High producing dairy cows in their second to fourth lactation more susceptible. In beef cows rare occurrence in individual cows pre-calving. Often exacerbated by a concurrent disorder (retained placenta, metritis, mastitis, hypocalcaemia, displaced abomasums, pregnancy toxaemia).

Aetiology
Overfeeding during the dry period is of particular importance for the development of the syndrome. The negative energy balance in postparturient cow results in excessive mobilisation of fat from the reserves by catabolism, transport into the liver, re-synthesis of triglycerides, inability to transport all out of the liver, accumulation in the hepatocytes, disturbance of their normal function.

Clinical findings
Obese well-conditioned cow, anorexia, depression, rapid weight loss, weakness, recumbency, rumen hypomotility, decreased milk production. Jaundice and other signs of hepatic injury rarely seen.

Diagnosis
Signs, liver biopsy. Biochemical tests: AST, NEFA's and Beta Hydroxy Butyrate will be increased.

Principal differential diagnosis
Ketosis, metritis, mastitis, displaced abomasums, hepatic disorders.

Treatment
Often unrewarding. Prognosis generally poor. Treat concurrent disorders. Recover rumen function. Correct negative energy balance. Supportive medication: intravenous glucose, propylene glycol, corticosteroids, glucagon, insulin.

Control
Avoid over-conditioning during the dry period. Optimise nutrition post-partum to decrease the effects of negative energy balance and encourage dry matter intake.

Femoral nerve paralysis

Disease Profile
Trauma is most common reason, particularly overstretching of the nerve in adult cattle that struggle to rise or 'hip-lock' at calving in new-borns. Posterior presenting calves, with dystocia and assisted calving with traction are at risk)

Clinical findings
Stifle is flexed (and usually all distal joints) and cannot be extended. Discrete quadriceps atrophy.

Frog like squatting standing posture.

Principal differential diagnosis
Other neurological disorders, femoral or pelvic fracture, tendon ruptures, hip dislocation; calves bilateral hip dislocation, bilateral luxation of patella. Fracture femoral neck.

Treatment
Supportive care, B-complex. Prognosis is good in cattle able to rise. The prognosis for calves should be guarded.

Fescue poisoning

Disease Profile
Endophyte-infected tall fescue (*Festuca arudinacea*). In cattle poisoning primary affects the cardiovascular and endocrine systems. Pastures and hay produced from infected pastures are equally dangerous.

Aetiology
Ergot-type and pirrolizidine-type alkaloids produced by endophytic fungus (*Neotyphodium coenophialum*).

Clinical findings
Fescue foot

Mild lameness (mainly hind limbs) that progresses into a severe form. Redness and swelling around coronary bands and coldness bellow the band. Necrosis of the digits, tips of ears and tail. Loss of body weight, rough, dull hair coat.

Summer slump

Slump in milk production. Hirsuitism, hyperpnoea, hyperthermia, reduced weight gain, reduced heat tolerance, diarrhoea, hypersalivation, photosensitivity, delayed puberty in heifers, decreased fertility, dystocia, reduced calf birth weight, hypogalactia to agalactia.

Fat necrosis form

Obstruction of abdominal organs (bloat, abdominal pain, constipation), reduced productivity.

Post-mortem findings
Fescue foot – Clearly demarcated distal necrosis of the digit.

Fat necrosis – Calcified fat in the omentum.

Diagnosis
Signs, history, detection of the fungus.

Treatment
Advanced cases no successful treatment. Early recognised cases – remove from fescue pasture, dilute with other feedstuffs, oral dosing with thiabendazole once weekly, feeding seaweed (*Ascophyllum nodosum*) extracts. Supportive treatment. Antimicrobials may be required for prevention of bacterial digital disorders.

Control
Avoid infected pastures. Grow 'endophyte-resistant' varieties. Practice pastures rotation.

Fluoride poisoning

Common synonyms
Fluorosis.

Disease Profile
Uncommon. Mainly chronic form associated with skeletal or dental abnormalities. Dental abnormalities occur only if toxic fluorides are ingested before teeth eruption. Acute form is rare. Cattle in poor condition may be more susceptible to fluorosis.

Aetiology
A chronic disorder associated with long-term ingestion of excessive levels of fluorine with feedstuffs or water (artesian wells, mining). Acute form is usually associated with inhalation or ingestion of highly toxic rodenticides.

Clinical findings
Chronic form – *Skeletal* – Weight, loss, lameness, particularly of forelimbs in early stages. Later hind limbs lameness in hip joint and abnormal hoof wear due to elongation of the pedal bones. Fractures of pedal bones. Palpation of long bones results in intense pain.

Dental – Mottled teeth, Problems with mastication and drinking cold water, weight loss, general illthrift.

Acute form – Constipation followed by diarrhoea, abdominal pain, dyspnoea, muscle tremors, tetany, collapse death.

Post-mortem findings
Skeletal abnormalities – periosteal hyperostosis, exostosis, roughened periosteal surface, osteosclerosis and arthritis.

Dental abnormalities – hypoplasia, dysplasia, yellow-brown discolouration of the enamel, pitting, chalking, mottling and abnormal tooth wear.

Diagnosis
Signs. History. Radiographic examination. Bone analysis.

Principal differential diagnosis
Coccidiosis, hypomagnesaemia, trauma, arthritis, osteoporosis, lead or copper poisoning.

Treatment
Remove from source. Recovery of skeletal abnormalities takes years. Dental abnormalities are usually irreversible. Supportive treatment. In acute cases prevent absorption.

Control
Avoid consumption of feedstuffs and water reach on fluorine. Adding substances that reduce fluorine absorption (aluminium and/or chloride, calcium aluminate and/or carbonate).

Fly-related dermatoses

Disease Profile
Two disorders are of importance in cattle: hypodematosis (warble fly) and screw worm. Nuisance by other flies (e.g. biting flies) may also be important.

Aetiology
Hypodermosis (*Hypoderma bovis, H. lineatum*). Screwworm (*Cochliomyia hominivorax, Chrysomuia bezzianna*), biting flies (black flies, send flies).

Clinical findings
Hypodermosis: soft swelling (usually in form of painful subcutaneous nodules) in spring each with a breathing hole, or reaction to larvae (bloat, anaphylaxis paralysis).

Screw worm infestation: extensive damage to the skin, copious brown discharge, and foul odour.

Biting flies: changes in behaviour, avoiding entry to milking shed, stumping, kicking, and flicking the tail.

Diagnosis
Detection of larvae, serology, clinical signs.

Treatment
Ectoparasiticides in spring or systemic antihelmintic in autumn.

Hypoderma: Do not treat systematically while larvae in spinal cord or around oesophagus.

Screw worm infestation: additionally symptomatic treatment.

Control
Specific eradication programmes.

Fog fever

Common synonyms
Acute Bovine Pulmonary Oedema and Emphysema (ABPEE).

Disease Profile
Animal introduced to new and lush pasture. Acute respiratory distress High prevalence in affected group. Some will die rapidly (1–2 days). Morbidity often >50% with up to 30% mortality in affected animals.

Aetiology
High levels of tryptophan in the grass is converted by rumen bacteria to 3-methylindole which is absorbed and causes severe irreversible lung damage.

Clinical findings
Usually, no fever. Loud breath sounds. On auscultation crackles. Expiratory dyspnoea of higher degree (Air hunger). Exercise intolerance. Death. Multiple animals affected.

Post-mortem findings
Pulmonary oedema, congestion and interstitial emphysema.

Diagnosis
History of exposure to lush pasture, multiple animals affected signs.

Important differentials include RSV and lungworm

Treatment
Mild cases may 'recover' others will remain debilitated. No specific treatment. Removal to reduce further exposure seems logical but stress of moving may exacerbate.

Control
Controlled access to new pasture by time or strip grazing. Monensin may reduce risk.

Foot and mouth disease

Disease Profile
Very contagious, viral disease of cloven-hoofed animals. Pigs are considered as amplifying host, goat and sheep maintenance host and cattle indicator host. Transmission by aerosol, ingestion, directs contact and animal products. Occurs as outbreaks, usually of large geographical areas. Morbidity up to 100%. Mortality 1–5%, but may be higher in calves. Endemic to Africa, Asia and parts of South America. North and Central America, Australia and New Zealand free for many years. Europe with occasional outbreaks. Low potential, zoonotic.

Aetiology
Picorna virus from genus Aphtovirus with 7 serotypes and more than 60 subtypes.

Clinical findings
Incubation 1–14 days. Clinical signs develop over 2–5 days. Runs it clinical course in 1–3 weeks.

Fever, lethargy, hypersalivation, lameness, inappetence. Short-lived vesicles in the mouth cavity, muzzle, nostrils, coronary band, interdigital space, heels and/or teats. Vesicles progress to erosions. Decrease milk production. In pregnant cattle abortion may occur.

Atypical forms:

Calves – myocardial degeneration and peracute death.

Nervous form –rare. During typical outbreak some cattle may show depression and ascending paralysis.

Alimentary form – rare. Dysentery.

Post-mortem findings
Detection of vesicles, erosion, 'tiger heart', denuded rumen papillae.

Diagnosis
Signs, virus isolation and identification.

Principal differential diagnosis
Other forms of stomatitis and teat lesions, foot rot, BVD, MCF, IBR, rinderpest, bluetongue.

Treatment
Not attempted. In foot-and-mouth free areas quarantine, test and slaughter usually evoked.

In endemic areas supportive treatment and improved milking hygiene. Surviving animals may become long-time shedders

Control
Biosecurity. Vaccination in endemic areas. No cross-protection between serotypes and often subtypes.

Fracture of distal phalanx

Disease Profile
Fracture of the distal phalanx is not uncommon in cattle.

Aetiology
Trauma. Offloading. Oestrus-riding of other cows.

Clinical findings
Severe lameness (sometimes bilateral). Cow assumes cross-legged stance, no swelling, but hot and painful on examination.

Diagnosis
Signs, radiography.

Principal differential diagnosis
Laminitis

Treatment
Avoid movements of the sole and leave the bone to heel spontaneously. Apply block on the sound claw. Time to heal is long – usually 2–3 months. Confine in yard.

Fusobacterium necrophorum abortion

Disease Profile
Little reported in Europe. May follow acidosis. Most abortion is around seven months.

Aetiology
Fusobacterium necrophorum infection.

Clinical findings
Abortion at about seven months. Cow may be in good condition.

Post-mortem findings
Exudation peritonitis and pleurisy, fibrinous pericarditis, consolidated lungs with fibrinous tags on liver. Histologically there is multifocal suppurative epicarditis and meningeal blood vessel infection.

Diagnosis
Isolation of bacterium from foetal stomach.

Principal differential diagnosis
Other causes of abortion.

Treatment
No advice at present available.

Control
Avoid over-feeding.

Granular vulvo-vaginitis

Common synonyms
Granular venereal disease, Granular vulvitis, Granular vulvitis complex.

Disease Profile
Reactive proliferation of lymphoid tissue. Relatively common. Under-diagnosed. Most common in heifers. Potentially zoonotic.

Aetiology
Not clear. *Ureaplasma* spp, *Mycoplasma* spp, *Chlamydophila* spp and *Histophilus somni* probably have role in development. Other pathogens include *Trueperella pyogenes*, *Escherichia coli*, *Streptococcus* spp, *Staphylococcus* spp and herpes virus.

Clinical findings
Onset of signs 3–5 days post coitus. Hyperaemia and whitish pustules of the vaginal and vulval mucosa. Straining, pollakiuria, mucopurulent discharge. Usually self-limiting within a month post service.

Diagnosis
Signs. Examination by speculum.

Principal differential diagnosis
Transmissible fibro-papilloma, infectious vulvo-vaginitis.

Treatment
Usually not required.

Haemorrhagic septicaemia

Disease Profile
Relatively common in tropical Asia and Africa. Buffaloes more susceptible than cattle. Transmitted by direct contact. In naïve populations high morbidity and mortality. Case fatality nearly 100%. Remote zoonotic risk.

Aetiology
Certain serotypes of *Pasteurella multocida*.

Clinical findings
Short incubation (18–36 hours). Peracute death (6–24 hours). Sometimes survival up to 3 days. Fever, depression, reluctance to move. Dyspnoea, hypersalivation and nasal discharge.

Post-mortem findings
Widely distributed haemorrhages. Signs of pneumonia. Oedematous swelling of cervical, parotid and pharyngeal region.

Diagnosis
Signs, post-mortem, detection of pathogen.

Principal differential diagnosis
Other causes of peracute death.

Treatment
Usually no time to start treatment. Antimicrobials in very early stages.

Control
Biosecurity. Vaccination. Isolation of affected cattle.

Heat stress

Disease Profile
Increased environmental temperature and/or temperature-humidity index (THI) affect milk production, reproduction and general health of dairy cattle. The termo-neutral zone for dairy cattle is between 5°C and 25°C. The temperature-humidity index should be less than 72. High producing lactating cows are more susceptible. Inadequate shademand overcrowding are important contributing factors. The effect is dependent on the degree of exceeded temperature and THI.

Aetiology
Ambient temperature exceeding 25°C of THI of above 72.

Clinical findings
Decreased activity, increased water intake, reduced DMI, hypersalivation, open mouth breathing, tachypnoea, seeking shade and wind. Rectal temperature increased. Decreased milk yield, decreased reproduction. Increased incidence of laminitis and associated disorders.

THI 72–78 results in heat stress and decreased reproduction. THI 78–82 results in heat stress, decreased reproduction and seriously decreased milk yield. THI above 82 results in heat stress, decreased reproduction, seriously decreased milk yield and is life threatening.

Treatment and control
Provide shade, improve ventilation, fans. Cooling down is more effective using sprinklers, feeding smaller portions more often and modifications of the diet (decreased fibre and protein; increased fats and minerals; adding extra bicarbonate).

Hepatitis

Disease Profile
Inflammatory disorder of the liver. In general term it usually encompasses also degenerative and diffuse liver pathology. It may be primary or secondary to a disorder in other body systems (e.g. omphalophlebitis in calves). Many hepatitis forms are characterised by photosensitivity (see appropriate headings).

Aetiology
Many factors; toxic (e.g. poisonous plants, inorganic and organic substances, mycotoxins), infectious (e.g. fluke, *Clostridium* spp, *Escherichai coli, Trueperella pyogenes, Chlamydia* spp, fungi, septicaemia, toxaemia), hypoxia (e.g. due to congestive heart failure), accumulation of photosensitive substances (e.g. porphyria).

Clinical findings
Icterus (despite hyperbilirubinaemia it may not be visible), liver enlargement, photosensitivity, emaciation, ventral oedema, diarrhoea or constipation, signs of hepatic encephalopathy.

Post-mortem findings
Enlarged liver, areas of focal necrosis and haemorrhages.

Diagnosis
Signs, ultrasonography, liver biopsy, raised liver enzymes (SDH, GGT, Alkaline phosphatise, AST), bilirubin, ammonia and bile acids assays.

Principal differential diagnosis
Signs of encephalopathy, myelopathy and meningitis. Other reasons for chronic weight loss.

Treatment
Provide soft, palatable feedstuffs. Changes in diet (decrease protein and fat; increase digestible carbohydrate). Supplement minerals, vitamins and methionine. Stop ingestion of toxic agents, charcoal. Antimicrobial treatment as required. Treat the primary disorder.

Control
Avoid exposure to toxic agents. Control liver fluke. Vaccination to prevent clostridial disorders.

Hip dislocation/luxation

Disease Profile
Common cause of upper lameness in younger dairy cattle (2–5 years old). Usually soon after calving or at mating. Usually traumatic. In calves – result of excessive traction during assisted parturition of a posterior presentation dystocia. The femoral head usually dislocated dorsal and cranial or less commonly ventral and caudal. The least common dislocation is ventral and cranial.

Clinical findings
Cranio-dorsal dislocation – affected limb appear shortened, held little forward and rotated outward. The greater femoral trochanter area is asymmetric. The stifle looks big and is rotated outwards whilst the hock is rotated inwards.

Caudo-ventral dislocation – These animals are usually recumbent.

Cranio-ventral dislocation – on rectal examination the femoral head can be palpated cranially to the pelvic brim.

Diagnosis
Signs.

Principal differential diagnosis
Pelvic fracture, proximal femoral fracture (trochanter, neck, proximal epiphysis), separation of the proximal femoral epiphysis, rupture of the round ligament, sacroiliac luxation, obturator nerve paralysis, atrophy or large muscles.

Treatment
The best prognosis is for standing animals attended within 8–12 hours from dislocation. The prognosis is not good for recumbent animals and those with being dislocated longer than 24hours or longer. The correction of the condition can be carried out by manipulative reduction or surgery.

Histophilus somni complex

Common synonyms
Neurologic form – Thrombo-embolic meningo-encephalitis (TEME, TME). Sleeper syndrome. Brainer.

Disease Profile
This complex may be characterised by infection of the respiratory, nervous, ophthalmic, cardiovascular and musculoskeletal systems in young cattle (predominantly 6–24 months of age) and the reproductive system in breeding-age cattle. The complex may be a significant cause of morbidity and mortality and feedlot cattle, with highest incidence in the first few weeks from arrival. The complex in young cattle (systemic form) is common in beef, while the reproductive from can be detected in beef and dairy and affects mainly females. The course may be anything from peracute to chronic.

Aetiology
Histophilus somni (formerly *Haemophilus somnus*)

Clinical findings
Systemic disease – Non-specific signs including fever, depression, lowered to loss of appetite.

Signs may differ dependent on the system affected. Combinations of signs of various systems are common. Usually the systemic form of the complex has high morbidity. The reproductive form is exception. It occurs usually alone, without involvement of other systems and is characterised mainly by sporadic abortion.

Peracute form – Sudden death.

Respiratory system – Signs of bovine respiratory disease complex. Reduced to absent appetite, dyspnoea, nasal discharge, epiphora, coughing, pneumonia (abnormal auscultation lung sounds), death.

Nervous system – Fever, although the temperature may be normal, severe depression, anorexia, ataxia, muscle weakness, proprioceptive deficits, recumbency and death in 12–24 hours. Sometimes with cerebellar and caudal brainstem lesions head tilt, opisthotonus, nystagmus, strabismus, uni- or bi- lateral blindness, hyperaesthesia, convulsions and coma.

Ophthalmic system – Conjunctivitis, epiphora, retinal haemorrhage. Usually associated with signs of infection in other systems.

Cardiovascular system – Myocarditis, pericarditis, septicaemia, congestive heart failure. Often seen after respiratory form.

Musculoskeletal system – Infection arthritis, swelling, pain, heat. Commonly seen in multiple joints.

Reproductive system – Sporadic abortion, usually with mild or without sings of disorder in the dam. It may cause infertility, endometritis, vaginitis, mastitis. In male cattle it may cause orchitis.

Post-mortem findings
Histopathology of affected tissues – Septic thrombi, vasculitis.

Respiratory system – Fibrinous to purulent pneumonia, fibrinous pleuritis mainly in cranioventral lobes.

Nervous system – Meningitis and encephalitis. Usually multifocal.

Ophthalmic system – Conjunctivitis and retinal haemorrhage.

Cardiovascular system – Sins consistent with myocarditis, pericarditis, and septicaemia. Myocarditis typically in papillary muscle of the left ventricle.

Musculoskeletal system – Serofibrinous arthritis in affected joints.

Reproductive system – Necrotising placentitis, signs of foetal septicaemia.

Diagnosis
Signs. History. Detection of the pathogen in CSF, synovial fluid or blood.

Principal differential diagnosis
Respiratory system – Other causes of bovine respiratory disease complex.

Nervous system – Polioencephalomalacia, Listeriosis, Viral encephalitis, Trauma, Lead or salt poisoning.

Ophthalmic system – Other causes of conjunctivitis and retinal haemorrhage.

Cardiovascular system – Other causes of myocarditis, pericarditis, septicaemia, congestive heart failure.

Musculoskeletal system – Other causes of infection arthritis.

Reproductive system – Other causes of abortion.

Treatment
Aggressive treatment with antimicrobials, non-steroidal anti-inflammatory drugs, low stress handling, supportive care. Severely affected and recumbent cattle humane euthanasia.

Control
Normal biosecurity measures. Good ventilation and hygiene. Avoid overcrowding and re-grouping. Pre-arrival and post-arrival vaccination. In face of outbreak metaphylaxis with antimicrobials, avoid stress.

Hydrancephaly

Disease Profile
Absence of brain hemispheres in normal cranium. More common than hydrocephalus.

Aetiology
BVDv, Akabane, bluetongue-intrauterine infection.

Clinical findings
At calving 'dummy syndrome' (depression, blindness), cerebellar signs and arthrogryposis.

Diagnosis
Post-mortem, pre-suckling serology.

Treatment
Euthanasia.

Control
Vaccination. Biosecurity measures.

Hydrocephalus

Disease Profile
Increased hydrostatic pressure of the cerebrospinal fluid. Rare.

Aetiology
Inherited or vitamin A deficiency.

Clinical findings
Stillborn or if alive depressed and blind. Sometimes 'domed' forehead and microphthalmia.

Diagnosis
Signs, ultrasonography.

Treatment
Euthanasia.

Control
Genetic selection/Vit A supplementation

Hypocalcaemia

Common synonyms
Milk fever, Parturient paresis.

Disease Profile
Relatively common. Sporadic. May occur as an outbreak due to improper transition cow management. Most common around calving within 1–3 days past calving. Predisposing factors – older cows, high producers, Channel Island breeds, cows with previous history.

Aetiology
Low serum calcium.

Clinical findings
Stage one – able to stand, hypersensitive and excitable, restless, bellowing, protruding tongue, in appetence, bruxism. Sometimes ataxia and reluctance to walk.

Stage two – unable to stand, maintain sternal recumbency, inappetence, dry muzzle, mydriasis, faint heart beats, tachycardia, hypotonic rumen, bloat, subnormal temperature and cold extremities, loss of swallowing reflex, depression, 'S'-shaped neck or head tucked into flank, constipation.

If pre-calving – no uterine contractions (e.g. dystocia).

Stage three – progressive loss of consciousness (to coma), unresponsive to stimuli, lateral recumbency, tachycardia, weak pulse, bloat. Lasts only few hours followed by death.

Diagnosis
Signs, Biochemistry: hypocalcaemia (+/– hypomagnesaemia +/– hypophosphatemia)

Principal differential diagnosis
Acute neurologic disorders, poisonings, acute mastitis, toxic metritis, acidosis, uterine rupture, trauma, nerve paralysis, acute haemorrhage, hypo-phosphataemia, downer cow.

Treatment
Restore calcium level to normal (injectable calcium), provide depot (oral calcium), prevent downer cow (nursing and supportive care).

Control
Proper transition cow management – maintain daily intake, provide adequate magnesium levels, low calcium content in ration pre-calving, reduce DCAD in the last few weeks pre-calving. Consider calcium supplementation after calving. Culling repeated offenders.

Hypokalaemia

Disease Profile
Relatively common. Underdiagnosed. Primary rare. Secondary due to shift of potassium ions to the intracellular fluid (e.g. metabolic alkalosis), increased loss via urinary (e.g. anorexia or previous treatment with steroids) or digestive (e.g. diarrhoea in mature cattle; NOTE: calves develop hyperkalaemia) tract. Can be seen in displaced abomasum due to metabolic alkalosis.

Aetiology
Primary (deficiency of potassium in diet) or secondary (increased loss of potassium).

Clinical findings
Muscle fasciculations, skeletal muscle weakness, progressing to recumbency. Head often tucked into flank.

Diagnosis
Signs. Biochemistry.

Principal differential diagnosis
Hypocalcaemia.

Treatment
Potassium (injectable and oral).

Hypomagnesaemia

Common synonyms
Grass tetany. Grass staggers. Transport tetany.

Disease Profile
One of common metabolic disorders. Most commonly detected in lactating beef cows in the first 2 months after calving. It may also occur in lactating dairy cows on pasture in spring or dry cows in autumn. Calves fed on all-milk diet are also at risk, particularly at age 2 to 4 months. Hypomagnesaemia predisposes lactating cows to hypocalcaemia. Clinical disorder is often precipitated by cold, stress, transport, lush pasture in spring and autumn, and lowered feed intake. It may have peracute, acute, subacute and chronic subclinical course.

Aetiology
A reduction in levels of magnesium in the blood and cerebrospinal fluid.

Clinical findings
Peracute – sudden death

Acute – Progression-early anorexia, separation from the herd in a bright, alert and hyperaesthetic cow. May charge. Muscle fasciculation, head and neck tremors, high-stepping forelimb gait. Ears are markedly erected and twitching. Sometimes bellowing, frenzy walk and ataxia. This stage progresses into a staggering form characterised by nystagmus, fluttering eyelids, lateral recumbency, paddling movements of the limbs, clonic convulsions or muscle spasm, opisthotonus, uncontrolled diarrhoea and urination, foaming at the mouth, hyperthermia, tachycardia, hyperpnoea, tachypnoea and loud heart sounds. Sometimes remission between staggers episodes. Any stimulus (clapping the hands) may provoke new episode. Death may occur during any of the episodes.

Subacute – similar signs but protracted over few days.

Chronic – Subclinical chronic form is common and may be undetected. Low magnesium levels in blood, dullness, lowered appetite, unthriftiness, odd facial expressions, slight changes in behaviour and decreased production. Common in autumn on pasture.

Calves – Similar to adults. In addition excessive ear movements, exophtalmia or enophtalmia, third eyelid prolapse, ataxia and difficulty feeding.

Post-mortem findings
Signs of staggering episode around the carcass, trauma and bruising, ecchymotic haemorrhages on mucosal and serous surfaces, aspirated rumen content into the trachea/lungs.

Diagnosis
Signs, history, detection of low levels of magnesium in blood, urine, cerebrospinal or ocular fluid.

Principal differential diagnosis
Mature – Hypocalcaemia, nervous ketosis, rabies, encephalitis, tetanus, lead, salt or arsenic poisoning.

Calves – nervous coccidiosis, lead poisoning, tetanus, encephalitis

Treatment
Muscle relaxants, sedation, magnesium therapy.

Control
Magnesium supplementation.

Hypophosphataemia

Common synonyms
Creeper cow.

Disease Profile
Relatively rare.

Periparturient hypophosphataemia in form of downer cow or periparturient haemoglobinuria).

Hypophosphataemia not associated with calving results in osteoporosis and pica; usually in lactating beef cows on phosphorus deficient pastures.

Hypophosphataemia in young growing cattle – rickets. Rare in calves with not fused epiphyses.

Hypophosphataemia in lactating dairy cows once the immediate post-calving period has passed is often associated with poor phosphorus diet or general malnutrition due to phosphorus and/or vitamin D deficiency.

Aetiology
Low phosphorus levels in food and/or excess of calcium, iron or aluminium.

Clinical findings
Periparturient hypophosphataemia in form of downer cow – often initially diagnosed and treated for hypocalcaemia. Become bright and alert, still unable to rise, pushes around on her sternum ('creeper' cow).

Osteomalacia-osteoporosis – cows ill-thriven, slab-chested, pica, gait abnormalities, increased incidence of pathologic fractures.

Cows with hypophosphataemia – ill thrift, decreased milk production, decreased fertility.

Rickets – uniform widening of epiphyseal-diaphyseal cartilage, enlargement of the ends of long bones, costo-chondral junctions.

Diagnosis
Signs. Blood chemistry. Measuring ash: Ca: P ratio of bone. Response to treatment or supplementation.

Principal differential diagnosis
Other metabolic disorders, chronic parasitism.

Treatment
Phosphorus supplementation. In downer cows initially injectable preparations.

Control
Correct diet.

Infectious bovine rhinotracheitis (IBR)

Common synonyms
Rednose.

Disease Profile
One of the components of the bovine respiratory disease complex. A mild to severe infection of the upper respiratory tract. Can also cause conjunctivitis, abortion, reproductive disorder (in Europe) and a nervous form. Latent infections. Most affected cattle are between 6 and 18 months of age. Morbidity may reach 100% with up to 10% mortality. Once infected, the affected animal is a life-long source of infection. In neonatal calves it may cause generalised form with gastrointestinal tract involvement.

Aetiology
Bovine herpes virus-1. Neurologic form is caused by its variant BHV-5. Strains that cause dermatitis, mastitis, abortion and encephalitis are rare.

Clinical findings
High fever, anorexia, depression.

Respiratory tract – Reddened muzzle, nasal discharge (serous to mucopurulent), petechial to ecchymotic haemorrhages, erosion to ulcerations, serofibrinous plaques in nasal and pharyngeal cavity. Inspiratory dyspnoea. Coughing. Drop in milk yield. Often combined with conjunctivitis. In case of bacterial complications bovine respiratory disease complex.

Conjunctivitis – usually bilateral. Opacity starting from the corneoscleral line and haemorrhagic conjunctivitis.

Abortion – occurs in the last trimester of gestation. Retained placenta and metritis are common sequel.

Reproductive disorder – In female infectious pustular vulvovaginatis (coital exanthema); in male infectious pustular balanoposthitis. Usually soon after service. Oedematous mucosa, small pustules on vulva and vagina/prepuce, penis and urethra. Surrounding mucosa is hyperaemic. Later pustules coalesce. Erosion and increased susceptibility to secondary bacterial infections. May result in purulent discharge for a few weeks.

Nervous form – Encephalitis and high mortality.

Neonatal calves/ Digestive from – Persistent mild fever, rhinitis, bronchitis, conjunctivitis, pustular palatitis, diarrhoea. Very high mortality.

Post-mortem findings
Respiratory form – nasal cavity, pharynx, trachea – petechial to ecchymotic haemorrhages, focal necrotic areas, serofibrinous plaques and exudates, damaged epithelium in trachea (sometimes spreading to bronchi).

Nervous form – non-suppurative meningoencephalitis, histopathology gliosis, infiltration with macrophages, particularly in anterior cerebrum and dorsal cortex.

Digestive from – erosions and ulcerations in the oral cavity, oesophagus and abomasum.

Diagnosis
Signs. Detection of the pathogen. Serology. Intranuclear inclusion bodies in livers of aborted foetuses.

Principal differential diagnosis
Other causes of bovine respiratory disease complex, abortion. For encephalitis – listeriosis, nervous ketosis, Aujezky, rabies and *Histophylus somni*.

Treatment
Supportive treatment. Antimicrobials to prevent secondary bacterial infection. Non-steroidal anti-inflammatory drugs.

Control
Usual biosecurity. Vaccination (maternal antibodies may interfere with early vaccination of calves).

Some vaccines enable differentiation of vaccinated and infected animals

Foul

Common synonyms
Infectious necrobacillosis of the foot, Foot rot.

Disease Profile
Contagious necrotising lesion of the interdigital skin. Bacterial infection caused by *Fusobacterium necrophorum*. Incidence usually low, but it may cause outbreaks. Continuous exposure to wet conditions, abrasions from rocks, mud and stones. Lack of nutrients (minerals and vitamins) can result in a weaker interdigital skin and increased risk of interdigital necrobacillosis.

Aetiology
Fusobacterium necrophorum. Some authors also include *Porphymonas levii, Bacteroides melaninogenicus* and *Dichelobacter nodosus*. Foot rot in cattle should not be confused with foot rot in sheep. These two disorders have different aetiology. It is believed that cross-infection does not occur.

Clinical findings
Sudden onset of lameness (mild to severe) of one limb and acute swelling of interdigital tissue. Milk production and body condition deteriorate rapidly. Symmetrical swelling of the foot. The interdigital skin cracks open, revealing foul smelling, necrotic, core-like material.

Diagnosis
Signs.

Principal differential diagnosis
Traumatic injuries, foreign bodies, toe abscess, sole abscess, vertical fissures, retro articular abscess, septic arthritis and abscess of distal interphalangeal joint, fracture of distal phalanx, FMD.

Treatment
Usually successful, provided instituted early.

Systemic antimicrobial therapy. NSAIDs.

For difficult, unresponsive cases regional intravenous administration of the antimicrobials may help.

Mild cases local treatment. Local treatment is also required for cases where the interdigital skin has sloughed. The local treatment consists of (cleaning, debridement of necrotic tissue and application of local products).

Control
Prevention of mechanical damage to the foot caused by frozen or dried mud, stones, brush and stubble and by minimising time that cattle spend standing in wet areas. Vaccine is available.

Inherited congenital porphyria

Disease Profile
Rare. More common in female cattle. The high tissue levels of porphyrin make the skin sensitive to light (photosensitive dermatitis).

Aetiology
Porphyrins are natural pigments that are present in higher than normal concentrations in affected cattle. Congenital. Recorded in Shorthorn, Holstein, Ayrshire, Danish Black and White and Jamaica Red and Black breed.

Clinical findings
Amber to port wine colour of the urine, pink to brown discolouration of the teeth and photosensitivity in cattle with retarded growth. On examination the visible mucosae are pale. Urine sample kept on light darkens.

Post-mortem findings
Brown to reddish purple discolouration of teeth and bones that fluoresce under illumination with ultraviolet light.

Diagnosis
Signs.

Principal differential diagnosis
Other causes of photosensitivity.

Treatment
No specific treatment available. Keep away from sunlight. Affected cattle should be culled.

Interdigital dermatitis

Common synonyms
Stable foot rot, Slurry heel

Disease Profile
Interdigital dermatitis is an acute or chronic inflammation of the epidermis of the interdigital skin extending commonly to the dermis. The morbidity can be high.

Aetiology
Dichelobacter nodosus.

Clinical findings
Thickening of the interdigital skin usually seen in the dorsal interdigital cleft. A pungent odour, pain to the touch and the concurrent presence of heel erosion. Often there is no lameness, except in advanced stages. The lesion is often painful to the touch. Affected cows show discomfort demonstrated as constant re-distribution of the weight from one foot to the other.

Diagnosis
Clinical signs.

Principal differential diagnosis
Interdigital necrobacillosis, heel erosion, digital dermatitis, some systemic viral diseases (FMD, BVD, MCF).

Treatment
Corrective trimming. Interdigital dermatitis should be treated topically (antimicrobial or copper sulphate).

Control
Proper management of manure and slurry removal.

Interdigital hyperplasia

Disease Profile
Proliferative reaction of the interdigital skin. Can be inherited or a result of chronic irritation/dermatitis. Common disorder in Holstein-Friesian and Hereford breed. Often hind feet.

Widespread claws at risk due to skin stretching. Bulls frequently affected.

Clinical findings
Lameness may be present, but not always.

The mass forming in the interdigital area is detected. Skin may be ulcerated and sometimes it oozes a purulent discharge. Secondary infection common in ulcerated lesions

Diagnosis
Signs.

Principal differential diagnosis
Interdigital foreign body, interdigital necrobacillosis, digital dermatitis.

Treatment
None in asymptomatic cases. Surgical removal of the mass indicated in severe cases. May recur

Ionophores toxicity

Disease Profile
Overdosing (miscalculation of the dose, mixing errors and rupture of an intraruminal capsule) with ionophores (used as bloat-, lameness- and acidosis-prevention, and for improved feed efficiency) may result in disorders of the cardio-vascular, musculo-skeletal, nervous, biliary and urinary systems. Respiratory system may also be affected. Poisoning can be acute or chronic. Deficiency of vitamin E and/or selenium result in aggravation of the inophores toxicity.

Aetiology
Ingestion of high doses of monensin, lasalosid, salinomycin and narasin. Concurrent treatment with sulphonamides, macrolides.

Clinical findings
Acute form: death, weakness, recumbency, tremors, ataxia, stiffness, tachycardia, arrhythmias, ruminal atomy. Often diarrhoea, myoglobinuria, dyspnoea, oedema of abdomen, legs and sometimes brisket. Death within 24–36 hours from ingestion.

Chronic form: arrhythmias, un-thriftness, poor exercise tolerance, dyspnoea, in-appetence, diarrhoea, ventral oedema, signs of congestive heart failure, death.

Post-mortem findings
Focal or extensive cardiac muscle pallor, epicardial and endocaridial haemorrhages, pulmonary congestion and oedema, yellow-to-grey streaks in skeletal muscles.

Diagnosis
History, clinical signs, increased CPK, AST, hypokalaemia, myoglobinuria, feedstuffs analysis, echocardiography of chronic cases.

Principal differential diagnosis
Vitamin E or selenium deficiency, poisoning by cardiotoxic plants (oleander, milkweed, digitalis, yews, rhododendron, death camas, avocado).

Treatment
No specific treatment. Evacuation of rumen content, activated charcoal or mineral oils and supportive care (oral electrolytes, prolonged stall rest, diuretics). Vitamin E and selenium.

Control
Prevention of ingestion of excessive doses. Cattle that survive acute toxicity are best culled due to myocardial damage.

Johne's disease

Common synonyms
Paratuberculosis.

Disease Profile
A chronic progressive disorder of cattle older than 2 years. More common in Chanel Island breeds. Most infections occur in calves less than a month old. Cattle start shedding 1–1.5 years before clinical signs.

Aetiology
Mycobacterium avium paratuberculosis.(MAP)

Clinical findings
Insidious onset. Cardinal signs are normal. Appetite maintained. Gradual weight loss progressing to emaciation, decrease in milk yield. Diarrhoea that develops gradually to watery, pipe-steam, without blood or mucin. Dependant oedema due to hypoproteinaemia.

Post-mortem findings
Thickened small intestine. Histopathology: MZN stained gut sections and intestinal lymph nodes.

Diagnosis
Suspicion on clinical signs. Detection of pathogen. Serology. Faecal culture. Faecal PCR.

Principal differential diagnosis
Parasitism, copper deficiency, bovine leucosis, salmonellosis, traumatic reticulo-peritonitis, amyloidosis.

Treatment
Unrewarding, as remission is common soon after treatment stopped.

Control
Culling of positive reactors. Remove calves from dams before suckling. Vaccination on some farms. Biosecurity to prevent introduction. Purchase from accredited herds (low risk)

Ketosis

Common synonyms
Acetonaemia

Disease Profile
Common, particularly early post calving (majority between 4 and 6 weeks, but can occur much earlier). Metabolic disorder, primarily of lactating dairy cows. Can be **primary** (underfeeding), **secondary** (decreased appetite due to a primary disorder) or **tertiary** (heavy consumption of ketogenic feedstuffs). **Pregnancy toxaemia** in beef and dairy cows carrying twins in the last 6 weeks of pregnancy also results in ketosis.

Aetiology
Negative energy balance associated with hypoglycaemia and β-oxidation of fats resulting in ketones in blood, milk, saliva and urine

Clinical findings
Wasting form – Commonest. Gradual reduction in milk yield and appetite, often acetone smell on breath, selective appetite (eats roughage but not concentrates), depressed rumen motility, firm faeces covered with mucus. Cardinal signs rarely altered. Loss of body condition.

Nervous form – Sudden onset, high excitability, muscle tremors, pica, apparent blindness, circling, aimless walking, sometimes incoordination and head pressing.

Post-mortem findings
Fatty infiltration of the liver.

Diagnosis
Signs, hypoglycaemia, acetonaemia, ketonuria,

Principal differential diagnosis
Traumatic reticulo-peritonitis, displaced abomasums, vagal indigestion, listeriosis, lead poisoning, hypomagnesaemia.

Treatment
Short term solution – IV glucose. Orally glucose precursors (e.g. propylene glycol, sodium propionate). Hormonal treatment – glucocorticoids, insulin, glucagon. Diet changes – increase in energy, energy substrates (e.g. molasses), balanced diet.

Control
Optimal body condition score at calving, proper transitional cow management and nutrition, balanced diet post calving, gradual changes in the diet. Some glucose precursors can be given preventatively. Prevent occurrence of primary disorders resulting in depressed appetite.

Early identification of at risk cows carrying twins.

Laminitis

Disease Profile
Acute form is uncommon but chronic form is very common. Often herd problem. Usually associated with feeding of high energy rations. Variable anoxia of hoof laminae with poor hoof formation.

Aetiology
Endotoxin released from rumen following adverse low pH from high energy feeds causing vascular anoxia in corium is postulated; occasionally an inherited trait.

Clinical findings
Acute – Pain in all four feet or just front feet.

Chronic – May follow the acute form. Poor quality horn produced by the corium. May produce sole ulceration, white line abscessation, horn separation, false sole and foot overgrowth. Ridges occur in hoof wall.

Diagnosis
Diet, signs. Eosinophilia may occur. Blood histamine levels may be raised.

Principal differential diagnosis
Foul of the foot, sole ulceration, white line abscessation.

Treatment
Remove cause or precipitating factor. Pare feet.

Hot water bathing to try to improve circulation.

NSAIDs, Nutritional supplements (Zn, biotin, methionine) – Supply methionine – 10g daily for one week (helps in normal hoof formation).

Control
Avoid rapid changes in feed from four weeks before to four weeks after calving. Include 1% sodium bicarbonate in the diet. Provide iodised ration. Down-calving heifers should enter concrete yards several weeks before calving. Give plenty of exercise in pre-partum month and after calving. Keep yards clean. Avoid large cattle groups. Provide adequate facilities for regular foot examination. Extra salt rations induce more salivation which contributes to buffering.

Lead poisoning

Disease Profile
More common in young cattle. Two forms, acute and subacute that are dose dependant. Acute form is characterised by encephalopathy. Subacute form is characterised by encephalopathy and gastrointestinal disorder. Common sources of lead include old batteries, motor oil, lead-bearing paints, machinery grease, pasture around lead factories, solder or leaded windows, and some defoliants.

Aetiology
Ingestion of lead.

Clinical findings
Acute form – Sudden onset and short duration. Death usually within 24 hours. Separation from the rest of the herd, depression, staggering, muscle tremors, clamping of jaws, snapping eyelids, hyperaesthesia, frothing at the mouth. Signs progress to ataxia, rolling eyes, cortical blindness, proprioceptive defects, head pressing, aggressiveness, bruxism, coma and convulsions. Sometimes aimless walking, running and bellowing.

Subacute form – dullness, anorexia, blindness, aimless walking and/or circling, muscle tremors, abdominal pain and gastrointestinal involvement (constipation, followed by foetid (very dark) diarrhoea, rumen atony).

Post-mortem findings
Acute form – no specific findings.

Subacute form – abomasitis, enteritis, degeneration of parenchymatous organs, evidence of ingested lead in the rumen content. Elevated concentration of lead in kidney, liver.

Diagnosis
Signs, history, increased concentrations in blood, milk, nucleated erythrocytes, response to treatment. Elevated tissue concentrations (kidney, liver)

Principal differential diagnosis
Hypomagnesaemia, hypovitaminosis A, brain abscess, listeriosis, polioencephalomalacia, thromboembolic meningoencephalitis, other poisoning (e.g. ergotism, mercury, arsenic).

Treatment
Removal from access to lead and from the gastrointestinal tract (rumenotomy and Epsom salt po), chelation therapy (iv calcium EDTA), thiamine, supportive care (nursing, fluid and nutritional support, anticonvulsants).

Control
Avoid sources. Cattle affected by lead poisoning should be withheld from slaughter for minimum 6 months. Monitoring of milk levels in dairy herd.

Leptospirosis

Common synonyms
Red water.

Disease Profile
Worldwide distribution. Important zoonosis. Infection through intact, moist or abraded skin and mucosa. Septicaemia (acute form) rarely important. Persistent (chronic) infections (agalactia, hepatitis, nephritis and abortion) more important. Leptospirae are fragile in dry environment.

Aetiology
Leptospirae of the serovars. Hardjo, Pomona. Less commonly Icterohaemorrhagiae, Canicola, Bratislava and Grippotyphosa.

Clinical findings
Acute form – short lasting septicaemia (4–7 days) followed by long-lasting hepatitis, nephritis, agalactiae, mastitis, blood-tinged milk and leptospiriuria. Abortion storms. Usually caused by non-host-specific serovars.

In calves – high fever, depression, haemolytic anaemia, petechial haemorrhages, haemoglobinuria, jaundice, dyspnoea. Sometimes meningitis and death.

Chronic form – usually due to the host-specific serovar (Hardjo). Abortion, stillbirths, infertility.

Post-mortem findings
Anaemia, icterus, haemoglubinuria, petechial haemorrhages, diffuse interstitial nephritis.

Diagnosis
Signs, detection of pathogen, serology.

Principal differential diagnosis
Other disorders characterised by intravascular haemolysis, abortions and infertility.

Treatment
Antimicrobials. Supportive care.

Control
Biosecurity, vaccination, minimise access to wildlife, rodents and contaminated water sources and pasture (do not graze for 2 months).

Lice

Common synonyms
Lice (infestation)

Disease Profile
Common. More common in winter in housed cattle.

Aetiology
Biting lice (*Damalinia bovis*) and sucking lice (*Haematopinus eurysternus, H. quadripertusus, Linognathus vituli, Solenopotes capillatus*).

Clinical findings
Pruritus, hair loss, roughened coat, anaemia, disrupted feeding patterns.

Diagnosis
Detection of adult lice or eggs on hairs (nits).

Principal differential diagnosis
Mange, pseudorabies.

Treatment
Ectoparasiticides. Particularly at housing or yarding (animals kept in close contact)

Control
Improved hygiene and nutrition, ectoparasiticides.

Listeriosis

Common synonyms
Circling disease.

Disease Profile
Relatively common. Mostly sporadic but it may occur in form of an outbreak. Common risk factor is feeding low quality silage and/or haylage. Most common neurological form. Other forms bovine iritis (see appropriate heading), septicaemia, abortion, mastitis. Neurological form due to formation of micro abscesses within the brain stem (multifocal cortical and cranial nerve deficits). Zoonotic risk from milk.

Aetiology
Listeria monocytogenes. Rarely *L. ivanovii.*

Clinical findings
Signs of cranial (facial) nerve deficits (e.g. drooped ear, eyelid, inability to close eyelids, strabismus, nystagmus, loss of facial sensation, inability to swallow, asymmetrical jaw), diminished arousal, circling, head tilt, loss of saliva, dehydration.

Pregnant cattle may abort (usually during late gestation).

Post-mortem findings
Micro abscesses in pons and medulla. Aborted foetuses usually autolysed.

Diagnosis
Signs, CSF analysis, post-mortem, detection of pathogen.

Principal differential diagnosis
Vestibular disease, bovine spongiform encephalopathy, brain abscess, polioencephalomalacia, nervous ketosis, lead poisoning.

Treatment
High doses of antimicrobials. Supportive treatment (correct dehydration, rumenotorics, transfaunation).

Control
Proper ensiling and storing of silage, avoid soil contamination.

Liver fluke

Common synonyms
Fasciolosis

Disease Profile
Common in geographical regions where the snails as intermediate host are distributed. Subclinical disorder is common. Clinical disorder is rare. Young cattle are more susceptible. Liver fluke is incriminated in facilitating salmonellosis (Dublin) and black disease.

Aetiology
Fasciola hepatica. Rarely *Dicrocoelium dendriticum, D. lanceolatum, F. gigantica,* and *Fascioloides magna*.

Clinical findings
Chronic form – Usually no signs. Decreased productivity and growth rates. Loss of condition, anaemia, sometimes diarrhoea, submandibular swelling.

Acute form – anaemia, abdominal pain recumbency.

Post-mortem findings
Chronic – hyperplastic cholangitis, adult flukes present in the bile ducts.

Acute – enlarged liver, haemorrhagic tracts, serosanguineous fluid in abdominal cavity.

Diagnosis
Signs, history, geographical location, raised liver enzymes (GGT and/or GLDH), demonstration of eggs in faeces (mature adult fluke present), ultrasonography, serology (ELISA).

Principal differential diagnosis
Gastro-intestinal parasitism, copper deficiency, Johne's disease.

Treatment
Flukicides.

Control
Avoid grazing of marshy areas, fencing off pastures with high potential to have intermediate hosts, improve pasture drainage, strategic deworming, regular faecal egg examination.

Lumpy skin disease

Disease Profile
Endemic in Africa. Occasional incursions in the Middle East. Morbidity higher in naïve populations and Channel Island breeds (up to 80%). Mortality low (usually less than 3%). Risk higher in young cattle. Transmitted by biting flies and mosquitoes. Outbreaks common during rainy season.

Notifiable disease.

Aetiology
Pox virus.

Clinical findings
Incubation 7–21 days.

Long-lasting fever. Development of skin nodules (1–5cm) that enlarge and affect surrounding tissue, tender, spread elsewhere (oral mucosa, generalised lymphadenitis). Nodules eventually necrotise centrally and often become complicated by bacterial secondary infection.

Lesions may persist up to 6 months. Loss of milk production, depressed growth, abortions and male sterility. Secondary infections of skin of skin around udder, joints, penis may cause serious complications.

Diagnosis
Signs, detection of pathogen, serology, histopathology.

Principal differential diagnosis
Insect bites, urticarial, hypodermosis, other skin infections.

Treatment
Antimicrobials of secondary bacterial infections.

Control
Vaccination, insect control.

Lungworm pneumonia

Common synonyms
Parasitic bronchitis, Parasitic bronchopneumonia, Verminous bronchitis, Verminous pneumonia, Verminous bronchopneumonia, Husk, Hoose, Dictiocauliasis, Parasitic pneumonia.

Disease Profile
Common in cattle on pasture. Most commonly in calves younger than 1 year. May also affect mature cattle with no previous exposure or after recent move to heavily contaminated pasture. Acute and subacute form. Acute form is common in calves been on the offending pasture 1–2 weeks.

Aetiology
Ingestion of infective larvae of *Dictyocaulus viviparus*. Prepatent period is around 7–25 days. Rarely aberrant infection with *Ascaris sum* larvae.

Clinical findings
Acute form: Rapid shallow respiration, fever, deep cough. On auscultation increased lung sounds and crackles. Excitement and exercise precipitate coughing and death. Sometimes subcutaneous emphysema from ruptured bullae of the lungs. Fever.

Subacute form: increased respiratory rate, paroxysmal cough, often diarrhoea. On auscultation increased lung sounds, crackles and areas of dullness (lung consolidation), rapid weight loss.

Mature cattle: sudden drop in milk production, frequent cough (particularly after exercise), harsh respiratory sounds.

Post-mortem findings
Adult worms in bronchi, signs of bronchopneumonia, interstitial emphysema.

Diagnosis
History, clinical findings, post-mortem findings, faecal sedimentation test for larvae (after approximately 4 weeks from infection), eosinophilia, tracheal aspirate for larvae.

Principal differential diagnosis
Fog fever, bovine respiratory disease complex.

Treatment
Anthelmintics. Remove cattle from offending pasture. Symptomatic treatment (antibiotics, NSAIDs, restricted exercise).

Control
Pasture management, parasiticides, vaccination (before exposure).

Lupine-associated poisoning

Disease Profile
Ingestion of lupines (*Lupinus* spp) may result in lupinosis, neurologic or teratogenic form of lupine poisoning. Lupine poisoning may occur after feeding lupines in increased amounts or at specific periods of the gestation.

Aetiology
Lupinosis – mycotic disorder caused usually by hepatotoxic phomopsin A (produced by fungus *Phomopsis leptostromiformis*). Lupine poisoning – alkaloids (piperidine and quinolizidine). Alkaloids are most concentrated in the seeds. Teratogenic effect is usually seen when feeding lupines day 40–100 of gestation.

Clinical findings
Lupinosis – anorexia, icterus, ketosis, epiphora, hypersalivation, sometimes photosensitisation (rare in cattle). Death in 2 days to 2 weeks.

Lupine poisoning neurologic form – anorexia, dyspnoea, violent neurologic signs, including great effort in movement, resisting to commands, convulsions, hyperexcitability, paralysis of different groups of muscles. Death due to paralysis of respiratory muscles.

Lupine poisoning teratogenic form – cleft palate, arthrogryposis, scoliosis, kyphosis, other contractures of muscles.

Post-mortem findings
Lupinosis – icterus, enlarge liver with orange-yellow discolouration and fatty infiltration. In chronic cases fibrosed liver with bronze- to tan-coloured. Often signs of ascites.

Lupine poisoning – no specific findings.

Diagnosis
History, signs, necropsy findings (lupinosis).

Principal differential diagnosis
Other mycotoxicoses, photosensitisation, other teratogenic disorders

Treatment
Stop feeding lupines. For lupinosis oral zinc administration may help the recovery.

Control
Controlled grazing (short periods). Check lupines for signs of fungal infestation. Avoid feeding lupines during teratogenic periods.

Malignant catarrhal fever

Common synonyms
Bovine malignant catarrh.

Disease Profile
Highly fatal viral disease with a low morbidity. Usually in cattle over a year old, individual animal, but herd outbreaks may occur. History invariably includes contact with sheep, goat or wildebeest. The disorder is characterised by widespread vasculitis, polyclonal T-lymphocytes hyperplasia and autoimmune phenomenon. The course of the disorder is 3 to 7 days, but peracute cases may occur.

Aetiology
At least two viruses, ovine herpes virus-2 (OHV-2) and alcelaphine herpes virus-1 (AHV-1).

Clinical findings
Incubation period is 3–10 weeks, sometimes longer (up to 6 months). Oral erosions, diarrhoea to dysentery, hypersalivation (ropy saliva), erosions and scabs on muzzle copious muco-purulent nasal discharge, severe kerato-conjunctivitis that spreads centripetally, hypopyon, epithelial, epiphora, dyspnoea, anorexia, high fever, marked lymphadenopathy, pronounced lameness, sloughing of the hooves and/or horns, ulcerations of the coronet, teat, vulva and perineum and haematuria. Nystagmus, weakness, tremors, paralysis and head pressing. A mild, chronic form may also occur. The affected animal remains chronically debilitated and does not thrive. Often misdiagnosed as persistently infected by bovine virus diarrhoea virus.

Post-mortem findings
Histology-disseminated vasculitis, degenerative epithelial lesions and infiltration with lymphoid in the tissues. Hyperaemia, haemorrhages, erosions in mouth, muzzle, upper respiratory tract and rumen to intestines, kidney often whitish raised foci in the capsule.

Diagnosis
History, serology, detection of pathogen, sporadic occurrence, clinical signs.

Principal differential diagnosis
Foot-and-mouth, rinderpest, vesicular stomatitis, mucosal disease, rabies, oral necrobacillosis, bluetongue, bovine iritis, severe infectious rhino-tracheitis.

Treatment
Therapy is unrewarding. A good response to antimicrobial therapy is indicative of misdiagnosis. Recovered animals become persistent carriers. Affected cattle should be euthanized.

Control
Separate cattle from sheep, particularly at lambing time.

Mange

Disease Profile
Common. Worldwide. Some forms of mange (e.g. sarcoptic) are zoonotic. More common in winter months in housed cattle.

Aetiology
Chorioptes bovis, Psoroptes ovis, P. communis, Sarcoptes scabiei var bovis, Psorergates bos, Demodex bovis.

Clinical findings
General – pruritus (except with Demodicosis), formation of crusts, scabs, papules, weight loss.

Chorioptic mange – usually base of tail; udder, thigh, perineum, scrotum, legs. Less pruritic.

Psoroptic mange – withers, neck, tail-head, backline. Papules, thickening of the skin. Very pruritic.

Sarcoptic mange – head, neck, shoulders, thighs. Papules, crusts, excoriation, broken hairs. Very pruritic.

Psorergatic mange – thorax, flanks, thighs. Patchy alopecia. Mildly pruritic.

Demodectic mange – face, neck, shoulder, sides, nodules, papules. Non pruritic.

Diagnosis
Skin scrapings, skin biopsy.

Principal differential diagnosis
Pediculosis, dermatophilosis, fly bite dermatitis, photosensitisation, pseudorabies, other causes of dermatitis, tuberculosis, ringworm.

Treatment
Ectoparasiticides. Steroids are contraindicated.

Control
Biosecurity, improve management, strategic use of ectoparasiticides.

Mastitis: coliform

Disease Profile
Environmental mastitis associated with faecal contamination directly or via bedding (sawdust, straw, other organic bedding) and contaminated water. More common in intensive dairying and during housing. Other important epidemiologic factors: high producers, around calving, most commonly in cows with slow mobilisation of somatic cells.

Peracute, acute and chronic.

Aetiology
Enterotoxins from many coliform bacteria (*Escherichia coli, Enterobacter* spp, *Klebsiella* spp, *Serratia* spp, *Citrobacter* spp) and *Pseudomonas* spp.

Clinical findings
Peracute – sudden onset of endotoxaemia, hypovolaemia, dehydration, depression, anorexia, fever, later hypothermia, recumbency, coma and death. Serous to sero-sanguineous secretion from the affected quarter.

Acute – slower progression, less severe. Additional signs – elevated pulse and respiratory rate, onset of diarrhoea, dehydration, affected quarter swollen and tender. Many have slight bluish discolouration.

Chronic – intermittent mastitis. Systemic effects mild or absent.

Post-mortem findings
Swollen, hyperaemic and cyanotic quarter. Dehydration.

Diagnosis
Signs, history, detection of pathogen.

Principal differential diagnosis
Metritis, hypocalcaemia, poisons.

Treatment
Per-acute/acute: Aims Treatment of endotoxaemia: correct dehydration and hypovolaemia (hypertonic saline commonly used), non-steroidal anti-inflammatories, fluids, systemic antimicrobials (bacteraemias due to endotoxaemia common) (+/– intra-mammary antimicrobial).

Frequent stripping out of udder (oxytocin facilitates). Pathogen in the gland often self-limiting once clinical signs present.

Control
Improve hygiene, good transitional cow management, use of internal teat sealants, vaccines.

Mastitis: gangrenous

Disease Profile
Least common. Severe form of mastitis caused by *Staphylococcus aureus*. Most commonly in freshly-calved cows.

Aetiology
Toxin producing Staphylococcus aureus (exotoxin).

Clinical findings
Secretion – usually difficult to strip. Blood-stained watery exudate, sometimes with gas.

Udder – initially swollen, hot, red and tender quarter. Later swollen, cold, cyanotic and non- sensitive quarter/s. Clearly demarcated blue-black (distally) to 'normal' udder colour (dorsally). In cows that recover sloughing of the affected quarter.

Cow – severe fever, depression, anorexia, no rumen activity followed by toxaemia and death.

Post-mortem findings
Udder changes relatively specific (necrotising distal portion of affected quarter).

Diagnosis
Signs. Detection of pathogen.

Principal differential diagnosis
Metritis, hypocalcaemia, toxic (coliform) mastitis.

Treatment
Early and aggressive. Systemic and local antimicrobials, non-steroidal anti-inflammatories, fluids. Supportive care. Incision of teat (allows toxin to be eliminated from affected quarter). Euthanasia may be the best option. Surgical debridement of affected quarter(s)

Mastitis

Disease Profile
Very common, particularly in dairy cattle. Clinical and subclinical. Underdiagnosed in beef underdiagnosed. Direct losses (treatment, discarded milk, labour). The highest loss is indirect (decreased milk quality and quantity, increased culling and associated health problems), often unrealised by farmer. Management plays significant role in the prevalence on a farm.

Aetiology
Most commonly bacteria (*Streptococcus* (*agalactiae, dysgalactiae* and *uberis*), *Staphylococcus aureus*, coagulase negative staphylococci, coliforms (*Escherichia coli, Klebsiella* spp), *Trueperella pathogens* and many others. Rarely other pathogens (viruses, algae, fungi) and trauma (mechanical, thermal, chemical). Environmental (environment reservoir of infection), Contagious (udder reservoir of infection)

Clinical findings
Peracute/acute – see Gangrenous and coliform-endotoxemic mastitis

Milk – change in colour, consistency, smell. Usually becomes clotted.

Udder – swollen, hot, reddened, tender. May become cyanotic and cold.

Cow – Systemic signs. Drop in milk production to agalactia.

Subclinical mastitis – no clinical signs or milk gross abnormalities but elevated SCC

Diagnosis
Signs, Swollen painful udder, Milk clots (in-line filters), increased SCC (cow-side tests (CMT), and detection of pathogen. Subclinical-somatic cell count.

Principal differential diagnosis

Treatment
Peracute/acute – see Gangrenous and coliform-endotoxemic mastitis

Depends on aetiology. Intra-mammary antimicrobials, NSAIDs. If systemic signs non-steroidal anti-i systemic antibiotics. Cull chronically infected older cows.

Control
Dry cow management important. Goals: prevent new infectious and eliminate existing infections.

Use of long acting antimicrobials (pathogen profile and sensitivity useful to inform selection) in infected cows. Combination of long acting antimicrobial and teat sealant reduced new infection rate. Uninfected cows defined on SCC treated with teat sealant only in some herds to prevent new intra-mammary infections.

Classification and identification of pathogens into environmental and contagious enables risk factors to be addressed in lactating herd. Environmental hygiene and teat cleaning important for environmental control, in parlour hygiene and post-milk teat dipping important for contagious.

Regular milk machine maintenance important.

Milk recording data invaluable in identifying high SCC (infected) cows.

Monitor +/– treat incoming cows for mastitis pathogens.

Megaoesophagus

Common synonyms
Megaoesophagus. Oesophageal dilation.

Disease Profile
Rare. Congenital or acquired. Acquired sequel to oesophageal stricture or blockage to external pressure (e.g. mediastinal mass, diaphragmatic hernia, pharyngeal trauma).

Clinical findings
Inappetence, dysphagia, regurgitation, mild bloat.

Diagnosis
Signs, passing a stomach tube, endoscopy, radiography.

Principal differential diagnosis
Oesophagitis, vagus indigestion.

Treatment
No treatment.

Meningitis (Bacterial)

Disease Profile
Most commonly seen in neonatal calves associated with septicaemia resulting from failure of passive transfer of maternal antibodies. In mature cattle associated with unskilful dehorning or docking and bacterial endocarditis.

Aetiology
Calves: Most frequently *Escherichia coli*. Less common *Klebsiella, Salmonella, Staphylococcus, Streptococcus*. Mature cattle *Trueperella pyogenes* and streptococci most common.

Clinical findings
Lethargy to depression, anorexia, loss of suckle reflex, ataxia, sometimes hyperesthesia, compulsive walking abnormal vocalisation, tremors, convulsions, opisthotonus, recumbency, coma and death.

Hypopyon in anterior chambers of eye is supportive sign. Fever may or may not be present.

Treatment
In cases of advanced neurologic signs treatment often unrewarding. Aggressive and long-term antimicrobial and supportive treatment. Anticonvulsants, sedatives (not acepromazine as it lowers the threshold for seizures). Nursing care.

Control
Ensure passive transfer. Proper dehorning and docking.

Metabolic acidosis – neonatal calves

Disease Profile
Common disorder of neonatal calves. In diarrhoea can occur independently of dehydration. Life threatening. Cause of death in diarrhoeic calves

Aetiology
Prolonged calving, dystocia, diarrhoea.

Clinical findings
Depressed, sternal to lateral recumbency, loss of suckling reflex.

Diagnosis
History, signs, blood pH of less than 7.38 and bicarbonate deficit of 8% or more.

Principal differential diagnosis
In utero infections, congenital abnormalities.

Treatment
Mild: oral electrolyte/Bicarbonate(or precursors)

Moderately to severe: treat intravenously. The best results achieved with i/v bicarbonate 200–400 mmol/calf. Correct dehydration.

Metritis

Disease Profile
Metritis is most common in peri-parturient period. It is an inflammation of all layers of the uterus (endometrium, myometrium, perimetrium). More common in dairy cows. Affected cows can become endotoxaemic. Metritis is associated with increased risk of endometritis, pyometra, ketosis, displaced abomasum, mastitis, decreased production and reduced fertility. Metritis is more common in cows with assisted calving, twinning dystocia, retained foetal membranes, abortion and delivery of a dead calf and hypocalcaemia. Somewhat higher incidence in primiparous heifers and over conditioned cattle.

Aetiology
Mixed bacterial population. Most common gram-positive bacteria *Trueperella pyogenes, Staphylococcus aureus, Clostridium* spp. Most common Gram-negative bacteria *Escherichia coli, Fusobacterium necrophorum, Bacteroides melaninogenicus, Pseudomonas* spp.

Clinical findings
Fever, depression, inappetence to anorexia, decreased milk yield. Vaginal discharge, serosanguineaus to sero-sanguineous and purulent (red-brown) with foetid odour. Signs of toxaemia. Sometimes recumbency. Secondary ketosis. Sometimes tenesmus and signs of abdominal pain (bruxism, rumen and intestinal stasis, gaunt). Congested mucous membranes. Uterine wall thickened, often tender on palpation and ultrasonography.

Post-mortem findings
Peritonitis, enlarged friable and gangrenous uterus. Signs of toxaemia.

Diagnosis
History clinical signs, vaginal examination.

Principal differential diagnosis
Normal locia, endometritis, ruptured uterus, reasons for downer cow.

Treatment
Antimicrobials (systemic and intrauterine). Little support for intrauterine antimicrobials. Supportive treatment (correction of electrolytes, ketosis, non-steroidal anti-inflammatory drugs). Monitor for development of ketosis, mastitis and displaced abomasum. Attempts to remove retained foetal membranes are contraindicated. Evacuation of uterine fluid by gentle uterine manipulation per rectum is frequently performed. The use of uterine flushing with sterile saline and evacuation is also performed but this may result in ascending/peritoneal contamination.

Control
Improved hygiene for assisted calvings. Proper management of transition period.

Milking machine-induced teat lesions

Disease Profile
Relatively common. Can be important contributing factor to high incidence of mastitis.

Forms: teat haemorrhage, teat-end oedema, hyperkeratosis and black spot (see appropriate heading), ringing at the teat base and other teat-end damage.

Most occur as herd outbreaks. More than 20% of examined teats affected.

Aetiology
Associated with improperly working milking machine (e.g. high vacuum, faulty pulsation, overstretched liners) or milking management (e.g. excessive over milking, mismatch between teat and teat-cup liner).

Clinical findings
Usually detected immediately after removal of the milking unit.

General – cows unwilling to enter milking shed, stepping, kicking, increase rate of clinical mastitis.

Teat haemorrhage – petechial or more extensive haemorrhage, particularly at teat end and teat base.

Teat-end oedema – oedema of teat end and sometimes whole teat barrel. Usually associated with bluish discolouration.

Teat-end hyperkeratosis – roughness, cornification and callosity of the teat end. Eversion, small; protruding filaments of keratin.

Ringing at teat base – oedema of teat base. Usually associated with bluish discolouration of teat.

Diagnosis
Signs.

Principal differential diagnosis
Infectious and environment-induced teat lesions.

Treatment
Correct milking machine faults or milking management. Emollients.

Mycotoxicosis

Disease Profile
Mycotoxins are secondary fungal metabolites produced by various moulds. Some moulds produce more than one mycotoxin and some mycotoxins are produced by many types of moulds. Mycotoxins of economic and clinical significance include aflatoxins, ochratoxins, trichothecens, fumonisins, zearalenone, tremorgenic toxins, and ergot alkaloids. Except fumonisins, mycotoxins are lipophilic and concentrate in lipid fraction of animals and plants. Mycotoxins in milk are of human health concern.

Aetiology
Ingestion of feedstuffs contaminated by mycotoxins.

Clinical findings
Aflatoxins: immunosuppression, reduced rumen motility, reduced appetite, reduced milk yield and milk quality. Liver damage with reduced blood clotting factors. Haemorrhages. Death.

Ochratoxins: probably not toxic to cattle.

Trichothecens: immunosuppression, late abortion, infertility, haemorrhagic syndrome, abomasal ulcers and in calves, sloughing of rumen papillae.

Zearalenone: infertility and decreased milk production, chronic hyperoestrogenisms.

Tremorgenic toxins: grass lend staggers (e.g. ryegrass, paspalum, phalaris)

Ergotism: ataxia, convulsions, abortion, decreased milk yield, lowered appetite and dry gangrene to extremities.

Diagnosis
Testing of feedstuffs.

Treatment
No specific treatment. Stop feeding offending feedstuffs or pasture and provide alternative. Some mycotoxins binders are available. Dilute affected feed with non-affected feedstuffs. Supportive treatment (e.g. treatment of liver failure, broad-spectrum antimicrobials).

Control
Avoid contaminated feedstuffs in the diet. Correct (dry) storage

Nasal granuloma

Common synonyms
Atopic rhinitis, Enzootic nasal granuloma.

Disease Profile
Allergic rhinitis common in Channel Island breeds between 6 months and 2 years at the first occurrence.

Aetiology
Various allergens (e.g. pollen, moulds). Some familial predisposition.

Clinical findings
Intense sneezing, pruritus (intense nose licking, rubbing the nose of the ground, using sticks to rub the nose), lodgement of foreign bodies in the nasal cavity, stertorious inspiration, dyspnoea, copious mucoid yellow to orange discharge (usually bilateral). The discharge may become purulent after lodgement of foreign body in the nasal cavity. Sometimes ocular signs of allergic reaction may also be present (swelling of the eyelids, excessive lacrimation, blepharospasm).

On examination multiple firm whitish nodules 1–2 mm scattered through the nasal cavity. Often foreign bodies (e.g. sticks).

Principal differential diagnosis
Other causes of rhinitis, neoplasia, foreign bodies.

Treatment
Removal of the affected cattle from the offending pasture, antihistamins, steroids (in non-pregnant cows).

Necrotic vaginitis, vestibulitis and vulvitis

Disease Profile
Sporadic. Individual female post-partum. Precipitated by hypoxia of the calving canal during dystocia. Most commonly seen in heifers. Common sequelae include permanent stricture and/or adhesions of the vagina and vaginal/perirectal abscessation.

Clinical findings
Onset 1–4 days after calving. Elevated tail, straining, dysuria, inappetence to anorexia, swelling of the calving canal. Often foetid discharge. May last 1–2 weeks.

Diagnosis
Signs. Examination by speculum.

Principal differential diagnosis
Puerperal endometritis, metritis.

Treatment
Antimicrobials, non-steroidal anti-inflammatories. Prevent clostridial myositis.

Necrotising enteritis

Common synonyms
Necrotic enteritis. Neonatal haemorrhagic enterotoxaemia.

Disease Profile
Rare. Occurs only in Great Britain. Outbreaks. Primarily neonatal and young cattle. In beef 2–4 months old calves on pasture. Morbidity low (<10%). Mortality high (>80%).

Aetiology
Most likely *Clostridium perfringens* type C although unknown aetiology.

Clinical findings
Peracute – sudden death. Rare form.

Acute – depression, failure to suck, fever, dehydration. Yellowish or more commonly haemorrhagic diarrhoea. Tenesmus. Often kidney failure. Oral and nasal ulcerations. Death in 7–10 days.

Post-mortem findings
Necrosis of mucosa of small intestines (particularly) jejenum.

Diagnosis
Signs.

Principal differential diagnosis
Salmonellosis, coccidiosis, mucosal disease

Treatment
Often unrewarding. Aggressive antimicrobial treatment. Supportive treatment (fluids, non-steroidal anti-inflammatories) and nursing care.

Control
Vaccination of dams. Early clostridial vaccination of calves.

Neonatal septicaemia

Disease Profile
An important cause of morbidity and mortality in calves. Failure of passive transfer and unhygienic environment are important risk factors. Other risk factors are dystocia, overcrowding and poor ventilation. Multiple organs often affected.

Aetiology
Escherichia coli most important. Other common pathogens include *Pasteurella* spp, *Klebsiella* spp and *Salmonella* spp. Less common pathogens are *Listeria monocytogenes, Streptococcus* spp, *Staphylococcus aureus, Clostridium* spp. Mixed infections are frequent.

Clinical findings
Starts with vague signs of lethargy, poor suckle reflex, weakness, recumbency, tachycardia, tachypnoea, and dehydration. Capillary refill time is usually increased and mucus membranes toxic.

The signs of the infection of various organs are related to the system affected and include: diarrhoea, omphalitis, arthritis, meningitis, pneumonia, cardiac murmurs, uveitis and septic shock.

Rectal temperature may be increased, normal or subnormal.

Diagnosis
Signs, detection of pathogen, blood count and biochemistry (normal white blood count to leucopoenia, toxic changes to neutrophils, hypoglycaemia, acidosis, IgG levels).

Treatment
Antimicrobials, fluid therapy, non-steroidal anti-inflammatory drugs, supportive care.

Control
Ensure adequate colostrum intake. Improved environmental conditions. Vaccination of dams.

Neosporosis

Common synonyms
Neospora. *Neospora caninum* infection. Neosporal abortion.

Disease Profile
Variable incidence and prevalence. In naïve herds may cause 'storm abortions'. More common in dairy cattle. Vertical and probably horizontal transmission. Definitive host is dog.

Aetiology
Neospora caninum – protozoan.

Clinical findings
Abortion, stillbirths, deformed calves or more commonly calves with neurologic signs (ataxia, weakness, tetraparesis). Many infected calves are clinically normal. Early embryonic losses.

Reduced milk production.

Diagnosis
Signs are only indicative. Serology. Detection of pathogen. Histopathology.

Principal differential diagnosis
Other causes of abortion and weak neonatal calves.

Treatment
No effective treatment.

Control
Biosecurity. Avoid contamination of cattle feedstuffs with dog faeces.

Nervous coccidiosis

Disease Profile
Calves and young cattle. Most commonly winter. More common in feedlot systems.

Aetiology
Heat-labile neurotoxin presumed to be produced by coccidian in the intestines.

Clinical findings
Ataxia, muscle tremors, hyperexitability, blindness and intermittent to continuous seizures (lateral recumbency, opisthotonos, snapping of eyelids, medial strabismus and tonic-clonic movement).

Diagnosis
Exam of cerebro-spinal fluid, rule out.

Principal differential diagnosis
Polioencephalomalacia, lead poisoning, salt poisoning, water poisoning and thromboembolic meningo-enecephalitis.

Treatment
Treatment for coccidiosis, anticonvulsants and (or tranquilisers) and nursing care. Prognosis poor. May need to correct iron and copper levels.

Control
Not known as aetiology not confirmed.

Nitrate and nitrite poisoning

Disease Profile
Usually occurs at pasture. Primary due to ingestion of nitrate-accumulating plants (e.g. sorghum, lucerne, stressed lush pasture, some weeds). Secondary due to contaminated hay or total mixed ratio. Nitrate concentration in plants higher in stress situations (sudden weather change, winter).

Peracute to acute poisoning. Rapid development of methaemoglobinaemia and lack of oxygen. Usually herd problem.

Aetiology
Ingestion of nitrate in high concentration. Conversion of nitrate to more toxic nitrite by rumen microorganism, absorption with metheamglobin formation.

Clinical findings
Peracute onset. Dyspnoea, weakness, recumbency, hypersalivation, muscle tremors, cyanotic to muddy mucous membranes. Chocolate brown colour of the blood.

Sudden death. Surviving pregnant cattle may abort.

Post-mortem findings
Muddy mucous membranes, signs of hypooxigenation.

Diagnosis
Signs, nitrate concentrations in blood, urine, peritoneal, pericardial or ocular humoural fluid.

Principal differential diagnosis
Other reasons for sudden death.

Treatment
Gentle handling, intravenous methylene blue, vitamin C.

Control
Avoid grazing of dangerous pastures in stressed times.

Oak poisoning

Common synonyms
Acorn poisoning, Acorn toxicity

Disease Profile
Ingested tannin from oaks are hydrolysed in the rumen to pyrogallae, gallic acid and other phenolic metabolites that are toxic to gastrointestinal and urinary systems. The main lesions are in the kidneys. The exposure is usually 1–2 weeks before first clinical signs. Ingestion of large amounts of acorns in mid pregnancy usually results in deformed calves at calving.

Aetiology
Ingestion of oak buds, stems, leaves and/or acorns.

Clinical findings
Peracute: found death.

Acute: ruminal stasis followed by bloat, anorexia, depression and constipation followed by haemorrhagic diarrhoea, polyuria and haematuria.

Chronic: dehydration, hydrothorax, ascites, ventral oedema, recumbency, polyuria, haematuria. Common complications are oral and gastro-intestinal ulcerations, bronchopneumonia and abscessation.

Post-mortem findings
Pale and enlarged kidneys with tubular necrosis and perirenal oedema, hydrothorax, ascites, multiple erosions, ulcerations and abscessation of the digestive system, acorns in the rumen content.

Diagnosis
History, time of year, casts in urine. Renal failure.

Principal differential diagnosis
Other causes of renal failure, urolithiasis, leptospirosis, clostridial disorders, type 1 ostertagiosis.

Treatment
No specific antidote. Restore adequate renal perfusion and urine production. Intravenous electrolytes. Add calcium hydroxide to the diet. Broad-spectrum antimicrobials.

Control
Avoid areas with oaks, particularly in autumn after storm.

Obturator nerve paralysis

Disease Profile
Common after dystocia (particularly hip-lock of the calf or oversized calf). Occasionally may occur after pelvic fractures or caudo-ventral dislocation of the femoral head.

Clinical findings
Cow is bright and alert.

Unilateral: one leg abducted .A common complication is hip dysplasia.

Bilateral: both legs abducted. Recumbent in frog-like position.

Diagnosis
Signs

Principal differential diagnosis
Split pelvic symphysis, rupture of adductor muscles, dislocated hip, femoral fracture.

Treatment
Downer cow physiotherapy. Lift, turn odd number of times a day, access to food and water, fly strike precautions, remove faeces and clean urine away. NSAIDs, B-complex, general care, hobbling the legs together.

Control
Avoid calves becoming 'hip-locked'. Do not apply excessive traction during calf delivery.

Oesophageal obstruction (intra-luminal)

Disease Profile
Most common sites of oesophageal blockage are the proximal cervical oesophagus, at the thoracic inlet and inside the thorax just around the heart base. Incomplete or complete partial oesophageal obstruction may occur as result of any swelling in the surrounding tissues (lymph nodes, neoplasm, abscess), oesophageal lesions or underlying neurological dysfunction. A complete oesophageal obstruction may occur as a result of root crops, potatoes or other foreign objects. Complete oesophageal obstructions in cattle may be fatal as a consequence of free gas bloat.

Clinical findings
Acute onset, severe distress sometimes frenzied, with extended head and neck. Drooling of saliva, rapidly worsening bloat, frequent attempts of swallowing and coughing are consistent signs.

Diagnosis
Attempts to pass a stomach tube, palpation.

Principal differential diagnosis
Oesophageal diverticula or paralysis, megaoesophagus, pharyngeal trauma, vagal indigestion, bloat, tetanus, botulism and rabies.

Treatment
Removal of the obstruction by manual manipulation if possible. Buscopan may be helpful in causing oesophageal relaxation. A probang or stiff stomach tube can be used to dislodge and propel the FB into the rumen. If unresolved trocharise the rumen and leave the trochar in position. Organic matter obstruction will decay and usually progress to the rumen with a few days. Oesophagoatomy is last resort and post-operative stricture is common.

Ocular squamous cell carcinoma

Common synonyms
Cancer eye

Disease Profile
One of the most common neoplasms in cattle. Important risk factors lack of pigmentation around the eye (Hereford, Simmental) and solar radiation, particularly the ultraviolet component. Viruses may have role in aetiology. Most common in outdoor cattle, particularly beef, cattle. Older cattle, usually older than 5 years, more commonly affected.

Clinical findings
Starting lesions is plaque anywhere on the conjunctiva or third eyelid. The plaque may progress into papilloma or regress. Classic cancer eye, resembling papillomas, with some necrotic and ulcerated mass with pale to salmon pink colour. Advanced lesions may be fly-blown and bleeding. Ocular discharge in advanced stages becomes purulent. Can be metastatic spread to adjacent lymphnodes.

Diagnosis
Signs.

Principal differential diagnosis
Trauma, foreign body, bovine infectious keratoconjuctivitis, lymphoma, fibripapillomata.

Treatment
Early stages can be excised but recurrence can occur. Eye enucleation if cannot be readily exceeded. Control, regular examination of the cattle and culling of affected animals are recommended.

Orchitis and epididymitis

Disease Profile
Sporadic disorders of bulls of any age, particularly mature. Usually unilateral, but can be bilateral. Result in temporary or permanent infertility. Can be traumatic or infectious. Usually haematogenous spread of bacteria, but can be retrograde from urogenital tract or from the peritoneum.

Aetiology
Bacteria (*Brucella abortus*, *Mycobacterium tuberculosis* and *M. bovis*, *Trueperella pyogenes*, *Actinomyces bovis*, *Escherichia coli*, *Histophilus somni*, *Staphylococcus* spp, *Yersinia* spp, viruses, herpesvirus III) and trauma (e.g. kick, stepped on, barbed wire, penetration).

Clinical findings
Acute – hot, tender swelling, scrotal oedema. Sometimes painful walking, reluctance to mate, stilted gait.

Chronic – usually no heat or tenderness. Permanent enlargement, misshapen or atrophy and fibrosis.

Diagnosis
Palpation, semen evaluation, semen culture, serology, ultrasonography, radiography, biopsy.

Principal differential diagnosis
Inguinal hernia, hydrocoele, haematocoele, spermatocoele, kariocoele, photosensitisation, neoplasia.

Treatment
Prognosis to return to full fertility is rarely good. Systemic antimicrobials 1–3 weeks. Unilateral trauma can be dealt with by unilateral castration. Check semen before use.

Control
Vaccines are available for some of the causative pathogens.

Organophosphate poisoning

Disease Profile
Relatively uncommon. Usually occurs as an outbreak. Accidental overdose or inadvertent exposure. Organophosphate acts as cholinesterase inhibitor. Affect sympathetic, peripheral and central nervous system.

Aetiology
Oral or percutaneous absorption of organophosphates.

Clinical findings
Sympathetic signs – miosis, hyper salivation, dacryorrhoea, increased gastro-intestinal tone (e.g. colic, diarrhoea) and bronchoconstriction (e.g. dyspnoea).

Peripheral signs – stiffness, fasciculations progressing to paralysis.

Central signs – ataxia, tremor, convulsions.

Rapid death soon after severe dyspnoea is detected.

Post-mortem findings
No grass lesions.

Diagnosis
Signs. History of exposure.

Principal differential diagnosis
Other poisonings, fog fever.

Treatment
Atropine. Supportive care.

Control
Following label recommendations. Proper storage and disposal of organophosphates.

Otitis externa

Disease Profile
Sporadic disorder. Usually individual beast. The most common reasons are improper or unhygienic application of ear tags and following otitis media/interna. Other reasons include ear mites, foreign bodies (e.g. grass awns).

Clinical findings
Head shaking. Drooped ear. Auditory canal contains exudate (usually purulent with offensive odour). Head may be intermittently (rarely persistently) rotated. Sometimes an abscess or haematoma around the ear tag.

Diagnosis
Clinical findings.

Principal differential diagnosis
Otitis media/interna, listeriosis.

Treatment
Systemic and topical antimicrobials. Drain the abscess. Treat ear mites.

Control
Hygienic application of ear tags. Prevent otitis media/interna.

Otitis media/interna

Disease Profile
Sporadic disorder. Seen occasionally in calves less than a month on some farms. Usually associated with navel ill or respiratory disorders as an ascending infection.

Aetiology
Mycoplasma spp, *Trueperella pyogenes* (may be over growth in late stages), ubiquitous bacteria, *Pasteurella multocida*.

Clinical findings
Head tilt, circling towards the side of infected ear, drooped ear, drooped eyelid, exacerbated when the head is lifted, sometimes horizontal (particularly in earlier stages of the disorder) nystagmus and strabismus, and signs of ipsilateral facial nerve paralysis. Tendency to fall towards the side of the infected ear. Early-head shaking, sometimes haematoma. Depression indicates involvement of the reticular formation. On otoscopy often ruptured ear membrane and purulent exudate in the external ear canal.

Diagnosis
Clinical signs, Otoscopy.

Principal differential diagnosis
Listeriosis, thrombo-embolic meningo-encephalitis.

Treatment
Systemic and topical antimicrobials continued for several weeks. Reasonable assumption is that antimicrobials effective for respiratory disorders should be the best choice (e.g. tetracyclines, macrolides, florfenicol).

Control
Proper colostrum management, prevention of respiratory disorders. Increased incidence on a dairy farm should prompt checking bulk milk samples for *Mycoplasma* mastitis and colostrum management.

Ovarian cystic degeneration

Common synonyms
Cystic ovarian disease

Disease Profile
Common. 5–25% of lactating dairy cows. Follicular or luteal. Cause infertility. High producing cows in the first 2 months of lactation at a higher risk. Other common risks dystocia, mastitis, metritis, lameness, poor body condition, mineral imbalance (some hereditary component). 70–80% acyclic, 20–30% nymphomaniac.

Aetiology
Unknown. Any reason that results in disruption of the hypothalamic-pituitary-ovarian axis.

Clinical findings
Cyst definition: >2.5cm in diameter

Follicular cysts – Presence of a cyst, absence of uterine tone or corpus luteum. Nymphomania, anoestrus. Elevated tail head. Rectally enlarged ovary, flaccid or spongy uterine wall, sometimes hydrometra.

Luteal cysts – The main feature is absence of cyclic activity. Chronic cyst may result in masculinisation of cow.

Ultrasonography: follicular cyst, thin-walled (follicular) often multiple or luteal cyst thick-walled (>3mm luteal)

Diagnosis
History, rectal examination, ultrasonography, low progesterone (follicular cysts)

Principal differential diagnosis
Pre-ovulatory follicle, corpus luteum.

Treatment
Luteal: GnRH, intra-vaginal progesterone devices, prostaglandin F2α

(Chronic cyst poor response to Tx)

Follicular: GnRH, intra-vaginal progesterone devices

Oxalate toxicity

Disease Profile
Dependent on amount and rate of ingested plants. Soluble oxalate form salts with calcium and magnesium.

Aetiology
Ingestion of plants reach on soluble oxalates (*Halogenon glomeratus, Sarcobastus vermiculatus, Oxalis, Pannicum*, etc.)

Clinical findings
Signs of hypocalcaemia within 12 hours from exposure. Dullness, anorexia, belligerence, stiffness, weakness, muscle tremors, paresis and recumbency. Coma, followed by death.

Oxalate crystal damage the kidneys and which can result in kidney failure following recovery from hypocalcaemic phase. Rumenitis is also reported.

Post-mortem findings
Acute: oedematous, hyperaemic kidneys, ruminitis.

Chronic: atrophic kidneys, oxalate crystals and uroliths.

Diagnosis
History, clinical findings.

Principal differential diagnosis
Hypocalcaemia, hypomagnesaemia, other reasons for kidney failure.

Treatment
Move herd from offending pasture, calcium supplementation in diet. Calcium iv for animals showing clinical signs of hypocalcaemia. Stimulate diuresis (fluids, mannitol, furosemide). Cattle with renal failure have grave prognosis.

Control
Avoid pastures with high concentrations of oxalate plants.

Papillomatosis

Common synonyms
Warts, Angle-berries, Fibro-papillomas

Disease Profile
Common skin disorder. More common in dairy breeds. Usually young cattle. Spontaneous regression (within 12 months) is common. Cutaneous and mucosal form. May progress to squamous cell carcinoma or bladder cancer. Widespread papillomatosis occur in immune-compromised cattle.

Aetiology
Infection with papilloma viruses (1 to 6). Each virus is antigenic ally distinct.

Clinical findings
Solid non-pruritic hairless epidermal growth. May be pendulous, cauliflower-like, and wide-based or rise grain-like. Can vary from single lump to hundreds. The most common skin locations are head, neck, dewlap and udder. The most common mucosal locations are genital, alimentary and urinary tract. Signs vary dependant on location from asymptomatic to interference with the normal physiology (e.g. lameness with interdigital, bloat with oesophageal or deceased milk production with teat papillomas).

Diagnosis
Signs, patho-histology.

Principal differential diagnosis
Squamous cell carcinoma, dermatophilosis, ringworm.

Treatment
Spontaneous regression, autogenous vaccine. Pendulous papillomas – rubber ring. Surgical excision, cryosurgery or thermocautery.

Control
Autogenous vaccine. Avoid usage of common equipment.

Parainfluenza

Common synonyms
PI–3

Disease Profile
Common. Most commonly in young cattle (2–12 months). Most infectious subclinical. Often complicated by secondary bacterial infection (see bovine respiratory disease complex). Overcrowding, inadequate ventilation and stress are predisposing factors.

Aetiology
Paramyxovirus, parainfluenza-3 virus infection.

Clinical findings
Subclinical. Sometimes coughing, slight fever, nasal discharge and spontaneous recovery in few days.

Diagnosis
Serology (paired serum samples 4–6 weeks appart , BAL wash,

Principal differential diagnosis
Other causes of BRDC.

Treatment
Correct environmental problems. Avoid stress. Spontaneous recovery in few days unless complicated with bacteria. Antimicrobials and NSAIDs.

Control
Vaccination. Avoid overcrowding environmental conditions. Avoid stress, proper environmental conditions.

Paralysis of the bladder

Disease Profile
Rare.

The most common reason for this type of neurologic disorder is careless tail restraint and neoplasia. Less common is 'crushed tail syndrome'.

Aetiology
Neurological disorders of lumbosacral spinal cord.

Clinical findings
Presence of other signs of lower motor neuron disorder.

Paralytic bladder indicated by continuous or intermittent urinary incontinence characterised by dribbling urine without straining. On rectal examination, the bladder is enlarged. It can be easily expressed manually.

Diagnosis
Signs.

Treatment
Treatment of primary disorder.

Administration of antimicrobials to prevent cystitis is advocated.

Prognosis depends on the prognosis of the primary disorder. Paralysis of the bladder without lower motor neuron signs is usually of poor prognosis.

Paralysis of the tongue

Common synonyms
Glossoplegia, Glossoparalysis.

Disease Profile
Rare. Can be primary (pathology to the glossopharyngeal nerve), or secondary (botulism, actinobacillosis). A false glossoplagia may result in paralysis of the masticatory branch of the trigeminal nerve (tongue protrudes, but pulled back in the oral cavity when touched).

Clinical findings
Passively protruding tongue, drooling, dysphagia, atrophy of the tongue muscles.

Diagnosis
Signs.

Principal differential diagnosis
Botulism, actinobacillossis, rabies, BSE.

Treatment
Non-steroidal anti-inflammatory drugs, soft food. Treat primary cause. In chronic cases culling.

Parasitic gastroenteritis

Disease Profile
Common in pasture-based, high density stocking groups of growing cattle. In calves usually affects groups, in 18–24 months old cattle individual cattle. In mature cattle often asymptomatic.

Parasite burden on pasture dependent upon time of year and weather.

Aetiology
Various cestodes and nematodes (*Bunostomum* spp, *Cooperia* spp, *Haemonchus* spp, *Moniezia* spp, *Ostertagia* spp, *Strongyloides* spp and *Trichostrongylus* spp.

Clinical findings
Common findings poor growth, loss of weight and body condition, poor coat quality and faecal staining of the tail and/or hocks in some or all animals in the group. In calves that are heavily infested there may be profuse diarrhoea, loss of appetite, dehydration and significant loss of body condition.

Type II ostertagiosis usually seen in individual cattle, 18–24 months of age (occasionally older). Usual clinical findings include rapid decline in body condition, rough hair coat, and sometimes dehydration and submandibular swelling. Sudden death may occur in some animals as a result of shock.

Post-mortem findings
Extensive inflammatory response in the abomasum and/or intestines.

'Morocco leather'-like appearance of abomasal mucosa, and presence of large numbers of parasites.

Diagnosis
Signs are only indicative. Faecal egg count, pepsinogen levels, post mortem worm count. All epidemiologic factors and farm or district history need to be considered.

Principal differential diagnosis
Other conditions causing ill-thrift (poor nutrition, mineral deficiencies, underfeeding, generalised conditions, mucosal disease, etc.) or diarrhoea (coccidiosis, salmonellosis, yersiniosis, etc.)

Treatment
Anthelmintics.

Calves and yearlings – treatment as a group. Adult cattle treatment of affected animals.

Treatment of type II ostertagiosis is often unrewarding and affected animals have poor prognosis.

Control
Reduce exposure and infection. Control may be carried out by use of antihelmintics alone or in combination with grazing strategy. The strategic use of antihelmintics based on faecal egg counts and faecal egg reduction tests for sensitivity or presence of resistance is desirable. Other strategies to minimise the use of antihelmintics and preserve their efficacy are described in the COWS program.

Penile deviation

Disease Profile
Common. A cause of concern when interferes with intromission (phalocamposis). Most common form is spiral (corkscrew) deviation. Less common are lateral, ventral and S-shaped.

Aetiology
Unknown.

Clinical findings
Bull repeatedly mounting but fails to thrust. The deviation is usually detectable after dismounting.

Diagnosis
Signs.

Principal differential diagnosis
Persistent frenulum, penile fibro papilloma.

Treatment
Surgical correction. Culling.

Penile haematoma

Common synonyms
Ruptured penis, Broken penis, Fractured penis.

Disease Profile
Relatively common. The most common presentation is penile haematoma. Later may progress to penile abscess or penile deviation. The most common place of penile haematoma is the dorsal aspect of the sigmoid flexure.

Aetiology
Rupture of the tunica albuginea when mounting cows or in homosexual attempts between bulls.

Clinical findings
Sudden cessation of service activity. Swelling of the preputium (most commonly just cranial to the scrotum). Sometimes tip of the penis or prepuce. The size of the haematoma increases with each attempt to mount.

Diagnosis
Clinical signs, ultrasonography.

Principal differential diagnosis
Preputial abscess, ruptured urethra.

Treatment
Surgical drainage and repair. Systemic antimicrobials Rest from service for at least 2 months.

Pericarditis

Disease Profile
Rare. Usually mature cattle. Most common a sequel to traumatic reticulo-peritonitis. Signs usually seen in late pregnancy and/or early postpartum can also spread from surrounding organs/tissue (e.g. pleuritis myocarditis, pleuropneumonia).

Aetiology
Trauma, hematogenous or direct spread, toxins, neoplasia.

Clinical findings
Signs of abdominal and thoracic pain, hyperpnoea, tachycardia, muffled heart sounds, sometimes pericardial friction rubs, washing machine murmurs, absence of lung sounds in ventral thorax, signs of congestive heart failure, sometimes fever. In chronic cases weakness, inappetence, weight loss (decreased production), signs of thoracic pain, abnormal auscultation findings and signs of right-sided congestive heart failure.

Diagnosis
Signs, history, ultrasonography, pericardiocentesis, radiography, auscultation.

Principal differential diagnosis
Other reasons for cardiac disorders, Hydropericardium, Pleuro-pneumonia and Lymph sarcoma.

Treatment
Often unrewarding. Systemic antimicrobials, surgery, pericardial lavage. Supportive treatment (e.g. NSAIDs, maintenance of hydration and acid-base balance). Prognosis not better than guarded (30%).

Control
Prevention of traumatic reticulo-peritonitis (remove wires, dose with magnets)

Peritonitis

Disease Profile
Relatively common. Traumatic reticulo-peritonitis, perforation of abomasal ulcer/s, uterine tears and following surgery of abdomen or dystocia are the most common causes.

Clinical findings
Localised peritonitis – signs of abdominal pain, mildly elevated body temperature, reluctance to move, depressed appetite.

Diffuse peritonitis – severe abdominal pain, reluctance to move, fever, scleral injection, loss of appetite, dehydration, sudden drop in milk production, rumen atomy, tachycardia, and initially abdominal dissention followed by gaunt.

Diagnosis
History, clinical signs, abdominal centesis, ultrasonography.

Principal differential diagnosis
Reasons for thoracic pain, toxic metritis, early stages of hypocalcemia.

Treatment
Diffuse peritonitis have grave prognosis. Restrict movement of the beast, systemic antimicrobials, NSAIDs, fluid therapy, ruminal magnet, rumenotomy, transfaunation, other surgical intervention.

Petroleum distillates poisoning

Disease Profile
Uncommon. Usually more than one animal affected at the same time.

Aetiology
Accidental access to highly volatile petroleum.

Clinical findings
Depression, ataxia, rumen stasis, bloat, diarrhoea, displaced abomasum, recumbency, sudden death. Some cattle appear to be anaesthetised. On physical examination oily nasal discharge, tachycardia, tachypnoea, petroleum odour on breath and faeces, absent menace response, decreased palpebral reflex. In pregnant cattle abortion.

Post-mortem findings
Consolidation of lungs, hyperaemic; corrosive damage to the gastrointestinal tract, strong petroleum odour of the content.

Diagnosis
History, clinical findings, gas chromatography.

Principal differential diagnosis
Lead poisoning, organophosphate poisoning.

Treatment
Rumenotomy, release bloat. Oral saline laxatives. Supportive treatment. Prognosis usually grave.

Pharyngeal trauma

Disease Profile
Trauma to the pharynx and retropharyngeal most commonly occurs from the incorrect use of a stomach tube. Using very stiff hoses (e.g. garden hose), sometimes with an angled and sharp end, increases the risk of misdirection and penetration of the soft tissues. Inappropriate administration of boluses, either the animal is too small or the applicator is misdirected can cause injury.

Clinical findings
Grossly enlarged pharyngeal (sub-mandibular and parotid) area. Copious drooling of saliva, pharyngeal pain, dysphagia, extended head and neck, in appetence, ruminal stasis, fever and dyspnoea. Affected cattle sometimes develop aspiration pneumonia (dull, anorexic and depressed).

Diagnosis
Signs, Gag and examine the pharynx using a plastic tube and a pen torch. The wound can often be visualised.

Principal differential diagnosis
Stomatitis, oral necrobacillosis, actinobacillosis.

Treatment
Aggressive broad spectrum antimicrobials, NSAIDs, and symptomatic supportive care over period of one to two weeks. Rumen fitulation may allow fluids and gruel to be administered

Control
Careful administration of oral medications

Prognosis
Guarded – Poor.

Photosensatisation

Common synonyms
Photodermatitis.

Disease Profile
May be **primary** ingestion of photodynamic substances or **secondary** hepatotoxic damage. More common in lightly coloured cattle. Muzzle is often affected. Mucocutaneous junctions, teats and scrotum common sites for visible changes.

Clinical findings
Attempt to seek shade. Early stages oozing dermatitis, erythema, oedema, pruritus and pain, followed by superficial necrosis of the skin and sloughing.

Diagnosis
Clinical findings, tests for hepatotoxic damage to differentiate primary and secondary.

Principal differential diagnosis
Congenital porphyria, facial eczema.

Treatment
Prevent exposure to sunlight, treat primary cause (e.g. prevent re-exposure), soothing topical ointments, anti-inflammatories. With severe hepatotoxic damage euthanasia. Systemic antibiotics may be required to prevent secondary bacterial infections.

Control
Prevent ingestion of photodynamic substances. Prevent liver damage.

Polioencephalomalacia (B1 deficiency)

Common synonyms
Cerebrocortial necrosis (CCN), PEM.

Disease Profile
Malacia of the grey matter of the brain. Excess sulphur consumption, altered metabolism of thiamine, grazing lush pasture, high-grain diet, sudden diet change, rumen-produced or ingested thiaminases and treatment with antithiamine drugs (e.g. amprolium) are predisposing factors. Often a herd problem. Acute and subacute form.

Aetiology
Deficiency of thiamine (B1)

Clinical findings
Acute form – Found recumbent and often comatose. Signs as sub-acute form.

Subacute form – cortical blindness, dorso-medial strabismus, nystagmus, dull separated from the group, may stagger, intermittent hyperaesthesia leading to recumbency, opisthotonus, paddling movements. Head pressing may be present.

Post-mortem findings
Fluorescence of freshly cut brain cortex exposed under UV light.

Diagnosis
Signs. Response to treatment

Principal differential diagnosis
Lead poisoning, sulphur toxicity, meningitis, nervous ketosis.

Treatment
Thiamine (B1) and supportive care (tranquilisers, mannitol, soft bedding).

Control
Prevent sudden diet change. If known to be prove to sulphur toxicity preventive oral thiamine administration.

Post-Partum Haemorrhage

Disease Profile
Occurs in cows with dystocia. May be peracute to acute.

Aetiology
Rupture of blood vessels in the brood ligaments, uterus or calving canal.

Clinical findings
Blood may be coming out (external haemorrhage) or not (internal haemorrhage). Weakness to recumbency. Pale mucous membranes, tachycardia, tachypnoea. Other signs of anaemia.

Diagnosis
Signs.

Treatment and management
Often unrewarding (with rupture of large blood vessels). Can try and locate with haemostats. Once clamped leave in place for 24 hours. Failing this a rolled towel to act as a tight fitting tampon can assist. Leave in place 12–24 hours. Blood transfusion may be needed. Adrenaline and oxytocin may help.

Control
Careful when assisting with dystocia although often difficult to prevent

Postparturient haemoglobinuria

Disease Profile
Sporadically in dairy and uncommon in beef cows. Usually small number of cows affected on a farm, of which half usually die. Disorder of adult high-producing cows. Characterised by a haemolytic syndrome usually in the period 2–4 weeks after calving. Associated with hypophosphataemia.

Aetiology
Phosphorus deficiency in North America, and copper and selenium deficiency in New Zealand.

Other possible agents are feeding cruciferous plants and ingestion of cold water.

Clinical findings
Haemoglobinuria, inappetence, weakness and severe depression. Urine is red to dark-brown. Pale mucous membranes, tachycardia and jugular pulse. Temperature may rise. Faeces dry and firm. Milk yield drops rapidly. Cattle slowly become recumbent. In later stages, in cows that survive the acute phase, jaundice develops. Recovery takes few weeks. Cattle in recovery often develop pica. Pica may also be detected in some of the herd-mates.

Post-mortem findings
Anaemia and jaundice through the body. Discoloured urine.

Diagnosis
Signs, low phosphorus, copper, selenium.

Principal differential diagnosis
Other causes of haemolytic anaemia.

Treatment
Immediate transfusion in severe cases. Delay of 12 hours may be fatal. Intravenous and oral fluid therapy to prevent nephrosis. Crystaloid fluids may be protective of kidneys when no blood transfusion is available.

Control
Control of phosphorus and copper. Elimination of plant toxins.

Pyelonephritis

Disease Profile
Common complication of infections to the lower urinary tract. The disorder is sporadic. Subclinical infection most common form. Infection can be iatrogenic in origin (careless catheterisation).

Mature cows most susceptible, particularly in early lactation. High producing dairy herds are at highest risk.

Aetiology
Secondary to lower urinary tract infections, embolic nephritis, associated with nephrolithiasis and specific infections (*Corynebacterium renale, C pilosum and C cystitiolitis). Escherichia coli* is the most common accompanying bacterial species. Other bacteria are usually various cocci, *Trueperella pyogenes.*

Clinical findings
The condition may develop over several weeks. The first sign is usually red urine or colic. Colic attacks last a few hours and rarely observed. Clinical form is more common. Temperature fluctuating. Capricious appetite, loss of body condition and depressed milk yield. Polyuria, stranguria and dribbling. The most obvious sign is changed urine. Urine, particularly later portions, is with evidence of haematuria, pyuria, mucosuria and increased tissue-based sediment. On rectal examination in later stages ureters are enlarged, the bladder is enlarged with thickened wall. The affected kidney is enlarged and painful on palpation. In protracted cases, ventral oedema (brisket, under the jaw) may develop.

Post-mortem findings
Enlarged kidneys with loss of lobulation. Ureters contain mucus pus and blood. Bladder and urethra may have thickened wall with oedematous and eroded to haemorrhagic mucous membranes. Renal pelvis similar to ureters.

Diagnosis
Signs, ultrasonography, urine analysis.

Principal differential diagnosis
Other causes of abdominal pain, cystitis, chronic endometritis, perivaginal abscessation, enzootic haematuria.

Treatment
Antimicrobial for a minimum of three weeks. A good prognosis is indicated by rapid improvement in body condition, return of appetite and milk yield, and clearing of the urine.

Advanced cases coupled with a cow in low BCS have guarded prognosis.

Control
Isolation of affected cattle, destruction of contaminated bedding, proper cleaning and sterilisation of instrument for catheterisation. In herds with increased prevalence of the disorder that use natural service, AI may result in a significant reduction in the number of cases. C. renale can be transmitted during natural mating.

Q-fever

Common synonyms
Coxiellosis, Queensland fever, Balkan grippe.

Disease Profile
Affects variety of animal species. Reservoirs are many wild and domestic mammals, and ticks. Often asymptomatic. In naïve herds abortion and infertility. Zoonotic. Excretion of pathogen in milk, urine, faeces, placenta, lochia.

Aetiology
Coxiella burnetii.

Clinical findings
Mostly asymptomatic.

Infertility, sporadic abortion, stillbirths, low calf weights, weak calves, retained placenta. In naïve herds abortion storm.

Diagnosis
Detection of pathogen, serology.

Principal differential diagnosis
Other causes of abortion and infertility.

Treatment
No effective treatment available.

Control
Segregate pregnant cows, disposal of placentas and still born calves appropriately, tick control, client education, vaccination available in some countries.

Rabies

Common synonyms
Hydrophobia

Disease Profile
Regional. Invariably fatal after appearance of clinical signs. Transmission through bite wounds or other methods of transdermal penetration. Remote zoonotic risk sporadic.

Aetiology
Rhabdovirus.

Clinical findings
Early signs nonspecific.

Furious forms – restlessness, excitability, exaggerated response to tactile and auditory stimuli, maniacal, often charge to herd mates, people and inanimate objects, starring eyes, erected ears, hypersalivaton, bruxism, and vocalisation with low pitched voice. Hydrophobia. Progressive ataxia, paralysis, coma and death.

Paralytic form – anorexia, shifting leg lameness, depression, fever, common attempts to bellow with no sound ('yawning), staggering gait, flaccid paralysis of tongue, masseters, pharynx, larynx, rapidly developing generalised paralysis, coma and death. Hypersalivation, inability to swallow, vocalisation. Can present as choke.

Post-mortem findings
Histopathology of brain (hypocampus) and finding Negrie's inclusion bodies.

Diagnosis
Signs, detection of pathogen, history, histopathology.

Principal differential diagnosis
Many neurologic disorders (e.g. nervous ketosis, hypomagnesaemia, encephalitis, pseudorabies, bovine spongiform encephalopathy, polioencephalomalacia, hypovitaminosis A, listeriosis).

Treatment
No effective treatment.

Repeated breeder cow

Disease Profile
Cow that has failed to become pregnant three or more serves at normal inter-oestrus intervals in an absence of obvious abnormalities. Common problem of the modern dairy industry. Incidence 5–20%. Can occur due to cow management, environment and bull factors. Can be a problem at cow or herd level.

Aetiology
Failure of fertilisation, early embryonic death, bull/semen quality, heat stress, incorrect insemination times, incorrect semen handling, various non-infectious and infectious disorders of the genito-urinary tract, malnutrition.

Clinical findings
Return to oestrus at regular interoestrus intervals and no detectable.

Diagnosis
When dealing with individual cow: examination of vaginal mucus cervix and ultrasonography on day of oestrus. When dealing with herd problem: bull examination, assessment of management, insemination and environment.

Treatment and management
Address bull soundness, ensure proper semen handling, retrain inseminator, improve oestrus detection, use hormonal aids, treat primary disorders, vaccination against infectious causes, use of mop-up (clean-up) bulls improve environmental conditions, cull repeated offenders.

Retained placenta

Common synonyms
Retained foetal membranes.

Disease Profile
Failure to pass the placenta after 12–24 hours post-partum. Incidence is farm-specific and ranges 1–10%, sometimes higher (some herds up to 40%). More common in dairy cattle. Common risk factors: deficiency of selenium, iodine and vitamin E, abortion, twinning, induced calving, dystocia, caesarean section, milk fever and prolonged recumbency. Increased risk of endometritis. Increase in calving to conception interval.

Aetiology
Failure of breaking down placental attachment.

Clinical findings
Usually putrid placenta visible hanging from the vulva. Sometimes straining. Rarely general illness-metritis, anorexia, fever, depressed milk yield.

Diagnosis
Signs.

Principal differential diagnosis
Retained foetus.

Treatment
Appropriate nursing care. Early treatment with oxytocin. Light manual traction after day 5. In case of systemic illness antimicrobials.

Control
Reduce or remove risk factors.

Rift Valley fever

Disease Profile
Endemic in Africa with occasional incursions in the Middle East. Associated with heavy rainfall and extended flooding. Transmission by mosquitoes. Often associated with mixing cattle and small ruminants. Abortion rate may reach 100%. Mortality 10–70% in calves and <10% in mature cattle. Zoonotic. Notifiable.

Aetiology
Phlebovirus.

Clinical findings
Short incubation period (0.5–1.5 days).

Calves – fever, depression, hepatitis, acute death (1–2 days).

Mature cattle – inapparent to fever, inappetence, weakness, hypersalivation, foetid diarrhoea, death.

Pregnant cattle – abortion and stillbirths.

Post-mortem findings
Hepatic necrosis, petechial haemorrhages.

Diagnosis
Signs, detection of pathogen, serology.

Principal differential diagnosis
Other causes for neonatal death and storm abortion.

Treatment
No treatment.

Control
Biosecurity, vector control. Vaccine with some side effects (abortogenic and teratogenic) also available in some countries.

Rinderpest (eradicated)

Common synonyms
Cattle plague.

Disease Profile
The world was declared to be officially free from **rinderpest i**nfection at the OIE General Session in May 2011.Historically caused pandemics with devastating outcomes. Naïve cattle of European breeds were most susceptible. Morbidity and mortality could exceed 90%.

Aetiology
Morbilli virus.

Clinical findings
Incubation 7–14 days.

Fever, depression, anorexia, drop in milk production. Inflammation of visible mucosa, followed by sloughing. Constipation followed by dysentery. Dehydration, prostration, recumbency, death.

Post-mortem findings
Ulceration of the oral mucosa. Necrotising enteritis. Ulcerations in other digestive organs.

Diagnosis
Signs, detection of pathogen, histopathology.

Principal differential diagnosis
BVD, MCF, IBR, FMD, Bluetongue, Bovine popular stomatitis, ingestion of corrosive chemicals.

Treatment
N/A

Control
Quarantine, restricted animal movement, biosecurity. Vaccination.

Ringworm

Common synonyms
Dermatophysosis

Disease Profile
Fungal infection of the fully keratinised skin and hair shafts. Most commonly young cattle. Particularly important in undernourished and immune-compromised calves. Moisture and micro trauma required start of an outbreak. Zoonosis.

Aetiology
Most commonly *Trychophyton verrucosum*. Sometimes *T. mentagrophytes* and *Microsporon* spp.

Clinical findings
Raised, grey, non-pruritic plaques with expanding alopecia. More commonly on head and neck. May extend over the body. When complicated with bacteria lesions are pruritic.

Diagnosis
Signs, detection of pathogen.

Principal differential diagnosis
Papillomatosis, skin lymphosarcoma, dermatophilosis, zinc-response skin disorder.

Treatment
Often self-limiting. Isolate affected cattle. Tropical antifungals. Improve nutrition and environmental conditions. The best treat all in-contact cattle.

Control
Vaccine available in some countries. Biosecurity.

Rotavirus infection

Disease Profile
The most common cause of diarrhoea in neonatal calves. Most affected calves are 5 to 14 days of age. Concurrent infection with *Escherichia coli* or other pathogens associated with calf diarrhoea (see appropriate heading) may result in diarrhoea in older calves

Transmission is primarily faecal-oral. Outbreaks with 50–100% morbidity. Large number of virus particles shed in diarrhoeic faeces. Mature cows may be subclinically infected and intermittent shedders, particularly around calving. Malabsorptive and secretion diarrhoea.

Common predisposing factor is failure of passive transfer.

Aetiology
Rotavirus. Mixes infection with other pathogens (see calf diarrhoea) are common.

Clinical findings
Incubation period is 1 to 3 days. Sudden onset of diarrhoea that spreads rapidly.

Mild to severe diarrhoea, dehydration, acidosis, depression, sometimes loss of sucking reflex. Usually distended or tense abdomen and sloshing on succession.

Frequency of cases increases as the calving season progresses.

Post-mortem findings
May be negative. Usually dehydration. On histopathology shortened villi.

Diagnosis
Signs. Detection of pathogen. History.

Principal differential diagnosis
Other causes of calf diarrhoea.

Treatment
Correct fluid loss (IV and oral fluids), correct acidosis (bicarbonate), supportive care (see calf diarrhoea).

Control
Proper hygiene, disinfection of environment, vaccination. Ensure intake of enough, good quality colostrum. Change calving paddock, calf-rearing facility.

Rumen alkalosis

Disease Profile
Rumen alkalosis may be a sequel of rumen inactivity (usually due to inappetence) or ingestion of toxic and alkalising substances. Rumen alkalosis associated with rumen inactivity is usually marginal (pH 7.0–7.5). Ingestion of toxic or alkalising substances (urea, biuret, ammonium phosphate, fertilizers containing ammonium) usually results in significant alkalosis (pH >7.5). Younger cattle are usually more susceptible to urea toxicity.

Clinical findings
Signs of toxicity may be observed soon after the ingestion of urea (within 20 minutes). Abdominal pain (kicking at the abdomen), fore-stomach stasis, dehydration, bloat, regurgitation, strong odour of ammonia in the breath, diarrhoea, excitation of the CNS (incoordination, hypersensitivity to sound, excessive salivation/frothing at the mouth, muscle tremors, sometimes tetany), increased respiratory rate, dyspnoea, weakness and bellowing. Death may occur in minutes to hours (usually less than 4 hours).

Diagnosis
Signs, bloods (dehydration, increased BUN, hypokalaemia, hypocalcaemia), rumen pH, no protozoal activity.

Principal differential diagnosis
Other forms of indigestion, hepatic encephalopathy, anaphylaxis, blue green algae toxicosis, hypomagnesaemia, salt poisoning and encephalitis.

Treatment
Empty the rumen via rumen lavage or rumenotomy. Acidifying the rumen using a weak acid like vinegar given repeatedly every half an hour helps prevent absorption of ammonia. Severe cases have a poor prognosis.

Control
Urea <3% of the concentrate. Ration should be mixed well. Cattle should have gradual adaptation period to urea.

Rye grass staggers

Common synonyms
Rye grass toxicity. Perennial ryegrass staggers.

Disease Profile
Common in certain regions. High morbidity, low mortality, slow onset. Risk factor grazing on perennial rye grass (*Lolium perenne*) or hybrid pasture infected with endophytic fungus *Neotyphodium lolii*. Late spring to early autumn.

Aetiology
Ingestion of lolitrems, mainly Lolitrem B, produced by symbiotic fungal endophyte. Probably other toxins.

Clinical findings
At rest no signs or only fine tremors. Excitement results in staggering (stiff spastic gait, hypermetria, nodding of the head, ataxia), falling opistothonus, nystagmus, extended limbs. Deaths are usually accidental.

Diagnosis
Signs, time of year, detection of hyphae on pasture samples.

Principal differential diagnosis
Annual rye grass staggers, Paspalum staggers, Phalaris poisoning, polioencephalomalacia.

Treatment
Not practical. Let cattle walk on their own to other paddocks. Recovery in 1–2 weeks.

Control
Prevent overgrazing. Mixed botanical species pastures. Improved perennial rye grass varieties.

Salmonellosis

Disease Profile
Very common. In mature cattle prevalence of infection usually high but incidence of clinical disease low. In calves incidence of clinical disease high. Mortality with clinical disease high.

Peracute, acute and chronic form.

Surviving and latently infected (Dublin) cattle often long-term shedders (up to 6 months or more).

Outbreaks often precipitated by stressor. In calves failure of passive transfer important. Can be a zoonosis (S. typhimurium).

Aetiology
Salmonella typhimurium (most common). *S. dublin* (cattle specific).

Signs often associated with endotoxaemia.

Clinical findings
Mature cattle peracute form – septicaemia, complete anorexia, foul-smelling diarrhoea (not always), meningitis, opisthotonus, convulsions, death.

Mature cattle acute form – the most common form. Septicaemia, anorexia, decreased milk yield, foul-smelling diarrhoea (blood, mucus and casts), dehydration, abortion, high mortality.

Mature cattle chronic form – less severe. Abortion. Failure to thrive. Growing animals stunted growth, poor hair coat. Rarely osteomyelitis.

Calves – fever, dullness, anorexia, diarrhoea, pneumonia, septicaemia, meningitis, joint ill, osteomyelitis. Usually 2 weeks to 2 months of age.

Post-mortem findings
Haemorrhagic enteritis, congested lungs, petechial haemorrhages on all serosas, sometimes meningitis, dehydration.

Diagnosis
Signs, detection of pathogen. Serology.

Principal differential diagnosis
Diarrhoea of other nature.

Treatment
Antimicrobials. Supportive care (fluids, correction of electrolyte imbalance, correction of acidosis) and nursing care.

Control
Biosecurity, isolation, vaccination. Avoid stressors and overcrowding. Improve hygiene and quarantine of new introductions.

Salt poisoning

Common synonyms
Salt toxicity.

Disease Profile
Associated with high drinking water with high salinity and water deprivation. Regional. Results in generalised oedema, including cortical oedema.

Aetiology
Ingestion of large quantities salt (e.g. salt-deprived cattle) or dehydration (e.g. water sources frozen).

Clinical findings
Nervous – ataxia, depression, nystagmus, muscle twitching, opisthotonus, intermittent convulsions, belligerent or aggressive behaviour. Anorexia, polydipsia and abdominal pain. Sometimes blindness and diarrhoea. Death common in convulsing cattle.

Diagnosis
Signs. Histopathology.

Principal differential diagnosis
Dehydration of other nature, meningitis, polioencephalomalacia, lead poisoning, rabies.

Treatment
Allow frequent access to limited amounts of water. Mannitol iv can reduce brain oedema but reserved for high value animals. Glucose iv has been used.

Control
Ensure adequate access to 'safe' water which has no or acceptable levels of salinity.

Schmallenberg virus disease

Disease Profile
Emerging disorder. May cause transient, clinical disorder in mature cattle. Main signs are associated with congenital malformations. Transmission through biting insects including midges (*Culicoides* spp).

Aetiology
Schmallenberg virus (family Bunyaviridae).

Clinical findings
Congenital malformations including torticollis, arthrogryposis, scoliosis, kyphosis, poor development of skeletal muscles and microencephaly or other changes affecting the central nervous system. Infection in first trimester of pregnancy may result in foetal death and abortion.

Signs of viraemia include fever, reduced milk yield, inappetence, loss of body condition and diarrhoea.

Diagnosis
Signs are only indication. Detection of pathogen.

Principal differential diagnosis
Other causes of congenital malformation, particularly Akabane.

Treatment
None.

Control
Vaccination. Control of biting insects. Biosecurity.

Sciatic nerve paralysis

Disease Profile
Damage most commonly seen at calving due to gross foeto-maternal disproportion or misdirected and inappropriate intramuscular injection in the gluteal muscle (chemical neuritis).

Clinical findings
Unilateral injury may cause dragging of the limb with flexed hip and attended stifle. Partial injury may cause intermittent knuckling of the digits. Analgesia of the limb distally of the stifle, with the exception of the medial surface. The tarsus partially flexed. Bilateral injury usually causes recumbency or sitting in frog-like position.

Diagnosis
Signs.

Principal differential diagnosis
Peroneal or tibial nerve paralysis, hypocalcaemia, hypophosphataemia, trauma.

Treatment
General care, splinting the distal limb to prevent rub sores. Prognosis is fairly good if affected cattle show signs of recovery within two weeks.

Seminal vesiculitis

Common synonyms
Vesiculitis seminalis, Vesiculitis, Adenitis of vesicular glands.

Disease Profile
Common. History of subfertility or infertility Underdiagnosed. Acute and chronic. Acute – most common in young bulls on high-energy diets. Chronic – older bulls. Most commonly diagnosis during bull soundness examination and semen evaluation. May occur as a sequel of infection elsewhere in the body.

Aetiology
Variety of bacteria (e.g. *Trueperella pyogenes, Staphylococci*), mycoplasma, chlamydia, viruses and fungi have been isolated.

Clinical findings
Often asymptomatic. History of subfertility or infertility. On rectal palpation: enlarged gland/s. Sometimes painful defecation, pain on rectal examination, reluctance to move and serve, stiff gait and tense abdomen. Cytology of semen may reveal inflammation and bacteria.

Diagnosis
Semen cytology and culture, ultrasonography.

Treatment
Prolonged antimicrobials. Sexual rest. Surgery. Prognoses guarded.

Septic Arthritis

Disease Profile
Septic arthritis may be:

primary (foreign body penetration), single joint, usually lower limb, adults

secondary (lateral spread), foot infections

tertiary (haematogenous spread). Septic polyarthritis in calves with failure of passive transfer.

Can affect any joint but limbs most commonly affected.

Aetiology
Bacteria, Mycoplasma, viruses and fungi can be causative organisms. Common causes are *Streptococcus, Salmonella, Proteus, Bacteroides, Mycoplasma spp, Trueperella pyogenes* and *Histophilus somni.*

Clinical findings
Severe lameness of sudden onset, shifting weight, swelling (synovial effusion), heat and pain on manipulation of affected joints, change in the general condition (fever, lethargy and often recumbency). Affected joints are tender on touch. In calves the umbilical scar may or may not show abnormality. Later stages a limited range of joint movement due to fibrosis.

Diagnosis
Signs. Elevated fibrinogen, leukocytosis. Radiography. Arthrocentesis. Culture.

Treatment
Treatment must be adapted to each individual case. Large doses of systemic antimicrobials for extended period, joint lavage, articular administration of antimicrobials. Chronic cases have unfavourable prognosis. Joint flushing in high value animals is recommended.

Control
Neonatal joint ill is associated with unhygienic calf rearing or insufficient colostrum intake. Therefore, hygiene of the rearing facilities should be improved, dipping of the novel in suitable disinfectants after birth and before moving to rearing facilities and ensuring sufficient intake of good quality colostrum.

Shipping fever

Common synonyms
Bovine pneumonic pasteurellosis. Transit fever.

Disease Profile
Common in intensively reared cattle. Probably the most important disorder associated with re-grouping, co-mingling and transport of cattle. Mainly in young cattle in feedlots within 4 weeks from arrival. Stress factors essential to development of the disorder. Usually explosive outbreak.**Aetiology**
The pathology associated with this condition is associated with lower airway infections of Mannheimia haemolytica +/− Pasteurella multocida. The condition is potentiated by stresses which lower the resistance and facilitate invasion of the lower airways. These stresses include physiological stresses (transport, handling, re-grouping) environmental stresses (dust) and other respiratory infections such as *Haemophilus somni, Mycoplasma* spp and viruses (BRSC, P13, IBR, BVD]).

Clinical findings
Decreased feed intake, separation from the group, tachypnoea, fever, evidence of bronchopneumonia, reluctance to move, keeping head and neck low, bilateral nasal discharge, with or without cough. Short duration 1–4 days, followed by death.

Post-mortem findings
Fibrinous pneumonia of cranio-ventral lobes, sometimes most of the lung.

Diagnosis
History, signs, post-mortem.

Principal differential diagnosis
Other causes of pneumonia (enzootic pneumonia, bovine respiratory disease complex, lungworm, viruses).

Treatment
Early treatment usually rewarding. Severe cases and delayed treatment may die or become ill-thrifty. Antimicrobials, non-steroidal anti-inflammatories, supportive treatment.

Control
Isolation of sick cattle. Minimise stress. Purchase already weaned cattle, vaccination. In case of outbreak or identified unavoidable risk-injectable metaphylaxis.

Simple indigestion

Disease Profile
Common in feed lot cattle changing the diet frequently. Usually individual cases, but outbreaks also occur. Predisposing factors are roughage of low quality, stress (e.g. transport, re-grouping), restricted access to water, prolonged antimicrobial therapy.

Aetiology
Sudden change in diet.

Clinical findings
Anorexia, reduced rumen motility. Cardinal signs normal to slightly elevate. Depression reduced faecal output of firmer character. Occasionally, loose malodorous faeces. Rumen fill usually normal, but rumen contents are fluid.

Diagnosis
Signs, history, examination of rumen fluid.

Principal differential diagnosis
Ketosis, traumatic reticuloperitonitis, vagus indigestion, rumen acidosis, displaced abomasum, rumen alkalosis, peritonitis.

Treatment and management
Provision of fresh, palatable feed stuffs. Rumenotorics. Transfaunation.

Control
Avoid sudden changes in diet.

Snake bite

Disease Profile
Fatal bites are rare. Usually sporadic cases. Calves at higher risk of fatality. Greater risk when envenomation around tongue, muzzle, directly into a large blood vessel, face and ventral thoracic wall. Venoms usually classified as haemotoxic and neurotoxic. Zoonotic potential – protective gloves required when treating the wound.

Aetiology
Bite by various venomous snakes.

Clinical findings
Rapidly developing swelling at the bite site. Apparent tissue necrosis. Hypersalivation, dysphagia, dyspnoea, lethargy, muscle fasciculations, reluctance to move, arrhythmias, shock.

With neurotoxic venoms – paresis, paralysis, respiratory distress.

Post-mortem findings
Swelling, tissue necrosis, sloughing.

Diagnosis
Signs. History

Principal differential diagnosis
Fracture, spider envenomations, abscess, haematoma, insect bites, lizard bites.

Treatment
Bite wound cleaning only. Maintain patency of airways, restore dehydration. Keep the beast calm and pain free. Antimicrobials, NSAIDs, clostridial protection. Specific treatment – specific antivenom. Some require use of steroids; for others steroids contraindicated. Neurotoxic venom may cause permanent damage.

Sole ulcer

Disease Profile
Sequel to laminitis.

Clinical findings
Usually acute onset of moderate to severe lameness. Often there is under-run of the sole extending dorsal (forward) and abaxial (lateral), and protruding granulation tissue. Early ulcers may often appear as nothing more than a circumscribed area of granulation tissue. A sole ulcer may be concealed. Frequent shifting of the weight. In cases of bilateral sole ulcers, the laying-down times significantly increased.

Diagnosis
Signs.

Principal differential diagnosis
Sole puncture, white line disease, bruised sole, exposed corium, acute laminitis.

Treatment
Therapeutic trimming. Antimicrobials. Block on the sound claw.

Spastic paresis

Common synonyms
Elso heel

Disease Profile
Inherited neuromuscular contracture disorder that causes progressive uni-or bi-lateral hyperextended posture and gait of the hock and stifles joints. Onset usually 2 weeks to 9 months. Some breed predisposition (Holstein, Hereford, Aberdeen Angus, Murray Grey, Ayrshire, Brown Swiss, Danish Red, Shorthorn) but in general it is sporadic.

Clinical findings
At rest. Lying down the limb is normal. On standing the hock becomes hyperextended although flexion on manipulation can be readily achieved. The walking is in a typical swinging motion (pendulum fashion). These animals do not graze well and do not grow or gain weight easily. Mobility can be severely restricted.

Diagnosis
Signs.

Principal differential diagnosis
Dorsal luxation of the patella, gonitis, tarsitis, luxation of biceps femoris muscle, fracture dislocation of calcaneus.

Treatment
Tenotomy of half of the tendons at the hock allows normal gait to return. Tibial neurectomy provide an alternative, permanent solution.

Control
Cull affected animals. Do not breed from affected bulls.

Spinal disorders

Disease Profile
Many various disorders (e.g. trauma, spinal abscess).

Clinical findings
Weakness decreased motor function, decreased sensory function and areflexia. Not all spinal disorders cause symmetrical loss of function. Septic disorders may be accompanied by fever.

Diagnosis
Signs. CSF cytology. Neurological examination

Treatment
Symptomatic. Supportive care (nursing, non-steroidal anti-inflammatories).

Sporadic bovine leukosis

Common synonyms
Sporadic leukaemia, Sporadic lymphoma.

Disease Profile
Usually individual cattle. Mostly in cattle younger than 3 years. Three forms: juvenile multicentric (mostly 4–8 months of age), thymic (0.5–2 years of age) and cutaneous lymphoma (1–3 up to 4 years of age).

Aetiology
The cause of SBL is not known

Clinical findings
Juvenile form – progressive to fatal weight loss, lymphadenopathy, depression, sometimes fever, dyspnoea, recurrent bloat, posterior paralysis. About half develop lymphoid leukaemia.

Thymic form – dyspnoea, bloat, jugular distention, local oedema, muffled heart sounds, fever. Sometimes swelling of the cervical thymus and/or lymphoid leukaemia.

Cutaneous form – cutaneous plaques (1–5 cm) on neck, back, rump, thighs. May regress spontaneously, followed by remission or death from generalised form.

Post-mortem findings
Lymphadenopathy.

Diagnosis
Signs, histopathology.

Treatment
No treatment.

Stomatitis

Disease Profile
Inflammation of oral cavity, including (inflammation of the mucosa of the tongue), palatitis (inflammation of the palate) and gingivitis (inflammation of the gums and surrounding mucosa). May be localised or a sign of a systemic disorder.

Aetiology
Infection can be caused by viruses (BVD, RMD, vesicular stomatitis, MCF, Rinderpest, popular stomatitis and bluetongue), bacteria (*Fusobacterium necrophorum*, *Actinobacillus lignieresi*) or fungi (*Candida* spp). Physical injury may be caused by abrasive feedstuffs, foreign bodies (sticks, rocks, pieces of wire), equipment for oral administration of drugs, dental equipment and gags. Chemical injury may be caused by ingestion of caustic or acidic substances (e.g. NaOH, HCL).

Clinical findings
Impaired mastication, pain, inappetence, difficult prehension, hypersalivation, malodorous lesions.

Drooling saliva.

Diagnosis
Signs.

Principal differential diagnosis
Actinomycosis, sialoadentis, other reasons of hypersalivation.

Treatment and management
Treat primary reason. Offer soft, palatable feed stuffs. Supportive treatment. For generalised conditions see appropriate headings.

Summer mastitis

Common synonyms
Dry cow mastitis, Heifer mastitis.

Disease Profile
Relatively common. Mainly pastoral dairy cattle near woods and bushes. Pregnant heifers and dry cows at highest risk. Spread by flies, particularly head fly (*Hydrotea irritans*).

Aetiology
Trueperella pyogenes, often mixed with other bacteria. Most common isolates include *Streptococcus dysgalactiae* and *Peptostreptococcus indolicus*.

Clinical findings
Very swollen gland, often unnoticed may be present for a few days before systemic signs develop. **Systemic signs** – peracute and severe. Fever, tachycardia, lethargy, weakness, lameness. Sometimes abortion. Calves born to cow/heifer that suffers summer mastitis often weak.

Affected quarter – very swollen, hard, tender. Initially watery secretion. Later purulent, green/yellow, foul smelling. Even if cow/heifer survives quarter will later rupture and often sloughs or is permanently damaged.

Often oedema and joint effusion of the ipsilateral hind limb.

Diagnosis
Signs, detection of pathogen.

Principal differential diagnosis
Other mastitis, fever and lameness.

Treatment
Treatment may be unrewarding. Systemic and local antimicrobials. Frequent stripping. Non-steroidal anti-inflammatories. Supportive care. Split teat longitudinally to facilitate drainage. Surgery to allow drainage.

Control
Avoid grazing high risk fields. Fly control. Use of teat sealants. Weekly application of Stockholm tar. Use of dry cow therapy. Long acting dry cow antimicrobials.

Sweet clover poisoning

Common synonyms
Sweet clover toxicity, Sweet clover coagulopathy.

Disease Profile
Sweet clover (*Melillotus* spp) common in North America. Rich in coumarines. Coumarines transformed into decoumarine by moulds (*Penicillium* spp, *Mucor* spp and *Aspergilus* spp).

Aetiology
Feeding mouldy hay or silage of sweet clover.

Clinical findings
Epistaxis, melaena, subcutaneous haematomas, prolonged bleeding after calving or injury. Lameness, stiffness. Peracute death by haemorrhage with minor injuries.

Post-mortem findings
Widespread haemorrhages.

Diagnosis
Signs, history, blood clothing profile, determination of prothrombin, chemical analysis of the diet.

Principal differential diagnosis
Warfarin poisoning, Purpura haemorrhagica, other reasons for sudden death.

Treatment
Discontinue offending diet, vitamin K1, blood transfusion. Recovery may take weeks.

Control
Do not feed mouldy sweet or feed it with breaks every second or third week.

Tarsal and carpal hygroma

Disease Profile
Both conditions associated with cattle of normal general condition and no lameness. If the conditions become infected, the infection may spread to the joint, causes lameness and heat. Associated with chronic trauma due to poorly designed stalls or lack of bedding. Herds with multiple cases of hygroma almost invariably have poor housing conditions.

Clinical findings
Carpal hygroma – painless, firm swelling, possibly fluctuating and up to several centimetres in diameter, located over the dorsal aspect of the carpus. The carpal bursa often involved. Occasionally, this condition may become infected and painful when touched.

Tarsal hygroma – starts as firm swelling at the lateral aspect of the hock that later shows soft spot that will eventually rupture to discharge pus. The joint mobility is not affected in early stages.

Diagnosis
Signs.

Principal differential diagnosis
Precarpal abscessation, perforating wounds, septic carpitis, septic tarsitis, serous tarsistis, septic tendosynovitis, localised phlegmon.

Treatment
General care important.

Transfer affected cattle to soft bedding or turn outside on pasture. Antimicrobial treatment is indicated in infected cases. If the animal is milking and eating well, hygromas should be left untreated. Most of the problems caused by carpal/tarsal hygromas are from unsuccessful treatment attempts (usually draining infusion with corticosteroids or attempted surgical removal of the affected tissues). Surgical incision and drainage is indicated, but the common breakdown of the surgical wound and septic inflammation make it unfavourable.

Control
Improve housing conditions. Prevent overcrowding.

Teat lesions: Environment-induced

Disease Profile
Relatively common.

Types – trauma, chapping, photosensitisation, thermal burns, sunburn, frostbite and chemical burns.

Chaps due to mud, wind and cold weather. Rarely excessive sucking or bites by older calves.

Photosensitisation usually due to ingestion of photodynamic agents.

Thermal burns usually due to accident fires and improper flaming of udder.

Frostbite most common on wet teats in very cold conditions.

Chemical burns – accidental overdosing of teat sprays or using wrong chemical, limestone bedding, too strong footbaths.

Clinical findings
Teat chaps – horizontal cracks of teat skin (barrel or junction to udder). Horizontal scabs. Often multiple. Painful milking.

Photosensitisation – initially marked erythema and oedema. Painful milking. Shade seeking. Later – skin necrosis, oozing of serum and scabs. Usually un-pigmented or lightly pigmented lateral and cranial surface of front and lateral and caudal surface of rear teats.

Burns – erythema, oedema, blisters, necrosis, oozing, scabs, signed udder hairs.

Sunburns – erythema, oedema, painful milking. Injuries only to one aspect of teat barrel.

Frostbite – oedema, discolouration, leathery texture, necrosis, sloughing.

Chemical burns – oedema, erythema, blisters, erosions, necrosis, oozing, scabs. Usually most of teat barrel, including pigmented teats. Painful milking. Usually many cows.

Diagnosis
Signs.

Principal differential diagnosis
Infectious and milking machine-induced teat lesions.

Treatment
General – teat disinfection using high-risk period concentrations. Emollients, Soothing creams. Sunscreens. Provision of proper bedding and shade. Nursing care. Stop milking or reduced milking frequency.

Teat chaps – increased emollient, creams.

Photosensitisation – sunscreen, creams, provision of shade, remove reason for photosensitisation.

Teat lesions

Disease Profile
Common. Some of zoonotic importance (e.g. FMD, ringworm, cowpox). Common contributing factors: milking machine (e.g. improper vacuum, pulsation and worn and overstretched of teats, improper biosecurity and milking management (e.g. over milking).

Can affect individual animals (e.g. photosensitivity), but more common out breaks (e.g. bovine herpes mammillitis, FMD, improper pulsation).

Infections fast spread. Superficial or deeper tissues involvement.

Aetiology
Various mechanical, thermal, weather and infectious (bacteria, viruses, fungi, ectoparasites) factors.

Clinical findings
Dependent on aetiology.

General – increased rate of clinical mastitis. Reluctance to be milked, kicking, stepping and brushing udder with hind limbs.

Superficial tissues – primary skin lesions (papillomas, nodules, vesicles, erosions), secondary skin lesions (crusts, scabs), altered circulation (erythema, cyanosis, oedema, petechiation). Everted teat orifices, hyperkeratosis, ringing at the teat base.

Deeper tissues – usually mechanical injury (lacerations, penetrating wounds, incisions, chapping).

Diagnosis
Signs. History. When applicable detection of pathogen. An outbreak present when more than 5% of teats affected.

Principal differential diagnosis
Various skin disorders, many infectious disorders.

Treatment
Dependent on aetiology.

General principles – prompt treatment, correct faults (milking machine or milking management), teat creams, improve teat disinfection, emollients, surgery, milking through a cannula, drying off.

Control
Avoid contributing factors. Use of emollients in high risk periods.

Teat trauma

Common synonyms
Teat lacerations.

Disease Profile
Common. From superficial abrasions that cause few problems to full thickness cuts and virtual amputation. Treading injuries, lacerations, bite wounds. Treading injuries at higher incidence in housed cattle with longer teats. Lacerations at higher risk in pasture-based cattle. Bite wounds most commonly due to improperly trained cattle dogs.

Clinical findings
Teat swelling, bleeding, pain during milking, blood in milk, visible breakage of the skin integrity.

Diagnosis
Signs.

Treatment
Superficial abrasions treat as environment-induced teat lesions. Deeper injuries require surgical repair. Wound breakdown common. Stop milking or reduce milking frequency. Milk through cannula. In severe cases drying off followed by surgery increases chance of successful repair.

Testicular degeneration

Disease Profile
Relatively common. The most common reason for infertility in mature bulls. Usually a sequel to primary disorder such as orchitis. May be of transient nature but often permanent

Aetiology
Usually secondary. Infection and orchitis, testicular hyperthermia.

Clinical findings
Often asymptomatic. Only sign may be infertility. On palpation sometimes smaller and/or softer testis. Calcification may occur in older bulls.

Diagnosis
Signs, semen evaluation, hormonal assay.

Principal differential diagnosis
Testicular hypoplasia, cryptorchism.

Treatment
Usually unrewarding. Occasionally self-cure may occur. Repeated semen evaluation every 10–12 weeks for 6 months may be required. Otherwise cull.

Testicular hypoplasia

Disease Profile
Unilateral or bilateral. Most common reason for congenital infertility in bulls. Hereditary.

Clinical findings
One or both testicles smaller than expected. Scrotal circumference less than 30cm by 12 months of age.

Unilateral testicular hypoplasia – asymmetrical scrotum. Reduced fertility.

Bilateral testicular hypoplasia – significantly reduced fertility to infertility.

Diagnosis
Scrotal circumference below standard. Semen test.

Principal differential diagnosis
Atrophied testis/testes.

Treatment
No treatment, culling.

Control
Avoid breeding of bulls with testicular hypoplasia.

Tetanus

Disease Profile
Rare, sporadic. A result of muscle hyper excitability. Usually associated with deep, anaerobic, puncture wounds. Introduction of spores. Can also occur after abortion and associated with injuries to the digestive system.

Castration and dehorning wounds. Bruising following calving/dystocia.

Aetiology
Endotoxin produced by *Clostridium tetani.*

Clinical findings
Slowly progressing.

Early signs – raised tail, bloat, erected ears, stiffness, difficulty walking. Progression to bulging eyes, protrusion of third eyelid, extended neck, low positioned head, locked jaw, profuse salivation, hyperexcitability to sound.

Late signs – opisthotonus and respiratory failure, recumbency in 2 to 5 days.

Post-mortem findings
No specific findings.

Diagnosis
Signs, detection of pathogen.

Principal differential diagnosis
Spastic paresis, white muscle disease, polioencephalomalacia, lead poisoning, reasons for chronic bloat, laminitis, meningitis, hypomagnesaemia.

Treatment
Antitoxin, high doses of antimicrobials, surgical debridement. Supportive care (relieve bloat, muscle relaxants, nursing). Very slow recovery (weeks).

Control
Vaccination. Improved hygiene.

Theileriosis

Disease Profile
Tick-transmitted blood-borne protozoal disorder.

Recently calved cows and young calves more susceptible. Naïve cattle at higher risk. Usually herd problem.

Two forms – anaemia (tropical theileriasis) and lymphoblastocytosis (East Coast fever).

Aetiology
There are six identified Theileria spp. that infects cattle; the two most pathogenic and

economically important are T. parva and T. annulata

T. parva occurs in Eastern and Southern Africa and causes East Coast fever (ECF or Corridor

disease). T. annulata causes tropical theileriosis (TT), also known as Mediterranean theileriosis and occurs in North Africa, southern Europe and Asia Theileria 'Benign' Theileriosis (T. Bufelli) strains can be associated with disease in naïve animals.

Clinical findings
Tropical theileriasis – signs of anaemia. Drop in milk production. Reduced activity. Sudden death.

East Coast fever – fever, anorexia, nasal and ocular discharge, swelling of lymph nodes, dyspnoea. Protracted disorder. Death.

Diagnosis
Signs. Detection of ticks. Detection of pathogen, blood smears, lymph node biopsies,

Treatment
Careful handling. Provide good quality feed stuffs. Blood transfusion.

Anti-protozoal treatment (e.g. parvoquinone or derivatives).

Control
Reliable vaccines of known efficacy have been developed for *T. parva* and *T. annulata* Tick control. Biosecurity

Tick paralysis

Disease Profile
Regional. Dependent upon the presence of tick species causing the condition. Relatively common in some regions of the world. Causes flaccid paralysis due to blockage of neuromuscular blockade.

Aetiology
64 species of ticks (Ixodid and Argasid genera) produce the neurotoxin.

Clinical findings
Progressive ascending ataxia and paralysis starting from the hindquarters. Paralysis of abdominal muscles results in dyspnoea. More cranial paralysis (thorax) may result in death.

Post-mortem findings
No specific findings.

Diagnosis
Signs. Presence of associated tick spp.

Principal differential diagnosis
Botulism.

Treatment
Remove all ticks. Supportive care. Recovery usually in 1–3 days. Untreated cattle die within 1–2 days.

Control
Tick control.

Tick-borne fever

Common synonyms
Ehrlichiosis, Rickettsial fever.

Disease Profile
Occurs in geographical regions where ticks are present. Mainly dairy cattle recently turned out to pasture. Transmitted by *Ixodes* ticks. Associated with immunosuppression – secondary infections common.

Aetiology
Anaplasma phagocytophilum (formerly *Ehrlichia phagocytophila*).

Clinical findings
Fever, depression, inappetence to anorexia, drop in milk yield, dyspnoea, cough, abortions (particularly in last trimester) and reduced semen quality. Death from uncomplicated disease rare. Self-limiting in period of 1–3 weeks.

Post-mortem findings
No macroscopic findings. Microscopically depletion of splenic lymphocytes, aggregation and apoptosis of macrophages in liver and para-cortical hyperplasia of lymph nodes.

Diagnosis
Signs. Detection of pathogen on blood smears. Necropsy and histopathology.

Principal differential diagnosis
Anaplasmosis. Babesiosis.

Treatment
Antimicrobials. Tetracyclines. Supportive treatment.

Control
Control of ticks.

Ticks

Disease Profile
Important in many tropical and subtropical countries. Important in the epidemiology of some disorders (babesiosis, anaplasmosis, tick-borne fever and theileriosis). Second most important blood-sucking ectoparasite for public health and veterinary importance.

Aetiology
Important genera are *Amblyomma, Boophilus, Dermatocentor, Haemophytalis, Hyalomma, Ixodes, Margorepus, Octobia, Rhipicentor, Rhipicephalus* and *Ornithodoros*.

Clinical findings
Anaemia, weight loss, decreased growth and productivity. Sometimes paralysis.

Diagnosis
Finding ticks on the host.

Treatment
Ectoparasiticides (acaricides)

Control
Avoid grazing in ticks-infected areas, acaricides, vaccination.

Toxic nephrosis

Disease Profile
Kidneys are highly susceptible to damage by various toxins due to the high blood perfusion rate and being a common excretion site for many toxins or haemodynamic insults.

Acute toxic nephrosis – oliguria, proteinuria and uraemia (in terminal stages).

Aetiology
Metals (arsenic, mercury, organic copper compounds, cadmium, chromium, lead, zinc), antimicrobials (benziminoglycosides, prolonged use of tetracyclines, monensis sulphonamides), antihelmintic (benzimidazoles), tannins (oak leaves, acorns), mycotoxins, oxalates (plants, fungi, ethylene glycol) oxalates, some plants (oak, philodendron, beets), overdose of vitamin C and D, overuse of non-steroidal anti-inflammatory drugs, haemoglobin and myoglobin. Haemodynamic reasons of tubular necrosis include any cause of reduced renal perfusion (blood loss, endotoxic shock).

Clinical findings
Toxic nephrosis usually not realised because of the prevailing signs of the toxic disorder of other body systems.

Acute – depression, dehydration, inappetence, slow or rapid heart rate, and in terminal stages hypothermia.

Sometimes – mild bloat, ileus, diarrhoea (may or may not be characterised by melaena) and severe dehydration. Diarrhoea may be with melaena.

Rarely – glycosuria and polyuria.

Post-mortem findings
Swollen kidney, wet on surface, on cut evident oedema, particularly perirenal.

Other signs characteristic of primary poisoning.

Diagnosis
Signs. Monitor renal function.

Treatment
Supportive care for acute renal disease. Antitoxic treatment. Prevention of further uptake of the toxin.

Tracheal oedema syndrome

Common synonyms
'Honker' syndrome.

Disease Profile
Sporadic. Feedlot cattle. Highest incidence in final stage of fattening. Risk factors heat and dust.

Aetiology
Unknown. Suspected viruses, bacteria, allergens, excessive fat accumulation and mycotoxins.

Clinical findings
Peracute – sudden death.

Acute – sudden onset of dyspnoea and loud inspiratory stretor. Sometimes open-mouth breathing, cyanosis, belligerence, recumbency and death. Exercise intolerance.

Subacute – persistent, hacking, non-productive coughs. Usually history of previous IBR. General ill thrift.

Post-mortem findings
Oedema, haemorrhagic thickening of dorsal wall of mid to distal trachea, sometimes with a complete obstruction of the tracheal lumen.

Diagnosis
Signs, post-mortem.

Principal differential diagnosis
Necrotic laryngitis, balling gun injury, tracheal collapse, laryngeal oedema, foreign body.

Treatment
Gentle handling, cooling fans and sprinklers, antimicrobials, corticosteroids. Prognosis poor to guarded.

Relapses very common.

Send to slaughter as soon as safe.

Control
Avoid movement of cattle in hot weather.

Traumatic injuries to the sole

Disease Profile
Common foreign bodies: broken glass, nails, wire and molar tooth. Over trimming of sole. FB stuck in sole or inter-digital space.

Clinical findings
Sudden onset of lameness of a high degree, detection of the foreign body, abscess, sole bruising and sole haemorrhages. Sometimes FB stuck in the interdigital space.

Diagnosis
Signs.

Principal differential diagnosis
For punctured sole: subacute laminitis, sole ulcer, toe ulcer, interdigital necrobacillosis.

Treatment
Excessive wear – rest, apply block or shoof, culling.

Foreign body – remove the foreign body, drain the abscess, apply block on sound claw. Antimicrobials may be required especially if the foreign body has reached the distal phalanx.

Control
When trimming the claw ensure >5mm of sole left. Keep tracks, pasture and yard clean.

Traumatic reticulo-peritonitis

Common synonyms
Hardware disease.

Disease Profile
Traumatic reticulo-peritonitis (TRP) is a disorder in adult cattle resulting from ingestion of sharp metal objects (e.g. nails, fence or tire wire, parts of farm machinery). The sharp objects penetrate the reticular wall and cause acute local peritonitis. In rare cases a generalised peritonitis may result. Further, migration of the foreign body may result in involvement of various surrounding organs (diaphragm, pericardium, lungs, mediastinum, liver and spleen).

Clinical findings
Acute clinical syndrome – at the onset of the disorder. It may be overlooked due to the short duration (usually only 24–36, rarely up to 72 hours). Signs of acute peritonitis (e.g. marked drop in milk production, complete inappetence, fore-stomach atony, slight impaction and bloating of the rumen, absence of rumination, reluctance to lie down, general rigidity, 'tucked up' belly, arched back and protruding neck). Temperature and pulse increased. Usually faeces firm and scant, dehydration and pain in the xyphoid area.

Sub-acute/chronic syndrome – Milk yield is decreased but not always easily detected. Appetite usually reduced. Rumination variable. Faeces regain the normal consistency. The back usually slightly arched. Spontaneous grunting rare finding. The pain usually requires to be elicited.

Diagnosis
Signs, radiography, metal detectors, blood (increased white blood cells (usually >10,000/ml) and neutrophil percentage (always >50%, usually 60–65%) with a left shift, increased plasma proteins (particularly fibrinogen)), abdominocentesis and exploratory laparotomy.

Principal differential diagnosis
Other causes of peritonitis: abomasal ulceration, other penetrating foreign bodies, other causes of cranial abdominal or caudal thorax pain, other causes of diffuse abdominal pain, other causes of ruminal impaction, other causes of ruminal tympany and other causes of stiffness of stance.

Treatment
The aim of treatment of acute TRP is to facilitate formation of adhesions and containment of the infection. Movement of the animals should be restricted and a systemic administration of antimicrobials combined with a reticular magnet may be effective. Surgical removal of reticular foreign bodies by rumenotomy is the preferred option to confirm the diagnosis and remove the offending wire.

Control

Control of TRP is often difficult. Passage of feed over a magnet prior to feeding, prophylactic administration of reticular magnets. The farm staff should be instructed to keep pasture and feeding areas free of foreign objects.

Trichomoniasis

Common synonyms

Trichomonosis.**Disease Profile**

Insidious, sexually transmitted, protozoal disorder. Worldwide but not present in all regions. Non-invasive infection of the epithelial surface of penis, prepuce, vagina, uterus and oviducts. Associated with natural service but also with contaminated semen. Bulls over 4 years more commonly infected. Pregnancy loss may reach 70%.

Aetiology

Trichomonas foetus.

Clinical findings

Asymptomatic. Discharge rarely detected.

Bulls – transient balanoposthitis may develop. Persistent source of infection.

Female cattle – repeated breeders. Mucopurulent vaginal discharge on return to oestrus. Pyometra. Abortion in first to second trimester. Females self-cure within a few months.

Diagnosis

Signs, history, detection of pathogen, trans-rectal ultrasonography in females.

Principal differential diagnosis

Campylobacter infection, poor nutrition, granular vuvlo-vaginitis.

Treatment

Imidazole. Treatment is difficult and poorly tolerated with reinfection from cows.

Control

Artificial insemination. Vaccination (Cows and bulls. Later bulls only) Biosecurity. Test incoming bulls (preputial washing).

Trypanosomiasis

Common synonyms

Tse-tse disease. African sleeping sickness, Nagana, Surra.

Disease Profile

Vector transmitted (e.g. tse-tse flies, biting flies and vampire bats). Subtropical and tropical areas of Africa. Central and South America. Acute, subclinical or chronic. In some countries notifiable. Some zoonotic risk.

Aetiology

Variety species of genus *Trypanosoma (brucei, congolense, vivax, simiae, evansi)*.

Clinical findings

Acute – anaemia, intermittent fever, stiff gait, drop in milk yield, ill thrift.

Chronic – chronic anaemia, marked jugular distention and positive jugular pulse, loss of body condition, dull hair coat. Protracted ill thrift. Dependent oedema. Death.

Post-mortem findings

Non-specific.

Diagnosis

Signs only suggestive. Detection of pathogen in blood smears.

Treatment

Antiprotozoal treatment (e.g. Diminazene aceturate)

Control

Vector control. Prophylactic drugs (e.g. isometamidium).

Udder impetigo

Common synonyms

Udder acne.

Disease Profile

Diffuse folliculitis of relatively hairless areas of udder (caudal and ventral aspects).

Aetiology

Staphylococcus aureus most commonly.

Clinical findings

Erythema, followed by modules and pustules at hair follicles. Sometimes spread to teats and/or coalesce into a shield-like crust.

Diagnosis

Signs.

Principal differential diagnosis

Chemical irritants, viral diseases, dermatophilosis.

Treatment

Local antimicrobial creams +/– systemic antimicrobials.

Udder: intertrigo and necrotic dermatitis

Common synonyms

Udder rot

Disease Profile

Two forms – intertrigo and necrotic dermatitis.

Intertrigo – rare. Necrotic dermatitis of the midline, particularly in heifers with severe udder oedema.

Necrotic dermatitis – relatively common. Udder skin where it contacts the medial thigh. Heifers with severe oedema and mature high-producing cows in hot, humid weather.

Aetiology
Most commonly *Staphylococcus* spp.

Clinical findings
Characteristic smell. Skin erythemathous, ezyematous, necrotic, oozing. Signs of skin-fold pyoderma.

Diagnosis
Signs.

Treatment
Gentle wash. Local and systemic antimicrobials.

Udder Oedema

Disease Profile
Common in periparturient heifers. Difficult to milk. Inconvenient.

Aetiology
Risk factors include high pre-partum diets high in salt

Clinical findings
Excessive swelling of the udder with pitting oedema which may extend forward along the abdomen and up to the vulva. The skin may stretch and crack. Increased pre-disposition to mastitis. Abnormal gait due to size of udder.

Diagnosis
Signs and signalment

Principal differential diagnosis
Mastitis

Treatment
NSAIDs, Diuretics. Corticio-steroids, Massage, Exercise

Control
Control salt in pre-partum diet.

Udder: skin disorders

Disease Profile
Relatively common. Physical, chemical and infectious nature. Also photosensitisation and skin parasitism.

Aetiology
Physical – sunburn, thermal burns, frost bite, pressure necrosis.

Chemical – irritant bedding (e.g. limestone), fly sprays, footbaths.

Infectious – bacteria (staphylococci), intertrigo dermatophilosis, viruses (bovine herpes mammillitis, pseudo-cowpox, foot-and-mouth); ringworm, Sarcoptic mange.

Clinical findings
Physical – oedema, erythema, oozing, necrosis or primary and secondary skin lesions (vesicles, erosions, ulcers, crusting).

Chemical – erythema, alopecia, pain. Sometimes vesicles, oozing and matting the hairs.

Infectious – erythema, oedema, pustules, necrosis, crusts, eczema (intertrigo)

Diagnosis
Signs.

Treatment
Physical – symptomatically.

Chemical – gentle wash, softening and protective creams. Removal of offending material from environment.

Infectious Bacterial: antimicrobials, gentle wash, creams and antimicrobials.

Umbilical infections

Disease Profile
This complex includes: omphalophlebitis (infection of umbilical veins), omphaloarteritis (infection of the umbilical arteries), omphalitis (infection of many structures, including tissues surrounding the umbilicus), urachal abscess and umbilical abscess. It can be primary (contaminated umbilicus) or secondary (focal infection somewhere else). Common in calves with failure of passive transfer.

Aetiology
Escherichia coli, Trueperella pyogenes, Enterococcus spp, *Proteus* spp.

Clinical findings
Fever, depression, decreased to absent sucking reflex. Umblical enlargement, swelling, painful, may or may not be hot. Sometimes purulent discharge. Deep abdominal palpation reveals pain, enlarged veins, sometimes arteries. Septicaemia. Urachal abscess – dysuria, frequent urination.

Diagnosis
Signs, ultrasonography.

Principal differential diagnosis
Umbilical hernia

Treatment
Prolonged antimicrobials. Surgical – debridement and resection.

Control
Neonatal umbilical care. Adequate colostrum management. Clean environment.

Umbilical hernia

Disease Profile
Common. Probably the most common congenital disorder in cattle. Some heritable component, other congenital or occur secondary to infection of umbilical remnants.

Clinical findings
Usually reducible swelling in the umbilical region and palpable hernia ring. Reducibility easier detected in lateral or dorsal recumbency. Strangulation of abdominal organs rare.

Most hernias detectable within 3 weeks from calving.

Diagnosis
Signs. Reducible swelling and hernia ring. Ultrasonography. Important to differentiate simple from complicated (concurrent localised infection) hernias.

Principal differential diagnosis
Infection of umbilical remnant, umbilical abscess, haematoma, cellulitis, omphalocoele.

Treatment
Small (<5cm in diameter) often close spontaneously. Hernias 5–10cm conservative bandaging may be enough for full recovery. Larger hernias surgical repair.

Control
Avoid breeding from cattle affected by umbilical hernias.

Urea/ammonia poisoning

Disease Profile
Excess blood ammonia. Most common risk factors urea used in feed or as fertiliser, ammoniated feeds, short rest of fertilised paddocks, inadequate mixing within the ration, unacclimated cattle, use of urea in low-energy ration, starving cattle and mixing with highly palatable supplements. Rapidly progressing. Can be highly fatal and cause economic losses. Younger cattle more susceptible. Can affect suckling calves through milk of the dam. Affected systems respiratory, gastrointestinal (see rumen alkalosis), musculo-skeletal and nervous.

Aetiology
Ingestion of urea and/or ammoniated feed stuffs.

Clinical findings
Usually shortly after exposure (minutes, sometimes hours). Sudden death. Early signs muscle tremors (ears, face), abdominal pain, bruxism, frothy salivation. Progression to tremors and weakness. Marked dyspnoea. Ataxia, bellowing, aggression. Development of bloat, tetanic spasms and convulsions followed by death.

Approaching and examining affected cattle may be dangerous.

Post-mortem findings
Rapid decomposition, bloat, generalised congestion, lung congestion and oedema, haemorrhages on the heart.

Diagnosis
Signs. History. Blood ammonia >0.5 mg/100mL, rumen alkalosis (pH>7.5).

Principal differential diagnosis
Nitrate/nitrite poisoning, lead poisoning, botulism, hypomagnesaemia, anthrax, clostridial disorders, bloat, grain overload, polioencephalomalacia and hepatic encephalopathy.

Treatment
Oral administration of vinegar, cold water, rumenotomy, supportive treatment (prevent self-injury, sedation, tranquilisation, magnesium, IV isotonic fluids).

Control
See rumen alkalosis.

Urolithiasis

Disease Profile
Common. Clinical form is urethral obstruction. Most common in feedlot steers castrated early in life. Contributing factors – low vitamin A, water deprivation, high-grain, high-phosphorus diet.

Aetiology
Urethral blockage (most commonly at sigmoid flexure of penis).

Clinical findings
Initially discomfort, abdominal colic-like syndrome, followed by relief (urethral or bladder rupture), stranguria, pollakiuria, crystals on preputial hairs. On rectal examination enlarged bladder and pulsating urethra before rupture. After rupture ascites (bladder) or ventral anasarca (urethra) and slowly progressing signs of uraemia. Progressive anorexia and lethargy.

Post-mortem findings
Finding uroliths, cystitis, signs of urethral obstruction, urethral and/or bladder rupture.

Diagnosis
Signs.

Principal differential diagnosis
Cystitis, constipation, abdominal pain due to other reasons.

Treatment
Medical (e.g. muscle relaxants) or surgical (urethrostomy). In expensive breeding bull ventral abdominal laparotomy and placement of a Foley catheter allows urine to be voided. Obstructive urethral uroliths fragment and patency may be restored over 7–10 days thus preserving future fertility.

Control
Water availability, adding salt to diet, proper calcium to phosphorus ratio, acidifying urine and adding ammonium chloride to diet. Increase roughage or long fibre in diet to promote increased saliva production (reduces blood and urine phosphate levels).

Urticaria

Common synonyms
Hives, Heat bumps, Feed bumps, Wheals.

Disease Profile
Relatively common. Underdiagnosed. Contact with allergen (contact, ingestion, iatrogenic) and auto-immune reaction (e.g. milk retention at drying off). Channel Island breeds at higher risk.

Can occur concurrently with anaphylactic reaction.

Aetiology
Allergic reaction to food, insects, vaccines, milk retention (milk allergy).

Clinical findings
Sudden onset of localised or generalised dermal oedema (wheals).

Some pitting evident. Pruritus may or may not occur.

Diagnosis
Signs.

Treatment
Self-cure in few days common. Avoid the allergen. In severe cases antihistamines and corticosteroids.

Uterine inertia

Disease Profile
Relatively common. Highest risk in obese and cow with hypocalcaemia. Other risks – hormonal imbalance, and uterine, foetal and placental pathology.

Aetiology
Failure of normal uterine contractions at parturition.

Clinical findings
Calving stops at the first-stage labour. Usually signs of restlessness and abdominal contraction. Cervix open. Calf death. Signs of primary disorder.

Diagnosis
Signs.

Principal differential diagnosis
Septicaemia, toxaemia, uterine rupture, foetal malpositioning, beef pregnancy toxaemia.

Treatment
Treat primary disorder. Caesarean section. When possible manual foetal extraction.

Control
Avoid primary disorders.

Uterine prolapse

Disease Profile
Incidence differs from farm-to-farm and year-to-year.

More common in multiparous cows. Predisposing factors: hypocalcaemia, hip-lock dystocia, stillborn calves. Holstein cows.

Clinical findings
Shortly after calving. Obvious prolapsed and everted uterus.

Prolonged prolapse – oedema, dehydration and superficial necrosis of the everted tissue; significant contamination. Placenta may or not be attached. Haemorrhage a risk which can be rapidly fatal.

Diagnosis
Signs.

Treatment
Isolate to avoid further damage by other cows. Epidural anaesthesia (inclusion of off label xylazine can reduce tenesmus 12–14 hours) +/– uterine relaxant. Debride and clean thouroughly before manual replacement. Ensure uterine horns are inverted (wine bottle can be used as a blunt probe to invert uterine horns once body of uterus is replaced to avoid recurrence). Suturing of vulval lips after replacement serves no purpose. After reposition administer calcium iv and oxytocin. Antimicrobials to prevent uterine infection and sepsis. Recurrence is possible. If the uterus is severely damaged amputation is possible.

Control
Avoid hypocalcaemia (sub-clinical) at parturition. Regular monitoring of the calving area.

Vagus indigestion

Common synonyms
Vagal indigestion. Hoflund's syndrome.

Disease Profile
The vagus indigestion syndrome refers to a group of motor disturbances that result in problems in the out flow of ingesta from the forestomachs and/or abomasum. Dysfunction of the vagus nerve is associated with less than 1/3 of all cases. Vagus indigestion has long duration and a slow progressive onset. It has grave prognosis even with aggressive treatment. There are four types of vagus indigestion: failure of eructation, failure of omasal transport, abomasal impaction and partial obstruction of the forestomachs in late pregnancy.

Aetiology
Vagal nerve damage due to: traumatic reticulo-peritonitis, localised abscess, neoplasia, adhesions, foreign body, pneumonia.

Clinical findings
Gradual abdominal enlargement and L-shaped rumen. Rumen becomes full of fibre. The abdomen is '10 to 4' distended or 'apple shaped'. Chronic rumen bloat. Intermittent episodes of indigestion. Gradual decrease in productivity and weight loss. Occasionally bradycardia. Early stages sometimes hypermotility with weak contractions progressing to atony. Rumen atony is a prognostically grave sign. Reduced faecal volume. Faeces are greasy or pasty and contain fibre with increased length. Animal may become recumbent with increasing abdominal weight and weakness.

Diagnosis
Signs, history, blood CBC, biochemistry, ultrasonography, laparotomy. Diagnosis of vagus indigestion is often based on exclusion.

Principal differential diagnosis
Simple indigestion, rumen acidosis, traumatic reticulo-peritonitis, other causes of decreased faecal volume, displaced abomasum, pregnancy, hydrops, frothy bloat, abdominal neoplasia. Rumen foreign body.

Treatment and management
Usually non-rewarding. Therefore, slaughter should be advised. Surgery (laparotomy. Supportive treatment (rumen transformation, rumenotorics, catharactics, exercise, fluid therapy, oral supplementation with minerals, induction of calving). Provide good quality, palatable feed stuffs.

Control
Difficult due to multifactorial nature. Rumen magnets to prevent traumatic reticulo-peritonitis prevent displaced abomasum, prevent access to indigestible substances (e.g. twine, plastics).

Vertebral body abscess

Disease Profile
Young cattle. Usually previous history of umbilical remnant infection or pneumonia.

Clinical findings
Depending on the spinal segment affected. Neck and/or back pain, ill thrift, paresis to paralysis, pathological fractures, sometimes heat, and swelling.

Diagnosis
Signs (neurological examination should enable the location to be established), complete blood sample, imaging. CSF sample may or may not be helpful.

Treatment
Unrewarding. Long term antimicrobials.

Vesicular stomatitis

Disease Profile
Viral disease that may cause sporadic outbreaks of vesicular-type disorder in cattle, equides, pigs. Mature cattle are most susceptible. Up to 90% of the herd may be affected in naïve herds. Lesions appear in the oral cavity, on the teats and interdigital space. Lesions start as vesicles that rupture fast, leaving erosions and ulcerations. Erosions may coalesce leaving large eroded areas. Zoonotic. Notifiable.

Aetiology
Rhabdovirus.

Clinical findings
Fever, anorexia, hypersalivation, weight loss. On oral examination typical lesions. Teat lesions are usually presented as erosions and predispose the cow to mastitis. Foot lesions are rare. Mild lameness is typical sign. Lesions heal slowly.

Diagnosis
Signs. Detection of pathogen.

Principal differential diagnosis
Foot-and-mouth, other stomatitis, bovine herpes mamillitis, parapox, foot rot, IBR, MCF, chemical or thermal burns.

Treatment and management
Supportive care. Soft palatable feed stuffs.

Control
Isolate infected cattle. Normal biosecurity measures. Disinfection.

Vitamin A deficiency

Common synonyms
Night blindness. Hyena disease.

Disease Profile
Rare. More common in younger cattle. Deficiency occurs after prolonged periods (3–6 months) insufficient intake. Congenital hypovitaminosis A may occur in calves from cows deficient of Vitamin A. More common in indoor on intensive cereal-based ration.

Aetiology
Prolonged insufficient intake of Vitamin A.

Clinical findings
Young growing cattle – Night blindness, non-responsive mydriasis, xerosis, xerophthalmia, stunted growth, weight loss, abnormal bone development, oral and nasal discharge, abnormal development of teeth, ataxia and convulsions.

Mature cattle – ophthalmic and neurologic signs similar to young cattle. Poor hair coat, presence of large bran-like scales, poor fertility stillbirths.

Stillborn calves – doming of the fore head, hydrocephalus, ophthalmic abnormalities.

Weak neonatal calves – neurological and ophthalmic signs.

Diagnosis
Signs. History. Blood, Vitamin A levels.

Principal differential diagnosis
BVD infection, meningitis, leads poisoning, polioencephalomalacia, hepatoencephalopathy, parasitic dermatoses.

Treatment
Parenteral Vitamin A. Bone, teeth and neurologic pathology irreparable. Blindness may be permanent.

Control
Proper supplementation (Vitamin A and/or ß-carotene).

White line disease

Disease Profile
Aseptic necrosis of the palmer/plantar third of the sole/bulb junction region of the hind limb (mature cows) or medial claw (heifers). This area of separation between the sole horn and wall horn allows entry of infection. This may result in ascending infections with swelling either appearing at the bulbs of the heel or the coronary band. Alternatively infection may spread laterally forming an abscess beneath the sole horn. Pre-disposing factors include the stress of calving, laminitis with weak horn formation, excessive walking, use of dogs, poorly constructed cow tracks and sharp turns with high forces being exerted at the white line.

Clinical findings
Lameness of various degrees (sometimes bilateral) depending on the infection present.

Swelling of the bulbs of the heel or coronary band or pain on the sole when tested with hoof tested

(solar abscess).

Diagnosis
Signs.

Principal differential diagnosis
Punctured sole, bruised sole, sole ulcer, laminitis, small coronary sand cracks, fracture of the distal phalanx.

Treatment
Facilitation of drainage by radical paring. Blocks may be required. Antibiotics should be considered.

Winter dysentery

Common synonyms
Vibrionic scour, Winter scour.

Disease Profile
Incidence varies from geographical location, farm and year. Outbreaks. Mainly mature, housed dairy cattle in winter. Morbidity may reach 100%. Mortality very rare. Herds with prior history at higher risk. Calves usually affected later than mature cattle on a farm.

Aetiology
Usually associated with corona virus.

Clinical findings
Acute onset of an outbreak of dark, bloody, liquid diarrhoea with no specific foetid odour.

Drop in milk yield, depression, inappetence to anorexia. Often nasolacrimal discharge, dyspnoea and cough. Protracted recovery over weeks.

Diagnosis
Signs.

Principal differential diagnosis
Other causes of diarrhoea (BVD, Johne's disease, coccidosis, salmonellosis and poisonings). Sudden diet change.

Treatment
No specific treatment. Provision of water +/– electrolytes.

Control
No practical control measures

Yersiniosis

Disease Profile
Relatively common. Usually sporadic but may cause outbreaks. Birds, rodents and deer believed to be the reservoir of infection. Mainly young cattle after weaning during inclement weather or other stress. Most commonly in cattle of good condition.

Aetiology
Yersinia pseudotuberculosis. Rarely *Y. enterocolitica*.

Clinical findings
Diarrhoea (usually subacute) sometimes with blood and/or mucin. Faeces not particularly malodorous. Cattle anorexic, depressed and dehydrated. Sometimes subclinical – stunted growth, wasting usually without diarrhoea.

Post-mortem findings
Ulcerative entero-colitis. Histopathology – villous atrophy, micro-abscessation of intestinal wall and mesenteric lymph nodes.

Diagnosis
Signs. Detection of pathogen. Post-mortem and histopathology.

Principal differential diagnosis
Salmonellosis, gastro-intestinal parasitism, undernourishment.

Treatment
Antimicrobials. Supportive treatment.

Control
Minimising stress.

Yew poisoning

Common synonyms
Taxus poisoning. Yew toxicity. Taxus toxicity, Ground hemlock.

Disease Profile
Usually outbreak. Many parts of the world. Most commonly associated with access to trimmings or non-grazed areas. Fresh and dry yew leaves are toxic. Very small quantities (0.1–0.5% of the body weight) cause sudden death. Plant very palatable to cattle.

Aetiology
Taxin – cardiotoxic alkaloid found in three yew varieties (*Taxus baccata, T. accata* and *T. cuspidata*).

Clinical findings
Sudden death soon after consumption (can be as fast as 15 minutes), occasionally preceded by tremors, weakness and collapse.

Rarely **prolonged form** – depression, dyspnoea, gastroenteritis, trembling, convulsions and death. On auscultation dysrhythmias, bradycardia, ventricular tachycardia.

Post-mortem findings
Evidence of plant within the rumen content.

Diagnosis
Signs. Examination of environment. Post-mortem.

Principal differential diagnosis
Other causes of sudden death.

Treatment
Usually too late. Treat all exposed cattle with activated charcoal or rumenotomy. Atropine. Supportive care. Handle exposed cattle with care.

Control
Avoid contact with yew plants or cuttings.

Index

Bovine Medicine, Third Edition. Edited by Peter D. Cockcroft.

Wiley The manufacturer's authorized representative according to the EU General Product Safety Regulation is Wiley-VCH GmbH, Boschstr. 12, 69469 Weinheim, Germany, e-mail: Product_Safety@wiley.com.

Printed and bound by CPI Group (UK) Ltd, Croydon, CR0 4YY
24/08/2026
02202109-0002